Spine Care

VOLUME TWO

VOLUME ONE
Diagnosis and Conservative Treatment

VOLUME TWO
Operative Treatment

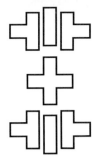

Spine Care

VOLUME TWO

Editor

Arthur H. White, M.D.

Medical Director
San Francisco Spine Institute
SpineCare Medical Group
Daly City, California

Associate Editor

Jerome A. Schofferman, M.D.

Director, Research and Education
San Francisco Spine Institute
SpineCare Medical Group
Daly City, California

with 1918 illustrations including 6 color plates

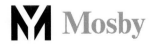

St. Louis Baltimore Boston Carlsbad Chicago Naples New York Philadelphia Portland
London Madrid Mexico City Singapore Sydney Tokyo Toronto Wiesbaden

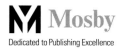

Publisher: Anne Patterson
Editor: Robert Hurley
Developmental Editor: Eugenia A. Klein
Project Manager: Barbara Bowes Merritt
Design, Editorial and Production: York Production Services
Manufacturing Supervisor: Theresa Fuchs

ONE EDITION

Copyright © 1995 by Mosby-Year Book, Inc.

All rights reserved. No part of this publication may be reproduced, stored in a retrieval system, or transmitted, in any form or by any means, electronic, mechanical, photocopying, recording, or otherwise, without prior written permission from the publisher.

Permission to photocopy or reproduce solely for internal or personal use is permitted for libraries or other users registered with the Copyright Clearance Center, provided that the base fee of $4.00 per chapter plus $.10 per page is paid directly to the Copyright Clearance Center, 27 Congress Street, Salem, MA 01970. This consent does not extend to other kinds of copying, such as copying for general distribution, for advertising or promotional purposes, for creating new collected works, or for resale.

Printed in the United States of America
Composition by York Graphic Services, Inc.
Printing/binding by Maple-Vail Book Manufacturing Group

Mosby-Year Book, Inc.
11830 Westline Industrial Drive
St. Louis, Missouri 63146

Library of Congress Cataloging in Publication Data
Spine care: editor, Arthur H. White; associate editor, Jerome A. Schofferman.
    p. cm.
   Includes bibliographical references and index.
   ISBN 0-8016-6328-8
   1. Spine—Diseases. 2. Spine—Wounds and injuries. 3. Backache.
I. White, Arthur H., II. Schofferman, Jerome A.
   [DNLM: 1. Spinal Diseases—therapy. 2. Spinal Diseases—diagnosis.
3. Back Pain—therapy. 4. Back Pain—diagnosis. WE 725 S75915 1995]
RD768; .S673 1995
617.3′75—dc20
DNLM/DLC   94-40833
for Library of Congress   CIP

95 96 97 / 9 8 7 6 5 4 3 2 1

Contributors

David J. Anderson, M.D.
Department of Psychiatry
SpineCare Medical Group
Daly City, California
Chapt 4: The Psychologic Cascade
Chapt 17: Psychiatric Evaluation of the Chronic
    Pain Patient
Chapt 38: Understanding the Chronic Spine Pain
    Patient: The Attachment Theory

Charles N. Aprill, M.D.
Magnolia Diagnostics
New Orleans, Louisiana
Chapt 14: Discography
Chapt 21: Diagnostic Blocks of Spinal Synovial Joints
Chapt 22: Epidural Steroid Injections

Bruce D. Beynnon, Ph.D.
Research Assistant Professor
Department of Orthopaedics and Rehabilitation
University of Vermont
Burlington, Vermont
Chapt 87: The Vermont Spinal Fixator for
    Posterior Application to Short Segments of the
    Thoracic, Lumbar, or Lumbosacral Spine

Ronald Blackman, M.D.
Director, Spinal Deformity Clinic
Kaiser Permanente Medical Center
Oakland, California
Chapt 73: Arthroscopic Microdiscectomy:
    Lumbar and Thoracic (section on "Endoscopic
    Thoracic Spine Surgery")

**Nikolai Bogduk, B.Sc. (Med), M.B. B.S., Ph.D.,
M.D., Dip Anat, Hon F.A.C.R.M.**
Professor of Anatomy
Director
Cervical Spine Research Unit
Faculty of Medicine
University of Newcastle
Newcastle, New South Wales, Australia
Chapt 14: Discography
Chapt 21: Diagnostic Blocks of Spinal Synovial Joints
Chapt 22: Epidural Steroid Injections
Chapt 60: Anatomy of the Spine

Richard S. Brower, M.D.
Instructor in Orthopaedic Surgery
Department of Orthopaedics
Northeastern Ohio Universities
College of Medicine
Akron, Ohio
Chapt 99: Cervical Spondylotic Radiculopathy and
    Myelopathy: Posterior Approach

Bobbi Buell
Documedics
San Bruno, California
Appendix: Practical Guide to Billing

Charles V. Burton, M.D.
Medical Director
Department of Neurosurgery
Institute for Low Back Care
Minneapolis, Minnesota
Chapt 79: The Controversy of "Large Vs. Small":
    The Present Role of Minimally Invasive Surgery
    of the Spine

Peter N. Capicotto, M.D.
Orthopaedic Surgeon
St. Vincent Hospital
Indianapolis, Indiana
Chapt 111: Clinical Cervical Deformity and Post
    Laminectomy Kyphosis

Kenichi Chatani, M.D., Ph.D.
Fellow
Department of Orthopaedic Surgery
Kyoto Prefectural University in Medicine
Kyoto City, Kyoto, Japan
Chapt 8: Anatomy, Biochemistry, and Physiology
    of Low-Back Pain

Andrew J. Cole, M.D.
Director
Spine Rehabilitation Services
The Tom Landry Sports Medicine and Research
    Center
Baylor University Medical Center
Dallas, Texas
Chapt 55: Swimming

Patrick J. Connolly, M.D.
Assistant Professor
Department of Orthopaedic Surgery
State University of New York
　　Health Science Center at Syracuse
Syracuse, New York
Chapt 101: Anterior Instrumentation of the
　　Cervical Spine
Chapt 104: Cervical Spine Fractures

Howard B. Cotler, M.D., F.A.C.S.
Clinical Associate Professor
Department of Orthopaedic Surgery
University of Texas
Houston, Texas
Chapt 100: Cervical Fusions: Arthrodesis and
　　Osteosynthesis of the Cervical Spine

Tracy P. Cotter, M.D.
Assistant Professor
Department of Anesthesiology
University of Wisconsin
Madison, Wisconsin
Chapt 68: Anesthesia in Cervical Spine Surgery

Ramon Cuencas-Zamora, Ph.D.
Behavioral Medicine Specialist
Department of Health Psychology and Behavioral
　　Medicine
Dallas Spine Rehabilitation Center
Dallas, Texas
Chapt 67: Pyschological Preparation for Surgery

P. Dean Cummings, M.D.
Department of Orthopaedics
Penn State
College of Medicine
The Milton S. Hershey Medical Center
Hershey, Pennsylvania
Chapt 102: Sports Injuries of the Head and
　　Cervical Spine

W. Bradford DeLong, M.D., F.A.C.S.
Assistant Clinical Professor
Department of Neurosurgery
University of California, San Francisco;
Neurological Consultant
St. Mary's Spine Center
San Francisco, California;
Neurological Consultant
SpineCare Medical Group
Daly City, California
Chapt 69: Positioning the Patient for Lumbar
　　Spine Surgery
Chapt 75: Microsurgical Discectomy and Spinal
　　Decompression

Richard Derby, Jr., M.D.
Chief
Department of Anesthesia, Diagnostic Spinal
　　Procedures
SpineCare Medical Group
Daly City, California;
Co-Founder
International Spinal Injection Society
Daly City, California
Chapt 14: Discography
Chapt 21: Diagnostic Blocks of Spinal Synovial Joints
Chapt 22: Epidural Steroid Injections

Susan J. Dreyer, M.D.
Diplomate
American Board of Physical Medicine
Clinical Assistant Professor
Department of Medicine and Rehabilitation
Emory University
Atlanta, Georgia
Chapt 56: Weight Lifting

James Dwyer, M.D.
Medical Director
New Jersey Spine Institute
Bedminster, New Jersey;
Clinical Assistant Professor
Orthopaedic Surgery
The New Jersey Medical School
Newark, New Jersey
Chapt 58: History of Spine Surgery

Richard A. Eagleston, M.A., P.T., A.T.C.
Strength Training and Rehabilitation Physical
　　Therapy
Redwood City, CA
Chapt 55: Swimming

Sanford E. Emery, M.D.
Assistant Professor, Spine Section
Department of Orthopaedics
Case Western Reserve University
University Hospitals of Cleveland
Cleveland, Ohio
Chapt 98: Cervical Spondylotic Radiculopathy and
　　Myelopathy: Anterior Approach and Pathology

William T. Evans, M.D.
Associate Medical Director
Center for Spine Rehabilitation
Colorado Neurological Institute
Englewood, Colorado
Chapt 23: Education: The Primary Treatment of
    Low-Back Pain

Frank J. E. Falco, M.D.
Physiatrist
Georgia Spine and Sports Physicians
Smyrna, Georgia
Chapt 56: Weight Lifting

Joseph P. Farrell, P.T., M.S.
Redwood Orthopaedic Physical Therapy, Inc.
Castro Valley, California;
Senior Clinical Faculty
Kaiser Hayward Physical Therapy Residency
Program in Advanced Manual Therapy
Kaiser Permanente Medical Center
Hayward, California
Chapt 30: The Role of Manual Therapy in Spinal
    Rehabilitation

John G. Finkenberg, M.D., D.C.
Spine Specialist
Department of Orthopedics
Johns Hopkins Hospital
Baltimore, Maryland
Chapt 110: Adult Scoliosis

Kevin S. Finnesey, M.D.
Attending Orthopedic Surgeon
Department of Orthopedics
Mills Peninsula Hospitals
San Mateo County General Hospital
San Mateo, California
Chapt 49: Golf
Chapt 93: The Use of Electrical Stimulation for
    Spinal Fusion

Joseph D. Fortin, D.O.
Clinical Assistant Professor
Department of Rehabilitation
Louisiana State University
New Orleans, Louisiana
Chapt 47: Figure Skating

Robert W. Gaines, Jr., M.D.
Professor
Department of Orthopaedic Surgery
University of Missouri Health Sciences Center
Columbia, Missouri
Chapt 109: Spinal Deformity in Children,
    Adolescents, and Young Adults

Robert J. Gatchel, Ph.D.
Professor of Psychiatry and Rehabilitation Science
Department of Psychiatry
University of Texas Southwestern Medical Center
Dallas, Texas
Chapt 36: Psychosocial Correlates of the
    Deconditioning Syndrome

Stanley D. Gertzbein, M.D.
Director
Department of Research and Education
Texas Back Institute;
Associate Professor
Department of Orthopaedics
University of Texas
Houston, Texas
Chapt 100: Cervical Fusions: Arthrodesis and
    Osteosynthesis of the Cervical Spine

Patricia H. Gibbs, M.D.
Medical Director
San Francisco Free Clinic
San Francisco, California
Chapt 46: Dance

Richard D. Gibbs, M.D.
Supervising Physician
San Francisco Ballet
San Francisco, California
Chapt 46: Dance

Richard G. Gillette, M.S., Ph.D.
Associate Professor
Department of Physiology
Basic Science Division
Western States Chiropractic College
Portland, Oregon
Chapt 9: Neurophysiology of Chronic Idiopathic
    Back Pain

Susan L. Goelzer, M.D.
Associate Professor
Departments of Anesthesiology and Internal
    Medicine
University of Wisconsin
Madison, Wisconsin
Chapt 68: Anesthesia in Cervical Spine Surgery

Erwin G. Gonzalez, M.D.
Director
Department of Physical Medicine and
    Rehabilitation
Professor
Department Rehabilitation Medicine
Mt. Sinai School of Medicine
Beth Israel Medical Center
New York, New York
Chapt 13: Somatosensory and Motor Evoked
    Potential

Matthew F. Gornet, M.D.
Department of Orthopaedic Surgery-Spine
DePaul Health Center
St. Louis, Missouri
Chapt 107: Spinal Infection

Serge Gracovetsky, M.D., Ph.D.
Associate Professor
Department of Electrical Engineering
Concordia University
President
Spinex Medical Technologies
Montreal, Quebec, Canada
Chapt 10: Biomechanics of the Spine

**Alexander G. Hadjipavlou, M.D., M.Sc.,
    F.R.C.S. (C), F.A.C.S.**
Professor
Department of Surgery
Section of Orthopedic Surgery
University of Arizona Health Sciences Center
Tucson, Arizona
Chapt 20: Principles of Assessment of
    Osteometabolic Bone Disease
Chapt 62: Osteoporosis of the Spine and Its
    Management
Chapt 113: Paget's Disease

John A. Handal, M.D.
Assistant Clinical Professor
Department of Orthopedic Surgery
University of Texas Southwestern Medical Center;
Dallas Spine Group
Dallas, Texas
Chapt 2: The Structural Degenerative Cascade
    The Cervical Spine
Chapt 96: Degenerative Disc Disease of the
    Cervical Spine: Degenerative Cascade and the
    Anterior Approach

Gregory A. Hanks, M.D.
Clinical Assistant Professor
Department of Orthopedic Surgery
Temple University
Philadelphia, Pennsylvania;
Pennsylvania Orthopedics, P.C.
Camp Hill, Pennsylvania
Chapt 102: Sports Injuries of the Head and
    Cervical Spine

Robert J. Henderson, M.D.
Spine Surgeon
Medical Arts Hospital
Dallas, Texas
Chapt 42: Use of the Morphine Pump for Pain
    Control
Chapt 82: Anterior Approach for Lumbar Fusions
    and Associated Morbidity

Harry N. Herkowitz, M.D.
Chairman
Department of Orthopaedic Surgery
William Beaumont Hospital
Royal Oak, Michigan
Chapt 99: Cervical Spondylotic Radiculopathy and
    Myelopathy: Posterior Approach

Robert H. Hines, Jr., M.D.
Psychiatrist
Department of Psychiatry
SpineCare Medical Group
Daly City, California
Chapt 38: Understanding the Chronic Spine Pain
    Patient: The Attachment Theory

Betsy A. Holland, M.D.
Co-Medical Director
San Francisco Neuroskeletal Imaging;
Medical Director
Marin Magnetic Imaging;
Assistant Clinical Professor
Department of Radiology
University of California
San Francisco, California
Chapt 11: Imaging of the Spine

Ken Y. Hsu, M.D.
Director of Orthopaedic Services
St. Mary's Spine Center
St. Mary's Hospital and Medical Center
San Francisco, California
Chapt 63: Bone Grafts and Implants

Susan J. Isernhagen, B.S., P.T.
President
Isernhagen and Associates, Inc.;
Isernhagen Clinics, Inc.;
Duluth, Minnesota
Chapt 16: Physical Therapy Approach to
    Diagnosing the Patient with Work Related Injury

Donald R. Johnson, II, M.D.
Medical Director
Carolina Spine Institute
Clinical Assistant Professor
Department of Orthopaedic Surgery
Medical University of South Carolina
Charleston, South Carolina
Chapt 58: History of Spine Surgery

Parviz Kambin, M.D.
Clinical Associate Professor
Department of Orthopaedic Surgery
University of Pennsylvania
School of Medicine;
Chief
Division of Spine Surgery
Director
Disc Treatment and Research Center
The Graduate Hospital
Philadelphia, Pennsylvania
Chapt 71: Selection of Surgical Treatment by
    Analysis of Pain Generators
Chapt 73: Arthroscopic Microdiscectomy
    Lumbar and Thoracic
Chapt 77: Arthroscopic Lumbar Interbody Fusion

Mamoru Kawakami, M.D., Ph.D.
Assistant
Department of Orthopedic Surgery
Wakayama Medical College
Wakayama City, Wakayama, Japan
Chapt 8: Anatomy, Biochemistry, and Physiology
    of Low-Back Pain

Gerald P. Keane, M.D.
Department of Sports Orthopaedics and
    Rehabilitation
Menlo Park, California;
Clinical Instructor
Department of Physical Medicine and
    Rehabilitation
Stanford University
Palo Alto, California
Chapt 18: Multidisciplinary Evaluation

Jeffrey A. Knapp, M.D.
Department of Orthopedics
Naval Hospital, Portsmouth
Portsmouth, Virginia
Chapt 2: The Structural Degenerative Cascade
    The Cervical Spine

Martin H. Krag, M.D.
Associate Professor
Department of Orthopaedics and Rehabilitation
University of Vermont
Burlington, Vermont
Chapt 87: The Vermont Spinal Fixator for
    Posterior Application to Short Segments of the
    Thoracic, Lumbar, or Lumbosacral Spine

Ronald C. Kramis, Ph.D.
Research Scientist
Department of Neurosurgery
Good Samaritan Hospital and Medical Center
Portland, Oregon
Chapt 9: Neurophysiology of Chronic Idiopathic
    Back Pain

Philip H. Lander, M.D.
Associate Professor
Department of Radiology
McGill University
Montreal, Quebec, Canada
Chapt 20: Principles of Assessment of
    Osteometabolic Bone Disease
Chapt 62: Osteoporosis of the Spine and Its
    Management
Chapt 113: Paget's Disease

Casey K. Lee, M.D.
Professor
Department of Orthopaedics
New Jersey Medical School
Newark, New Jersey
Chapt 61: Clinical Biomechanics of the Lumbar
Spine

Jonathan P. Lester, M.D.
Georgia Spine and Sports Physicians
Atlanta, Georgia
Chapt 56: Weight Lifting

Michael J. Martin, M.D.
Orthopaedic Spine Surgeon
Puget Sound Spine Institute
Tacoma, Washington
Chapt 45: Bicycling

Tom G. Mayer, M.D.
Clinical Professor
Department of Orthopedic Surgery
Southwestern Medical School
University of Texas;
Medical Director
PRIDE
Dallas, Texas
Chapt 35: Physical Correlates of the
Deconditioning and Dehabilitation Cascade

C. E. McCoy, M.D.
Chairman of the Board
Dallas Spinal Rehabilitation Center
Dallas, Texas
Chapt 67: Psychological Preparation for Surgery

**Marion McGregor, B.Sc., D.C., F.C.C.S.(c),
M.Sc.**
Associate Professor
Department of Research
National Course of Chiropractic
Lombard, Illinois
Chapt 29: Validity and Basis of Manipulation

Frances A. McManemin, Ph.D.
Psychologist
Department of Behavioral Medicine
Dallas Spinal Rehabilitation Center
Dallas, Texas
Adjunct Professor (Biofeedback)
Department of Psychology
University of North Texas
Denton, Texas
Chapt 67: Psychological Preparation for Surgery

John N. McMillin, M.D.
Battlefield Orthopedics, Inc.
Springfield, Missouri
Chapt 81: Posterior Lumbar Interbody Fusion:
Biomechanical Selection for Fusions

Henrik Mike-Mayer, M.D.
Orthopaedic Spine Surgeon
Altoona, Pennsylvania
Chapt 100: Cervical Fusions: Arthrodesis and
Osteosynthesis of the Cervical Spine

Fujio Mita, M.D.
Chairman
Mita Orthopaedic Clinic;
Assistant Professor
Jichi Medical School
Department of Orthopaedic Surgery;
Joysan Orthopaedic Association
Tokyo, Japan
Chapt 78: Myeloscopy and Endoscopic
Nucleotomy

Vert Mooney, M.D.
Professor
Department of Orthopaedics
University California, San Diego;
Medical Director
USCD OrthoMed Center
LaJolla, California
Chapt 15: Diagnostic Tests for the Patient with
Work Related Injuries

David B. Morris, Ph.D.
Associate Editor
Literature and Medicine
Kalamazoo, Michigan
Chapt 33: Pain and Its Meaning: A Biocultural
Model

Marilou Moschetti
Executive Director
AquaTechnics Consulting Group
Aptos, California
Chapt 55: Swimming

Michael H. Moskowitz, M.D., M.P.H.
Psychiatry and Psychosomatics
Department of Psychiatry
SpineCare Medical Group
Daly City, California
Chapt 39: Transcutaneous Electrical Nerve
Stimulation, Acupuncture, Biofeedback,
Hypnotherapy, and Spine Pain

Eugene J. Nordby, M.D.
Associate Clinical Professor
Department of Orthopaedics
University of Wisconsin Medical School
Madison, Wisconsin
Chapt 72: Chemonucleolysis

Richard B. North, M.D.
Associate Professor
Department of Neurosurgery
Johns Hopkins Hospital
Baltimore, Maryland
Chapt 41: Neurosurgical Approaches to Chronic
    Pain

Paul J. Nugent, M.D.
Orthopaedic Spine Surgeon
Fresno, California
Chapt 103: Surgical Treatment of Spinal Tumors

Kelly O'Neal, M.D.
Department of Surgery
Kaiser Permanente Medical Center
Oakland, California
Chapt 73: Arthroscopic Microdiscectomy: Lumbar
    and Thoracic (section on "Endoscopic Thoracic
    Spine Surgery")

Gary M. Onik, M.D.
Chairman
Department of Minimally Invasive Therapy
Princeton Hospital
Orlando, Florida
Chapt 74: Automated Percutaneous Lumbar
    Discectomy

Yoshio Ooi, M.D., Ph.D.
Professor and Chairman
Department of Orthopaedic Surgery and
    Rehabilitation Center
Jichi Medical School
Tochigi Pref., Japan
Chapt 78: Myeloscopy and Endoscopic
    Nucleotomy

John H. Peloza, M.D.
Clinical Assistant Professor
Department of Orthopedic Surgery
University of Texas Southwestern Medical Center;
Dallas Spine Group
Dallas, Texas
Chapt 86: Instrumented Posterior Lumbar Surgery

Mark S. Pfeil, B.S., P.T.
Physical Therapist—Trainer
Department of Sports Medicine
Milwaukee Bucks
Milwaukee, Wisconsin
Chapt 44: Basketball

George Picetti, III, M.D.
Clinical Instructor
Department of Orthopaedic Surgery
University of California, Davis
Sacramento, California
Chapt 73: Arthroscopic Microdiscectomy: Lumbar
    and Thoracic (section on "Endoscopic Thoracic
    Spine Surgery")

Peter B. Polatin, M.D.
Associate Clinical Professor
Department of Psychiatry
University of Texas
Southwest Medical Center at Dallas;
Associate Medical Director
PRIDE
Dallas, Texas
Chapt 32: Work Simulation, Work Hardening, and
    Functional Restoration

Steven C. Poletti, M.D.
Assistant Clinical Professor
Department of Orthopaedic Surgery
Medical University of South Carolina;
Carolina Spine Institute
Charleston, South Carolina
Chapt 2: The Structural Degenerative Cascade
    The Cervical Spine
Chapt 96: Degenerative Disc Disease of the
    Cervical Spine: Degenerative Cascade and the
    Anterior Approach

Carol P. Prentice
Alexander Technique Teacher
Alexander Training Institute
San Francisco, California
Chapt 28: Cervicothoracic Muscular
    Stabilization Techniques

Joel M. Press, M.D.
Director
Sports Rehabilitation Program
Rehabilitation Institute of Chicago;
Assistant Professor
Department of Clinical Physical Medicine and
    Rehabilitation
Northwestern University Medical School
Chicago, Illinois
Chapt 12: Electrodiagnostic Evaluation of Spine
    Problems
Chapt 26: The Physiologic Basis of Therapeutic
    Exercise
Chapt 44: Basketball

Charles D. Ray, M.S., M.D., F.A.C.S.
Chief
Department of Neuroaugmentive Surgery
Associate Director
Institute for Low Back Care;
Minneapolis, Minnesota
Past President
North American Spine Society
Chapt 65: Graft Materials to Prevent Lumbar
    Spine Postoperative Adhesions
Chapt 69: Positioning the Patient for Lumbar
    Spine Surgery
Chapt 80: Lumbar Spinal Stenoses: Reliable
    Methods of Decompression
Chapt 88: Posterior Lumbar Interbody Fusions by
    Implanted Threaded Titanium Cages
Chapt 90: Lumbar Pathoanatomy: Soft- and Hard-
    Tissue Decompression

R. Charles Ray, M.D.
Director
Scoliosis Program
Mary Bridge Children's Hospital
Tacoma, Washington
Chapt 85: Anatomic Strategies of Internal Fixation

Thomas S. Renshaw, M.D.
Professor
Department of Orthopaedic Surgery
Yale University
New Haven, Connecticut
Chapt 108: Congenital Spinal Deformity

James B. Reynolds, M.D.
Orthopedic Surgeon
SpineCare Medical Group
Daly City, California
Chapt 91: Degenerative Spondylolisthesis
Chapt 92: Spondylolisthesis: Isthmic, Congenital,
    Traumatic, and Post-Surgical

William J. Richardson, M.D.
Assistant Professor of Surgery
Department of Orthopaedic Surgery
Duke University Medical Center
Durham, North Carolina
Chapt 9: Neurophysiology of Chronic Idiopathic
    Back Pain
Chapt 95: Surgical Approaches to the Cervical
    Spine

**William J. Roberts, Ph.D.,
    M.S.**
Senior Scientist
R.S. Dow Neurological Sciences Institute
Good Samaritan Hospital and Medical Center
Portland, Oregon
Chapt 9: Neurophysiology of Chronic Idiopathic
    Back Pain

**Robin S. Robison, M.S.,
    B.S.**
Spine Coordinator
Department of Physical Therapy
HEALTHSOUTH
Outpatient Services
Stanford University
Menlo Park, California
Chapt 27: Low-Back School and Stabilization:
    Aggressive Conservative Care

Thomas E. Rudy, Ph.D.
Associate Professor
Departments of Anesthesiology and Psychiatry
University of Pittsburgh Medical Center
Pittsburgh, Pennsylvania
Chapt 37: Cognitive-Behavioral Treatment of the
    Chronic Pain Patient

Damon C. Sacco, M.D.
Diagnostic Radiologist
Department of Magnetic Resonance Imaging
California Advanced Imaging
San Francisco, California
Chapt 11: Imaging of the Spine

Richard M. Salib, M.D.
Associate Medical Director
Institute for Low Back Care
Minneapolis, Minnesota
Chapt 83: Anterior Lumbar Interbody Fusion and
    Combined Antero-posterior Fusion

Yukichi Satoh, M.D., Ph.D.
Lecturer
Jichi Medical School
Chief
Tsowa Hospital
Department of Orthopaedic Surgery
Jichi Medical School
Yakushiji, Minamikawachi-Machi,
Kawachi-Gun, Tochigi Prefecture,
Japan
Chapt 78: Myeloscopy and Endoscopic
    Nucleotomy

J.A. Sazy, M.D.
Spine Fellow
Chicago Spine Fellowship
Rush-Presbyterian-St. Luke's Hospital
Rush Medical College of Rush University
Chicago, Illinois
Chapt 76: Laser Surgery

Jonathan L. Schaffer, M.D.
Instructor, Orthopedic Surgery
Orthopedic Surgery
Harvard Medical School and Brigham & Womens
    Hospital
Boston, Massachusetts
Chapt 78: Myeloscopy and Endoscopic
    Nucleotomy

Guido F. Schauer
Founder
LifeWell™
San Francisco, California
Chapt 51: Spine Defense and the Martial Arts

John D. Schlegel, M.D.
Associate Professor
Division of Orthopedic Surgery
University of Utah School of Medicine
Salt Lake City, Utah
Chapt 89: Anterior Lumbar Instrumentation and
    Fusion
Chapt 105: Thoracolumbar Fractures

Rand L. Schleusener, M.D.
Assistant Professor
Division of Orthopedic Surgery
University of Utah Medical Center
Salt Lake City, Utah
Chapt 89: Anterior Lumbar Instrumentation and
    Fusion
Chapt 105: Thoracolumbar Fractures

Carson Schneck, M.D., Ph.D.
Professor of Anatomy and Cell Biology
Professor of Diagnostic Imaging
Department of Anatomy and Cell Biology
Temple University
Philadelphia, Pennsylvania
Chapt 94: Clinical Anatomy of the Cervical Spine

Jerome A. Schofferman, M.D., F.A.C.P.M.
Pain Management and Internal Medicine
SpineCare Medical Group
Director
Research and Education
San Francisco Spine Institute
Daly City, California
Chapt 1: Introduction
Chapt 2: The Structural Degenerative Cascade
    Applied Neurophysiology of Pain
Chapt 5: Diagnostic Decision Making
Chapt 6: Lumbar Spine Disorders: Taking and
    Interpreting the History
Chapt 7: Physical Examination
Chapt 24: Evaluation of Outcome Studies
Chapt 34: Use of Medications for Pain of Spinal
    Origin

David K. Selby, M.D.
Dallas Spine Group
Dallas, Texas
Chapt 2: The Structural Degenerative Cascade
    The Lumbar Spine
Chapt 86: Instrumented Posterior Lumbar Surgery

Henry H. Sherk, M.D.
Professor and Chief
Division of Orthopedic Surgery
Medical College of Pennsylvania
Philadelphia, Pennsylvania
Chapt 76: Laser Surgery

Robert M. Shugart, M.D.
Orthopaedic Surgery and Spine
Fort Wayne Orthopaedics
Fort Wayne, Indiana
Chapt 48: Football

Chris C. Shulenberger, M.S. Engr.
Ergonomist
Occupational Management Systems, Inc.
Pleasant Hill, California
Chapt 31: Ergonomic Intervention for the
    Prevention and Treatment of Spinal Disorders

Edward D. Simmons, M.D., B.Sc., C.M., M.Sc., F.R.C.S.(C)
Clinical Assistant Professor
Department of Orthopaedic Surgery
Buffalo General Hospital
State University of New York at Buffalo
Buffalo, New York
Chapt 111: Clinical Cervical Deformity and Post
    Laminectomy Kyphosis

Edward H. Simmons, M.D., B.Sc. (Med), F.R.C.S. (C), M.S. (Tor), F.A.C.S.
Professor of Orthopaedic Surgery
Head, University Orthopaedic Spine Service
State University of New York at Buffalo
Buffalo, New York
Chapt 112: Arthritic Spinal Deformity: Ankylosing
    Spondylitis

James W. Simmons, Jr., M.D., F.A.C.S.
Spinal Surgeon
Alamo Bone and Joint Clinic
San Antonio, Texas
Chapt 64: Bone Banking
Chapt 72: Chemonucleolysis
Chapt 81: Posterior Lumbar Interbody Fusion:
    Biomechanical Selection for Fusions

Dennis R. Skogsbergh, D.C.
Assistant Professor
Chairman
Department of Diagnostic Imaging and Clinical
    Orthopedics
National College of Chiropractic
Lombard, Illinois
Chapt 29: Validity and Basis of Manipulation

Paul J. Slosar, M.D.
Spine Surgeon
Mercy Hospital and Medical Center
Chicago, Illinois
Chapt 50: Ice Hockey
Chapt 53: Snow Skiing
Chapt 91: Degenerative Spondylolisthesis
Chapt 92: Spondylolisthesis: Isthmic, Congenital,
    Traumatic, and Post-Surgical

George F. Smith, M.D.
Departments of Pain Management, Spinal
    Diagnostics, and Internal Medicine
SpineCare Medical Group
Daly City, California
Chapt 19: Medical Evaluation of the Spine Patient
Chapt 70: Perioperative Care of the Spine Patient

Janet Y. Soto, B.S. P.T.
Private Practitioner
Berkeley Physical Therapy
Berkeley, California
Senior Faculty Member
Physical Therapy Residency
Program in Advanced Orthopedic Manual Therapy
Kaiser Permanente Medical Center
Hayward, California
Chapt 30: The Role of Manual Therapy in Spinal
    Rehabilitation

Robert J. Spinner, M.D.
Resident
Division of Orthopaedic Surgery
Duke University Medical Center
Durham, North Carolina
Chapt 95: Surgical Approaches

E. Shannon Stauffer, M.D.
Professor and Chairman
Department of Surgery
Division of Orthopaedics and Rehabilitation
Southern Illinois University
School of Medicine
Springfield, Illinois
Chapt 106: Management of the Spinal Cord-
    Injured Patient

Lisa A. Steinkamp, M.S., P.T.
Director and Owner
Functional Rehabilitation and Sports Therapy
Palo Alto, California
Chapt 54: Soccer

Tara B. Sweeney, P.T.
Physical Therapist
Precision Biomechanics
Goleta, California
Chapt 28: Cervicothoracic Muscular
    Stabilization Techniques

Charles S. Szabo, M.D., Ph.D.
Associate Director
San Francisco Center for Comprehensive Pain
    Management
San Francisco, California
Chapt 40: Pain Management by Electrical Implant

James R. Taylor, M.D., Ph.D.
Professor
Department of Anatomy and Human Biology
University of Western Australia
Nedlands, Australia
Chapt 59: Development and Growth of the
    Cervical and Lumbar Spine

Carol Jo Tichenor, M.A., P.T.
Director
Physical Therapy Residency Program in Advanced
    Orthopedic Manual Therapy
Kaiser Permanente Medical Center
Hayward, California
Chapt 30: The Role of Manual Therapy in Spinal
    Rehabilitation

William W. Tomford, M.D.
Associate Professor
Orthopaedic Surgery
Harvard Medical School
Director
Massachusetts General Hospital Bone Bank
Department of Orthopaedic Surgery
Massachusetts General Hospital
Boston, Massachusetts
Chapt 64: Bone Banking

John J. Triano, M.A., D.C., Ph.D.
Staff Physician
Texas Back Institute
Plano, Texas
Chapt 29: Validity and Basis of Manipulation

Dennis C. Turk, Ph.D.
Professor
Department of Psychiatry, Anesthesiology, and
    Behavioral Science
Director
Pain Evaluation and Treatment Institute
University of Pittsburgh
School of Medicine
Pittsburgh, Pennsylvania
Chapt 37: Cognitive-Behavioral Treatment of the
    Chronic Pain Patient

**Lance Twomey, B.A.pp.Sc. (WAIT), B.Sc.
    (Hons), Ph.D. (WAust), T.T.C., M.A.P.A.**
Deputy Vice-Chancellor and Professor
Department of Physiotherapy
Curtin University of Technology
Perth, Western Australia, Australia
Chapt 59: Development and Growth of the
    Cervical and Lumbar Spine

Mark W. Van Dyke, D.O., M.P.H.
Medical Director
Department of Occupational Medicine
Center for Occupational Health
St. Margaret Memorial Hospital
Pittsburgh, Pennsylvania
Chapt 18: Multidisciplinary Evaluation

Paul P. Vessa, M.D.
Somerset Orthopaedic Associates
Bridgewater, New Jersey
Chapt 57: Wrestling

Robert G. Watkins, M.D.
Associate Clinical Professor
Department of Orthopaedics
University of Southern California School of
    Medicine;
Kerlin-Jobe Orthopaedic Clinic
Los Angeles, California
Chapt 43: Baseball
Chapt 84: Results of Anterior Interbody Fusion

James N. Weinstein, D.O.
Professor
Department of Orthopaedic Surgery
Director
Spine Diagnostic and Treatment Center
University of Iowa College of Medicine
Iowa City, Iowa
Chapt 8: Anatomy, Biochemistry, and Physiology
    of Low-Back Pain

F. Todd Wetzel, M.D.
Associate Professor and Director
Department of Orthopaedics and Rehabilitation
University of Chicago Spine Center
University of Chicago
School of Medicine
Chicago, Illinois
Chapt 97: Degenerative Disc Disease of the
    Cervical Spine: Posterior Approach
Chapt 102: Sports Injuries of the Head and
    Cervical Spine

Arthur H. White, M.D.
Medical Director
San Francisco Spine Institute
SpineCare Medical Group
Daly City, California
Chapt 1: Introduction
Chapt 3: The Socioeconomic Cascade
Chapt 18: Multidisciplinary Evaluation
Chapt 25: Conservative Care—Pulling It all
    Together
Chapt 52: Running
Chapt 63: Bone Grafts and Implants
Chapt 66: Surgical Decision Making for
    Degenerative Disease
Appendix: Dynamic Lumbar Stabilization Exercises

Robert E. Windsor, M.D.
President
Georgia Spine and Sports Physicians, P.C.
Smyrna, Georgia
Chapt 56: Weight Lifting

Jeffrey L. Young, M.D., M.A.
Assistant Professor
Department of Physical Medicine and
    Rehabilitation
Northwestern University Medical School;
Attending Physician
Sports Rehabilitation Program
Rehabilitation Institute of Chicago
Chicago, Illinois
Chapt 12: Electrodiagnostic Evaluation of Spine
    Problems
Chapt 26: The Physiologic Basis of Therapeutic
    Exercise
Chapt 44: Basketball

Hansen A. Yuan, M.D.
Professor
Departments of Orthopaedic Surgery and
    Neurological Surgery
Chief
Division of Spinal Surgery
SUNY Health Science Center at Syracuse,
    New York
State University of New York Health Science
    Center at Syracuse
Syracuse, New York
Chapt 89: Anterior Lumbar Instrumentation and
    Fusion
Chapt 101: Anterior Instrumentation of the
    Cervical Spine
Chapt 104: Cervical Spine Fractures
Chapt 105: Thoracolumbar Spine Fractures

James F. Zucherman, M.D.
Director
Department of Orthopaedics
St. Mary's Spine Center
San Francisco, California
Chapt 63: Bone Grafts and Implants

Foreword

Leon L. Wiltse

There are many books on spinal disorders. What to do about any given situation is well documented. I have found none, however, which offers a better framework from which to view the entire patient with all of his complexities than does this one.

The spine specialist needs to be a total doctor, not just a surgical technician or rehabilitationist. Spine medicine is extremely complex. In order to be a good spine specialist, the physician must be well-schooled in many subspecialities, including rehabilitation, surgery, psychiatry, internal medicine, radiology and diagnostics.

Because of the wide range of subjects covered, especially the non-operative, this book will have a strong appeal to all health care professionals who treat the spine. The formation of the International Society for the Study of the Lumbar Spine in 1973 was a landmark in the development of spine medicine and surgery. This organization pioneered the idea of comprehensive care. It selected its members from all health care disciplines which have an interest in the spine. Its membership includes the following: orthopedic surgeons, neurosurgeons, neuroradiologists, neurologists, physiatrists, psychologists, psychiatrists, rheumatologists, epidemiologists, pathologists, engineers, basic scientists, statisticians, chiropractors, and physical therapists.

Other spine organizations which have come along since, in particular, the North American Spine Society, have carried on the same tradition. This book is the embodiment of that concept.

Patient education in the care of the spine is stressed and a neck school is described as well as the more traditional low back school. There is a chapter on the basic theories of spinal manipulation and a chapter on clinical manipulation.

Chapters 43 to 57 are interesting. This section is devoted to sport-specific injuries, including those associated with baseball, basketball, ballet, skating, football, golf, hockey, martial arts, running, skiing, soccer, swimming, lifting, and wrestling. The editors have obviously been very aware of the fact that for conditions in the spine, but especially in the lumbar and cervical spines, pain is the thing that brings the patient to the doctor. But for pain, few would come near us. As a result, a fairly large share of the book is devoted to the treatment of pain, both the basic science of pain, e.g., neurophysiology, and the clinical management of pain.

We are all familiar with Dr. Kirkaldy-Willis' degenerative cascade, but the idea of a socioeconomic cascade (Chapter 3) and a psychological cascade (Chapter 4) would seem unique.

This book gives the reader a framework and a philosophy on which to base his practice. The practice of spine care that this book advocates works. It has been derived from many decades of many spine specialists' lifetime practice experiences.

I have watched this practice style develop out of the teachings of our leading spine luminaries; Philip Newman, Bill Kirkaldy-Willis, Homer Pheasant, Harry Farfan, Harry Crock, Bernie Finneson, and Vert Mooney (to name just a few). These men and many others have progressively added to our current concept of the practice of spinal medicine, which is brought to you in this book.

Foreword

Scott Haldeman

The treatment of patients with spinal symptoms used to be easy, enjoyable, and satisfying. If one was a family physician, most patients seemed to get better with anti-inflammatory medications and bed rest. If one was a chiropractor, one simply looked for subluxations and adjusted them. If one was a surgeon, most patients were diagnosed as having disc herniations and, when unresponsive to other treatments, underwent laminectomy and discectomy. If one was a consultant in neurology, rheumatology, or psychiatry, one simply examined the patient and proclaimed the presence or absence of disease within one's specialty and where appropriate treated (or more likely, declared untreatable) the disease. Unlike this book, textbooks on the topic were small and simplistic, usually concentrating on unproven and often unquestioned theories and then describing the technical method of treatment preferred by the author. Since clinicians from different specialties and professions rarely spoke to each other or attended meetings outside their specialty, everyone was comfortable with the situation and assumed that their method of managing patients was the most effective.

This level of comfort has been gradually eroding over the past two decades. The primary motivation for the change has been the realization that, at least in the Western industrialized nations, back pain disability has reached epidemic proportions. The number of patients claiming disability as a result of spinal problems has increased each year. This has occurred despite a proliferation in the number of clinicians and increased complexity and sophistication of the methods of diagnosing and treating this problem. This text brings these specialties and philosophies together in a usable fashion.

There has also been a rapid, almost exponential, increase in the cost of both treatment and indemnity associated with back pain disability. This, in turn, has been the motivating factor for the growing importance of research into all aspects of spine pathophysiology and management. Whereas there were virtually no scientific peer-reviewed journals devoted to publishing research on spinal disorders in 1976 when "Spine" was first established, it is no longer possible for clinicians, or even scientists, to keep abreast of the twenty or more journals which publish original scientific papers which relate to the spine and its associated structures. The international societies on the lumbar spine, cervical spine and scoliosis used to be the only forums for the presentation of original research for peer review. These organizations must now compete with the North American Spine Society and other national associations with much larger membership, for the best research papers. Furthermore, most of these societies have become interdisciplinary, accepting membership from clinicians and scientists with greatly differing backgrounds and experience.

All this research and debate has resulted in serious questioning of prior theories and models for back pain. Prior simplistic concepts have given way to complex models which combine the increasing number of factors which seem to influence and predict the disability that patients are likely to experience when their back hurts. The new models are attempts to incorporate current knowledge obtained from laboratory experimentation, epidemiology, sociology, psychology and clinical outcome studies. The concept of a structural degenerative cascade, a socioeconomic cascade and a psychological cascade as outlined in the early chapters of this text represent modern efforts at interpreting this data. These modes, in turn, are increasingly being used as a basis for the management of patients with back pain.

Recent emphasis on so-called managed care and costs of health care has forced clinicians to justify the effectiveness of their diagnosis and treatment methods. In the past, the simple observation that a patient or group of patients felt better following a particular treatment approach was sufficient to justify that treatment. In order to be compensated, it has become increasingly important to prove, by means of controlled clinical trials, that a treatment is successful. In the same way a diagnosis test used to be considered important if it revealed information about a patient. It is now necessary to demonstrate that a test will influence the outcome of a patient's treatment for it to be considered reasonable. Professional and governmental expert panels have been convened to provide guidelines on the management of patients with back pain. They have inevitably relied on controlled clinical trials and outcome studies rather than case reports, anecdotal observations, and uncontrolled or retrospective studies when issuing recommendations. This has caused somewhat of a panic among clinicians, but at the same time, has led to the establishment of increasingly sophisticated clinical trials on a wide variety of diagnostic tests and treatment methods. The documentation in this text parallels these scientific directions.

Recent research has also challenged some of the more classic concepts of treatment. There are a large number of studies which have shown a breakdown in the previously perceived relationship between spinal abnormalities on x-rays, MRI and other imaging studies and symptoms. This has changed the emphasis on ordering routine x-rays and early expensive testing unless the study is likely to influence management. The observation that patients with well-defined disc herniations can and do respond to non-surgical approaches not only with reduction of symptoms, but also in the size of the herniation, has led to a de-emphasis of the surgical approach to these patients. At the same time, research on the intervertebral disc as a primary source of pain through the release of inflammatory agents has resulted in an increase in the use of surgery for the treatment of discogenic pain.

More than anything, however, the research has lead to greater understanding of the role of patient social attitudes and habits as a predictor of disability. Increasingly, rehabilitation and preventative interventions are focusing on changing the lifestyle of the patient with back pain. The impact of smoking, exercise and a well-designed work site is being recognized. Patient habits and attitude also appear to influence the response to treatment. For example, the fusion rates following surgery are diminished if the patient is a smoker, while effects of motivation, psychological depression and litigation on the rehabilitation process is the subject of an increasing number of studies. This knowledge is now being incorporated in work- and sports-related activities in an attempt to reduce the frequency and severity of back injuries. The fact that this text has a whole section of sports-specific injuries reflects the importance of these issues.

It is no longer possible to state that the treatment of back pain is easy. The complexity of the issue has reduced the comfort level and, to some extent, the confidence of many clinicians in dealing with patients with these problems. Furthermore, as this text illustrates, the books on the topic have gotten considerably thicker and more detailed. There is, however, no doubt that spine care has become more interesting and challenging to both the clinician and the scientist. Those of us, including many of the authors in this text, who have had the privilege of watching and participating in the expansion of knowledge on the spine over the past two decades recognize that our understanding of the spine is far from complete. The hope is that by laying out everything we do know in a text such as this, we can begin to see the areas of future research which will clarify and consolidate current knowledge. This is expected to lead to more well-defined and clear-cut models for the understanding and management of patients with spinal problems. At that time, spine care should, once again, become satisfying and enjoyable while, at the same time, more scientifically valid, cost-effective and beneficial to our patients.

Preface

The practice of spinal medicine is in chronic disarray and facing serious jeopardy. This is due to the disorganized and unscientific fashion in which the subspecialties deal with the vague etiologies of back pain and the impatience of the managed care organizations, the government, and the public, with our inefficient, expensive, and disorganized care.

As a result, there may be mandatory restructuring of the spinal medicine delivery system which may set back the quality of spine care twenty years. If we can present a unified approach to a high quality and efficient practice of spine care, we can salvage our subspecialty and have a more rewarding, successful, and enjoyable practice than we now have.

This book presents an answer to our dilemma. It brings together all subspecialty philosophies into a common concept of total spine care. It offers systematic methods of diagnosis and treatment which are efficient and already acceptable to the demands of managed care and government agencies.

We present strong scientific evidence for the source and preferred treatment of back pain. Rather than a compilation of individual opinions, we provide a model which is complete and easy to follow. It takes into consideration not only the physical structural sources of low-back pain, but the psychological, social, and cultural ramifications.

We hope that this book will serve as a catalyst for a unified approach to spine care which will be more beneficial for our individual patients and for society, as a whole.

Arthur H. White, M.D.
Jerome A. Schofferman, M.D.

Acknowledgements

All of the authors of the chapters in this book have devoted considerable time and effort to produce palatable, state of the art spine care information for you, the reader. Several of the authors deserve special thanks because of their voluminous contributions, each of which could have been separate books on their own. These authors are Nicholas Bogduk, M.D., Charlie Ray, M.D., and Jerome Schofferman, M.D. I would like to thank Robert Gaines, for creating at the last minute, a chapter on spinal deformity in children, adolescents, and young adults, which is a distillation of an entire field of spinal medicine. In future revisions of this book he will hopefully expand that chapter to the multiple chapters the subject deserves. Dr. Ken Hsu from San Francisco deserves special thanks for many of the drawings that are found throughout this book.

Most of all I would like to thank Eugenia Klein for the years of effort and consultation that she has provided as well as her valuable editorial support concerning the design and organization of this work.

Arthur H. White, M.D.

I would like to thank Arthur White, MD, who first gave me the opportunity to work with spine patients many years ago and thereby introduced me to an area of medicine that has been so enjoyable and fruitful. I would like to thank the patients with whom I have worked for teaching me the lessons that are not in any book and challenging me to search for better ways to do things. I thank my colleagues and staff at SpineCare whose support allowed me the time and energy to work on this book. Most of all I thank my wife, Sally, for her love and support as well as the encouragement to explore better ways to live. It is perhaps too easy in life to remain static, to accept things as they are, to "gel." Working on this book has kept me fluid professionally. Living with Sally has kept me fluid personally.

Jerome A. Schofferman, M.D.

Contents

VOLUME ONE
Diagnosis and Conservative Treatment

PART I

The Multidisciplinary Approach to Spine Practice

1   Introduction   2

Arthur H. White, M.D.

Jerome A. Schofferman, M.D.

2   The Structural Degenerative Cascade
The Lumbar Spine   8

David K. Selby, M.D.

The Cervical Spine   16

John A. Handal, M.D.

Jeffrey A. Knapp, M.D.

Steven C. Poletti, M.D.

Applied Neurophysiology of Pain   23

Jerome A. Schofferman, M.D.

3   The Socioeconomic Cascade   27

Arthur H. White, M.D.

4   The Psychologic Cascade   35

David J. Anderson, M.D.

5   Diagnostic Decision Making 41

Jerome A. Schofferman, M.D.

6   Lumbar Spine Disorders: Taking and Interpreting the History   52

Jerome A. Schofferman, M.D.

7   Physical Examination   71

Jerome A. Schofferman, M.D.

PART II

Basic Science

8   Anatomy, Biochemistry, and Physiology of Low-Back Pain   84

Mamoru Kawakami, M.D., Ph.D.

Kenichi Chatani, M.D., Ph.D.

James N. Weinstein, D.O.

9   Neurophysiology of Chronic Idiopathic Back Pain   104

Ronald C. Kramis, Ph.D.

Richard G. Gillette, M.S. Ph.D.

William J. Roberts, M.S., Ph.D.

xxvi   Contents

10   Biomechanics of the
      Spine   116

      Serge Gracovetsky, Ph.D.

PART III

Diagnostic Measures

11   Imaging of the Spine   140

      Betsy A. Holland, M.D.

      Damon C. Sacco, M.D.

12   Electrodiagnostic Evaluation of
      Spine Problems   191

      Joel M. Press, M.D.

      Jeffrey L. Young, M.D., M.A.

13   Somatosensory and Motor
      Evoked Potentials   204

      Erwin G. Gonzalez, M.D.

14   Discography   219

      Nikolai Bogduk, M.D., Ph.D.

      Charles N. Aprill, M.D.

      Richard Derby, Jr., M.D.

15   Diagnostic Tests for the
      Patient with Work Related
      Injuries   239

      Vert Mooney, M.D.

16   Physical Therapy Approach to
      Diagnosing the Patient with
      Work-Related Injury   250

      Susan J. Isernhagen, B.S., P.T.

17   Psychiatric Evaluation of the
      Chronic Pain Patient   259

      David J. Anderson, M.D.

18   Multidisciplinary Evaluation
      265

      Mark Van Dyke, D.O., M.P.H.

      Gerald P. Keane, M.D.

      Arthur H. White, M.D.

19   Medical Evaluation of the Spine
      Patient   272

      George F. Smith, M.D.

20   Principles of Assessment of
      Osteometabolic Bone
      Disease   281

      Alexander G. Hadjipavlou, M.D., F.R.C.S. (c)

      Philip H. Lander, M.D.

PART IV

Diagnostic and Therapeutic Blocks

21   Diagnostic Blocks of Spinal
      Synovial Joints   298

      Nikolai Bogduk, M.D., Ph.D.

      Charles N. Aprill, M.D.

      Richard Derby, Jr., M.D.

22   Epidural Steroid
      Injections   322

      Nikolai Bogduk, M.D., Ph.D.

      Charles N. Aprill, M.D.

      Richard Derby, Jr., M.D.

PART V

Conservative Treatment and Rehabilitation

Section 1

The Patient with Structural Degenerative Disease

23   Education: The Primary Treatment of Low-Back Pain   347

William T. Evans, M.D.

24   Evaluation of Outcome Studies   359

Jerome A. Schofferman, M.D.

25   Conservative Care—Pulling It all Together   367

Arthur H. White, M.D.

26   The Physiologic Basis of Therapeutic Exercise   375

Jeffrey L. Young, M.D., M.A.
Joel M. Press, M.D.

27   Low-Back School and Stabilization: Aggressive Conservative Care   394

Robin S. Robison, B.S., M.S.

28   Cervicothoracic Muscular Stabilization Techniques   413

Tara B. Sweeney, P.T.
Carol P. Prentice

29   Validity and Basis of Manipulation   437

John J. Triano, M.A., D.C., Ph.D.
Dennis R. Skogsbergh, D.C.
Marion McGregor, D.C., M.Sc.

30   The Role of Manual Therapy in Spinal Rehabilitation   451

Joseph P. Farrell, M.S., P.T.
Janet Y. Soto, B.S., P.T.
Carol Jo Tichenor, M.A., P.T.

Section 2

The Patient within the Socioeconomic Cascade

31   Ergonomic Intervention for the Prevention and Treatment of Spinal Disorders   472

Chris C. Shulenberger, M.S. Engr.

32   Work Simulation, Work Hardening, and Functional Restoration   486

Peter B. Polatin, M.D.

Section 3

The Chronic Pain Patient within the Psychologic Cascade

33   Pain and Its Meaning: A Biocultural Model   496

David B. Morris, Ph.D.

34   Use of Medications for Pain of Spinal Origin   509

Jerome A. Schofferman, M.D.

35   Physical Correlates of the Deconditioning and Dehabilitation Cascade   528

Tom G. Mayer, M.D.

36   Psychosocial Correlates of the Deconditioning Syndrome in Patients with Chronic Low-Back Pain   537

Robert J. Gatchel, Ph.D.

37   Cognitive-Behavioral Treatment of the Chronic Pain Patient   546

Thomas E. Rudy, Ph.D.
Dennis C. Turk, Ph.D.

38   Understanding the Chronic Spine Pain Patient: The Attachment Theory   558

David J. Anderson, M.D.
Robert H. Hines, Jr., M.D.

39   Transcutaneous Electrical Nerve Stimulation, Acupuncture, Biofeedback, Hypnotherapy, and Spine Pain   564

Michael H. Moskowitz, M.D., M.P.H.

40   Pain Management by Electrical Implant   573

Charles S. Szabo, M.D., Ph.D.

41   Neurosurgical Approaches to Chronic Pain   584

Richard B. North, M.D.

42   Use of the Morphine Pump for Pain Control   599

Robert J. Henderson, M.D.

Section 4

Sport-Specific Structural Injuries

43   Baseball   608

Robert G. Watkins, M.D.

44   Basketball   627

Joel M. Press, M.D.
Mark S. Pfeil, B.S., P.T.
Jeffrey L. Young, M.D., M.A.

45   Bicycling   635

Michael J. Martin, M.D.

46   Dance   641

Richard D. Gibbs, M.D.
Patricia H. Gibbs, M.D.

47   Figure Skating   649

Joseph D. Fortin, D.O.

48   Football   667

Robert M. Shugart, M.D.

49   Golf   675

Kevin S. Finnesey, M.D.

50   Ice Hockey   683

Paul J. Slosar, M.D.

51   Spine Defense and the Martial Arts   687

Guido F. Schauer

52   Running   711

Arthur H. White, M.D.

53   Snow Skiing   716

Paul J. Slosar, M.D.

54   Soccer   721
      Lisa A. Steinkamp, M.S., P.T.

55   Swimming   727
      Andrew J. Cole, M.D.
      Richard E. Eagleston, M.A., P.T., A.T.C.
      Marilou Moschetti

56   Weight Lifting   746
      Robert E. Windsor, M.D.
      Susan J. Dreyer, M.D.
      Jonathan P. Lester, M.D.
      Frank J. E. Falco, M.D.

57   Wrestling   762
      Paul P. Vessa, M.D.

VOLUME TWO

Operative Treatment

PART VI

Surgical Treatment

Section 1

General Considerations

58   History of Spine Surgery   773
      James Dwyer, M.D.
      Donald R. Johnson, II, M.D.

59   Development and Growth of
      the Cervical and Lumbar
      Spine   792
      Lance T. Twomey, Ph.D.
      James R. Taylor, M.D., Ph.D.

60   Anatomy of the Spine   809
      Nikolai Bogduk, M.D., Ph.D.

61   Clinical Biomechanics of the
      Lumbar Spine   837
      Casey K. Lee, M.D.

62   Osteoporosis of the Spine and
      Its Management   847
      Alexander G. Hadjipavlou, M.D., F.R.C.S. (c)
      Philip H. Lander, M.D.

63   Bone Grafts and
      Implants   870
      Ken Y. Hsu, M.D.
      James F. Zucherman, M.D.
      Arthur H. White, M.D.

64   Bone Banking   891
      James W. Simmons, Jr., M.D., F.A.C.S.
      William W. Tomford, M.D.

65   Graft Materials to Prevent
      Lumbar Spine Postoperative
      Adhesions   899
      Charles D. Ray, M.S., M.D., F.A.C.S.

66   Surgical Decision Making for
      Degenerative Disease   908
      Arthur H. White, M.D.

67   Psychological Preparation for
     Surgery   915

     C. E. McCoy, M.D.

     Frances A. McManemin, Ph.D.

     Ramon Cuencas-Zamora, Ph.D.

68   Anesthesia in Cervical Spine
     Surgery   939

     Tracy P. Cotter, M.D.

     Susan L. Goelzer, M.D.

69   Positioning the Patient for
     Lumbar Spine Surgery   950

     W. Bradford DeLong, M.D., F.A.C.S.

     Charles D. Ray, M.S., M.D., F.A.C.S.

70   Perioperative Care of the Spine
     Patient   964

     George F. Smith, M.D.

71   Selection of Surgical Treatment
     by Analysis of Pain
     Generators   984

     Parviz Kambin, M.D.

Section 2

Minimally Invasive Surgery of the Lumbar Spine

72   Chemonucleolysis   991

     James W. Simmons, Jr., M.D., F.A.C.S.

     Eugene J. Nordby, M.D.

73   Arthroscopic Microdiscectomy:
     Lumbar and Thoracic   1002

     Parviz Kambin, M.D.

74   Automated Percutaneous
     Lumbar Discectomy   1017

     Gary M. Onik, M.D.

75   Microsurgical Discectomy and
     Spinal Decompression   1028

     W. Bradford DeLong, M.D., F.A.C.S.

76   Laser Surgery   1046

     John A. Sazy, M.D.

     Henry H. Sherk, M.D.

77   Arthroscopic Lumbar Interbody
     Fusion   1055

     Parviz Kambin, M.D.

78   Myeloscopy and Endoscopic
     Nucleotomy   1067

     Yoshio Ooi, M.D., Ph.D.

     Yukichi Satoh, M.D., Ph.D.

     Fujio Mita, M.D.

     Jonathan L. Schaffer, M.D.

Section 3

Open Surgery of the Lumbar Spine

79   The Controversy of "Large Vs.
     Small": The Present Role of
     Minimally Invasive Surgery of
     the Spine   1075

     Charles V. Burton, M.D.

80   Lumbar Spinal Stenoses:
     Reliable Methods of
     Decompression   1084

     Charles D. Ray, M.S., M.D., F.A.C.S.

81   Posterior Lumbar Interbody
     Fusion: Biomechanical Selection
     for Fusions   1100

     James W. Simmons, Jr., M.D., F.A.C.S.

     John N. McMillin, M.D.

82   Anterior Approach for Lumbar Fusions and Associated Morbidity   1112

Robert J. Henderson, M.D.

83   Anterior Lumbar Interbody Fusion and Combined Anteroposterior Fusion   1126

Richard M. Salib, M.D.

84   Results of Anterior Interbody Fusion   1135

Robert G. Watkins, M.D.

85   Anatomic Strategies of Internal Fixation   1157

R. Charles Ray, M.D.

86   Instrumented Posterior Lumbar Surgery   1173

John H. Peloza, M.D.
David K. Selby, M.D.

87   The Vermont Spinal Fixator for Posterior Application to Short Segments of the Thoracic, Lumbar, or Lumbosacral Spine   1196

Martin H. Krag, M.D.
Bruce D. Beynnon, Ph.D.

88   Posterior Lumbar Interbody Fusions by Implanted Threaded Titanium Cages   1123

Charles D. Ray, M.S., M.D., F.A.C.S.

89   Anterior Lumbar Instrumentation and Fusion   1233

John D. Schlegel, M.D.
Rand L. Schleusener, M.D.
Hansen A. Yuan, M.D.

90   Lumbar Pathoanatomy: Soft- and Hard-Tissue Decompression   1250

Charles D. Ray, M.S., M.D., F.A.C.S.

91   Degenerative Spondylolisthesis   1266

Paul J. Slosar, M.D.
James B. Reynolds, M.D.

92   Spondylolisthesis: Isthmic, Congenital, Traumatic, and Post-Surgical   1280

James B. Reynolds, M.D.
Paul J. Slosar, Jr.

93   The Use of Electrical Stimulation for Spinal Fusion   1296

Kevin S. Finnesey, M.D.

Section 4

Open Surgery of the Cervical Spine

94   Clinical Anatomy of the Cervical Spine   1306

Carson D. Schneck, M.D., Ph.D.

95   Surgical Approaches to the Cervical Spine   1335

William J. Richardson, M.D.
Robert J. Spinner, M.D.

96   Degenerative Disc Disease of the Cervical Spine: Degenerative Cascade and the Anterior Approach   1351

Steven C. Poletti, M.D.
John A. Handal, M.D.

97   Degenerative Disc Disease of the
      Cervical Spine: Posterior
      Approach   1358

      F. Todd Wetzel, M.D.

98   Cervical Spondylotic
      Radiculopathy and Myelopathy:
      Anterior Approach and
      Pathology   1368

      Sanford E. Emery, M.D.

99   Cervical Spondylotic
      Radiculopathy and Myelopathy:
      Posterior Approach   1379

      Richard S. Brower, M.D.

      Harry N. Herkowitz, M.D.

100   Cervical Fusions: Arthrodesis
      and Osteosynthesis of the
      Cervical Spine   1394

      Henrik Mike-Mayer, M.D.

      Howard B. Cotler, M.D., F.A.C.S.

      Stanley D. Gertzbein, M.D.

101   Anterior Instrumentation of the
      Cervical Spine   1428

      Patrick J. Connolly, M.D.

      Hansen A. Yuan, M.D.

102   Sports Injuries of the Head and
      Cervical Spine   1437

      F. Todd Wetzel, M.D.

      Gregory A. Hanks, M.D.

      P. Dean Cummings, M.D.

PART VII

Tumor, Trauma, Infection, Deformity, and Other Conditions

Section 1

Tumors

103   Surgical Treatment of Spinal
      Tumors   1457

      P. James Nugent, M.D.

Section 2

Trauma

104   Cervical Spine Fractures   1486

      Patrick J. Connolly, M.D.

      Hansen Yuan, M.D.

105   Thoracolumbar Spine Fractures
      1510

      John D. Schlegel, M.D.

      Hansen Yuan, M.D.

      Rand L. Schleusener, M.D.

106   Management of the Spinal Cord-
      Injured Patient   1529

      E. Shannon Stauffer, M.D.

Section 3

Infection

107   Spinal Infection   1543

      Matthew F. Gornet, M.D.

Section 4

Deformity

108   Congenital Spinal
      Deformity   1554

      Thomas S. Renshaw, M.D.

109   Spinal Deformity in Children,
       Adolescents, and Young
       Adults   1557

       Robert W. Gaines, Jr., M.D.

110   Adult Scoliosis   1612

       John G. Finkenberg, M.D.

111   Clinical Cervical Deformity
       and Post Laminectomy
       Kyphosis   1632

       Edward D. Simmons, M.D., F.R.C.S. (c)
       Peter N. Capicotto, M.D.

Section 5

Other Conditions

112   Arthritic Spinal Deformity:
       Ankylosing Spondyliltis   1652

       Edward H. Simmons, M.D., F.R.C.S. (c)

113   Paget's Disease   1720

       Alexander G. Hadjipavlou, M.D., F.R.C.S. (c)
       Philip H. Lander, M.D.

Appendix

A   Dynamic Lumbar Stabilization
       Exercises   1738

       Arthur W. White, M.D.

B   Practical Guide to
       Billing   1746

       Bobbi Buell

       Index I-1

Color Plates

Color plate I follows   94

Color plate II follows   986

Color plate III follows   1008

Color plate IV follows   1056

Color plate V follows   1072

Color plate VI follows   1376

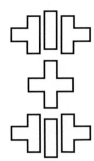

PART VI

Surgical Treatment

Section 1
General Considerations

58 History of Spine Surgery

James Dwyer
Donald R. Johnson, II

59 Development and Growth of the Cervical and Lumbar Spine

Lance T. Twomey
James R. Taylor

60 Anatomy of the Spine

Nikolai Bogduk

61 Clinical Biomechanics of Lumbar Spine

Casey K. Lee

62 Osteoporosis of the Spine and Its Management

Alexander G. Hadjipavlou
Philip H. Lander

63 Bone Grafts and Implants

Ken Y. Hsu
James Zucherman
Arthur H. White

64 Bone Banking

James W. Simmons, Jr.
William W. Tomford

65 Graft Materials to Prevent Lumbar Spine Postoperative Adhesions

Charles D. Ray

66 Surgical Decision Making

Arthur H. White

67 Psychological Preparation for Surgery

C. Eddie McCoy
Frances A. McManemin
Ramon Cuencas-Zamora

68 Anesthesia in Cervical Spine Surgery

Tracy P. Cotter
Susan L. Goelzer

69 Positioning the Patient for Lumbar Spine Surgery

W. Bradford DeLong
Charles D. Ray

70 Perioperative Care of the Spine Patient

George F. Smith

71 Selection of Surgical Treatment by Analysis of Pain Generators

Parviz Kambin

Chapter 58
History of Spine Surgery

James Dwyer
Donald R. Johnson, II

Laminectomy

Arthroscopic and Percutaneous
   Discectomy

Stenosis

Spondylolisthesis

Fusion

Posterior Interbody Fusion

Anterior Interbody Fusion

Circumferential Lumbar Fusion

Internal Fixation

Cervical Spine

Thoracic Spine

Summary

Low back pain and sciatica have plagued humans since ancient time. As early as five thousand years ago, The Edwin Smith papyrus from Ancient Egypt document a detailed account of traumatic quadriplegia. In Shakespeare's *Timon of Athens,*[176] there is a literary description of sciatica. Then, in 1764, Cotugno[36] noted an incidence of sciatica, in which he made a correlation, for the first time in medical history, between the sciatic nerve and severe leg pain. In the first surgical papers, Imhoptep Viser of Djoser described many musculo-skeletal lesions and stated that spinal cord injury causes paralysis.

As early as 460 B.C., Hippocrates referred to the sciatic nerve, with detailed descriptions of its existence, but had no clue as to its origin. Similarly, a Persian miniature dating from 1400 B.C., depicts a dissection of the human figure, which revealed a surprising knowledge of spinal anatomy. Galen, physician to Marcus Aurelius, describes scoliosis, kyphosis, and spinal deformity. Paul of Agena,[141] a Greek physician, performed the first laminectomies for fractures of the spine.

Knowledge came in isolated bursts. Osseous pathology was diagnosed early, in 1782, by Herbinaux,[73] who identified a case of spondylolisthesis. More than half a century later, in 1841, Valleix[198] pinpointed sciatica, by identifying tender spots along the course of the sciatic nerve, named for him as Valleix's points.

Spinal surgery bears its own unique history. The first attempt at performing a laminectomy was apparently made by Henry Cline of England in 1841. His unsuccessful attempt was followed by another similarly unsuccessful endeavor, by a surgeon at St. Thomas's Hospital in London on October 17, 1822. The 30-year-old patient died of peritonitis 12 days postoperatively, and because of the repeated mortality in these procedures, laminectomy was abandoned.

Six years later, however, Alban Gilpin Smith[182] of America repeated the attempt, and in 1828, the first successful laminectomy was performed. The surgical procedure, which involved the removal of multiple lamina, was performed to treat traumatic paraplegia, secondary to spinal fracture. The patient, who had fallen from a horse, survived the surgery and achieved partial neurologic recovery. The success of this case and its findings was published in the *North American Journal of Medicine and Surgery* in 1829.

Later, in 1857, the first clinical descriptions of disc pathology were made by Virchow,[205] who identified a fracture disc at autopsy. Quickly following this finding, Von Lushka,[206] in 1858, reported a posteriorly protruded disc. Then, in 1896,

Kocher[104] isolated a traumatic rupture of the disc at L1-L2 during autopsy. The first steps in diagnosing back disorders were now underway.

The first inroads in the area of claudication were made in 1858, when Charcot[25] described a traumatic aneurysm of the iliac artery in a French Legionnaire, which resulted in limited ambulation. This observation led Joseph Jules Dejeuine[44] to propose the concept of spinal claudication in 1911, when he utilized Charcot's research in diagnosing three cases of activity-related limb weakness.

Degenerative vertebral subluxation was first identified in 1893, when William Lane[109] observed the condition after operating on a 34-year-old woman who had become progressively paraparetic.

In Glasgow in 1911, physician George Middleton and pathologist John Teacher[128] diagnosed the first case of disc extrusion, clinically resulting in paraplegia and urinary tract dysfunction. An autopsy showed disc extrusion at L1, with compression of the spinal cord. They, and others, however, still failed to correlate disc problems with back pain or sciatica.

A breakthrough was made in the same year, however, when Goldthwaite[69] made the first leap in determining the clinical association between disc rupture and back pain. His report on this finding also analyzed the direct influence of posterior disc displacement in paraplegia, another key discovery that was never before suspected. Goldthwaite showed how the nucleus pulposus could project posteriorly and cause paralysis as illustrated in his article, which shows a disc protrusion at L5.

Goldthwaite's findings were further substantiated by Sacks and Frankel[161] later in 1911, when they hypothesized that sciatic pain was due to pinched nerves in the spinal canal. They recommended laminectomy to treat the condition, and their hypothesis was proven correct when Bailey and Casamajor[3] successfully performed a laminectomy for spinal nerve symptoms secondary to bony stenosis. In 1925, Danforth and Wilson[42] believed that the spinal nerve root could be compressed laterally in the neuroforamen, causing sciatica.

However, true knowledge of the spine and the functioning of the central nervous system remained a mystery until the modern age. In 1921, Siccard[177] became one of the first pioneers to probe the mysteries of the body's spinal anatomy. He observed that the lumbar nerve root could be compressed by ruptured discs and give rise to sciatica. He confirmed the presence of the disc rupture by lumbar myelography, using poppyseed oil.

A year later, Putti[147] observed that the entrapment of the emerging nerve root in the subarticular gutter could be produced by overgrowth of the superior articular facet. Then, in 1927, drawing on the work of Siccard, who performed laminectomies from the third lumbar vertebra to the sacrum to relieve retractable sciatic pain, Putti successfully treated a patient by conducting a laminectomy and facetectomy for decompression of the L5-S1 nerve roots.

A year earlier, in 1926, Schmorl[167] conducted one of the largest scientific research studies in spinal anatomy to date, performing five thousand spinal autopsies. As a result of his work, Schmorl discovered that 15% of the bodies he examined exhibited signs of posterior protrusion of the intervertebral disc at the spinal canal. Treatment for such conditions led to advancements in the use of laminectomies, which until this time were used only to treat decompression of the spinal canal, or in some cases, to relieve sciatic pain.

In 1929, a deeper understanding of sciatica was made when Walter Dandy[41] determined that nodules of discal material could produce this condition. As he observed, their removal relieved sciatic pain. However, he incorrectly diagnosed these nodules as tumors, and hence, failed to indicate disc material as the pain-producing culprit.

It was not until 1932 that the full picture came together. In this year, Schmorl and Junghanns[166] of Dresden, published "The Human Spine in Health and Disease," in which they included detailed descriptions of the intervertebral disc. It was this report that contained the first true connection between pathologic disc material and back and leg pain.

Drawing on Schmorl's work, Dr. Jason Mixter and Dr. Joseph Barr[130] of Massachusetts General Hospital performed a laminectomy in 1933, and after removing a number of "intraspinal tumors," which they examined under a microscope, the two physicians observed that their operative specimens were identical to the photomicrographs pictured in Schmorl's book. Inspired by their findings, Mixter and Barr conducted further study of these "intraspinal tumors" and determined that they were actually disc material. In 1934, they demonstrated that excising a herniated disc by laminectomy and discectomy was a surgical cure for sciatica. These findings were reported to the New England Surgical Society on September 30, 1933, and subsequently published in the *New England Journal of Medicine* in 1934.

By 1937, Charles Elsberg[53] had performed 60 consecutive laminectomies at the New York Neurological Institution and Mount Sinai Hospital. Twenty-two of these operations were performed for

tumors; nine for sectional posterior sensory fibers for control of pain; four for inflammatory bone disease; five for old fractures; two for syringomyelia; one for intermedial cyst; one for aneurysm; and three for what was described as a "peculiar disease of the nerve roots." In 13 cases, no pathology was found.

Laminectomy

Not long after Mixter and Barr published their findings on the pathology of herniated discs in the *New England Journal of Medicine,* new approaches in spinal surgery evolved. The initial method was transdural, but in 1939, Love[117] introduced a hemilaminotomy approach that was extradural.

However, in the five-plus decades that have passed since the initial success of these noteworthy discoveries, laminectomies have evolved to include a number of different forms. Seems and Love developed a laminectomy approach that consisted of removing ligamentum flavum, a swell as the caudal margin of the proximal lamina on one side. Others, such as Herron[74] and Pheasant later reported a series of patients who were treated with bilateral decompressive laminectomies and radical partial discectomy. This approach also included partial facetectomies and foraminotomies. Herron and Pheasant believed that the advantage of this "new" procedure was the ability to recognize and surgically address all components of neural compression with maintenance of segmental stability.

Robert Williams,[212] a neurosurgeon from Las Vegas, was the first to advocate microsurgical discectomy, in 1978. This technique involves use of the operating microscope during all the procedures, but its application has taken on numerous variations over the years. Some surgeons who use this approach advocate a purely interlaminar approach, while others conduct complete laminectomies. In his initial experience, Williams treated a total of 530 patients, with a follow-up that ranged from 6 to 18 months. When treating these patients, Williams adopted a purely interlaminar technique, without removing bone, which yielded a 91% success rate among patients who underwent one surgical procedure. Patients who failed to show improvement underwent a second microsurgical discectomy, of which 2.1% still failed to improve. In analyzing the repeated surgical failure in this small group of 37 patients, Williams observed that eight of these patients suffered recurrent herniations at the same level, four suffered recurrent herniations at the same level but on the opposite side, and six experienced adhesions only. The average operative time for this procedure was 37 minutes, with an average hospital stay of 3.1 days.

Success rates for these procedures ranged from 46% to 90%, depending on the outcome criteria selected by their authors. Optimizing the outcome of the laminectomy procedure would seem to involve the following:

- Addressing the correct pathologic lesion
- Adequately removing disc material, with minimal reaction of the nerve root
- Maintaining meticulous hemostasis
- Determining the presence of concomitant pathology
- Preserving spinal stability
- Minimizing epidural fibrosis

By conducting failure analysis, Burton et al.[20] evaluated 225 discectomy patients and found that 56% experienced concomitant lateral recess stenosis or lateral recess stenosis alone. In a year long interinstitutional study of 800 patients with failed back surgery, Burton also observed that lateral recess stenosis or central stenosis accounted for 65% to 70% of the failures, and that postoperative arachnoiditis and epidural fibrosis were responsible for an additional 12% to 24% of the failed cases. In another study, approximately 30% of patients presenting with lateral recess stenosis in addition to disc disease, required a limited medial foraminotomy at the time of surgery.

After long analysis of these findings, two key factors responsible for spinal surgery failure have been determined. The first is a lack of adequate exposure and incomplete evaluation of the lumbar spine, where part of the pathology may remain undetected. The second involves overmanipulation of the neural tissue, which results from a more radical surgical approach. These two findings seem to be diametrically opposed, since complete evaluation of the lumbar spine can lead to overmanipulation of neural tissue. However, it is this very contradiction that has led to the two current, but diverging, schools of thought regarding spinal surgery approaches. Some surgeons are inclined toward a "minimal intervention technique," while others opt for a more comprehensive, definitive surgical technique.

Adopting Williams' microdiscectomy technique, Goald[5] conducted surgery and a 2-year follow-up study on 116 patients, reporting a surgical cure rate of 96% following a single procedure. This revealed a marginal increase in success over Williams' study, and after a 1-year follow-up, no complications were

evident in his patients. All noncompensation patients were back on the job, as well as 80% of his compensated ones.

Influenced by the success of Williams and Goald, Hudgins performed microsurgical discectomy on 200 cases, with a 1-year follow-up. However, in his case, Hudgins removed sufficient bone and ligamentum flavum to visualize the lateral edge of the nerve root. His rationale for this more extensive exposure was based on the fact that the interlamina technique appeared to result in greater traction injuries and inadequate decompression. By applying this new technique, Hudgins reported that 68% of his patients achieved excellent results, 20% good, 8% fair, and only 4% poor. Recurrent herniation developed within a year in only 11 of the 200 patients.

To further understand what these new surgical findings implied, Wilson and Harbaugh[4] compared a series of microlumbar discectomies with standard discectomy cases on a retrospective basis. After a 2-year follow-up, they concluded that the microsurgical technique was superior to the standard operation. However, analysis of the data revealed an excessive number of dural tears in their early experience. Still, even in the presence of these dural tears, the microdiscectomy patients returned to work in less than half the time of those who underwent the standard approach, and were less inclined to require subsequent operations. However, more recent papers have disputed these findings. Tullberg et al.'s randomized prospective study of 1993[197] found no advantage to the microscopic technique.

Arthroscopic and Percutaneous Discectomy

Valls et al.[199] first described a percutaneous posterolateral approach in 1948, but it was not until 1954 that Hult[87] reported on a successful anteriolateral decompression of a lumbar disc herniation.

Similar research for minimal intervention and spinal canal entry began long before Wilson and Harbaugh's report. In 1954, Hult[87] reported on anterior lateral decompression of herniated discs through use of a retroperitoneal approach. In contrast to laminectomy and lumbar discectomy, the percutaneous approach to the lumbar intervertebral disc does not violate the spinal canal and its contents.

This fact was first observed by Craig,[39] who determined that anatomical soundness of the percutaneous procedure by conducting research on the posterior lateral approach to the spine for biopsy purposes. Once applied, this approach was subsequently used for discography and chemonucleolysis.

Later, in 1983, Kambin and Gellman[96] initiated experimental work with percutaneous lumbar discectomy. Their first patient was a 60-year-old man with right-sided sciatica, who presented with disc protrusion at the L3-L4 and L4-L5 levels. To treat him, Kambin and Gellman excised the L3-L4 disc following an open laminectomy, then decompressed the L4-L5 disc and evacuated it through a Craig needle that was inserted dorsolaterally.

In 1975, Hijikata et al.[77] reported the first known series of percutaneous discectomies, in which they used a 5-mm cannula to approach the lateral anulus to achieve an 80% success rate among the patients treated. This surgical technique varies, however. The port of entry is made approximately 10 cm from the midline and an 18-gauge needle is inserted with the tip lying just lateral to the superior articular process of the inferior vertebra. This gains access to the "triangular working zone," allowing entry to the anulus and the disc, where injury to the nerve root can be avoided.

Advancing on the technique, Onik et al.[136] developed the automated percutaneous lumbar discectomy procedure, which involved the placement of a cutting device, via the posterior lateral approach, into the center of the disc. With the automated needle positioned at the central disc, a debulking of the disc occurs. This approach yielded a 78% success rate among 200 patients. Proponents of this technique believed that the advantage of an indirect approach was that it eliminated epidural bleeding associated with subsequent development of epidural scarring or (epidural) fibrosis. The fenestration of the anulus also tends to decrease intradiscal pressure as well as creating a "weak portal" for future reherniations.

The indirect extrapedicular approach does, however, have limitations. It limits the surgeon's ability to evacuate sequestered fragments and to decompress the spinal canal on a lateral recess. Complications have been reported as well. Surgeons such as Friedman,[63] who have used a far lateral approach have encountered complications involving abdominal viscera. Markhoff and Morris[123] later demonstrated on cadavers that anulus fenestration led to a marked decrease in compressive stiffness and increase in the creep and relaxation rate when the segments were exposed to compressive force. Later, Sakamoto[163] performed a percutaneous lumbar discectomy to relieve intradiscal pressure and observed a 40% decline in pressure in the patients he treated. The reduced pressure was still observed 21 months after surgery.

Despite these limitations, indirect approaches still offer certain advantages, including the ability to eliminate epidural bleeding, scarring, and epidural fibrosis.

With a wealth of surgical options to choose from, it is not surprising that a controversy regarding treatment exists. Onik et al.[136] emphasize central nucleotomy using the nucleotome. Kambin and Gellman,[96] however, insist that posterolateral placement of the instrumentation and nucleus evacuation are essential for producing successful results. Success rate comparisons reveal a satisfactory outcome of 72% for Hijikata et al.'s[77] approach and 87% to 90% for Kambin and Gellman's.[96]

Stenosis

As with many other spinal conditions, spinal stenosis as a symptom-producing entity has only recently been described. This condition apparently was not a common one in antiquity. This probably can be explained by the relatively short average life span. As we now know, spinal stenosis is a degenerative condition that occurs primarily in elderly patients. Portal,[145] in 1880, was the first to relate the size of the spinal canal to severe cord compression with paraplegia. He thought that curvature of the spine itself could produce such a situation. However, he did not contribute any clinical reports or studies. In the late 1800s and early 1900s, there were several isolated reports of cures of ill-defined conditions that responded when the posterior structures, namely the lamina, were removed. In 1893, William A. Lane[109] described a case of a 35-year-old woman who became progressively paraplegic. His operative report on this case described incidents of degenerative spondylolisthesis, which appeared to cause cauda equina compression. Lane decompressed a degenerative spondylolisthesis, decreasing the pain of his patient. Sachs and Frankel in 1900[161] described the classical clinical symptoms of the patient who could walk in a flexed-forward position but had excruciating pain on extension of the spine. They described the case of an 48-year-old tailor in whom progressive lower limb weakness developed associated with pain on lumbar extension over a 2.5 year period. After undergoing surgery, which proved successful, the patient showed no evidence of a mass or tumor, but an unusual thickness of the lamina. Surgery eventually relieved most of this patient's pain; however, pathologic lesion and diagnosis were not established. DeJeune, in 1911,[44] was the first to introduce the concept of spinal claudication. He described three cases in which activity was followed by limb weakness and the appearance of long-tract signs, which decreased with rest. Elsberg, in 1913,[51] described several cases in which claudication was relieved with wide laminectomy. Parker and Adson,[138] of the Mayo Clinic, reported a case of longstanding, intermittent left lower extremity pain and weakness. Surgery for this patient involved laminectomy from T12 to L5. At the time of the operation, edema of the cauda equina was noted, and the surgeons removed the lamina, which was nearly three times as thick as normal. Putti, in 1927,[147] described similar conditions in the neural foramen, namely, hypertrophic arthritis-sciatica, which was partially relieved with facetectomy. Kramer, in 1934,[6] was the first to coin the term *cauda equina radiculitis.* He further suggested that this unusual condition was secondary to arthritic changes of the posterior spinal elements. Sarpyenyer, in 1945,[165] described a congenital stricture of the vertebral canal. Interestingly, he also found a number of cases with narrowing and no developmental abnormality whatsoever. Sumita, in 1910,[192] described a spinal condition seen in achondroplastics.

Verbeist,[201] in 1949, was the first to tie together many of these concepts, which predated him. He described the syndrome of disturbance of the cauda equina on walking that decreased when a patient was recumbent. He included myelograms, which showed areas of stricture of the dye column. He suggested that the symptoms were indeed due to the narrowing of the spinal canal not only by thickened lamina but also ligamentum flavum and the articular facets. He further followed a large number of patients after decompressive laminectomy and clearly showed the relief of their symptoms. Although many of his concepts were considered to be radical when they first appeared, he is now credited with more clearly elucidating the condition of spinal stenosis than probably anyone else.

Epstein and Malis, in 1955,[58] published the first series noting the existence of stenosis in achondroplastic dwarfs. Further papers more clearly elucidated the more exact anatomic areas of stenosis and refined the definitions thereof. In 1973, Epstein et al.[57] described stenosis of the lateral recesses. They noted nerve entrapment in 15 patients in areas beneath the lamina adjacent to pedicles and extending underneath the superior articular facet (the so-called lateral recess). In 1974, Kirkaldy-Willis et al.[103] divided spinal stenosis into that involving centrally the vertebral canal, more laterally the nerve root canal, and even more laterally the neural foramen. Getty[66] in 1980, published a series recommending undercutting the facet for relief of foraminal stenosis. In 1988, Lee et al.[11] further defined the pathology of

the lateral spinal canal. They proposed three zones of the lateral canal based on the pars and the facet joints. He described these as the entrance, mid, and exit zones. Simmons and Jackson in 1991[178] and San Martino et al. in 1983[164] described spinal stenosis caused by scoliosis in the adult patient. Both recommended surgical treatment, with Simmons et al. recommending wide decompression followed by pedicle instrumentation and fusion. They reported relief of pain in 93% of the 40 patients in their series.

Current areas of exploration involve increasing spinal stability after destabilizing decompressive procedures for stenosis, either centrally or laterally. Questions of when to fuse, whether to fuse, and with which instrumentation, if any, to fuse have yet to be clearly defined. These issues become more important particularly with older patients who already have conditions causing mechanical imbalance, such as scoliosis.

Spondylolisthesis

The first description of this condition is attributed to Herbinaux[73] in 1782. He noted a bony prominence of the sacrum obstructing labor in one of his patients. The actual term *spondylolisthesis,* from the Greek meaning "vertebra to slide" was used by Kilian[101] in 1854. The first surgical attempt to treat this condition was reported by Burns in 1933.[19] This first anterior lumbar interbody fusion was performed with an autogenous tibial strut from the fifth lumbar vertebra into the sacrum. In 1936, Jerkins[93] reported a similar case, in which he first attempted to reduce the spondylolisthesis using traction with the patient in extension. In 1936, Mercer[126] reported similar techniques with attempts at reduction. In 1971, Freebody et al.[62] reported in situ fusions even for high-grade slips at L5-S1. They advocated several weeks of postoperative bed rest and reported good results. This became widely adopted in the 1970s for high-grade L5-S1 spondylolisthesis.

In 1976, Wiltse[223] proposed the now-accepted classification system for spondylolisthesis. In 1977,[219] he reported a large series of in situ fusions with a 94% fusion rate for one level and 48% fusion for two levels. In 1983, Wiltse[220] further defined the terminology and techniques of measurement that are commonly used in assessing spondylolisthesis. In 1989, Peek et al.[142] recommended in situ fusion for high-grade slips even with neurological deficit. All in all they reported good fusion rates with relief of most of the neurologic symptoms. Unfortunately, others have not been able to attain such excellent results. Boxall et al. in 1979,[11] Bohlman and Cook in 1982,[9] Dewald et al. in 1981,[46] and van Rens and van Horn in 1982[200] all reported high rates of nonunion with in situ fusions for high-grade L5-S1 spondylolisthesis. Dewald et al.[46] and Smith and Bohlman in 1990[183] advocated combined anterior and posterior fusion in limited cases with severe grade slips and neurologic deficits. Although Steffee and Sitkowski[190] recommended reduction of high-grade slips in 1988, the papers of Kostuik in 1988,[105] Bradford in 1979,[12] and Seitsalo et al.[170] in 1988 should always be kept in mind, as they report major complications in 10% to 60% of the cases in which reduction was attempted.

In 1984, Wiltse et al.[218] described the "far-out" syndrome. In this condition, the fifth lumbar root is compressed between the transverse processes and the ala of the sacrum laterally, secondary either to lumbar scoliosis or spondylolisthesis.

Degenerative spondylolisthesis is different from other types of spondylolisthesis in a number of ways. Listhesis in the absence of a pars defect was first described in 1930 by Junghanns.[34] This condition usually occurs at L4-L5 level and is thought to be due to facet hypertrophy and incompetence. It is now well recognized that adequate decompression, centered in the lateral recesses and in the foramen, is the procedure of choice. What is less clear is exactly why arthrodesis is needed. Epstein et al.[56] reported good results with decompression only. Davis and Baily[43] and Reynolds and Wiltse,[151] however, noted further progression with unsatisfactory results after decompression alone. Feffer et al.[59] and Kaneda et al.[97] have published more recently, espousing the need for arthrodesis. It is hoped that this area will be more clearly delineated in the future.

Fusion

Stabilization of the spine has been a key concept since surgery of the spine began. In fact, the first attempts at surgery were for scoliosis, poliomyelitis, Pott's disease, and deformity secondary to fractures. In 1891, Hadra[70] was the first to report the use of internal fixation when he wired the spinous processes together in a fracture dislocation of an infant. In his article, however, he gave credit to Wilkins[211] for a similar procedure done for a thoracolumbar fracture dislocation in a newborn. In 1896, Chipault[27] made mention of this technique in his first neurosurgical journal. In 1910 Fritz Lanke[110] was the first to devise a procedure for using celluloid and then steel bars fixed to the spinous process of the spine. In 1911, Hunie used bone struts similarly wired to the spine for support. However, in all these attempts at internal fixation, the most important point is that at the time there was no concept of fusion. The materials used were thought to be simply a support for spinal problems.

When Russel A. Hibbs[75] was appointed Director and Chairman of the New York Orthopedic Dispensary and Hospital in 1900 at the age of 29, he observed that some cases of spinal tuberculosis spontaneously resolved with the appearance of fused vertebra. After successfully obtaining a spinal fusion in canines, he performed the first human spinal fusion on January 9, 1911, and eventually expanded his theory to indicate fusion for treatment of spinal deformities.

Fred Albee,[2] another pioneer in fusion research was appointed to the staff at the Hospital for Rupture and Crippled. Later, at the age of 32, he was appointed chairman of Orthopedic Surgery at Cornell Medical College. On May 15, 1911, Albee reported his fusion technique to the American Orthopedic Association in Cincinnati. Hibbs published his research on fusion 13 days after Albee reported his results in a verbal presentation. There has been controversy ever since. In 1911, almost simultaneously, Hibbs and Albee described their fusion procedure. Both had previously recognized that with tuberculosis at the major point, after spontaneous fusion, the disease was eradicated. Hibbs reported such a procedure in the knee in 1991. Hibbs used no bone graft; however, he layered the lamina and sought posterior and facet joint fusions with the processes placed in the interlaminal space. Both procedures gained popularity in the second and third decade of the twentieth century. Hibbs presented a landmark paper in 1945, in which he described 59 cases of fusion for scoliosis; this eventually led to his procedure becoming the more widely practiced one. Albee's method of fusion involved splitting the spinous processes and laying a strip of autologous tibia between the split processes. Hibbs' method included decortication of the lamina with feathering of the bone, overlapping the local bone.

Other adaptations quickly followed. McKenzie-Forbes, in 1920, described the use of slivers of cortical bone over cancellous surfaces of the lamina. Cancellous strips were also used. Ghormley[67] published an article in 1933 that advocated the use of iliac crest bone in lumbar fusion. This has subsequently become the standard source of graft material for most surgeons. In 1922, Kleinberg supplemented McKenzie-Forbes' slivering techniques with beef bone grafts. In 1927, Campbell[21] used strips of iliac crest graft over the intertransverse processes to obtain fusion from the fourth lumbar vertebra to the sacrum. Campbell apparently was before his time, as it was many years before his technique was widely adopted. In 1939, Campbell described a method of fusion in the lumbar spine, in which he placed bone out of the tips of the transverse processes—a procedure that has become the basis of the standard intertransverse fusion.

In 1948, Cleveland[30] recommended repairing pseudarthrosis by exposing the transverse processes on one side. It then became common to reexplore both sides for pseudarthrosis and graft. In 1953, Watkins[208] described the so-called lateral approach to the transverse process and used a large slab of iliac crest fixed with screws for L5-S1 lumbosacral fusions. Fourteen years later, in 1953, Watkins approached the transverse processes lateral to the sacrospinalis and erector spinae, using a full-thickness graft from the iliac wing. In 1968, Wiltse et al.[217] described the sacrospinalis-splitting approach to the transverse processes and simply used the iliac crest bone placed between the transverse processes. Their transsacrospinalis approach to the transverse processes obtained a 97% fusion rate. Based on Watkins' success,[208] Truchley and Thompson[195] modified the procedure using slivers of bone graft, inserted with two separate incisions. Solid fusions were obtained in 100% of lumbosacral fusions and in 92% of two-level fusions.

Adkins[1] used a midline approach with subperiosteal dissection to the tips of the transverse processes. He then placed autogenous tibial grafts, obtaining fusion in 82% of his patients.

Stauffer and Coventry[186] treated 177 patients with posterolateral fusion across the transverse processes and lamina, reporting clinical success in 81% of their patients and a fusion rate of 90%.

Currently transverse process fusion, or posterolateral fusion, is widely accepted and practiced. Unfortunately, the indications for this procedure have not been clearly delineated, nor have the results been critically analyzed. A natural progression then allowed fusions to be considered in the intervertebral area.

Posterior Interbody Fusion

It has long been realized that the primary weight-bearing axis of the vertebral column lies not posteriorly or posterolaterally, but rather anterior to the canal itself in the intervertebral area. Particularly when procedures necessitated removal of large amounts of disc material, concerns of subsequent instability arose. The concept of an interbody fusion

done posteriorly then gradually gained popularity. In 1946, Jaslow[93] created such an interbody using chips off the spinous processes. This created a semisolid fusion posteriorly after discectomy. Cloward[32,33] published a large series on interbody fusions. He reported his first case in 1945. In 1952, he reported a large series using a dowel graft. During this time, he developed specialized instrumentation to make the procedure technically easier. In 1944, Briggs and Milligan[18] also described a "chip fusion." Interestingly, they noted good fusion only when the interbody fusion was combined with a posterior fusion. They also used posterior elements cut out and packed into the disc space.

Since that time, there have been many adaptations of this procedure. Although this is a technically demanding procedure, it has gained wide support. In 1967, LeVay[113] reported that the posterior lumbar interbody fusion is favored by neurosurgeons in the United Kingdom for treatment of a lumbar disc prolapse. Other notable contributions include Ma and Paulson in 1982,[120] who devised chisels for the PLIF procedure. Lin et al.,[114] in 1973 described technical modification of the Cloward's PLIF procedure. Selby, in 1985,[171] adapted the Crock systems for posterior lumbar interbody fusion. Hutter in 1985[89] and Branch in 1987[17] described a keystone configuration to the graft in the hope of preventing retropulsion. A time line appears in the box to follow.

Anterior Interbody Fusion

The first series of this procedure was actually reported as being a treatment for spondylolisthesis. In 1945, Capener[22] described a transperitoneal approach using a tibial graft. In 1934, Ito[90] described 10 cases of interbody debridement for Potts disease through an anterior approach. No fusion was done, however. Ito followed with a technique for sympathetic ganglionectomy that he had developed and reported in 1923.[99] Wilkinson, in 1950, described an anterior approach for curettage of vertebral tuberculosis. Importantly, however, he made no attempt at fusion. In 1952, Wiltbarger,[216] using Ito's approach, debrided and applied cancellous graft to adjacent vertebral bodies and was the first to describe fusion for this problem. Finally, in Hong Kong in 1956 and later in 1960, Hodgson and Stock[82,84] described extension of the anterior approach in the thoracic and lumbar spine for debridement of tuberculous abscess with subsequent interbody fusion. Obviously, the impact of this on Western work was immediately felt, and subsequently, many English-speaking surgeons visited Hodgson's Hong Kong

Cloward	1945[33]	Devised treatment of ruptured lumbar disc by intervertebral fusion. Results reported in 1947.
	1952[32]	Reported an 85% cure rate in 321 patients.
	1963	100 cases: 84% asymptomatic; 12% good, with occasional minor symptoms
	1982[34]	100 cases: evaluated by orthopedist. 90% good/excellent; 60% > 10 year follow-up; 73% solid fusion
Lin	1982	50 consecutive cases: 82% fusion rate, 69% good/excellent
	1983	500 cases: 5% neurologic; 5% deep venous thrombosis; 2 cases incontinent; 4 cases immediate reoperation with 2 graft displacements
Ma and Paulson	1982[120]	74% good/excellent; 69% graft extrusion; 15% pseudarthrosis
Hutter	1983[89]	90% fusion; 83% good/excellent results; 5% technical difficulties; 18 cases of residual paresis
Collis	1987[35]	950 levels in disc replacement procedure 750 patients: even fusion graft material becomes osseous/fibrosis matrix that sustains distraction

center to learn these techniques. In 1944, Iwahara[91] demonstrated the extraperitoneal approach to be just as convenient as the transperitoneal approach and had none of the disadvantages of opening the peritoneum. Further reports of anterior interbody fusions came from Harmon in 1960,[71] who reported 244 cases with 90% good results after 3- to 5-year follow-ups. Further good results were reported by Goldner in 1969,[68] Sacks in 1965,[162] Suzuki in 1967,[193] Hodgson et al. in 1968,[83] and Leong et al. in 1983,[112] all with relatively good results with anterior interbody fusions. In 1989, Selby and Henderson[172] described their refinement of the exposure using a non-muscle-splitting approach using Crock instrumentation.

With time, the complications reported with this procedure have decreased. There had been some

concern regarding retrograde ejaculation. The best article on this appears to be from Flynn and Hogue in 1979,[61] who reported a very small incidence of sterility secondary to retrograde ejaculation.

Circumferential Lumbar Fusion

Combined anterior and posterior lumbar fusion, the so-called 360, was first described in a series by Stauffer and Coventry in 1972.[185,186] Their series showed a nonunion rate of 44% with salvage procedures using anterior and posterior fusions. This was mentioned briefly, but overall they discouraged its use. Hoover, in 1968,[85] reported six circumferential fusions; three were single-staged and three were separated stages. Four of the six had good results. He advocated 360 anterior-posterior procedures only in insurmountable case. Goldner, in 1969,[68] suggested a second-stage posterior fusion if the anterior fusion did not appear to be healing well.

First in 1983 and then in 1986, O'Brien et al.[134,135] reported a series of patients with disabling back pain who were treated simultaneously with anterior and posterior fusions. In 1990, Kozak and O'Brien[108] showed that "360s" can be done safely. They reported a 90% fusion with one or two levels and 78% fusion with three levels. They had 80% acceptable clinical results in their series. Interestingly, levels of fusion were identified using discographic pain provocation, and internal fixation was initially achieved using Harrington and Knodt's rods. Several centers have reported the use of circumferential fusion, most recently with pedicle fixation. The most recent results and series at this time are still pending.

Internal Fixation

Ever since the first spinal procedures were performed, stabilization has been a concern. In 1888, Wilkins[211] wired together the pedicles of T12 and L1 in a fracture dislocation of a newborn, using carbolized silver suture. In 1891 Hadra[70] reportedly wired the posterior spinous processes of C5 and C6 for fracture dislocation. In 1910, Lanke[110] initially stabilized the spine with celluloid bars. He then progressed to steel rods, which were tied to the sides of the spinous processes first with silk and later with wire. Similarly Albee,[2] in 1911, used strips of bone as a type of internal fixation. After both Albee and Hibbs simultaneously devised their concepts of spinal fusion, posterior fusions became the standard for stabilizing the spine. Over the years, as it became apparent that a simple posterior fusion did not always succeed, attention turned to different types of internal fixation for additional support. King,[102] in 1948, fastened facet joints with screws. He reported a 90% fusion from L5 to S1 in over 40 patients. In 1952, Wilson and Straub[214] attempted bolting plates on either side of the spinous process. This process unfortunately never worked well. In 1959, Boucher[10] placed facet screws more medially. This probably was the first use of bone screws for fixation. These were aimed out far laterally from the facets through the pedicle to the anterior base of the transverse process.

During the 1950s and 1960s, Paul Harrington[72] devised his techniques of treating the paralytic scoliosis of many polio patients with internal fixation using hooks and rods. His rods thereafter quickly gained wide recognition and success and were essentially the gold standard for many years in this country. They continue to be used. In 1963, Roy-Camille et al. began using bone screws attached to plates, thinking that this added a greater degree of stability. They reported this in 1970.[157] Luque[118,119] reported on his use of sublaminar wires and rods primarily for scoliotic deformities. In 1986, Arthur Steffee[188] reported his use of bone screws and plates, although he had used these since the late 1960s. He later also added posterior lumbar interbody fusions to his procedure. Magerl, in 1982,[121] described techniques of placing the bone screw percutaneously in combination with the external fixator. Dick et al. in 1985,[47] internalized this fixation using many of the principles espoused by Magerl. Cotrel and Dubousset in 1985,[37] described their techniques of using rods and screws attached to malleable rods, primarily in cases of deformity. Edwards, in 1985,[50] described his system, which combined a type of bone screw with the Harrington rod construct. He felt this added additional transverse control.

Certainly, of the past 15 years, pedicle fixation with posterior stabilization of the spine has become fairly common. Currently, there are 12 companies with some type of bone screw system, and 17 systems are in various phases of approval. Almost all these systems have screws with plates or rods, and several include hooks also. It appears to be more widely accepted that shorter fusions should be performed when possible, thus sacrificing fewer mobile intervertebral levels when possible.

As the anterior approaches to the lumbar spine became more widely used, so began an evolution of internal fixation of the anterior lumbar spine. In 1969, Dwyer et al.[48] described a system of screws placed into intervertebral bodies with cable attachment for curvature correction. First used in 1964, this was a major breakthrough in the anterior correction of deformity. Unfortunately, in many series, it had an unacceptable complication rate. In 1986, Zielke and Strempel[223] modified the Dwyer system and attached the screws to a threaded rod. This allowed compression across the apex of the curve. This system has now been used in several series for adult degenerative scoliosis. In 1974, Werlinich[209] described the use of a serrated staple. Even though he reported relatively good results in over 120 patients, this technique never gained popularity.

Anteriorly in the lumbar spine, the use of a plate attached to screws has enjoyed more popularity. In 1959, Humphries et al.[88] described a slotted plate attached with screws; their results, however, were poor. In 1986, Ryan et al.[160] described a bolt-plate-type fixation. Lack, in 1988, described a low-profile longitudinal plate with multiple holes. He reported on seven patients, with encouraging results. Yuan, in 1988,[9] described a so-called Syracuse I plate. He reported on 16 cases with relatively good results; although there was some difficulty with deformity. In 1986[106] and 1988,[105] Kostuik described an anterior modification of the Harrington instrumentation. In 1989, he described its use for kyphotic deformities in almost 300 patients with good results.[107] In 1986, Kaneda et al.[97] described the use of their system; essentially, two vertebral plates screwed into the bodies of interconnected with rods, providing a very rigid system anteriorly. In 1987, both Mann[10] and McGowan[11] compared several anterior constructs. They found that both the Kaneda plate and the I-plate provided the greatest stiffness. Interestingly however, they felt that if posterior disruption of any type was present, anterior instrumentation alone did not provide adequate support.

Cervical Spine

The earliest history of cervical spine disorders seems to stem from the treatment of cervical spine trauma. The Egyptians in the Edwin Smith papyrus considered an acute neck injury "an ailment not to be treated." By the time of Hippocrates, traction had come into some use, although no truly efficacious treatment for cervical spine trauma was even approached. With time, the value of cervical traction had been demonstrated. In 1877, Boutecou[12] was among the first to reduce fractures with weight attached by adhesive tape to the patient's face. Taylor[194] introduced head-halter traction in 1929, which was improved by Crutchfeld[40] in 1933 with the introduction of his head-holding tongs. To

Nickel et al.[133] goes the distinction of the concept and refinement of the use of halo immobilization. The halo's use during operations for deformity and/or stability as well as its postoperative stabilizing effects are still in wide use.

The first individual to propose a more aggressive treatment of cervical spine trauma was probably Hildanus,[78] who in 1672 described a technique for reducing fracture dislocations of the neck. As early as the seventh century, Paul of Agena, suggested surgical excision of fractured spinous processes for treating traumatic spinal disorders.[141] However, this certainly never came into the mainstream of surgical thinking. As late as the latter half of the nineteenth century, there was much argument over the efficacy of open surgical laminectomy in the face of trauma. Few were attempted and even fewer succeeded. A French surgeon, Chipault,[26-28] in 1894 published perhaps the first textbook on spinal surgery, presenting the most complete survey of past and current spinal surgery. Interestingly in 1856, he started a specialist yearbook, *Travaux de Neurologie Chirurgicale,* which became the first neurosurgical journal in the world. In 1904, he published *Manuel de Orthpedie Vertebrale,* which dealt primarily with the orthopedic treatment of spinal disorders. His doctoral thesis was based on the anatomic relationship between spinous processes and spinal nerve roots, thus allowing a determination of the levels of spinal cord lesions based on disturbances observed in myotonal or dermatomal areas. In a 14-year period, he published several books as well as over 90 original manuscripts. Unfortunately, in 1905 at the age of 39, he developed a slowly progressive paraplegia of unknown origin, which finally led to his demise in 1920. He certainly was at least one of the first to combine orthopedic and neurosurgical interests and thus is one of the pioneers of spinal surgery.

The use of anesthetic agents (ether, 1846; and chloroform, 1848) and the principles of antisepsis (Lister, 1867[115]; and Semmelweiss, 1861[173,174]) made possible a new era in all fields of surgery. The success of postlaminectomy surgery was now much higher. By the early 1900s many surgeons observed localized tumefaction extending into the ventral portion of the spinal canal, which was reported as neoplasms under such names as chondroma, enchondroma, and fibrochondroma. Brian Stookey,[191] read a paper entitled, "Compression of the Spinal Cord Due to Ventral Extradural Cervical Chondromas" at the fifty-third annual meeting of the American Neurologic Association. He described syndromes based on the anatomic location of these lesions. Although he termed these "chondromas," had he had the benefit of Schmorl's microscopic postmortem findings, he probably would have recognized the true nature of this lesion. However, it was not until 1934 that Mixter and Barr[130] noticed the true connection between the herniated disc (previously called "chondromas") and radicular compression as a cause of sciatica. In fact, of Mixter and Barr's 19 original cases, four were cervical herniated discs. This series was enlarged by Mixter and Ayer to seven cases involving cervical cord compression and one case of radiculopathy due to herniated cervical disc. The concept of cervical disc disease at that time was that most ruptured discs in the cervical spine produced cord pressure and very rarely radicular symptoms. Simmons and Murphy, in 1943, argued however, that radicular symptoms were probably more common and that ruptured cervical discs may cause no sign of cord compression. Their interesting paper, published in 1943, consisted of a series of four patients, two of whom were physicians and all of whom had a unilateral rupture of the sixth cervical disc with seventh cervical root symptoms. They further believed that many patients with pain in the precordium, shoulder, and arm who previously had been thought to have diagnoses that were noncervical in origin, indeed would be found on close examination to have a rupture of the cervical disc with radicular symptoms. In 1950, Schultz and Semmes[168] published an article in the journal *Laryngoscope* espousing that much head and neck pain is of cervical disc origin. This concept is indeed not as novel as many today would think.

For some time, it was thought that the proper surgical approach for cervical herniated disc was a posterior laminectomy. In 1951, Scoville et al.[169] reported on 150 cases in which they advocated limited decompression of the root posteriorly by removal of the medial half of the facet and small portion of the lamina. Frykholm in 1951[64] also described a posterior foraminal decompression. It is unclear why attention to anterior cervical surgical approaches began. Undoubtedly, there were many clear results with posterior surgery and root and/or cord manipulation. As early as 1894, Chipault[28] in his textbook described the surgical approach. In 1930, Wright wrote of using his approach to attempt anterior drainage of tuberculous abscesses. This approach was also described in the otolaryngology literature for removing anterior osteophytes that make swallowing difficult.

The anterior approach for the surgical treatment of cervical spine disease was developed almost simultaneously in three different parts of the world. Robinson and Smith[154] at Johns Hopkins University in 1955 were the first to report an anterior disc removal with interbody fusion. Dereymaker et al. published his work on this approach in Brussels, Belgium in 1965.[45] However, they first began using this operation in 1956. Ralph Cloward[31] published his first work in 1958, having first done the surgery in 1956, presenting his paper to the Harvey Cushing Society in April 1957. There were, however, philosophical differences in the treatment of cervical disc disease. Robinson and Smith, for instance, felt that there was no need for aggressive removal of posterior osteophytes because they would, with time, disappear after a solid interbody fusion was obtained. Cloward, however, created a larger opening in the disc space using his circular dowel cutters. This allowed direct access to the posterior osteophytes and more lateral disc lesions. In 1960, Hirsch[80] advocated discectomy alone without fusion. This seemed to be particularly useful for "softer" herniations. Wilson and Campbell in 1977[215] and Robertson in 1978[152] reported large series of patients who underwent anterior cervical discectomy without bone graft. These surgeons also espoused the use of the operating microscope. Robertson,[152] however, proposed removing the cartilaginous end plate, and in his series of 40 patients, all interspaces undergoing disc removal achieved bony or fibrous union. Wilson, however, removed the disc without disturbing the cartilaginous end plates. In their series of 71 cases, 68 patients had good or excellent results.

Linesford reported in over 250 cases in 1988, that postoperative complications were more frequent and hospitalizations longer in patients undergoing fusion. In regard to the necessity of fusion after disc excision, review of the results in the literature shows no discernible difference between fusion and disc excision without fusion. It is the authors' opinion, however, that with the advent of readily available banked bone and the common postoperative complaint of neck and interscapular pain in procedures done without fusion, that interbody fusion will become more popular.

Bailey and Badgley[4] described a procedure in 1960 to treat instability by fusion with iliac crest graft. Their initial series consisted of 20 patients with instability due to trauma, tumor, or infection. Their technique involved creating an anterior trough in the vertebrae. The canal was not routinely opened. It should be noted that this series did not include degenerative disc disease.

For multilevel decompression of the canal with deformity, several techniques have been devised. Verbeist et al.[204] in 1966 espoused using autogenous

cortical bone. Simmons and Bhallia[179] in 1969 described a "keystone" graft of the iliac crest. Whitecloud and LaRocca[210] in 1976 advised the use of cortical fibula.

Cervical spondylosis is the cause for cord compression and myelopathy. It has been espoused only since the midtwentieth century. In 1947, Kahn[95] thought that compression was caused by the dentate ligament. Murphy[131] presented a paper in 1985 with a compelling argument that the cord was compressed posteriorly by the sharp edge of the lamina and by a hard bar of the disc anteriorly. This paper was so thoroughly ridiculed by his contemporaries that he never bothered to publish it. Brain and his colleagues,[14,15] however, as early as 1952, wrote of the neurologic manifestations of cervical spondylosis in his textbook of 1967. He made a definitive case for the distinction between the chronic protrusions of cervical spondylosis responsible for cord progression in the acute more lateral herniated cervical disc with radicular symptoms. The syndrome of cervical myelopathy by cervical spondylosis has more recently been ably covered by multiple authors in the journal *Spine*.

As far as the surgical approaches for this entity, there are proponents for both anterior and posterior surgical approaches. In 1983, Raynor[149] published an anatomic comparison of both approaches to the cervical spine and pointed to leaving 50% of the cervical facets intact to avoid gross postoperative instability. Epstein and Epstein[55] in a thorough review of the literature concluded there was no statistical evidence establishing the superiority of the anterior or posterior approach. It appears, in the authors' opinion, that most surgeons prefer a posterior approach for three or more intervertebral levels, with anterior decompressions and fusion reserved for lesser numbers of levels.

What is known of ossification in the posterior longitudinal ligament primarily comes from the Japanese. Although compression of the cord with ossified posterior ligament was reported by Key in 1838 in Britain,[99] it was much later that ossification of the posterior longitudinal ligament (OPLL) was recognized as a distinct clinical entity. In 1967, Onji et al.[137] reported a series of 18 patient in which posterior ossification of ligaments caused cervical myelopathy. In 1974, the Japanese ministry of Public Health and Welfare appointed a special investigational committee to study ossification of the posterior longitudinal ligament thoroughly. Readers are referred to the excellent review article by Tsuyami.[196] Expansive open-door laminoplasty, described by Hirabayashi in 1983,[81] would seem to be the current procedure of choice for multilevel involvement with this malady.

Verbeist[202] had done extensive work with a lateral approach to the cervical intertransverse space paraspinally. This can be extended medially into the disc space and canal. This might be particularly helpful for far lateral disc extrusions, osteophytes, or where vertebral artery compression exists. These are areas that would be particularly hard to reach by a transdiscal approach. In reviewing the English literature, its use seems to be somewhat limited. The use of internal fixation in the cervical spine has certainly been less expansive when compared to work in the dorsal and lumbar spine. It is well accepted that fusion rates in the cervical spine are much higher than in other areas. In 1891, Hadra[70] performed a spinous process wiring of C6 and C7 for a fractured dislocation in a baby, with a reportedly good result. In 1910, Pilcher[144] reduced a C1-C2 dislocation and obtained a good result after spontaneous fusion occurred. William Rogers[155] in 1942 established many of the principles of modern cervical spine surgery. These included operating under traction, reduction of fracture as necessary, fixation with wires around spinous processes, and then fusion. Many of his general techniques are still in use today. Robinson and Southwick[153] in 1960 suggested using rods wired to the facets, with not uniformly good results.

Roy-Camille et al.,[158] in France in the 1970s, began developing techniques of posterior screw fixation in the lateral masses with plate stabilization. In 1982, Magerl and Seeman[122] published their work on lateral screw fixation attached to plates. In 1982, Bohler[7] published work on anterior stabilization using odontoid fracture fixation. In 1986, Caspar[24] published a series on anterior cervical plating using bicortical fixation. This has not gained wide popularity to this date. For the rare patient who needs support for pseudobasilar invagination, dorsal occipital cervical internal fixation has been shown to be possible by both Ransford et al. using loop fixation[148] and Roy-Camille et al. using posterior plating and screws.[159] Lastly, osteotomy of the cervical spine is rarely necessary except in ankylosing spondylitis with severe flexion deformity as first suggested by Mason et al. in 1953.[124] Edward Simmons of New York in 1972[180] published the most comprehensive explanation of the surgical technique, complications, and results to date.

Thoracic Spine

The evolution of surgery in the thoracic spine was undoubtedly first proposed by Paul of Agena[141] when he suggested removing the depressed posterior elements for treatment of thoracic fracture and dislocations. The first formal laminectomy in the thoracic spine was performed by Cline in 1814. Unfortunately, however, the patient died. The first laminectomy was done with some success by Smith[182] in 1829 for a fracture dislocation at T4.

The next real impetus for the development of surgical techniques in the thoracic spine was the treatment of spinal tuberculosis. In 1900, Menard[125] was the first to describe a posterolateral costotransversectomy for abscess drainage. In 1954, Capener,[23] modified this approach with the removal of an additional rib out laterally and improved this exposure for decompression of central lesions. Hodgson and Stock in Hong Kong in 1956[82,84] reported a transthoracic approach. This allowed abscess drainage radicular curettage of any avascular bone, direct anterior decompression of the spinal cord and interbody fusion. In 1960, they reported their first 100 cases using this approach with results that were much superior to any series using posterior or posterolateral approaches.

The first description of the thoracic discs as a pathologic entity came in 1911 with Middleton and Teacher's[127] description of a traumatic disc herniation, which led to subsequent paraplegia and death. As in the lumbar spine, the first thoracic disc herniations were thought to be some type of tumor. Elsberg[52,53] described a series of "extradural ventral chondromas." After Mixter and Barr identified lumbar herniations, thoracic disc herniations were described by both Muller in 1950 and Logue in 1952.[116] Both advocated a posterior approach as a surgical procedure choice. However, in Logue's series of 11 patients, 6 were left paraplegic. The overall failure rate with the posterior approach approached 50% to 65%. Crafford et al., in 1958,[38] were the first to try an anterior approach to address these problems. They described an anterolateral fenestration of the protruded thoracic disc in a case report. In 1960, Hulme[86] described a costotransversectomy approach as "the surgical approach" for thoracic herniated disc. The first widely acclaimed series using an anterior transthoracic approach for thoracic herniated disc came from Perot and Monro in 1969.[143] This has subsequently been followed by many others with an overall improvement rate of 85% or greater. Even with the advent of the operating microscope and improved diagnostic techniques, the series of Benjamin in 1983[6] and Singounas and Karvounis in 1977[181] have not shown a substantial improvement with the posterior approach to thoracic disc herniations. There has been some enthusiasm for a transpedicular approach to the thoracic herniated disc and series by Patterson and Arbit in 1978[140] and Epstein in 1983[54] have shown satisfactory results. Some are concerned that the removal of an entire pedicle and facet may predispose to problems with stability; others feel that it may be difficult to remove very central disc lesions through this approach.

The use of posterior techniques for anterior thoracic pathology, regardless of etiology, has all too frequently led to unfavorable results. Enough experience has now been gained with anterior approaches to the thoracic spine to show that vascular compromise, while a theoretic possibility, in fact rarely occurs. For the vast majority of surgical procedures in this area, the direct posterior approach has now been abandoned.

Summary

Today, sciatica and low-back pain are common conditions seen in medical practice. So common in fact that the cost for treatment in the United States alone has soared to a staggering 60 billion dollars. It is currently estimated that 80% of all adults will experience a significant episode of low-back pain and an additional 40% of these individuals will suffer from bouts of sciatica.

Back pain is the leading cause of nonsurgical hospitalizations. Admission for spinal surgery now rank third among all surgical procedures.

Current findings estimate that 10 million Americans suffer from chronic symptoms of low-back pain. Approximately 5.2 million people are disabled by the condition, half of whom suffer on a permanent basis. An additional 9 million individuals are impaired due to other back disorders. Taken as a whole, back and neck disorders are the most common causes of disability in the population younger than 45 years of age.

Given these startling statistics, it is interesting to note that standard surgical treatment for these disorders did not develop until the twentieth century. As a result of their tremendous prevalence and the contrasting short history of their medical understanding, this chapter has attempted to chronicle the evolution of spinal surgery techniques, while tracing the process by which knowledge regarding back disorders was acquired.

The authors hope that a thorough understanding of the history of this problem will help us to develop a rational approach to spinal disease.

References

1. Adkins EWD: Lumbosacral arthrodesis after laminectomy; *J Bone Joint Surg* 37B:308, 1955.
2. Albee FH: Transplantation of a portion of skin into the spine for Pott's disease, *JAMA* 37:885, 1911.
3. Bailey P, Casamajor C: Orthordesis of the spine as a cause of compression of the spinal cord and its roots, *J Nerv Ment Dis* 36:588, 1911.
4. Bailey RW, Badgley CR: Stabilization of the cervical spine by anterior fusion, *J Bone Joint Surg* 42A:565, 1960.
5. Barr JS: Lumbar disc lesions in retrospect, *Clin Orthop* 129:48, 1977.
6. Benjamin V: Diagnosis and management of thoracic disc disease, *Clin Neurosurg* 30:577, 1983.
7. Bohler J: Anterior stabilization for acute fractures and non-unions of the dens, *J Bone Joint Surg* 64A:18, 1982.
8. Bohlman BHH: Acute fractures and dislocations of the cervical spine, *J Bone Joint Surg* 61A:1119, 1979.
9. Bohlman HH, Cook SS: One-stage decompression and posterolateral and interbody fusion for lumbosacral spondylotosis through a posterior approach, *J Bone Joint Surg* 64:415, 1982.
10. Boucher HH: A method of spinal fusion, *J Bone Joint Surg* 41B:248, 1959.
11. Boxall D, Bradford D, Winter R, et al.: Management of severe spondylolisthesis in children and adolescents, *J Bone Joint Surg* 61A:479, 1979.
12. Bradford DS: Treatment of severe spondylolisthesis, *Spine* 4:423, 1979.
13. Brain R: Spondylosis: the known and unknown, *Lancet* 3:689, 1954.
14. Brain WR, Wilkinson JL: *Cervical spondylosis and other disorders of the spine*, Philadelphia, 1967, W.B. Saunders.
15. Brain WR, Northfield D, Wilkerson M: The neurological manifestations of cervical spondylosis, *Brain* 75:187, 1952.
16. Breasted JH: *The Edwin Smith surgical papyrus*, vol. 1, Chicago, 1930, University of Chicago, p. 316.
17. Branch CL: Posterior lumbar interbody fusion with the keystone graft techniques and results, *Surg Neurol* 27:449, 1987.
18. Briggs H, Milligan PR: Chip fusion of the low back following exploration of the spinal canal, *J Bone Joint Surg* 26A:125, 1944.
19. Burns DH: An operation for spondylolisthesis, *Lancet* 1:1233, 1933.
20. Burton C, et al.: Causes of failure of surgery on the lumbar spine, *Clin Orthop* 157:191, 1981.
21. Campbell WC: An operation for extra-articular fusion of sacroiliac joint, *Surg Gynecol Obstet* 45:218, 1927.
22. Capener N: Spondylolisthesis, *Betsin J Surg* 19:374, 1945.

23. Capener N: The evolution of lateral rhachotomy, *J Bone Joint Surg* 36B:173, 1954.

24. Caspar W: *Anterior cervical fusion and interbody stabilization with the trapezial osteosynthetic plate technique,* Tuttlinge, West Germany, 1986, Aesculap-Werke AG.

25. Charcot JJ: Sur la caludication intermittente: dans un can d'obliteration complete de lune des arteres iliaques primitives, *C R Soc Seances Soc Biol Fil* 5:225, 19.

26. Chipault A: *Manuel d'orthopedic vertebrale,* Paris, 1904, Maloine.

27. Chipault A: L'orthopedie rachidienne operatoire: ligature et suture des vertebres; quatre interventions, l'une contre une luxation cervicale ballante, trois autres contre des gibbosites pottiques rapidement croissantes, *Trav Neurol Chir* 1:222, 1896.

28. Chipault A: Etudes de chirurgie medullaire, Paris, 1894, Alan.

29. Chipault A: Les rapports des apophyses epineuses avec la moelle, les racines medullaires et les meninges, Paris, 1894, Universite de Paris.

30. Cleveland M, et al.: Pseudoarthrosis in lumbosacral spine, *J Bone Joint Surg* 30A:302, 1948.

31. Cloward RB: The anterior approach for removal of ruptured cervical discs, *J Neurosurgery* 15:602, 1958.

32. Cloward RB: The treatment of ruptured intervertebral disc by vertebral body fusion, *Ann Surg* 136:987, 1952.

33. Cloward RB: A new treatment for intervertebral disc herniations, Presented at the Hawaiian Territorial Medical Association meeting, 1945.

34. Cloward RB: The history of posterior lumbar interbody fusion, Springfield, 1982, Charles C Thomas.

35. Collis JS: Posteral lumbar interbody fusion disc replacement (TDR), Presented at the 3rd international PLIF symposium, Cleveland, 1987.

36. Cortugno D: De ischiade nervosa canmentarius, Naples, 1764, Simonocos Brothers.

37. Cotrel Y, Dubousset J: The use of pedicle screws and universal instrumentation for spinal fixation, Presented to the AO Trauma Course, Davos, Switzerland, December 1985.

38. Crafford C, Hiertonn T, Lindbloom K, et al.: Spinal cord compression caused by a protruded thoracic disc: report of a case treated with anterolateral fenestration of the disc, *Acta Orthop Scand* 28:103, 1958.

39. Craig FS: Vertebral body biopsy, *J Bone Joint Surg* 38A:93, 1956.

40. Crutchfield WG: Skeletal traction for dislocation of cervical spine, *South Surg* 2:156, 1933.

41. Dandy WE: Loose cartilage from the intervertebral disc simulating tumor of the spinal cord, *Arch Surg* 19:660, 1929.

42. Danforth MS, Wilson PD: The anatomy of the lumbrasacral region in relation to sciatic pain, *J Bone Joint Surg* 7A:109, 1925.

43. Davis IS, Baily RW: Spondylolisthesis: long-term follow-up study of treatment with total laminectomy, *Clin Orthop* 88:46, 1972.

44. DeJeune JJ: La claudication intermittente de la moelle epiniere, *Presse Med* 19:981, 1911.

45. Dereymaker A, Chosez JP, et al.: Les traitment chirurgical de la discopathic cervicale, *Clin Orthop* 40:113, 1965.

46. Dewald RI, Faut MM, Tadonio RF, Neuwirth MG: Severe lumbosacral spondylolisthesis in adolescents and children, *J Bone Joint Surg* 63A:619, 1981.

47. Dick W, Kluger P, Magerl F, et al.: A new device for internal fixation of the thoracolumbar and lumbar spine fractures: the fixateur interne, *Paraplegia* 23:225, 1985.

48. Dwyer AM, Newton NC, Sherwood AA: An anterior approach to scoliosis: a preliminary report, *Clin Orthop* 62:192, 1969.

49. Edwards CC: Prospective evaluation of a new method for complete reduction of L5-S1 spondylolisthesis using corrective forces alone, *Orthop Trans* 14:549, 1990.

50. Edwards WC: *The sacral fixation device: a new alternative for lumbosacral fixation,* Presented at the North American Spine Society meeting, Laguna Niquel, California, July 1985.

51. Elsberg CA: Experiences in spinal surgery, *Surg Gynecol Obstet* 16:117, 1913.

52. Elsberg CA: Extradural spinal tumors. Primary, secondary, metastatic, *Surg Gynecol Obstet* 46:1, 1928.

53. Elsberg CA: The extradural ventral chondromes (ecchondroses), their favorite sites, the spinal cord and root symptoms they produce and their surgical treatment, *Bull Neurol Inst N Y* 1:359, 1931.

54. Epstein JA: Thoracic disc herniation: operative approaches and results, *Neurosurgery* 12:305, 1983.

55. Epstein JA, Epstein NE: The surgical management of cervical spinal stenosis and myeloradiculopathy, In editor: The cervical spine. Philadelphia, 1989, J.B. Lippincott.

56. Epstein NE, Epstein JA, Carras R, et al.: Degenerative spondylolisthesis with an intact neural arch: a review of 60 cases with an analysis of clinical findings and the development of surgical management, *Neurosurgery* 13:555, 1983.

57. Epstein JA, Epstein BS, et al.: Sciatica caused by nerve root entrapment in the lateral recess: the superior facet syndrome, *J Neurosurg* 39:362, 1973.

58. Epstein JA, Malis LI: Compression of spinal cord and cauda equina in achondroplastic dwarfs, *Neurology* 5:875, 1955.

59. Feffer HL, Wiesel S, Cuckler JM, et al.: Degenerative spondylolisthesis—to fuse or not to fuse, *Spine* 10:287, 1985.

60. Flynn JC, Price CT: Sexual complications of anterior fusion of the lumbar spine, *Spine* 9:489, 1984.

61. Flynn JC, Hoque MA: Anterior fusion of the lumbar spine: end-result study with long term follow up, *J Bone Joint Surg* 61A:1143, 1979.

62. Freebody D, Bendall R, Taylor RD: Anterior transperitoneal lumbar fusion, *J Bone Joint Surg* 53B:617, 1971.

63. Friedman WA: Percutaneous discectomy: an alternative to chemonucleolysis? *Neurosurgery* 13:542, 1983.

64. Frykholm R: Cervical nerve root compression resulting from disc degeneration and root sleeve fibrosis, *Acta Chir Scand* suppl 160:1951.

65. Garrison F: *Introduction to the history of medicine,* 4th ed., Philadelphia, 1929, W.B. Saunders.

66. Getty CJM: Lumbar spinal stenosis, *J Bone Joint Surg* 64B:481, 1980.

67. Ghormley RK: Low back pain with special reference articular facets with presentation of an operative procedure, *JAMA* 101:1773, 1933.

68. Goldner JL, et al.: *Anterior disc excision and interbody spine fusion for chronic low back pain,* American Academy of Orthopaedic Surgeons symposium on the spine, St. Louis, 1969, Mosby.

69. Goldthwaite JE: The lumbosacral articulation, *Boston Med Surg J* 164:365, 1911.

70. Hadra BE: Wiring the spinous processes in Pott's disease, *Trans Am Orthop Assoc* 4:206, 1891.

71. Harmon PH: Anterior extraperitoneal lumbar disc excision and vertebral body fusion, *Clin Orthop* 18:169, 1960.

72. Harrington PR: Treatment of scoliosis: correction and internal fixation body spine instrumentation, *J Bone Joint Surg* 44A:591, 1962.

73. Herbinaux G: Traite sur diverse accouchemens laborieux et sur les polypes de la matrice, *Bruxelles,* 1782, De Boubers.

74. Herron J: Bilateral laminectomy and discectomy for segental lumbar disc disease, *Spine* 8:86, 1983.

75. Hibbs RA: An operation for progressive spine deformities, *N Y State J Med* 93:1013, 1911.

76. Hijakata SA: A method of percutaneous nuclear extraction, *J Toden Hosp* 5:39, 1975.

77. Hijikata SA, Yamagishi M, Nakayama T, et al.: Percutaneous discectomy: a new treatment method for lumbar disc herniation, *J Toden Hosp* 5:5, 1975.

78. Hildanus F: *Opera.* In Walker AE, editor: *A history of neurosurgical surgery,* New York, 1672, Hatner Publishing Company, p. 366.

79. Hirabayski K, Watambe K, Wakano K, et al.: Expansive open-door laminoplasty for cervical spinal stenotic myelopathy, *Spine* 8:693, 1983.

80. Hirsh C: Cervical disc rupture: diagnosis and therapy, *Acta Orthop Scand* 30:172, 1960.

81. Hirabayashi K, Watanabe K, Wakano K, et al.: Expansive open-door laminoplasty for cervical spinal stenoic myelopathy, *Spine* 8:693, 1983.

82. Hodgson AR, Stock FE: Anterior spine fusion for treatment of tuberculosis of the spine, *J Bone Joint Surg* 42A:295, 1960.

83. Hodgson AR, Stock FE, Wong SK: A description of a technique and evaluation of anterior spinal fusion for deranged discs and spondylolisthesis, *Clin Orthop* 56:133, 1968.

84. Hodgson AR, Stock FE: Anterior spinal fusion: a preliminary communication on the radical treatment of Pott's disease and Pott's paraplegia, *Br J Surg* 44:266, 1956.

85. Hoover NW: Methods of lumbar fusion, *J Bone Joint Surg* 50A:194, 1968.

86. Hulme A: The surgical approach to thoracic intervertebral disc protrusions, *J Neurol Neurosurg Psychiatry* 23:133, 1960.

87. Hult L: *The Munkfors investigation, Acta Orthop Scand Retroperitoneal Disc Fenestration in Low Back Pain and Sciatica.*

88. Humphries AW, Hawk WA, Berndt AL: Anterior fusion of the lumbar spine using an internal fixation device, *J Bone Joint Surg* 41A:371, 1959.

89. Hutter CG: Posterior intervertebral body fusion: a 25 year study, *Clin Orthop* 179:86, 1983.

90. Ito H, et al.: A new radical operation for Pott's disease, *J Bone Joint Surg* 16:499, 1934.

91. Iwahara T: A new method of vertebral body fusion, *Surgery* (Jpn) 8:271, 1944.

92. Jaslow IA: Intercorporal bone graft in spinal fusion after disc removal. *Surg Gynecol Obstet* 82:215, 1946.

93. Jerkins JA: Spondylolisthesis, *Br J Surg* 24:80, 1936.

94. Junghanns H: Spondylolisthesen ohne Spalt in Swischengelenkstijck *Archiv fur Orthopedische and Unfall-dehirurgie* 29:118, 1930.

95. Kahn EA: The role of the dentate ligaments in spinal cord compression and the syndrome of lateral sclerosis, *J Neurosurg* 4:191, 1947.

96. Kambin P, Gellman H: Percutaneous lateral discectomy of the lumbar spine: a preliminary report, *Clin Orthop* 174:127, 1983.

97. Kaneda K, Kazama H, et al.: Follow-up study of medial facetectomies and posterolateral fusion with instrumentation in unstable degenerative spondylolisthesis, *Clin Orthop* 203:159, 1986.

98. Kaneda K, Abumi K, Fujiya M: Burst fractures with neurologic deficits of the thoracolumbar-lumbar spine, *Spine* 9:788, 1984.

99. Key CA: On paraplegia depending on disease of the ligaments of the spine, *Guys Hosp Rep* 3:17, 1838.

100. Key DC, Compere LE: Normal and pathological physiology of the nucleus pulposus and intervertebral disc, *J Bone Joint Surg* 14A:897, 1932.

101. Kilian JF: *Schilderungen neuer backen formen and ihrev verhalten im leben,* Manuheim, 1854, Bassermann und Mathy.

102. King D: Internal fixation for lumbosacral fusion, *J Bone Joint Surg* 30A:560, 1948.

103. Kirkaldy-Willis WH, Paine KW, Cauchoix J, et al.: Lumbar spinal stenosis, *Clin Orthop* 99:30, 1974.

104. Kocher T: Die Verletzungen der Wirbelsaule zubleich als Beitung zur Physiologie des menschlichen Ruckenmarks, *Mitt Grenzgeb Med Chir* 1:415, 1896.

105. Kostuik JP: Anterior Kostuik-Harrington distraction systems for the treatment of kyphotic deformities, *Iowa Orthop J* 69:77, 1988.

106. Kostuik JP, Erico TJ, Gleason TF: Techniques of internal fixation for degenerative conditions of the lumbar spine, *Clin Orthop* 203:219, 1986.

107. Kostuik JP, Carl A, Ferron S: Anterior Zielke instrumentation for spinal deformity in adults, *J Bone Joint Surg* 71A:898, 1989.

108. Kozak JA, O'Brien JP: Simultaneous combined anterior and posterior fusion, *Spine* 15:322, 1990.

109. Lane WA: Case of spondylolisthesis associated with progressive paraplegia: laminectomy, *Lancet* 1:991, 1893.

110. Lanke F: Support for the spondylitic spine by means of buried steel bars, attached to the vertebrae, *Am J Orthop Surg* 8:344, 1910.

111. Lee CK, Rauschning, Glenn W: Lateral lumbar spinal canal stenosis: classification, pathology anatomy and surgical decompression, *Spine* 13:3, 1988.

112. Leong JCY, Chun SY, Grange WJ, et al.: Long-term results of lumbar intervertebral disc prolapse, *Spine* 8:793, 1983.

113. Levay D: A survey of surgical management of lumbar disc prolapse in the United Kingdom and Eire, *Lancet* 1:1211, 1967.

114. Lin PM, Cantilli RA, Joyce MF: Posterior lumbar interbody fusion, *Clin Orthop* 180:154, 1977.

115. Lister J: On the antiseptic principle in the practice of surgery, *BMJ* 2:246, 1867.

116. Logue V: Thoracic intervertebral disc prolapse with spinal cord compression, *J Neurol Neursurg Psychiatry* 15:227, 1952.

117. Love JG: Removal of intervertebral discs without laminectomy, *Proc Staff Meet Mayo Clin* 14:800, 1939.

118. Luque ER: The anatomic basis and development of segmental spinal instrumentation, *Spine* 7:256, 1982.

119. Luque ER: Interpeduncular segmental fixation, *Clin Orthop* 203:54, 1986.

120. Ma G, Paulson J: *Interbody fusion of the lumbar spine with the use of box chisels,* Presented at the Western Orthopaedic Association meeting, October 1982.

121. Magerl F: *External skeletal fixation of the lower thoracic and lumbar spine: current concepts of external fixation of fractures,* Berlin, 1982, Springer-Verlag.

122. Magerl F, Seemann P: Stable posterior fusion of the atlas and axis by transarticular screw fixation. In Kehi P, Weidner A, editors: *Cervical Spine I,* New York, 1987, Springer Verlag, p. 322.

123. Markhoff KL, Morris JM: The structural components of the intervertebral disc, *J Bone Joint Surg* 56A:675, 1974.

124. Mason C, Cozen L, Adelstein L: Surgical correction of flexion deformity of the cervical spine, *Calif Med* 79:244, 1953.

125. Menard V: Couses de la paraplegie dansle mal de Pott: son treatment chirurgical par l'ouverture directe du foyer tuberculeux des vertebres, *Rev Orthop* 5:47, 1894.

126. Mercer W: Spondylolisthesis, *Edinb Med J* 43:545, 1936.

127. Middleton GS, Teacher JH: Extruded disc at the T12-L1 level—microscopic exam showed it to be nucleus pulposus, *Glasgow Med J* 1

128. Middleton GS, Teacher JH: Injury of the spinal cord due to rupture of an intervertebral disc during muscular effort, *Glasgow Med J* 76:1, 1911.

129. Miller R: Protrusion of the thoracic intervertebral discs with compression of the spinal cord, *Acta Med Scand* 139:99, 1951.

130. Mixter WJ, Barr JS: Rupture of the intervertebral disc with involvement of the spinal canal, *N Engl J Med* 211:210, 1934.

131. Murphy F: The early days of neurosurgery as I remember them, with emphasis on disc surgery, *Neurosurgery* 17:370, 1985.

132. Murphy F: Experience with lumbar disc surgery, *Clin Neurosurg* 20:1, 1973.

133. Nickel VL, Perry J, Garrett A, et al.: The halo: a spinal skeletal traction fixation device, *J Bone Joint Surg* 50A:1400, 1968.

134. O'Brien JP, Dawson MHO, Heard CW, et al.: Simultaneous combined anterior and posterior fusion, *Clin Orthop* 203:191, 1986.

135. O'Brien JP: The role of fusion for chronic low back pain, *Orthop Clin North Am* 14:639, 1983.

136. Onik G, Helms CA, Ginsbergh, et al.: Percutaneous lumbar discectomy using a new aspiration probe, *AJNR Am J Neuroradiol* 6:290, 1985.

137. Onji Y, Akiyama H, et al.: Posterior paravertebral ossification causing cervical myelopathy: a report of eighteen cases, *J Bone Joint Surg* 49A:1314, 1967.

138. Parker, Adson: Quoted in Reynolds F, Katz S: Herniated lumbar intervertebral disc, American Academy of Orthopaedic Surgeons symposium on the spine, St. Louis, 1969, Mosby.

139. Patterson AM: Fractures of the cervical spine, *J Anat Lond* 24:ix, 1890.

140. Patterson RH, Arbit E: A surgical approach through the pedicle to protruded thoracic discs, *J Neurosurg* 48:768, 1978.

141. Paul of Agena: Collected works, translated by F Adams, Sydenman Society, London, 1834, et seq.

142. Peek RD, Wiltse LL, Reynolds JB, et al.: In situ arthrodesis without decompression for grade III or IV isthmic spondylolisthesis in adults with severe sciatica, *J Bone Joint Surg* 71A:63, 1989.

143. Perot PL, Munro DD: Transthoracic removal of midline thoracic disc protrusions causing spinal cord compression, *J Neurosurg* 31:452, 1969.

144. Pilcher LS: Alto-axoid fracture dislocation, *Ann Surg* 51:208, 1910.

145. Portal A: Cours d'anatomie medicle ou elements de l'anatomie de l'homme, vol. 1. Paris, 1803, Baudouin.

146. Potts P: Remarks on that kind of palsy frequently found to accompany curvature of the spine, London. Also in Medical Classics, vol. 6, no. 4, December 1936.

147. Putti V: New conceptions in pathogenesis of sciatic pain, *Lancet* 2:53, 1927.

148. Ransford AO, Crockard HA, Pozo JL, et al.: Craniocervical instability treated by contoured loop fixation, *J Bone Joint Surg* 68B:173, 1986.

149. Raynor RB: Anterior or posterior approach to the cervical spine: an anatomical and radiographic evaluation and comparison, *Neurosurgery* 12:7, 1983.

150. Raynor RB, Pugh J, Shapiro I: Cervical facetectomy and its effect on spine strength, *J Neurosurg* 63:278, 1985.

151. Reynolds JB, Wiltse LL: Surgical treatment of degenerative spondylolisthesis, *Spine* 4:148, 1979.

152. Robertson JT: Anterior operations for herniated cervical discs and for myelopathy, *Clin Neurosurg* 25:245, 1978.

153. Robinson RA, Southwick WO: Indications and techniques for early stabilization of the neck in some fracture dislocation of the cervical spine, *South Med J* 53:565, 1960.

154. Robinson RA, Smith GW: Anterolateral cervical disc removal and interbody fusion for cervical disc syndrome, *Bull Johns Hopkins Hosp* 96:223, 1955.

155. Rogers WA: Treatment of fracture-dislocation of the cervical spine, *J Bone Joint Surg* 24A:245, 1942.

156. Roy-Camille R, Saillant G, Mazel C: Internal fixation of the lumbar spine with pedicle screw plating, *Clin Orthop* 203:7, 1986.

157. Roy-Camille R, Roy-Camille M, Demeulenaere C: Osseosynthesis of dorsal, lumbar and lumbosacral spine with metallic planes screwed into vertebral pedicles and articular apophyses, *Presse Med* 78: 1446, 1970.

158. Roy-Camille R, Saillant G, Mazel CH: *Treatment of cervical spine injuries by a posterior osteosynthesis with plates and screws.* In Kehr P, Weidner A, editors: *Cervical spine* I, New York, 1987, Springer Verlag, p. 163.

159. Roy-Camille R, Gagna G, Lazennec JY: *L'arthrodese occipito-cervicale.* In Roy-Camille, editor: *5 emes journees d'orthopedic de la pitie: rachis cervical superieur,* Paris, 1986, Masson, p. 49.

160. Ryan MD, Taylor TKF, Sherwood AA: Bolt-plate fixation for anterior spinal fusion, *Clin Orthop* 203:196, 1986.

161. Sachs B, Frankel J: Progressive ankylotic rigidity of the spine, *J Nerv Ment Dis* 27:1, 1900.

162. Sacks S: Anterior interbody fusion of the lumbar spine, *J Bone Joint Surg* 47B:211, 1965.

163. Sakamoto T: *A study of percutaneous lumbar nucleotomy and lumbar intradiscal pressure,* Presented at the International Symposium of Percutaneous Nucleotomy, Bruxelles, March 1989.

164. San Martino A, D'Andria FM, San Martino C: The surgical treatment of nerve root compression caused by scoliosis of the lumbar spine, *Spine* 8:261, 1983.

165. Sarpyenyer MA: Congenital stricture of the spinal canal, *J Bone Joint Surg* 27:70, 1945.

166. Schmoral G, Junghanns H: *The human spine in health and disease,* New York, 1971, Grune & Stratton, p. 22.

167. Schmorl G: Die Pathalogische Anatomie der Wirbelsaule, *Verh Dtsch Orthop Ges* 21:3, 1926.

168. Schultz EC, Semmes RE: Head and neck pains of cervical disc origin, *Laryngoscope* 60:338, 1950.

169. Scoville WB, Whitcomb BB, McLaurin R: The cervical ruptured disc: report of 115 operative cases, *Trans Am Neurol Assoc* 76:222, 1951.

170. Seitsalo S, Osterman K, Poussa M: Scoliosis associated with lumbar spondylolisthesis: a clinical survey of 190 young patients, *Spine* 13:899, 1988.

171. Selby D: *Lumbar spine surgery,* 1985, Arthur H. White, p. 383.

172. Selby D: Personal communication,1985.

173. Semmelweiss IG: *The concept of child-bed fever,* In Thomas H, editor: *Selected readings in obstetrics and gynecology,* Springfield, IL, 1861, Charles C Thomas.

174. Semmelweis IP: The etiology, the concept and the prophylaxis of childbed fever, translated by FP Murphy. In: *Medical Classics* 4:350, 1941.

175. Semmes RE, Murphey F: Syndrome of C-6 disc, *JAMA* 121:1209, 1943.

176. Shakespeare W: Timon of Athens, Act 4, Scene 1, line 23.

177. Siccard JA, Forestier J: Methode radiographique d'exploration de la cavité epidurale par le lipiodoi, *Rev Neurol* 37:1264, 1921.

178. Simmons EH, Jackson RP: The management of nerve root entrapment syndromes associated with the collapsing scoliosis of idiopathic lumbar and thoracolumbar curves, *Spine* 4:533, 1979.

179. Simmons EH, Bhallia SK: Anterior cervical discectomy and fusion: a clinical and biomechanical study with eight year follow up, *J Bone Joint Surg* 51B:225, 1969.

180. Simmons EH: The surgical correction of flexion deformity of the cervical spine in ankylosing spondylitis, *Clin Orthop* 86:132, 1972.

181. Singounas EG, Karvounis PC: Thoracic disc protrusion, *Acta Neurochir* 29:251, 1977.

182. Smith AG: Account of a case in which portions of three dorsal vertebrae were removed for the relief of paralysis from fracture, with partial success, *North Am J Med Surg* 1829.

183. Smith MD, Bohlman HH: Spondylolisthesis treated by a single stage operation decompression with in situ posterolateral and anterior fusion, *J Bone Joint Surg* 72A:415, 1990.

184. Stauffer RN, Coventry MB: Symposium: low back and sciatic pain, *J Bone Joint Surg* 50A:167, 1968.

185. Stauffer RN, Coventry MB: Anterior interbody lumbar spine fusion, *J Bone Joint Surg* 54A:756, 1972.

186. Stauffer RN, Coventry MB: Posterolateral lumbar spine fusion, *J Bone Joint Surg* 54A:1195, 1972.

187. Steffee AD, Sitkowski DJ: Posterior lumbar interbody fusion and plates, *Clin Orthop* 227:99, 1988.

188. Steffee AD: Segmental spine plates with pedicle screw fixation, *Clin Orthop* 203:45, 1986.

189. Steffee AD, Biscup RS, Sitkowski DJ: Segmental spine plates with pedicle screw fixation, *Clin Orthop* 203:45, 1986.

190. Steffee AD, Sitkowski DJ: Reduction and stabilization of grade IV spondylolisthesis, *Clin Orthop* 227:82, 1988.

191. Stookey B: Compression of the spinal cord due to ventral extradural cervical chondromas, *Arch Neurol Psychiatry* 20:275, 1928.

192. Sumita M: Beitrage zur Lehre von Derchondrodystrophia Foetalis (Kaufmann) und Osteogenesis Imperfecta (Vrolik) mit Besomderer Berucksichtingung der Anatomischen und Klinischen Differential Diagnose, *Dtsch Z Chir* 107:1, 1976.

193. Suzuki J: Anterior spinal fusion, *Annu Cong Jpn Orthop Assoc* 40:6, 1967.

194. Taylor AR: Fracture dislocation of cervical spine, *Ann Surg* 90:321, 1929.

195. Truchley G, Thompson WA: Posterolateral fusion of the lumbosacral spine, *J Bone Joint Surg* 44A:505, 1962.

196. Tsuyami N: Ossification of the posterior longitudinal ligament of the spine, *CORR* 184:71, 1984.

197. Tullberg T, Isacson J, Weidenhielm L: Does microscopic removal of the lumbar disc herniation lead to better results than the standard procedure? *Spine* 18:24, 1993.

198. Valleix: Quoted in Reynolds F, Katz S: *Herniated lumbar intervertebral disc,* American Academy of Orthopaedic Surgeon symposium on the spine, St. Louis, 1969, Mosby.

199. Valls J, Ottolenghi EC, Schajowicz F: Aspiration biopsy in diagnosis of lesions of vertebral bodies, *JAMA* 136:376, 1948.

200. van Rens TJ, van Horn JR: *Long-term results in lumbosacral interbody fusion for spondylolisthesis,* 1982.

201. Verbeist H: *Sur certaines formes rares de compression de la queue de cheval hommage a clovis vincent,* Paris, 1949, Malouie.

202. Verbeist H: A lateral approach to the cervical spine: technique and indications. *J Neurosurg* 28:191, 1968.

203. Verbeist H: *Neurogenic intermittent claudication,* Amsterdam, 1976, North Holland Publishing Co.

204. Verbeist H, Paz Y, Geuse HD: Anterolateral surgery for cervical spondylosis in cases of myelopathy or nerve root compression, *J Neurosurg* 25:611, 1966.

205. Virchow R: *Untersuchunger fiber die enwickelung die Schadelgrunder,* Berlin, 1857, G. Reimer.

206. Von Lushka H: *Die Hagelenke des Menschlichen Korpers,* vol. 4, Berlin, 1858, G. Reimer.

207. Walsh J: Galen's second sojourn in Italy and his treatment of the family of Marcus Aurelius, *Med Life* 37(9) [120], September 1930.

208. Watkins MB: Posterolateral fusion of the lumbar and lumbosacral spine, *J Bone Joint Surg* 35A:1014, 1953.

209. Werlinich M: *Anterior interbody fusion and stabilization with metal fixation,* 1974.

210. Whitecloud TS III, LaRocca SH: Fibular strut graft in reconstructive surgery of the cervical spine, *Spine* 1:33, 1976.

211. Wilkins BF: Separation of the vertebrae with protrusion of hernia between the same-operation-cure, *St Louis Med Surg* 54:340, 1888.

212. Williams RW: Microsurgical lumbar discectomy: report to American Association of Neurology and Surgery, 1975, *Neurosurgery* 4:140, 1979.

213. Wilson PD, Danford MS: The anatomy of the lumbosacral region in relation to sciatic pain, *J Bone Joint Surg* 7A:109, 1925.

214. Wilson PD, Straub LR: *The use of metal plate fastened to the spinous processes,* American Academy of Orthopaedic Surgeons Instructional Course Lecture. Ann Arbor, MI, 1952.

215. Wilson DH, Campbell DD: Anterior cervical discectomy without bone graft: report of 11 cases, *J Neurosurg* 47:551, 1977.

216. Wiltbarger BR: The dowel intervertebral-body fusion as used in lumbar disc surgery, *J Bone Joint Surg* 39A:284, 1957.

217. Wiltse LL, Bateman JG, Hutchinson RA: The paraspinal sacrospinalis-splitting approach to the lumbar spine, *J Bone Joint Surg* 50A:919, 1968.

218. Wiltse LL, Guyer RD, Spencer CW, et al.: Alter transverse process impingement of the L5 spinal nerve: the far-out syndrome, *Spine* 9:31, 1984.

219. Wiltse LL: *Spondylolisthesis and its treatment: conservative treatment, fusion, with and without reduction. In* Ruge D, Wiltse LL, editors: *Spinal disorder:* diagnosis and treatment, Philadelphia, 1977, Lea & Febiger, p. 193.

220. Wiltse LL, Winter R: Terminology and measurement of spondylolisthesis, *J Bone Joint Surg* 65A:768, 1983.

221. Wiltse LL, Newman PH, Macnab I: Classification of spondylolysis and spondylolisthesis, *Clin Orthop* 117:23, 1976.

222. Wiltse LL, Bateman JG, Hutchinson RA: The paraspinal sacrospinalis—splitting approach to the lumbar spine, *J Bone Joint Surg* 50A:919, 1968.

223. Zielke K, Strempel AV: Posterior lateral distraction spondylodesis using the twofold sacral bar, *Clin Orthop* 151, 1986.

Chapter 59

Development and Growth of the Cervical and Lumbar Spine

Lance T. Twomey

James R. Taylor

Development and Adult Structure

Contrast Between Cervical and Lumbar Motion Segments

Development of the Vertebral Column

    blastemal stage
    cartilaginous stage
    osseous stage
    important factors controlling
      early development
    variation in segmental number and at
      junctional regions

Disc and Vertebral Body Development and Growth

    intervertebral discs
    changes in disc nutrition with growth and
      their consequences

Facet (Zygapophyseal) Joints

    coronal component (anteromedial third of
      joint)
    sagittal component (posterior two thirds
      of joint)

Growth in Length of the Vertebral Column as a Whole

    regional differences in maturation
    mechanical and postural influences
      on growth
    sexual dimorphism in vertebral body growth
    vascular and notochordal influences on
      the development of Schmorl nodes

Developmental and Growth-Related Pathology: A Summary

Development and Adult Structure

The embryonic development of the human vertebral column is a relatively rapid phenomenon. During a few short weeks the morphologic pattern of a normal or abnormal spine, on which normal or abnormal spinal function (stability or instability) depends, will be established. However, as the fetus, infant, and child continue to develop, further important changes in the dimensions and tissues of the spine render it vulnerable to abnormal genetic and environmental influences. Normal development and growth of the spine produces a complex series of bones and joints that support and move the trunk and protect the spinal cord. If these processes go wrong, congenital anomalies, growth-related deformities and malfunction of the vertebral column will result. An account of the whole range of development and growth up to maturity is therefore highly relevant to an understanding of normal and abnormal adult spinal structure and function.

Growth is a measurable increase in size by increase in cell numbers, in cell size, and in cell products of matrix and fibers. Prenatal growth is characterized principally by cell multiplication and postnatal growth principally, but not entirely, by increases in cell size and cell products. Development also involves cell differentiation. Cells become specialized and less versatile as they multiply and differentiate. Connective-tissue cells differentiate depending on their genetic programs. The tissues they form are also affected by their position in the developing embryo, by their contact and interaction with other cells, and by vascular, hormonal, and mechanical influences. Some cells produce diffusible products that influence the development of neighboring tissues, but many of the growth control mechanisms remain incompletely understood. Malformations may result from abnormal genetic or intrauterine environmental influences.

There have been few comprehensive studies of the growth and development of the human spine in the past three decades. The major hindrance to such studies is the difficulty in collecting sufficient human material across the whole range of development and maturation. The following account is based on an extensive review of the literature and on four major studies of our own.[31,33,37,43] Taylor's[31] study provides a histologic and measurement amount of the prenatal and postnatal development of vertebrae and intervertebral discs, while Twomey's[43] study provides additional data on childhood and adolescent development plus data on age-related changes in the dimensions of spinal elements and changes in movement, posture, and biomechanics of the lumbar spine. The former study considered 67 embryos, fetuses, infants, and children, with a cumulative total of 272 discs, and in addition, radiographic measurements were recorded from 29 cervical, 196 thoracic, and 321 lumbar radiographs of children and adolescents.[31] The second study[43] sectioned, examined, and measured all vertebral elements (vertebrae, discs, and posterior elements) in fresh cadaveric material from more than 200 spines with an age range of 1 day to 97 years. Taylor's[33] study examined over 100 spinal columns of juveniles in Natural History museums in Washington, London, and Paris. Our more recent study of the cervical spine is based on 70 postmortem cervical spines of children and adults that have been x-rayed, sectioned, and examined microscopically.

Contrast Between Cervical and Lumbar Motion Segments

Although many clinicians make the assumption that the anatomy of the cervical motion segments is virtually identical (although smaller in size) with those in the lumbar region, they are clearly mistaken. Not only are there easily apparent differences in the size and shape of the vertebral elements, there are clear structural differences in the morphology of the intervertebral joints.

In normal erect standing, the intervertebral disc (IVD) and zygapophyseal (facet) joints in the neck bear approximately equal vertical compressive forces,[21] whereas in the lumbar spine, the discs bear about 85% of the axial load, with the facet joints sharing the remaining 15% of the compressive load.[17]

The zygapophyseal joint facets in the cervical spine are usually flat and oriented at about 45 degrees to the horizontal plane,[36] thus facilitating movement in all directions. The principal restraint to motion at end range is increased tension in the soft tissues and ligaments of the neck. However, in the low back, the facets are biplanar in transverse section and vertically oriented, parallel to the long axis of the spine.[24,36] This arrangement provides articular restraint to limit motion in the horizontal and coronal planes, facilitating motion in the sagittal plane only. Even flexion is limited by facetal compressive loading more than it is by increasing soft-tissue ligamentous tension.[45] The zygapophyseal joints in the lumbar spine protect the IVDs from considerable strain, particularly from torsion movement.[9,50]

The cervical discs differ in a number of important respects from the discs of the lumbar spine. These

Delayed Development in Cervical Region in a 30cm CRL 34 week fetus

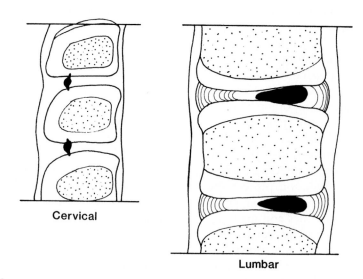

Cervical

Lumbar

Fig. 59-1

Delayed development of notochordal segment (*black*) in the cervical discs of premature stillborn fetus, compared to rapid growth of notochordal nucleus in lumbar discs of same fetus. Note also that cervical centra have not yet extended to anterior and posterior margins of cartilage model of vertebral body.

differences are based on developmental features unique to cervical discs. Notochordal tissue plays a less important and an inconsistent role in the development of the cervical nucleus pulposus compared to its major role in development of the nucleus pulposus of lumbar discs. The original cervical notochordal segments are very small (Fig. 59-1); their increase in size is delayed or even absent in many fetal discs, and the cervical nucleus is formed largely from the precartilaginous mesenchyme around the notochord.[31,36] Both notochordal cells and fetal cartilage cells form glycosaminoglycans, but the fetal cartilage cells also produce plentiful collagen. Consequently, the cervical nucleus of the infant and young child has a higher collagen content than the lumbar nucleus.[27]

With the growth of the uncus on each side of a cervical vertebral body in later childhood, lateral uncovertebral clefts appear in the discs, which spread transversely as fissures through the center of each disc in young adults. This also results in increased fibrous change in the disc and loss of some of the disc proteoglycans, which are necessary to ensure a high water content in intervertebral discs. These developmental features of the cervical spine mean that the cervical nucleus pulposus has a relatively short existence as a soft central gel, and it soon changes through the 20s and 30s to firm fibrocartilage.[14,31] Cervical discograms in patients over 30 years of age

show spread of centrally injected contrast material to both uncovertebral joints, and not infrequently there is a leakage of contrast into the anterior epidural space. A firm fibrocartilaginous nucleus is less likely to prolapse than a soft gel, so cervical disc herniation is less frequent than lumbar disc herniation. The presence of an uncus forms a barrier to prolapse of nuclear material into cervical intervertebral foramina, but the transverse fissures across the posterior parts of cervical discs may favor extrusion of fragments into the spinal canal, particularly as a consequence of a traumatic incident. In degenerative disease of the cervical spine it is uncovertebral osteophytes that invade the intervertebral foramen and posterior osteocartilaginous bars that protrude into the cervical spinal canal.

The development of the *uncovertebral joints* in the cervical spine requires specific description. From the age of 8 or 10 years, the cervical IVD is partly protected by the presence of the posterolaterally placed uncovertebral joints. This additional protection is important since the cervical facet joints are designed to allow free movement in all planes, rather than to limit movement and protect the discs. The uncovertebral joints are also known as the "lateral interbody joints" or the joints of von Luschka.

The lateral parts of a cervical body are formed from the neural arch centers of ossification and not from the centrum. In the fetus and infant the IVD

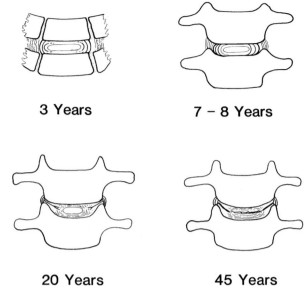

3 Years   **7 – 8 Years**

20 Years   **45 Years**

Fig. 59-2

Diagrammatic coronal sections through midcervical discs at four stages. At 3 years there are no uncinate processes, neurocentral growth plates are not fused, and there is gelatinous nucleus contained by intact anulus. At 4 to 8 years uncus has grown on each side and clefts are about to be formed in lateral anulus. At 20 years uncovertebral clefts are well formed but nucleus remains gelatinous. At 45 years clefts extend right across disc and center of disc is fibrocartilaginous.

does not extend to the whole transverse extent of the vertebral body. The outer edge of the anulus fibrosus extends only just lateral to the line of fusion of the centrum and vertebral arches. From the superior aspect of each lateral vertebral body margin, an uncinate process grows upward toward the vertebral body above, in the loose vascular fibrous tissue lateral to the anulus (Fig. 59-2). This process (or uncus) has grown enough by about 8 years to form a kind of adventitious joint, the uncovertebral joint, on each side of the disc. There is some doubt as to whether this "joint" or pseudoarthrosis develops within true disc tissue or whether it appears as a cleft in the looser connective tissue immediately lateral to the anulus.[11,12,23,42] The tip of the uncus and the groove in the lateral margin of the vertebra above are lined by fibrocartilage that may be derived from the outer anulus; a thin fibrous capsule limits each joint cleft laterally. The formation of the uncovertebral joints effectively narrows the horizontal band within which the translatory movements accompanying flexion take place; it "concentrates" the plane of shear to a narrow horizontal band within the lat-

eral anulus because of the gliding movements in the adjacent uncovertebral joints. This appears to result in medial extension of horizontal fissures into the anulus from the uncovertebral joints (see Fig. 59-2).

This fine fissuring, which begins developmentally from the uncovertebral joints, gradually extends, in the adult, right through the IVD, leaving only the anterior anulus and longitudinal ligaments intact. As a consequence, movements of the cervical IVD change from rolling and gliding around a soft central nucleus in young adults of 20 years to a combined gliding and deformation in middle-aged or elderly cervical discs; a bipartite, fibrocartilaginous disc would allow translation between its upper and lower parts. This cervical motion segment is much less stable than thoracolumbar motion segments and is heavily dependent for its stability on the integrity of the posterior joints, muscles, and ligaments. The additional loading of the uncovertebral joints that accompanies disc fissuring concentrates degenerative change in them much more than in the facet joints. This leads to lateral osteophytosis from the uncovertebral joints into the intervertebral canals. This relates as much to their distinctive developmental morphology as it does to the stresses to which they are subject.[13]

In *lumbar discs* by contrast, the notochordal phase of development of the nucleus pulposus is much more dramatic, with rapid expansion of the notochordal segment to fill the center of fetal lumbar discs (see Fig. 59-1). Notochordal cells continue to multiply in infant lumbar discs,[31] and a notochordal nucleus pulposus with its large soft central gel occupies three quarters of the anteroposterior extent of a lumbar disc in 1-year-old infants. Notochordal tissue remains the dominant tissue in a lumbar nucleus pulposus until 3 or 4 years. It is gradually replaced by a different cell population of fibroblasts and chondrocytes by the end of the first postnatal decade, but the soft central gel persists within an envelope formed by the anulus fibrosus and the cartilage plates that cap the vertebral bodies. This lumbar nucleus remains soft until a much later stage than a cervical nucleus because its collagen content is relatively lower and its proteoglycan content (and therefore its water content) remain higher than in cervical discs. Lumbar disc fissuring occurs much later and as part of an aging process rather than a developmental process. The first fissures are circumferential in the inner anulus and even when radial fissures appear they seldom extend through the whole anulus.[48]

Development of the Vertebral Column

Before there is any vertebral column, in the third week of embryonic life, the axis of the flat embryonic disc is defined by the appearance and "headward growth" of the notochord from the primitive node (Hensen node), between the ectoderm and the endoderm. At about the same time, mesoderm, the third primary layer of the embryo, develops from the primitive node and primitive streak, spreading laterally to separate the ectoderm from the endoderm on each side of the notochord.

The notochord induces the thickening of the neuroectoderm on its dorsal aspect, forming a neural plate that then folds longitudinally to form the neural tube. The mesoderm thickens on each side of the notochord and the neural tube to form bilateral longitudinal columns of paraxial mesoderm. The *notochord* and the *neural tube,* with the columns of *paraxial mesoderm* on each side, extend approximately from the level of the primitive mouth to the primitive anus, with the primitive aorta ventral to them (Fig. 59-3). These are the essential components for the formation of the vertebral column. As the embryo grows in length and width, it curls up and bends by ventrally directed growth of its head and tail, becoming convex on its dorsal aspects. The dorsal axial structures are now curved in a bow around the ventral gut tube. The columns of paraxial mesoderm divide into a large number of segments or *somites,* which will form the vertebral column with its associated muscles around the notochord and the neural tube.

The vertebral column will pass through three developmental stages: the blastemal stage, the cartilaginous stage, and the osseous stage. These are discussed below.

Blastemal stage

The *blastemal* column is first formed by the medial migration of mesoderm from the ventromedial portions of the somites to surround the notochord. Although formed from segmented mesoderm, this original mesodermal condensation around the notochord is itself continuous and unsegmented. The aorta, which lies immediately in front of the blastemal column, gives off dorsolateral "intersegmental branches" at regular intervals. The continuous blastemal column "resegments" into alternate light and dark bands all the way along its length. The *intersegmental arteries* are now seen to pass

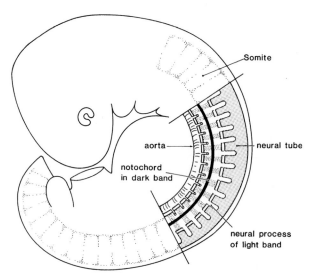

7mm embryo showing axial structures

Fig. 59-3

External structure, showing somites, is removed in central part of embryo to show axial structures. Notochord is continuous and unsegmented within blastemal vertebral column, which has differentiated into alternate light and dark bands. Intersegmental branches of aorta pass around light bands on each side; neural processes are growing backward around neural tube on each side.

around the center of each light band, which is a primordial vertebra. Neural processes grow dorsally around the neural tube from each light band. The light bands, or primordial vertebrae, grow much more rapidly than the dark bands, soon becoming four times thicker than the dark bands, which are the primordia of the intervertebral discs.

Cartilaginous stage

The cells of the light bands with their neural processes differentiate into fetal chondroblasts. The chondroblasts change the light bands into clearly recognizable cartilage models of vertebrae. Meanwhile, the peripheral cells of the dark bands differentiate into fibroblasts, which arrange themselves in concentric layers and begin to lay down the collagen fibers of the primitive annulus fibrosus.

The rapid growth of the fetal cartilage models of vertebral bodies is accompanied by notochordal segmentation. Notochordal cells disappear from the cartilaginous vertebral bodies and aggregate in the centers of the dark bands. Each notochordal segment forms a nucleus pulposus at the center of a dark band, which now becomes recognizable as an intervertebral disc, as fibroblasts and collagen bundles appear in lamellar form at its periphery (Fig. 59-4).

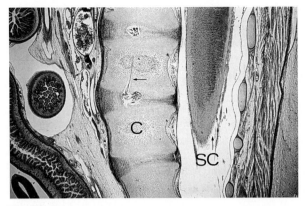

Fig. 59-4
Median sagittal section of lower lumbar spine of an 11-week fetus, showing developing centra (*c*), notochordal segment in intervertebral disc, and mucoid streak (*arrow*). At this stage of development spinal cord (*SC*) extends into lumbar region.

The cartilaginous stage of vertebral development is a relatively short one.

Osseous stage

Primary centers of ossification soon begin to appear—three centers in the cartilage model of each vertebra. The paired centers in the vertebral arches appear first, then the centra appear in the vertebral bodies. The paired primary centers of the arches appear, one on each side, at the vertebral canal aspect of what will be the junction of the pedicle and lamina (Fig. 59-5). The earliest vertebral arch centers are seen in the cervicothoracic region, and the subsequent sequential appearance of primary centers of ossification, with the processes of chondrocyte swelling and calcification then ossification of the matrix, extend rapidly up and down the column. Cervical arch centers appear from 8 to 10 weeks' and lumbar centers from 10 to 12 weeks' gestation. While the appearance of vertebral arch centers is generally sequential, midthoracic centers are an exception, as their appearance is delayed until all cervical, lower thoracic, and lumbar centers have appeared; finally, sacral centers are the last to appear.[2,19,33]

A single primary center for each vertebral body forms the "centrum." The centra appear first near the thoracolumbar junction and then appear in sequence up and down the column. The process of ossification extends from the primary centers through the cartilage model of each vertebra, but growth plates persist bilaterally between the arch and the centrum and as a single dorsal growth plate between the two halves of the vertebral arch in the median plane. The two halves of each vertebral arch fuse at about

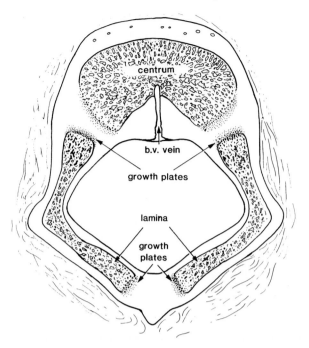

Fig. 59-5
Diagram based on transverse section of lumbar vertebra from 32-week fetus showing centrum and ossification of arches from paired centers of ossification. Growth plates between three centers ensure growth of spinal canal.

1 year postnatally; the neurocentral growth plates continue to grow until 3 to 7 years, depending on the segmental level (see Fig. 59-5). These growth plates provide growth of the vertebral canal to accommodate the growing spinal cord and cauda equina. Growth plates at the cephalic and caudal surfaces of the centrum ensure growth in height of the vertebral body. These growth plates remain active until completion of growth in height of the vertebral bodies at 15 to 17 years. They join the cartilage plates or "cartilaginous epiphyses," which cap the cephalic and caudal surfaces of each vertebral body to the bony "diaphysis." Each cartilage plate remains unossified throughout life, except at its circumference, where a bony ring apophysis is formed. This appears between 9 and 12 years and fuses with the vertebral body at 16 to 19 years, forming its bony rim.

Important Factors Controlling Early Development

Both the neural tube and the notochord have the potential to induce formation of a blastemal column around themselves,[49] and the first "blastemal" condensation is formed around the notochord by the medial migration of the ventromedial portions of the somites. The original, continuous, unsegmented, blastemal column resegments in such a way that the cartilaginous vertebrae are formed at intersegmental levels. Thus, the muscles derived from the myotomes of the paraxial somites alternate with the vertebrae and are attached to the upper and lower vertebra borders, rather than the middle of each vertebra. This alternation of muscles and bones is essential to the proper function of the locomotor system.[47]

The *intersegmental branches of the dorsal aorta* (see Fig. 59-3) have an important influence in vertebral column resegmentation by virtue of their situation at the centers of the light bands, where they provide the nutrition for the more rapid growth of the primitive vertebrae.[40] They are the only constant and regularly recurring structures in the blastemal vertebral column, and vascular anomalies may result in anomalies of segmentation.[28] A hemivertebra results if the bone of one side of the vertebral body fails to develop. Since there is normally only one center of chondrification in each vertebral body and only one primary ossification center for each centrum, the anomaly must originate at a preosseous or even a precartilaginous stage of development. Absence of an intersegmental vessel on one side may give rise to a hemivertebra.

The light bands grow much more rapidly than the dark bands, and their rapid growth appears to expel notochordal tissue into the more slowly growing dark bands, which will become intervertebral discs. Each notochordal segment forms a nucleus pulposus (or interacts with mesenchyme to do so in cervical discs). Notochordal cells multiply, produce matrix, and grow rapidly in the fetal discs of the thoracic and lumbar regions. Absence of a notochordal segment may give rise to congenital block vertebrae if no nucleus pulposus is formed to separate the centra. In the fetus and infant the notochordal nucleus pulposus grows by multiplication of its cells and liquifaction of the surrounding matrix. Notochordal cells are invasive and appear to produce substances that loosen and digest the inner layers of the surrounding envelope, incorporating these tissues into the expanding nucleus. It is appropriate that such invasive cells should not survive the end of the period of rapid growth.[31]

The acellular notochordal track persists for a while as a longitudinal "mucoid streak" in the cartilage models of the vertebrae, but it is usually obliterated when ossification commences. It has a temporary inhibiting effect on ossification, and a developing centrum sectioned along the mucoid streak has a bilobed appearance. Persistence of parts of the mucoid streak through the centrum is quite common

until infancy[31] but rare after that. If the notochordal track does persist until later stages of growth, a "butterfly vertebra" may be the result.

Vascular Influences and Asymmetric Growth

Taylor[34] hypothesized that in the fetal circulation, there is a delay in mixing of the blood pumped from the left ventricle through the aortic arch, with the blood entering the distal aortic arch through the ductus arteriosus. This would give asymmetric oxygenation to the right and left sides of developing fetal vertebrae. The poorly oxygenated blood from the ductus would pass from the convexity of the aortic arch into the left intersegmental branches and the well-oxygenated blood from the left ventricle would supply the right intersegmental branches. This could explain the observation that right and primary centers often appear before corresponding left arch centers, particularly in midthoracic vertebrae.[31] This primary asynchrony in appearance of paired ossification centers correlates with measured asymmetry in "pedicle lengths" in infants, in whom right pedicles are longer than left pedicles, and with the observation that when thoracic scoliosis is seen in infancy, the vertebral bodies are usually twisted to the left and the scoliosis is convex to the left.

The asynchrony in maturation and growth of vertebral arches seen in fetuses and infants persists until the time of closure of the neurocentral growth plates (6 to 7 years in the midthoracic spine) but reverses its direction in older children by catch-up growth and by the influence of aortic pressure on the left side. In children and adolescents, left pedicles tend to be longer than the corresponding right pedicles (measured to the lines of neurocentral fusion). The consequent vertebral body asymmetry and rotation of T5 to T10, when viewed from the front, gives a twist of the thoracic spine to the right. This change in the direction of asymmetry takes place from 7 years onward (Fig. 59-6). It is associ-

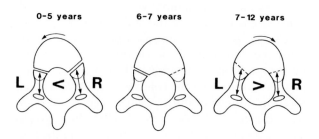

Fig. 59-6

Schematic diagram illustrating types of pedicle-length asymmetry found before and after asynchronous fusion of the neurocentral growth plates.

ated with the flattening of the anterior left surfaces of midthoracic vertebrae where they are in contact with the aorta. Aortic pressure also exerts a force tending to rotate thoracic vertebral bodies to the right.[7,30] It is also possible that the different position of the aorta on the lumbar vertebrae may favor left rotation in the lumbar spine.[8,34] These asynchronous events on right and left and the measured pedicle-length asymmetries accompany normal growth and may cause a physiologic scoliosis. They probably also determine the side of curvature of all forms of scoliosis, whatever other causes operate in the multifactorial etiology of progressive forms.[34]

Neural Influences on Vertebral Arch Growth

Just as growth of the brain is the primary influence on growth of the vault of the skull (e.g., in hydrocephalus), the growth of the spinal cord is an important influence on the growth of the vertebral arch. Watterson et al.[49] showed, in experiments on chick embryos, that experimental reduction or enlargement in the size of the neural tube resulted in corresponding changes in the size of the spinal canal. The rate of growth of the spinal canal in human development appears to adapt itself to the rate of growth of the spinal cord, but the control mechanisms remain unknown.

Spina Bifida Failure of closure of the neural arch results in a persistent cleft between the two halves of the arch. This common skeletal congenital anomaly, as an isolated phenomenon is called "spina bifida occulta." It is a common defect, which usually affects L5 or S1 vertebrae, occasionally the posterior arch of the atlas, or rarely, the arches of lower cervical vertebrae. It is generally an innocuous condition, though its presence in L5 is associated with a higher incidence of spondylolysis. In symptomatic forms of spina bifida there are varying degrees of malformation of the meninges and spinal cord. In rachischisis the neural folds fail to fuse and the cord develops as a flattened structure rather than as a closed cylindrical tube. The neural processes of affected vertebrae remain atrophic and do not grow together, leaving a wide open gap in the vertebral arches, overlying muscles and skin. The abnormal cord may project through this gap into a cystic swelling formed by the meninges, or the meninges themselves may be deficient, with leakage of cerebrospinal fluid to the exterior. This condition (occurring in 1 per 1000 births) may now be diagnosed antenatally by ultrasonography from 12 to 16 weeks gestation, and from the presence of increased α-fetoprotein in the amniotic fluid. Spina bifida cystica is most common in the lumbosacral region and then in the neck.

Variation in Segmental Number and at Junctional Regions

Normal segmentation produces 7 cervical, 12 thoracic, 5 lumbar, and 4 coccygeal segments in 65% to 95% of different population groups.[18,26] The remainder show either an extra segment or one segment less. Alternatively, there may be variations at the occipitocervical, cervicothoracic, thoracolumbar, or lumbosacral junctional regions—e.g., there may be an unfused odontoid, a cervical rib of variable size attached to C7, 6 lumbar and 11 thoracic vertebrae, or sacralization at the lumbosacral transition. The reported incidence of transitional anomalies varies widely. In 8 studies cited by Schmorl and Junghanns[26] lumbosacral transitional anomalies were present in from 4% to 22% of spines.

Disc and Vertebral Body Development and Growth

Anatomic texts describe the intervertebral disc as being composed of an outer anulus fibrosus and a central nucleus pulposus.[25,51] The disc and particularly its nucleus undergo continuous change during development, maturation, and decline (Fig. 59-7). Similarly, the vertebral bodies change remarkably in their shape, form, and function through the whole of the life cycle, while the zygapophyseal joints are coronally oriented in fetuses and infants, but change their early orientation to become biplanar joints in children, by posterior growth from the lateral margins of the facets. In adults, the major posterior parts of the joints approximate to the sagittal plane.[24,36]

Intervertebral Discs

Histologic examination of the fetal and infant disc shows it to consist of three elements: the notochordal *nucleus pulposus*, encapsulated by the *anulus fibrosus* and the *cartilage plates* (see Fig. 59-7). The expansion and multiplication of notochordal cells in the center of the developing disc forms the fetal notochordal nucleus pulposus. Around this, the anulus fibrosus is constructed by fibroblasts in the form of concentric lamellae of fibrocartilage. Between the notochordal nucleus and the anulus, a zone of primitive "fetal cartilage" is gradually absorbed into the

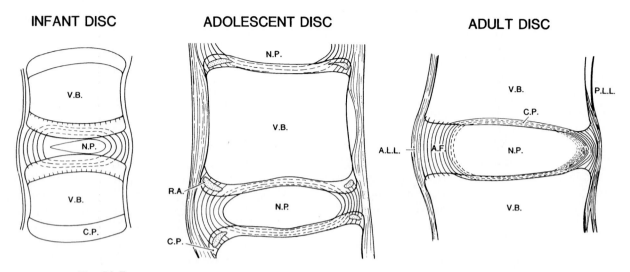

Fig. 59-7

Three stages of disc development showing continuity of lamellae of anulus with lamellar structure of cartilage plates (*CP*). When ring apophysis (*RA*) appears to form rim of vertebral body (*VB*), outer half of anulus is anchored to bone but inner half of anulus remains continuous with CPs. *NP* = nucleus pulposus; *ALL* = anterior longitudinal ligament; *PLL* = posterior longitudinal ligament.

expanding nucleus. During fetal life and infancy all three discal elements grow rapidly.[31]

The notochordal cells of the nucleus pulposus are among the most active cells of the rapidly growing fetus and infant.[30] This is confirmed by their rapid multiplication during the growth period, by their active production of proteoglycans, and by their ability to liquefy and digest the inner margins of their surrounding envelope.[31,35,38]

The cartilage plates have been described as "unossified epiphyses" of the vertebral bodies, but they are also integral parts of the disc. Polarized light studies reveal the continuity of the lamellae of the anulus with the lamellar structure of the cartilage plates. Thus, the anulus fibrosus and the cartilage plates together form an envelope containing the nucleus pulposus.[38]

In the fetus and infant this envelope is highly vascular (Fig. 59-8). Vascular canals enter the periphery of the cartilage plates from the periosteum around the vertebral body and end in multiple capillary loops. These approach very close to the anulus fibrosus and nucleus pulposus without ever penetrating the nucleus. At all stages of development, the nucleus pulposus remains avascular. Vessels from the intervertebral foramen enter the fetal anulus postero-laterally and supply its outer third. The anular vessels gradually disappear in infancy, leaving only a few surface vessels, and the vascular canals of the cartilage plates atrophy during the first few postnatal years.

The usual description of the *intervertebral disc* as comprising an anulus fibrosus and a nucleus pulposus is too simplistic, both in the immature and the older disc for the following reasons: (1) *Transitional zone in the developing disc:* Peacock[22] describes a "transitional zone" of randomly orientated fibrocartilage in the fetal disc, lying between the lamellar anulus fibrosus and the viscous fluid nucleus pulposus. This "inner cell zone" disappears after infancy but it makes an important contribution to the formation of the nucleus especially in cervical discs. (2) *The continuity of the anulus fibrosus and cartilage plates:* The lamellar structure of the anulus fibrosus in infants and children is not just confined to the anulus, but continues around, above, and below the nucleus, completely encapsulating it as shown in Fig. 59-7.[10,31] Within the lamellar anulus fibrosus, there are two parts. The lamellae of the outer third are almost entirely fibrous. These lamellae are continuous with the longitudinal ligaments of the vertebral column or inserted into the peripheral parts of the vertebral bodies. The fibrocartilaginous layers of the inner two thirds of the anulus are directly continuous with the cartilage plates, forming a complete "envelope" for the nucleus pulposus.

The anulus fibrosus in young adult intervertebral discs has a similar structure to that in children. The outer lamellae of the anulus fibrosus are anchored into the vertebral rim, formed from the ring apophysis by Sharpey fibers and the inner lamellae are continuous with the cartilage plates. The outermost

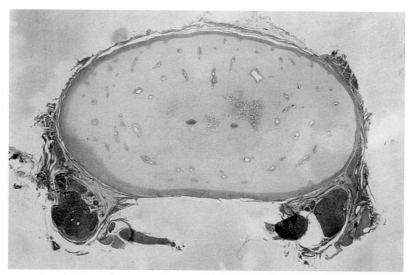

Fig. 59-8
Transverse section of lumbar disc from infant showing vascularity of cartilage plate.

lamellae of the anulus fibrous are difficult to distinguish from the longitudinal ligaments. Inner fibers of the longitudinal ligaments also attach to the vertebral rims. Transverse sections of fresh young adult discs show a white glistening appearance with regular concentric anular lamellae. While there are few changes in the anulus with maturation (other than those already described in the cervical discs) there are dramatic changes in the nucleus pulposus, with a complete change in its cells during the first 5 to 10 postnatal years and a more gradual change in its matrix with increased collagen formation and reduction in its water content. The nucleus of the older child and young adult remains rich in proteoglycans, but the nature of the proteoglycans change.[6,35]

Vertebral Body Shape Changes

Each vertebral body is formed mainly from the centrum, but a small posterolateral part of the lumbar vertebral body and a large lateral part of each cervical vertebral body are ossified from the vertebral arch. In the fetus and infant the cephalic and caudal end plates are convex, but the lumbar vertebral end plates become concave as the child assumes an erect posture. These changes in lumbar vertebrae are closely related to the growth in size and the change in position of the nucleus pulposus as the column changes from the fetal curve to a lordotic posture. Changes in shape of the central parts of cervical vertebral end plates are less dramatic, as the cervical lordosis develops much earlier and the weight-bearing forces are much smaller. The notable changes in

shape of cervical vertebrae are due to the growth of uncinate processes in childhood. As the lumbar lordosis develops, the large, fluid nucleus pulposus moves from its fetal position in the posterior half of the disc to a central position, where it acts as a central fluid cushion for weight bearing and as an axis around which movements take place. Thus, compressive loading on the central end plates inhibits central growth, while traction on the peripheral end plates may stimulate growth, resulting in the change of shape described.[32] This change is dependent on erect posture weight-bearing (see Fig. 5-2).

Changes in Disc Nutrition with Growth and Their Consequences

Nutrition of the IVD during growth and development is derived from vertebral blood vessels ramifying close to the annulus fibrosis and nucleus pulposus within the cartilage plates, and also from blood vessels entering the periphery of the annulus fibrosis. The vascularity of the disc gradually decreases in the infant and growing child, resulting in a change in the cell population of the nucleus pulposus. Notochordal cells cannot survive in the relatively avascular disc of the older child (Fig. 59-9). Fibroblasts and chondrocytes from the inner annulus begin to "colonize" the nucleus pulposus, since these cells can survive and work in conditions of lower oxygen tension. This new cell population continues to provide proteoglycans, but it also produces collagen, which progressively increases in the nucleus pulposus, making it less fluid and gelatinous but firmer and more viscous.

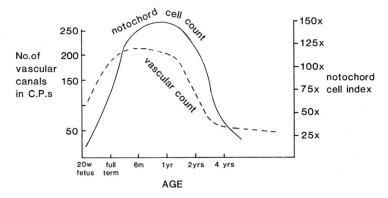

Fig. 59-9

Close correlation of notochordal cell count with disc vascularity shows that notochordal cells cannot survive in rapidly growing avascular disc.

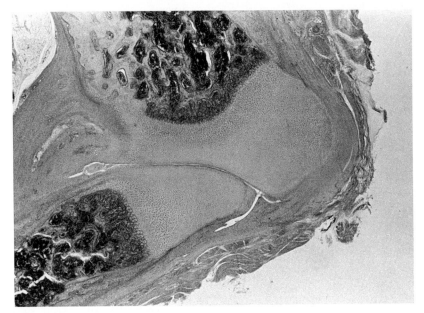

Fig. 59-10

Lumbar facet joint from 1-month-old child, demonstrating its coronal orientation and incomplete ossification.

The growth in the volume of the disc, combined with the disappearance of most of its blood vessels by the age of 4 or 5 years[31] makes the lumbar disc one of the largest avascular structures in the human body. In addition to the changes in cell population in the nucleus, this avascularity results in changes in the nature of proteoglycans in the disc.[35] The chondroitin sulfates are progressively replaced by keratan sulfate during growth. This change is rapid in infancy and childhood and virtually complete by the age of 10 years. Studies have shown that the rise in the keratan sulfate:chondroitin sulfate ratio, previously regarded as a feature of aging, occurs predominantly during growth. Keratan sulfate is used

by the body as a functional substitute for chondroitin sulfate in conditions of oxygen lack.[35]

After the regression of blood vessels from the anulus fibrosus and cartilage plates, intervertebral discs are dependent on diffusion of nutrients over considerable distances. This diffusion takes place through the cartilage plates from the vertebral vessels and through the anulus fibrosus from the blood vessels around the periphery of the disc. The rate of nutrient diffusion is dependent on the concentration gradients of the molecules involved, the resistance offered to diffusion by the cartilage plates and anulus, by the resistance to diffusion offered by the proteoglycans in the nucleus and by the amount of

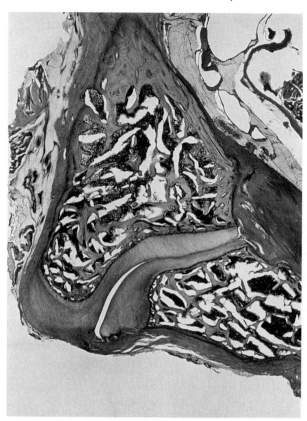

Fig. 59-11

The L3-4 facet joint from a 3-year-old male child demonstrating the biplanar nature of the joint.

spinal movement.[3] The compression and relaxation of the intervertebral disc during movement acts as a fluid pump, assisting the movement of fluid in and out of the disc. Vascular contacts penetrating from the vertebral marrow as small vascular buds into the calcified zone of the cartilage plates, occupy about 10% of the interface,[15,16] but an increased vascularization in the region of newly forming Schmorl nodes in adolescents increases this to 30%. This increased vascularity may weaken the end plate and contribute to the deformity of juvenile kyphosis.[16]

Facet (Zygapophyseal) Joints

The facet, or zygapophyseal, joints develop from the mesenchyme of the vertebral arches. Rudimentary articular processes appear in the mesenchyme after about 32 days of development, while chondrification begins at about 50 days.[20] There are definitive joints present at birth,[42] although the articular processes are flat, incompletely ossified, and oriented in the coronal plane (Fig. 59-10).[36] From the time the child begins to stand and walk, growth of the joints

occurs largely in the sagittal plane in the lumbar spine. This growth is in a posterior direction from the lateral margins of the lumbar facets, changing their shape to the typical biplanar lumbar facet joint (Fig. 59-11) by about 11 years of age.[24,36] In the cervical and thoracic regions, facetal growth continues in a coronal direction.[42] Thus, the lumbar facet joints start out very similar in shape to those in the cervical and thoracic regions, and it is only with growth and maturation that they achieve their distinct regional characteristics.

Development of the biplanar joints proceeds through childhood and adolescence, reaching skeletal maturity about the age of 16 years in females and 18 years in males, when the small epiphyses in the mamillary processes fuse with the main mass of the superior articular processes. The changes in lumbar facet shape and structure continue through adolescence into the young adult and appear to be dependent on their function and the loads to which they are subject.

Coronal Component (Anteromedial Third of Joint)

The loading stress imposed on the anteromedial third of the joints is reflected by a progressive thickening of the underlying subchondral bone plate of the superior articular process (mainly in adolescence), and by changes to the articular cartilage in young adults.[36,46] From the beginning of the fourth decade or earlier, the articular cartilage lining this thicker part of the subchondral bone plate shows cell hypertrophy and increased staining of chondrocytes and matrix. These articular cartilage changes occur in the concave superior articular facet first and in the coronal component of the convex facet soon afterward. Generally, they do not affect the sagittal components of either facet and they progress in many joints in the fourth decade of life to splitting of the full thickness of the cartilage, perpendicular to the subchondral bone plate. The changes in bone and cartilage both appear to be reactions to compressive loading of the anteromedial parts of the joint, which occurs in flexion as a result of forward-translational movement of the inferior process of the vertebra above, against the superior facet of the vertebra below. In many respects these changes are analogous to patellofemoral chondromalacia, where the stress also involves gliding movement accompanied by compression of the patella against the trochlea of the femur.

Sagittal Component
(Posterior Two Thirds of Joint)

The age changes in the posterior, sagitally oriented two thirds of the facet joints are quite different in character, and tend to occur later than the pressure changes described in the coronal component and at the center of the articular facets. The posterior, sagitally oriented pats of the subchondral plates are relatively thin, suggesting less pressure stress. However, in the fourth decade or later, the sagittal components of a number of joints show splitting of the articular cartilage at or parallel to the subchondral plate near the posterior joint margin, where the posterior fibrous capsule attaches to the posterior margin of the articular cartilage. Multifidus muscle is also partly inserted through the capsule in this region at the upper half of each joint. It is suggested that the shearing force of attempted axial rotation, especially under conditions in which the joint surfaces are compressed tightly together, is the force that tears the cartilage parallel to the joint surface.[36,37,44]

There have not as yet been comprehensive studies of the lifecycle of the facet joints of the cervical and thoracic spines to complement those of the lumbar region.

Growth in Length of the Vertebral Column as a Whole

Growth is most rapid prenatally, decreasing exponentially throughout infancy and childhood. As the spine contributes 60% of sitting height, this measure is often used to gauge growth in the length of the spine. We have used both sitting height and thoracolumbar spine length as measures of postnatal growth in length of the spine.[40]

Our own data and the data of Anderson[1] show that the growth rate in sitting height is virtually the same in males and females during childhood, but there are marked sex differences from about 9 years onward. The rate of growth declines from 5 cm per year between 1 and 2 years of age, to 2.5 cm per year at 4 years. Growth in sitting height continues at this rate until 7 years, then the rate declines further to 1.5 cm per year just before adolescence. A preadolescent spinal growth spurt begins at 9 years in females, continuing through adolescence until 14 years and peaking at 12 years with a growth velocity of 4 cm per year. In males there is no significant preadolescent spurt in spine length, and the adolescent growth spurt lasts from 12 to 17 years, with a peak growth rate of 4 cm per year at 14 years of age. Growth spurts in the thoracolumbar spine begin slightly earlier than for sitting height as a whole, and growth and maturation vary both regionally and by gender. The lumbar spine grows more rapidly than the thoracic spine in both sexes before puberty, but the thoracic spine grows more rapidly after puberty. The cervical and sacral regions mature latest in all humans. The female spine grows in length much more rapidly than the male spine, between the ages of 9 and 13 years, and reaches its maximum length 1.5 years earlier in Australian adolescents. On average, sitting height reaches 99% of its maximum by 15 years in girls and 16.5 in boys, but individual variation is so wide that Risser sign (appearance, excursion, and fusion of the iliac apophyses) is required to judge individual completion of spinal growth.[35]

Regional Differences in Maturation

It is interesting that different regions of the vertebral column mature at different rates throughout the period of growth and development. In the normal sequence of appearance of the primary centers of ossification, the arch centers appear first at the cervicothoracic and thoracolumbar junctional areas. Midthoracic centers appear quite late, and sacral centers appear last. The appearance of centra has a different sequence from the arches, and the cervical centra are the last to appear in the presacral column. The extension of ossification to the anterior surface of the cartilage models is much later in cervical vertebral bodies than in lumbar vertebral bodies. In the discs, the maturation of the notochord is also delayed in the cervical region compared to other regions so that when the notochordal nucleus pulposus is large and well formed in lumbar and thoracic discs at birth, it may remain small and rudimentary in cervical discs. In these cases the cervical nucleus is principally formed from other connective-tissue cells. It is not surprising, therefore, that collagen levels are higher in the nucleus of cervical discs than in lumbar discs throughout development and growth.[27]

Neurocentral fusion also occurs at different times in the different regions. It occurs earliest in cervical vertebrae (about 3 years), next in lumbar vertebrae (about 4 years), and last in midthoracic vertebrae (not until 7 years).

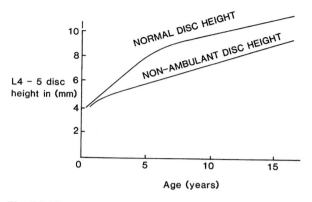

Fig. 59-12

Graphs, based on x-ray measurements in large number of normal spines and spines from children with cerebral palsy,[32] show the influence of erect posture on central disc height.

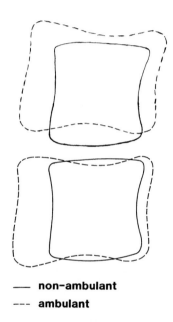

—— **non-ambulant**
--- **ambulant**

Fig. 59-13

Comparison of vertebral body outlines traced from x-ray films of adolescent spines, showing persistence of immature shape and absence of normal horizontal growth in nonambulant person with cerebral palsy.

Mechanical and Postural Influences on Growth

Studies of lumbar vertebral postnatal growth[32] show that normal development with changes in shape during childhood are dependent on weight bearing in erect posture. Fetal and infant vertebral bodies have convex vertebral end plates. The end plates flatten and may become concave in childhood. The normal concavities of the vertebral end plates do not develop in the absence of weight bearing. The normal childhood increases in transverse and anteroposterior ver-

tebral growth do not take place in children who are unable to stand and bear weight. In addition, the intervertebral discs do not develop normally in height (or thickness) in children who are bedridden or confined to wheelchairs (Fig. 59-12).[32] In these nonweight-bearing children the vertebral bodies are slender and "square" in outline on lateral x-ray films. This appearance is due to lack of horizontal growth, rather than increased vertical growth. It is as though assumption of the erect posture and the associated muscular activity on the vertebrae "stimulate" new growth in predominantly horizontal directions, giving them a shape that confers better stability in the erect vertebral column (Fig. 59-13).

Sexual Dimorphism in Vertebral Body Growth

Sexual dimorphism in vertebral body shape has been demonstrated in radiographic and anthropometric measurement studies by Brandner[5] and by Taylor and Twomey.[39] It has been suggested that the relative slenderness of the female column may contribute to the greater likelihood of the progression of scoliosis in females than in males. Taylor and Twomey showed that during the growth spurt male and female vertebral bodies develop different shapes. There is greater growth in vertebral height in females than in males due to another earlier, preadolescent growth spurt in females, affecting thoracic and lumbar vertebrae. During the later adolescent male growth spurt there is a greater transverse growth of vertebral bodies in males than in females. As a consequence, female vertebral bodies and discs are more slender than in males from the age of 8 years onward. This, together with the stronger muscle support provided for the male column[29] would make the female column more susceptible to buckling under axial loads than the male column.

Vascular and Notochordal Influences on the Development of Schmorl Nodes

Vascular canals grow into the cartilage plates of infants from the adjacent vertebral periosteum. These radially arrange canals in each cartilage plate to bring nutrition to the rapidly growing intervertebral disc. The central ends of the vascular arcades approach close to the growing notochordal nucleus pulposus. When these vessels undergo attrition during childhood, the connective-tissue canals that contained them are plugged by a loose amorphous matrix, forming channels of reduced resistance from near the nucleus to the peripheral vertebral spongiosa. These

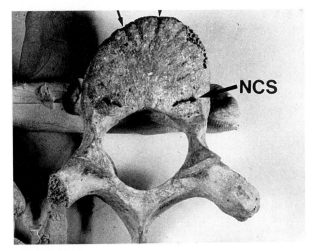

Fig. 59-14

Thoracic vertebra from 8- to 9-year-old child showing radial grooves (*arrows*) in end plate, where vascular canals were situated, and neurocentral fusion lines (*NCS*). Note flattening of anterior left surface of vertebral body due to aorta.

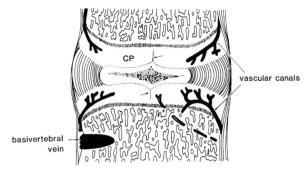

Fig. 59-15

Diagrammatic median sagittal section of newborn infant disc; cartilage plates (*CP*) capping ends of each vertebral body contain vascular canals and central triangular dimples where notochord originally passed through column.

radially arranged connective-tissue structures, arching around the advancing ossification fronts of the centrum, inhibit ossification locally, causing radial grooves to appear on the surfaces of adolescent vertebral end plates (Fig. 59-14).

The cartilage plates also show a consistently situated funnel-shaped defect on their nuclear aspect, where the longitudinal notochordal track formerly penetrated the developing disc (Fig. 59-15). This reduces the local thickness of the cartilage plate by as much as 50%. These notochordal and vascular weak points are the sites of two varieties of central and peripheral (mainly anterior) Schmorl nodes, which occur as frequently in adolescents as in adults (P164).[26,36] Schmorl nodes occur in the thoracic and lumbar vertebrae of 38% of all spines, more often in males than females. The nodes related to the

SCHMORL'S NODES

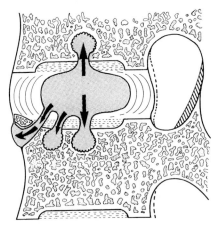

limbus vertebra   central anterior

Fig. 59-16

Diagrammatic median sagittal section of young adult spine. Position of nuclear prolapses is determined by "weak channels" left by notochord (centrally) and by vascular canals (peripherally). "Central" nodes are very common, and peripheral (anterior) nodes are relatively unusual.

notochordal weakness in cartilage plates are nearer the posterior than the anterior surface of the vertebral body. They may not cause any symptoms, but anterior nodes in the vertebral spingiosa, which probably follow vascular canal tracks, are often associated with an identifiable traumatic incident and may be painful. The prolapse may stretch the pain-sensitive anterior longitudinal ligament, and the patient may report localized "somatic" back pain (Fig. 59-16).

Multiple Schmorl nodes, both large and small, are seen in Scheuermann kyphosis, with a radiologic appearance of irregularity of the vertebral end plates and anterior vertebral body collapse with wedging. There may be associated vascular increase[16] or an associated osteoporosis of the underlying bone.[4]

Developmental and Growth-Related Pathology: A Summary

A number of developmental factors influence both congenital and other developmental variations and pathologies. The roles of the notochord and the neural tube in inducing formation of the blastemal vertebral column from the adjacent somites have been described. The role of the notochordal segments in forming a nucleus pulposus and the disappearance of notochordal cells during childhood have also been outlined.

Occasionally, groups of notochordal cells persist in vertebral bodies or cartilage plates; we have seen what appear to be viable notochordal cell clumps in the region of Schmorl nodes in 13- and 17-year-old subjects at autopsy.[41] Rarely, chordomas develop from notochordal restes (in about two per million of population per year), usually at the cephalic or caudal ends of the original notochordal track (i.e., above the tip of the dens or in the sacrococcygeal region).

Rarely, abnormal development of the notochord or of the intersegmental blood vessels is associated with anomalies of vertebral column segmentation, or anomalous vertebral development.[28]

As a universal phenomenon, weak areas are left in the central and peripheral parts of the cartilage plates of developing vertebrae when the notochord and cartilage plate blood vessels disappear. Schmorl nodes are frequently found at these sites (in 38% of adults).

Growth of the spinal cord and cauda equina exercise a powerful influence on growth of the spinal canal. Incomplete growth of the blastemal neural arches results in spina bifida. This varies from the innocuous spina bifida occulta to complete rachischisis. In severe forms of spina bifida, a neural abnormality accompanies the skeletal defect. In these cases, the abnormal development of the neural tube is probably the primary event, and the skeletal defects are secondary to the neural defects.

Physiologic asynchrony of appearance of the bilateral primary centers in vertebral arches and asynchrony of fusion in the neurocentral growth plates are associated with physiologic asymmetries of the right and left halves of the vertebral arches. Unequal pedicle lengths produce mild twisting of midthoracic anterior elements to the left in infancy and to the right in adolescence. This physiologic asymmetry probably influences the direction of curvature in all forms of scoliosis.[33,34]

In the absence of erect posture and weight bearing with normal muscular activity, the discs do not develop their normal thickness, the vertebral end plates do not change from their infantile convexity to a flat or concave shape, and the vertebral bodies become abnormally slender due to the absence of normal horizontal growth.

Irregular growth at the vertebral end plates in adolescence is associated with the presence of multiple Schmorl nodes and possibly with increased vascularity of the vertebral end plates and with juvenile osteoporosis. These changes would contribute to the development of juvenile kyphosis.[16]

References

1. Anderson MGT: Growth of the normal trunk in boys and girls during the second decade of life. *J Bone Joint Surg* 47A:1554, 1965.
2. Bagnall KM, Harris PF, Jones PRM: A radiographic study of the human foetus spine, *Anat* 124:791, 1977.
3. Bogduk N, Twomey LT: *Clinical anatomy of the lumbar spine*, Melbourne, Australia, 1987, Churchill-Livingstone.
4. Bradford DS, Brown DM, Moe JH, et al.: Scheuermann's kyphosis: a form of osteoporosis, *Clin Orthop* 118:10, 1976.
5. Brandner MF: Normal values of the vertebral body and intervertebral disc index during growth, *Am J Roentgenol* 110:618, 1970.
6. Buckwalter JA, Pedrini-Mille A, Pedrini V, Tudisco C: Proteoglycans of human infant intervertebral disc, *J Bone Joint Surg* 67A:284, 1985.
7. Dale-Stewart TD, Kerley ER: *Essentials of forensic anthropology*, Springfield, IL, 1979, Charles C Thomas.
8. Dickson R, Bradford DS: *Orthopaedics 2: management of spinal deformities*, London, 1984, Butterworths and Co.
9. Farfan HF: *Mechanical disorders of the low back*, Philadelphia, 1973, Lea & Febiger.
10. Franceschini M: Inner layers of PAF may be convex towards N.P., *Atti Accad Sci Med Nat Ferrara* 26:1, 1947.
11. Hayashi K, Yakubi T: Origins of the uncus and of Luschka's joint in the cervical spine, *J Bone Joint Surg* 67:788, 1985.
12. Hirsch C, Schajowicz F, Galante J: Structural changes in the cervical spine, *Acta Orthop Scand Suppl* 109:1, 1967.
13. Johnson RM, Crelin ES, White AA, et al.: Some new observations on the functional anatomy of the cervical spine, *Clin Orthop Relat Res* 109:85, 1975.
14. Kramer J: *Intervertebral disc lesions: causes, diagnosis, treatment and prophylaxis*, Stuttgart, Germany, 1981, Georg Thieme Verlag.
15. Maroudas A, Nachemson A, Stockwell RA: Factors involved in the mutation of the adult human intervertebral disc, *J Anat* 120:113, 1975.
16. McFadden KD, Taylor JR: End-plate lesions of the lumbar spine, *Spine* 14:867, 1989.
17. Miller JAA, Haderspeck KA, Schultz AB: Posterior element loads in lumbar motion segments, *Spine* 8:331, 1983.
18. Moore KL: *Before we are born: basic embryology and birth defects*, ed 3, Philadelphia, 1989, W.B. Saunders Co.
19. Noback CR, Robertson GA: Sequences of appearance of ossification centers in the human skeleton during the first five pre-natal months, *Am J Anat* 89:1, 1951.
20. O'Rahilly R, Meyer DB: The timing and sequence of events in the development of the human vertebral column during the embryonic period proper, *Anat Embryol* 157:167, 1979.
21. Pal GP, Sherk HH: The vertical stability of the cervical spine, *Spine* 13:447, 1988.

22. Peacock A: Observations on the pre-natal development of the intervertebral disc in man, *J Anat* 85:260, 1951.

23. Penning L: *Functional pathology of the cervical spine*, Baltimore, 1968, Williams & Wilkins.

24. Reichmann S: Motion of the lumbar articular processes in flexion-extension and lateral flexions of the spine, *Acta Morphol Neerl Scand* 8:261, 1971.

25. Romances CJ: *Cunningham's textbook of anatomy*, ed 11, Oxford, 1972, Oxford University Press.

26. Schmorl G, Junghanns H: *The human spine in health and disease*, ed 2, New York, 1971, Grune & Stratton.

27. Scott JE, Bosworth TR, Cribb AM, Taylor JR The chemical morphology of age related changes in human intervertebral disc glycosaminoglycans from cervical, thoracic and lumbar nucleus pulposus and annulus fibrosus. *J Anat* 184:73-82, 1994.

28. Tanaka T, Uhthoff HK: The pathogenisis of congenital vertebral malformations, *Acta Orthop Scand* 52:413, 1981.

29. Tanner JM, et al.: *Assessment of skeletal maturity & prediction of adult height*, London, 1975, Academic Press.

30. Taylor JR: The development and adult structure of lumbar intervertebral discs, *J Man Med* 5:43, 1990.

31. Taylor JR: *Growth and development of the human invertebral disc*. Ph.D. dissertation, Edinburgh, 1973, University of Edinburgh.

32. Taylor JR: Growth of human I/V discs and vertebral bodies, *J Anat* 120:49, 1975.

33. Taylor JR: Scoliosis and growth, *Acta Orthop Scand* 54:596, 1983.

34. Taylor JR: Vascular causes of vertebral asymmetry and the laterality of scoliosis, *Med J Aust* 144:533, 1986.

35. Taylor JR, Scott JE, Cribb A, Bosworth TR: *Maturation in human intervertebral discs*. In Proceedings of Combined Meeting of the Physiological Society of New Zealand, Australian Neuroscience Society and Anatomical Society of Australia and New Zealand, Auckland, New Zealand, 1991, p 18.

36. Taylor JR, Twomey LT: Age changes in lumbar zygapophyseal joints: observations on structure and function, *Spine* 11:739, 1986.

37. Taylor JR, Twomey LT: Bone and soft tissue injuries in postmortem lumbar spines, *Paraplegia* 28:119, 1990.

38. Taylor JR, Twomey LT: *Development of the human intervertebral disc*. In Ghosh P, editor: *Biology of the intervertebral disc*, Boca Raton, FL, 1968, CRC Press, p 39.

39. Taylor JR, Twomey LT: Sexual dimorphism in human vertebral body shape, *J Anat* 138:281, 1984.

40. Taylor JR, Twomey LT: Vertebral column development and its relation to adult pathology, *Aust J Physiother* 3113:83, 1985.

41. Taylor JR, Twomey LT: *Cervical spine anatomy and pathology*. Unpublished Data, 1994.

42. Tondury G: Functional anatomy of the small joints of the spine, *Ann Med Phys* 15:2, 1972.

43. Twomey LT: *Age changes in the human lumbar spine*, Ph.D. thesis, 1981, University of Western Australia.

44. Twomey LT, Taylor JR: *Joints of the middle and lower cervical spine: age changes and pathology*. In Proceedings of the MTAA, Adelaide, Australia, 1989, 215.

45. Twomey LT, Taylor JR: *Physical therapy of the low back*, New York, 1987, Churchill-Livingstone.

46. Twomey LT, Taylor JR: Sagittal movements of the human lumbar vertebral column: a quantitative study of the role of the posterior vertebral elements, *Arch Phys Med Rehab* 64:322, 1983.

47. Verbout AJ: A critical review of the neugliederung concept in relation to the development of the vertebral column, *Acta Biotheor* 25:219, 1976.

48. Vernon-Roberts B, Pirie CJ: Degenerative changes in the intervertebral discs of the lumbar spine and their sequelae, *Rheumatol Rehab* 16:13, 1977.

49. Watterson RL, Fowler I, Fowler BI: The role of the neural tube and notochord in the development of the axial skeleton of the chick, *Am J Anat* 95:337, 1954.

50. White AA, Panjabi MM: The clinical biomechanics of the occipitoatlantis-axial complex, *Clin Orthop Rela Res* 9:867, 1978.

51. Williams PL, Warwick R, Dyson M, Bannister LH: *Gray's Anatomy,* ed 37, Edinburgh, 1989, Churchill-Livingstone.

Chapter 60
Anatomy of the Spine
Nikolai Bogduk

The Vertebral Column

    regions of the vertebral column
    thoracic vertebrae
    typical cervical vertebrae
    axis and atlas
    lumbar vertebrae
    sacrum
    coccyx
    homologies

Spinal Joints

    the intervertebral disc
    the zygapophyseal joints
    craniocervical joints
    sacrococcygeal joints
    uncovertebral joints
    costovertebral joints
    sacroiliac joint

Muscles of the Vertebral Column

    unisegmental muscles
    lateral cervical muscles
    quadratus lumborum
    the diaphragm
    psoas major
    prevertebral muscles
    postvertebral muscles

Nerves of the Vertebral Column

    the spinal cord and nerve roots
    spinal nerves
    dorsal rami
    ventral rami
    sympathetic trunks
    dermatomes and myotomes

The term *spine* has no formal status in anatomic nomenclature. However, in colloquial usage it refers to that part of the body that surrounds the vertebral column. Thus, the spine can be defined as the vertebral column and its contents, and immediate adnexae, the latter being the muscles, nerves, and blood vessels of the vertebral column.

The Vertebral Column

The vertebral column is a series of individual bones—the vertebrae, which when articulated constitute the central, axial skeleton of the body. Its primary function is to endow the body with longitudinal rigidity—the hallmark of all vertebrates. Secondarily, the vertebral column constitutes a firm base from which structures can be suspended, such as the ribs and abdominal muscles, which allow the body to maintain cavities of relative constant size and shape.

Textbooks of anatomy emphasize the role of the vertebral column in protecting the spinal cord, but this is not a primary role; its primary role is musculoskeletal, as outlined above. The relationship between the spinal cord and vertebral column is only adventitious: the vertebral column constitutes a convenient route for the spinal cord to follow in order to gain access to distant parts of the trunk and to the limbs. Fortuitously, the vertebral column protects the spinal cord through its various components, but these components are designed primarily to subserve mechanical functions.

Weight-bearing is not a primary function of the vertebral column; fish have a vertebral column, but being buoyant they have no call for weight-bearing. Similarly, quadrupeds only occasionally use their vertebral column in weight-bearing; otherwise the vertebral column constitutes an arched, horizontal bridge between the four limbs that suspends the abdominal and thoracic cavities, with the cervical spine constituting a cantilever extension that allows the head to be moved around in space. Only human beings habitually use the vertebral column in an upright fashion. Consequently, in humanbeings, the basic vertebrate design of individual vertebrae and of the column as a whole has been adapted to accommodate weight-bearing, and to maximize stability while not excessively compromising useful mobility.

Regions of the Vertebral Column

Along its length the vertebral column is divided into distinct regions, each having different functions and demands (Fig. 60-1). The most cephalad region constitutes the axial skeleton of the neck and is known

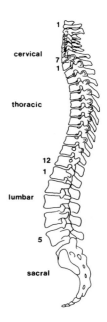

Fig. 60-1

The vertebral column and its regions viewed from the side, with the vertebrae numbered.

as the *cervical region*. It is responsible for supporting and moving the head. The next region is the *thoracic region,* distinguished by having ribs suspended from it. Its role is to support the thoracic cavity; that is, the respiratory cavity. Next in sequence is the *lumbar region,* which lies opposite the abdominal cavity. It allows for mobility between the thoracic portion of the trunk and the pelvis. The fourth region of the vertebral column is the *sacral region,* which is strongly incorporated into the pelvis. It unites the vertebral column with the bones of the lower limb girdle. The terminal portion of the vertebral column is the *coccyx:* a rudimentary structure in humanbeings, representing a vestigial tail, but a structure that nevertheless retains a function in supporting the pelvic floor.

Typically the cervical region is made up of seven vertebrae, the thoracic region of 12 vertebrae, the lumbar region of five, the sacral region of five fused vertebrae, and the coccyx of about four fused segments that constitute rudimentary vertebrae. In each region the vertebrae are named by a number from above downwards: C1 to C7, T1 to T12, L1 to L5, S1 to S5.

When fully articulated, the vertebral column exhibits four curves; the cervical and lumbar regions are lordotic (convex forward, and the thoracic and sacral regions are kyphotic (concave forward). The two kyphotic curves are primary, being present at birth, and are dictated largely by the shape of the constituent vertebrae; they lie opposite the thoracic

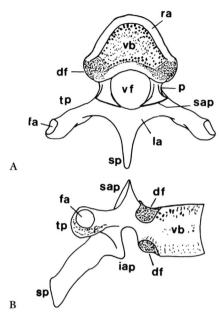

Fig. 60-2

A top view (**A**) and a side view (**B**) of a thoracic vertebra. vb = vertebral body; ra = ring apophysis; p = pedicle, la = lamina, sp = spinous process; tp = trasverse process; sap = superior articular process; iap = inferior articular process: fa = costal facet; df = demi-facet; vf = vertebral foramen.

and pelvic visceral cavities respectively. The two lordotic curves are secondary, arising during infancy as weight-bearing is assumed; they characterize the regions of the vertebral column with the greatest mobility. The lordotic curves enhance the compliance of the vertebral column in weight-bearing. Compressive loads exerted through these regions tend to accentuate the curve, whereupon the compressive load can be resisted, in part, by tension developed in ligaments along the convex aspect of the curve; variations or oscillations in compressive loads can therefore be partly buffered by variations in ligamentous tension, instead of being wholly absorbed by the crystalline (bony) structure of the vertebrae.

Thoracic Vertebrae

The thoracic vertebrae exhibit most faithfully the archetypical structure of vertebrae. Vertebrae from other regions can be considered as having been modified from the basic thoracic form (Fig. 60-2).

The quintessential element of any vertebra is the *vertebral body*. This is a block of bone rounded in perimeter in top view, with flat top and bottom surfaces but with relatively concave sides in lateral and front views. The perimeter of each top and bottom surface is marked by a slightly elevated rim of bone—the *ring apophysis*.

Projecting from the posterior surface of the vertebral body is the neural arch, a semicircular ring of bone supported by two stout pillars of bone—the *pedicles*, and completed by two plates of bone—the *laminae*, which unite in the midline posteriorly.

Projecting backward and laterally from the junction of the pedicle and lamina on each side is a *transverse process*. Projecting dorsally from the junction of the two laminae is a *spinous process*. Projecting from the lateral corners of the laminae are *articular processes*—a superior pair and an inferior pair. The transverse and spinous processes constitute levers to which muscles are attached, while the articular processes form joints connecting consecutive vertebrae. The articular surface of each articular process is known as the *articular facet* and is covered by hyaline cartilage.

The body and transverse processes of thoracic vertebrae are marked by facets that allow for the articulation of the ribs. Each rib articulates by its head to the column of vertebral bodies and by its tubercle to a transverse process (see below).

The transverse and spinous processes and the articular processes sustain forces exerted by gravity and by muscles, and serve to stabilize the vertebral column as it stands or moves in the earth's gravitational field. The neural arch primarily serves to transmit the stabilizing forces from the articular and muscular processes to the vertebral bodies. However, in forming an arch it produces an aperture through which the spinal cord is transmitted. In a single vertebra the aperture surrounded by the neural arch and the posterior surface of the vertebral body is known formally as the *vertebral foramen* (Fig. 60-2). When a series of vertebrae are connected their neural foramina are aligned to form a longitudinal canal known as the *vertebral canal* (Fig. 60-3).

Each vertebra is typically articulated to the next by three joints—one anteriorly between the vertebral bodies and a pair posteriorly between the articular processes (Fig. 60-3). The interbody joint is a secondary cartilaginous joint incorporating an *intervertebral disc*. The posterior joints—known formally as *zygapophyseal joints*—are synovial joints formed by the inferior articular process of one vertebra and the superior articular process of the next.

Spinal nerves leaving the spinal cord emerge from the vertebral column by passing between consecutive vertebrae. They do so through an aperture known as the *intervertebral foramen*, which is bounded superiorly by the pedicle of the upper vertebra, inferiorly by the pedicle of the lower vertebra, anteriorly by the intervertebral disc and adjacent vertebra bodies, and posteriorly by the joint formed be-

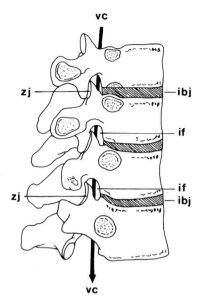

Fig. 60-3

A side view of an articulated series of thoracic vertebrae showing the vertebral canal (vc) and intervertebral foramina (if), and the zygapophyseal joints (zj) and interbody joints (ibj).

tween the inferior and superior articular processes of the two vertebrae.

Externally, all the surfaces of a vertebra are formed by compact, cortical bone. Internally, the vertebra is formed by trabeculated, cancellous (or spongy) bone. In the vertebral body the trabeculae are arranged basically as vertical and transverse struts whose arrangement reinforces the surfaces and walls of the vertebral body to allow it to sustain large weights with a minimum of expenditure of bone. From the vertebral body, trabeculae sweep into the posterior elements forming buttresses that reinforce the articular processes and transverse processes in a manner corresponding to the direction of forces that these processes habitually sustain.

The upper and lower surfaces of the vertebral bodies are flat because the vertebral bodies are the essential weight-bearing elements of the vertebra. The flat design presents a maximal surface area dedicated to withstanding longitudinal compression forces. However, the legacy of this design is that the vertebral bodies themselves provide no bony features to stabilize them against sliding and axial rotatory movements. This missing stability is provided by the posterior elements of the vertebrae. The inferior articular processes of each vertebra constitute hooks that engage the superior articular processes of the next lower vertebra. The resistance to forward sliding offered by the superior articular processes is transmitted through the inferior articular processes

via the laminae and pedicles to the upper vertebral body, thereby preventing forward sliding between vertebral bodies.

Typical Cervical Vertebrae

A typical cervical vertebra has a short vertebral body which in top view is ovoid in outline with the long axis running transversely (Fig. 60-4). The superior surface of the vertebral body exhibits two flanges projecting upward from its lateral and posterolateral edges. These are the *uncinate processes*. They endow the upper surface of the vertebral body with a transverse concavity. The anterior lip of the lower surface of the vertebral body projects inferiorly, endowing the lower surface with a slight concavity along the sagittal plane. The interbody joint between typical cervical vertebrae therefore accommodates two orthogonally opposed concave surfaces; the typical form of a saddle joint. (The significance of this saddle shape is emphasized below in the context of the joints of the cervical vertebrae.)

The pedicles of a typical cervical vertebra project posterolaterally and the laminae curve toward the midline. This results in the vertebral foramen assuming a broad, ovoid shape, flattened against the vertebral body, designed to accommodate the width and thickness of the ovoid, cervical enlargement of the spinal cord.

The transverse processes project from the pedicle and vertebral body and are U shaped in cross sec-

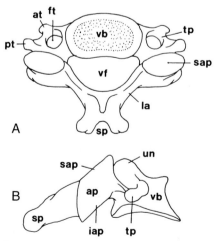

Fig. 60-4

A top view (**A**) and a side view (**B**) of a typical cervical vertebra. vb = vertebral body; la = lamina; sp = spinous process; tp = transverse process; at = anterior tubercle; pt = posterior tubercle; ft = foramen transversarium; ap = articular pillar; sap = superior articular process; iap = inferior articular process; vf = vertebral foramen; un = uncinate process.

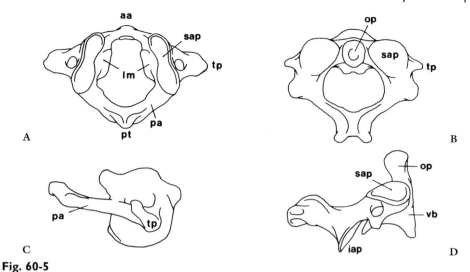

Fig. 60-5

Top views (**A** and **B**) and side views (**C** and **D**) of the atlas and axis. aa = anterior arch; pa = posterior arch; tp = transverse process; lm = lateral mass; pt = posterior tubercle; sap = superior articular process; iap = inferior articular process; vb = vertebral body; op = odontoid process.

tion. This shape forms a gutter that accommodates the ventral ramus that emerges above the vertebra. Proximally the floor of the transverse process exhibits a large *foramen transversarium,* which at levels C1 to C6 transmits the vertebral artery. The foramen transversarium of C7 usually transmits only the vertebral veins.

The foramen transversarium divides a cervical transverse process into three parts: a ventral bar in front of the foramen, ending in an anterior tubercle; a dorsal bar behind the foramen, ending in a posterior tubercle; and an intertubercular lamella, lying lateral to the foramen.

The junction of the pedicle and lamina on each side is marked by a stout column of bone whose long axis runs longitudinally. This is the *articular pillar;* its ends constitute the superior and inferior articular processes. The superior articular facets face up and backward while the inferior articular facets face down and forward. This obliquity allows the articular processes to exert two types of resisting force. By facing partly up a superior articular process is able to take compression loads from the downward-facing inferior articular process above. Thus the cervical zygapophyseal joints share the weight borne by the neck. By facing partly forward an inferior articular process can lock against the superior articular process of the vertebra below, thereby preventing a forward slip of the upper vertebra in any pair.

Axis and Atlas

The first and second cervical vertebrae, known respectively as the *atlas* and *axis,* are greatly modified from the typical form of a cervical vertebra in order to subserve their particular function (Fig. 60-5). The atlas carries the skull and the axis forms a pivot around which the atlas and skull can rotate.

The inferior half of the axis resembles that of a typical cervical vertebra. The vertebral body bears an anterior lip, and the neural arch supports an inferior articular process that faces down and forward.

The superior half of the axis is modified to accommodate the atlas. The axis lacks a typical superior articular process. Instead, it bears on each side a superior articular facet on the upper lateral edge of its vertebral body. This facet is large and flat, circular or ovoid in outline, and faces up and slightly laterally. From the superior surface of the vertebral body anteriorly a pillar of bone projects upward, curving slightly backward. This is the *odontoid process.* It constitutes a pivot around which the atlas can rotate.

The atlas vertebra resembles no other vertebra. It lacks a vertebral body and is basically a ring with a thickened *lateral mass* on each side. Each lateral mass bears on its superior surface a concave facet that articulates with the ipsilateral condyle of the skull, forming the *atlantooccipital joint.* On its inferior surface, the lateral mass bears a flat inferior articular facet that articulates with the axis and through which the weight of the head is transmitted to the axis. This joint is formally known as the *lateral atlantoaxial joint.*

A transverse process projects from the lateral aspect of the lateral mass. This process bears a foramen transversarium for the vertebral artery but bears only a posterior tubercle. The anterior tubercle is represented only by a faint bump absorbed into the anterior surface of the lateral mass.

The two lateral masses are joined anteriorly and posteriorly by arches of bone. The *posterior arch* bears at its middle a tubercle that represents a rudimentary spinous process. A corresponding tubercle is found anteriorly on the *anterior arch.* When the axis and atlas are articulated the anterior arch of the atlas lies in front of the odontoid process and a joint is formed between them—the *median atlantoaxial joint.* Consequently, the anterior arch bears on its posterior surface a small articular facet, and reciprocally the odontoid process bears an articular facet on its anterior surface.

The atlas is so distinctly different from other cervical vertebrae that it is hard to conceive of it as a cervical vertebra. Arguments have been raised in the past that the odontoid process of the atlas constitutes the vertebral body of the atlas that has been incorporated into the axis, but the embryology of this process is not consistent with this view. A radical view, but one that satisfies the incongruence of morphology of the atlas, is that the atlas should be regarded not as a cervical vertebra but as a separate "ring" vertebra interposed between the occiput and the true cervical vertebrae.

Lumbar Vertebrae

The lumbar vertebrae are robust bones designed to bear the weight of the trunk and to control its movements on the pelvis in the upright posture. Each consists of a large vertebral body endowed with stout posterior elements (Fig. 60-6).

The vertebral bodies are broad transversely and deep in an anteroposterior direction. Each has a reniform outline in top view, the posterior surface being somewhat concave. The laminae are narrow transversely but tall rostrocaudally and bear a thick, but short, rectangular spinous process that exhibits a tubercle at its caudal, posterior corner. The articular processes are designed to resist forward translation and axial rotation of the vertebrae, and their facets are orientated accordingly.

The articular facets may be flat or curved. Flat facets on superior articular processes face backward and medially to engage the facets of inferior articular processes that reciprocally face forward and laterally. The backward orientation of the superior facets resists forward displacement of the vertebra above while the medial orientation prevents the posterior elements of the vertebra above from swinging laterally during axial rotation of that vertebra. Curved

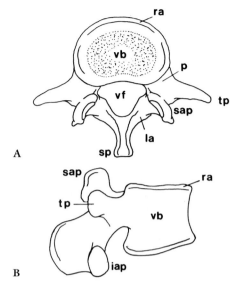

Fig. 60-6

A top view (**A**) and a side view (**B**) of a lumbar vertebra. vb = vertebral body; ra = ring apophysis; p = pedicle; la = lamina; sp = spinous process; tp = transverse process; sap = superior articular process; iap = inferior articular process; vf = vertebral foramen.

facets on superior articular processes are concave and have an anterior portion that faces backward while the posterior portion faces medially. They engage reciprocally curved, convex facets on inferior articular processes, with the two portions of the facet respectively resisting forward displacement and axial rotation of the upper vertebra in any consecutive pair.

The transverse processes of a lumbar vertebra are long, narrow and thin. They project transversely with only a slight backward orientation. Each bears on its posterior surface near its root a bony prominence known as the *accessory process.* Nearby, the superior articular process bears a rounded tubercle called the *mamillary process* at the caudal end of its dorsal edge. The mamillary and accessory processes constitute special sites of attachment for certain muscles. The transverse processes of the lumbar vertebrae typically project from the junction of the pedicle and lamina, but the transverse process of L5 is distinct in that its base extends across the entire lateral surface of the pedicle onto the vertebral body. This feature allows the fifth lumbar vertebra to be recognized on CT scans without having to resort to scout films.

Sacrum

The sacrum is a mass of five fused vertebrae. It is triangular or shield-like in shape, slightly concave anteriorly, broad superiorly, and tapering inferiorly

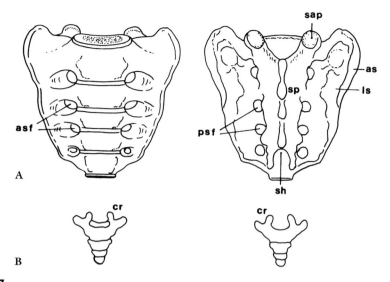

Fig. 60-7

Anterior (A) and posterior (P) views of the sacrum and coccyx. asf = anterior sacral foramen; psf = posterior sacral foramen; sh = sacral hiatus; sp = spinous process; sap = suprior articular process; as = articular surface: ls = ligamentous surface; cr = cornu.

(Fig. 60-7). Each sacral segment presents what can be recognized as a vertebral body, a transverse projection forming a lateral mass on each side and a neural arch posteriorly that supports a rudimentary spinous process.

The vertebral bodies of the sacrum are completely fused to one another, each line of fusion being marked by a slight transverse ridge at the location of what would have been an intervertebral disc. At their ends the lateral masses of the first four sacral segments extend caudally to fuse with the next lower segment. This results in foramina being formed anteriorly and posteriorly between the fused lateral masses and the fused vertebral bodies. The anterior sacral foramina transmit the sacral ventral rami; the posterior sacral foramina transmit the sacral dorsal rami. The lateral mass of the fifth sacral segment does not project caudally and leaves only a notch at the caudolateral corner of the sacrum.

Opposite the first three sacral segments the lateral portion of the sacrum is thickened and bears an auricular (ear-shaped) surface on its lateral aspect, which constitutes the articular surface of the sacroiliac joint. Posterior to this, mainly opposite the first sacral segment, lies a large pitted area for the attachment of the interosseous sacroiliac ligament.

The top of the first sacral vertebral body resembles the upper surface of a lumbar vertebra, and supports the lumbosacral intervertebral disc. Posteriorly the first sacral segment presents a superior articular process on each side that articulates with the inferior articular process of the fifth lumbar vertebra.

Laterally, the lateral mass of the first sacral segment is expanded like a wing and is referred as the *ala* of the sacrum.

The neural arches of the first four sacral segments are fused to one another, forming a continuous roof to the sacral portion of the vertebral canal. The sacral spinous processes are developed only on the first three sacral segments and vary in size and in the extent to which they are fused to one another. The fifth sacral segment lacks a complete neural arch, and presents only what constitutes a rudimentary pedicle and inferior articular process on each side. These prominences constitute the *cornua* of the sacral. The sacral canal opens onto the posterior aspect of the bone through an aperture known as the *sacral hiatus*, which is bounded by the sacral cornua and the caudal edge of the neural arch of the fourth sacral segment. The caudal surface of the fifth sacral vertebral body is flattened to articulate with the coccyx.

Coccyx

The coccyx consists of the fused vertebral bodies of four or more small coccygeal vertebrae (Fig. 60-7). The first two segments carry rudimentary transverse processes, and the first carries rudimentary superior articular processes.

Homologies

Although the cervical, lumbar and, sacral vertebrae are distinctly different from the archetypical thoracic

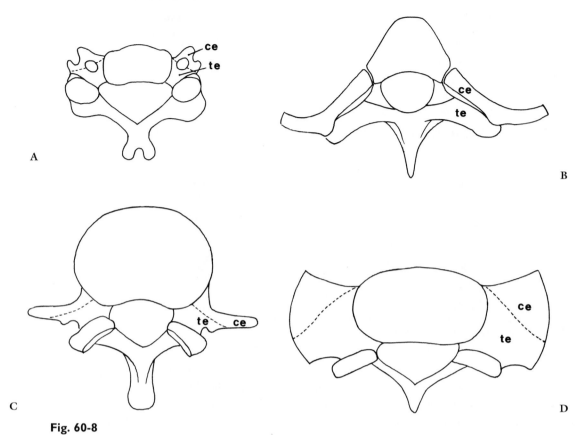

Fig. 60-8

Homologous parts of the cervical (**A**), thoracic (**B**), lumbar (**C**) and sacral (**D**) vertebrae. ce = costal element (rib); te = transverse element (true transverse process).

vertebrae, various of their parts are equivalent on embryologic grounds to the standard parts of a thoracic vertebra. Certain elements in the cervical, lumbar, and sacral vertebrae have the same embryology as the ribs that connect to the thoracic vertebrae, but these have been incorporated into other parts of the vertebra (Fig. 60-8). Consequently, in nonthoracic vertebrae it is possible to identify parts that correspond to the costal elements of a thoracic vertebra and parts that correspond to what are equivalent to the true transverse processes of a thoracic vertebra. Recognition of these homologies serves to clarify the systematic nature of the attachments of the various back muscles and the courses of the dorsal rami of spinal nerves.

The costal element in a cervical vertebra is absorbed as the anterior half and lateral end of the transverse process. The true transverse element is represented only by the proximal dorsal half of the transverse process. If these homologies are recognized it becomes evident that the foramen transversarium is equivalent to the space between a thoracic transverse process and the neck of the adjacent rib. A cervical rib would be generated if the anterior tu-

bercle were drawn laterally and forward to complete a more substantial shaft.

The costal element in a lumbar vertebra forms most of what is named as the transverse process. The true transverse element is represented by the accessory process and the layer of bone that extends from the accessory process across the superior articular process up to and including the mamillary process.

The costal elements in the sacrum form the anterolateral sectors of the ala and lateral masses. The true transverse element is represented by the posterior and more medial sector of the lateral mass.

It will be seen below that whereas the back muscles seem to assume various and confusing attachments along the vertebral column to articular processes, transverse processes, and accessory processes, these attachments become systematic and simple when interpreted in terms of costal elements and true transverse elements.

Spinal Joints

Each vertebra is typically united to the next by three joints. The joint between the vertebral bodies is

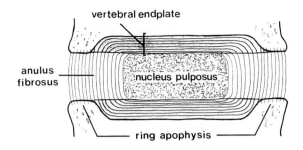

Fig. 60-9

The structure of a lumbar intervertebral disc, as revealed in sagittal section.

formed by an intervertebral disc; the joints between the articular processes are typical synovial joints.

The Intervertebral Disc

The intervertebral disc subserves several functions. Foremost, it separates the vertebral bodies, allowing them to bend with respect to one another. For this function it must be pliable. Meanwhile, it must also sustain the compression loads exerted on the interbody joint by the weight of the body above the joint and by the back muscles when they act. For this function the intervertebral disc must also be strong.

An intervertebral disc typically consists of a nucleus pulposus surrounded by an anulus fibrosus, both sandwiched between superior and inferior vertebral end plates (Fig. 60-9). Our knowledge of the detailed structure of the intervertebral disc is based on studies of lumbar discs.[3] There is a tendency to extrapolate or assume that discs in other regions of the vertebral column are similar in structure, but sufficient differences have been noted to caution against unreserved assumptions. Ongoing studies are set to reveal significant differences in structure particularly between cervical discs and lumbar discs that render assumed equivalence between the two unjustified.

The nucleus pulposus of a lumbar intervertebral disc consists of a central core of a well-hydrated proteoglycan matrix surrounded by fibrocartilage. The anulus fibrosus consists of 10 to 12 concentric lamellae of collagen fibers. In any given lamella the collagen fibers run in parallel at an angle of about 65 degrees to the vertical, but the direction of this angle alternates in successive layers.

Within the anulus fibrosus one can identify two portions. The outermost lamellae are attached to the ring apophysis of the two vertebrae and constitute the "ligamentous" portion of the anulus fibrosus.[3] The inner lamellae of the anulus fibrosus do not at-

tach to bone. Instead, they pass into the vertebral end plates above and below the nucleus pulposus, forming a complete spheroidal envelope around the nucleus. Because of its bony attachments the ligamentous portion of the anulus fibrosus is designed primarily to limit movement between the vertebral bodies. By forming a capsule around the nucleus pulposus, the internal lamellae of the anulus fibrosus function to resist radial expansion of the nucleus pulposus under pressure.

The vertebral end plates are layers of cartilage that bind the disc to the vertebral body. Toward its vertebral surface each end plate consists of hyaline cartilage, but toward its discal surface it consists of fibrocartilage because of the collagen fibers of the anulus fibrosus embedded in it.

The disc sustains weight-bearing through both the anulus fibrosus and the nucleus pulposus. Although designed to sustain tensile loads, the anulus fibrosus constitutes a mass of tissue sandwiched between two vertebral bodies, which can act passively to sustain compression loads. Its liability, however, is that under sustained loading an isolated anulus fibrosus will creep; its lamellae will buckle inward and outward and the vertebral bodies will approximate one another. To prevent such buckling, in an intact disc the nucleus pulposus braces the anulus fibrosus. When compressed, the nucleus pulposus tends to expand radially but is prevented from doing so by tension developed in the encircling anulus fibrosus. As long as the anulus fibrosus remains intact, the nucleus pulposus behaves essentially as a mass of incompressible fluid. The pressure developed in the nucleus pulposus braces the anulus fibrosus to prevent it from buckling and acts on the vertebral end plates to prevent the vertebral bodies from approximating.

Bending movements between vertebral bodies are possible because the disc is deformable. When bending occurs in any direction the anulus fibrosus on that side is compressed and bulges outward, while the anulus fibrosus on the opposite surface of the disc is stretched and tensed. Meanwhile, the nucleus pulposus is deformed; it is compressed on the side to which bending occurs and is expanded on the opposite side.

Twisting movements between vertebral bodies are limited by tension in those layers of collagen in the anulus fibrosus that are inclined in the direction of movement. Because of the alternating orientation of the lamellae of the anulus fibrosus, half its fibers are set to limit rotation in one direction; the remainder to limit the opposite movement.

Regional Differences

Little is known of the detailed structure of thoracic intervertebral discs. The extent to which they conform or differ from the structure of lumbar discs is unknown. The normal anatomy of cervical discs has only recently started to be studied and conspicuous differences from lumbar discs have been noted.

Foremost, the nucleus pulposus of a cervical disc constitutes a much smaller component of the disc than in the lumbar region. The nucleus pulposus of the lumbar disc constitutes about 50% of its cross-sectional area and volume whereas, in a cervical disc, it is closer to 25%.[16] Secondly, only in infants, children, and adolescents is the nucleus pulposus of a cervical disc mucoid in nature like that of lumbar discs. Beyond the age of 20 the nucleus pulposus of a cervical disc becomes quite fibrous.[12] Consequently, in young adults and into middle age a cervical disc is more like a fibrous, interosseous ligament than a buoyant, hydrodynamic structure like a lumbar disc of the same age. Thirdly, emerging evidence suggests that transverse fissures across the posterior half of a cervical disc occur increasingly often with age, and so regularly that they constitute a normal feature.[17] This feature is of significance in the context of the so-called *uncovertebral joints* and the movements of the cervical vertebrae.

The Longitudinal Ligaments

The interbody joints are reinforced by the anterior and posterior longitudinal ligaments. The *anterior longitudinal ligament* consists of collagen fibers of various lengths that bridge the anterior edges of the vertebral bodies, spanning either one, two, or three joints. The anterior longitudinal ligament is most obvious and best developed in the thoracic region where it forms a thin but wide band over the anterior and anterolateral aspects of the thoracic vertebral bodies and intervertebral discs. In the cervical region this ligament is attenuated to a narrow, thin strip lying between the prevertebral muscles of the neck, terminating as a tapering cord attached to the anterior tubercle of the atlas. In the lumbar region the anterior longitudinal ligament appears robust, but much of its apparent mass consists of prolongations of the tendons of the crura of the diaphragm.[3]

The *posterior longitudinal ligament* is peculiar in form throughout most of its length. Over the backs of the lumbar and thoracic vertebral bodies this ligament is quite narrow and thin, but over each intervertebral disc it expands to take on a serrated outline. Its fibers blend with the posterior anulus fibrosus and are virtually indistinguishable from those of the disc. The serrated form of the posterior longitudinal ligament renders it unlikely to have any substantial mechanical role. Rather, it seems more like a carpet along the floor of the vertebral canal that separates the basivertebral plexus from the dural sac of the spinal cord. In the upper cervical region the posterior longitudinal ligament expands to form a uniform, wide sheet: the *membrana tectoria*, that covers the atlantoaxial region and attaches to the anterior margin of the foramen magnum. Despite its size, the membrana tectoria is of little mechanical significance and seems to function more like a membranous barrier between the spinal cord and the odontoid process.

The Zygapophyseal Joints

The zygapophyseal joints are formed by the inferior articular process of one vertebra and the ipsilateral superior articular process of the next. Each articular facet is covered by hyaline cartilage and the joint is enclosed by a fibrous capsule. A variety of intraarticular inclusions occur in each joint: intraarticular fat pads, fibroadipose meniscoids, and capsular rims. Each of these is covered by a synovial membrane that lines the deep surface of the capsule.

Intraarticular fat pads and fibroadipose meniscoids typically occur at the poles of the joint where the capsule is relatively loose to accommodate the subluxation that the joint undergoes during normal movement. The fat pads appear to act as fillers of the variable space deep to the capsule but outside the articular space. The fibroadipose meniscoids intervene between the joint surfaces. Their function appears to be to cover the articular cartilage when it subluxates during movement, and to maintain a film of synovial fluid over the cartilage. Capsular rims are simply adventitious thickenings of the joint capsule that fill the recess between the curved edges of the articular cartilage. They occur typically around the medial and lateral edges of the joint where the capsule is more closely applied than at the poles.

Regional Differences

Regional differences occur in several features of the zygapophyseal joints that reflect the different functions and demands placed on them (Fig. 60-10).

In the cervical region the articular facets are relatively flat, and the plane of the joint runs up and forward. Because of this oblique orientation the articular facets participate in weight-bearing and serve to restrict anterior translation of the upper vertebra

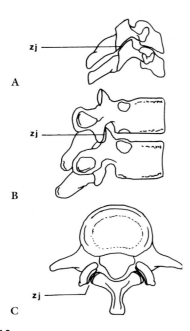

Fig. 60-10

Regional differences in the orientation of the zygapophyseal joints (zj) as seen in lateral views of cervical and thoracic joints (**A** and **B**), and in a top view of a pair of lumbar joints (**C**).

in any pair. Otherwise, gliding movements are possible between the articular processes to enable flexion, extension, and axial rotation of the intervertebral joint to occur.

The cardinal regional difference of thoracic zygapophyseal joints lies in the orientation of their facets. The plane of the joint is basically coronal but faces slightly laterally. This design precludes any forward translation of the thoracic vertebrae but does not impede axial rotation.

The zygapophyseal joints of the lumbar spine are designed to prevent forward translation and rotation of the upper vertebra.[3] The superior articular process faces backward and medially and the plane of the joint runs in a longitudinal direction. From L1 to L5 the average orientation of the articular facets changes. At upper lumbar levels the facets are aligned along an oblique plane that is almost sagittal in orientation. In lower lumbar vertebrae the facets approach a coronal orientation, but on the average have an orientation of 45° to the sagittal plane. This difference in orientation indicates that upper lumbar facets are designed more to restrict axial rotation of the vertebrae while lower lumbar facets are designed to resist both axial rotation and forward sliding of the vertebrae.

Thoracolumbar zygapophyseal joints assume a lumbar configuration, and the transition from thoracic to lumbar features typically occurs gradually between segments T10-T11 and T12-L1.[14]

The Posterior Ligaments

Insofar as the zygapophyseal joints are the joints of the vertebral arches, they are said to be reinforced by the ligaments of the vertebral arches: the ligamentum flavum, the interspinous ligament, and the supraspinous ligament. However, these ligaments offer insubstantial support for these joints and, indeed, paradoxically, the strongest of the posterior spinal ligaments prove to be the capsules of the zygapophyseal joints themselves.

The *ligamentum flavum* is represented from between the C2-C3 level to the L5-S1 level and consists largely of elastic fibers that connect consecutive laminae. In the lumbar region the most lateral fibers of the ligamentum flavum pass ventral to the zygapophyseal joints at each level and replace the fibrous capsule of the joint. While offering some resistance to separation of the laminae in flexion of the vertebral column, the ligamentum flavum is too distensible because of its elastic nature to limit this movement. Its function is to provide a smooth posterior wall to the vertebral canal that accommodates large changes in interlaminar distance during flexion and extension of the vertebral column without buckling.[3]

In the lumbar region, the *interspinous ligament* is formed by collagen fibers passing caudoventrally between adjacent spinous processes. Only the anterior two thirds of each ligament is truly ligamentous. The posterior third represents terminal tendons of the erector spinae muscle finding attachment to a spinous process.[3] The detailed structure of the interspinous ligament in the thoracic region is not known but is assumed to be similar to that seen in the lumbar region. In the cervical region a definitive interspinous ligament is lacking. A cervical interspinous space is typically filled with fascial tissue derived from the so-called *ligamentum nuchae.*

Classical descriptions of the ligamentum nuchae seem to have been influenced by observations of the structure of this ligament in quadrupeds, in which it is well developed. However, in human beings it has a different, considerably reduced, structure. Dorsally the ligamentum nuchae consists of a raphe formed by the interlacing tendinous fibers of the trapezius, splenius, and rhomboid minor. The fibers of this raphe are oriented transversely and obliquely along a coronal plane, and the raphe itself forms a thin narrow strip of tissue extending from the external occipital protuberance to the tip of the C7 spinous process.

Ventrad of this dorsal raphe, the ligamentum nuchae consists of a sheet of relatively loose fascia oriented in the sagittal plane. Dorsal to the tips of the cervical spinous processes this fascial sheet forms a

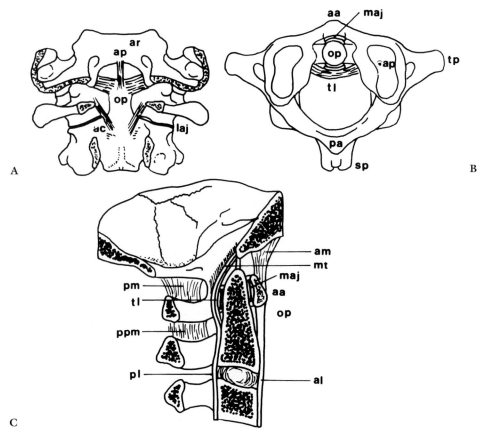

Fig. 60-11

The craniocervical joints. **A,** Posterior view. **B,** Top view. **C,** sagittal section. ap = apical ligament; ar = alar ligament; op = odontoid process; tp = transverse process; ac = accessory atlantoaxial ligament; laj = lateral atlantoaxial joint; aa = anterior arch of atlas; pa = posterior arch of atlas; sap = superior articular process; maj = median atlantoaxial joint; tl = transverse ligament; sp = spinous process of axis; mt = membrana tectoria; pl = posterior longitudinal ligament; am = anterior atlantooccipital membrane; pm = posterior atlantooccipital membrane; ppm = posterior atlantoaxial membrane; al = anterior longitudinal ligament.

septum that separates the two semispinalis capitis muscles. Near the tips of the spinous processes this septum splits into three layers: a lateral division on each side that reflects laterally to form the fascia between semispinalis capitis dorsally and the semispinalis cervicis and multifidus ventrally; and a median division that occupies the interspinous spaces and constitutes what otherwise would have been the cervical interspinous ligaments. This interspinous tissue, however, is distinctly fascial in nature and does not constitute a true ligament in the conventional sense.

Traditional descriptions of the ligamentum nuchae misrepresent this structure as a firm ligament anchoring the posterior neck muscles to the cervical spinous processes. In reality, only the raphenous portion of the ligament affords any attachment to muscles. The septal portion is distinctly fascial in nature and provides no definitive anchorage of any muscles to the cervical spinous processes.

Craniocervical Joints

The head is connected to the neck by a series of unique joints involving the atlas and axis vertebrae (Fig. 60-11). The atlas constitutes a platform that supports the skull through the atlantooccipital joints. In turn, this platform is supported by the axis, which is designed to permit axial rotation of the atlas and head.

The atlantooccipital joints are paired synovial joints in which the concave facets of the superior articular processes of the atlas form stable sockets that accommodate the condyles of the occiput. The occiput and atlas are held together by the capsules of the atlantooccipital joints, which constitute the only substantial ligamentous connection between the skull and atlas. The curvature of the sockets permits nodding movements of the head on the atlas but largely precludes other movements. A tiny amount of axial rotation is possible at the atlantooccipital joints but requires the ipsilateral condyle of the occiput to move backward and upward in its socket while the opposite condyle moves forward and upward. Tension in the capsules of the joints restricts the upward displacement of each condyle and thereby limits the available range of axial rotation. Consequently, during axial rotation of the head, the head and atlas move essentially as a single unit on the axis, and ligaments stabilizing the movement of axial rotation are connected not between the atlas and skull or between the atlas and axis but between the skull and the axis. Accordingly, during axial rotation of the head the atlas lies and moves like a passive washer interposed between the head and the axis.

The atlas is supported on the axis by the lateral atlantoaxial joints formed between the inferior articular processes of the atlas and the superior articular processes of the axis. These are essentially planar, synovial joints, which allow a large range of gliding movements. Rotation is achieved by the ipsilateral inferior articular process of the atlas sliding backward and medially on the axis while the opposite inferior articular process slides forward and medially. During this movement, the anterior arch of the atlas slides around the anterior surface of the base of the odontoid process. This movement is accommodated and lubricated by the median atlantoaxial joint at this site.

The atlantoaxial joints are designed to eliminate all sliding movements between the atlas and axis, other than axial rotation. The presence of the odontoid process prevents the axis sliding backward. Any attempt at backward movement results in the anterior arch of the atlas being impacted against the odontoid process. The reverse movement is prevented by the *transverse ligament* of the atlas, which constitutes a strong belt passing behind the odontoid process and connecting the left and right lateral masses of the atlas. To lubricate movement between the transverse ligament and the odontoid process during axial rotation of the atlas a synovial joint is formed between an articular facet on the anterior surface of the transverse ligament and a facet on the back of the odontoid process. The transverse ligament of the atlas is the most important structure stabilizing the atlantoaxial joint.

The next most major ligaments in this region are the *alar ligaments,* which pass laterally and slightly upward from the posterolateral surface of each side of the odontoid process to the lateral margin of the foramen magnum (see Fig. 60-11). Because of their orientation the alar ligaments prevent distraction of the head from the axis, and each prevents ipsilateral gliding of the head and atlas on the axis. Each also limits the range of contralateral axial rotation of the head.[8] Because it is attached to the posterolateral surface of the odontoid process, an alar ligament must wrap around the perimeter of the odontoid process when the head is turned to the opposite side. This consumes the available strain in the ligament and limits the amplitude of movement. The alar ligaments are also sufficiently strong that, if the transverse ligament of the atlas is disabled, they can limit forward sliding of the skull with respect to the axis.[9] Complete forward dislocation of the skull and atlas therefore requires destruction of both the transverse ligament and the alar ligaments.

Other ligaments in the craniocervical region are not of any known mechanical significance. Classically the transverse ligament is considered to be the transverse portion of what is known as the *cruciate ligament*. The longitudinal band of this ligament passes from the back of the vertebral body of the axis to the occipital bone. At most, this ligament may serve to limit the range of flexion of the head insofar as during this movement the ligament is drawn over the tip of the odontoid process. The tip of the odontoid process is connected to the rim of the foramen magnum by the apical ligament of the dens, which simply constitute the rostral remnant of the embryonic notochord.

No substantial ligaments connect the atlas and axis other than the capsules of the atlantoaxial joints. The accessory atlantoaxial ligaments are sometimes highlighted, but these constitute bands of fibrous tissue passing from the back of the vertebral body of the axis to the lateral mass of the atlas, which convey blood vessels to the region of the lateral atlantoaxial joint. Sheets of fascial tissue known as the *anterior* and *posterior atlantooccipital membranes* connect the occiput and the respective arches of the atlas, and similar sheets connect these arches to the axis. These membranes constitute fascial septa separating the vertebral canal from the exterior regions of the vertebral column rather than structures of any dynamic mechanical importance.

Sacrococcygeal Joints

The sacrum is united to the body of the coccyx by a rudimentary intervertebral disc in the form of a symphysis. Posteriorly, the superior articular processes of the coccyx are united to the cornua of the sacrum by fibrous joints reinforced by the posterior sacrococcygeal ligaments. The sacrococcygeal joint is mobile only in children, adolescents, and young adults. With increasing age it undergoes ankylosis. In some individuals, particularly women, a mo-

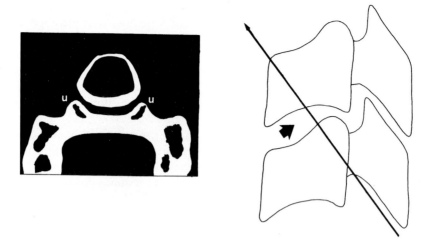

Fig. 60-12

The uncovertebral region. Sections through the joint taken along the plane of the zygapophyseal joints reveal an ellipsoid shape to the interbody joint, formed by the uncinate process (u).

bile fibrous joint may persist between the first and second coccygeal segments.

Uncovertebral Joints

The uncinate processes of the cervical vertebrae are a fascinating and hitherto mysterious feature of the vertebral column. They have been portrayed as forming a synovial joint with the vertebral body above—the so-called *uncovertebral joints,* but anatomic evidence refutes this interpretation. No such joints are present in embryos, infants, or children. Rather, what develops in this region are adventitious clefts in the annulus fibrosus of the cervical intervertebral disc. What has been misrepresented as articular cartilage in these clefts are in fact reflected layers of split collagen fibers of the annulus fibrosus that have undergone cartilaginous metaplasia.

Insights into the functional nature of the uncovertebral clefts have been provided by the studies of Penning[13] who used unconventionally oriented CT scans and anatomic sections to study this region. If CT scans are taken through the uncovertebral region along the plane of the cervical articular facets, that is, at about 45° to the usual transverse section, a fascinating view of the cervical intervertebral joints is revealed (Fig. 60-12).

In such views, the lower vertebral body and its uncinate processes present an upwardly concave articular surface while the upper vertebral body presents a reciprocally curved convex articular surface. Together the two articular surfaces assume the appearance of an ellipsoid joint. This suggests that the uncinate processes and the upper surface of a cervi-

cal vertebral body are designed to allow a swinging, rotatory movement of the vertebra above, but in the plane of the zygapophyseal joints.

CT scans at right angles to the plane of the zygapophyseal joints reveal a similar ellipsoid shape of the interbody joint but movement in this plane is not possible for it results in direct, face-to-face impaction of the zygapophyseal joints.

Given these perspectives, it is evident that the cervical interbody joints can undergo gliding rotation across an ellipsoid joint in the plane of the zygapophyseal joints but not at right angles to this plane. Meanwhile, the vertebral body freely undergoes flexion and extension in the sagittal plane. The arcuate nature of this latter movement is reflected by the anterior lip of the cervical vertebral bodies and their slightly concave inferior surfaces (see Fig. 60-12).

If these observations are coupled, it transpires that the design of a cervical intervertebral joint satisfies the criteria for a saddle joint, with concave surfaces facing one another but in orthogonal planes, allowing gliding and rotatory movements in each of these two planes but no movement in the third plane. Thus, the cervical interbody joints are saddle joints. Translating these observations into conventional terminology, the cervical intervertebral joints are designed to allow flexion and extension in the sagittal plane, and axial rotation in the plane of the zygapophyseal joints. Under these conventions lateral flexion does not occur in the neck. What appears to be lateral flexion is a composite of axial rotation of lower cervical vertebrae coupled with contralateral rotation of the atlas.

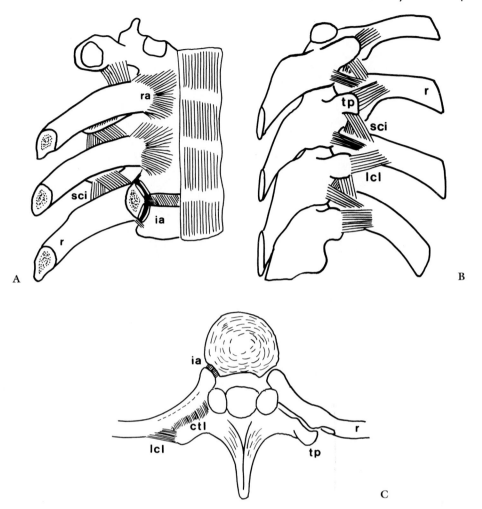

Fig. 60-13

Anterolateral (**A**), posterolateral (**B**), and top (**C**) views of the costovertebral joints. r = rib; tp = transverse process; ra = radiate ligament; ia = intraarticular ligament; sci = superior costotransverse ligament; lcl = lateral costotransverse ligament; ctl = costotransverse ligament.

Costovertebral Joints

Each rib forms two synovial joints as it articulates with the vertebral column. A costotransverse joint joins the tubercle of the rib with the transverse process of the ipsisegmental vertebra, while a costovertebral joint joins the head of the rib either with one vertebral body or with two vertebral bodies and the intervening intervertebral disc (Fig. 60-13).

At upper thoracic levels the costotransverse joints are small ball-and-socket joints, but at progressively lower levels these joints become more planar with the articular facet on the transverse process facing forward and up.

The first, eleventh, and twelfth ribs, and frequently the tenth, form costovertebral joints with singular facets on the upper, lateral surface of the ipsisegmental vertebral body. The other ribs form joints centered on the intervertebral disc but incorporating demi-facets on the upper edge of the ipsisegmental vertebral body and the lower edge of the vertebral body above. In these joints the synovial cavity is divided into an upper and a lower half by an intraarticular ligament that connects the apex of the head of the rib to the intervertebral disc.

The costovertebral joints are reinforced by a radiate ligament that covers the anterior aspect of the joint. The costotransverse joints are reinforced by the costotransverse and lateral costotransverse ligaments, which connect the rib to its ipsisegmental transverse process, and by the superior costotransverse ligament, which suspends the rib from the transverse process above.

The nature and movements expressed by different ribs is governed by the structure of their costotransverse joints. The ball-and-socket design of the

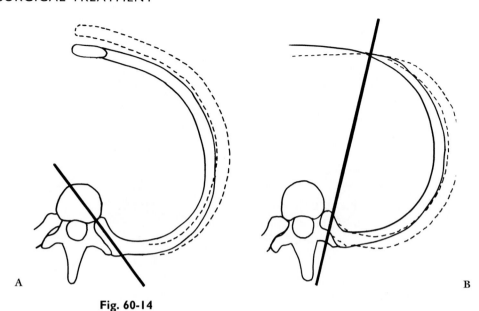

Fig. 60-14

The axes and movements of upper ribs (**A**) and lower ribs (**B**).

first six costotransverse joints firmly fixes the tubercle of the rib against its transverse process. Otherwise, the rib is held firmly in place at the costovertebral joint. The axis of movement of each rib therefore runs between the two sites of fixation: the head and the tubercle. The movement expressed by an upper rib is therefore a rotation about this axis, which results in the anterior end of the rib being raised up and forward. This type of movement raises the sternum and increases the anteroposterior diameter of the chest (Fig. 60-14, *A*).

The planar design of the lower six costotransverse joints allows the tubercle to glide upward on its transverse process. Therefore, these tubercles are not fixed. The points of maximum fixation of the lower six ribs are at their costovertebral joints and at their costal cartilages. Their axis of movement consequently runs between the head and the costal cartilage. Movement about this axis maximally raises the lateral aspect of the shaft of the rib, which increases the lateral diameter of the lower chest wall (Fig. 60-14, *B*)

Sacroiliac Joint

The sacroiliac joint is a synovial joint between the sacrum and ilium on each side. The joint cavity is auricular in shape and reaches the anterior margin of the sacrum. The joint is designed to connect the vertebral column firmly to the lower limb girdle but also to allow obligatory movements that occur during gait.

The stability of the sacroiliac joint lies in the nature of its articular surfaces and ligaments (Fig.

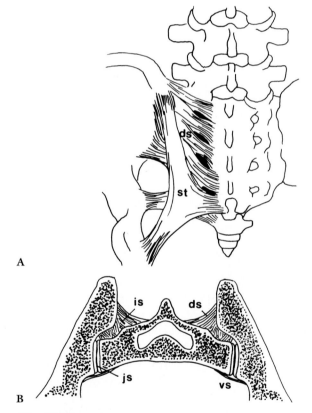

Fig. 60-15

The sacroiliac joints in posterior view (**A**) and in coronal section (**B**). st = sacrotuberous ligament; ds = dorsal sacroiliac ligament; is = interosseous sacroiliac ligament; vs = ventral sacroiliac ligament; js = joint space of the sacroiliac joint.

60-15). The sacral articular surface is corrugated: a depression occurs opposite the second sacral segment, whereas the first and third segments exhibit

FLEXION   **EXTENSION**

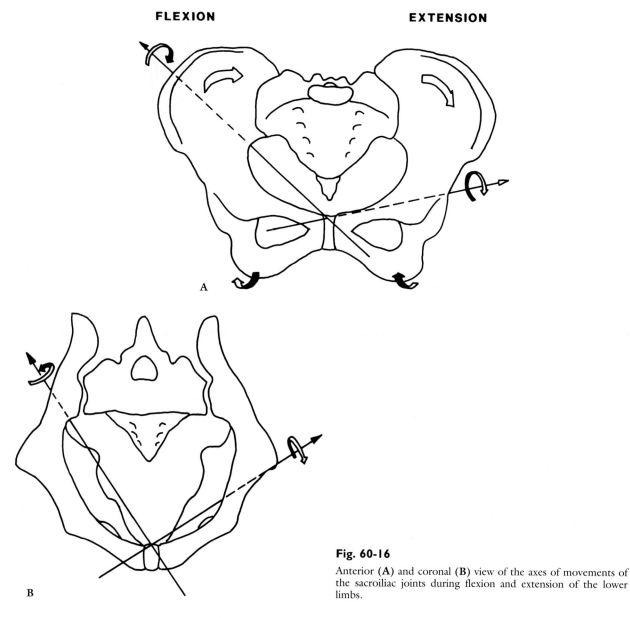

Fig. 60-16

Anterior (**A**) and coronal (**B**) view of the axes of movements of the sacroiliac joints during flexion and extension of the lower limbs.

prominences. These are matched by reciprocal prominences and depressions on the articular surface of the ilium. If the two ilia are clamped against the sacrum, the irregularities in the articular surfaces lock the sacrum in place, preventing it from sliding down between the two ilia, under the influence of body weight, and restricting its ability to rotate in the sagittal plane. This clamping effect is achieved by the dense interosseous sacroiliac ligaments that occupy the space between the two bones, dorsal to the sacroiliac joint, and by the ventral sacroiliac ligament, which covers the anterior aspect of each joint. The dorsal sacroiliac ligament is a supplementary ligament that bridges the posterior superior iliac spine and the posterior surface of the sacrum, covering the interosseous sacroiliac ligament.

Rotation of the sacrum in the sagittal plane, otherwise known as "nutation," is limited by the clamping effect of the sacroiliac ligaments; its amplitude is not more than about one or two degrees.[15] Nutation is also restricted by the sacrotuberous and sacrospinous ligaments, and symptoms may develop in these ligaments if the intrinsic sacroiliac ligaments are disabled.

Movements that do occur in the sacroiliac joint are those of the pelvis as a whole. During flexion and extension of the hips, particularly during gait, each hemipelvis rotates about an axis that passes from the pubic symphysis to the greater sciatic notch (Fig. 60-16). During extension, each hemipelvis turns downward about this axis, and during flexion it turns upward.[11] The resultant movement of the sacroiliac joint is a complicated, compound one. In extension of the lower limb it involves an upward gliding of the ilium on the sacrum coupled with an element of distraction between the two bones superiorly and anteriorly. A converse coupling occurs during flexion.

The complexity of movements at the sacroiliac joint can, perhaps, be better appreciated in a different way. During gait the flexion of one hip coupled with the extension of the upper hip imposes severe twisting forces on the pelvis as a whole. Were the pelvis a solid, single ring of bone it would suffer stress fracture under these conditions. The sacroiliac joint consequently serves as a stress-relieving joint, the tension that otherwise would have been imposed upon bone being absorbed by the sacroiliac ligaments, at the expense of slight distracting and sliding movements between the sacrum and ilium.

Muscles of the Vertebral Column

The muscles of the vertebral column can be addressed according to topographic location and size. Small unisegmental muscles connect consecutive vertebrae, but these are covered by muscles of various lengths lying posterior, anterior, and lateral to different regions of the vertebral column. The entire vertebral column is endowed with muscles posteriorly, but only the cervical and lumbar regions are covered by muscles anteriorly and laterally. The thoracic region lacks any lateral or prevertebral musculature.

Unisegmental Muscles

The unisegmental muscles are the interspinales, connecting consecutive spinous processes, and the intertransversarii, connecting consecutive transverse processes. These are best developed in the cervical and lumbar regions (Fig. 60-17). The rectus capitis anterior and rectus capitis lateralis are homologues of the intertransverse muscles at the craniocervical junction.

These unisegmental muscles are too small to contribute significantly to the power required to move the vertebral column, which raises questions as to their function. Contemporary evidence is conducive to the suggestion that they function as proprioceptors. Of all muscles of the body, third only to those of the eye and hand, the unisegmental muscles of the vertebral column carry the highest density of muscle spindles.[3]

A unique set of short muscles occurs in the suboccipital region (see Fig. 60-17). These muscles control the movements of the skull in nodding and ro-

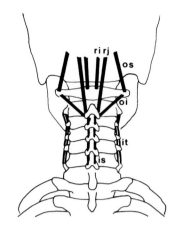

Fig. 60-17

The disposition and attachments of the intersegmental and suboccipital muscles of the neck. ri = rectus capitis posterior minor; rj = rectus capitis posterior major; os = obliquus superior; oi = obliquus inferior; it = intertransversarii; is = interspinales.

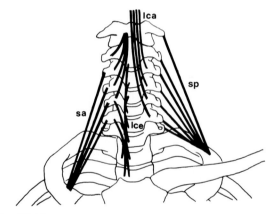

Fig. 60-18

The disposition and attachments of the scalene muscles and prevertebral muscles of the neck. lca = longus capitis; lce = longus cervicis; sp = scalenus posterior; sa = scalenus anterior.

tation. They are the rectus capitis posterior major, passing from the C2 spinous process to the skull; rectus capitis posterior minor, passing from the posterior tubercle of the atlas to the skull; obliquus inferior, joining the C2 spinous process and the transverse process of the atlas; and obliquus, superior joining the transverse process of the atlas to the skull.

Lateral Cervical Muscles

The lateral cervical muscles are the scalenus, anterior, medius, and posterior (Fig. 60-18). These arise from the transverse processes of the cervical vertebrae and are anchored to the first and second ribs. Acting from above, they act as muscles of respiration in raising the first two ribs. Acting from below these muscles can bend the neck sideways or stabilize it against contrary movements when the opposite limb is used in carrying or lifting weights.

Quadratus Lumborum

Quadratus lumborum is portrayed as a lateral flexor of the lumbar spine. However, its actual structure is not particularly consistent with this view. Most of its fibers arise from the ilium and the lumbar transverse processes and insert into the twelfth rib. This emphasizes its role as a respiratory muscle that stabilizes the twelfth rib and thereby the diaphragm. Only a small portion of the quadratus lumborum passes between the ilium and the lumbar transverse processes, and only these fibers are oriented to generate lateral flexion of the lumbar spine.[3]

The Diaphragm

The crura of the diaphragm take origin from the front of the upper three lumbar vertebrae. Their tendons can be traced inferiorly, forming most of what is depicted as the anterior longitudinal ligament of the lumbar spine.[3]

Psoas Major

The psoas major arises from the transverse processes of the lumbar vertebrae and from the T12-L1 to L4-L5 intervertebral discs and the adjoining vertebral bodies. This attachment to the vertebral column is only adventitious, forming a firm base for the muscle to act as a flexor of the hip. The psoas major effects no primary movement on the lumbar vertebral column. Its fascicles lie too close to the axes of rotation of the lumbar vertebrae for them to exert any appreciable moment.[2] However, when psoas major contracts it does exert substantial compressive force on the lumbar intervertebral discs, measuring up to the equivalent of four times body weight upon maximum contraction of both muscles.

Prevertebral Muscles

The prevertebral muscles of the neck are the longus cervicis and longus capitis (see Fig. 60-18). The longus cervicis consists of three portions disposed in a triangular fashion. The superior portion passes between the middle cervical transverse processes and the upper cervical vertebral bodies. The inferior portion passes between the middle cervical transverse processes and the lower cervical and upper thoracic vertebral bodies. The vertical portion connects up-

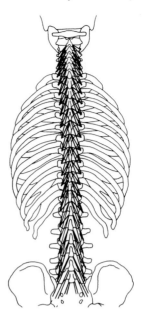

Fig. 60-19

The disposition and attachments of the multifidus muscle.

per and lower cervical vertebral bodies. The longus capitis covers the longus cervicis and passes between the upper cervical transverse processes and the occipital bone anterior to the foramen magnum.

The longus cervicis and capitis are not well-developed muscles and their lines of action lie close to the axes of sagittal rotation of the cervical vertebra. Consequently, they are not particularly strong flexors of the neck. At best they control small-amplitude movements of the head and neck in the sagittal plane. Forced flexion of the neck is achieved by sternocleidomastoid.

Postvertebral Muscles

The postvertebral muscles are those lying behind the plane of the transverse processes of the vertebral column. They are best considered in groups: multifidus, semispinalis, erector spinae, and splenius.

Multifidus

The multifidus is a series of multipennate muscles covering the laminae of the vertebral column, each stemming from a spinous process from level C2 to L5 (Fig. 60-19). Each spinous process is subtended by up to three or four fascicles, each of which assumes a distinct caudal attachment. Those fascicles from cervical spinous processes are anchored to the cervical articular processes and to the bases of the cervical transverse processes. In the thoracic region

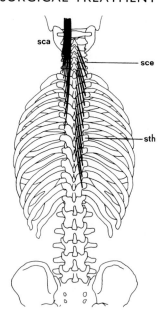

Fig. 60-20

The disposition and attachments of the semispinalis muscles. sca = semispsinalis capitis; sce = semispinalis cervicis; sth = semispinalis thoracis.

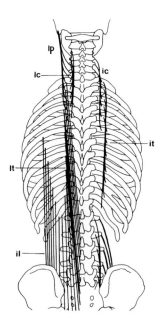

Fig. 60-21

The disposition and attachments of the erector spinae. Il = iliocostalis lumborum.

fascicles of multifidus are anchored to the bases of the transverse processes. In the lumbar region they are anchored to the mamillary processes, while the lowest fibers of multifidus, from the L3 to L5 spinous processes, are large in size and are anchored to the entire posterior surface of the sacrum and to the posterior superior iliac spine.[3]

The fibers of multifidus act to pull down on the spinous process from which they arise. Through this action they execute posterior sagittal rotation of their vertebra of origin. The multifidus has been represented as a rotator of the vertebral column. However, the orientation of its fibers is such that any such rotation must occur simultaneously with extension, with extension being by far the dominant movement.[3] In the lumbar region, such rotation is precluded by the orientation of the zygapophyseal joints.

Semispinalis

The semispinalis system of muscles is characterized by fibers that arise from transverse processes and insert into spinous processes or their equivalent (Fig. 60-20). These fibers arise lateral to the attachments of multifidus and cover this muscle.

Three divisions of the semispinalis are recognized along the length of the vertebral column. *Semispinalis thoracis* arises from lower thoracic transverse processes and inserts into thoracic spinous processes. *Semispinalis cervicis* arises from upper thoracic transverse processes and inserts into cervical spinous processes. *Semispinalis capitis* arises from upper thoracic and cervical transverse processes and inserts into the occipital bone below the superior nuchal line. This latter muscle constitutes the largest and strongest of the posterior neck muscles. Semispinalis thoracis and semispinalis cervicis are disposed to execute posterior sagittal rotation of the vertebrae to whose spinous processes they are attached, while the semispinalis capitis executes extension of the head.

Erector Spinae

The erector spinae consists of a minor portion: the spinalis, and two major portions: longissimus and iliocostalis. The spinalis connects spinous processes, while the longissimus and iliocostalis connect homologous portions of the costal and transverse elements of the lumbar, thoracic, and cervical vertebrae and skull (Fig. 60-21).

The *spinalis* is developed only in the thoracic region where its fibers connect middle thoracic spinous processes to lower thoracic and upper lumbar spinous processes. Its fibers characteristically circumvent the T10 spinous process, to which none are attached.

The *longissimus* consists of a staggered series of overlapping segmental fascicles that overlie the costotransverse regions of the vertebral column. The largest division of longissimus is *longissimus thoracis.* Its fibers arise from thoracic and lumbar levels and lie lateral to the semispinalis thoracis and lumbar multifidus. In the lumbar region they arise from the junction of the transverse and costal elements of the lumbar vertebrae, viz. from the accessory processes and the adjacent portion of the ipsisegmental transverse process. These fibers converge to a common tendon that inserts into the medial aspect of the posterior superior iliac spine.[3]

The lumbar fibers of longissimus thoracis are covered by its thoracic fibers, which arise from the thoracic transverse processes and the adjacent portion of the ipsisegmental rib. From each segmental level a short, small muscle belly arises that in turn forms a long caudal tendon. Collectively, these tendons of the longissimus thoracis form the medial half of the erector spinae aponeurosis: a broad tendinous sheet that is attached to the lumbar and sacral spinous processes, to the sacrum, and to the posterior superior iliac spine.[3]

Two smaller divisions of longissimus are *longissimus cervicis* and *longissimus capitis.* The longissimus cervicis rises in the thoracic region and inserts into the lower cervical transverse processes at the junction of the costal and transverse elements of these processes. The longissimus capitis rises in the thoracic region and inserts into the mastoid process of the skull, which, by analogy with the remainder of the attachments of longissimus, may be regarded as the costal equivalent of the posterior skull.

The iliocostalis lies lateral to the longissimus and may be regarded as connecting costal elements of the vertebral column. It has three divisions: iliocostalis lumborum, iliocostalis thoracis, and iliocostalis cervicis.

The fibers of the *ilicostalis lumborum* stem from the ilium and attach to the costal elements of the lumbar vertebrae, that is, their transverse processes, and to the angles of the lower eight ribs. Above their attachment to the ilium the more superficial fibers of iliocostalis lumborum are tendinous and collectively they constitute the lateral half of the erector spinae aponeurosis.[3]

Ilicostalis thoracis consists of fibers that connect the lower ribs to the upper ribs near their angles. *Iliocostalis cervicis* is a small muscle that connects the upper ribs to the costal elements of the lower cervical vertebrae.

Spinalis is topographically distinct from the rest of erector spinae and really should not be consid-

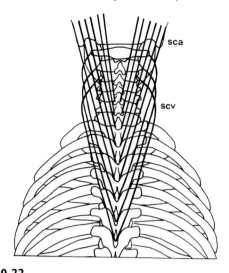

Fig. 60-22

The disposition and attachments of the spienius muscles. scv = splenius cervicis; sca = splenius capitis.

ered part of it. Its fibers are disposed to extend that portion of the vertebral column over which its fibers span.

Collectively and acting bilaterally those fibers of the longissimus thoracis and iliocostalis lumborum that span the lumbar region are the most powerful extensors of the trunk, accounting for up to 80% of the extensor moment at L1-L2 and about 40% of the moment at L5 (at lower lumbar levels multifidus is the major extensor). Acting unilaterally the longissimus thoracis and iliocostalis lumborum control lateral flexion of the lumbar spine.

The functions of iliocostalis thoracis, longissimus cervicis, iliocostalis cervicis, and longissimus capitis have not been determined formally. They are all disposed to be extensors of their particular regions of the vertebral column but they are relatively very small in size. Their seemingly obscure and perhaps subtle function in the company of much stronger extensors such as semispinalis capitis has yet to be revealed.

Splenius

The splenius muscle arises from the cervical and upper thoracic spinous processes and wraps around the posterior and lateral aspects of the neck, covering all the other posterior neck muscles (Fig. 60-22). It consists of two parts: *splenius cervicis,* consisting of those fibers that insert into the cervical transverse processes, and *splenius capitis,* which inserts into the superior nuchal line and mastoid process of the skull. Collectively, the splenius acts as an extensor of the neck and head. Unilaterally, the splenius acts syner-gistically with the opposite sternocleidomastoid to rotate the head and neck.

Nerves of the Vertebral Column

The Spinal Cord and Nerve Roots

The spinal cord occupies the upper four fifths of the vertebral canal. It extends from the foramen magnum to the upper lumbar region. Its caudal end usually lies opposite the L1-L2 intervertebral disc but may lie one vertebral level above or below this. Its surface is intimately covered by the pia mater.

The spinal cord is enclosed by the dural sac, otherwise referred to as the theca, which extends from the foramen magnum as far as the S2 segment of the sacrum. The internal surface of the dural sac is lined by the arachnoid mater, and cerebrospinal fluid in the subarachnoid space bathes the spinal cord. The spinal cord is attached to the dural sac by the ligamentum denticulatum, which consists of 21 pairs of triangular extensions of pia mater whose apices are anchored to the dural sac. Within the vertebral canal the dural sac is attached to the vertebral column by fibrous ligaments that connect the ventral surface of the dural sac to the bodies and pedicles of the vertebrae.

The spinal cord consists of 31 segments—eight cervical, 12 thoracic, five lumbar, five sacral, and one coccygeal. Each gives rise to a pair of dorsal and a pair of ventral nerve roots. Each set of ventral and dorsal roots aims to converge and leave the dural sac as a spinal nerve. The cervical spinal nerves lie above their ipsisegmental vertebrae except for the C8 spinal nerve, which lies below the seventh cervical vertebra. All other spinal nerves lie below their ipsisegmental vertebra.

Within the dural sac the upper cervical nerve roots tend to pass upward toward their spinal nerve. Lower cervical nerve roots pass transversely or slightly downwards. Thoracic, lumbar, and sacral nerve roots assume a progressively steeper, downward course from the spinal cord to their respective spinal nerves. Below the caudal end of the spinal cord the lumbar, sacral, and coccygeal nerve roots are aggregated in the dural sac as a leash of nerves known as the *cauda equina*. Within the cauda equina the nerve roots assume a constant topographic relationship. Those destined for more caudal locations lie medially and dorsally, while those about to leave the dural sac lie laterally and ventrally.

As each set of ventral and dorsal roots leaves the dural sac, it draws with it a sleeve dura mater and arachnoid mater, which distally blends with the

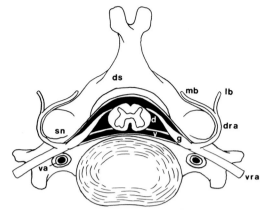

Fig. 60-23

A top view of the course and relations of typical cervical nerve roots. ds = dural sac; d = dorsal root; g = gaglion; v = ventral root; sn = spinal nerve; dra = dorsal ramus; vra = ventral ramus; mb = medial branch; lb = lateral branch; va = vertebral artery.

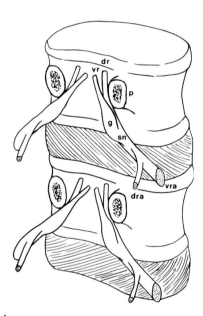

Fig. 60-24

A posterior view of the course and location of the lumbar nerve roots in the vertebral canal and intervertebral foramina. p = pedicle; dr = dorsal root; g = ganglion; vr = ventral root; sn = spinal nerve; vra = ventral ramus; dra = dorsal ramus.

epineurium of the spinal nerve. The dorsal root ganglia typically lie at the distal end of the dorsal root inside the apex of the dural sleeve.

Spinal Nerves

Spinal nerves are mixed nerves consisting of motor fibers leaving the spinal cord in the ventral roots, and sensory fibers passing to the spinal cord along the dorsal roots. Some sensory fibers also enter the spinal cord along the ventral roots, and at segmen-

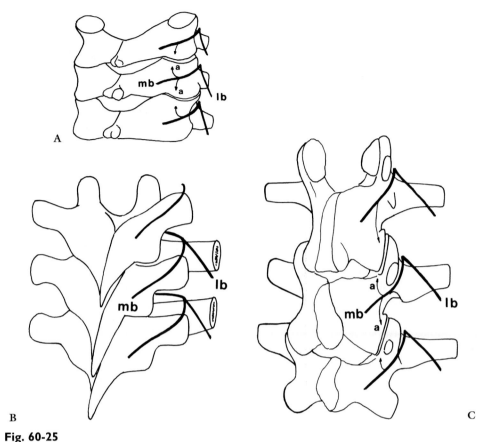

Fig. 60-25

Posterolateral views of the courses and branches of the dorsal rami of the spinal nerves. **A**. Cervical, **B**, Thoracic, **C**, Lumbar. mb = medial branch; lb = lateral branch; a = articular branch to zygapophyseal joint.

tal levels T1 to L2 the ventral roots convey preganglionic sympathetic efferent fibers, while the S2 and S3 ventral roots convey preganglionic parasympathetic efferents.

At typical cervical levels the spinal nerves occupy the intervertebral foramen resting on top of the ipsisegmental pedicle (Fig. 60-23). In this location they lie below the level of the intervertebral disc. The C1 spinal nerve rests on the posterior arch of the atlas, while the C2 spinal nerve lies behind or slightly below the lateral atlantoaxial joint.

At thoracic and lumbar levels, the nerve roots forming a given spinal nerve pass around the medial aspect of the ipsisegmental pedicle, and the spinal nerve is formed slightly below the pedicle (Fig. 60-24). Each spinal nerve therefore lies behind the lower end of its ipsisegmental vertebra and consequently above the intervertebral disc at that level. At each lumbar level, the dorsal root ganglion typically lies directly below the center of the pedicle. At sacral levels the spinal nerves occupy the sacral canal above and medial to the sacral foramina of the same segmental number.

Each spinal nerve is very short, being not longer than the intervertebral foramen is wide. At the lateral margin of the intervertebral foramen, the spinal nerve divides into a ventral ramus and a dorsal ramus. The C1 spinal nerve undergoes its branching on the posterior arch of the atlas; the sacral spinal nerves divide inside the sacral canal.

Dorsal Rami

The dorsal rami of the spinal nerves are distributed to the posterior elements of the vertebral column and to the postvertebral muscles.[1,5,6] Upon leaving the intervertebral foramen each dorsal ramus enters the posterior compartment of the spine by crossing the top edge of the transverse element of the subjacent vertebra. This means that in the thoracic region the dorsal ramus reaches the superior, lateral corner of the transverse process, but at cervical and lumbar levels the dorsal ramus reaches only the top edge of the base of the so-called transverse process in which the true transverse element constitutes only the proximal end of this process (Fig. 60-25). In the sacrum the equivalent sites are the posterior sacral foramina.

Upon reaching the transverse element, each dorsal ramus typically divides into medial and lateral branches, although in the lumbar region a third, intermediate branch is frequently formed. The C1 dorsal ramus is atypical. This dorsal ramus leaves the posterior arch of the atlas to enter the suboccipital triangle, and innervates the suboccipital muscles.

The lateral branches of the dorsal rami are distributed to the more lateral of the postvertebral muscle: those with attachments to costal elements—splenius, longissimus, and iliocostalis in the neck, and longissimus and iliocostalis in the thoracic and lumbar regions. At lumbar levels the intermediate and lateral branches of the dorsal rami are distributed respectively to the longissimus and iliocostalis. The lateral branches of the sacral dorsal rami have no muscular distribution and become only cutaneous.

The medial branches of the dorsal rami innervate the posterior joints of the vertebral column and the more medial of the back muscles, namely those that attach to the transverse elements of the vertebral column: multifidus and semispinalis. Upon crossing the transverse element, each medial branch typically passes medially onto the lamina of the vertebra, running between two consecutive zygapophyseal joints. Articular branches are distributed to each of these joints.

The medial branch of the C2 dorsal ramus is distinctive in that it forms the greater occipital nerve, which winds around the inferior border of the obliquus inferior. This nerve enters and supplies semispinalis capitis before becoming cutaneous over the occiput.[1] The C3 dorsal ramus forms two medial branches: a deep medial branch conforming to the pattern of typical cervical medial branches, and a superficial medial branch, which is the third occipital nerve. The third occipital nerve wraps around the C2-C3 zygapophyseal joint which it supplies, and innervates the semispinalis capitis before becoming cutaneous over the suboccipital region.[1] The medial branches of the sacral dorsal rami are tiny; they have no muscular distribution and ramify in the posterior sacroiliac ligament.

As a rule, at lower thoracic, lumbar, and sacral levels, the lateral branches of the dorsal rami become cutaneous, the lateral branches of the S1, S2, and S3 dorsal rami forming the medial clunial nerves of the buttock. At cervical and upper thoracic levels the medial branches of the dorsal rami provide the cutaneous distribution, save that the dorsal rami of C5, C6, and C7 typically have no cutaneous branches.

Ventral Rami

The thoracic ventral rami simply leave their intervertebral foramen and become intercostal nerves, each supplying the muscles of that intercostal space and the overlying skin. The lower six intercostal nerves are prolonged beyond the costal margin to supply the muscles and skin of the lateral and anterior abdominal wall in a segmental fashion.

The cervical, lumbar, and sacral ventral rami form plexuses before being distributed peripherally. The cervical plexus is formed by the C1-C4 ventral rami and supplies the sternocleidomastoid, trapezius, levator scapulae, the upper scalenes, and the prevertebral muscles of the neck, and cutaneous branches to the side of the face, auricle, and neck.

The brachial plexus is formed by the C5-C8 and the T1 ventral rami, and supplies the lower scalenes, the muscles of the shoulder girdle, and the muscles and skin of the upper limb. The lumbar plexus is formed by the L1-L4 ventral rami; it innervates the lower abdominal wall and groin, psoas major, and quadratus lumborum, and gives rise to the femoral and obturator nerves of the lower limb.

The lumbosacral plexus is formed by the L4, L5 and S1, S2, S3 ventral rami, and gives rise to the nerves of the lower limb and lower limb girdle. The sacral plexus is formed by the S3, S4, S5 and coccygeal ventral rami, and innervates the pelvic floor and perianal skin.

Proximally, each ventral ramus participates in the innervation of the anterior elements of the vertebral column. The C1 ventral ramus innervates the atlantooccipital joint and the C2 ventral ramus innervates the lateral atlantoaxial joint. Otherwise, the ventral rami innervate the vertebral bodies and intervertebral discs in conjunction with the sympathetic nervous system.

Sympathetic Trunks

The sympathetic trunks run along the entire length of the vertebral column, spanning from the carotid canal superiorly to the ganglion impar in front of the tip of the coccyx. In the thoracic region each sympathetic trunk is located anterior to the heads of the ribs where they join the vertebral column. In other regions, the sympathetic trunks assume a homologous location—anterior to the proximal ends of the costal elements of the respective vertebrae, viz. medial to the anterior sacral foramina, and in front of the roots of the cervical and lumbar transverse processes; although, in the cervical and lumbar re-

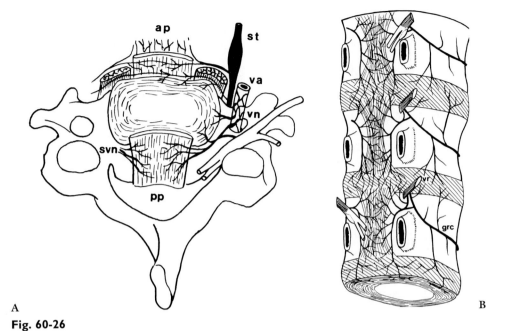

Fig. 60-26

The plexuses of the anterior elements of the cervical (**A**) and lumbar (**B**) vertebral column. st = sympathetic trunk; va = vertebral artery; vn = vertebral nerve; svn = sinuvertebral nerve; ap = anterior longitudinal plexus; pp = posterior longitudinal plexus; grc = grey ramus communicans; vr = ventral ramus. (Based on Groen and colleagues.[10])

gions, the sympathetic trunk is displaced from its bony relations by the prevertebral muscles and psoas major, respectively.

Each sympathetic trunk receives white rami communicantes from the T1 to L2 ventral rami, but provides a grey ramus communicans to each and every ventral ramus. Grey rami communicantes pass directly from the sympathetic trunk to the thoracic and lumbar ventral rami in their intervertebral foramina and to the sacral ventral rami opposite the anterior sacral foramina. At upper cervical levels, grey rami communicantes reach the ventral rami in the cervical plexus. At lower cervical levels grey rami communicantes from the stellate ganglion pass through the foramina transversaria to join the lower cervical ventral rami in their intervertebral foramina. These are supplemented by direct branches from the middle cervical ganglion and cervical sympathetic trunk that reach the cervical ventral rami through their intertransverse spaces. In the foramina transversaria and intertransverse spaces, these grey rami communicantes accompany the vertebral artery, constituting what is referred to as the "vertebral nerve."

The anterior elements of the vertebral column are innervated by extensive, fine plexuses covering the anterior, lateral, and posterior aspects of the vertebral bodies and intervertebral discs, and derived from the sympathetic trunks, grey rami communicantes, vertebral nerve, and ventral rami (Fig. 60-26). From these plexuses nerve fibers penetrate the depths of the vertebral bodies in company with intraosseous blood vessels, and penetrate the outer layers of the anulus fibrosus of the intervertebral disc at all levels.[10]

The posterior plexus lies along the floor of the vertebral canal. It supplies the anterior internal vertebral venous plexus, the posterior longitudinal ligament, the ventral surface of the dural sac, and the posterior aspects of the intervertebral discs. Within this plexus, major branches are frequently present, which constitute what in the past have been identified upon dissection as the sinuvertebral nerves.[4,7] However, the sinuvertebral nerves are only large representatives of what is otherwise a dense microscopic plexus in the vertebral canal. At atlantoaxial levels the C1, C2, and C3 sinuvertebral nerves innervate the transverse ligament of the atlas and the alar ligaments before entering the skull to supply the dura mater over the clivus.

Dermatomes and Myotomes

Each segment of the spinal cord, and by the same token, each spinal nerve, is distributed to particular structures in the periphery. This segmental relationship is established in the embryo before the peripheral nerves and their plexuses are formed. All those

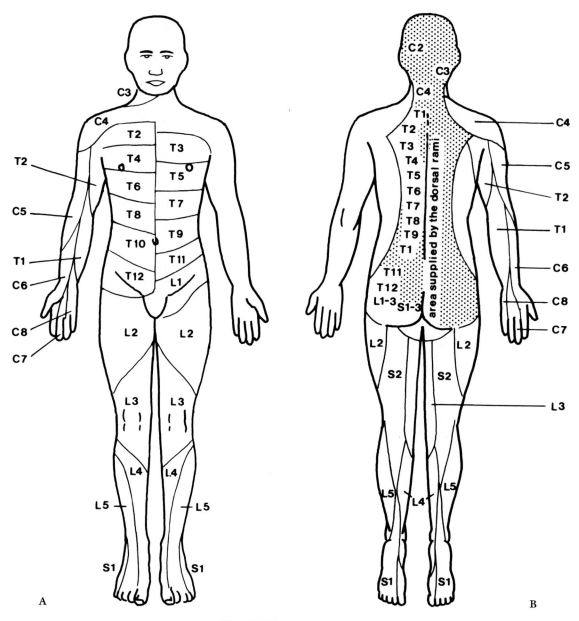

Fig. 60-27

The dermatomes of the body.

muscles fibers supplied by a given spinal cord segment constitute the *myotome* of that segment. The region of skin supplied by a segment is the *dermatome* of that segment.

A concept that has been floated in the past is that of the sclerotome. This concept seeks to refer to the segmental, sensory innervation of deep structures. However, unlike myotomes and dermatomes, sclerotomes have not been defined on objective electrophysiological or anatomical grounds. Rather, they are inferences drawn from the subjective reports of the distribution of referred pain in volunteers undergo-

ing experimental noxious stimulation of deep structures. Consequently, they reflect central patterning of nociceptive pathways more than any actual peripheral distribution of segmental nerves. There is no need to adopt a poorly based concept such as sclerotomes when a more firmly based body of information can serve the same purpose. For clinical purposes, such as the interpretation of referred pain patterns, the segmental distribution of muscle nerves provides sufficient information. For practical purposes one can assume that the segmental sensory distribution to muscles is the same as that of their mo-

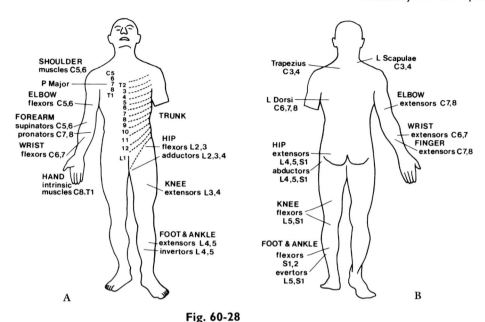

Fig. 60-28

The myotomes of the body.

tor distribution; and joints are supplied by the same segments as the principal muscles that act on them.

The basic pattern of dermatomes is depicted by the thoracic spinal nerves. Each nerve supplies the skin overlying the ipsisegmental intercostal space, with the addition that lower intercostal nerves project in the direction of their ribs onto the anterolateral abdominal wall. In the limbs this basic parallel pattern of dermatomes is stretched and distorted by the longitudinal growth and rotation of the limb bud in the embryo. The systematic pattern is nonetheless evident insofar as consecutive segments are represented in order from proximal to distal along the cephalic border of the limb and then from distal to proximal along the caudal border of the limb (Fig. 60-27).

The myotomes of the body follow a similar systematic pattern. The muscles of the trunk are supplied by consecutive segments represented in the intercostal and first two lumbar nerves. In the limbs, two relationships apply. More proximal muscles are innervated by higher segments, and ventral muscles acting on a given joint are innervated by higher segments than the dorsal muscles acting on the same joint. The actual distribution of myotomes varies from individual to individual, but the modal pattern is summarized in Fig. 60-28.

This pattern can be used as the basis for clinical testing of segmental motor deficits, but it serves equally well for the interpretation of deep and referred pain. Pain perceived in a region occupied by a particular muscle or joint does not necessarily imply an origin in that muscle or joint. Rather, it may indicate a source in any of the deep, somatic structures innervated by the same segments that innervate the muscle or joint in question.

For example, levator scapulae lies above the scapula and is innervated by C3 and C4. Pain overlying the levator scapulae may reflect an origin in levator scapulae but also may reflect a source in any structure innervated by C3 or C4. The posterior scapular muscles and the glenohumeral joint are both supplied by C5 and C6, but pain in the shoulder or over the scapula may reflect an origin in any of the structures innervated by C5 or C6, which includes not only the shoulder muscles and shoulder joints but also the C5-C6 segments of the vertebral column.

The anterior chest wall provides a further illustrative example. Deeply, the upper chest wall is supplied by the T1-T4 segments, but it is covered by the pectoralis major, which is supplied by C5, C6, C7, and C8. Consequently, chest-wall pain may indicate an origin anywhere in the tissues supplied by C5 to T4. The T1-T4 component invites a consideration of the thoracic viscera, but the C5-C8 component invites a consideration of referred pain from the neck.

References

1. Bogduk N: The clinical anatomy of the cervical dorsal rami; *Spine* 7:319, 1982.

2. Bogduk N, Pearch MJ, Hadfield G: The anatomy and biomechanics of the psoas major, *Clin Biomech* 7:109, 1992.

3. Bogduk N, Twomey LT: *Clinical anatomy of the lumbar spine,* ed 2, Melbourne, 1991. Churchill Livingstone.

4. Bogduk N, Tynan W, Wilson AS: The nerve supply to the human lumbar intervertebral discs, *J Anat* 132:39, 1981.

5. Bogduk N, Valencia F: *Innervation and pain patterns of the thoracic spine.* In Grant R, ed: *Physical therapy of the neck and thorax,* New York, 1988, Churchill Livingstone, p27.

6. Bogduk N, Wilson AS, Tynan W: The human lumbar dorsal rami, *J Anat* 134:383, 1982.

7. Bogduk N, Windsor M, Inglis A: The innervation of the cervical intervertebral discs, *Spine* 13:2, 1988.

8. Dvorak J, Panjabi MM: Functional anatomy of the alar ligaments, *Spine* 12:183, 1987.

9. Fielding JW, and others: Tears of the transverse ligament of the atlas, *J Bone Joint Surg* 56A:1683, 1974.

10. Groen GJ, Baljet B, Drukker J: Nerves and nerve plexuses of the human vertebral column, *Am J Anat* 188:282, 1990.

11. Lavignolle B and others: An approach to the functional anatomy of the sacroiliac joints in vivo, *Anat Clin* 5:169, 1983.

12. Oda J, Tanaka H, Tsuzuki N: Intervertebral disc changes with aging of human cervical vertebra, *Spine* 11:1205, 1988.

13. Penning L: Differences in anatomy, motion, development and aging of the upper and lower cervical disc segments, *Clin Biomech* 3:37, 1988.

14. Singer KP, Breidahl PD, Day RE: Posterior element variation at the thoracolumbar transition: a morphometric study using computed tomography, *Clin Biomech* 4:80, 1989.

15. Sturesson B, Selvik, G, Uden A: Movements of the sacroiliac joints: a roentgen stereophotogrammetric analysis, *Spine* 14:162, 1989.

16. Taylor JR: *Growth and development of the human intervertebral disc,* PhD Thesis, University of Edinburgh, 1973.

17. Taylor JR, Milne N: *The cervical mobile segments.* Proceedings of Whiplash Symposium. Adelaide: Orthopaedic Special Interest Group, Australian Physiotherapy Association, South Australian Branch, 1988, p21.

Chapter 61
Clinical Biomechanics of Lumbar Spine

Casey K. Lee

Historical Review

Physiologic Pain Mechanism

The Disc

Surgical Procedures, Disc Degeneration, Stability, and Low-Back Pain

spinal instability and mechanical low-back pain
posterior spinal decompression and spinal instability

Biomechanics of Spinal Fusion

Internal Fixation of the Lumbosacral Spine

Historical Review

Clinical biomechanics for lumbosacral spine surgery has evolved around the following:

1. To fuse or not to fuse the lumbosacral spine for idiopathic low-back pain (LBP).
2. Iatrogenic instability after disc excision.
3. Determination of degenerative instability of a spinal motion segment.

These questions emerged many decades ago and have remained unanswered.

Before the report of successful treatment of LBP and sciatica by surgical excision of the herniated disc by Mixter and Barr,[40] spinal fusion was a commonly accepted procedure for patients with LBP caused by structural anomalies or facet tropism of the lumbosacral spine.[*] Until recently, enthusiasm for spinal fusion has diminished as the disc excision procedure became popular. The herniated disc problem was known to be a manifestation of a degenerative process of the disc, and the disc excision for herniated disc was generally thought to cause further mechanical instability of the spine. Although the combined procedure of disc excision and spinal fusion was advocated by many surgeons,[†] its efficacy for pain relief was questioned by some.[8,17,52] Is mechanical instability of a spinal motion segment caused by degenerative processes of the disc, by the surgical procedure of partial excision of the disc, or by the combination of both?

A biomechanical study of a partial excision of the disc demonstrated no significant alterations of biomechanical behavior of the disc.[27,28,39,55] This study suggests that the disc excision procedure does not contribute to the instability of the motion segment.

Others[15,25,41] observed that instability of the lumbosacral spine was occasionally associated with degenerative changes of the disc and was a common cause for chronic LBP. In these patients satisfactory relief of low back pain was obtained by spinal fusion.[41,53,54]

In recent years spinal surgeons, not having answers to these fundamental questions, are confronted with further problems as we are performing more complicated surgical procedures such as extensive decompression for spinal stenosis, use of various internal fixation devices, and choices of different types of fusion procedures.

Physiologic Pain Mechanism

Three common causes for idiopathic LBP are ligamentous sprain causing nociceptive irritation, neural compression as in disc herniation or spinal stenosis, and biochemical irritation of nociceptive endings by inflammation-provoking degenerative byproducts. These three pain mechanisms are all closely related to the structural integrity, external loads, structural response to the applied loads, and kinematics of spinal motion segment. Further explanations of this relationship between pain mechanisms and biomechanics of a spinal motion segment are made in the subsequent paragraphs.

The anulus fibrosus, various ligamentous structures of the spinal motion segments, and joint capsules of the facet joint are richly innervated by nociceptive endings and are common sources for idiopathic low back pain. The physical deformations of these structures (strain) beyond their physiologic limit is defined as sprain (excessive strain)[‡] in clinical practice. Therefore sprain of various structures, including the anulus fibrosus, depends largely on two factors—applied load and structural response to the applied load. The applied load to a specific ligamentous structure about a joint causes two significant biomechanical changes—forces acting on the structure (stress) and deformation of the structure (strain). These two biomechanical factors caused by external loads are closely related to the movement patterns of the joint (kinesiology).

Normal structures of the anulus fibrosus, joint capsules of the facet joint, and various ligaments of a spinal motion segment require greater amounts of force (stress) to make these structures deform beyond the physiologic limit (sprain). Degenerated and attenuated structures of annulus, ligaments, or capsules have altered biomechanical response to the applied forces. In this circumstance a physiologic loading condition can become an abnormal loading condition to these structures, causing abnormal excessive strain (sprain). Abnormal motion pattern (hypermobility or irrational motion) can also alter the stress and strain responses of these structures to external loads.

Clinical biomechanics for diagnosis and treatment of idiopathic low back pain encompasses studies on loads to the spine; stress/strain characteristics of

---

[*]References 2, 5, 9, 10, 14, 24, 29, 30, 48, and 56.
[†]References 3, 4, 21, 59, and 60.

[‡]The biomechanical term *strain* refers to the deformation of structures caused by forces applied on them (stress). The clinical term *strain* refers to the excessive deformation of the muscle–tendon unit (sprain of ligaments vs. strain of muscle).

normal and degenerated structures of anulus, ligamentous structures, and joint capsule; and motion studies.

A spinal motion segment is a compound joint that is made of a three-joint complex. The posterior two joints are the facet joints, which are true synovial joints. The anterior joint is the intervertebral disc. The disc has many similarities, as well as dissimilarities, with a synovial joint; it is a highly specialized joint to accommodate specific physiologic requirements—movements, stability, load-bearing capacity, and protective mechanism to the neural contents.

The structural specifications of the disc are designed to provide maximum stability with a relatively small but important amount of motion and load transmission. In a typical large weight-bearing synovial joint such as the knee joint, the movement is primarily guided by geometric configuration of the articulating surfaces, joint capsule, and surrounding ligaments (probably in the order of significance). In the disc the articulating surface of the joints, the "vertebral end plates," are simple and made of two relatively flat and parallel surfaces. The guidance of motion of the disc is therefore heavily dependent on the anulus fibrosus (capsular component of a synovial joint) and the adjacent facet joints. The anterior and posterior longitudinal ligaments are important for flexion and extension of a motion segment in the saggital plane but do not significantly contribute to guidance and stabilization for torsion, side bending, and horizontal translation. In a large weight-bearing synovial joint, most of the weight-bearing function is provided by the articular cartilage. This function of a synovial joint is transformed into a very special design arrangement in the disc as a form of anulus fibrosus and nucleus pulposus.

The spinal motion segment is a functional unit of the spinal column that is made of a three-joint complex—one disc and two facet joints. The concept of a three-joint complex is not new but is very important to understanding LBP problems. Historically, we have been conditioned to think only of the disc problems whenever we are faced with patients with LBP and sciatica, and we have neglected problems arising from the other two joints—facet joints.

The Disc

The disc is a nonsynovial joint and the largest avascular structure in the human body. A disc is made of three component structures: the vertebral end plates, the anulus fibrosus, and the nucleus pulposus.

The vertebral end plate provides a comparable function to the subchondral bone plate in a synovial joint to disperse the load to the adjacent nucleus pulposus and anulus fibrosus. However, the vertebral end plate, unlike the subchondral bony plate in which no fluid exchanges between the joint cavity and subchondral bony sinusoid, permits fluid diffusion between vertebral sinusoids and the nucleus pulposus and anulus fibrosus.[43] This fluid exchange through the vertebral end plates plays a major role in the nourishment of the largest avascular structure of the disc. When the disc is loaded on axial compression, the vertebral end plate is the weakest structure among the three component structures of the disc.[7,43]

The nucleus pulposus, which has no cells, consists of a three-dimensional network of collagen fibers (mainly type II) embedded in a mucoprotein gel.[27] It is located near but slightly posterior to the geometric center of the disc. Acid mucopolysaccharide is the main component of the ground substance. Water content of the nucleus pulposus is about 80% in a young adult and decreases with age.[47] The nucleus pulposus is incompressible material, and it bulges out when the disc is cut through the nucleus pulposus. In physiologic status in vivo, the nucleus pulposus is compressed by the elastic properties of the ligamentum flavum, maintaining the disc height. It also acts like a ball bearing when the vertebral bodies roll in flexion and extension. The center of rotation within the disc changes instantaneously, depending on the position of the spine during flexion and extension.[28,49] In the degenerated disc the instant center of rotation tends to move posteriorly,[13] and an increased stress is applied to the facet joints. The nucleus pulposus transforms the vertebral compression forces into tangential stresses (hoop stress) in the anulus fibrosus.[42]

The nucleus pulposus has no nociceptive endings. Therefore any biochemical or morphologic change of the nucleus pulposus does not set up direct nociceptive stimulation. However, these changes can produce secondary changes of the biomechanical behaviors of the motion segments and can set up nociceptive stimulation. Degeneration of the nucleus pulposus may lead to loss of disc height and altered load transmission across the disc and the facet joints.

The anulus fibrosus is made of concentric lamellae of collagen fibers (type II and I), which expand obliquely across the disc space between vertebral end plates. The fibers in each lamella run obliquely 30° to the end plate. Thus, two adjoining lamellae run in the opposite direction and fibers cross each other at 120°. The anulus is stiffest and has lowest deformation and energy dissipation in this arrangement.[18,19]

The interlamellar spaces are filled with abundant amounts of proteoglycan. The mechanical properties of the anulus for these physiologic functions are from mechanical behavior of the composite material (collagen fibers and proteoglycan). The proteoglycan component of the composite material binds collagen fibers and lamellae and provides water-binding capacity. Abnormal biomechanical behaviors of degenerated discs are commonly associated with changes in composition of proteoglycan, which cause changes in collagen-binding capacity and water-binding capacity of the disc. Whether these changes are secondary to repetitive trauma to the disc or are the primary cause for disc disruption is not clear. Nevertheless, changes in biochemical composition caused by aging produces susceptibility of the disc to trauma by delamination of the anulus fibrosus and abnormal strain to the collagen fibers.

The anulus fibrosus is the most important component structure in a spinal motion segment for biomechanical stability and for transmitting vertical weight-bearing forces.[49] The viscoelastic behavior of the anulus fibrosus in relation to the load-bearing ability and stability of a spinal motion segment in normal and abnormally degenerated discs has been extensively studied with static or dynamic compression tests.[*]

Under the axial compressive load the disc fails at the vertebral end plate. The normal anulus fibrosus can withstand much greater stress than the failure stress of the vertical end plate, and it does not fail first under the axial load. The vertical compressive load applied on the vertebral body is transmitted to the anulus fibrosus as the tangential hoop stress through the end plate and the nucleus pulposus.

Studies on the disc bulge and intradiscal pressure have been frequently quoted subjects in the literature in attempts to correlate back pain to pathologic conditions of the disc degeneration and to various physiologic postures and activities. The amount of disc bulge under controlled axial loads was higher in the degenerated disc.[26] In the degenerated disc the amount of disc bulge under controlled axial loads was much higher (30%), and the anulus was subjected to higher vertical stress and lower tangential forces because of loss of hydrostatic behavior of the degenerated nucleus pulposus. However, it is not clear that the lateral bulge of the anulus fibrosus under the axial load produces abnormal strain on the anulus fibers and causes pain by stimulation to the nociceptive endings within the outer layers of the anulus. An abnormal amount of bulge beyond a certain critical level may exert direct pressure on the nerve root, causing radiculopathy.

Bulging of a disc under a given amount of axial compressive load can be manifested as two very different phenomena, depending on the status of component structures of composite material of the anulus fibrosus-proteoglycan and collagen framework.

When the disc is loaded externally, the external load is counterbalanced by an internal resistive force of the disc (joint reaction force). Two main components of the internal resistive force of the disc are osmotic pressure and solid structural stiffness (networks of the anulus fibrosus). The osmotic pressure is provided by the proteoglycan component of the anulus fibrosus and nucleus pulposus.

When the applied axial compressive load causes disc-space narrowing by less internal resistive pressure of the disc caused by changes in proteoglycan components with low osmotic pressure, the outer layer of the anulus will bulge out by the buckling phenomenon. In this case the bulged anulus does not have any significantly increased stress or strain. This situation is similar to a deflated balloon between two solid objects. When two solid objects are squeezed together, the balloon will bulge out but the balloon's wall will not be stretched much.

When external compressive load is applied to the disc with a good osmotic pressure mechanism but weaker solid structural frame, the disc wall (anulus) will bulge out with increased stress and strain (stretched out wall). When the same load is applied to a disc with normal osmotic pressure mechanism and intact solid structure force, the disc bulge and increased stress and strain of the wall will be minimal, but the intradiscal pressure will become very high. The intradiscal pressure in the disc with normal osmotic pressure mechanism but weak solid structure frame will have only a moderate level. The intradiscal pressure in the disc with low osmotic pressure but normal solid structural frameworks will be lower than the above cases, and the intradiscal pressure in the disc with low osmotic pressure and weak solid structure frame will be the lowest among all.

Therefore, abnormal bulge of the anulus fibrosus does not necessarily mean increased stress and strain on the fibers of the anulus or the overlying posterior longitudinal ligament, and it does not necessarily cause stimulation to nociceptive endings contained in these structures. This may be a reason why some patients with bulging disc are asymptomatic as long as the disc bulge is not causing direct radicular compression.

Intradiscal pressure may not necessarily represent the stress or strain status of the fibers of the anulus fibrosus. The relationship between the factors (intradiscal pressure and stretch of outer layer of the

---

[*]References 7, 39, 42, 49, 59, and 62.

anulus) is also greatly influenced by the integrity of the solid structures. The results of measurements of intradiscal pressure have been applied to clinical care for patients with LBP to guide postures and activities for less pain. The relationship between the intradiscal pressure and pain in various stages of disc degeneration and in various postures and activities is not completely understood.

The anulus fibrosus provides maximal stability against horizontal displacement.[19] It also provides a very significant amount of torsional stability of a motion segment (40% to 50%), and an approximately equal amount of torsional stability is provided by the posterior lumbar facet joints.[13] The anulus fibrosus provides minimal resistance in tension to angular motion of the motion segment.

The two posteriorly located facet joints are the other part of the three-joint complex of a motion segment. The facet joint is a true synovial joint and is richly innervated by nociceptive endings. The primary function of the lumbar facet joint is to provide torsional stability of a motion segment.[13] The facet joints have very small amounts (less than 20%) of the weight-bearing capacity in normal physiologic conditions. The resection of the facet joints (partial or complete) as a part of posterior spinal decompression for spinal stenosis can compromise the torsional stability of the whole motion segment and probably place extra burdens on the anulus fibrosus.

Surgical Procedures, Disc Degeneration, Stability, and Low-Back Pain

Low-back pain in degenerative disc disease is commonly caused either by abnormal strain (sprain of ligaments and capsules) of the anulus fibrosus and the posterior longitudinal ligament or by mechanical or chemical irritation of the degenerative facet joints. The abnormal strain on the anulus fibrosus, posterior longitudinal ligament, and facet joints capsule is produced either by nonphysiologic external overloading to the normal structures (common cause of injury to normal healthy structures) or by physiologic loading to the degenerated abnormal structures.

In biologic systems the degenerative process is almost always accompanied by the biologic reparative system. The identifiable evidences of reparative processes in the degenerated spinal motion segments are increased surface area of the vertebral end plates by local or circumferential ridging or osteophyte formation, increased surface areas of the facet joints with change of geometric joint configuration, and scarring or thickening of the outer layer of the anulus fibrosus, ligamentum flavum, and facet joint capsule. Accurate measurements of the degree of the negative effect (structural weakness, destabilization) of degenerative processes and of the degree of the positive effect (structural enhancement, self-stabilization) of the reparative, processes have not been obtained.

The three most common pathologic conditions for treatment by spinal surgeons are disc herniation, spinal instability, and spinal stenosis.

Disc herniation is a manifestation of a spectrum of degenerative processes of the disc. The successful choice of surgical procedures for a herniated disc depends on the proper evaluation of biomechanical function of the whole motion segment. Partial excision of a herniated disc (degenerated nucleus pulposus and inner layers of the anulus) through a laminotomy does not appear to cause serious biomechanical derangement of the motion segment, if the herniated disc is a relatively isolated pathologic condition. A biomechanical study on fresh human cadaver lumbar spine demonstrated a self-sealing effect of the disc after a simulated procedure of disc excision on the motion segment.[39] The mechanism of pain relief of sciatica after disc excision is probably due to removal of mechanical pressure and the source of chemical irritation to the nerve root. The relief of back pain in disc herniation is not often predictable either by surgical excision or discolysis. A possible mechanism for back pain relief by discolysis is decreased intradiscal osmotic pressure and decreased strain on the outer layer of the anulus fibrosus.

Spinal Instability and Mechanical Low-Back Pain

Clinical stability is defined as "the ability of the spine under physiologic loads to limit patterns of displacement so as not to damage or irritate the spinal cord or nerve root and, in addition, to prevent incapacitating deformity or pain due to structural changes."[57] Clinical instability for LBP can be caused by abnormal displacement under physiologic loading (hypermobility) and also by structural changes without evidence of hypermobility.

Clinicians in practice use the term *spinal instability* to designate the condition of painful hypermobility, and the term *mechanical low-back pain* to designate the condition of LBP caused by abnormal structural behavior under physiologic loading without evidences of hypermobility.

Spinal hypermobility caused by degenerative processes (degenerative spondylolisthesis) has long been recognized as an important cause of LBP. The hypermobility of the motion segment can be manifested in any plane of motion. The most commonly observed type is translation in the horizontal plane. In a normal spinal motion segment there is no translation of one vertebral body on the other in the horizontal plane throughout the physiologic ranges of motion of the lumbosacral spine. Translation in excess of 2 to 3 mm in either extension or flexion is considered to be clinically significant for instability.[41,46]

The most common type of hypermobility observed in practice is excessive angular displacement in the saggital plane. Excessive disc space angle, greater than 9° above the normal (1{deg for L5-S1) is considered to be significant for clinical instability.[46] Farfan[11] reported that the principal pathomechanics of degenerative spondylolisthesis is the torsional translation of a vertebra to the adjacent vertebra. Pearcy and his associate[45] performed an in vivo motion study of degenerative spondylolisthesis and reported that there is no detectable movement across the segment of the degenerative spondylolisthesis. It is quite common in clinical practice, however, for definitive hypermobility to be detected on flexion and extension roentgenograms of the lumbosacral spine of patients with degenerative spondylolisthesis, especially during the early stage.

It is probable that the end stage of many hypermobile segments reaches static equilibrium between the degenerative and reparative processes. Any disturbances in this equilibrium will result in a dynamic instability with hypermobility. Such unstable hypermobility is frequently observed after decompressive surgery for spinal stenosis caused by degenerative spondylolisthesis.

The term *mechanical low-back pain* was discarded either because it lacks precision in meaning or because it does not describe a verifiable condition. Can any abnormal pattern (erratic motion but within the magnitude of movements that can be detected by conventional evaluation techniques of the lateral flexion-extension roentgenogram) be the cause of pain from the degenerated motion segment? An erratic motion pattern within a motion segment may produce abnormal strain in certain parts of the motion segment without producing hypermobility that can be detected by conventional techniques of lateral flexion-extension roentgenogram. Clinicians have occasionally observed patients with chronic LBP whose symptoms were thought to be due to abnormal movements, although there are no signs of hypermobility and their symptoms are relieved successfully by a spinal fusion procedure alone.

Unfortunately, no reliable technique to diagnose this condition exists. Some clinicians use a conventional trial method of external immobilization of the lumbosacral spine by applying a pantaloon-type cast. This technique is useful but lacks specificity for establishment of nonhypermobile instability. The presence of traction osteophytes was thought to be indicative of segmental instability,[37] but when it becomes significant for production of pair symptoms is not known. I could establish no significant relationship between the size of the traction spur and biomechanical characteristics of the motion segment (kinematic and load-bearing capacity) in a preliminary study on fresh human cadaveric spine. The presence of traction spurs indicates the past biomechanical history of the motion segments, but it does not tell us the current status regarding load-bearing capacity of the motion segment.

Nonhypermobile abnormal motion patterns may be detected by special techniques. A very minute degree of abnormal motion patterns may be detectable by stereophoto-roentgenography, and an erratic motion pattern may be detected by determination of a locus of instantaneous centers of rotation of a motion segment.[20] However, the clinical relevance of these new techniques of detecting fine movement patterns is not established.

Discometric evaluation of the disc can provide useful information concerning the clinical relevance of disc degeneration. The acceptance capacity of volume and pressure increase within a disc, its pain production, and morphologic grading of the disc degeneration can provide us physiologic responses of the disc and their pain production mechanism. Pain from the outer layers of the anulus fibrosus caused by abnormal strain (stretching) due to increased disc volume and/or pressure is probably a good indicator of the structural integrity of the disc, providing that there is a constant relationship between the disc pressure and volume and the anulus strain. As mentioned in the discussion of disc pressure, the responses of the anulus to these tests are probably variable depending on the types of degeneration (solid framework vs. ground substance), leakage of the anulus, and the biomechanical property of scarred outer layers of the anulus fibrosus.

The diagnosis of clinical instability of a spinal motion segment can be established when pain is caused by demonstrable hypermobility. The diagnosis of clinical instability is very difficult to establish when pain is caused by nonhypermobile abnormal motion and/or abnormal biomechanical response of structures to a physiologic loading situation. In this case, the physician may use other criteria based on empirical experiences, traction spur and other roentgenographic findings,[18] discogram, and trial immobilization.

Posterior Spinal Decompression and Spinal Instability

How much of posterior spinal structures can the surgeon remove and yet maintain stability of the motion segment? The question has been asked frequently since the extensive posterior decompressive procedure became popular for the treatment of spinal stenosis.

Posner and associates[46] found that a functional spinal motion segment failed under simulated flexion loading conditions when all the posterior components plus one anterior component had been destroyed during laboratory testing on fresh human cadaveric spines. This suggests that no immediate disastrous instability of a motion segment will result when all posterior structures are surgically removed as long as the anterior structures have normal biomechanical load-bearing functions. Two unknown factors for the postdecompression instability in clinical practice are structural integrity of the anterior structures (amounts of degenerative and reparative processes) and fatigue behavior of the anterior structures with increased stress by removal of posterior structures.

The incidence of post-decompression spondylolisthesis is reported to be 2% among 182 patients reviewed by White and Wiltse[58] and 10% among 59 patients reviewed by Shenkin and Hash.[51] In a study group of patients with no preoperative evidence of olisthesis, the postdecompression incidence of olisthesis was 3.7%.[33] Progressive spondylolisthesis after decompressive laminectomy in those patients with preoperative degenerative spondylolisthesis was observed in all cases. The two most important factors for stability after posterior decompression are the extent of decompression in width and the functional integrity of the other remaining structures.

Incremental loss of functional stability of a spinal motion segment can be expected when more posterior spinal structures are surgically removed. Clinical experience[11,33] suggests that no gross instability is expected when a less than bilateral one-half facetectomy is performed on a motion segment provided that the anterior spinal structures are able to provide a relatively normal load-bearing function. However, it is not known whether the increased stress on the anulus fibrosus and posterior longitudinal ligament by loss of posterior supporting structures can produce nociceptive irritation without detectable gross instability. Fractures of pars interarticularis or the inferior articular process have been observed[11] in those patients who were treated with bilateral medial one-half process fracture, indicating stress concentration of the remaining structures. Multilevel decompression was reported to have a higher incidence of post-compression olisthesis,[49] but the true incidence rate per level is not clearly known. Four levels of decompression will have approximately a four times higher incidence rate of post-decompression olisthesis, but the per level incidence rate will be constant. There is no clear biomechanical understanding of how multiple levels of decompression will affect one level within the multiply decompressed levels, in comparison to one level of decompression alone.

The determination of functional integrity of the anterior structure is very difficult (see the discussion on segmental instability). The normal disc height of the motion segment to be decompressed was considered to be a contributing factor for postdecompression olisthesis.[58] The normal height of the disc space does not always mean that the disc has normal load-bearing capacity. I have found no consistent relationship between the disc height and the incidence of post-decompression olisthesis. Narrow disc space with exuberant osteophyte formation may be indicative of reparative effects. The literature indicates that these patients with sufficient preoperative amounts of reparative processes with self-stabilizing segmental instability will most probably have further instability after a posterior decompressive procedure. Spinal fusion with internal stabilization may be necessary in these cases.

Post-decompression spinal instability can be expected in the following circumstances: (1) the presence of preoperative segmental instability (either static or dynamic hypermobility, and pain by abnormal biomechanics of the motion segment even in the absence of gross hypermobility) and (2) posterior decompression involving more than bilateral one-half facetectomies and disc excision combined with extensive posterior decompression.

Biomechanics of Spinal Fusion

The rationale for spinal fusion procedures for treatment of LBP was based on the thought that painful symptoms can be relieved by elimination of the degenerated or unstable spinal motion segment by fusion. Some authors[8,17] reported that spinal fusion offered few benefits in the management of lumbar disc disease. Spinal fusion, however, has become important for the treatment of LBP. The effectiveness of spinal fusion for LBP can be measured on the parameters of relief of the pain symptoms, achievement of stabilization of the fused segments, and the incidence of adverse effects. Failure of pain relief by spinal fusion may be from several sources: (1) poor indication, (2) failure of stabilization of the fused segments, and (3) complications of fusion.

A poor indication for spinal fusion is probably the most common cause for poor results. The best indication for spinal fusion is clinical spinal instability due to degeneration, trauma, or surgical decompression. In all of these cases the achievement of successful spinal fusion is usually difficult because of the presence of inherent instability and abnormal shear stress across the segment to be fused. Other indications of spinal fusion for idiopathic LBP are poor, such as for herniated disc or chronic LBP without localizing signs and recurrent disc herniation without signs of clinical instability. Spinal fusion is occasionally well indicated even with no definitive hypermobility on flexion-extension lateral roentgenogram of the lumbosacral spine, when there is sufficient indirect evidence of spinal instability identified by physical examination, plain x-ray films, and discographic examination.[12]

Failure to achieve adequate stabilization of the segments to be fused is another important source for poor results. The inadequate stabilization may be due to failure of fusion (pseudoarthrosis) or inadequate mechanical support by the fusion mass. Pseudoarthrosis has been considered generally to be a leading cause for poor results, although its significance for persistent symptoms after spinal fusion has been questioned.[50] The two most common causes for pseudoarthrosis are (1) the presence of preexisting instability with a significant amount of shear stress across the segment to be fused and (2) inadequate technique. The successful achievement of spinal fusion in cases with grossly hypermobile degenerative spondylolisthesis is often very difficult, unless the abnormal shear stress of the segment is neutralized with either an internal or external immobilization or fixation system. The common technical errors responsible for pseudoarthrosis are inadequate preparation of the graft bed (insufficient amount of graft bed or inadequate decortication) and poor availability of the graft material (inadequate amount, poor osteogenic or osteoconductive graft).

Inadequate mechanical support by the fusion mass may result in continuous motion of the diseased parts within the fused segments and may produce persistent symptoms. The posterior spinal fusion is observed to allow a significant amount of

detectable motion across the disc of the same segment under compression and torsional loadings.[36,39] Both the anterior fusion and bilateral lateral intertransverse processes fusion provide adequate stabilizing efforts on the segment to be fused.[36,49]

Complications of lumbosacral spinal fusion are spondylolysis acquisita and spinal stenosis. The incidence of postfusion spinal stenosis has ranged from 11% to 41%.[6,38] The most common type of postfusion spinal stenosis is associated with posterior spinal fusion and is usually found within the fused segment. However, I find that posterior fusion also causes a high incidence of spinal stenosis at the adjacent free level. Postfusion stenosis and spondylolysis acquisita at the level above the fusion segments (juxtafused) are indicative of clinical manifestations of abnormal stress increase at the juxtafused level. Biomechanical fusion studies on fresh human cadaveric spines and mathematic analysis of the stress redistribution due to various types of spinal fusion procedures revealed abnormal stress concentration at the juxtafused segment after all types of fusion procedures.[36] Posterior fusion gave highest abnormal stress at the juxtafree segment, especially about the facet joints.

Internal Fixation of the Lumbosacral Spine

The internal fixation system is used during the surgical treatment of LBP to prevent or correct deformity such as spondylolisthetic slip and to neutralize normal shear stress across the segment to fuse and to achieve solid fusion.

Because of the anatomic arrangement of the greater vessels anterior to the lumbosacral spine, most of internal fixation systems are designed for posterior spinal fixation. The use of the internal fixation system for the lumbosacral spine has not been popular until recently, because the lumbosacral joints are highly mobile joints with high stress and also because of shorts-segments fixation, problems of secure fixation of the device to the sacrum, and the lumbosacral angle.

Various types of internal fixation systems have been used for lumbosacral spinal fusion: Harrington rods, Knodt rods, Luque rods, Luque rectangular rods, Harrington rods with sublaminar wiring, and a few systems using bone screws with plates, rods, or cables.

Harrington rods are biomechanically unstable systems in flexion and torsion, and they cannot be readily contoured for the lumbrosacral angle.[23] The sacral hooks for Harrington rods or Knodt rods are not well tolerated and often cause painful symptoms under high stress. The Knodt rods system provides very poor stabilization in flexion and poor torsion.[1,23,35] Although the posterior Harrington distraction rods and Knodt rods can provide flexion posture of the lumbosacral spine, clinical evidence of benefit is doubtful.[34] For a short-segment fusion at the lumbosacral junction, it is very important to maintain the proper lumbosacral angle to minimize untoward effects on the juxtafused free segments. The Luque rectangular system with sublaminar wiring or wiring around transverse processes or with bone screws provides much more stable fixation and provides better clinical results.[23,32] Other systems using bone screws with plates or rods (Zielke, Steffee, and Wiltse) can also provide more rigid internal fixation.

The use of rigid fixation systems for spinal fusion is best indicated when any significant amount of posterior decompression is contemplated on the segment with preoperative gross instability. In such cases successful achievement of solid fusion becomes very difficult because of increased instability and reduced graft bed size due to decompression. Failure to obtain solid fusion after repeated bone grafting for pseudoarthrosis is an additional indication for the use of internal fixation devices. Another indication is correction (reduction) of deformities caused by trauma or degeneration. Although the rigid fixation of a short segment can provide good stabilization of the segment to be fused, it can also produce increased untoward effects on the juxtafused segment. Only prudent indications of various internal fixation systems can provide the maximal benefit of stabilization and minimal adverse effects.

References

1. August AC and others: A bimechanical comparison of methods of posterior fixation in lumbosacral spine fusion. Transactions of the Thirty-First Annual Meeting, *Orthop Res Soc* 10:333, 1985.
2. Ayers CE: Further case studies of lumbosacral pathology with considerations of the involvement of the intervertebral discs and facets, *N Engl J Med* 213:713, 1935.
3. Barr JS: Low back and sciatic pain: results and treatment, *J Bone Joint Surg* 33A:633, 1951.
4. Barr JS: Ruptured intervertebral disc and sciatic pain, *J Bone Joint Surg* 29:429, 1947.
5. Brailsford JF: Deformities of the lumbosacral region of the spine, *Br J Surg* 16:562, 1928-1929.
6. Brodsky AE: Post-laminectomy and post-laminectomy and post-fusion stenosis of the lumbar spine, *Clin Orthop* 115:130, 1970.
7. Brown T and others: Some mechanical tests on the lumbosacral spine with particular reference to the intervertebral disc, *J Bone Joint Surg* 39A:1135, 1957.
8. Caldwell GA, Sheppard WB: Criteria for spinal fusion following removal of protruded nuclear pulposus, *J Bone Joint Surg* 39A:1971, 1948.
9. Chandler FA: Spinal fusion operations in the treatment of low back and sciatic pain, *JAMA* 93:1447, 1929.
10. Danforth MS, Wilson PD: The anatomy of lumbosacral region in relation to sciatic pain, *J Bone Joint Surg* 6:109, 1925.
11. Farfan H: The pathological anatomy of degenerative spondylolistheses: a cadaver study, *Spine* 5:412, 1980.
12. Farfan H: *The use of mechanical etiology to determine the efficacy of active intervention in single joint lumbar intervertebral joint problems: surgery and chemonucleolysis compared,* Unpublished manuscript, 1986.
13. Farfan HF and others: The effects of torsion on the lumbar intervertebral joints: the role of torsion in the production of disc degeneration, *J Bone Joint Surg* 52A:468, 1970.
14. Ferguson A: The clinical and roentgenographic interpretation of lumbosacral anomalies, *Radiology* 22:548, 1934.
15. Friberg S, Hirsch C: Anatomical and clinical studies on lumbar disc degeneration, *Acta Orthop Scand* 19:222, 1950.
16. Frymoyer JW and others: Disc excision and spine fusion in the management of lumbar disc disease: a minimum ten-year follow-up, *Spine* 3:1, 1978.
17. Frymoyer JW: The role of spine fusion: question 3, *Spine* 6:248, 1981.
18. Fung YB: Biomechanics: its scope, history and some problems of centenuum mechanics in physiology, *Appl Mech Rev* 21:1, 1968.
19. Galante JL: Tensile properties of the human lumbar annulus fibrosus, *Acta Orthop Scand Suppl* 100, 1967.
20. Gertzbein SD and others: Determination of a locus of instantaneous center of rotation of the lumbar disc by Moire fringes: a new technique, *Spine* 9:409, 1984.
21. Ghormley RK and others: The combined operation in low back and sciatic pain, *JAMA* 120:1171, 1942.
22. Goldworth JE: The lumbosacral articulation: an explanation of many cases of lumbago, ischias and paraplegia, *Boston Med Surg J* 164:365, 1911.
23. Guyer D and others: *Biomechanical comparison of seven internal fixation devices for the lumbosacral junction.* Paper presented to the second NASA meeting, Laguna Niguel, Calif., July 25-27, 1985.
24. Hibbs R, Swift W: Development abnormalities at the lumbosacral juncture causing pain and disability (a report of 147 patients treated by the spine fusion operation), *Surg Gynecol Obstet* 48:604, 1929.
25. Hirsch C: Studies on the mechnism of low back pain, *Acta Orthop Scand* 20:261, 1951.
26. Hirsch C, Naehemson A: New observations on the mechanical behavior of lumbar discs, *Acta Orthop Scand* 23:254, 1954.
27. Hirsch C and others: Biophysical and physiological investigation on cartilage and other mesenchymal tissues. Vl. Characteristics of human nuclei pulposi during aging, *Acta Orthop Scand* 22:179, 1952.

28. Hoag JM and others: Kinematic analysis and classification of vertebral motion, *J Am Osteopath Assoc* 59:899, 982, 1960.

29. Key AJ, Ford LT: Experimental intervertebral disc lesion, *J Bone Joint Surg* 30A:621, 1948.

30. Kimberly AG: Low back pain and sciatica, *Surg Gynecol Obstet* 65:195, 1937.

31. Knutsson F: The instability associated with disc degeneration in the lumbar spine, *Acta Radiologica* 25:593, 1944.

32. Lee CK: *A clinical comparison study for internal fixation systems for lumbosacral spinal stenosis.* Paper presented at the Annual Meeting of the International Society for the Study of the Lumbar Spine, Dallas, May 29-June 1, 1985.

33. Lee CK: Lumbar spinal instability (olisthesis) after extensive posterior spinal decompression, *Spine* 8:429, 1983.

34. Lee CK, DeBari A: Lumbosacral spinal fusion with Knodt distraction rods, *Spine* 11:373, 1986.

35. Lee CK Langrana NA: *Biomechanical study of the Knodt rods in fresh human cadaveric lumbosacral spines,* Unpublished manuscript.

36. Lee CK, Langrana NA: Lumbosacral spinal fusion: a biomechanical study, *Spine* 9:574, 1984.

37. MacNab I: The traction spur: an indicator of segmental instability, *J Bone Joint Surg* 53:663, 1971.

38. MacNab I Dall D: The blood supply of the lumbar spine and its application to the technique of intertransverse lumbar fusion, *J Bone Joint Surg* 53B:130, 1970.

39. Markoff KL, and Morris JM: Structural component of the intervertebral disc, *J Bone Joint Surg* 56A:675, 1974.

40. Mixter WJ, Barr JS: Rupture of the intervertebral disc with involvement of the spinal canal, *N Engl J Med* 211:210, 1934.

41. Morgan FP, King T: Primary instability of lumbar vertebrae as a common cause of low back pain, *J Bone Joint Surg* 39B:6, 1957.

42. Nachemson A: Lumbar intradiscal pressure: experimental studies on postmortem material, *Acta Orthop Scand Suppl* 43, 1960.

43. Nachemson A and others: In-vitro diffusion of dye through the end plate and the annulus of human lumbar intervertebral disc, *Acta Orthrop Scand* 41:589, 1970.

44. Overton LJ: Arthrodesis of the lumbosacral spine (a study of end results), *Clin Orthop* 5:97, 1955.

45. Pearcy M, Sheperd J: Is there instability in spondylolisthesis? *Spine* 10:175, 1985.

46. Posner I and others: A biomechanical analysis of the clinical stability of the lumbar and lumbosacral spine, *Spine* 7:374, 1982.

47. Puschel J: Der wssergehald normalerr und degenerieter zweischenwirbel scheiben, *Bietr Path Anat* 84:123, 1930 (quoted by Galante).

48. Putli V: New conceptions in the pathogenesis of sciatic pain, *Lancet* 2:53, 1927.

49. Tollander SD: Motion of the spine with special reference to stabilizing effect of posterior fusion, *Acta Orthop Scand Suppl* 90, 1966.

50. Rothman RH, Booth R: Failure of spinal fusion, *Orthop Clin North Am* 6:299, 1975.

51. Shenkin HA, Hash CJ: Spondylolisthesis after multiple bilateral laminectomies and facetectomies for lumbar spondylosis: follow-up review, *J Neurosurg* 50:45, 1979.

52. Spurling RG, Grantham EG: Ruptured lumbar discs in lower lumbar region, *Am J Surg* 75:140, 1948.

53. Unander-Scharin L: On low back pain with special reference to the vlue of operative treatment with fusion, *Acta Orthop Scand Suppl* 5, 1950.

54. Unander-Scharin L: Spinal fusion in low back pain, *Acta Orthop Scand* 20:335, 1951.

55. Virgin W: Experimental investigation into the physical properties of the intervertebral disc, *J Bone Joint Surg* 33B:607, 1951.

56. Wagner LC: Congenital defects of the lumbosacral joints with associated nerve symptoms, *Am J Surg* 27:311, 1935.

57. White AA Panjabi MM: *Clinical biomechanics of the spine,* Philadelphia, 1978, J.B. Lippincott.

58. White AH, Wiltse LL: *Spondylolisthesis after extensive lumbar laminectomy.* Paper presented at the Forty-Third Annual Meeting of the American Academy of Orthopaedic Surgeons, New Orleans, February 1976.

59. Wu HC, Yao RF: Mechanical behavior of the human annulus fibrosus, *J Biomech* 9:127, 1976.

60. Young HH, Walsh AC: *Combined operation for low back and sciatic pain: follow-up study,* Collected papers of the Mayo Clinic and Mayo Foundation, 39:475, 1948.

61. Young HH and others: Low back and sciatic pain: long term results after removal of protruded intervertebral disc with or without fusion, *Clin Orthop* 5:128, 1955.

62. Zie N: Load capacity of the low back, *J Oslo City Hosp* 16:75, 1966.

Chapter 62
Osteoporosis of the Spine and Its Management

Alexander G. Hadjipavlou

Philip H. Lander

The Magnitude of the Problem

Classification and Etiology of Osteoporosis

Decay of the Skeleton

Pathophysiology of Bone Mass Reduction

Pathology

Biomechanics

Clinical Presentation

Laboratory Assessment

> radiography
> densitometry
> ultrasonography

Management of Osteoporosis

> prevention
> surgical treatment
> management of back pain

It is ironic that advances in medicine make it possible to prolong life, yet as we grow older, our skeleton decays and its medical rejuvenation is still beyond our reach. Our bones do not have a "lifetime guarantee" as we age; therefore, despite an increased life span, we are unable to preserve our skeletal mass for our golden age. Osteoporosis is an age-related disorder, defined by the National Institutes of Health (NIH) Consensus Conference[152] as decreased bone mass and increased susceptibility to fractures in the absence of other recognizable causes of bone loss. A reduction in bone mass denotes osteopenia, which is frequently but not always equivalent to osteoporosis. According to Frost[64,65,67,68,70] osteoporosis can be defined as an absolute decrease in the amount of bone mass (osteopenia), associated with a skeletal biomechanical incompetence, leading to fracture after minimal trauma. Ostopenia is the result of defective remodeling units in which there is predominance of bone resorption over reformation, leading to a net decreased bone mass, producing a weaker skeleton. Biomechanical incompetence is defined by Frost[67] as the accumulation of mechanical micro damage from normal daily biomechanical demands, the repair of which is retarded by defects in basic multicellular unit (BMU) remodeling. This microdamage consists of a fatigue-like process in both compact and cancellous osteopenic bone,[14,39,64,67,69] analogous to the micro-cracks that occur in any structural material subjected to repetitive loading. These microscopic cracks in bone have been demonstrated *in vivo*.[1,69,70] The BMUs normally repair this bone micro-damage. However, defective remodeling units allow the micro damage to accumulate and propagate to the point that bone fails under trivial loading, resulting in fractures (disease osteoporosis). The remodeling units in osteoporosis are characterized by slow and prolonged cycles, which are unable to keep pace with the propagation of micro-damages incurred every day by physical activity.[66] According to Frost, remodeling normally lasts 3 to 4 months. In osteoporosis, this value may range from 2 to 4 years.[105]

The Magnitude of the Problem

Osteoporosis is considered to be one of today's most serious public health problems; this can best be seen by quoting some pertinent statistics. In the United States, $6.1 billion are spent annually for osteoporosis-related problems,[96] and if loss of productivity is included in these figures, the cost rises to about $10 billion. Approximately 20 million Americans suffer from osteoporosis (National Osteoporosis Foundation). About 1.2 million fractures are caused directly or indirectly by osteoporosis annually in the United States; of these, 538,000 cases occur in the vertebrae (44.8%), 225,000 in the hip (18.9%), 172,000 in the distal forearm (14.3%), and 283,000 in other sites (23.5%).[109,167] It is estimated that over 5 million Caucasian women in the U.S. have one or more vertebral fractures,[109,133] and of this number, 83,000 patients with vertebral fracture are treated medically each year.[96] Vertebral fractures from osteoporosis are probably at least 10 times as common in women as they are in men. Epidemiologic studies in the U.S. reveal that 18% of women over 50 years of age, and 27% of women over 65 years of age, have one or more vertebral fractures.[130,131] This suggests that one of every three women over the age of 65 may be expected to have a vertebral fracture.[167] It has been reported that crushed vertebrae occur in 6.6% of women over the age of 68 in the United States[59]; this occurs in 4% of women over the age of 60, and 8% over the age of 80 in Great Britain.[40,72] More than 40 million American women are menopausal, and an additional 35 million women will be reaching the climacteric during the next decade. These women have a life expectancy of 30 years after menopause.[177] Therefore, osteoporosis will be a significant cause of morbidity and mortality in the elderly, and as the population of the U.S. becomes older, the magnitude of the problem will become greater.

Classification and Etiology of Osteoporosis

Osteoporosis can be classified as either primary (evolutional osteoporosis) or secondary. The most common type of osteoporosis is evolutional or primary osteoporosis which, according to Riggs and Melton,[166,167] has been subdivided into two types: Type I and Type II. Type I, or postmenopausal, osteoporosis occurs in females aged 51 to 75 years old. Estrogen deficiency has been implicated as the primary causative factor. It affects mainly trabecular bone and is characterized by vertebral and Colles' fractures. Parathyroid function is not increased. Type II, or senile, osteoporosis is age-related and is seen in both women and men over the age of 70 and affects both cortical and cancellous bone. The pathogenesis of this disorder is attributable to aging, chronic calcium deficiency, estrogen deficiency, decreased vitamin D activity, increased parathyroid hormone production, and other genetic and environmental factors. It is characterized by fractures of the hip, pelvis, proximal humerus, and proximal tibia. This difference in the two types of osteoporosis has been confirmed by Härmä and associates,[87] who observed that in postmenopausal osteoporosis the degree of osteopenia in the spine is disproportionate to, and more extensive than, the osteopenia of the hips. Additionally, there is a tendency for increased bone turnover in these patients, as opposed to postmenopausal patients suffering from fractures of the appendicular skeleton. These studies support the view that spinal osteoporosis and osteoporosis of the hip may be two different forms of osteoporosis.

Several factors predispose a person to osteoporosis, and these can be considered in the appropriate clinical setting as "risk factors" to identify potential osteoporotic patients, as seen in the boxed material. Consumption of alcohol predisposes to osteoporosis[42,95,140] by directly depressing osteoblastic activity.[20] There is a higher incidence of osteoporotic hip and spinal fractures among smokers. Smoking may increase the risk of osteoporosis by enhancing the degradation of estrogen[47,209,210] or by decreasing calcium absorption.[110] Caffeine has also been shown to increase the risk of osteoporotic fractures in middle-age women.[95] Lack of exercise and decreased physical activity also predispose to osteopenia.[113] Calcium deficiency,[123,141] lactase deficiency with calcium malabsorption,[21] and decreased calcium absorption after gastrectomy[71] lead to loss of bone mass. The inhabitants of communities with a high calcium intake have a lower incidence of fractures and higher bone mass than those of similar communities with a lower calcium intake.[123]

Decay of the Skeleton

In the period between birth and skeletal maturity, factors such as heredity, nutrition, sex, physical activity, race, and toxic-metabolic elements have a large role in determining bone mass, which peaks about the third decade. It has been demonstrated that blacks[196] have a larger bone mass at maturity than whites. After the fourth decade, bone loss is continuous throughout life. This loss of cortical bone has been estimated at approximately 0.3% to 0.5% per year for both men and women. At menopause, women exhibit an accelerated cortical bone loss at the rate of 2% to 3% per year, which lasts about 10 years.[121,124,164,187] Accelerated bone loss has also been observed in men after 68 years of age.[197] More recently it has been shown that after menopause compact bone is lost at the rate of 1% to 3% annually.[58] The annual bone loss at the mid-radius is approximately 1.63% and at the ultradistal radius

Risk Factors for Osteoporosis

- Women
- Caucasian or Asian
- Early menopause
- Sedentary lifestyle
- Nutritional factors
    Lactose intolerance, low calcium
    High intake of protein, alcohol, caffeine, phosphate
- Underweight
- Cigarette smoking
- Family history of osteoporosis
- Blonde or red hair, freckles
- Steroid therapy
- ?Scoliosis
- ?Hypermobility, poor teeth, easy bruisability
- Gastric or small bowel resection
- Thyrotoxicosis
- Long-term glucocorticoid therapy
- Hyperparathyroidism
- Long-term anticonvulsant therapy

(Modified from Riggs BL, Melton LJ: Involutional osteoporosis, N Engl J Med 26:1676, 1986.)

1.0%.[81] Sowers and colleagues[190] confirmed these findings by showing that 65% of women may lose in excess of 1% of radial bone mineral density (BMD) as measured by single-photon absorptiometry, whereas 30% of women may lose at least 2% of BMD per year. In postmenopausal women, the mean rate of trabecular bone loss is approximately 5% to 8% per year, but after 10 to 15 years the rate of bone loss decreases to premenopausal levels.[58,111]

Pathophysiology of Bone Mass Reduction

An inadequate supply of building material to the skeleton, such as calcium or collagen, or loss of building material (calcium, protein, etc.), has a negative influence on bone mass. In addition, osteoporosis is affected not only by abnormal calcium kinetics such as an insufficient calcium supply and loss of skeletal calcium secondary to hormonal or vitamin factors, but also by abnormalities of the remodeling units. The rate of bone turnover is determined by the frequency of activation of newborn remodeling units. Defects in the remodeling units with uncoupling can increase the osteoclast resorption phase over the osteoblast formation phase, leading to loss of bone mass.

Apart from gonadal deficiency, the actual role of calciotropic hormones and their relationship to estrogen in the production of primary osteoporosis is still not clear. After menopause, serum estradiol levels fall from 120 pg/ml to 14 pg/ml. Estrogen deficiency leads to an increase in bone turnover, with resorption dominating over formation (at least a twofold increase in bone turnover follows estrogen deficiency) as measured by histomorphometric studies.[10] Each cycle of remodeling activity after menopause puts back less bone than it takes out, resulting in decreased bone mass. The total annual bone loss (both cancellous and cortical) with estrogen deficiency is about 2% to 3% for 6 to 10 years.[125] Gnudi and colleagues[81] compared bone loss among three groups of patients: ovariectomized patients, patients with natural menopause, and patients with normal ovarian function. They concluded that estrogen deficiency is the principal factor responsible for 52.5% to 66.4% of bone mineral loss, with the remaining amount being attributable to causes related to aging. Estrogen may exert a tonic inhibitory effect on the skeletal action of parathormone.[90,91] Estrogen deficiency therefore makes the bone more sensitive to the resorbogenic effect of parathyroid hormone. Estrogen deficiency may also impair the 1-hydroxylation of vitamin D in the kidney[193] by not stimulating 1-hydroxylase, to convert 25-hydroxyvitamin D_3 (25-OH-D) to $1,25(OH)_2D$ and also lead to decreased vitamin D levels. Impaired renal function associated with aging is another factor that fails to promote the conversion of vitamin 25(OH)D to $1,25(OH)_2D$. Serum levels of $1,25(OH)_2D$ are decreased by about 50% with aging.[13,73,198] Postmenopausal women also show a rise in renal tubular resorption of plasma levels of inorganic phosphate,[149] which is reversible with estrogen administration. This hyperphosphatemia, in turn, may inhibit 1,25-dihydroxyvitamin D synthesis. The reduced levels of vitamin D lead to decreased intestinal absorption of calcium and renal resorption of calcium, which result in low serum calcium levels. This in turn will stimulate the production of parathyroid hormone, which promotes bone resorption and loss of skeletal mass. Serum levels of immunoreactive parathyroid hormones have been shown to increase with age,[51,101] as does the level of urinary and nephrogenous cyclic AMP,[51,101,122] reflecting the biologic action of parathormone. However, no clear distinction exists between osteoporotic patients and controls.[78] Ten percent of osteoporotic patients have secondary hyperparathyroidism, according to Riggs and co-workers.[172]

High phosphorus intake in man[162] and in animals[108] results in a rise in serum phosphate, a fall in ionized calcium, and an increase in serum parathyroid hormone. The rate of bone loss is greater in omnivores than in ovo-lacto-vegetarians, who avoid meat, which is the main source of dietary phosphate.[56] Calcitonin acts on bone by opposing the activity of parathyroid hormone, thus inhibiting osteoclastic activity and bone resorption. For this reason calcitonin deficiency has also been implicated in the development of osteoporosis.[77] Decreased levels of calcitonin have been found in the elderly,[50] in normal women,[50,92] and in oophorectomized women,[184] and increased levels have been demonstrated with estrogen therapy.[184] Calcitonin deficiency has been implicated as a causative factor in osteoporosis[128] because patients who underwent total thyroidectomy and who were presumably calcitonin-deficient had lower bone density than controls. Thus, calcitonin and estrogen may be linked in the pathogenesis of osteoporosis. Calcitonin may be considered as a mediator of estrogen action on bone.[77] However, the role of calcitonin in the development of osteoporosis in postmenopausal women has also been questioned.[22,195]

Pathology

Examination of sections of osteoporotic vertebrae reveals a definite pattern of atrophy. The horizontal trabeculae are strikingly deficient, whereas there is a tendency for preservation of vertically oriented trabeculae. Evidence of vertebral trabecular micro fractures and healing micro fractures have been reported in cadaver spines. Nodular enlargements were found on the vertically oriented trabeculae, especially adjacent to the end plates, suggesting that the propagation of fracture starts from the end plates. With aging, the degree of osteopenia is greater and micro fractures are found more frequently.[200]

Biomechanics

Bone mineral density is important in the strength of the vertebral body. It has been shown that reduction of mineral density to one third of normal reduces compressive strength of the vertebral body to one ninth of normal, whereas reduction of bone mineral density to one half of normal brings about reduction of compressive strength to one quarter of normal.[85] The mineral content in the more cephalad vertebrae is less than that of the more caudad-placed vertebrae, which predisposes these vertebrae to fractures.[85] Vertebrae with relatively high bone mineral content are more prone to central compression fractures, whereas wedge compression fractures have a predilection to occur in vertebrae with low mineral content.[86]

Clinical Presentation

According to Frost,[65,68,70] an acute fracture in the lower thoracic spine is associated with severe regional pain that usually lasts 3 to 4 weeks. This results in accentuation of the patient's thoracic kyphosis, compensated a few months later by increased lumbar lordosis, which alters the spinal biomechanics and induces low-back pain, most likely of facetogenic origin. This cascade of events lasts about 9 months, after which the patient becomes asymptomatic. Osteoporosis per se does not predispose to back pain before the age of 80.[61] However, the prevalence of back pain was greater (50%) in women who lost over 2 cm of height than in those (20%) who lost less than 2 cm of height, a statistically significant difference ($p < 0.001$). Stooping of the back, which reflects mainly compression fracture, also predisposes to back pain (54.2%) compared with a straight back (24.5%). Previous observations have suggested that spinal deformity caused by osteoporosis is a contributory factor to back pain. A past history of hip fracture or Colles' fracture has no correlation with osteoporotic back pain.[61] The clinical picture of osteoporosis was also studied by Patel and associates,[151] who found that after an acute fracture pain radiated into the flank or anteriorly in the majority of patients (66%). Radiation of pain into the lower extremities was rare and was reported in 6% of patients. Other associated symptoms were nausea (26%), abdominal pain (20%), chest pain (30%), and strain exacerbated pain (60%). Positions that improved pain were recumbency (43%), sitting (36%), and standing and walking (16%). Although back pain in osteoporotic patients has been theoretically attributed to micro fractures, it has been shown that sudden and severe fractures can produce pain, whereas gradual fractures may remain asymptomatic. This finding suggests that micro-fractures, when they occur, might not be a contributory factor to pain.[200] There is no scientific clinical data to support micro fractures as the cause of back pain, and therefore, the concept of micro fractures as the origin of back pain is not proven, except in severe osteopenia and after the age of 80.

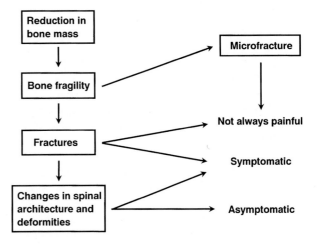

Fig. 62-1
Model of pain in osteoporosis.

A reduction in bone mass is not always painful, although this reduction in bone mass may lead to bone fragility, predisposing to painful or even asymptomatic (silent) fractures. Bone fragility and fractures may culminate in spinal structural changes that can become so severe as to be almost indistinguishable from idiopathic scoliosis.[89] These structural changes may then predispose these patients to mechanical low-back pain that will be unresponsive to osteoporotic drug treatment (Fig. 62-1).

Laboratory Assessment

Osteoporosis is the result of heterogeneous pathologic conditions, and investigation should aim at detecting the primary cause. Figure 62-2 is a flow chart outlining the various tests to investigate the origin of osteoporosis and to assess the severity of the osteopenic condition and its resulting structural changes.

According to Baillie and associates,[16] an underlying cause of osteoporosis was found in 54% of vertebral fractures in men, and therefore, an appropriate investigation should be carried out in these patients. Osteoporosis was secondary to hypogonadism with low levels of testosterone in 16% of these patients, and neoplastic disease was found in 9% of patients. Osteoporotic pathologic fractures were attributed to malabsorption secondary to gastrectomy (1%), to steroid therapy (13%), or to a combination of factors contributing to osteoporosis (10%). Alcoholism should also be suspected in this situation and was actually present in 6% of their cases.

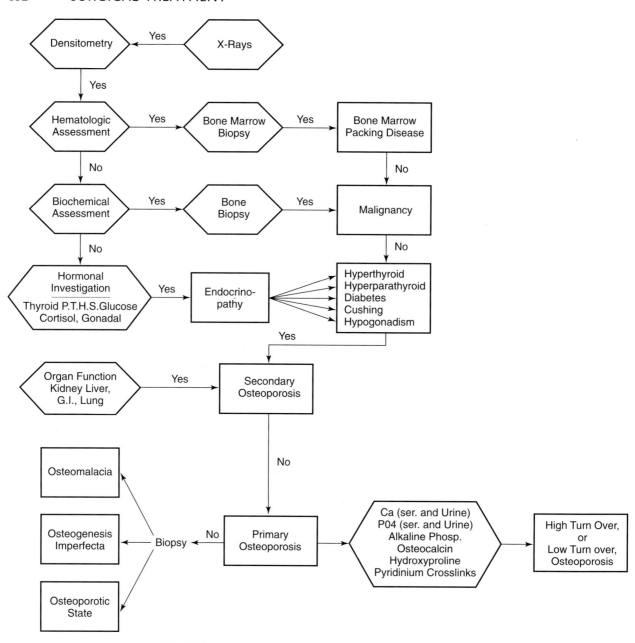

Fig. 62-2

Algorithm to determine origin and severity of osteopenic condition.

Radiography

Radiography is a poor indicator of bone density, since the apparent density may be influenced by a number of technical factors. However, morphometric radiographic studies are important in evaluating the spine when looking for early structural changes caused by osteopenia (disease osteoporosis), and baseline data should be obtained for later comparison. Biconcavity and wedging of the vertebrae can be assessed on lateral films of the thoracic and lumbar spine, and lat-

eral films should be taken as a baseline during the initial evaluation of the patient at risk for vertebral fracture, and at 12-month intervals thereafter. According to Gallagher and associates[74] both the anterior and posterior height of the normal vertebral body increases from T3 to L3, with a mean increase in anterior height of 1 mm from T3 to T8 and 1.2 mm from T8 to L3. In the thoracic spine the anterior height of the vertebral body is about 10% less than the posterior height, whereas the height of the bodies of L3 and L4 are the same, and at L5 the ante-

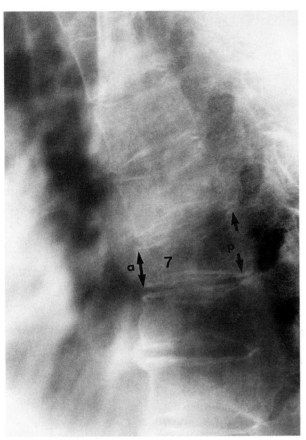

Fig. 62-3

Lateral radiograph of the thoracic spine. There is a wedge fracture of the body of T7 with the ratio of anterior height of the body (a) to the posterior height (p) equal to 0.6. Osteoporosis is present if the ratio is less than 0.8.

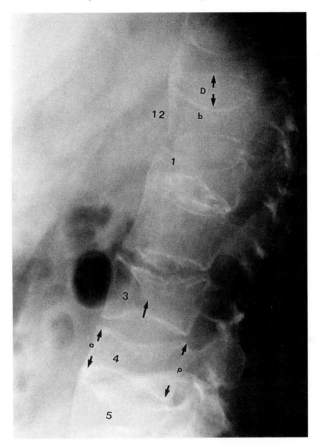

Fig. 62-4

Lateral radiograph of the lumbar spine. The body of T12 has a biconcave configuration with increased disc space height. The ratio of the disc height (D) to the adjacent vertebral body height (b) is 0.7. Osteoporosis is present if the ratio is ≥ 0.4. Note the inferior end-plate fracture of L1, the superior end-plate fracture of L3, as well as an anterior wedge fracture of L4 and a posterior wedge fracture of L5. The ratio of the anterior to the posterior height of the body of L4 = 0.7.

rior height is greater than the posterior height. These measurements of vertebral height include the articular facet of the rib. According to Davies and co-workers,[48] the posterior height of L4 is smaller than the posterior height of the L3 vertebral body. The lower limits of the difference between the anterior height of the vertebral body and the posterior height are 18% for the upper thoracic spine and 25% for the midthoracic spine (Fig. 62-3).

Vertebral biconcavity is found mainly in the lumbar spine and thoracolumbar region and can be measured as a ratio between the height of the midportion of the vertebral body and the height of the anterior vertebral margin. A ratio of less than 80% is suggestive of osteoporosis.[18] Another sensitive morphometric study is to measure the vertical dimension of the vertebral body and the disc spaces. The height of the disc spaces in the upper lumbar area should not exceed 35% of the height of the adjacent vertebral body.[100] With this method it is possible to predict osteoporosis even if the increased concavity

of the vertebral end plate is not apparent. The diagnosis of osteoporosis is entertained when the vertical measurement of the adjacent intervertebral disc above exceeds 40% of the vertical measurement of the midvertebral body (Fig. 62-4).

Another feature of osteopenia is prominence of the vertebral end plates. This appearance is not just an increased contrast of the end plates caused by resorption of the adjacent trabecular bone, but may also reflect an absolute increase in the mineral content of the cortical bone with aging.[156] Osteophytes are frequently absent,[191] and the vertebral body may demonstrate vertical striations secondary to loss of horizontal trabeculae and preservation of the vertical trabeculae, which may in some instances actually become thicker than normal.[191] A thick dense band of increased horizontal density or pseudocallus adjacent to the fractured end plates caused by persis-

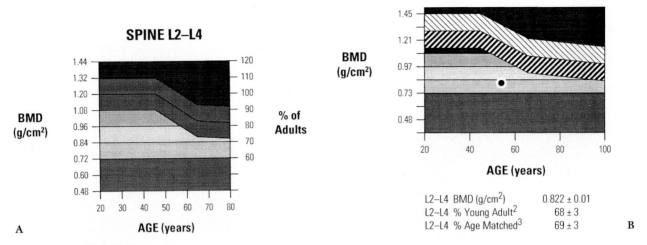

Fig. 62-5

A. Dual energy x-ray absorptiometry (DEXA) of the lumbar spine. This female reference graph demonstrates the bone mineral density (BMD) of the lumbar spine (L2-L4) in g/cm² on the y axis, and age on x axis. Each horizontal bar below the thick horizontal bar at the top of the graph is one standard deviation (S.D.) below the mean for young adults. The thick sloping regression bar is the average value of BMD adjusted for age, height, weight, and race. *(Courtesy of LUNAR Corporation).* **B.** The BMD of this 54-year-old female patient is 0.822 g/cm² (black dot), which is 3 S.D. below the bone density for age-matched and young female patients. This represents a sixfold greater risk of fracture than a young adult female. The percentage young adult value of 68% compares the BMD with the expected peak bone mass for a female 20 to 40 years old. The percentage age-matched value of 69% compares the BMD with the expected values of the same age and sex (represented within the hatched regression bar).

tence of calcified cartilage has been described with Cushing's syndrome.[135] According to Sartoris and colleagues,[178] a concave deformity in the thoracolumbar spine is indicative of benign osteopenia, whereas an angular deformity is more likely to denote an underlying malignancy.

Densitometry

Bone densitometry studies measure the patient's BMD and reflect osseous strength. Densitometry is indicated when osteoporosis is suspected clinically or after morphometric radiographic studies, as well as in high-risk patients who are placed on estrogen replacement therapy and as a base line before any drug therapy for osteoporosis.

Single-Photon Absorptiometry

Single-photon absorptiometry (SPA) measures bone density of the appendicular skeleton and is a good indicator of its cortical bone density, but may not reflect the bone density of the axial skeleton. Single-photon absorptiometry usually measures the distal third of the radius, which is composed of 95% cortical bone and 5% trabecular bone. At this site, the reproducibility error is 2% to 3% and the accuracy is 6%. At the ultradistal radius, the amount of trabecular bone is 40%, but it is sensitive to positioning errors and precision may be poor. Calcaneus measurements reflect 90% to 95% trabecular bone and have been introduced more recently because the calcaneus is a weight-bearing structure. The precision error is about 1% to 2%.[179,189]

Quantitative Computed Tomography

Quantitative computed tomography (QCT) scan selectively measures the trabecular bone density of the lumbar vertebral bodies. It is generally accurate; however, increase in marrow fat can lead to overestimation of bone loss. This can be eliminated by dual energy QCT.[76] Unfortunately, this procedure entails a high radiation dose (50-100 μSv) and is expensive. The precision is 2% to 5% and the accuracy is 5% to 20%.[175]

Dual-Photon Absorptiometry

Dual-photon absorptiometry (DPA) uses radioactive gadolinium as a source to measure bone and soft-tissue densities of the lumbar spine in the antero-posterior plane. The precision error is 2% to 4%, the radiation dose is 2 to 5 MREM, and the scan time is 30 minutes.[54] The radioactive source has been recently superseded by low-energy x-ray tube (dual-energy x-ray absorptiometry—DPX, DXA, or DEXA). The scan time is reduced to less than 10 minutes, radiation dose to 1 MREM, and precision error to 1% to 2% with an accuracy of 3% to 5%. The DEXA may give false high values of bone mineral concentration when vertebral osteophytes or a calcified aorta is present. This can be eliminated by obtaining a DEXA of the vertebral body in the lateral plane or the total body BMD.[81a]

The BMD is expressed in g/cm² and reflects both cancellous and cortical bone. Figure 62-5, *A* represents a female reference graph of normative DEXA values of BMD of the lumbar spine at L2-L4 (courtesy of Lunar Corp.). The thick horizontal bar at the top of the graph represents the range of BMD values for a young adult. Each horizontal bar below the young adult value reflects a 10% change in BMD below the mean and is approximately 1 standard deviation (S.D.) for the anteroposterior spine. A reduction of 1 S.D. doubles the fracture risk. The thick sloping lines represent the age-matched regression bar, with the middle of the bar marking the average BMD value and the area above and below the middle line indicating 1 S.D. above and below this average. This regression bar shows an abrupt decrease in value with the onset of menopause.

The absolute level of bone density is also predictive of fracture risk.[86,127,133] As BMD decreases, the fracture risk increases, regardless of age. In Fig. 62-5, *B* the BMD of a 54-year-old patient is 0.822 g/cm². This is 3 S.D. below the young adult peak value; and since fracture risk doubles with each decrease of 1 S.D., the risk in this patient is six times greater than that of a young adult female.[125]

Tables 62-1 and 62-2 demonstrate the relationship between BMD changes and fractures as reported by two different groups of investigators.[19,125] A fracture threshold for the spine has been specified for BMD values below 0.9 g/cm².[125] Melton and associates[133] found that when the BMD was 0.6 g/cm², the prevelance of vertebral fracture was 54%. Davis and associates,[49] after studying 1000 postmenopausal women ranging from 43 to 80 years of age with single- or dual-photon absorptiometry and lateral roentgenograms, developed the following predictive fracture risk values for osteopenic patients. A single base-line fracture increases the risk of new fracture five times, whereas two or more fractures increases the risk 12 times. The combination of low bone mass and the presence of two fractures increases the risk 75-fold.

Table 62-1

Relationship between fracture of the spine and BMD*

BMD (g/cm²)	No. Studied	Percent with Spinal Fracture
> 1.10	100	6.0
1.00-1.09	111	9.9
0.09-0.99	159	17.0
0.80-0.89	134	23.1
0.70-0.79	20	40.8
0.60-0.69	49	50.0

*From Mazess RB, Barton HS: *DPX reference data*, University of Wisconsin Department of Medical Physics and Lunar Radiation Corporation, Madison, WI, 1989.

Table 62-2

Prevalence of spinal fractures in post-menopausal women as related to BMD*

BMD (g/cm²)	Percent with Spinal Fractures
0.8-0.9	26
0.7-0.8	33
0.6-0.7	51
0.5-0.6	63

*From Barth RW, Lane JM: Osteoporosis, *Orthop Clin North Am* 19:845, 1988.

Ultrasonography

Recently, broadband ultrasound attenuation (BUA) of the calcaneus has been shown to be a safe, effective, and reliable tool for diagnosing osteoporosis.[46,153]

Management of Osteoporosis

The primary aim of treatment is prevention of osteoporosis; in established osteoporosis it is to improve bone mass and thereby prevent further deformities and fractures. Several drugs can be used in osteoporosis. Estrogen, bisphosphonates (etidronate, clodrinate), and calcitonin can be considered to be antiresorbogenic drugs because they act primarily on osteoclastic resorption. Calcium can also be considered a weak antiresorbogenic agent. Four drugs are available for stimulation of osteoblasts: fluorides, parathyroid hormone, growth hormone, and anabolic steroids. Figure 62-6 is an algorithmic approach for the management of osteoporosis.

Prevention

Prevention of bone loss should be the main goal in osteoporosis. Specific measures should be taken during adolescence and young adulthood to both prevent bone loss and promote bone formation when the body is naturally building bone. Intervention in the younger age group should be aimed at both preventing bone loss and maximizing the peak bone mass through a combination of exercise, proper nutrition, calcium, Vitamin D, and lifestyle changes such as avoiding alcohol, cigarettes, and sodas.

Exercise

It is well known that lack of activity is associated with decreased bone mass as measured by densitometric studies,[23] and it is therefore logical to include exercise in prevention and treatment programs for osteoporosis. Exercises should aim to maintain good posture, cardiorespiratory fitness, and endurance and should include low-impact aerobics, walking, and stationary exercise bicycle, stretching, and body extension exercises. Flexion exercises should be avoided in established osteoporosis. Exercises should not be considered as a substitute for drug treatment, but an adjunct to drug management in osteoporosis.

Although there are some conflicting reports as to the beneficial effects of exercise for osteoporotic patients, it is apparent that in the majority of reported cases, a well conducted exercise program can improve bone mass as measured by densitometric studies.

Accumulated data have shown a significant correlation between the level of exercise activity and bone density of the spine, but not of the radius if the latter is not subjected to stresses by the exercise.[8,112,154] However, if the radius is subjected to dynamic bone loading exercises, it will increase its density.[15] In athletes such as tennis players the radius of the dominant extremity has a distinct bone hypertrophy[107] and higher bone density.[99,102] The femoral bone density is also shown to be higher in athletes as opposed to controls, and there is a direct relationship between femoral bone density and intensity of exercises.[139] These observations suggest that in order for physical activity to increase bone mass, it should have some sort of loading effect on the skeleton. A greater bone mass has been found in a group of marathon runners as compared with a sedentary control group.[9] Williams and associates[208] have demonstrated that there was a definite direct relationship between the number of miles run by the athletes and the bone mass.

How much and what kind of specific exercises are required to prevent bone loss in postmenopausal women? It has been demonstrated that an aerobic dance exercise program was more successful than a walking program in inhibiting radial bone loss as measured by SPA in 73 recently postmenopausal females.[206] Brisk walking for 15 to 40 minutes three times a week for 42 weeks failed to prevent bone loss of the axial skeleton in early postmenopausal women.[29] However, more intense exercises were shown to have an unequivocal beneficial effect on bone mass. According to Chow and co-workers,[30] a 30 minute exercise consisting of walking, jogging, or dancing, or an exercise strengthening program (10 to 15 minutes of isometric or isotonic muscle contracture of the extremities, or trunk muscles with weights attached to the ankles and wrists) can improve bone density. One hour of aerobic exercises per day, three times a week[6] or twice a week[113] can prevent bone loss. The beneficial effect of aerobic exercises on the skeleton has also been reported by others.[43,188]

Estrogen

Arresting bone loss has proven to be much more effective than rebuilding a depleted skeleton. After menopause, decreased levels of estrogen induce increased bone remodeling with osteoclastic bone resorption dominating over osteoblastic bone reformation, resulting in decreased bone mass and osteoporosis. Estrogen replacement therapy (ERT) restores the premenopausal level of bone mass, as has been shown by densitometric studies (SPA, DPA, DPX, QCT). Quigley[157] and Riis,[175] and their colleagues demonstrated that estrogen users show an annual average bone loss ranging from 0.0% to 0.9% depending on the age of the group examined. However, there is no doubt that in the majority of the reported studies ERT increases bone mass. The reported increase in bone density with ERT ranges from 1% to 1.65% per annum, whereas bone loss in the nontreated patient has been reported to range between 2% to 5%.* More recently, in a double-blind study,[134] combined estrogen and progesterone treatment were shown to result in substantial bone mass gain of both the appendicular and axial skeleton. The net gain in vertebral bone density amounted to 6.4% per year, and in the appendicular skeleton 3.6% per

*References 2, 5, 32, 34, and 209.

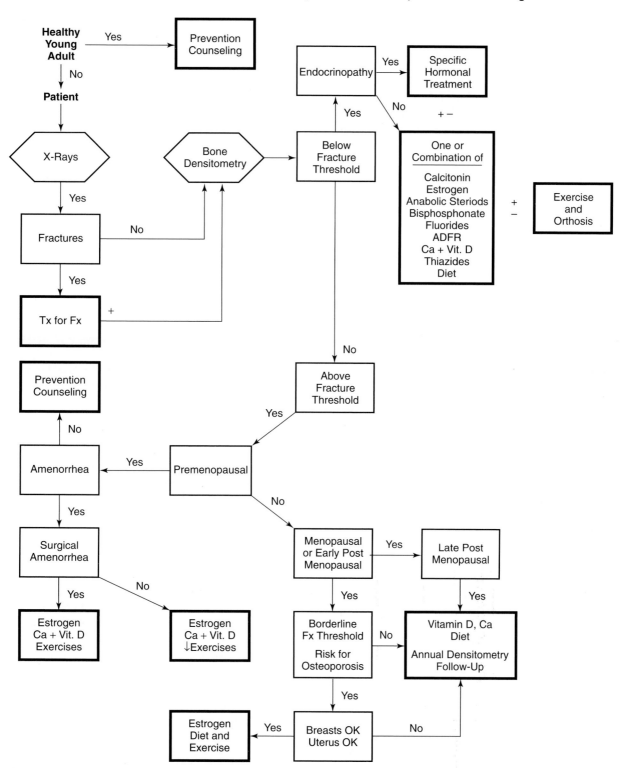

Fig. 62-6

Algorithm for the management of osteoporosis.

year, with continuous supplementation of estrogen and progestogen. With sequential supplementation of this hormone, the net gain was 5.4% for the axial skeleton and 3.7% for the appendicular skeleton. Transdermal ERT not only normalizes the total skeletal turnover but also promotes bone formation within 12 months, as pointed out by Williams and associates.[209] Long-term users (17.6 years) showed a 54% greater spinal BMD as measured by QCT, 19% greater forearm BMD as measured by SPA, and 16% greater metacarpal cortical thickness as measured by x-ray.[59]

Estrogen users also demonstrate an almost 50% decrease in the incidence of fractures as compared with control groups.[59] Estrogen replacement therapy should be administered close to menopause to obtain maximum beneficial effect. Some even suggest that ERT may even start during menopause if the FSH level is elevated. Because ERT is associated with an increased risk of endometrial carcinoma,[106] progesterone should also be prescribed. Progesterone induces endometrial sloughing, thus reducing the risk of cancer. Various forms of estrogen and progesterone are prescribed for postmenopausal hormonal replacement therapy. Estrogen replacement therapy should be continued for 10 to 15 years, beginning after menopause. A generally accepted daily oral estrogen replacement dose is 0.625 mg of conjugated estrogen, or 1 to 2 mg of estrogel valerate, or 25 μg of ethinyl estradiol, or 1 mg of 17 estradiol, or 1.25 mg of piperazine estrone sulfate. This should be supplemented with a low dose of progestin (5 mg medroxyprogesterone acetate) rather than supplementing with a higher dose (10 mg) on days 15 to 25. The addition of progestogen to estrogen therapy may even result in further increase of bone formation and decreased bone absorption.[34] Long-acting medroxyprogesterone acetate (MPA, Depo-provera) seems to stimulate osteoblastic activity as suggested by sustained increase in osteocalcin and alkaline phosphatase and also enhances production of calcitonin by the C cells of the thyroid.[82] It has also been suggested that even smaller doses of conjugated estrogen (0.3 mg) may be sufficient in some women if combined with high calcium supplementation of 1500 mg daily. However, 0.3 mg conjugated estrogen without calcium supplementation was not effective.[120] The continuous ethanyle estrogel-norethidron (estrogen–progesterone replacement therapy) tablet, even at the low doses (0.5 μg respectively), provided the same beneficial effects on bone, endometrial tissue, and postmenopausal symptoms as sequential therapy (conjugated estrogen 0.625 mg on days 1 to 25, and methoxyprogesterone acetate, 10 mg on days 16 to 25) while minimizing annoying vaginal bleeding and spotting.[209] Transdermal estrogen is not as widely used in the United States as it is in Europe. However, low doses of transdermal estrogen (0.55 mg per day, for three weeks a month) have been found to be sufficient treatment to relieve menopausal symptoms and also to be effective in preventing postmenopausal bone loss.[163] In this study, an oral estrogen was given for 10 days per month, resulting in regular withdrawal bleeding. Although the addition of progestins may reduce the risk of endometrial cancer, progestins may have some adverse affects on serum lipids, thus negating the potential beneficial cardiovascular effect of estrogens. Estrogens are believed to be protective against coronary mortality, by improving serum atherosclerotic risk factors. Total cholesterol and low-density lipoprotein cholesterol are reduced, while high-density lipoprotein cholesterol is increased.[26] Estrogen treatment is contraindicated in the presence of breast cancer, endometrial cancer, and osteosclerosis. There are also conditions in which estrogen is relatively contraindicated and must be used with care, such as a history of jaundice or liver disease, diabetes mellitus, hypertriglyceridemia, hypertension, history of phlebothrombosis, endometriosis or uterine fibrosis, obesity, tobacco use, or family history of breast cancer.[203] Since 1 in 12 American women will develop breast cancer in her lifetime, even a slightly increased risk, especially if hormone replacement therapy is prescribed for longer than 15 years, is worrisome.[25,94,203] The risk of breast cancer resulting from administration of estrogen for osteoporosis is still controversial. Gambrell[75] is of the opinion that ERT does not increase the risk factor. He claims that the addition of progestogen may even decrease the risk factor.

In the United States, there are three widely recognized indications for postmenopausal hormonal replacement: postmenopausal symptoms, dyspareunia, and osteoporosis.[177] The United States Preventive Services Task Force recommends that estrogen therapy should be considered for symptomatic women who are at increased risk for osteoporosis, who have received adequate counseling about potential risks and benefits, and who lack known contraindications.[117] Routine postmenopausal ERT is not recommended for asymptomatic patients who are at low risk for osteoporosis.

Calcitonin

Calcitonin action on bone consists of inhibiting osteoclastic activity and thus decreasing bone resorption. This appears to have a direct action on bone. Calcitonin also acts on the renal tubule, decreasing resorption of calcium, phosphate, sodium, and water.[84] Long-term calcitonin therapy in postmenopausal osteoporosis has shown significantly increased total body calcium and trabecular bone mass as measured by iliac crest biopsy.[83] A controlled double-blind clinical study by Mazzuoli and colleagues[126] demonstrated that postmenopausal osteoporotic women who are treated with salmon calcitonin at a dose of 100 MRC units every other day over 12 months had a significant increase in distal radius bone mineral content (13%) as opposed to controls. Calcitonin has also been used in coherent treatment with phosphates with a 36% increase in the trabecular bone mass in eight patients with postmenopausal osteoporosis.[158] Kuntz and associates[115] believe that phosphate in the combination treatment with intermittent calcitonin increases the recruitment of bone remodeling units as calcitonin decreases the rate of bone resorption. The indicated dose for treatment of osteoporosis with calcitonin is 50 to 100 MRC units every other day. Because of antibody formation to salmon calcitonin, the period of efficacy may be limited to only a few months. Synthetic human calcitonin may therefore be more effective. One of the objections to calcitonin treatment is the need for self-administered injection of the hormone by the patient. This, however, may be overcome with the introduction of nasal spray calcitonin. Preliminary data on nasal salmon calcitonin treatment are encouraging and demonstrate a more beneficial effect on spinal bone mass than on the appendicular skeleton.[194] The bioequivalence of calcitonin by intranasal insufflation is low as compared with parenteral use,[143] and should be taken into consideration when electing this form of treatment. Calcitonin treatment appears to be particularly indicated for patients with high-turnover osteoporosis. Civitelli and colleagues[35] have shown that calcitonin promotes a net gain of bone mineral in the axial skeleton and a slowing of bone loss in the appendicular skeleton.

Bisphosphonates

Bisphosphonates are analogs of pyrophosphates, which are used to inhibit bone resorption in hypercalcemia of malignancy and in Paget's disease of bone. For more details regarding their mode of action, see Chapter 113, Bisphosphonates in Paget's Disease. Bisphosphonates, previously known as diphosphonates, bind to mineral surfaces where they act to prevent crystal growth and dissolution. They also have a cytotoxic effect on the osteoclast. Etidronate and other bisphosphonates whose action as crystal poisons exceeds their toxic effects will produce a predominant mineralization defect; those such as Cl_2 MDP (dichloromethyldiphosphonates) that are cytotoxic at concentrations that do not significantly inhibit crystal growth, primarily inhibit osteoclastic resorption.[63] Bisphosphonates have been used mainly in cyclical coherence programs. The goal of coherence therapy, or ADFR (activate, depress, free, and repeat), is to circumvent the coupling of the bone remodeling unit's resorption and formation processes. Osteoprogenitor cells are activated with phosphate (2 to 3 g daily) for 3 days. This stimulates the osteoprogenitor cells of both the osteoclastic and osteoblastic cell lines in the skeleton to come to a common temporal phase. Subsequently, for 14 days resorption is suppressed with the administration of etidronate at a dose of 400 mg per day for 14 days. Although this suppresses the resorption phase, the signal for bone formation has already been expressed and remains uninhibited during the subsequent 74 days of the treatment-free phase (without etidronate treatment). Calcium may be given during the second month of the cycle. Then the entire regimen is repeated, thereby blocking the resorption phase and free reformation phase and leading to a net increase in bone formation. Anderson and associates[11] first used this type of therapy, and they coined the term ADFR. In their studies they found that this treatment increased the trabecular volume of iliac crest bone as seen in biopsies. However, Pacifici and colleagues,[145] in their experience with coherence therapy, were unable to duplicate the same successful results. Subsequently, two studies by Watts[205] and Storm[192] and their colleagues demonstrated that intermittent cyclical therapy with etidronate with or without the addition of phosphate significantly increased spinal bone mass and reduced the incidence of new vertebral fracture in women with postmenopausal osteoporosis, after approximately 1 year of treatment. More recently, disodium clodronate was successfully used in the treatment of osteoporosis in chronic juvenile arthritis, where the bone loss is multifactorial.[118] We have treated osteoporosis over the past 5 years with bisphosphonate in our clinic and we have found that cyclical etidronate treatment as described by Anderson increases the DEXA bone mineral density of the spine.

Calcium

Some data suggest that women in their early postmenopausal years may benefit from a high calcium intake[41] with the effect primarily on cortical bone[98]; it has no effect on trabecular bone loss.[78] Patients with osteoporosis treated with calcium have shown a significant reduction in urinary hydroxyproline, although the action of calcium as a weak resorbogenic agent has not been definitely substantiated. It has been proposed that this fall in bone resorption might be secondary to reduction in circulating parathyroid hormone, although parathormone was not measured.[97] However, a calcium intake of 1500 mg per day might significantly reduce bone loss if combined with a low estrogen dose (0.3 mg estrogen per day) instead of the usual dosage of 0.625 mg per day. A certain minimal intake of calcium is highly recommended.[120] The recommended dose of calcium is 1000 mg per day for patients on estrogen therapy, and 1500 mg per day for a woman who does not receive estrogen. There is greater bioavailability of calcium from calcium citrate than from calcium carbonate.[138] In the presence of achlorhydria calcium citrate is recommended because it is better absorbed; otherwise, calcium carbonate is prescribed.[146] Calcium pidolate at a dose of 1 g per day may inhibit bone resorption but does not influence bone formation.[165]

Vitamin D

Vitamin D is indicated when there is calcium malabsorption or coexisting vitamin D deficiency. Pharmacologic doses of vitamin D (7000 to 50000 IU per day) cause symptoms of hypervitaminosis with elevated hypercalcemia and chronic renal failure, and should not be used with estrogen, calcium, fluoride, or any other form of therapy for osteoporosis.[183] Long-term calcitriol therapy (Rocaltrol or 1,25-$(OH)_2D$, or D hormone) at a dose ranging from 0.8 μg per day to 1.0 μg per day was shown to increase bone density of the appendicular skeleton, stabilize the bone density of the spine, increase calcium absorption, increase serum osteocalcin levels (presumably due to osteoblastic activity), and improve pain and mobility in patients.[7,27,28] However, there are also reports of hypercalcemia, especially when combined with calcium. Care, therefore, must be taken to limit calcium supplementation and to control the dose of vitamin D.[104] Other investigators, especially when using a low dosage of calcitriol (0.25 μg per day or 0.50 μg per day), failed to demonstrate fore-

arm bone loss as measured by SPA.[32,103] Calcitriol or 1,25-$(OH)_2D$ acts on the intestine, kidney, bone, skin, and female reproductive tract. In the intestine, vitamin D improves calcium and phosphate absorption and promotes renal tubular absorption of calcium and phosphate in the kidneys. On bone, calcitriol stimulates both osteoblastic and osteoclastic activity and mobilizes calcium and phosphates. Vitamin D directly suppresses the action of parathyroid hormone and promotes the recruitment of osteoclastic linkage cells for osteoblast formation.[52] Calcitriol therapy is still experimental and may be used in the future for promotion of appendicular bone formation.

Anabolic Steroids

Anabolic steroids are chemically related to natural androgens, with, however, little adrogenic effect but with a powerful protein anabolic effect. They may promote bone formation by stimulating collagen synthesis in osteoporosis. The most widely used anabolic steroid for osteoporosis treatment is nandrolon decanoate, which is a 19-nontesterone. In addition to its beneficial effect on bone, it may also increase muscle mass. The side effects of anabolic steroids are atherogenic changes in plasma lipoprotein, liver dysfunction, hoarseness of voice, male-pattern baldness, hirsutism, and muscularization. Anabolic steroids are contraindicated in cardiorenal failure, liver disease with impaired bilirubin excretion, and in male patients with carcinoma of the prostate or breast. Anabolic steroids are indicated in osteoporosis with renal osteodystrophy, corticoid use, and in advanced end-stage osteoporosis. The recommended dose for treatment of osteoporosis is 50 mg IM every 3 to 4 weeks. At this low dose there are fewer side effects and it is well-tolerated by the patient.[79,80,142,161]

Fluoride

Fluoride may stimulate increased production of osteoblasts and increased bone formation,[60] but mineralization of the matrix produced with fluoride may be reduced.[114,180] Some authorities recommend vitamin D and calcium be added to fluoride treatment. However, Riggs and associates[171] cautioned that the addition of vitamin D may increase the risk of hypercalciuria and hypercalcemia. Eriksen and colleagues[57] suggested that a cyclic regimen of fluoride and fluoride-free periods may prevent mineralization defect. Fluoride treatment for osteoporosis is widely used in Europe, but it is still considered experimental in the United States. The recommended dose is 0.5 to 1.0 mg per kilogram of body weight (30 to 80 mg per day) and should only be used carefully, as an experimental drug.

Fluoride treatment, by stimulating osteoblastic activity, increases serum alkaline phosphatase[60] and osteocalcin. These bone markers can be used as an index of therapeutic response to fluoride treatment.[147] The newly generated trabecular structure with fluoride treatment leads to increased bone between trabeculae (connectivity) without significant increase in the midtrabecular thickness, resulting in increased strength of trabecular bone.[201] Fluoride therapy increases cancellous BMD in the axial skeleton.* The effects on cortical bone are not encouraging and there may even be resorption of cortical bone leading to skeletal fragility.[17,45,172] An increased incidence of fracture of the hip in patients treated with fluoride has been reported by several investigators.[88,156,170,181] However, fractures of the femoral neck were less common in populations drinking fluoridated water than in people consuming nonfluoridated drinking water.[185] Although it has been shown that there is a decrease in the fracture rate of the spine with fluoride treatment,[24,44] recently Riggs and associates[168] demonstrated that the number of new vertebral fractures was similar in both placebo and treatment groups, but the number of nonvertebral fractures was higher in the treatment group. Thus, they concluded that the fluoride-calcium regimen was not effective treatment for postmenopausal osteoporosis. Bone fragility occurred in 37.5% of patients treated with sodium fluoride, calcium, and vitamin D for 2.5 years. Trabecular stress fractures tended to occur in the first 18 months of treatment and cortical stress fractures after 30 months of therapy.[181] According to Power and Gay,[155] sodium fluoride protection against compression vertebral fractures was provided in only 30% of patients who demonstrated vertebral fluorosis by radiography.

Side effects include extraaxial bone formation at sites that are subjected to significant mechanical stresses, such as calcaneus femoral neck and metatarsals, when treatment exceeds 6 months.[182] Bone pain is not uncommon with fluoride treatment and is attributed to increased bone turnover and stress fractures, mainly at the juxtaarticular region.[119,144,181] According to La Roche and Maziere,[116] the incidence of stress fractures and arthralgia is up to 30%,

although they do not cause a significant disability and follow a benign course.

Other side effects are on the gastrointestinal system and are usually mild, including nausea, vomiting, epigastric pain, and diarrhea.[119,146] The new enteric-coated, slow-release sodium fluoride preparation introduced recently greatly reduces the incidence of gastrointestinal side effects by limiting the amount of fluoride released in the stomach.[146]

Thiazide Diuretics

Thiazides have been shown to have a salubrious effect on bone mass and on fractures.[160,204] When thiazide is combined with estrogen the effect seems to be additive.[202] Thiazides may be indicated in patients with osteoporosis who suffer from hypertension, where estrogen is contraindicated, in renal hypercalciuria, and especially in hypercalciuria following corticosteroid therapy.[37] The administration of thiazides is associated with higher bone mineral (by DPA), and reduces the incidence of fracture as compared with controls. However, these results were inferior to those obtained with estrogen use.[202] Heidrich and colleagues[93] found that thiazide use does not protect against hip fractures. Hip fractures, however, should not be considered solely as osteoporotic in origin. More controlled clinical trials are needed to establish the effect of thiazides on bone mass and prevention of fractures. The adverse effects such as glucose intolerance, hyperuricemia, hypokalemia, and precipitation of azotemia in patients with renal disease are well known and require caution. The recommended dose is 25 mg per day.

Parathyroid Hormone

Parathyroid hormone can stimulate both bone formation and bone resorption. In small doses bone formation may dominate over resorption. Daily small doses of parathyroid hormone combined with daily ingestion of $1,25\text{-}(OH)_2$ vitamin D can significantly increase trabecular bone density in the spine and improve intestinal calcium and phosphate absorption in middle-aged men with idiopathic osteoporosis.[186]

Growth Hormone

Growth hormone has been used in a few clinical trials. It is indicated in the treatment of osteoporosis caused by growth-hormone deficiency. Administration of growth hormone in combination with calci-

*References 44, 53, 55, 88, 168, and 171.

tonin in the growth hormone–deficient adult patient results in an increased bone mass.[199]

Ipriflavone

Recently a new medication, ipriflavone (7-isoproxy-3-phenyl-4h-1-benzopyran-4-one), which is an isoflavone, was successfully used in the treatment of osteoporosis. Patients receiving 600 mg of oral ipriflavone per day were examined at 7 and 12 months following the beginning of treatment. At these points, significant increase in BMD was determined by DPA.[4,129,136,150] Apparently, ipriflavone stimulates the secretion of calcitonin,[136] thus indirectly suppressing bone resorption. Apart from some mild side effects such as gastrointestinal intolerance, the drug was well tolerated.[150]

Surgical Treatment

It has been reported in the literature that spontaneous crush fracture in osteoporotic patients is never complicated by spinal cord compression.[148] This has been challenged by others who have reported spinal-cord compromise by spontaneous crush fractures in osteoporotic patients necessitating decompression of the spinal cord.[12,176] The principle treatment in this situation is urgent decompression, fusion, and stabilization. Certain technical problems related to osteopenic bones should be kept in mind. If decompression is deemed necessary, especially in the presence of kyphosis, an anterior corpectomy is indicated. The defect can be bridged either with tricortical bone graft from the ilium, fibular graft, or titanium mesh filled with cancellous bone and interposed between the vertebrae. Methylmethacrylate cement should be avoided unless there is superimposed malignancy. The spine should also be stabilized by anterior instrumentation (Kaneda, Kostuik, Harrington, Armstrong, or AMS plate). If vertebral screw purchase is precarious because of osteopenia, it can be augmented by polymethylmethacrylate (PMMA) cement. The screws should also purchase the opposite cortex for better fixation. If the cement is introduced anteriorly and without pressurization, it usually does not extravasate into the spinal canal; however, we do not recommend a blind transpedicular cement augmentation without laminectomy when a posterior approach is used, for we have witnessed, and it has been reported by others (A. Steffee, personal communication), that the cement may extravasate into the spinal canal. Anterior stabilization usually suffices; if not, it can be augmented posteriorly. Sometimes posterior stabilization using the

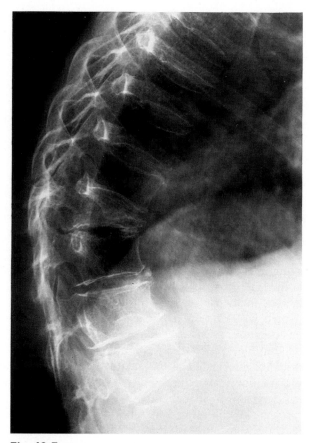

Fig. 62-7

Lateral radiograph of the thoracic spine showing a severe wedge fracture of the body of T10 with severe dorsal kyphosis.

current devices (Steffee, C-D instrumentation, Isola, etc.) can be used before anterior decompression. For a burst fracture of the lumbar spine with symptomatology of spinal stenosis without impending cauda equina or paraplegia and with evidence of marked atherosclerosis of the aorta, we advise a posterior decompression, reduction, and transpedicular instrumentation and fusion. With laminectomy a transpedicular fixation can better control the reduction than laminar hooks, which apply only distraction. Again, if the bone screw fixation is not solid, the fixation should be augmented by means of PMMA cement. This technique has been supported scientifically by Zindrik and associates,[211] who found that the force needed to pull out a bone screw doubled when screw purchase was augmented with PMMA cement. Because triangulation also can resist the pull-out force directed posteriorly, we strongly recommend the addition of a cross-link device to posterior instrumentation. It has been suggested that laminar hooks or claws should be avoided because osteoporotic bones are fragile; we suspect they lead to weakening of the lamina with excessive

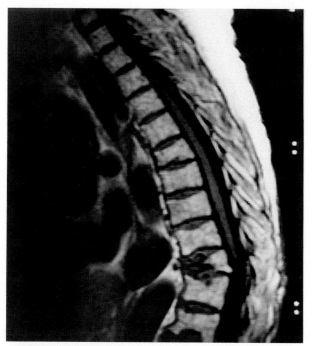

Fig. 62-8

Sagittal T_1-weighted MRI image of the thoracic spine, demonstrating the retropulsed posteroinferior margin of the body of the T10 vertebra impinging upon the thecal sac and the spinal cord.

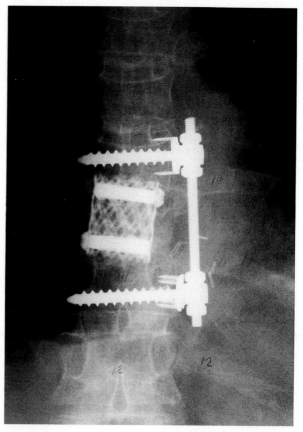

Fig. 62-9

Anteroposterior radiograph showing replacement of the T10 vertebral body by a titanium cage (filled with autologous bone graft) and stabilized by a rod attached to two screws, one inserted into the vertebra cephalad and the other in the vertebra caudad to the cage.

decortication for fusion preparation. In one of our cases, a claw was pulled out and fractured the thoracic lamina because of excessive decortication of the lamina. Careful application of hooks and claws can be successful and can even be combined with transpedicular fixation if necessary. Recently, Coe and associates[36] tested four different implants: laminar hooks, Steffee transpedicular screws, Drummond spinous process wire and button, and Cotrel-Dubousset transpedicular screws, and found that laminar hooks were more resistant to failure from posteriorly directed forces. The difference between the loads to failure for laminar hooks and the other implants was significant ($p < 0.05$).

We have treated six patients with spontaneous osteopenic fracture compromising the neural elements of the spinal canal. One of our patients developed complete paraplegia from crush fracture of the T7 vertebra, and a delayed anterior decompression with Kostuik-Harrington instrumentation and stabilization was done. This patient did not recover from this surgery. A second patient with a T10 fracture (Figs. 62-7 and 62-8) developed severe Brown-Sequard syndrome with increasing paraparesis and spasticity and finally became wheelchair-bound. An anterior vertebrectomy and reconstruction with a titanium cage filled with cancellous bone graft taken from the rib excised during thoracotomy was performed (Fig.

62-9). The spine was then stabilized anteriorly with a rod attached to two screws inserted in the body of the vertebrae adjacent to the cage. Following this operation, the patient's strength in her lower extremities improved. Four other fractures resulted in spinal stenosis with neurologic compromise. Two crush fractures in the lumbar vertebrae were treated by posterior instrumentation—one in the thoracic spine was treated by anterior corpectomy and posterior stabilization with an Isola device; the other, an osteoporotic burst fracture compromising the thecal sac in the thoracolumbar spine, was treated by corpectomy through an anterior approach and reconstruction with an iliac crest tricortical bone graft and stabilization with a Kaneda device.

Management of Back Pain

Pain that originates from altered spinal biomechanics should be treated by orthosis and physical therapy aimed at restoring spinal posture. Low-back pain that is persistent and is facetogenic in origin can be relieved by radiofrequency percutaneous rhizotomy. We have successfully treated a few patients with osteoporosis with this method.[159]

References

1. Aaron JE and others: Frequency of osteomalacia and osteoporosis in fractures of the proximal femus, *Lancet* 1:229, 1974.
2. Abdalla HI and others: Prevention of bone mineral loss in postmenopausal women by norethisterone, *Obstet Gynecol* 66:789, 1985.
3. Agnusdei D and others: Effects of ipriflavone on bone mass and calcium metabolism in postmenopausal osteoporosis, *Bone Min (Suppl)* 19:43, 1992.
4. Agnusdei D and others: Short-term treatment of Paget's disease of bone with ipriflavone, *Bone Min (Suppl)* 19:35, 1992.
5. Al-Azzawi F, Hart DM, Lindsay R: Long term effect of oestrogen replacement therapy on bone mass as measured by dual photon absorptiometry, *BMJ* 294:1261, 1987.
6. Aloia J, Cohn S, Babu T: Skeletal man and body competition in marathon runners, *Metabolism* 27:1793, 1978.
7. Aloia J and others: *Calcitriol in the treatment of postmenopausal osteoporosis.* In Cohn VD, Martin TJ, Meunier PJ, editors: *Calcium regulation and bone metabolism: Basic and clinical,* New York, 1987, Elsevier.
8. Aloia J and others: Premenopausal bone mass is related to physical activity, *Arch Intern Med* 148:121, 1988.
9. Aloia J and others: Prevention of involutional bone loss by exercise, *Ann Intern Med* 89:356, 1978.
10. Anderson C: Personal communication, 1990.
11. Anderson C and others: Preliminary observations of a form of coherence therapy for osteoporosis, *Calcif Tissue Int* 36: 341, 1984.
12. Arciero RA, Leung KYK, Pierre JH: Spontaneous unstable burst fracture of the thoracolumbar spine in osteoporosis: a report of two cases, *Spine* 14:114, 1989.
13. Armbrecht HJ, Zenser TV, Davis BB: Effect of age on the conversion of 25-hydroxyvitamin D_3 to 1,25-dihydroxyvitamin D_3 by kidney of rat, *J Clin Invest* 66:1118, 1980.
14. Arnold JS: *The quantitation of bone mineralization as an organ and tissue in osteoporosis.* In Pearson OH, Joplij JF, editors: *Dynamic studies of metabolic bone disease,* Philadelphia, 1964, F.A. Davis, p 59.
15. Ayalon J and others: Dynamic bone-loading exercises for postmenopausal women: effect on density of distal radius, *Arch Phys Med Rehabil* 68:280, 1987.
16. Bailie SP and others: Pathogenesis of vertebral crush fractures in men, *Age Aging* 24:139, 1992.
17. Bang S and others: *Morphometric and biophysical study of bone tissue in industrial fluorosis.* In Courvoisier B, Donath A, Baud CA, editors: *Fluoride and bone,* Bern, Switzerland, 1978, Hans Huber, p 168.
18. Barnett E, Nordin BEC: The clinical and radiologic problem of thin bones, *Br J Radiol* 34:683, 1961.
19. Barth RW, Lane JM: Osteoporosis, *Orthop Clin North Am* 19:845, 1988.
20. Bikle DD and others: Bone disease in alcohol abuse, *Ann Intern Med* 103:42, 1985.
21. Birge SJ and others: Osteoporosis, intestinal lactose deficiency, and low dietary calcium intake, *N Engl J Med* 276:443, 1967.
22. Boddy J-J, Heath H III: Estimates of circulating monometric calcitonin: physiological studies in normal and thyroidectomized man, *J Clin Endocrinol Metab* 57:897, 1983.
23. Bohr H and others: Measurements of bone mineral content in patients with spinal cord injuries, *Acta Orthop Scand* 57:184, 1986.
24. Briancon D, Meunier PJ: Treatment of osteoporosis with fluoride, calcium, and vitamin D, *Orthop Clin North Am* 12:629, 1981.
25. Buring JE and others: A prospective cohort study of postmenopausal hormone use and risk of breast cancer in U.S. women, *Am J Epidemiol* 125:939, 1987.
26. Bush TL, Miller VT: *Effects of pharmacologic agents used during menopause: impact on lipids and lipoproteins.* In Mishell DR Jr, editor: *Menopause: physiology and pharmacology,* Chicago, 1987, Year Book Medical Publishers, p 187.
27. Caniggia A and others: Effect of long-term treatment with 1,25-dihydroxyvitamin D_3 on osteocalcin in postmenopausal osteoporosis, *Calcif Tissue Int* 38:328, 1986.
28. Caniggia A and others: The hormonal form of vitamin D in the pathophysiology and therapy of postmenopausal osteoporosis, *J Endocrinol Invest* 7:373, 1984.
29. Cavanaugh D, Cann C: Brisk walking does not stop bone loss in women, *Bone* 9:201, 1988.
30. Chow R, Harrison J, Notarins C: Effect of two randomized exercise programs on bone mass of healthy postmenopausal women, *BMJ* 295:1441, 1987.
31. Christiansen C: Photon absorptiometry studies in osteoporosis, *Acta Obstet Gynaecol Scand Suppl* 130:67, 1985.
32. Christiansen C and others: Effect of 1,25-dihydroxyvitamin D_3 in itself or combined with hormone treatment in preventing postmenopausal osteoporosis, *Eur J Clin Invest* 11:305, 1981.
33. Christiansen C and others: Factors in response to treatment of early menopausal bone loss, *Calcif Tissue Int* 33:575, 1981.
34. Christiansen C and others: Uncoupling of bone formation and resorption by combined oestrogen and progestagen therapy in postmenopausal osteoporosis, *Lancet* 2:800, 1985.
35. Civitelli R and others: Bone turnover in postmenopausal osteoporosis: effect of calcitonin treatment, *J Clin Invest* 82(4):1268, 1988.
36. Coe JD and others: Influence of bone mineral density on the fixation of thoracolumbar implants: a comparative study of transpedicular screws, laminar hooks, and spinous process wires, *Spine* 15(9):902, 1990.

37. Condon JR and others: Possible prevention and treatment of steroid-induced osteoporosis, *Postgrad Med J* 54:249, 1978.

38. Corghi E and others: Basal plasma levels of calcitonin and bone mineral mass in normal and uremic women: effect of menopause, *Biomed Pharmacother* 38:263, 1984.

39. Courpron P: Bone tissue mechanics underlying osteoporosis, *Orthop Clin North Am* 12:513, 1981.

40. Crilly R and others: Prevalence, pathogenesis, and treatment of post-menopausal osteoporosis, *Aust N Z J Med* 9:24, 1979.

41. Cumming RG: Calcium intake and bone mass: a quantitative review of the evidence, *Calcif Tissue Int* 47(4):194, 1990.

42. Dalen N, Feldreich AL: Osteopenia in alcoholism, *Clin Orthop* 99:201, 1974.

43. Dalsky G and others: Weight-bearing exercise training and lumbar bone mineral content in postmenopausal women, *Ann Intern Med* 108:824, 1988.

44. Dambacher MA, Ittner J, Rnegsegger P: Long-term fluoride therapy and postmenopausal osteoporosis, *Bone* 7:199, 1986.

45. Dambacher MA and others: *Long-term effects of sodium fluoride in osteoporosis*. In Courvoisier B, Donath A, Baud CA, editors: *Fluoride and bone*, Bern, Switzerland, 1978, Hans Huber, p 238.

46. Damilakis JE, Dretakis E, Gourtsaylannis NC: Ultrasound attenuation of the calcaneus in the female population: normative data, *Calcif Tissue Int* 51:180, 1992.

47. Daniel HW: Osteoporosis of the slender smoker: vertebral compression fracture and loss of metacarpal cortex in relation to postmenopausal cigarette smoking and lack of obesity, *Arch Intern Med* 136:298, 1976.

48. Davies KM, Redker RR, Heaney RP: Normal vertebral dimensions and normal varieties in serial measurements of vertebrae, *J Bone Min Res* 4:341, 1989.

49. Davis JW, Epstein RS, Wasnich RD: Pre-existing fractures and bone mass predict vertebral fracture incidence in women, *Ann Intern Med* 114:919, 1991.

50. Deftos LJ and others: Influence of age and sex on plasma calcitonin in human beings, *N Engl J Med* 302:1351, 1980.

51. Delmas PD and others: Increase in serum boney carboxyglutemic acid protein with aging in women: implications for the mechanism of age-related bone loss, *J Clin Invest* 71:1316, 1983.

52. DeLuca HF: New concepts of vitamin D functions, *Ann NY Acad Sci* 30:669, 1992.

53. Devogelaer JP and others: The effect of therapy with sodium fluoride and calcium supplements on bone mineral content of the lumbar spine and the radius in the vertebral crush fracture syndrome, *J Bone Min Res* 1(suppl 1):264, 1986.

54. Dunn WL, Wahner HW, Riggs BL: Measurement of bone mineral content in human vertebrae and hip by dual photon absorptiometry, *Radiology* 136:485, 1980.

55. Duursma SA and others: Responders and non-responders after fluoride therapy in osteoporosis, *Bone* 8:131, 1987.

56. Ellis FR, Holesh S, Ellis JW: Incidence of osteoporosis in vegetarians and omnivores, *Am J Clin Nutr* 25:555, 1972.

57. Eriksen EF, Mosekilde L, Melsen F: Effect of sodium fluoride calcium phosphate and vitamin D₂ on trabecular bone and remodeling in osteoporosis, *Bone* 6:381, 1985.

58. Ettinger B: Prevention of osteoporosis: treatment of estradiol deficiency, *Obstet Gynecol* 72(suppl 5):125, 1988.

59. Ettinger B, Genant HK, Cann CE: Long-term estrogen replacement therapy prevents bone loss and fractures, *Ann Intern Med* 102:319, 1985.

60. Farley JR, Mergedal JE, Baylink DJ: Fluoride directly stimulates proliferation and alkaline phosphatase activity of bone-forming cells, *Science* 222:330, 1983.

61. Finsen V: *Back pain among the old: the relevance of osteoporosis, Osteoporosis*, 65-67. In Christiansen C, Johansen JS, Riis BJ, editors: International Symposium on Osteoporosis, Denmark, 1987.

62. Finsen V: Osteoporosis and back pain among the elderly, *Acta Med Scand* 223:443, 1988.

63. Flanagan AM, Chambers TJ: *The mechanism of inhibition of bone resorption by diphosphonates, Osteoporosis*, 1987. In Christiansen C, Johansen JS, Riis BJ, editors: International Symposium on Osteoporosis, Denmark, 1987.

64. Frost HM: *Bone dynamics in osteoporosis and osteomalacia*, Springfield, IL, 1966, Charles C Thomas.

65. Frost HM: *Bone remodeling and skeletal modeling errors*, Springfield, IL, 1973, Charles C Thomas.

66. Frost HM: *Bone remodeling dynamics*, Springfield, IL, 1963, Charles C Thomas.

67. Frost HM: Coherence treatment of osteoporosis, *Orthop Clin North Am* 12:649, 1981.

68. Frost HM: Managing the skeletal pain and disability of osteoporosis, *Orthop Clin North Am* 3:561, 1972.

69. Frost HM: Presence of microscopic cracks in *in vivo* bone, *Henry Ford Hosp Med J* 8:25, 1960.

70. Frost HM: The spinal osteoporosis: mechanism of pathogenesis and pathophysiology, *J Clin Endocrinol Metab* 2:257, 1973.

71. Fujita T and others: Age-dependent bone loss after gastrectomy, *J Am Geriatr Soc* 19:840, 1971.

72. Gallagher JC, Nordin BEC: *Oestrogen and calcium metabolism*. In Van Keep PA, Lauritzen C, editors: *Aging and estrogen*, Basel, 1973, Karger, p 98.

73. Gallagher JC and others: Internal calcium absorption and serum vitamin D metabolites in normal subjects and osteoporotic patients: effect of age and dietary calcium, *J Clin Invest* 64:729, 1979.

74. Gallagher JC and others: Vertebral morphometry: normative data, *Bone Min* 4:18, 1988.

75. Gambrell BD Jr: Update on hormone replacement therapy, *Am Fam Physician (Suppl)* 46:875, 1992.

76. Genant HK, Boy D: Quantitative bone mineral analysis using dual energy computed tomography, *Invest Radiol* 12:545, 1977.

77. Gennari C, Agnusdei D: Calcitonin, estrogens and bone, *J Steroid Biochem Biol* 37:451, 1990.

78. Gennari C and others: Comparative effects on bone mineral content of calcium and calcium plus salmon calcitonin given in two different regimens in postmenopausal osteoporosis, *Curr Ther Res Clin Exp* 38:455, 1985.

79. Geusens P, Dequeker J: Long-term effect of nandrolone decanoate 1α-hydroxyvitamin D$_3$ or intermittent calcium infusion therapy on bone mineral content, bone remodeling and fracture rate in symptomatic osteoporosis: a double-blind controlled study, *Bone Min* 1:347, 1986.

80. Geusens P and others: Bone mineral content, cortical thickness, and fracture rate in osteoporotic women after withdrawal of treatment with nandrolone decanoate, 1-alpha hydroxyvitamin D$_3$ or intermittent calcium infusions, *Maturitas* 8:281, 1986.

81. Gnudi S and others: Evaluation of the relative rates of bone mineral content loss in postmenopause due to both estrogen deficiency and aging, *Boll Soc Ital Biol Sper* 66(12):1153, 1990.

81a. Grampp S and others: Radiologic diagnosis of osteoporosis. Current methods and perspectives, *Radiol Clin North Am* 31: 1133, 1993.

82. Grecu EO and others: Effects of medroxyprogesterone acetate on some parameters of calcium metabolism in patients with glucocorticoid-induced osteoporosis, *Bone Min* 13(2):153, 1991.

83. Gruber HE and others: Long-term calcitonin therapy in postmenopausal osteoporosis, *Metabolism* 33:295, 1984.

84. Hadjipavlou A, Brooks EC: Etude de l'action de la calcitonin sur le rein, *L'Union Med Canada* 105:915, 1976.

85. Hanson T, Roos B, Nachemson A: The bone mineral content and ultimate compressive strength of lumbar vertebrae, *Spine* 5:46, 1980.

86. Hanson T, Roos B: The relation between bone mineral content, experimental compression fractures, and disc degeneration in lumbar vertebrae, *Spine* 6:147, 1981.

87. Härmä M and others: Bone density, histomorphometry and biochemistry in patients with fractures of hip or spine, *Ann Clin Res* 19(6):378, 1987.

88. Harrison JE and others: The relationship between fluoride effects on bone histology and on bone mass in patients with postmenopausal osteoporosis, *Bone Min* 1:321, 1986.

89. Healy JH, Lane JM: Structural scoliosis in osteoporotic women, *Clin Orthop* 195:216, 1985.

90. Heaney RP: *Unified concept of the pathogenesis of osteoporosis.* In DeLuca HF and others, editors: *Osteoporosis: recent advances in pathogenesis and treatment*, Baltimore, 1981, University Park Press.

91. Heaney RP, Recker RP, Saville PD: Menopausal changes in calcium balance performance, *J Lab Clin Med* 29:953, 1978.

92. Heath H III, Sizemore GW: Plasma calcitonin in normal man: differences between men and women, *J Clin Invest* 60:1135, 1977.

93. Heidrich FE, Stergachis A, Gross KM: Diuretic drug use and the risk for hip fracture, *Ann Intern Med* 15:1, 1991.

94. Henderson BE, Ross R, Berstrein L: Estrogen as a cause of human cancer: The Richard and Hinde Rosenthal Foundation Award Lecture, *Cancer Res* 48:246, 1988.

95. Hernandez-Avila M and others: Caffeine, moderate alcohol intake, and risk of fractures of the hip and forearm in middle-aged women, *Am J Clin Nutr* 54(1):157, 1991.

96. Holbrook TL and others: The frequency of occurrence, impact, and cost of musculoskeletal conditions in the United States, *Am Acad Orthop Surg*, Chicago, 1984.

97. Horowitz M and others: Effect of clacium supplementation on urinary hydroxyproline in osteoporotic postmenopausal women, *Am J Clin Nutr* 39:857, 1984.

98. Horsman A and others: Prospective trial of oestrogen and calcium in postmenopausal women, *BMJ* 2:289, 1977.

99. Huddleston A and others: Bone mass in lifetime tennis athletes, *JAMA* 244:1107, 1980.

100. Hurxthel LM: Measurement of anterior vertebral compression and biconcave vertebrae, *Am J Roentgenol* 103:635, 1968.

101. Insogna KL and others: Effect of age on serum immunoreactive parathyroid hormone and its biological effects, *J Clin Endocrinol Metab* 53:1072, 1981.

102. Jacobson P: Bone density in woman college athletes and older athletic women, *J Orthop Res* 2:328, 1984.

103. Jensen GF, Christiansen C, Transbol I: Treatment of postmenopausal osteoporosis: a controlled therapeutic trial comparing oestregen/gestagen, 1,25-dihydroxyvitamin D$_3$ and calcium, *Clin Endocrinol* 16:515, 1982.

104. Jensen GF and others: Does 1,25(OH)$_2$D accelerate spinal bone loss?, *Clin Orthop Rel Res* 192:215, 1985.

105. Jett SWK, Frost HM: Tetracycline based histological measurement of cortical endosteal bone formation in normal and osteoporotic rib, *Henry Ford Hosp Med J* 15:325, 1967.

106. Jick A and others: Replacement estrogens and endometrial cancer, *N Engl J Med* 300:218, 1979.

107. Jones H and others: Humeral hypertrophy in response to exercise, *J Bone Joint Surg* 59A:204, 1977.

108. Joycy JR and others: Clinical study of nutritional secondary hyperparathyroidism in horses, *J Am Vet Med Assoc* 158:2033, 1980.

109. Kelsey JF: *Osteoporosis: prevalence and incidence.* In Proceedings of the NIH Consensus Development Conference, April 2-4, 1984.

110. Krall EA, Dawson-Hughes B: Smoking and bone loss among postmenopausal women, *J Bone Min Res* 6(4):331, 1991.

111. Krolner B, Nielsen SP: Bone mineral content of the lumbar spine in normal and osteoporotic women: cross-sectional and longitudinal studies, *Clin Sci* 62:329, 1982.

112. Krolner B, Toft B: Vertebral bone loss: an unheeded side effect of therapeutic bed rest, *Clin Sci* 64:537, 1983.

113. Krolner B and others: Physical exercise as prophylaxis against involutional vertebral bone loss: a controlled trial, *Clin Sci* 64:541, 1983.

114. Kuntz D and others: Extended treatment of primary osteoporosis by sodium fluoride combined with 25-hydroxychole-calciferol, *Clin Rheumatol* 3:145, 1984.

115. Kuntz D and others: Treatment of postmenopausal osteoporosis with phosphate and intermittent calcitonin, *Int J Clin Pharmacol Health* VI:157, 1986.

116. Laroche M, Maziere B: Side effects of fluoride therapy, *Baillieres Clin Rheumatol* 5(1):61, 1991.

117. Lawrence SR, Chairman: *Estrogen prophylaxis: guide to clinical preventive services*, Report of the US Preventive Services Task Force, 1989, p 255.

118. Lepore L and others: Treatment and prevention of osteoporosis in juvenile chronic arthritis with disodium chondrate, *Clin Exp Rheumatol* 9(suppl 6):33, 1991.

119. Libanti CR and others: *Fluoride in the treatment of osteoporosis*. In Genant HK, editor: *Osteoporosis update*, Berkeley, 1987, University Press.

120. Lindsay R, Hart DM, Clark DM: The minimum effective dose of estrogen for prevention of postmenopausal bone loss, *Obstet Gynecol* 63:759, 1984.

121. Lindsay R and others: Prevention of spinal osteoporosis in oophorectomized women, *Cancer* 2:21151, 1980.

122. Marcus R, Medvig P, Young G: Age-related changes in parathyroid hormone action in normal humans, *J Clin Endocrinol Metab* 58:223, 1984.

123. Matkovic V and others: Bone status and fracture rates in two regions of Yugoslavia, *Am J Clin Nutr* 32:540, 1979.

124. Mazess RB: On aging bone loss, *Clin Orthop* 165:239, 1982.

125. Mazess RB, Borden HS: *DPX reference data*, University of Wisconsin, Department of Medical Physics, and Lunar Radiation Corporation, Madison, WI, 1989.

126. Mazzuali GF and others: Effect of salmon calcitonin in postmenopausal osteoporosis: a controlled double-blind study, *Clin Calcif Tissue Int* 38:3, 1986.

127. McBroom RJ and others: Prediction of vertebral body compression fracture using quantitative computed tomography, *J Bone Joint Surg* 67A:1206, 1985.

128. McDermott MT and others: Reduced bone mineral content in totally thyroidectomized patients: possible effect of calcitonin deficiency, *J Clin Endocrinol Metab* 56:936, 1983.

129. Melis GB and others: Ipriflavone and low doses of estrogen in the prevention of bone mineral loss in climacterium, *Bone Min (Suppl)* 19:49, 1992.

130. Melton LJ: *Epidemiology of vertebral fractures, osteoporosis*. In Christiansen O, Johansen JS, Riis BJ, editors: International Symposium on Osteoporosis, Denmark, September 27-October 2, 1987.

131. Melton LJ III, Riggs BL: *Epidemiology of age-related fractures*. In Avioloi LV, editor: *The osteoporotic syndrome*, 1987, Grune & Stratton.

132. Melton LJ, Riggs BL: Risk factors for injury after a fall, *Clin Geriatr Med* 1:525, 1985.

133. Melton LJ and others: Epidemiology of vertebral fracture in women, *Am J Epidemiol* 129:1000, 1989.

134. Munk-Jensen N and others: Reversal of postmenopausal vertebral bone loss by oestrogen and progestogen: a double-blind placebo controlled study, *BMJ* 296(6630):1150, 1988.

135. Murray RO: Radiological bone changes in Cushing's syndrome and steroid therapy, *Br J Radiol* 33:1, 1960.

136. Nakamura S and others: Effect of ipriflavone on bone mineral density and calcium related factors in elderly females, *Calcif Tissue Int (Suppl)* 1:30, 1992.

137. National Osteoporosis Foundation: A Special Topic Conference, Osteoporosis, Washington DC, 1987.

138. Nicar MJ, Pak CYC: Calcium bioavailability from calcium carbonate and calcium citrate, *J Clin Endocrinol Metab* 61:391, 1985.

139. Nilsson BE, Westlin NE: Bone density in athletes, *Clin Orthop* 77:179, 1971.

140. Nilsson BE, Westlin NE: Changes in bone mass in alcoholics, *Clin Orthop* 90:229, 1973.

141. Nordin BEC: Osteomalacia, osteoporosis, and calcium deficiency, *Clin Orthop* 17:235, 1960.

142. Nordin BEC and others: New approach to the problem of osteoporosis, *Clin Orthop* 200:181, 1988.

143. O'Doherty DP and others: A comparison of the acute effects of subcutaneous and intranasal calcitonin, *Clin Sci* 78(2):215, 1990.

144. O'Duffy JD and others: Mechanism of acute lower extremity pain syndrome in fluoride-treated osteoporotic patients, *Am J Med* 80:561, 1986.

145. Pacifici R and others: Coherence therapy does not prevent axial bone loss in osteoporotic women: a preliminary comparative study, *J Clin Endocrinol Metab* 66:747, 1988.

146. Pak CYC, Avioli LV: Factors affecting the absorbability of calcium from calcium salts and food, *Calcif Tissue Int* 43:55, 1988.

147. Pak CY and others: Attainment of therapeutic fluoride levels in serum without major side effects using a slow-release preparation of sodium fluoride in postmenopausal osteoporosis, *J Bone Min Res* 1(6):563, 1986.

148. Parfitt AM, Duncon H: *Metabolic bone disease affecting the spine*. In Rothman R, Simeone F, editors: *The spine*, ed 2, Philadelphia, 1982, W.B. Saunders.

149. Parfitt AM, Kleerekoper M: *Clinical disorders of calcium, phosphorus, and magnesium metabolism*. In *Clinical disorders of fluid and electrolyte metabolism*, ed 2, New York, 1980, M. Maxwell & C.R. Kellerman.

150. Passeri M and others: Effect of ipriflavone on bone mass in elderly osteoporotic women, *Bone Min (Suppl)* 19:57, 1992.

151. Patel U and others: Clinical profile of acute vertebral compression fractures in osteoporosis, *Br J Rheumatol* 30(6):418, 1991.

152. Peck WA and others: Osteoporosis, consensus conference, *JAMA* 252:799, 1984.

153. Petley GW and others: Comparison between broadband ultrasonic attenuation and single photon absorptiometry of the calcaneus. In Christiansen C, Johansen JS, Riis BJ, editors: *Osteoporosis,* Copenhagen, Denmark, 1987.

154. Pocock N and others: Physical fitness is a major determinant of fenoral neck and lumbar spine bone mineral density, *J Clin Invest* 78:618, 1986.

155. Power GRI, Gay JDL: Sodium fluoride in treatment of osteoporosis, *Clin Invest Med* 9:141, 1986.

156. Pridie RB: The diagnosis of senile osteoporosis using a new bone density index, *Br J Radiol* 40:251, 1967.

157. Quigley MET and others: Estrogen therapy averts bone loss in elderly women, *Am J Obstet Gynecol* 156:1511, 1987.

158. Rasmussen H and others: Effect of combined therapy with phosphate and calcitonin on bone volume in osteoporosis, *Metab Bone Dis Relat Res* 2:107, 1980.

159. Ray C: Facet syndrome pathophysiology: clinical picture and treatment, *Giorn Int Ant* 1:80, 1991.

160. Ray WA and others: Long-term use of thiazide diuretics and risk of hip fracture, *Lancet* 1:687, 1989.

161. Reid DM and others: Treatment of corticosteroid-induced osteoporosis with anabolic steroids and microcrystalline calcium hydroxyapatite, *Br J Rheumatol* 25(suppl 2), 1986, (abstract 74).

162. Reiss E and others: The role of phosphate in the secretion of parathyroid hormone in man, *J Clin Invest* 49:2146, 1970.

163. Ribot C and others: Preventive effects of transdermal administration of 17-beta-estradiol on postmenopausal bone loss: a 2-year prospective study, *Gynecol Endorcinol* 3(4):259, 1989.

164. Richelson LS and others: Relative contributions of aging and estrogen deficiency to postmenopausal bone loss, *N Engl J Med* 311:1273, 1984.

165. Rico H and others: Effect of calcium pidolate on biochemical and hormonal parameters in involutional osteoposoris, *Maturitas* 12(2):105, 1990.

166. Riggs BL, Melton LJ III: Evidence for two distinct syndromes of involutional osteoporosis, *Am J Med* 75:899, 1983.

167. Riggs BL, Melton LJ III: Involutional osteoporosis, *N Engl J Med* 314:1676, 1986.

168. Riggs BL and others: Effect of fluoride treatment on the fracture rate of postmenopausal women with osteoporosis, *N Engl J Med* 322(12):802, 1990.

169. Riggs BL and others: Effect of the fluoride/calcium regimen on vertebral fracture occurrence in postmenopausal osteoporosis, *N Engl J Med* 306:446, 1982.

170. Riggs BL and others: Incidence of hip fractures in osteoporotic women treated with sodium fluoride, *J Bone Min Res* 2:123, 1987.

171. Riggs BL and others: Rates of bone loss in the axial and appendicular skeletons of women: evidence of substantial vertebral bone loss prior to menopause, *J Clin Invest* 77:487, 1986.

172. Riggs BL and others: A syndrome of osteoporosis, increased serum immunoreactive parathyroid hormone, and inappropriately low serum 1,25-dihydroxy vitamin D, *Mayo Clin Proc* 53:701, 1978.

173. Riis BJ, Thomensen K, Christiansen C: Does calcium supplementation prevent postmenopausal bone loss? *N Engl J Med* 316:173, 1987.

174. Riis BJ and others: The effect of percutaneous estradiol and natural progesterol on postmenopausal bone loss, *Am J Obstet BGynecol* 156:61, 1987.

175. Rosenthal DI and others: Quantitative computed tomography for spine mineral density: factors affecting precision, *Invest Radiol* 20:306, 1985.

176. Salomon C, Chopin D, Benoit M: Spinal cord compression: an exceptional complication of spinal osteoporosis, *Spine* 13:222, 1988.

177. Sarrel PM: Estrogen replacement therapy, *Obstet Gynecol* 72(suppl):25, 1988.

178. Sartoris DJ and others: Vertebral body collapse in focal and diffuse disease: patterns of pathological processes, *Radiology* 160:479, 1986.

179. Schlenker RH, Von Seggen WW: The distribution of cortical and trabecular bone mass along the lengths of the radius and ulna and the implications for *in vivo* bone mass measurements, *Calcif Tissue Int* 20:41, 1976.

180. Schnitzler CM, Solomon L: Trabecular stress fracture during fluoride therapy for osteoporosis, *Skeletal Radiol* 14:276, 1985.

181. Schnitzler CM and others: Bone fragility of the peripheral skeleton during fluoride therapy for osteoporosis, *Clin Orthop* 261:268, 1990.

182. Schulz EE and others: Radiographic detection of fluoride-induced extra-axial bone formation, *Radiology* 159:457, 1986.

183. Schwartzman, MS, Franck WA: Vitamin D toxicity complicating the treatment of senile, postmenopausal, and glucocorticoid-induced osteoporosis: four case reports and a critical commentary on the use of vitamin D in these disorders, *Am J Med* 82:224, 1987.

184. Shamonki IM and others: Age-related changes of calcitonin secretion in females, *J Clin Endocrinol Metab* 50:437, 1980.

185. Simonen O, Laitinen O: Does fluoridation of drinking water prevent bone fragility and osteoporosis? *Lancet* 2:432, 1985.

186. Slovik DM and others: Restoration of spinal bone in osteoporotic men by treatment with human parathyroid hormone (1-34) and 1,25-dihydroxy-vitamin D, *J Bone Min Res* 1(4):377, 1986.

187. Smith DM, Khairi MRA, Johnston CC: The loss of bone mineral with aging and its relationship to risk of fracture, *J Clin Invest* 56:311, 1975.

188. Smith E and others: Deterring bone loss by exercises: intervention in premenopausal and postmenopausal women, *Calcif Tissue Int* 44:312, 1989.

189. Smith MC and others: *Bone mineral measurement: experimental MO78.* In Johnston RS, Dredlein LF, editors: *Biomedical results from Skylab,* NASA, Washington, DC, 1977.

190. Sowers M and others: Prospective study of radial bone mineral density in a geographically defined population of postmenopausal Caucasian women, *Calcif Tissue Int* 48(4):232, 1991.

191. Steinbach HL: The roentgen appearance of osteoporosis, *Radiol Clin North Am* 2:191, 1964.

192. Storm T and others: Effect of intermittent cyclic etidronate therapy on bone mass and fracture rate in women with postmenopausal osteoporosis, *N Engl J Med* 322:1265, 1990.

193. Tanaka Y, Castillo L, De Luca HF: *Sex hormonal control of the renal hydroxylation of vitamin D.* In Norman AW and others, editors: *Vitamin D, biochemical, chemical, and clinical aspects related to calcium metabolism,* New York, 1977, A. De Gruyter.

194. Thomsborg G and others: Effect of different doses of nasal salmon calcitonin on bone mass, *Calcif Tissue Int* 48(5):302, 1991.

195. Tiegs RD, Body JJ, Wehner HW: Calcitonin secretion in postmenopausal osteoporosis, *N Engl J Med* 312:1097, 1985.

196. Trotter M, Broman GE, Peterson RR: Densities of bone of white and negro skeleton, *J Bone Joint Surg* 42A:50, 1960.

197. Trouerbach WT and others: A cross-sectional study of age-related loss of mineral content of phalangeal bone in men and women, *Skeletal Radiol* 17(5):338, 1988.

198. Tsai K-S and others: Impaired vitamin D metabolites with aging in women: possible role in pathogenesis of senile osteoporosis, *J Clin Invest* 73:1668, 1988.

199. van der Veen EA, Netelenbos JC: Growth hormone (replacement) therapy in adults: bone and calcium metabolism, *Horm Res* 33(suppl 4):65, 1990.

200. Vernon-Robert B, Pirie CJ: Healing trabecular microfractures in the bodies of lumbar vertebrae, *Ann Rheum Dis* 32:406, 1973.

201. Vesterby A and others: Mazzow space star volume in the iliac crest decreases in osteoporotic patients after continuous treatment with fluoride, calcium, and vitamin D for five years, *Bone* 12(2):99, 1991.

202. Wasnich RD and others: Differential effect of thiazide and estrogen upon mineral content and fracture prevalence, *Obstet Gynecol* 67:457, 1986.

203. Wasnich RD and others: *Osteoporosis: critique and practicum,* 1989, Banyan Press, p 59.

204. Wasnich RD and others: Thiazide effect on the mineral content of bone, *N Engl J Med* 309:344, 1983.

205. Watts NB and others: Intermittent cyclical etidronate treatment of postmenopausal osteoporosis, *N Engl J Med* 323:73, 1990.

206. White MK and others: The effects of exercise on the bones of postmenopausal women, *Int Orthop (SCIOT)* 7:209, 1984.

207. Williams AR and others: Effect of weight, smoking, and estrogen use on the risk of hip and forearm fractures in postmenopausal women, *Obstet Gynecol* 60:695, 1982.

208. Williams J and others: The effect of long-distance running upon appendicular bone mineral content, *Med Sci Sports Exer* 16:223, 1984.

209. Williams SR and others: A study of combined continuous ethinyl estradiol and norethindrone acetate for postmenopausal hormone replacement, *Am J Obstet Gynecol* 162(2):438, 1990.

210. Wilson DWF, Garisson RJ, Castell WP: Postmenopausal estrogen use, cigarette smoking and cardiovascular morbidity in women over 50: The Framingham study, *N Engl J Med* 313:1038, 1985.

211. Zindrick MR and others: A biomechanical study of interpedicular screw fixation in the lumbar spine, *Clin Orthop* 203:99, 1986.

Chapter 63
Bone Grafts and Implants

Ken Y. Hsu
James Zucherman
Arthur H. White

The Autograft

anterior iliac crest grafts
posterior iliac crest grafts

Complications

nerve injuries
severe donor-site pain (chronic)
vascular injuries
hernia
pelvic instability

Graft Sites

the tibia
the fibula
free-vascularized bone grafts

Allografts

freezing and freeze drying
biomechanical properties
radiation, heat, and chemical treatment of
allografts and xenografts
bone morphogenetic protein

Xenografts (Heterologous Bones, Heterografts)

Synthetic Implants

Nonmetallic Synthetic Implants

Collagen and Other Matrix Proteins

Methylmethacrylate Cement

Advances in both fusion techniques and instrumentation have markedly facilitated the treatment of spinal disorders. Yet a significant number of patients exist who continue to have pseudarthroses. Despite the surgical advances, the essentials of a successful spinal fusion still appear to be the effective application of sound bone-grafting principles. These principles, along with the techniques, problems, and complications associated with bone grafting, are reviewed in this chapter.

The loss of bone in the spine often presents serious difficulties not seen in other areas. The most favorable replacement would still be a bone graft that fills the defect and becomes incorporated into the spine. However, the availability of appropriate bone to replace the loss is a significant problem. Also surveyed in this chapter are alternatives to autogenous bone grafts, or autografts, including allografts, xenografts, and synthetic bone substitutes as well as other implants used to stabilize the spine.

Bone grafts have often played the roles of scaffolds, bridges, spacers, defect fillers, and bone-loss replacements. Immobilization of multiple motion segments is frequently necessary in the spine; great demands are made on bone grafts. In the lumbosacral spine, body weight and muscular forces impart loads equal to three or four times body weight.[149] It is not surprising that the highest rate of bone-graft failure is seen in the lumbosacral spine. Hence, the following is a discussion of technical problems and the biomechanical and physiologic characteristics of bone grafts, bone substitutes, and implants. Since our last edition on this subject in 1987,[62] significant progress has been made, and this updated chapter reflects the additional knowledge we have gained. At this time, the exact mechanisms controlling the physiologic processes of bone-graft incorporation and remodeling are still not completely understood. Yet, we may be able to improve our clinical results in spine surgery by appreciating the principles and information already known regarding this subject.

The Autograft

Autograft, or bone graft transplanted from one site to another in the same individual, is considered to be the most biologically suitable type of graft. Its advantages include

1. Superior osteogenic capacity
   a. Contributes cells capable of immediate bone formation

   b. Allows for bone induction by recipient bed where nonosseous tissue is influenced to change its cellular function and become osteogenic
2. Lack of histocompatibility differences or immunologic problems
3. Ease of incorporation
4. Lack of disease transmission

Autogenous cancellous bone has osteogenic, osteoinductive, and osteoconductive properties owing to the surviving bone cells, collagen, mineral, and matrix proteins, as well as a large trabecular surface area that is joined together as new bone forms.[72] The disadvantages of autografts include

1. Additional incision or wider exposure, prolonged operative time, and increased blood loss and trauma
2. Increased postoperative morbidity from pain and potential infection or deformity
3. Sacrifice of normal structure and weakening of donor bone
4. Risks of significant complications
5. Limitations in size, shape, quantity, and quality (the supply is limited, especially in children)

For optimum results harvest autogenous cancellous bone in the following manner:

1. Harvest graft in thin strips (not exceeding 5 mm in thickness[59,125])
   a. To provide maximum exposure of superficial cells
   b. To allow rapid vascularization
2. Wrap graft in a gauze soaked in patient's blood
   a. Avoid exposure to high-intensity lights
   b. Maintain temperature less than 42°C[59]
   c. Do not store in saline or antibiotic solution[3,130]
   d. Do not use chemical sterilization[130]
3. Transfer graft to the recipient bed as soon as possible
   a. To avoid exposure to air for more than 30 minutes[59]
   b. To protect the viability of the surface cells
4. Place graft
   a. In well-vascularized bone bed
   b. In well-decorticated bone surface (cancellous site is superior)
   c. With healthy soft-tissue coverage
5. Minimize surgical trauma (e.g., high-speed burring and inadequate irrigation retard healing[1,143])
6. Position cancellous surface
   a. On opposing cancellous surface
   b. On surrounding soft tissue with good blood supply
   c. So that total mass of graft is not too thick to prevent nutrient diffusion from recipient bed

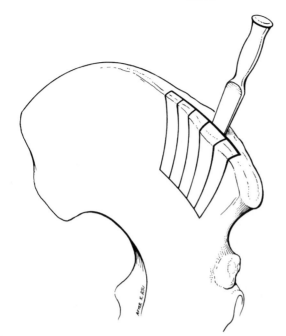

Fig. 63-1

Corticocancellous bone graft is obtained from the lateral iliac surface using longitudinal parallel cuts with an osteotome or chisel.

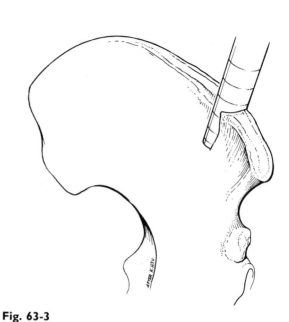

Fig. 63-3

Dowel-cutting instrument is used to obtain an iliac graft with two tooled cancellous surfaces and cortical faces on three sides for anterior spinal interbody fusion.

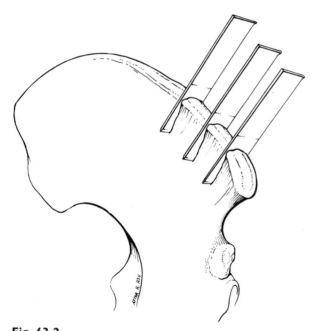

Fig. 63-2

Horseshoe-shaped corticocancellous bone graft is obtained from the iliac crest using osteotomes positioned to each other.

7. Avoid
a. Dead space
b. Hematoma
c. Interposition of necrotic tissue
8. Minimize risk; be aware of
a. Anatomy
b. Potential complications

The iliac crest is the most versatile bone graft reserve. It is subcutaneous and easy to harvest in prone, supine, lateral, or other positions. It is expendable, and has a large reserve of cortical and cancellous bone. In addition, it allows creation of different shapes and sizes.

Anterior Iliac Crest Grafts

Anterior iliac crest bone grafts are used for anterior interbody fusion of the cervical, thoracic, or lumbosacral spine. The subcutaneous anterosuperior iliac spine and iliac crest are easily palpable. The iliac tubercle is the widest portion, and is where a large quantity of corticocancellous bone is found (see Fig. 63-8).

A skin incision is made parallel to, or in line with, the iliac crest. It is advantageous to center the incision over the iliac tubercle. The incision is carried down to the bone of the crest, and the muscles are elevated subperiosteally to expose the wing of the ilium.

The tensor fascia latae, gluteus medius, and gluteus minimus originate from the lateral aspect of the ilium. They are innervated by the superior gluteal nerve. The abdominal muscles are also attached to the iliac crest and are segmentally innervated. The

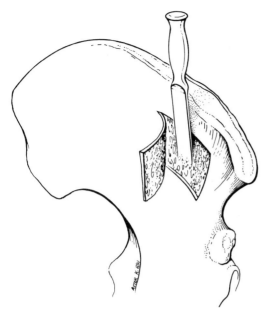

Fig. 63-4
Cortical "trap door" is used to gain access to iliac cancellous bone.

incision over the crest is, therefore, "internervous" and safe.

An appropriate osteotome or chisel may be used to outline a cortical window in the lateral iliac surface from which to procure the bone graft. Longitudinal parallel cuts may be made (Fig. 63-1). Strips of cancellous bone may be removed with a curved gauge. Care must be taken not to violate the inner table of the iliac wing, where hernia is a significant potential complication.

Bone graft may be obtained from the inner table of the iliac wing. However, there are risks of peritoneal perforation and significant bleeding with formation of hematoma in the retroperitoneal space.

It is important not to carry the incision to, or anterior to, the anterosuperior iliac spine. Injury to the lateral femoral cutaneous nerve or the inguinal ligament must be avoided. Detachment of the inguinal ligament may result in inguinal hernia. If bicortical bone is taken too close to the anterosuperior iliac spine, fracture may occur (see Fig. 63-6). Avulsion of the anterosuperior iliac spine may occur by the action of the attached muscles, such as the tensor fascia lata or sartorius.

Bone may be removed in the form of block, dowel, strips, or by way of a cortical window or "trap door" (Figs. 63-1 to 63-4). The iliac-crest contour can be preserved by removing the bone deep to the crest, or by temporarily detaching and repositioning it later (Fig. 63-5). The anterosuperior iliac spine should be left intact to maintain normal appearance. The region of the iliac spine should not be weakened by removing bone adjacent to it. Fracture and displacement of the inguinal ligament may result (Fig. 63-6).

The wound should be closed properly. The muscles and fascia must be sutured to their original anatomic positions and the defects closed; an effective drain should be used.

Posterior Iliac Crest Grafts

The posterior iliac crest provides a large quantity of cortical cancellous bone graft. The posterosuperior iliac crest is palpable under the skin dimple in the superior medial aspect of the gluteal region. The iliac crest curves cephalad and laterally from the posterosuperior iliac spine.

An oblique, curved, or vertical incision may be made over the posterior iliac crest or in line with it.

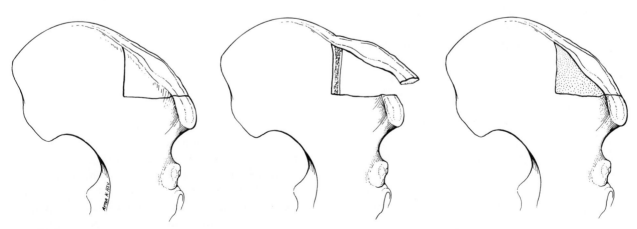

Fig. 63-5
Large iliac graft is obtained with preservation of the iliac contour.

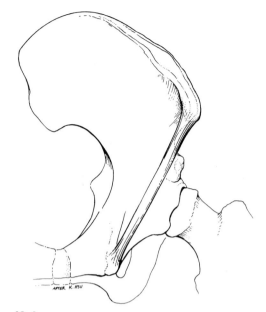

Fig. 63-6

Illustration of attachment of inguinal ligament to anterior superior iliac spine. Detachment of inguinal ligament may lead to inguinal hernia. Injury to lateral femoral cutaneous nerve should be avoided.

The cluneal nerves cross the iliac crest 7 to 12 cm anterolateral to the posterosuperior iliac spine (see discussion under Complications) and must be protected (see Fig. 63-13).

A midline spine incision may be extended distally and the posterior iliac crest approached laterally under the skin and subcutaneous fat. This avoids the use of a second skin incision.

The incision is carried down to the bone of the crest, and the muscles are elevated subperiosteally from the posterolateral surface of the ilium. This approach does not denervate the muscles. The gluteus maximus, medius, and minimus originate from the lateral surface of the ilium. The superior gluteal nerve innervates the gluteus medius and minimus, and the inferior gluteal nerve innervates the gluteus maximus. The paraspinal musculature innervated segmentally originates from the iliac crest.

It is very important to remember the following rules:

1. Stay on bone and work subperiosteally.

2. Avoid the sciatic notch and protect the sciatic nerve.

3. Protect the superior gluteal vessels (see discussion under Complications) and protect the pelvic stability.

4. Avoid the sacroiliac joint.

5. Protect the posterior sacroiliac ligaments.

The removal of bone in the vicinity of the sciatic notch can weaken the thick bone that forms the notch. This can produce instability of the pelvis. It is important to stay cephalad to the sciatic notch and remove bone only from the false pelvis. For a landmark, an imaginary line dropped anteriorly from the posterosuperior iliac spine with the patient in the prone position can be used as the caudal limit of bone removal (see Fig. 63-15, *A* and *B*). Care must be taken not to enter the sacroiliac joint, which may become a source of persistent pain and instability when injured.

A sharp surgical instrument (e.g., an osteotome or tip of Taylor retractor) may injure the sciatic nerve deep to the sciatic notch. Laceration of the superior gluteal vessels is a significant danger in this region. The vessels leave the pelvis via the sciatic notch. A divided vessel can easily retract into the pelvis and present a very alarming complication (see discussion under Complications [Fig. 63-14]).

Nutrient vessels supplying the ilium found in the mid-portion of the anterior gluteal line may present troublesome bleeding and should be controlled with Gelfoam, Surgicel, bone wax, or electrocoagulation.

A less painful bone-graft donor site for lumbar spine fusion is possible by applying the following technique. A separate incision over the iliac crest is *not* made through the skin. The fascia is grasped with Kochers clamps and pulled medially through the wound of the lumbar surgical site. The subcutaneous tissue is carefully elevated off the fascia laterally and caudally until the fascia immediately above the posterior iliac crest and posterosuperior iliac spine is reached. A Taylor retractor is placed in the subcutaneous tissue lateral to the crest over the ilium posteriorly. The periosteum is not dissected from the ilium except from the medial aspect of the crest. The fascia is incised along the medial edge of the crest, and an elevator is used to scrape the medial surface of the crest free of periosteum to bare bone. After a window is made in the medial cortex with an osteotome, gouges are used to remove the cancellous bone between the cortical layers (Fig. 63-7), leaving the cortices intact laterally and posteriorly with their soft-tissue attachments. This technique minimizes postoperative donor-site pain and prevents formation of uncomfortable scar tissue over the ilium, as when the lateral cortices are removed.

When limited quantity of cancellous bone is required, the following methods may be advantageous:

1. Currettage allows harvest of cancellous graft with least morbidity through a small round cortical window using a sharp curette as shown in Fig. 63-8. Cancellous bone is most abundant in the pos-

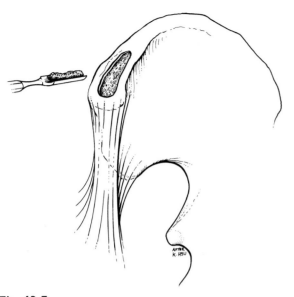

Fig. 63-7

A gouge is used to remove the posterior "roof" of the illium and the cancellous bone between the cortical layers.

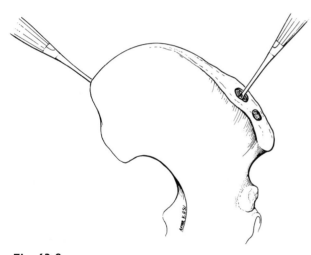

Fig. 63-8

Cancellous bone is removed from the iliac tubercle in the anterior or posterior iliac spine region through a small cortical opening.

terior aspect of the iliac crest, followed by the iliac tubercle and anterosuperior iliac spine areas.

2. A "trap door" cut in the anterior or posterior outer table of the ilium and hinged on muscles can be opened to allow access to cancellous bone. The trap door is closed at the end. Postoperative pain appears to be less with this technique. Cosmetic deformity is minimal (see Fig. 63-4).

Wolfe and Kawamoto[153] reported a technique of obtaining full-thickness bone graft from the anterior ilium. An incision is made through the iliac crest. The outer ridges of the iliac crest are split obliquely

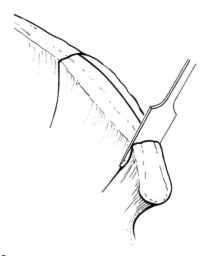

Fig. 63-9

Wolfe and Kawamoto's technique of obtaining full-thickness bone graft from the anterior ilium. A sharp osteotome is used to make appropriate cuts shown above and in Fig. 63-10.

with the muscular and periosteal attachments remaining. All the iliac bone beneath this split can then be removed. The edges of the crest may be reapproximated, thus minimizing cosmetic deformity, hernia, hematoma, and postoperative morbidity (Figs. 63-9 to 63-12).

Complications

Complications involving the iliac bone-graft donor site are not uncommon. Although some of these complications may not be serious, they add to the patient's discomfort and prolong the convalescence. Complications secondary to graft removal from the ilium include

1. Major blood loss
2. Hematoma
3. Nerve injury (neuroma formation)
4. Severe pain (chronic pain)
5. Hernia
6. Cosmetic deformity
7. Fracture
8. Necessity for sacroiliac joint surgery
9. Pelvic instability
10. Hip subluxation
11. Gait disturbance
12. Peritoneal injury
13. Ureteral injury
14. Heterotopic bone formation
15. Infection

Cockin[28] reviewed 118 cases of iliac crest bone-graft procedures and found major complications in

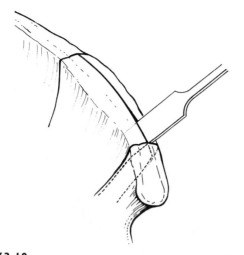

Fig. 63-10

The ridges of the iliac crest are split obliquely with the osteotome. The muscular and periosteal attachments should remain.

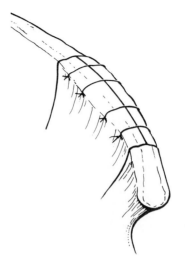

Fig. 63-12

Wolfe and Kawamoto's technique of reapproximating the two fragments of the crest using wires or sutures. Figure-eight wire or suture may be passed through the bone with an awl and fixed to adjacent bone.

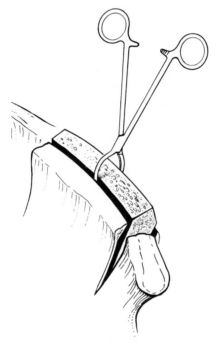

Fig. 63-11

A large full-thickness bone graft can be removed as shown, using Wolfe and Kawamoto's method.

3.4% of the cases and minor complaints in 6%. There were two cases of meralgia paresthetica, one of hernia, and one of hip subluxation after extensive removal of the iliac crest. The minor complaints included wound pain, hypersensitivity, and buttock anesthesia.

Younger and Chapman reviewed the medical records of 239 patients with 243 bone grafts.[155] The overall major complication rate was 8.6% and in-

cluded infection (2.5%), prolonged wound drainage (0.8%), large hematomas (3.3%), reoperation (3.8%), pain greater than 6 months (2.5%), sensory loss (1.2%), and unsightly scars. The minor complication rate was 20.6% and included superficial infection, minor wound problems, temporary sensory loss, and mild or resolving pain. A significantly higher major complication rate of 17.9% occurred if the surgical incision was also used to harvest the bone graft.

Nerve Injuries

Possible nerve injuries include the following:
1. Lateral femoral cutaneous nerve[28,85,144]
2. Iliohypogastric (lateral cutaneous branch) nerve
3. Superior cluneal nerve (cutaneous branches of dorsal rami L1, L2, L3)[29,39]
4. Middle cluneal nerve (cutaneous branches of dorsal rami S1, S2, S3)
5. Sciatic nerve
6. Ilioinguinal nerve[14]
7. Femoral nerve
8. Superior gluteal nerve

Superior cluneal nerves are lateral branches of the posterior primary division of the upper three lumbar nerves that run posteriorly through the lumbosacral fascia at the lateral origin of the sacrospinatus muscle. They cross over the dorsal aspect of the posterior iliac crest and provide sensation to the skin of the buttocks. They are found 7 to 12 cm anterolateral to the posterosuperior iliac spine in the

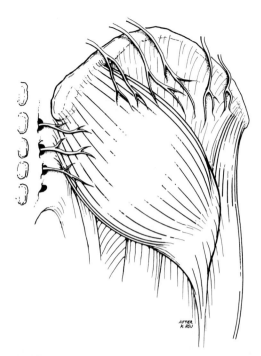

Fig. 63-13

Illustration of the nerves that may be injured during the procedure to remove bone graft from the iliac crest.

adult. When an incision is made across or parallel to the posterior iliac crest, the cluneal nerves may be injured (Fig. 63-13).

Painful neuritis of the buttocks has been reported.[29,39] That these nerves are a cause of disability can be demonstrated by the relief of symptoms after the nerves have been infiltrated with local anesthetics. Permanent relief can be obtained by resection of the nerves with the transected ends being allowed to retract into the soft tissue.

A possible complication of anterior iliac bonegraft procurement is injury to the lateral femoral cutaneous nerve.[85,144] This nerve arises from the dorsal branches of the second and third lumbar nerve roots, crosses the ilium obliquely, and passes medial to the anterosuperior iliac spine under the inguinal ligament. Then it courses toward the sartorius muscle and divides into anterior and posterior branches. The anterior branch passes through the fascia lata and provides sensation to the anterior and lateral aspects of the thigh. The posterior branch penetrates the fascia lata and provides sensation from the region of the greater trochanter to the mid-thigh. Sometimes the nerve may have an anomalous route lateral to the anterosuperior iliac spine.[53] Therefore, when dissection is carried out in the region of the anterosuperior iliac spine the nerve may be injured. It can also be entrapped in postsurgical scar tissue.

Excessive retraction of the iliacus muscle when the medial wall of the ilium is exposed may also injure this nerve. Compromise to the lateral forward cutaneous nerve presents as meralgia paresthetica, which may involve numbness, paresthesias, burning, and/or pain over the anterior and lateral thigh. Most of the time meralgia paresthetica causes minor symptoms or resolves spontaneously after the local causes are corrected. For some severe and resistant symptoms, nerve injections or surgical intervention may be necessary. Surgery may involve neuroma excision or freeing the nerve from the scar tissue entrapment.

The sciatic nerve may be injured when the dissection is extended down to the sciatic notch. A surgical instrument such as an osteotome may be passed deep to the sciatic notch to cause this injury. The bony rim of the notch should be palpated before the dissection is carried to this area. An imaginary plumb line dropped from the posterosuperior iliac spine with the patient in the prone position will pass through the bony rim of the sciatic notch. This serious complication can be avoided by staying cephalad to this line (Figs. 63-14 and 63-15).

The ilioinguinal nerve may be injured when the abdominal wall is retracted medially from the anterior iliac crest. The nerve may be compressed beneath the retractor on the inner part of the wall of the ilium. It occurs when the inner cortex of the anterior ilium is exposed for removal of bone grafts. Ilioinguinal neurologic injury is characterized by pain radiating from the iliac toward the inguinal and genital areas. This complication is well-discussed by Smith and associates.[121]

The iliohypogastric nerve (lateral cutaneous branch, L1 ventral rami) is found over the midlateral aspect of the iliac crest. It should be protected when working in this region (see Fig. 63-13).

Severe Donor-Site Pain (Chronic)

Chronic donor-site pain from the ilium was reported in 25% of 290 patients who had undergone anterior spine fusion in Summers' and Eisenstein's study.[126] Fernyhough and co-workers explored the relationship between surgical approach and chronic posterior iliac crest donor-site pain in 151 harvests.[47] No difference was observed in the incidence of chronic donor-site pain between harvests performed through a primary midline incision versus a separate lateral oblique incision (28% vs. 31%). Twice as many donor sites harvested for reconstructive spinal procedures were reported to have chronic pain as compared with those harvested for spinal trauma, regardless of the approach used (39% vs. 18%). Summers and Eisen-

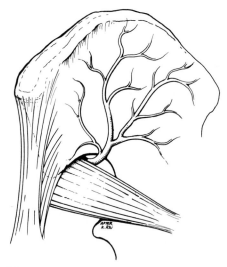

Fig. 63-14

Illustration of the superior gluteal artery, curving around the rim of the sciatic notch as it leaves the pelvis.

stein reported the highest prevalence of donor-site pain to be in patients who had a tricortical full-thickness graft taken through a separate incision overlying the iliac crest.[126] Patients with a clinically unsatisfactory result from spine fusion also had a significantly higher prevalence of donor-site pain.[126]

Vascular Injuries

Vascular injuries may include the superior gluteal artery (and vein),[45,66] the deep circumflex iliac artery, the iliolumbar artery, and the fourth lumbar artery.

The superior gluteal artery is a branch of the internal iliac artery that curves around the rim of the sciatic notch as it leaves the pelvis. It may be injured when dissection is carried close to the sciatic notch. An osteotome or the sharp point of a Taylor retractor may enter the notch and pose similar danger to the artery. This complication can become alarming, since the divided vessel easily retracts into the pelvis (see Fig. 63-14).

If the superior gluteal vessel is lacerated, it can be compressed locally and exposed for ligation or clipping. A finger may be used to apply direct pressure to the vessel against the bone. Kahn[66] discussed the use of a Raney-modified Kerrison rongeur to remove the upper margin of the sciatic notch to expose the bleeding vessel. If the bleeding vessel is still not accessible, the patient may be positioned for a retroperitoneal or transperitoneal exposure of the vessel. Arterial occlusion by embolization or by use of a Fogerty catheter is another option.

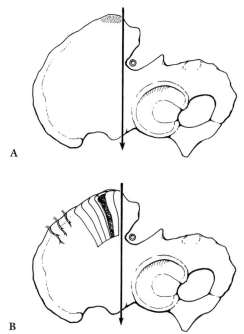

Fig. 63-15

A, The bony origin of the gluteus maximus or the roughened area anterior to the posterosuperior iliac crest is a good landmark and can be used as the caudal limit of bone removal. An imaginary plumb line dropped from the posterosuperior iliac spine with the patient in the prone position will pass through the bony rim of the sciatic notch. The superior gluteal artery is adjacent to the bony rim. **B,** A large amount of bone graft can be removed safely if the surgeon stays cephalad to the posterosuperior iliac spine, the sciatic notch, and the imaginary line joining them.

Injury to the superior gluteal vessels can be prevented if the surgeon is aware of the anatomy in this region. The bony origin of the gluteus maximus or the roughened area anterior to the posterosuperior iliac spine is a good landmark and can be used as the caudal limit of bone removal (see Fig. 63-15, *A* and *B*). An imaginary plumb line dropped from the posterosuperior iliac spine with the patient in the prone position will pass through the bony rim of the sciatic notch. It is important to stay cephalad to this line.

Escalas and DeWald[45] reported a case of combined traumatic superior gluteal arteriovenous fistula and ureteral injury complicating removal of a bone graft from the posterior ilium. The tip of a Taylor retractor accidentally dislodged and penetrated into the sciatic notch to cause this unusual injury.

The deep circumflex iliac artery, the iliolumbar artery, or the fourth lumbar artery may cause troublesome bleeding when working on the inner table of the ilium. Occasionally, peritoneal perforation accompanies the arterial injury. The anatomic position of the arteries are illustrated in Figs. 63-16 and

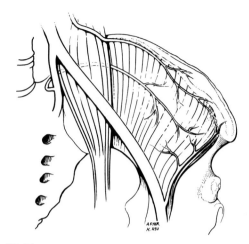

Fig. 63-16

Illustration of the anatomic positions of the arteries that may cause troublesome bleeding when working on the inner table of the ilium.

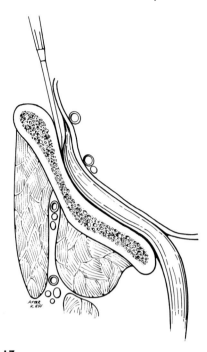

Fig. 63-17

The anatomic locations of the peritoneal wall and the vulnerable arteries are shown relative to the iliacus muscle and the inner wall of the ilium.

63-17. It is very important to stay subperiosteal and carefully elevate the abdominal wall muscles off the crest and the iliacus muscles off the inner table of the ilium (Fig. 63-18).

Hernia

A hernia through the iliac bone-graft donor site may occur after the removal of a full-thickness bone graft from that site. It may appear as an iliac swelling, sometimes associated with pain or symptoms of bowel obstruction.[51,78,96,106,109] Strangulated hernia and valvulae are very rare occurrences.[25] Symptoms have been reported to have occurred from 24 days[25] to 15 years[141] after the formation of the iliac defect.[31]

Treatment requires the reduction of the hernia and repairing the defect by

1. Using soft-tissue[9,25,78,96,109] advancement, imbrication, flaps, or fascial flaps

2. Using a prosthesis[106] (tantalum or Marlex mesh)

3. Using methylmethacrylate cement to reconstruct the iliac wall[79] (Figs. 63-19 to 63-21)

4. Using the Bosworth technique[9,31]: removing the remaining wings of the ilium on either side of the defect, followed by layered soft-tissue closure

Pelvic Instability

Removal of a large quantity of bone graft from the posterior ilium may disrupt the mechanical keystone effect of the sacroiliac joint and the posterior sacroil-

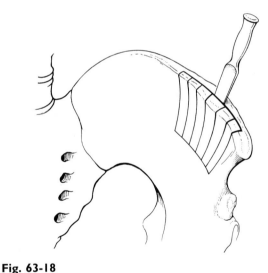

Fig. 63-18

It is very important to stay subperiosteally and carefully elevate the abdominal wall muscles off the crest and the iliacus muscle off the iliac wall before removing the bone from the inner table of the ilium.

iac ligament, causing instability. Lichtblau[76] first reported such complications after a bone-grafting procedure in which the posterior sacroiliac ligaments were postulated to be interrupted. The ensuing instability transferred the stress forces to the pelvic

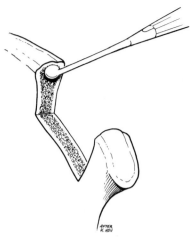

Fig. 63-19

The large defect left in the iliac wall may be repaired and the iliac contour restored using bone cement. Anchoring holes are made with a curette before the cement is applied.

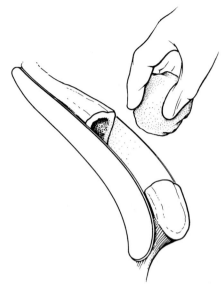

Fig. 63-20

The iliac wing defect is filled with bone cement. Malleable blades are used to repair the iliac wall as shown.

ring, causing fractures of the superior and inferior pubic rami. Coventry and Tapper[30] reported six cases of pelvic instability following removal of bone graft from the ilium. The patients with such instability often developed symptoms indistinguishable from other spinal disorders. History of clicking or thudding, as well as pain in the thigh and gluteal region, is characteristic.

Sacroiliac stability is maintained by formation of the sacrum as a keystone with interlocking eminences and depressions, along with ligamentous support mostly in the posterior and superior aspect.[14] Multiparous women with lax ligaments and anatomic variations in the sacroiliac joints are more prone to develop such pelvic instability. Radiologic examination of the entire pelvic ring is important. Changes in the sacroiliac joint, the pubic rami, and the symphysis pubis should be looked for.

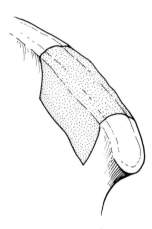

Fig. 63-21

The iliac wall is reconstructed with bone cement.

Graft Sites

The Tibia

The tibia provides strong full-thickness cortical graft material and is occasionally used in spine fusion. The subcutaneous anteromedial aspect of the tibia is a convenient donor site. The periosteum should be left intact and sutured over the defect. The condyles also supply cancellous bone. However, significant risks exist when using the tibia as a donor site. Biomechanically, the tibia is changed from a closed section to an open one when a bone graft is obtained. It is markedly weakened and much less able to resist torsional and bending loads.

Frankel and Burstein[48] discussed the effect of cortical graft removal from the tibia. They described the torque and angular deformation owing to failure of the tibia to be reduced to 30% of normal, and energy absorption capacity to 10% of normal. Even when the corners of the cutout are rounded, open section overshadows any reduction in stress concentration gained.

Fatigue fractures are fairly common, and the tibia should be immobilized in a cast for 6 to 12 months after the bone graft is obtained.[41] Thus, the disadvantages of autogenous tibial graft far outweigh the benefits.

The Fibula

Although the upper two thirds of the fibula may be removed as a bone graft, the middle one third provides the best cylindric cortical bone graft. The fibula graft is strongest in resisting compressive loading and can be depended on for longer periods of structural support in interbody fusion. For large defects in the vertebral bodies, fibula struts may be used to achieve stability. Because of the small amount of cancellous bone in the fibula, iliac cancellous graft should be supplemented to enhance osteogenesis.

Peroneal nerve injuries may occur when obtaining the graft from the proximal one third of the fibula. Valgus deformity of the ankle is a serious risk when the lower one third is violated. Significant donor-site pain and compartment syndrome have also been reported.

Ribs have been used for thoracic spine fusion. However, their modest cortex and porous cancellous bone are rarely appropriate for lumbar spine fusion.

Free-Vascularized Bone Grafts

Free-vascularized bone grafts may be used to circumvent the disadvantage of large cortical grafts, most of which become necrotic.[89,107] Progress in microsurgical techniques is making this type of graft possible.[35,127,145] Of the different patterns of blood supply to cortical bone, nutrient artery enters the diaphysis and divides into ascending and descending branches. The diaphyseal cortex is supplied by the radially oriented branches. Specific arteries also supply the epiphyseal and metaphyseal areas. A periosteal blood supply from the surrounding muscles enters the outer third of the cortex.[54] Continuing circulation and increased viability of the bone grafts facilitate the problem of fracture healing. Vascularized grafts are less dependent on the recipient bed for survival, and their use is advantageous in a poorly vascularized bed with deficient soft tissue after previous surgery, trauma, infection, or irradiation. The fibula, rib, and anterior or posterior ilium may be used. However, their application is usually limited by the small size and need for time-consuming, highly specialized microvascular techniques. Superior results have been reported in clinical cases in which a vascularized fibula graft was transplanted into a segmental bony defect, larger than 6 cm.[35,54] Rapid healing and hypertrophy of the graft were noted.

The use of free-vascularized bone graft may be advantageous in spine fusion in special circumstances. Bradford[11] reported favorable results with vascularized rib pedicle grafts used in patients with posttraumatic kyphotic deformity. The superiority of vascularized rib grafts in bridging vertebral bodies was also demonstrated in canine experiments.[119] Free-vascularized fibular grafts have been applied clinically in spine fusions.[38,67]

Dupuis and co-workers[38] successfully used a free-vascularized fibular graft in a case of progressive congenital kyphosis, following the work of O'Brien and Ostrup.[100] In a similar situation, an avascular strut graft becomes weaker to the point of mechanical failure as it is replaced by creeping substitution, which may take 2 or more years to complete.

Muscle-pedicle bone grafting procedures were reported by Hartman and associates for failed lumbosacral spinal fusion.[57] An iliac crest autograft with an intact quadratus lumborum muscle pedicle was used in this case.

Allografts

Allografts are the most frequently used alternatives to autografts in spine surgery. They are bones transplanted from one individual to another and are used to circumvent the problems encountered with autografts.[13,44,95,146] Fresh, frozen, lyophilized, and demineralized bone matrix from allografts are used clinically.

Allografts are readily available and come in a wide variety of shapes and sizes. They can provide immediate support and minimize the use of stabilization hardware or braces. Bone allografts can replace missing structures and become incorporated into the spine. They provide biologic scaffolding that is gradually replaced with the patient's own bone.

Major problems lead to the decreased effectiveness of allografts.[19-21,58] Immunologic rejection of implanted graft,[7,120] delayed union, nonunion, and fracture of the graft are not uncommon. Incorporation of allografts by the host is slower. Vascular penetration is slower and less dense. There is less perivascular new bone formation when compared with autografts. Transmission of disease from allografts is also a serious concern.

The major weakness of the allograft is that it is *dead* and cannot contribute directly to osteogenesis, as do fresh autografts. Burwell[18] found a way around this problem by combining the osteogenic potential of autogenous marrow with allografts. The use of autogenous marrow to provide superior osteogenic capability in allografts and xenografts, as well as autografts, is finding greater clinical application (see further discussion on xenograft and synthetic implants). The use of bank bone would be very advantageous if storage problems, immunologic reactions, and infection could be eliminated. The allograft must be aseptically obtained soon after death or properly sterilized and processed early to

1. Minimize its antigenicity
2. Prevent degradation by proteolytic enzymes
3. Maintain the mechanical structure
4. Preserve the osteogenic induction property

Freezing and Freeze Drying

Freezing and freeze drying are the most widely used preservation methods that allow storage of bone in a biologically useful (but nonviable) state.*

Allograft freezing is carried out as soon as possible after procurement. The length of safe storage for bone is not currently known. However, based on the knowledge of autolysis retardation by cold, lower temperatures are expected to extend the "shelf life" of allografts.[49] At −15° C to −30° C, using a home-type mechanical freezer, long-term storage of bone is difficult. This form of freezing is not advisable because ice crystals grow rapidly in this temperature range and mechanically destroy the tissue viability.[83] Freezing at −76° C is achieved in dry ice. At −60° C to −90° C, using a laboratory-type mechanical deep freezer, and at −150° C or colder, using a refrigerator with cryogenic gases, more effective preservation of bone is possible. At temperatures near −70° C, ice crystal formation is slower.[83] Bones frozen to −70° C have been stored for several years and successfully applied clinically.[49] Freezing in a cryoprotective agent such as glycerol at controlled cooling velocity may be a more effective option.

Freeze drying is a process in which the bone is first frozen to −70° C and then sublimated in a high vacuum. The bone is freeze dried until the water content is reduced to 5% or less. The freeze-dried bone graft can then be shipped and stored conveniently and indefinitely at room temperature in a vacuum container. Since freeze-dried bone is very brittle, it must be reconstituted by immersion in normal saline before use.[84] The reconstitution time depends on the size and shape of the graft. Chips of bone may not require any rehydration, whereas larger cortical-bone may require up to 24 hours for reconstitution.[49]

In the clinical application of freeze-dried allografts in spine fusion, Malinin and Brown[83] reported that the union rate of such allografts under compression load (interbody or strut grafts) was not delayed by low-grade immunologic response. This is in contrast to a high incidence of resorption with cortical graft placed under tension posteriorly in the spine.

*References 15, 49, 71, 74, 82, and 83.

Biomechanical Properties

Biomechanical properties of bone grafts may be changed by the techniques used for preservation, although Sedlin's study showed that freezing and thawing do not significantly alter the mechanical properties of bone.[117]

Bright and Burstein,[12] as well as Triantafyllou and co-workers,[129] studied the biomechanical properties of freeze-dried and irradiated bones. Komender[70] found that freezing to −78° C does not alter the mechanical properties of bone. Pelker and associates[103] also concluded that freezing allograft bone to temperatures as low as that of liquid nitrogen (−196° C) does not significantly alter its biomechanical properties. They showed that freeze drying does diminish the torsional and bending strength but not the compressive strength. The data of Pelker and co-workers indicate that frozen bones are better suited than freeze-dried bones when they are subjected to torsional loads.[102,103]

Both frozen and freeze-dried bones are acceptable when compressive forces are the primary concern. It must be remembered that the initial biomechanical properties of the bone graft will change with resorption, incorporation, and remodeling by the host. Surgical technique, internal fixation, and postoperative management must therefore be planned accordingly.

Radiation, Heat, and Chemical Treatment of Allografts and Xenografts

Although most of the aseptically procured cadaver bones do not require sterilization, allografts or xenografts have been sterilized by physical means such as high-energy radiation and heat (boiling, autoclaving); and by chemicals such as thimerosal (Merthiolate), ethylene dioxide, propiolactone, or antibiotic solutions. Some of these sterilization methods were used in the past and are discussed for historic interest only.

Radiation of at least 2 megarads is required to kill bacteria; 4 megarads inactivates some viruses.[83] The same dose of radiation (2 to 4 megarads) needed to sterilize or destroy antigens also significantly impairs the inductive repair capacity of the bone graft.[16,132,133] Increased solubility of collagen and glycosaminoglycan, destruction of the bone matrix fibrillar network,[16,22] and discoloration[83] of irradiated bone have been reported. In cobalt-60 irradiated bone, Ostrowski[99] reported free radicals of unusual stability to be present, although their effect on the host tissue is unclear.[83]

The effect of radiation on the biomechanical properties of bone is not well defined at this time. The effect seems to be minimal with low-level radiation. Radiation doses exceeding 3 megarads are known to destroy bone matrix fibrillar network.[16,22] There appears to be a significant drop of breaking strength of bone with more than 3 megarads. This effect is magnified when radiation is combined with freeze drying. Komender noted that 6 megarads of radiation reduced the strength in bending, compression, and torsion.[70] Irradiation of freeze-dried bone with only 3 megarads markedly diminished the bending strength, but not the strength in compression or torsion.

Boiled bones have been used for graft material since the early part of this century.[52] Although some good clinical results have been reported,[77,152] boiled allografts and xenografts have generally produced undesirable results. Boiling destroys all inductive capacity.[152] Heat may be intended to destroy transplantation antigen, but it only denatures the antigenic proteins into another unacceptable material.

It may be tempting to use autoclaved contaminated bone in the operating room, but this produces haversian canal coagulation and denaturation of bone protein,[16,83] which severely retard host incorporation. Autoclaving destroys bone morphogenic protein activity.

Chemical processing of bone graft may present significant problems such as potential carcinogenesis and difficulty of penetration into bone. Propiolactone (1% solution) has been found to be more bacteriocidal than ethylene dioxide, which is more difficult to use.[83]

Merthiolate-treated grafts have, in general, produced poor results; 30% of the grafts failed in the study by Reynolds and co-workers,[110] with apparently three times as many failures as with autografts. Reduced callus formation and osteogenesis have been noted. When the graft fractured, there was minimal healing. When washed before use, no significant host sensitivity to Merthiolate was noted in Merthiolate-treated bone graft.[83]

Benzalkonium chloride completely destroys the osteogenic inductive capacity of bone, according to Urist and associates.[135] Antibiotic solutions do not penetrate completely into bone. Their germicidal effect in bone graft is variable. In general, antibiotics appear to inhibit the osteogenic inductive capacity of bone.[3,83]

A prospective study evaluating the radiographic appearance of demineralized bone matrix (DBM) chemosterilized with ethylene oxide in posterolateral lumbar spine fusion in human beings was presented by Zucherman and associates.[156] Sixty-eight levels of bilateral posterolateral lumbar spinal fusions were performed using combinations of autologous bone graft (ABG) and DBM. Patients were randomly assigned to three groups: Group 1[20] (the control) consisted of bilateral placement of the ABG/DBM mixture, Group 2[30] consisted of ABG on one side with the ABG/DBM mixture on the other, and Group 3[30] consisted of ABG on one side and DBM on the other. Mean follow-up was 15 months. An orthopedist and a radiologist blinded to the content of the fusion masses rated the fusions on a scale from zero (resorption) to three (confluence) on the basis of appearance of consolidation on an anteroposterior radiograph of the lumbar spine. Results of this prospective series suggest that in posterolateral spine fusion in human beings, it is less effective than autologous bone graft.[156]

Bone Morphogenetic Protein

Urist states that allograft bone must be removed from the donor within 4 to 8 hours after death or within the minimal biodegradable time.[132] Radiation sterilization with more than 2 megarads; heating over 60° C; exposure to chemicals such as hydrogen peroxide, betapropriolactone, or benzalkonium chloride; cryolysis; immediate freeze drying; and prolonged storage at 0° C to 30° C must be avoided to preserve the inductive properties of the bone. Urist and co-workers have extensively studied osteogenic induction and discovered the biologically active factor that they called bone morphogenetic protein (BMP), which modulates recruitment of mesenchymal stem cells that differentiate into osteoblasts from surrounding tissues.[131,132,135,136,139] Bone morphogenetic protein has been extracted from bone-forming tumors, dentin, and diaphysis of cortical bone. Studies demonstrated a number of highly active proteins with molecular weights of approximately 30,000.[80,115,154] To date, seven BMP proteins have been isolated from bone-inducing preparations using high-resolution protein purification techniques and recombinant DNA technology.[6] Four proteins (BMP-2, BMP-3, BMP-4 and BMP-7) have been shown to induce bone formation in animals.[6,142] Their clinical application has been evaluated in the form of an injectable substance linked to different delivery systems.[137]

A chemosterilized bone that is an autodigested, antigen-extracted allograft (AAA) has been developed and clinically tested by Urist and co-workers. It is an allogeneic bone of high osteogenetic property and low immunogenicity prepared in five basic steps. Urist believes that BMP is also preserved by these measures.[132,138,139]

Urist and Dawson[134] reported 40 intertransverse-process fusions in 36 cases of degenerative joint and disc disease including spinal stenosis and spondylolisthesis, as well as four cases of thoracolumbar fracture dislocation. A composite of AAA cortical bone strips and local autologous bone was used in all cases. There were over 80% excellent and good results, with a nonunion rate of 12%.

Xenografts (Heterologous Bones, Heterografts)

Xenografts, or bones transplanted from other species, have been used in spine surgery.[64,86] The advantages of xenografts are the almost unlimited supply from animal sources; wide range of sizes, shapes, and strength; and cortical-cancellous ratio. The application of ivory,[63,81] animal horns,[63] corals,[60,61] and other exotic materials has been explored. Animal horns and ivory are very resistant to incorporation into the host bone.[112] Fresh xenograft bones have been shown to be unacceptable. Due to the antigenicity of the foreign tissue they are unable to generate satisfactory bony repair. Invariably, they produce inflammation, fever, sequestration, resorption, or other manifestations of rejection.[16] Fibrous envelopment occurs as over a metal plate. Even when fusion takes place, sequestration of the xenograft is observed. Urist believes that xenografts should not be used in patients.[132]

Partially deproteinated and defatted xenografts[43] were reported to have markedly decreased antigenicity resulting in a minimized immune response. However, the osteoinductive capacity is reduced by the denaturing process that destroys BMP and other osteoinductive proteins.

Bovine bones have been popular because they incorporate and remodel with less difficulty.[112] Different types of preserved bovine bone have been tried since the nineteenth century, including

1. Frozen calf bone
2. Freeze-dried calf bone (Boplant)[104]
3. Decalcified ox bone[55] (as well as decalcified calf and sheep bone) was evaluated experimentally and clinically, but found to be unsatisfactory.

Deproteinized xenografts, including "os purim," "anorganic bone," "Oswestry bone," and "Kiel bone,"[86,112-114] have also been tried.

Kiel bone, partly deproteinized bone from freshly killed calf, sterilized either by ethylene dioxide or by gamma radiation, is commercially available. Experimental studies showed that it is weakly antigenic and does not possess active bone-inducing capacity.[114] Since its introduction in 1957, Kiel bone has been used in almost every possible bone-graft site, and varying success rates have been reported clinically.[64,86,112]

In spinal fusion, Jackson[64] noted that Kiel-bone implant became surrounded by autogenous bone with time. For larger defects, he recommended the use of an autogenous and Kiel bone composite. McMurray[92] presented clinical, radiologic, and histologic data on the fate of Kiel-bone implants in four anterior spine fusions that failed. Biopsies of the Kiel-bone implants showed invasion by fibrous tissue. There was no ossification and no incorporation into the surrounding bone. Such deproteinized bone could be invaded by host new bone when placed in an excellent vascular bed with potentially osteogenic cells. When impregnated with autogenous bone marrow cells, it may prove to be an excellent scaffolding with good bone-conduction property.[112,114] Plenk and associates,[105] Salama,[112] and Salama and co-workers[113,114] reported good results using autogenous bone marrow and Kiel bone as composite grafts in patients. The red marrow can be easily aspirated from the patient's own iliac crest. The bone marrow is protected from the action of the adjacent tissues when the deproteinized bone is present to serve as an osteoconductive supportive structure.

Synthetic Implants

Synthetic implants can be prepared to fit any size or shape, but they have traditionally been considered to be subject to wear and not incorporate biologically into the host bone.[16] Metals such as titanium, ceramics, and polymers (e.g., polyethylene with porous surfaces) could allow ingrowth of bone when the interface between the implant and living bone is stable. When significant motion is present between the implant and the bone, fibrous ingrowth occurs. A number of implants fashioned from metals have been tried as replacement for bone in the spinal column (see, for example, Steffee's titanium vertebral replacement: "Total Vertebral Body and Pedicle Replacement"[124] [Steffee A: personal communication, 1991]).

Metal scaffolds in the shape of the bone being replaced may be covered by ground autologous bone grafts of small particle size. In animal experiments, ingrowth of bone occurred over the total surface area of fiber metal implants and bone penetrated deep into the composite.[2]

Titanium mesh implants have been clinically applied by Leong[75] (Leong JCY: personal communication, 1984) and co-workers for anterior spinal fusion after discectomy in the lumbar spine. This porous implant allows ingrowth of bone and appears to obviate the use of bone graft. It acts as a spacer and can provide immediate stability, while allowing time for the slow ingrowth of bone and long-term stability.

Experimentally, porous titanium mesh blocks with a 50% void allow rapid ingrowth of bone in canine long bone. A 12-year follow-up was possible in two patients who are asymptomatic, and the implants have remained unchanged and undisplaced; 10 patients had a follow-up of more than 5-years. Of these, seven patients were asymptomatic, two had more than 70% symptomatic relief, and one retained a very stiff back. Radiologic analysis showed that disc height was maintained at 5 years with no movement between the adjacent vertebral bodies, often with bony overgrowth anterior to the implant.

Steffee and co-workers[124] reported a total vertebral body replacement and artificial pedicle replacement with the aid of a special segmental spine plate fixation[123,124] (Steffee A: personal communication, 1991). Their system allows immediate and rigid fixation after extensive decompressions and radical tumor excisions. Theoretically, the total vertebral replacement may be performed using metallic or nonmetallic implants with a porous structure that allows bony ingrowth.

Nonmetallic Synthetic Implants

A growing number of other synthetic implants are being used as bone substitutes. These biosynthetic bone-graft substitutes address the disadvantages of both autogenous bone harvest and allograft problems.[72] According to Osborn and Nemesley[98] the chemical nature of the implant determines the biodynamics and reaction of the recipient bed in the interaction with living bone. They considered the following materials[23,98]:

1. Bone cement and stainless steel are biotolerant, resulting in *distance osteogenesis* with a fibrous layer separating the implant from bone.

2. Alumina and carbon materials are bioinert, resulting in *contact osteogenesis*.

3. Glass ceramic, calcium phosphate ceramics, and hydroxyapatite ceramics are bioactive, resulting in *bonding osteogenesis*.

Bioinert porous ceramics of alumina were noted by Benum and associates[4] to be bound to bone by the ingrowth of bone 3 to 4 mm thick in regions exposed to compressive forces.

Evidence suggests that porous calcium phosphate ceramics are the most biocompatible synthetic-bone substitute, with the ability to become chemically bonded by living bone and with a chemical composition devoid of toxicologic liabilities.[65] They are shown to be superior to biodegradable polymers, such as polylactic acid and polyglycolic acid, which have been considered as bone substitutes.[24,65] The implants may be dense or porous. The minimum pore size for ingrowth of bone is shown to be 100 μm.[68] Corals provide such porous structures.[60,61]

Holmes and co-workers[61] performed histologic and biomechanical studies in dogs using hydroxyapatite converted from sea coral calcite as bone substitute. The material was incorporated in bone and became almost as strong as the native bone. They also reported encouraging clinical application with fractures in 18 patients. Hydroxyapatite is the natural bone mineral. There is great potential of developing or discovering minerals so close to human bone that normal bone turnover would occur in a physiologic environment. Such porous mineral structure would undergo appropriate gradual and timely biodegradation and eventually be replaced by living bone. Tricalcium phosphate, for example, has the potential to undergo slow biodegradation and be replaced by bone in the living system.[88]

Another material, replam hydroxyapatite-porites (RHAP), is a ceramic with three-dimensional interconnected porous material of calcium hydroxyapatite from the exoskeleton of porites (coral). It may be carved by the surgeon before implanting. Replam hydroxyapatite-porites was approved for evaluation in spinal fusion in several centers under Mooney and associates.[88]

Bioactive and biodegradable porous ceramics of hydroxyapatite or tricalcium phosphate have been studied. Jarcho[65] stated that they are usually well tolerated and become chemically bonded to bone by natural bone-cementing mechanisms.

Porous hydroxyapatite ceramics have been used in canine experiments for the spine[33] and other skeletal defects. Porous ceramics and autologous marrow composites were studied by Nade and associates.[91] Porous alumina, calcium aluminate calcium hydroxyapatite, and tricalcium phosphate were placed with bone marrow into intermuscular sites. Bone was found to adhere to the ceramics and to penetrate the interior if the pore size was greater than 100 μm. The marrow cells were shown to play a significant part in new bone formation into the framework. Nade and co-workers believe that the appropriate histocompatible, biodegradable ceramic material would act as a scaffold by virtue of its porosity for retention of bone-marrow cells, and provide mechanical strength while bone ingrowth progresses. This type of bone substitute would also allow a wide selection of sizes and shapes in sterile form. More recently, Ohgushi and co-workers[94] demonstrated improved biomechanical properties with increased bone growth when porous ceramics were combined with bone marrow.

Porous biodegradable ceramic and BMP composites were evaluated by Urist and co-workers.[137] They reported that an aggregate of B-tricalcium phosphate and bone morphogenetic protein (TCP/BMP) induced the differentiation of cartilage in 8 days and in lamella bone in 21 days. The yield of new bone was more than 12 times greater from the TCP/BMP than from the BMP alone. It is possible that a porous ceramic acts as a slow-release delivery system to distribute BMP more favorably and to potentiate its activity.

Calcium phosphate–coated metallic implants showed superior bone-bonding characteristics according to Ducheyne and associates.[36] Such implants may solve the problem of weak mechanical strength of ceramics, particularly the porous ones. Ceramic implants by themselves are probably unsuitable for restoration that would have to withstand significant impact, or torsional or bending stresses,[65] as in the spinal column.

Calcium phosphate–containing bone cements are also being developed. Calcium hydroxyapatite in powder form was used as an expander of a patient's own cancellous bone graft. It has been used in spine fusion, especially in children, when sufficient autologous bone graft is unavailable (Luque ER: personal communication, 1985). In general, the various synthetic hydroxyapatite and tricalcium phosphate ceramic or crystalline preparations have been shown to be nontoxic and biocompatible, and to have the potential to form intimate bonding with the host bone.[50] They are osteoconductive and usually not osteoinductive by themselves. These synthetic preparations have the greatest potential as a vehicle for bone marrow, BMP, and other bone-inducing agents.[50]

Collagen and Other Matrix Proteins

Major constituents of demineralized bone matrix are collagen and other matrix proteins. The mineralization process relies on the extracellular organic matrix. It is believed that fibrillar collagen, the main component of this matrix, has the capacity to serve as the structural osteoconductive scaffolding for the mineralization. Osteonectin, a noncollagen matrix protein, is complex with collagen.[128] Proteolipids and calcium acidic-phospholipid phosphate com-

plexes,[128,140] as well as bone and dentin phosphoprotein, were demonstrated to cause hydroxyapatite formation in vitro.[8,10,93,128,140] Fibronectin, a matrix and cell membrane protein, is believed to act as a binder for mesenchymal-cell attachment to collagen matrix, which in turn allows the osteoinductor to contact cell-surface receptors.[147] Wernts and co-workers demonstrated that soluble fibrillar collagen and marrow composite is more effective than even cancellous bone for bridging large bone defects.[148] However, without the marrow, the collagen by itself is inferior to cancellous bone.[72] A combination of soluble fibrillar collagen, marrow, and ceramic of 40% tricalcium phosphate and 60% hydroxyapatite with the ceramic constituting 25% to 50% of the volume is effective in healing rat femoral segmental defects.[72,73] With further studies, similar synthetic composites may prove to be clinically useful.

Methylmethacrylate Cement

Knight[69] was the first to report the use of acrylic cement to fix the cervical spine with chronic fracture dislocation, atlantoaxial subluxation, and cervical spondylosis. He also stabilized the lumbar spine using the cement in one patient with disc disease. Scoville and co-workers[116] reported the use of acrylic plastic for vertebral replacement or fixation in metastatic tumor destruction of the spine.

Harrington[56] documented the use of methylmethacrylate for vertebral body replacement and anterior stabilization of the spine with metastatic tumor. His series included 14 patients treated by anterior decompression and stabilization using metal and bone cement. The strength of methylmethacrylate is about one half that of bone.[151] Attempts have been made to strengthen the cement by adding fibers,[87] but clinical data are still unavailable. After polymerization, methylmethacrylate becomes a rigid and brittle solid that can withstand significant compression. However, it fails under tension or shear forces. It is reasonable to use in the replacement of a vertebral body where compression is the predominant force present. It is important to remember that when used alone, the outer part of the cement mass is still subject to tension when bending, and will fail with time in a clinical setting. The primary indication for application of methylmethacrylate in spinal stabilization is in patients with malignant disease and limited life expectancy.[42,90] It should not be expected to provide long-term support of the spine.[37]

In the spinal column, methylmethacrylate cement should be used with secure metal fixation. It may be used as reinforcement for screws and hooks in cancellous bone. The cement does enhance fixation of implants by increasing the contact area, especially in osteoporotic bone.

References

1. Albrektsson T: The healing of autologous bone grafts after varying degrees of surgical trauma, *J Bone Joint Surg* 62B:403, 1980.

2. Andersson GBJ and others: Segmental replacement of the femur in baboons with fiber metal implants and autologous bone grafts of different particle size, *Acta Orthop Scand* 53:349, 1982.

3. Bassett CAL: Clinical implications of cell function in bone grafting, *Clin Orthop* 87:45, 1972.

4. Benum P and others: Porous ceramics as a bone substitute in the medial condyle of the tibia: an experimental study in sheep: long-term observations, *Acta Orthop Scand* 48:150, 1977.

5. Blakemore ME: Fractures at cancellous bone graft donor sites, *Injury* 14:519, 1983.

6. Bolander ME: *Inducers of osteogenesis.* In *Bone and cartilage allografts: biology and clinical applications,* Park Ridge, IL, 1991, American Academy of Orthopedic Surgeons, p 75.

7. Bonfiglio M, Jetter WS: Immunological response to bone, *Clin Orthop* 87:19, 1972.

8. Boskey AL, Posner AS: The role of synthetic and bone extracted Ca-phospholipid-PO4 complexes in hydroxyapatite formation, *Calcif Tissue Res* 23:251, 1977.

9. Bosworth DM: Repair of herniae through iliac crest defects, *J Bone Joint Surg* 37A:1069, 1955.

10. Bovan-Salvars BD, Boskey AL: Relationship between proteolipids and calcium phospholipid phosphate complexes in calcification, *Calcif Tissue Int* 30:167, 1980.

11. Bradford DSL: Anterior vascular pedicle bone grafting for the treatment of kyphosis, *Spine* 5:318, 1980.

12. Bright R, Burstein A: Material properties of preserved cortical bone, *Trans Orthop Res Soc* 3:210, 1978.

13. Brown KLB, Cruess RL: Bone and cartilage transplantation in orthopaedic surgery, *J Bone Joint Surg* 64A:270, 1982.

14. Brown LT: The mechanics of the lumbosacral and sacroiliac joints, *J Bone Joint Surg.* 19:770, 1937.

15. Brown MD and others: A roentgenographic evaluation of frozen allografts versus autografts in anterior cervical spine fusions, *Clin Orthop* 119:231, 1976.

16. Burchardt H: The biology of bone graft repair, *Clin Orthop* 174:28, 1983.

17. Burchardt H and others: Freeze-dried allogenic segmental cortical-bone grafts in dogs, *J Bone Joint Surg* 60A:1082, 1978.

18. Burwell RG: A study of homologous cancellous bone combined with autologous red marrow after transplantation to a muscular site, *J Anat* 95:613, 1961.

19. Burwell RG: Studies in the transplantation of bone. V. the capacity of fresh and treated homografts of bone to evoke transplantation immunity, *J Bone Joint Surg* 45B:386, 1963.

20. Burwell RG: Studies in transplantation of bone. VIII. treated composite homo-autografts of cancellous bone, *J Bone Joint Surg* 48B:532, 1966.

21. Burwell RG: The fate of bone grafts. In Apley AG, editor: *Recent advances in orthopaedics,* Baltimore, 1969, Williams & Wilkins.

22. Burwell RG: The fate of freeze-dried bone allografts, *Transplant Proc.* (suppl 1) 8:95, 1976.

23. Burwell RG: The function of bone marrow in the incorporation of a bone graft, *Clin Orthop* 200:125, 1985.

24. Cameron HU: Evaluation of a biodegradable ceramic, *J Biomed Mater Res* 11:179, 1977.

25. Challis JH and others: Strangulated lumbar hernia and volvulus following removal of iliac crest bone graft, *Acta Orthop Scand* 46:230, 1975.

26. Chalmers J, Rush J: Observations on the induction of bone in soft tissues, *J Bone Joint Surg* 57B:36, 1975.

27. Cobey ML: A national bone bank survey, *Clin Orthop* 110:333, 1975.

28. Cockin J: Autologous bone grafting-complications at the donor site, *J Bone Joint Surg* 53B:153, 1971.

29. Cooper JW: Cluneal nerve injury and chronic postsurgical neuritis, *J Bone Joint Surg* 49A:199, 1967.

30. Coventry MB, Tapper EM: Pelvic instability: a consequence of removing iliac bone for grafting, *J Bone Joint Surg* 54A:83, 1972.

31. Cowley SP, Anderson LD: Brief note: hernias through donor sites for iliac-bone grafts, *J Bone Joint Surg* 65A:1023, 1983.

32. Curtiss PhH and others: Immunological factors in homologous bone transplantation, *J Bone Joint Surg* 41A:1481, 1959.

33. Dawson E: *The fate of bone substitution with porous hydroxyapatite implants in the dog spine.* In Transactions of the 27th Annual Meeting, Orthopaedic Research Society Vol 6, 1981.

34. deBoer HH: The history of bone grafts, *Clin Orthop* 226:292, 1988.

35. Doi K and others: Anterior cervical fusion using the free vascularized fibular graft, *Spine* 13:1239, 1988.

36. Ducheyne P and others: Effect of hydroxyapatite impregnation on skeletal bonding of porous coated implants, *J Biomed Mater Res* 14:225, 1980.

37. Dunn EJ: The role of methylmethacrylate in the stabilization and replacement of tumors of the cervical spine, *Spine* 2:15, 1977.

38. Dupuis PR and others: Anterior free vascular transplant of the fibula for the treatment of kyphosis, *J Bone Joint Surg* 64B:259, 1982.

39. Drury BJ: Clinical evaluation of back and leg pain due to irritation of the superior cluneal nerve, *J Bone Joint Surg* 49A:199, 1967.

40. Bone harvesting and transplantation, *Lancet* 2:730, 1981 (editorial).

41. Edmonson AS and others: *Campbell's operative orthopaedics,* ed 6, St. Louis, 1980, Mosby.

42. Eftekhar NS, Thurston CW: Effect of irradiation on acrylic cement with special reference to fixation of pathological fractures, *J Biomech* 8:53, 1975.

43. Elves MW, Salama R: A study of the development of cytotoxic antibodies produced in recipients of

xenografts (heterografts) of iliac bone, *J Bone Joint Surg* 56B:331, 1974.

44. Enneking WF and others: Autogenous cortical bone grafts in the reconstruction of segmental skeletal defects, *J Bone Joint Surg* 62A:1039, 1980.

45. Escalas F, Dewald RL: Combined traumatic arteriovenous fistula and ureteral injury: a complication of iliac bone-grafting, a case report. *J Bone Joint Surg* 59A:270, 1977.

46. Evarts CM: *Surgery of the musculoskeletal system,* New York, 1983, Churchill Livingstone.

47. Fernyhough JC and others: Chronic donor site pain complicating bone graft harvesting from the posterior iliac crest for spinal fusion, *Spine* 17:1474, 1992.

48. Frankel VH Burstein AH: *Orthopedic biomechanics,* Philadelphia, 1970, Lea & Febiger.

49. Friedlander GE: Current concepts review - bone-banking, *J Bone Joint Surg* 64A:307, 1982.

50. Friedlander G, Huo M: *Bone grafts and bone graft substitutes.* In Frymoyer JW, editor: *The adult spine: principles and practice.* New York, 1991, Raven Press, p 565.

51. Froimson AI, Cummings AG, Jr: Iliac hernia following hip arthrodesis, *Clin Orthop* 30:89, 1971.

52. Gallie WE: The use of boiled bone in operative surgery, *Am J Orthop Surg* 16:373, 1918.

53. Ghent WR: Further studies on meralgia paresthetica, *Can Med Assoc J* 85:871, 1961.

54. Goldberg VM, Shaffer JW, Stevenson S: *Biology of vascularized bone grafts. Bone and cartilage allografts: biology and clinical applications,* Park Ridge, IL, 1991, American Academy of Orthopedic Surgeons, p 13.

55. Gupta D and others: Bridging large bone defects with a xenograft composited with autologous bone marrow: an experimental study, *Int Orthop (SICOT)* 6:79, 1982.

56. Harrington KD: The use of methylmethacrylate for vertebral body replacement and anterior stabilization of pathological fracture dislocations of the spine, due to metastatic disease, *J Bone Joint Surg* 63A:36, 1981.

57. Hartman JR and others: A pedicle bone grafting procedure for failed lumbosacral spinal fusion, *Clin Orthop* 178:223, 1983.

58. Heiple KG and others: A comparative study of the healing process following different types of bone transplantation, *J Bone Joint Surg* 45A:1593, 1963.

59. Heppenstall RB: *Fracture treatment and healing,* Philadelphia, 1989, W.B. Saunders.

60. Holmes RE: Bone regeneration within a coraline hydroxyapatite implant, *Plast Reconstr Surg* 63:626, 1979.

61. Holmes R and others: A coralline hydroxyapatite bone graft substitute: preliminary report, *Clin Orthop* 188:252, 1984.

62. Hsu K, Zucherman J, White A: *Bone grafts and implants in spine surgery.* In White AH, Rothman RH, Ray CD, editors: *Lumbar spine surgery: techniques and complications,* St. Louis, 1987, Mosby, p 343.

63. Hughes CW: Rate of absorption and callus stimulating properties of cow horn, ivory, beef bone and autogenous bone, *Surg Gynecol Obstet* 76:665, 1943.

64. Jackson JW: Surgical approaches to the anterior aspect of the spinal column, *Ann R Coll Surg Engl* 48:83, 1971.

65. Jarcho M: Calcium phosphate ceramics as hard tissue prosthetics, *Clin Orthop* 157:259, 1981.

66. Kahn BP: Superior gluteal artery laceration: a complication of iliac bone graft surgery, *Clin Orthop* 140:204, 1979.

67. Kaneda K, Kurakami C, Minami A: Free vascularized fibular strut graft in the treatment of kyphosis, *Spine* 13:1273, 1988.

68. Klawitter JJ, Hulbert SF: Application of porous ceramics for the attachment of load bearing orthopaedic applications, *J Biomed Mater Res* 2:161, 1971.

69. Knight G: Paraspinal acrylic inlays in the treatment of cervical and lumbar spondylosis and other conditions, *Lancet* 2:147, 1959.

70. Komender A: Influence of preservation on some mechanical properties of human haversian bone, *Mater Med Pol* 8:13, 1976.

71. Kreuz FP and others: The preservation and clinical use of freeze-dried bone, *J Bone Joint Surg* 33A:297, 1974.

72. Lane JM and others: *Clinical application of biosynthetics - bone and cartilage allografts: biology and clinical applications,* Park Ridge, IL, 1991, American Academy of Orthopedic Surgeons.

73. Lane JM, Sandhu HS: Current approaches to experimental bone grfting, *Orthop Clin North Am* 18:213, 1987.

74. Langer F and others: The immunogenicity of fresh and frozen allogeneic bone, *J Bone Joint Surg* 57A:216, 1975.

75. Leong JCY and others: *The use of porous titanium mesh implant after discectomy in patients with deranged lumbar intervertebral disc—the five-year results of a prospective trial,* Twelfth Annual Meeting of the International Society for the Study of the Lumbar Spine, 1985 (abstracts).

76. Lichtblau S: Dislocation of the sacro-iliac joint: a complication of bone-grafting, *J Bone Joint Surg* 44A:193, 1962.

77. Lloyd-Roberts GC: Experiences with boiled cadaveric bone, *J Bone Joint Surg* 34B:428, 1952.

78. Lotem M and others: Lumbar hernia at an iliac bone graft donor site: a case report, *Clin Orthop* 80:130, 1971.

79. Lubicky JP, Dewald RL: Methylmethacrylatae reconstruction of large iliac crest bone defect donor site, *Clin Orthop* 164:252, 1982.

80. Luyten FP and others: Purification and partial amino acid sequence of osteogenin, a protein initiating bone differentiation, *J Biol Chem* 264:13370, 1989.

81. Magnusson PB: Holding fractures with absorbable materials—ivory plates and screws, *JAMA* 61:1514, 1913.

82. Malinin TI: University of Miami tissue bank: collection of postmortem tissues for clinical use and laboratory investigation, *Transplant Proc* (suppl) 8:53, 1976.

83. Malinin TI: *Cadaver bone allografts—bone banks.* In Turek SL, editor: *Orthopaedics, principles and their application,* Philadelphia, 1984, Lippincott.

84. Malinin TI, and Brown MD: Bone allograft in spinal surgery, *Clin Orthop* 154:168, 1981.

85. Massey EW: Meralgia paresthetica secondary to trauma of bone graft, *J Trauma* 20:342, 1980.

86. McMurray GN: The evaluation of Kiel bone in spinal fusions, *J Bone Joint Surg* 64B:100, 1982.

87. Mittelmeier JH and others: PMMA cement with carbon fiber reinforcement and apatite ingredients: mechanical properties and tissue reaction in animal tests, First World Biomaterials Congress, Bade, Austria, 1980.

88. Mooney J, Derian C: *Synthetic bone graft, lumbar spine surgery: techniques and complications.* In White AH, Rothman RH, Ray CD, editors: *Lumbar Spine Surgery Techniques and Complications.* St. Louis, 1987, Mosby, p 471.

89. Moore JB and others: A biomechanical comparison of vascularized and conventional autogenous bone grafts, *Plast Reconstr Surg* 73:382, 1984.

90. Murray JA and others: Irradiation of polymethylmethacrylate: in vitro gamma radiation effect, *J Bone Joint Surg* 56A:311, 1974.

91. Nade S and others: Osteogenesis and bone marrow transplantation, the ability of ceramic materials to sustain osteogenesis from transplanted bone marrow cells: preliminary studies, *Clin Orthop* 181:255, 1983.

92. Nade S, Burwell RG: Decalcified bone as a substrate for osteogenesis: an appraisal of the interrelation of bone and marrow in combined grafts, *J Bone Joint Surg* 59B:189, 1977.

93. Nawrot CJF and others: Dental phosphoprotein-induced formation of hydroxylapatite during in vitro synthesis of amorphous calcium phosphate, *Biochemistry* 15:3445, 1976.

94. Ohgushi H, Goldberg VM, Caplan AI: Heterotopic osteogenesis in porous ceramics induced by marrow cells, *J Orthop Res* 7:568, 1989.

95. Oikarinen J, Korhonen LK: The bone inductive capacity of various bone transplanting materials used for treatment of experimental bone defects, *Clin Orthop* 140:208, 1979.

96. Oldfield MD: Iliac hernia after bone grafting, *Lancet* 248:810, 1945.

97. Osborn JF, Newesely H: Dynamic aspects of the implant-bone-interface, *Dental Implants* 111:123, 1980.

98. Osborn JF, and Newesely H: The material science of calcium phosphate ceramics, *Biomaterials* 1:108, 1980.

99. Ostrowski K: Current problems of tissue banking, *Transplant Proc* 1:126, 1969.

100. Ostrup LT: Distant transfer of a free living bone graft by microvascular anastomoses, and experimental study, *Plast Reconstr Surg* 54:274, 1974.

101. Pappas AM: Current methods of freezing and freeze-drying, *Cryobiology* 4:358, 1968.

102. Pelker RR and others: Biomechanical properties of bone allografts, *Clin Orthop* 174:54, 1983.

103. Pelker R and others: The effects of preservation on allograft strength, *Trans Orthop Res Soc* 7:283, 1982.

104. Pierson AP and others: Bone grafting with Boplant: results in thirty-three cases, *J Bone Joint Surg* 50B:364, 1968.

105. Plenk H Jr, Hollmann K, Wilfert KH: Experimental bridging of osseous defects in rats by the implantation of Kiel bone containing fresh autologous marrow, *J Bone Joint Surg* 54B:735, 1972.

106. Pyrtek LJ, Kelly CC: Management of herniation through large iliac bone defects, *Ann Surg* 152:998, 1960.

107. Ray RD: Vascularization of bone grafts and implants, *Clin Orthop* 87:43, 1972.

108. Ray RD, Holloway JA: Bone implants, *J Bone Joint Surg* 39A:1119, 1957.

109. Reid RL: Hernia through an iliac bone-graft donor site: a case report, *J Bone Joint Surg* 50A:757, 1968.

110. Reynold CF and others: Clinical evaluation of the merthiolate bone bank and homogenous bone grafts, *J Bone Joint Surg* 33A:873, 1951.

111. Rhinelander FW: Tibial blood supply in relation to fracture healing, *Clin Orthop* 105:34, 1974.

112. Salama R: Xenogeneic bone grafting in humans, *Clin Orthop* 174:113, 1983.

113. Salama R, Weissman SL: The clinical use of combined xenografts of bone and autologous red marrow: a preliminary report, *J Bone Joint Surg* 60B:111, 1978.

114. Salama R and others: Recombined grafts of bone and marrow, *J Bone Joint Surg* 55B:402, 1973.

115. Sampath TK, Coughlin JE, Whetstone RM and others: Bovine osteogenic protein is composed of dimers of OP-1 and BMP 2A, two members of the transforming growth factor Beta superfamily, *J Biol Chem* 265:13198, 1990.

116. Scoville WB and others: The use of acrylic plastic for vertebral replacement or fixation in metastatic disease of the spine, *J Neurosurg* 27:274, 1967.

117. Sedlin E: A rheologic model for cortical bone, *Acta Orthop Scand* (suppl) 36:83, 1965.

118. Seres JL: Fusion in the presence of severe metastatic destruction of the cervical spine (case report), *J Neurosurg* 28:592, 1968.

119. Shaffer JW and others: The superiority of vascularized compared to nonvascularized rib grafts in spine surgery shown by biological and physical methods, *Spine* 13:1150, 1988.

120. Smith RT: The mechanism of graft rejection, *Clin Orthop* 87:15, 1972.

121. Smith SE and others: Ilioinguinal neuralgia following iliac bone-grafting, *J Bone Joint Surg* 66A:1306, 1984.

122. Spence WT: Internal plastic splint for stabilization of the spine, *Clin Orthop* 92:325, 1973.

123. Steffee A, Biscup R, Sitkowski D: Segmental spine plates with pedicle screw fixation: a new internal fixation device for disorders of the lumbar and thoracic spine, *Clin Orthop* 203:45, 1986.

124. Steffee A, Sitkowski D, Topham L: Total vertebral body and pedicle replacement, *Clin Orthop* 203:203, 1986.

125. Stringa G: Studies on the vascularization of bone grafts, *J Bone Joint Surg* 39B:395, 1957.

126. Summers BN, Eisenstein SM: Donor site pain from the ilium, a complication of lumbar spine fusion, *J Bone Joint Surg* 71B:677, 1989.

127. Taylor GI and others: The free vascularized bone graft: a clinical extension of microvascular techniques, *Plast Reconstr Surg* 64:745, 1979.

128. Termine JD, Kleinman HK, Whitson SWK and others: Osteonectin: a bone-specific protein linking mineral to collagen, *Cell* 26:99, 1981.

129. Triantafyllou N and others: The mechanical properties of the lyophilized and irradiated bone grafts, *Acta Orthop Belg* 41:35, 1975.

130. Turek SL: *Orthopaedics, principles, and their application,* Philadelphia, 1984, Lippincott.

131. Urist MR: Bone: formation by autoinduction, *Science* 150:893, 1965.

132. Urist MR: *Practical applications of bone research on bone graft physiology.* In *Instructional course lectures,* American Academy of Orthopaedic Surgeons, vol 25, St. Louis, 1976, Mosby.

133. Urist MR: Surface-decalcified allogenic bone implants, *Clin Orthop* 56:37, 1968.

134. Urist MR, Dawson E: Intertransverse process fusion with the aid of chemosterilized autolyzed antigen-extracted allogeneic (AAA) bone, *Clin Orthop* 154:97, 1981.

135. Urist MR, Nogami H: Morphogenetic substratum for differentiation cartilage in tissue culture, *Nature* 225:1051, 1970.

136. Urist MR, Strates BJS: Bone morphogenetic protein, *J Dent Res* 50:1392, 1971.

137. Urist MR and others: B-tricalcium phosphate delivery system for bone morphogenetic protein, *Clin Orthop* 187:277, 1984.

138. Urist MR and others: A chemosterilized antigen-extracted autodigested allo-implant for bone banks, *Arch Surg* 110:416, 1975.

139. Urist MR and others: Human bone morphorgenic protein (BMP), *Proc Soc Exp Biol Med* 173(2):194, 1983.

140. Veis A: *The role of acidic proteins in biological mineralization: ions in macromolecular and biological systems.* In Everett DH, Vincent B, editors: *Colston paper 29,* Bristol, England, 1978, Society Technica, p 259.

141. Verheugen P and others: Hernie illique apres prelevement osseux: subobstruction, *Acta Chir Belg* 1051:1056, 1965.

142. Wang EA, Rosen J, D'Alessandro JS and others: Recombinant human bone morphogenetic protein induces bone formation, *Proc Natl Acad Sci USA,* 87:2220, 1990.

143. Watson-Jones R: *Transplantation of bone.* In *Fracture and joint injuries,* vol 1, ed 4, Baltimore, 1955, Williams & Wilkins.

144. Weikel AM, Habal MB: Meralgia paresthetica: a complication of iliac bone procurement, *Plast Reconstr Surg* 60:572, 1977.

145. Weiland AJ: Current concept review: vascularized free bone transplants, *J Bone Joint Surg* 63A:166, 1981.

146. Weiland AJ, Phillips TW, Randolph MA: Bone grafts: a radiologic, histologic, and biomechanical model comparing autografts, allografts, and free vascularized bone grafts, *Plast Reconstr Surg* 74:368, 1984

147. Weiss RE, Reddi AH: Role of fibronectin in collagaenous matrix induced mesenchymal cell proliferation and differentiation in vivo, *Exp Cell Res* 133:243, 1981.

148. Werntz J, Lane JM, Piez C and others: The repair of segmental bone defects with collagen and marrow, *Orthop Trans* 10:346, 1986.

149. White AA III, Panjabi MM: *Clinical biomechanics of the spine,* Philadelphia, 1978, Lippincott.

150. White AA III and others: *Spinal stability: evaluation and treatment,* Instructional course lectures. The American Academy of Orthopaedic Surgeons, vol 30, St. Louis, 1981, Mosby.

151. Wilde AH, Greenwald AS: Shear strength of self-curing acrylic cement, *Clin Orthop* 106:126, 1975.

152. Williams G: Experiences with boiled cadaveric cancellous bone for fractures of long bones, *J Bone Joint Surg* 46B:398, 1964.

153. Wolfe SA, Kawamoto HK: Taking the iliac-bone graft: a new technique, *J Bone Joint Surg* 60A:411, 1978.

154. Wozney JM, Rosen J, Celeste AJ and others: Novel regulators of bone formation: molecular clones and activities, *Science* 242:1528, 1988.

155. Younger EM, Chapman MW: Morbidity at bone graft donor sites, *J Orthop Trauma* 3:192, 1989.

156. Zucherman JF, Brack S, Hsu KY and others: *Radiographic comparison of autogenous and freeze-dried ethylene oxide sterilized demineralized cortico-cancellous allograft bone in posterolateral spine fusion—a prospective study* (Submitted for publication).

Chapter 64
Bone Banking

James W. Simmons, Jr.
William W. Tomford

Tissue Banking

Donor Selection and Screening

Tissue Recovery

Processing of Bone

Secondary Sterilization

Freeze Drying

Freezing (Fresh Frozen)

Demineralized Bone

Summary

*"The art of progress is to preserve order amid change
and to preserve change amid order."*

Alfred North Whitehead

Ancient works of art and early medical records show that over the centuries physicians have sought to replace the damaged bones of their patients with bones from other human beings or from animals.[11] It is claimed that the first bone allograft transplant, represented in numerous Renaissance artistic renderings, was performed in the 6th century as a "miraculous" limb replacement performed by Saints Cosmas and Damian.[27] The first written record of a bone transplant occurs in Russian church records of 1682 when Meekren successfully used a piece of dog skull to repair a defect in the skull of a soldier.[6]

The first "modern" report of an allograft transplant is credited to Macewen[20] who began the systematic use and study of bone grafts in the mid-1800s. Since then, improved surgical skills and aseptic techniques have enabled surgeons to use bone for filling bony defects, creating spinal fusions, treating fracture nonunions, reshaping craniofacial deformities, and performing limb-sparing tumor resections.[4,17,22]

Throughout the first half of the 20th century, three sources of bone graft were used: the patient's own body (autograft), another human body (allograft), and other species (xenograft). Although many methods of bone storage and sterilization were tried,[8,19] until the 1950s, the effectiveness of bone grafting was limited by a high rate of complication and allograft failure that most likely was a result of insufficient understanding of graft preparation and handling.[28]

As modern freezing technology became widely available, it was discovered that adverse immunological responses could be significantly reduced if bone was deep frozen before transplantation. The success of long-term bone storage has led to the development of modern bone banking methods and techniques.[28]

Today, bone grafting is a common procedure, and approximately 250,000 bone and bone-tendon grafts are performed in the United States each year.[10] The increased number of procedures requiring bone has led to a concomitant increase in the demand for banked bone. Although fresh autogenous bone is considered to be biologically more effective,[11] banked allograft bone obviates the sacrifice of normal bone tissue and eliminates potential donor-site morbidity.[6,11] Autogenous bone is available only in limited quantity, whereas banked bone can be ordered by size, shape, and quantity for each surgical procedure.

Although a perceived risk of disease transmission exists with allograft use, such an occurrence is rare.[10,30] Public awareness and fear of HIV infection is high, but the small number of documented cases indicates that the incidence of HIV transmission is extremely rare with bone transplants.[28] The rate of complications for procedures using allograft compare favorably with those using autograft.[10,31]

Tissue Banking

Responding to the demand for allograft tissues, the number of tissue banks in the United States has increased rapidly. To meet the needs of these banks for a national organization or forum, the American Association of Tissue Banks (AATB) was formed in 1976 to establish legal, moral, ethical, and medical guidelines for organs and tissues used in transplantation. The AATB publishes standards for tissue banking[1,2] to help ensure that tissue banks follow accepted technical and ethical standards. Because these standards are not federally regulated, well planned protocols, validated procedures, and ongoing quality assurance systems must be in place in a tissue bank if the safety and efficacy of allografts are to be ensured.[28] In order to have confidence in the source and quality of the allograft, the surgeon must have a working knowledge of how the supplying tissue bank operates.

Donor Selection and Screening

It is the responsibility of each tissue bank to use current banking knowledge to protect the potential graft recipient and provide biologically functional grafts.[12] Part of this responsibility involves careful donor selection. Scrupulous attention must be paid to evaluating the donor's complete medical picture and lifestyle. This requires an objective perspective and strict adherence to exclusionary criteria.[28] Additionally, the medical history, physical examination or autopsy, and laboratory test results should be closely scrutinized to provide safe tissue for transplantation.

Permission for anatomical donation must be given by the legal next of kin. The AATB recommends a policy of informed consent and the explicit listing of the tissues to be removed. Donor cards and appropriately marked drivers' licenses are not sufficient to allow an automatic anatomical donation; rather, they are a mechanism for donors to express their wishes.[28]

Because a family may not have discussed the possibility of anatomic donation, it is important to approach the family of the deceased with sensitivity to their grief. If more than one transplant organization is seeking permission for tissue donation from the same donor, it is best to assign one person to represent the group of organizations, thereby protecting the family from being contacted several times.

When a family is approached, an effort also should be made to obtain information for the donor screening form. Such information should include the donor's medical history as well as information about the donor's lifestyle and the situation leading to death. High-risk behavior for HIV and other communicable diseases is an absolute contraindication.[7,10] Institutionalization in a prison, mental health facility, or other environment with a high incidence of communicable disease is also a contraindication.[28] Medical histories provide information about medical and sociologic conditions that may eliminate a donor from consideration.[11,12,28,32] A completed donor information form can be a valuable tool for prequalifying a potential donor.

Because infection is the most common complication of bone allograft transplantation,[10,32] the donor's medical or hospital record should be evaluated carefully for elevated temperatures, white cell counts, infected wounds, and culture results. The presence of antibiotics may mask underlying infection. Use of a respirator for more than 72 hours may produce septicemia and be a cause for excluding the donor.

Carcinoma (other than basal-cell carcinoma of the skin) is an exclusionary condition because of the potential for metastasis to donated tissues. Other exclusionary conditions include viral diseases (HIV, hepatitis, etc.), rheumatoid arthritis, metabolic bone disease, disease of the connective tissue, insulin-dependent diabetes, alcoholism or drug abuse (including the presence of any toxic substance), long-term steroid use, tuberculosis, malaria, and conditions of unknown etiology such as Alzheimer's disease.[28] A history of sexually transmitted disease warrants serious evaluation and may be an exclusionary condition.[28]

The risk factor for transmissible disease may be increased by the donor's transfusion history. A false-negative result of a donor's serologic status may result from hemodilution secondary to fluid therapy following a traumatic accident.[28] In addition, some blood banks suggest that donors receiving more than six units of blood products are not acceptable unless they are also organ donors.[28]

Finally, in making a decision about the acceptability of a donor, a physical examination of the donor's body and consideration of the circumstances leading to the donor's death must be taken into account. Ultimately, the evaluating physician would do well to ask, "Would I want this donor's tissue placed into my body?"[28]

Tissue Recovery

After permission for anatomic donation has been obtained, it is necessary to arrange procurement with any other transplant organizations that may be involved. Eye and skin tissues are normally the first to be retrieved after viable organs have been removed. If the coroner or medical examiner is in charge of the case, it is necessary to obtain his or her approval before tissues are recovered.

Tissue retrieval may be performed with sterile technique in an operating room or in a comparable environment. It is also possible to retrieve tissue in a nonsterile environment such as a morgue, autopsy room, or funeral home. While the nonsterile method of procurement allows a tissue bank to consider more potential donors, tissues that are not retrieved sterilely must undergo terminal sterilization. To avoid the cartilage cell death that results from secondary sterilization, sterile procurement is the method of choice when large osteochondral grafts are to be transplanted.

Cultures should be performed on each piece of tissue retrieved.[12] It is advisable to use at least two different culture media[25] in aerobic and anaerobic conditions for at least fourteen days of incubation. When large bones are cut into smaller graft specimens, the procedure must take place under aseptic conditions and additional cultures must be made of each of the specimens produced.

In its guidelines, the AATB requires screening for HIV antibodies (Ab), hepatitis B surface antigen, ABO/Rh, and syphilis (VDRL or RPR).[2] Additional recommended tests include hepatitis C antibodies, hepatitis B core antibody, cytomegalovirus, and HIV-PCR.[18,29] No tissue should be distributed for clinical use unless all laboratory reports are negative.

After all desired tissues have been retrieved, the donor's body should be reconstructed to prevent disfigurement and provide a cosmetically acceptable appearance for the funeral; arrangements for the funeral are made by the donor's family.

Processing of Bone

Bone that has been procured under sterile conditions may be used without processing provided tissue cultures are negative and donor serum tests are nonreactive. Tissue processing is achieved most effectively when "clean room" technology is used to avoid air-borne contamination.[28] A major advantage of this technique is that a reduced rate of positive cultures results in a lower discard rate. Pyrogenicity and endotoxin levels also may be decreased.[34,35]

It is a common practice at both the retrieval and processing of donor tissues to use antibiotics as a means of inhibiting growth of bacterial contaminants. Polymyxin and bacitracin are used most often. While the concentration of these substrates in the final graft may be low, notice of their use should be included on the label accompanying the tissue.[28]

Bone that has been procured under nonsterile conditions may be processed in a clean facility but must be sterilized before distribution to prevent or eliminate contamination. This secondary sterilization is generally achieved through the use of ethylene oxide or gamma irradiation.

Before cutting the bone, all soft tissue is removed to reduce the potential for immunologic response and transmission of disease. Various types of saws may be used to cut the bone into the desired sizes and shapes. The cut specimens are then washed to remove blood and bone marrow.

Table 64-1 outlines examples of specimens that may be produced from various procured bones to produce the highest yield of transplantable tissues.

Secondary Sterilization

Several methods of secondary sterilization have been used with varying degrees of success. Urist found that

Table 64-1
Commonly used banked allograft bone and their procurement sites

Procured Bone	Specimens Produced
Ilium	Tricortical blocks for spinal fusions
	Bicortical blocks for spinal fusions
	Cortical-cancellous strips of various sizes
	Crock dowels for lumbar fusions
	Ilium matchsticks
Femur	Cervical fusion dowels
	Whole femoral heads
	Femoral head cross sections
	Cancellous chips
	Cortical bone powder
	Crushed cortical bone
	Ground cancellous bone
Tibia	Cervical fusion dowels
	Cancellous chips
	Cancellous blocks
	Cortical struts
	Ground cancellous bone
	Cortical bone powder
	Crushed cortical bone
Fibula	Cross sections
	Crushed cortical bone
Humerus, radius, ulna, clavicle	Cross sections
	Crushed cortical bone
	Cortical struts
Ribs	Whole ribs
	Split ribs
	Rib matchsticks
Mandible	Whole mandible
	Hemimandible

β-propiolactone and hydrogen peroxide are effective sterilizing agents but may decrease the bone-forming capacity of a graft.[40] Reynolds and associates reported clinical results that showed approximately 30% of implants treated with Merthiolate (thimerasol) failed.[26] Bonfiglio reported that Merthiolate-treated grafts demonstrated poor osteogenic stimulus in host tissues and fractured grafts; vascularization of these grafts seldom occurred.[3]

Today, most bone banks sterilize grafts with the use of Cobalt-60 gamma radiation or ethylene oxide gas. Bone is usually exposed to 2.0 to 3.0 megarads to achieve sterilization. Urist and Hernandez suggested that these dosages may affect the ability of a bone graft to initiate a morphogenic response in host tissue.[38] However, if irradiated grafts are placed in contact with normal host bone in young patients, they compare favorably with autogenous bone in osteoconductive function.[36,38]

Ethylene oxide gas has been shown to be an effective sterilizing agent for tissues.[25] Some concern has been expressed regarding the residual levels of ethylene oxide, ethylene glycol, and ethylene chlorohydrin in tissues that have been sterilized with this gas. Prolo conducted an investigation to determine the levels of each of these residues in bone, dura mater, and fascia that had been sterilized with ethylene oxide gas followed by aeration and lyophilization. Results showed that aeration and lyophilization were effective in reducing residual levels to within acceptable limits. Bone that is not lyophilized should be well aerated before clinical use.[9,32] Soaking bone in a saline solution before implantation also is effective in reducing residue levels.[24,25]

Freeze Drying

Freeze-dried tissues are generally those that have been cut into small pieces such as chips, wedges, or dowels. Freeze drying, or lyophilization, is a process in which frozen bone is dehydrated by sublimation. Tissue moisture passes directly from the solid phase to the vapor phase and is converted to ice on the condenser of the freeze dryer. A vacuum is maintained in the freeze dryer during the process, ensuring that bottles of bone grafts are sterilely sealed. This process allows tissues to be maintained at room temperature for at least 5 years, as long as the vacuum seal remains unbroken.

Bone tissues are prepared for freeze drying by thorough rinsing with high pressure water to remove marrow elements. They also are treated with ethanol and sonic cleaning to defat and remove cellular debris.[28]

Depending on the types of tissue to be processed, the freeze-dry cycle may take up to 16 days to reduce residual moisture content to no more than 5%, as determined by gravimetric methods.[21] Some tissues cannot be freeze dried because there is inaccessible moisture within the matrix.

Although the normal proteins found in bone have proved to be stable chemically, antigenically, and electrophoretically after freeze drying,[5] a reduced or undetectable immune response in the recipient has been reported following the use of freeze-dried grafts.[13-15] The mechanism of this reduced antigenicity is unclear.

Deleterious effects of freeze drying have been reported; these include diminished torsional and bend-ing strength in cortical grafts. If bone is freeze dried in addition to being sterilized by irradiation, a significant decrease in breaking strength occurs.[23] Other studies have shown decreased osteogenesis and callous production, delayed revascularization and collection of lymphocytes around freeze-dried grafts as well as changes in biomechanical characteristics caused by microfractures thought to be secondary to dehydration.[5]

Dr. Cloward's 45 years of experience using cadaver bone for interbody spinal fusions has led to the development of a specialized bone graft. Bone removed unsterilely from fresh cadavers is cut into appropriate sizes and shapes, washed clean, packaged, sterilized with ethylene oxide gas, aerated, and stored at room temperature.[9]

When ordering banked bone, it is important to know the effects of various preservation methods on bone strength and to evaluate the effects of these changes in view of the type and magnitude of the load to which a graft will be subjected.[23] When used in appropriate cases, freeze-dried bone appears to serve well by retaining sufficient biologic potential and providing a nonviable structure on which new bone can be built.

Freezing (Fresh Frozen)

Although most allograft bone is stored by freeze drying, some bones are easier to store by freezing to $-80°$ C. Either storage method reduces or stops bone tissue degradation.

Enzymes such as collagenase, which are present in organic tissue, actively destroy structural proteins within a graft. Through freeze drying, water is removed and the activity of the enzymes is reduced. Storing bone in a freezer reduces or stops the molecular motion of the active enzymes in the bone tissue. When the bone is packaged properly to prevent freezer burn, and the temperature is monitored and maintained carefully, frozen tissue can be preserved without degradation for at least 5 years.[28]

The lower the temperature, the greater the reduction of molecular activity, including enzymatic activity. At $-160°$ C, the temperature of liquid nitrogen, essentially all molecular motion is stopped and theoretically tissue can be stored indefinitely. While some bone banks prefer to store tissues at this temperature, there are several reasons liquid nitrogen is infrequently used for storage. First, storing tissues by liquid nitrogen is more expensive than conventional mechanical methods. Second, other methods of storage essentially are as effective as liquid nitrogen, and rapid turnover of tissues makes it unnecessary to store them indefinitely. Third, liquid nitrogen may increase the brittleness of bone due to the immediate crystallization of water that occurs upon rapid exposure to very low temperatures. For these reasons, most tissue banks choose to keep tissues in a frozen state in electrical freezers set to $-80°$ C.

Storing a bone by freezing as compared to freeze drying has advantages and disadvantages. The main advantage of freezing is that long bones, such as femurs and tibias, may be stored without lyophilization. Lyophilizing a long bone requires several weeks to remove water. In addition, because of their bulk, it is difficult and expensive to package long bones in a large vacuumized container. For these reasons, instead of freeze drying, long bones are usually stored in a freezer in plastic bags that are watertight but not airtight.

The major disadvantage of storage by freezing is the cost of purchasing, operating, and maintaining a freezer. Large freezers are expensive to operate, require periodic maintenance, and must be monitored constantly. In contrast, bone that has been freeze dried may be kept at room temperature, making it less costly to store.

Beyond simple storage issues, there are important differences between frozen and freeze dried bone that determine application and clinical use in transplantation.

Frozen bone has superior strength. The process of freezing minimally affects the bending strength, torque strength, and modulus of elasticity, whereas freeze drying substantially reduces these properties of cortical bone.[23] Long bones stored by freezing are preferred when replacing sections of long bones resected for bone tumor or replacement of bones affected by osteolysis in failed joint replacement.

Frozen bones are used also as osteoarticular allografts to replace articular cartilage with cryopreserved chondrocytes. Freeze-dried cortical struts may sometimes be substituted for frozen long bones in situations where a buttress is required to support weak portions of a long bone. In general, however, frozen long bones are used when skeletal or structural stability is required.

A major disadvantage in the use of a frozen bone is that it may transfer disease more easily than a freeze-dried bone because usually it is not processed before freezing. Freeze-dried bone is always processed by washing it free of marrow and blood. As a result, freeze-dried bone can be virtually sterilized by washing.

Frozen bones are transplanted usually with their marrow intact, and it is generally in the cells of the marrow, blood, and serum that viruses are carried. Although the bone can be washed by the surgeon at the time of use, this requires extra operative time and may introduce contamination into the operative field. Therefore, frozen bone usually is not used where bone is needed for packing, such as for the treatment of benign cysts, or for a graft to supplement autograft bone.

In conclusion, allograft bones are banked by freezing for use in fairly specific applications. Frozen bone, because it usually contains blood and marrow, implies a risk of disease transfer that must be considered by the surgeon and the patient. With careful donor screening by the tissue bank that supplies frozen bone, and judicious use of this type of allograft, bone stored by freezing is a very reliable biological graft.

Demineralized Bone

Demineralized or autolysed antigen-extracted allogeneic bone (AAA) consists chiefly of collagen and fiber-entrapped insoluble noncollagenous proteins. Demineralized bone is prepared by extraction of mineral with 0.6 NHCl followed by several washes with distilled water and sequential washes in absolute ethanol and anhydrous ether.[17] It is stabilized by dehydration and defatting in chloroform-methanol followed by freeze drying and packaging. Though clinical use of demineralized or AAA bone is limited, results demonstrate that the organic matrix is more rapidly resorbed with less cell-mediated local immune reaction and more rapid incorporation of the donor tissue in the recipient bed.[39]

When rehydrated and before implantation, demineralized bone is pliable and can be trimmed with scissors to the desired shape. Cancellous bone becomes sponge-like in texture and is ideal for use in filling defects. Types of demineralized bone specimens available from tissue banks include crushed cortical bone powder, cortical struts, femoral head cross sections, ribs, fibula cross sections, and bone chips.

Rapid bone formation has been demonstrated with demineralized implants.* This process is called "osteoinduction" and is described as the differentiation of migratory mesenchymal cells into osteoprogenitor cells (chondroblasts) with subsequent bone formation. The presence of a growth factor, bone morphogenetic protein (BMP), is believed to stimulate this process.[40] Nondemineralized allografts

*References 16, 17, 22, 33, and 37.

undergo a process termed "osteoconduction" that involves the ingrowth of capillaries, perivascular tissue, and osteoprogenitor cells from the recipient bed. Resorption of both the allograft and surrounding living bone with subsequent new bone formation takes place to bring about incorporation of the graft.[37]

The clinical advantages or benefits of demineralized bone implants compared to other allograft bone grafts include ease of manipulation and insertion and decreased late resorption, rapid healing of skeletal defects, induction of large quantities of new bone, elimination or avoidance of a surgical procedure to collect donor bone, and a potentially unlimited supply of banked material that increases treatment options.[16] Demineralized bone implants may be the favored allotransplant for the future where fairly immediate return to normalcy of bone structure and stability are desired but where support is not a prerequisite. Nondemineralized allografts will be used clinically when support and weight bearing are essential.

Summary

The advantages of using allogeneic bone include a reduction of morbidity, an excellent means of physical stabilization and prevention of collapse, a good matrix for new bone growth, and a means of stimulating induction by host tissues.

Bone banking methods will change as more knowledge is gained about the biomechanical and biologic aspects of bone grafting. Sterilization methods, cleaning of bone, storage, preservation, and packaging are all subject to improvement when better methods are discovered. Bone banks have a responsibility to surgeons and to recipients to provide grafts of highest quality in a timely and efficient manner.

References

1. American Association of Tissue Banks: *Standards for tissue banking*, McLean, VA, 1989, AATB.
2. American Association of Tissue Banks: *Technical manual for tissue banking*, McLean, VA, 1991, AATB.
3. Bonfiglio M: Repair of bone-transplant fractures, *J Bone Joint Surg [Am]* 40:446, 1958.
4. Brown KL and others: Bone and cartilage transplantation in orthopaedic surgery, *J Bone Joint Surg [Am]* 64:270, 1982.
5. Burchardt H: The biology of bone graft repair, *Clin Orthop* 174:28, 1983.
6. Burchardt H, Enneking WF: Transplantation of bone, *Surg Clin North Am* 58:403, 1978.
7. Center for Biologics and Research: *Revised recommendations for prevention of human immunodeficiency virus (HIV) transmission by blood and blood products*, Letter to registered blood establishments, Bethesda, MD, Dec. 5, 1990, Food and Drug Administration.
8. Cloward RB: Creation and operation of a bone bank, *J Neurosurg* 33:682, 1980.
9. Cloward RB: Gas-sterilized cadaver bone grafts for spinal fusion operations: a simplified bone bank, *Spine* 5:4, 1980.
10. Eastlund T: Infectious disease transmission through tissue transplantation: reducing the risk through donor selection, *J Transplant Coordination* 1:23, 1991.
11. Friedlaender GE: Current concepts review: bone banking, *J Bone Joint Surg [Am]* 64:307, 1982.
12. Friedlaender GE: *Guidelines for banking osteochondral allografts*. In *Osteochondral allografts, biology, banking, and clinical applications*, Boston/Toronto, 1983, Little Brown.
13. Friedlaender GE: *Immune responses to preserved bone allografts in humans*. In *Osteochondral allografts, biology, banking, and clinical applications*. Boston/Toronto, 1983, Little Brown.
14. Friedlaender GE, Mankin HJ: *Bone banking: current methods and suggested guidelines*. In *Instructional course lectures, The American Academy of Orthopaedic Surgeons*, vol 30, St. Louis, 1981, Mosby.
15. Friedlaender GE and others: Studies on the antigenicity of bone, I. freeze-dried and deep frozen bone allografts in rabbits, *J Bone Joint Surg [Am]* 58:854, 1976.
16. Glowacki J: Application of the biological principle of induced osteogenesis for craniofacial defects, *Lancet* 8227:959, 1981.
17. Glowacki J and others: Fate of mineralized and demineralized osseous implants in cranial defects, *Calcif Tissue Int* 33:71, 1981.
18. Holoidniy M and others: Detection and quantification of human immunodeficiency virus RNA in patient serum by use of the polymerase chain reaction, *J Infect Dis* 163:862, 1991.
19. Inclan A: The use of preserved bone grafts in orthopaedic surgery, *J Bone Joint Surg* 24:81, 1942.
20. Macewen W: The growth of bone: Chapter III. Osteogenic power of bone bereft of periosteum, *Clin Orthop* 174:5, 1983.
21. Malinin TI and others: *Freeze-drying of bone for allotransplantation*. In *Osteochondral allografts, biology, banking, and clinical applications*, Boston/Toronto, 1983, Little Brown.
22. Mulliken JB, Glowacki J: Induced osteogenesis for repair and construction in the craniofacial region, *Plast Reconstr Surg* 65:553, 1980.
23. Pelker RR and others: Biomechanical properties of bone allografts, *Clin Orthop* 174:54, 1983.
24. Prolo DJ: The neurosurgeon in transplantation: provision and use of cadaver tissues and organs, *Neurosurg* 6(3):342, 1980.
25. Prolo DJ and others: Ethylene oxide sterilization of bone, dura mater, and fascia lata for human transplantation, *Neurosurg* 6:529, 1980.

26. Reynolds FC and others: Clinical evaluation of the merthiolate bone bank and homogenous bone grafts, *J Bone Joint Surg [Am]* 33:873, 1951.

27. Rinaldi E: The first homoplastic limb transplant according to the legend of Saint Cosmas and Saint Damian, *Ital J Orthop Traumatol,* 13:394, 1987.

28. Scarborough NL: Allograft bones and soft tissues. current procedures for banking allograft human bone, *Orthop* 15(10):1161, 1992.

29. Sninsky JJ, Kwok S: Detection of human immunodeficiency virus by the polymerase chain reaction, *Arch Pathol Lab Med* 114:259, 1990.

30. Strong DM, Sayers MH, Conrad EU: *Screening tissue donors for infectious markers.* In Friedlaender GE, Goldberg VM, editors: *Bone and cartilage allografts,* Parkridge, IL, 1991, American Academy of Orthopaedic Surgeons.

31. Tomford WW and others: A study of the clinical incidence of infection in the use of banked allograft bone, *J Bone Joint Surg* 63A:244, 1981.

32. Tomford WW and others: 1983 Bone bank procedures, *Clin Orthop* 174:15, 1983.

33. Tuli SM, Singh AD: The osteoinductive property of decalcified bone matrix: an experimental study, *J Bone Joint Surg [Br]* 60:116, 1978.

34. United States Pharmacopeia XXII: *Bacterial endotoxins test,* Rockville, MD, 1990, p 1493.

35. United States Pharmacopeia XXII: *Pyrogen test,* Rockville, MD, 1990, p 1515.

36. Urist MR: *Practical applications of basic research on bone graft physiology.* In *Instructional course lectures, The American Academy of Orthopaedic Surgeons,* St. Louis, 1976, Mosby.

37. Urist MR: Surface-decalcified allogeneic bone (SDAB) implants: a preliminary report of 10 cases and 25 comparable operations with undecalcified lyophilized bone implants, *Clin Orthop* 56:37, 1968.

38. Urist MR, Hernandez A: Excitation transfer in bone, *Arch Surg* 109:486, 1974.

39. Urist MR and others: A chemosterilized antigen-extracted autodigested alloimplant for bone banks, *Arch Surg* 100:416, 1975.

40. Urist MR and others: Human bone morphogenetic protein (BMP), *Proc Soc Exp Biol Med* 173(2):194, 1983.

Chapter 65
Graft Materials to Prevent Lumbar Spine Postoperative Adhesions

Charles D. Ray

Sources of Fibrosis and Indications for Barriers

Free-Fat Grafting

the nature of fat grafts
the fate of free-fat grafts

Obtaining a Fat Graft

Paratenon, Ligamentum Flavum, and Other Tissues Used as Barriers

Experimental Use of Other Tissues and Agents

Synthetics as Barriers to Fibrosis

Sources of Fibrosis and Indications for Barriers

Postoperative fibrosis in the spinal canal around the dura and nerves can never be prevented entirely, nor would this be desirable; fibrosis formation is an essential part of postoperative tissue repair. Furthermore, most investigators assert that there is no proof that postoperative scarring alone, in virtually any part of the body, produces dysfunction or pain. Evidence does not support that scar tissue can produce a true compressive mass effect in the spine, although it may grow to fill a void. However, scarring may produce adhesive anchoring between the dissected bone and other tissues or between adjacent soft tissues themselves, that is, ligaments, muscle, the dura, or nerves.

It is well established in spine surgery that the primary source of fibrosis arises from the outpouring of fibroblasts from the undersurface of injured muscle (muscle that has been stripped away from the bone and then laid back against the remaining tissues). The muscle is often damaged from cutting or tearing during dissection, by coagulation techniques to control blood loss, and by application of prolonged retraction, leading to circulatory occlusion and subsequent hypoxia.*

To reduce the likelihood of postoperative massive epidural and perineural fibrosis, three basic conditions must be met: (1) little or no remaining fluid should accumulate after wound closure (good hemostasis, watertight repair of any dural leaks); (2) little or no unfilled tissue void (dead space) should be present; and (3) a mechanical barrier to the ingrowth of the fibroblasts must exist. We should add to this criteria gentle handling and retraction of tissues and intermittent release of firm retraction to promote return of circulation to the muscle.

Barbera and associates discovered experimentally that a solid barrier is necessary to prevent effectively the classic "sheet" of scar tissue, the so-called "laminectomy membrane," from forming.[1] The term *solidity* means continuity in the barrier material, that is, without a break in its physical integrity. Long, in an editorial review of a paper by Bryant and co-workers about fat grafting,[2] noted that determining the ultimate value of routine fat grafting to block scar tissue formation after lumbar spine surgery would have to await clear proof that epidural scarring produces definite, often chronic, postoperative problems, especially pain.[15] Although any operation in the epidural space produces some degree of scarring, few patients become disabled from pain after spine surgery except where direct nerve trauma or spinal instability has occurred. On the other hand, this concept appears to counter the anecdotal experience and the position taken by many surgeons. Several clinicians have reported many cases in which they believe that lysis of adhesions and opening entrapments assumed to be caused by scarring have restored function and reduced pain. However, this belief is dwindling as the preponderant evidence is now to the contrary in that removal of bulk epidural scar tissue provides little, if any, help. Notwithstanding, clear tethering or constriction of neural elements, regardless of cause, can produce irritation and interfere with normal neuronal function. These complications may arise from interference with circulation to the nerve or perhaps with its axonal transport, where the entrapment or tethering is severe.

Triano and Luttges have shown in mice that chronic, mild mechanical irritation of sciatic nerves by soft silastic plugs (affixed adjacent to the living nerve) significantly altered nerve conduction velocity and refractoriness.[28] In addition, histologic evidence of chronic irritation was documented, and the animals exhibited objective signs of pain-like behavior. Interestingly, they found objective evidence of compression neuropathy in the absence of gross mechanical entrapment. It would be reasonable to believe, therefore, that a clump of inflexible scar tissue or a small, partly calcified mass in the appropriate location may act in a similar way.

Clearly, the issues related to possible entrapment and pain by scar tissue will be debated for some time, but meanwhile prevention of massive epidural and perineural scar tissue formation will continue to be a goal of spine surgeons and researchers.

Adhesive arachnoiditis is an entirely different matter than epidural fibrosis. This internal entrapment, postinflammatory state is literally a "gluing together" of delicate, essentially unmyelinated, intradural rootlets.[3] The sometimes bizarre clinical pain presentation and dysesthetic disturbances associated with this disorder are most likely related to a short circuiting of nerve signals between essentially uninsulated (unmyelinated) rootlets that are normally separated but now are permanently stuck together.

Free-Fat Grafting

The Nature of Fat Grafts

Of all the substances investigated to date for use as a barrier to the fibrous invasion of epidural structures in spine surgery, autogenous (or autologous)

*References 2, 6, 8, 12, 13, 31, and 32.

free-fat grafts are the most often used.* Fat is a remarkable tissue, normally serving both mechanical and metabolic functions throughout the body. Peer discussed the differences between two types of body fat: white, subcutaneous fat has its nuclei located around the cell's periphery (the signet ring cells), while brown fat (extensively developed in hibernating animals) has central nuclei.[19] The latter type is not used in grafting as it is too dense, too scarce, and too difficult to harvest. The most consistent location of this highly metabolic, body warming, brown fat is along the shoulders near the base of the neck. This fat may be abundant in some animals, especially those that hibernate, and is sometimes referred to as a hibernation "gland." White fat, containing the largest cells of the body, provides roundness to the whole body and typically fills intermuscular fossae; thus, it is ordinarily rather plentiful. A considerable variation of white fat exists among patients, with differences in consistency, color (content of lipochrome and exogenous vs. dietary fat contribution), size of globules, content of fibrous substrate, and friability. Organized fatty tissues thus vary in respect to firmness, depending, in part, on their supporting or padding functions in a particular body location.

Free-fat grafts, that is, those globules detached from their original beds, resemble lipomas. Tethered (pedunculate or pedicle) fat grafts must retain a vascular stalk from the originating bed, making the graft more difficult to obtain and the elongated donor site potentially more disfiguring. Both these graft types forever reflect the metabolism of their origin, similarly changing fat content with diet and so on. Peer stressed that following the harvest of a fat graft and before it is transplanted to the recipient site, one should avoid cutting through it randomly, handling it roughly, or permitting it to dry. To do otherwise may lead to breakage of the fragile cell walls, leading to atrophy of the graft.[20] If infection occurs, the entire graft will probably be lost; therefore, it is reasonable to protect the patient with antibiotics at least before surgery and perhaps afterwards. Peer also makes an interesting point that is mentioned by other authors; it may be an advantage for patients to be on a fat-restricted diet for some time before surgery. This diet ensures that specific fats synthesized from the patient's own carbohydrates and protein will predominate in the fat-graft cells, that is, they will contain a lower content of directly absorbed dietary fats. Since approximately 30% or more of fat cells in the graft will atrophy and release complex oils, a high content of one's own specific fats may

*References 3, 4, 6, 8, 9, 17, 19-22, 24, 30, and 32.

be less irritating in the recipient site than grafts with a high content of dietary or "exogenous" fat.[19] A fat-free diet also reduces the fat content of fat cells; this may allow them to withstand better the trauma and manipulation of harvest and transplantation. Fat grafts in lean patients lose less bulk by atrophy than those in obese patients since the latter's cells are more easily damaged during dissection. Thus, one should avoid the use of the super-large globular, areolar fat cells found deep in the buttocks of obese patients.

The Fate of Free-Fat Grafts

Burton[3] and I did a limited retrospective study using CT scanning to estimate the viability of fat grafts placed during lumbar decompression. After approximately 2 years, no discernible difference was present in the extent of epidural fibrosis formation between patients having had small, particulate fat grafts (fat collected from the walls and depths of the decompression) and those having had no grafts at all. However, in a cohort of 183 patients receiving large (20 to 30 ml) fat grafts taken from the superior gluteal region, Burton found significant graft still present in about two thirds of the cases (Fig. 65-1). He also estimated with the use of serial CT scanning of selected patients that approximately one third of the transplanted fat underwent shrinkage (necrosis with absorption) over a matter of some months or years.[3] Although a clear positive correlation exists between the viability of the fat graft and the reduction of postoperative epidural fibrosis, no comparison was made among them regarding clinical outcome. Further, since the fat was placed dorsal to the nerve structures, no visible protection against adhesions ventral to the dura could be seen. In fact, more recently, Burton and his associates have virtually eliminated the use of large, full-thickness free-fat grafts; a small number of patients in whom the grafts proved too large or were stuffed beneath a neural arch developed cauda equina syndromes shortly after surgery. They required immediate surgery for removal of a major portion or all of the graft (personal communication). This potentially devastating effect also has been reported by other authors.[4]

Bryant and co-workers also reported the use of serial CT scans to follow the progress of fat graft viability.[2] They found that fat grafts greater than 1 cm in thickness are easily identified in scans. This presents a convenient means to follow the progress of such grafts. MRI scans are even better for this purpose.

Peer reported from an extended animal study and some scattered observations of human beings that

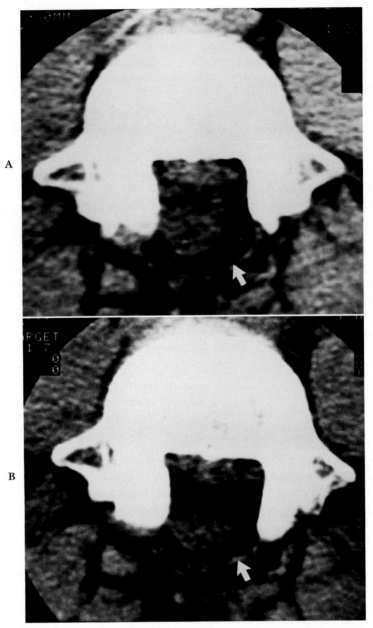

Fig. 65-1

Postoperative CT scans after extensive lumbar decompression. Note surviving fat graft and formation of an outer fibrous tissue capsule *(arrow)*. **A,** 6 months after surgery. **B,** 2½ years after surgery. Note small difference between this scan and A, made 2 years earlier.

fat allografts completely disappear following transplantation.[19] This study serves to rule out the use of cadaver fat as a graft source. He also found that human autogenous fat grafts lose about 45% of weight or volume in 1 or more years after transplantation. A composite (particulate) graft made of multiple small pieces of autogenous fat loses a larger percentage of its weight and volume than does an intact piece of equal size; that is, about 79% of the particulate fat mass is lost over 1 year or more, sim-

ilar to Burton's finding.[3] In general, areas of fat degeneration are always scattered within grafts, but the margins show the greatest loss, as a result of both cell disruption injuries from dissection and drying before insertion. Surviving graft cells appear as normal fat, whereas degenerating cells become fibrotic, showing mixed types of connective tissue formation (scar) or free oil.*

*References 9, 12, 13, 24, 29, and 30.

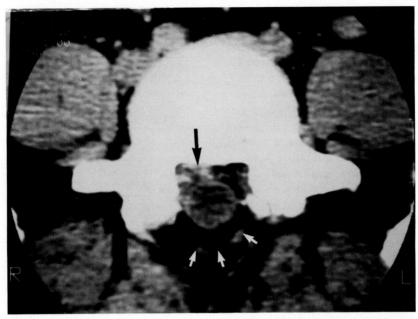

Fig. 65-2

Postoperative CT scan 3 years after removal of HNP showing fat graft with overlying, encapsulating membrane (*short arrows*) and recurrent disc fragment (*long arrow*). Presence of fat simplified diagnosis by scanning and also in removal of fragment.[15]

In a related vein, experimental and clinical work with autologous fat sewn directly into the margins of a dural defect has for many years enjoyed excellent results as a means to close the gap.[10,21,22,24] Mayfield reported success with the use of fat both as a material for the protection of dura and as a graft for dural repair.[17] Indeed, where the dura cannot be closed (because of inaccessibility or impracticality), a fat graft placed over the defect (sewn in or not) is one of the preferred methods for dealing with such lesions and has no potential for viral transinfection that a homologous dural donor source might have.

Rather than suturing the fat graft in place, a stamp of free fat can be attached to the dura by using "tissue glue."[27] This is a mixture of topical thrombin with sludge, or cryogenic precipitate, obtained from the bottom cloudy layer of thawing, previously frozen human plasma. The two ingredients (cryoprecipitate and thrombin) are separately but simultaneously injected onto the site, each in small quantity, using parallel syringes and long needles tied together near their tips. The thrombus gelling occurs instantly so the fat graft must be placed over the injected components quickly to cement the graft in position. This tissue glue leaves no residual and is totally absorbed, as would be a blood clot. Of course, the donated human plasma may expose the recipient patient to the donor's possibly undesirable viruses, if present.[10]

If there were no other major reason for the use of fat grafts, Long and other authors have observed facilitation of reexploration or repeat decompression.* Without question, when repeat surgery at the same level is required, a good-sized, intact fat graft lying over the surface of the dura and nerves is ordinarily a distinct advantage (Fig. 65-2).

Gill and co-workers reported the use of pedicled (attached) fat grafts taken from the wound margins and passed downward to the recipient site.[6] In my experience, since paraincisional fat is sparse in slender or average-weight patients, it is technically unacceptable to try to establish a good pedicle; such grafts can only be obtained in overweight patients. Furthermore, one must be careful not to close the deep fascia of the wound too tightly, otherwise the already marginal blood supply to the graft will become strangulated and lose the advantage of pedunculation. In addition, nothing in the literature indicates that this method is more effective than a simple free-fat graft alone.

Obtaining a Fat Graft

If a fat graft is planned, the usual volume required (large graft) is 20 to 30 ml (as measured intraoperatively in a sterile medicine glass) per bilateral lum-

*References 3, 12, 14, 15, and 32.

bar level decompressed. Proportionately less graft is used following a hemilaminotomy or hemilaminectomy. For such a volume, the superior gluteal region is the best donor site. The surgeon must make the incision approximately a hand's width from the midline to avoid the cluneal nerves in the deeper layers (Fig. 65-3). If this is not done, an area that is more painful than that of the decompression itself may result; that is, regrowth dysesthesia or small, painful neuromas might develop in the injured sensory nerves. The more superficial layers of fat around the buttocks, arising in Camper's fascia, have smaller globules than the deeper ones, which come from around Scarpa's layer (Fig. 65-4).[3] Either of these is quite acceptable, although generally, the smaller the globules, the less likely the cells will be transected or injured during the harvest.

A simple incision, 5 to 8 cm in length, is placed roughly 12 to 15 cm from the midline. Immediately beneath the skin the dissection is angled, sloping laterally (using Metzenbaum scissors and rat-tooth forceps) so that the graft resembles a shortened canoe. A few singular globules are also good to take if they are apparently intact. One must be careful not to pass so deeply that a muscle biopsy might be included. The donor bed must have good hemostasis,

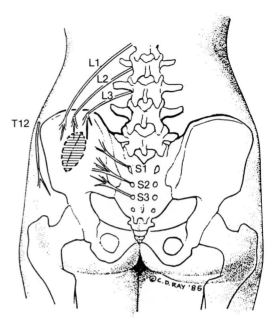

Fig. 65-3

Sketch of relative location of usual fat graft site, gluteal area *(shaded ellipse)*. Note approximate location of the iliohypogastric (T12), cluneal (L1 to L3), and sacral nerves relative to midline and to location of fat graft incision. Generally, fat is obtained from side opposite radiating leg pain so that patient will not confuse postoperative laminotomy pain from that arising from fat donor site.

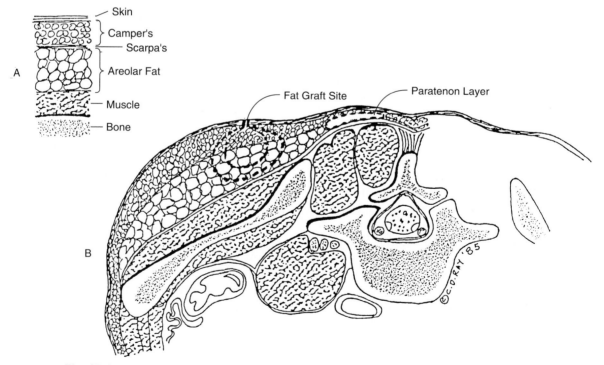

Fig. 65-4

A, Diagram of cross section of skin, fat, fascia, and muscle layers of the gluteal area and midline at the L5-S1 spinal level. **B,** The approximate location of the fat donor site, laterally, is defined by two dashed-line circles. The Paratenon donor site is defined by a flat, dashed-line oval, closer to the midline, just above the muscle fascia.

else it will likely accumulate a hematoma, which may produce a painful lump or possibly act as a pocket for infection.

Deep, space-obliterating, 2.0 absorbable sutures are used to reapproximate the cavity in two or more layers. A subcuticular skin closure, reinforced with skin margin adhesive tape, helps prevent skin-stretch scarring. Although most of the posterior and lateral fat may be missing, especially in slender males, often some fat is present in the lumbodorsal triangle, further laterally. This may be approached by tunneling under the skin from the wound laterally in the direction of the iliac crest, similar to dissection toward the posterior superior iliac crest for a bone graft. The surgeon may also progress downward to extract some of the retrosacral fat pad. In obese patients, a satisfactory graft may be obtained in the paraincisional area, perhaps during the initial opening of the wound. This is also the easiest location from which to obtain a fat graft with a pedicle attached, if this is desired. In any case, the piece of fat removed directly beneath the incision should not be large, as the remaining cavity may be hard to close and the cosmetic result poor. Interestingly, clinical and experimental evidence demonstrates that almost all fat donor sites will regenerate to some extent with time.[29]

In preparation of the precursor book (*Lumbar Spine Surgery* by Arthur H. White, Richard H. Rothman, and Charles D. Ray, Published by Mosby—1987), the several contributing authors were asked to comment on their use of fat grafts. The group was about equally divided: those who never used them, those who sometimes used them, and those who regularly used them. At least half the authors who had used such grafts commented on rare but significant complications, such as cauda equina compression, discussed previously. In addition, fat grafts were sometimes found to be attached firmly to the dura, rendering subsequent dissection as difficult as postoperative scar tissue itself. Many authors found no increase in operative success rate and therefore reported that they were not willing to use a fat graft if it required a significant increase in surgical time, a separate incision, or resulted in a cosmetic or painful deformity.

Paratenon, Ligamentum Flavum, and Other Tissues Used as Barriers

Clearly, using virtually any intact autologous tissue, that is fat, fascia, ligament, omentum, dermis, or other tissue having both a low metabolism and a reduced capability for fibroblastic proliferation as compared with injured muscle, might make that tissue acceptable as a graft for the prevention of adhesions. For example, Yong-Hing and associates showed that the ligamentum nuchae or flavum (containing about 80% elastin and 20% collagen fibers, much like all elastic ligaments and tendons) makes a good free-graft barrier material.[31,32] In many cases, I have successfully used carefully harvested, virtually intact ligamentum flavum, split or shaved into layers about 2 mm thick, to cover the exposed dura and noted, by repeat scanning, that the tissue had survived and reattached to the original lamina site. Such barriers preferably should be an unbroken blanket of tissue. Furthermore, they must produce only a small mass effect, otherwise compression of nerve structures after wound closure might result.

Stark and associates reported the practical use of paratenon as a graft material to prevent adhesions in hand tendon reconstruction.[26] Paratenon is a thin layer of loose areolar tissue that covers the deep fascia overlying muscle compartments, as seen closer to the midline in Fig. 65-4 *B*.[14] Usually, it has many, smaller fat cells inside the loose tissues. Using this tissue in a few hundred cases, Paratenon has become my graft of choice for covering exposed nerve or dura in small to medium sized decompressions. Even in thin individuals, this tissue is easily located near the midline incision, extending out over the dorsal fascia that overlies the lateral spinal erector muscles. It can be dissected, along with substantial fat cells, from its loose attachment to the fascia. It immediately contracts into a lump that can be stretched out into its original, limp, membranous, sheet-like form. As a continuous tissue with a low metabolic rate, it meets the criteria for an adhesion barrier that also has some volume-filling effect.

Almost all tissue grafts present a problem in the interpretation of immediate postoperative scans (CT, MRI, or radionuclide). The shadows generally resemble mature or active scar tissue and thus may be misinterpreted as a disc reherniation or an infection.

Experimental Use of Other Tissues and Agents

A 2-year study by O'Neal and Booth reported that in 28 human cases, porcine dermis was successfully used to wrap lumbar nerve roots after discectomies or decompressions. Extradural adhesions were minimal, and foreign-body inflammatory responses were not found.[18] Glutaraldehyde-tanned umbilical veins have been reported as useful in covering the median nerve after carpal tunnel decompression; this biologically acceptable material might prove useful in preventing scar formation in the spine as well.[16] Other reports indicate the potential use of saphenous veins or glutaraldehyde-tanned bovine or equine pericardium or peritoneum as coverings for exposed neural tissues (data from Bio-Vascular, Inc., 2670 Patton Rd., St Paul, MN 55113). A gel made of cultured cellular material has been reported as valuable for replacing blood vessels, and such an application for scar prevention in various body sites is currently under investigation.[11] High-molecular-weight polysaccharides, various polymer gels (such as polyvinylpyrillidone or polyacrylonitrile), and semisynthetic carbohydrate polymers are also enjoying some current investigation for inhibition of epidural and other scar formation.[23]

Other materials have been tried. For example, in a study of inhibitory action on postlaminectomy scar formation in animals, Jacobs and associates compared a variety of hemostatic agents, antiinflammatory drugs, and mechanical barriers.[8] The study showed that for inhibitory purposes, microfibrillar collagen (Avitene) was superior to gelatin foam (Gelfoam). These investigators extended their work to 50 human cases and noted that microfibrillar collagen also was superior to gelatin foam as a hemostatic agent, as well as a barrier to fibrosis. Nonetheless, they found that free-fat grafts proved to be the preferred means for preventing scar formation. Schuerman and colleagues found that Gelfoam did not inhibit ingrowth of fibrosis.[25] Keeler and associates also obtained this result, but autogenous fat grafts clearly proved to be the best protector.[10] Incidentally, among the hemostatic agents, I prefer SuperStat, as it has a tissue response about the same as Avitene and is significantly less costly. However, its use to prevent scar formation in the epidural space has not yet been reported.

Cortisone injected into the experimental wounds of laminectomized mongrel dogs delayed healing and often resulted in abscess formation with an eventual filling of the wound with considerable scar tissue.[32] On the other hand, Williams reported that oral or parenteral cortisone given for 9 days postoperatively had no particular effect on the ultimate outcome of homografts.[30] Jacobs and co-workers further found that bone wax as a barrier was also moderately responsible for both scar formation and protracted inflammation.[8] Free-fat grafts proved the superior material in all criteria.

Recombinant tissue-plasminogen activator (rt-PA) gel, a naturally occuring fibrinolytic protein found in most human organs and secretions, has also been tried as a means to reduce the postlaminectomy membrane.[7] Unfortunately, this method also has failed and was less effective compared with dogs who had free-fat grafts. Control animals that had no implants showed less reaction than the rt-PA but more than the fat grafts.

Synthetics as Barriers to Fibrosis

Unfortunately, after dissections in the central canal, it is extremely difficult, if not impractical, to place a significant fat graft on the ventral surface, between the dura and nerves and the dorsum of the anulus or vertebral body. The use of fat and tissue glue, as discussed above, might be useful here but has the significant considerations mentioned above. An inert-material shield may have a role in ventral and perhaps dorsal dural placement as a barrier. Many materials have been tried and reported, such as plastic polymer sheets, rubbers, and gelatin foam, but the early expectations have not held with time.[23] Keeler and co-workers studied several dural substitute materials and found that polyester fiber mesh was effective.[10] However, Dacron polyester, with or without a silicone coating, produced connective tissue encapsulation; this encapsulation was sufficient, in some animals, to produce compression of the underlying spinal cord. Feild and McHenry fabricated a plastic shield of Dacron-supported silicone and placed it either ventral or dorsal to the dura and nerve through a laminotomy window.[5] To date, even though such synthetic membranes might act to prevent or hinder ingrowth of fibrosis (the evidence is not well established, however), they do not help to fill voids created by the resection.

It appears that the preferred barrier membrane must retain some permeability to fluids and nutrients.[8,10, 17,28] The ideal synthetic material, acting as both a barrier and a void/filler, has yet to be developed.

References

1. Barbera J and others: Prophylaxis of the laminectomy membrane, *J Neurosurg* 49:419, 1978.
2. Bryant MS and others: Autogenic fat transplants in the epidural space in routine lumbar spine surgery, *Neurosurgery* 13:367, 1993.
3. Burton CV: *Diagnosis and treatment of lateral spinal stenosis: implications regarding the "failed back surgery syndrome."* In Genant HK, editor: *Spine update 1984,* San Francisco, 1983, Radiology Research and Education Foundation.
4. Carbezudo JM, Lopez A, Bacci F: Symptomatic root compression by a free fat graft transplant after hemilaminectomy, *J Neurosurg* 63:633, 1985.

5. Feild JR, McHenry H: The lumbar shield: a progress report, *Spine* 5:264, 1980.

6. Gill GG and others: Pedicle fat grafts for the prevention of scar formation after laminectomy, *Spine* 4:176, 1979.

7. Henderson R and others: Attempted experimental modification of the postlaminectomy membrane by local instillation of recombinant tissue-plasminogen activator gel, *Spine* 18:1268, 1993.

8. Jacobs RR, McClain O, Neff J: Control of postlaminectomy scar formation, *Spine* 5:223, 1980.

9. Keeler JT and others: The fate of autogenous grafts to the spinal dura, *J Neurosurg* 49:412, 1978.

10. Keeler JT and others: Repair of spinal dura defects: an experimental study, *J Neurosurg* 60:1022, 1984.

11. Kobayashi H and others: An artificial blood vessel with an endothelial-cell monolayer, *J Neurosurg* 77:397, 1992.

12. Langenskiold A, Kivuluoto O: Prevention of epidural scar formation after operations on the lumbar spine by means of free fat transplants, *Clin Orthop* 115:92, 1976.

13. Langenskiold A, Valli M: Epidurally placed free fat grafts visualized by CT scanning 15–18 years after discectomy, *Spine* 10:97, 1985.

14. Lexer E: *Die freien Transplantation. I. Neue Deutsche Chirurgie 26,* Stuttgart, 1919, Ferdinand Enke.

15. Long DM: Free fat graft in laminectomy (letter), *J Neurosurg* 54:711, 1981.

16. Masear VR, Tulloss J, Meyer RD: *Venous wrapping of nerves to prevent scarring,* Presented at the American Society of Surgeons of the Hand, Annual Meeting, Seattle, Sept 15, 1989.

17. Mayfield FH: Autologous fat transplants for the protection and repair of the spinal dura, *Clin Neurosurg* 27:349, 1980.

18. O'Neill P, Booth AE: Use of porcine dermis as a dural substitute in 72 patients, *J Neurosurg* 61:351, 1984.

19. Peer LA: Loss of weight and volume in human fat grafts, *Plast Reconstr Surg* 5:217, 1950.

20. Peer LA: The neglected free fat graft, *Plast Reconstr Surg* 18:233, 1956.

21. Rehn E: Die Fetttransplantation, *Arch Klin Chir* 98:1, 1912.

22. Rehn E: Die Verwendung der autoplastischen Fett-transplantation bei Dura und Hirndefecten, *Arch Klin Chir* 101:962, 1913.

23. Robertson JT and others: The reduction of postlaminectomy fibrosis in rabbits by a carbohydrate polymer, *J Neurosurg* 79:89-95, 1993.

24. Saunders MN and others: Survival of autologous fat grafts in humans and in mice, *Connect Tissue Res* 8:85, 1981.

25. Schuerman WG and others: The use of Gelfoam film as a dural substitute, *J Neurosurg* 8:608, 1951.

26. Stark HH and others: The use of Paratenon, polyethylene film or silastic sheeting to prevent restricting adhesions to tendons in the hand, *J Bone Joint Surg* 59:908, 1977.

27. Stechison MT: Rapid polymerizing fibrin glue from autologous or single donor blood: preparation and indications, *J Neurosurg* 76:626, 1992.

28. Triano JJ, Luttges MW: Nerve irritation: a possible model of sciatic neuritis, *Spine* 7:129, 1982.

29. Van RLR, Roncari DAK: Complete differentiation in vivo of implanted cultured adipocytic precursors from adult rats, *Cell Tissue Res* 225:557, 1982.

30. Williams RG: Studies of autoplastic and homoplastic grafts in rabbits, *Am J Anat* 93:1, 1853.

31. Yong-Hing K and others: The ligamentum flavum, *Spine* 1:226, 1976.

32. Yong-Hing K and others: Prevention of nerve root adhesions after laminectomy, *Spine* 5:59, 1980.

Chapter 66

Surgical Decision-Making for Degenerative Disease

Arthur H. White

Nonsurgical Decisions

Political and Social Issues

Conservative Care and Physical Conditioning

Accurate Diagnosis

Basic Surgical Concepts

Surgical Decisions

is surgery necessary?
when to operate?
on whom to operate?
what surgery to perform?

Summary

Nonsurgical Decisions

Surgical decision-making for degenerative disc disease is considerably different than for deformity, tumor, trauma, and infection. The latter conditions require mainly a structural evaluation and decision as to the biomechanically best surgical procedure for the structural disease at hand. Surgical decisions for degenerative disease, however, include many other multidisciplinary ramifications that revolve around pain and function. It is important that the pain that we are operating on is not predominantly psychosocially induced or simply part of the normal aging process. Many surgeons are not specialists in diagnosing and treating psychosocial disease. It therefore is usually necessary to consult specialists in other fields of medicine to be sure that the surgery anticipated is for an appropriate reason and of a type that has the highest likelihood to benefit the patient (see Chapters 4 and 18).

Political and Social Issues

Many political and socioeconomic controversies surround surgery for degenerative disease. While most spine specialists agree that surgery is indicated when there is neurologic loss and disabling leg pain, many well-meaning individuals believe that surgery is rarely if ever indicated when there is back pain only, without neurologic loss or leg pain. Others, however, who deal with an elderly population, or many patients with low-back pain (LBP), especially athletes, realize that back pain without neurologic involvement can be very disabling and can, when properly evaluated, respond quite well to a surgical procedure. Decision-making in such individuals is critical to avoid the great cost of excessive and unnecessary surgery. Diagnostic testing may include such things as scans, diagnostic blocks, discograms, psychologic testing, functional capacity evaluations, and extensive general medicine evaluations.

If surgery is deemed necessary, the type of surgery should take into consideration not only the physical diagnosis but many other factors related to the psychologic and socioeconomic cascades (see Chapters 3 and 4). Information such as the patient's occupation, athletic activities, overall conditioning, training level, pain tolerance, and other existing medical conditions are important.

The spine specialist has to make decisions daily as to which patients are surgical candidates and what surgery is most appropriate. This is no mean task. Patients arrive in the examining room with all variations of pain behavior, neurologic deficit, and structural, psychologic, and socioeconomic cascade symptoms. The seasoned spine specialist may be able to sort out these infinite variations by himself, but the patient is much better served by a multidisciplinary team (see Chapter 18).

Conservative Care and Physical Conditioning

Patients in top physical condition frequently require less surgery and have better results than patients with the same disease process who are in poor physical condition. Aggressive conservative care that includes high levels of exercise, education, and training will compensate for many underlying structural abnormalities by improving the alignment and function of a diseased spinal segment through strength, flexibility, and movement patterns (see Chapter 25). Patients who have had aggressive conservative care have a more rapid recovery from surgery and are more likely to maintain the benefits of surgery rather than destroying it by returning to bad habits of poor posture and movement patterns. We therefore prefer that patients have aggressive conservative care prior to surgery, and expect the patient to continue a similar type of training postoperatively. Surgery is only one step in the rehabilitation process.

Accurate Diagnosis

To choose the appropriate surgical procedure it is important to have an accurate diagnosis. In addition, it is imperative that we do not operate on patients who could get better with less expensive and non-invasive means. All reasonable conservative care should be exhausted and documented prior to surgical intervention.

Basic Surgical Concepts

Several concepts may help the general spine specialist avoid operating on the wrong patient. Such surgeries can create extreme consternation in the daily life and practice of a spine specialist, and puts patients into a multi-operative environment, responsible for the billions of dollars that are being wasted on inappropriate spinal management.

Those concepts are as follows:

1. Determine the level of disability and function of the patient.

2. Arrive at a specific diagnosis by doing as much diagnostic testing as necessary to be absolutely certain.

3. Determine whether the level of function is consistent with the working diagnosis.

4. Determine and apportion the structural, psychologic, and socioeconomic cascade diagnoses for each patient.

5. If the proportion of psychologic or socioeconomic cascade involvement is greater than the structural involvement, treat the psychosocial affects before considering surgery.

6. Be sure that all reasonable conservative measures have been exhausted before considering elective surgery.

7. Obtain second and third opinions, especially from multidisciplinary spine specialists, to obtain a universally acceptable diagnosis and plan.

8. Use the agreed-upon diagnosis, which includes the structural and psychosocial aspects, to select the most appropriate surgical procedure.

9. Enlist the patient in a contract with the understanding that surgery is only one step in the rehabilitation process. They must understand that elective surgery for degenerative disease is not a cure but an attempt at slowing a degenerative (aging) process that is likely to continue unabated unless the patient changes longstanding habits and other activities that affect the health of the spine.

Surgical Decisions

The major surgical decisions that need to be made are as follows.

  Is surgery necessary?
  When should we operate?
  On whom should we operate?
  What surgery should we do on which patient?

Is Surgery Necessary?

Surgery is necessary only when there is a correctable physical abnormality that would otherwise lead to neurologic loss, significant deformity, or long-term pain. Tumor, trauma, infection, and developmental deformities are universally accepted conditions that frequently require spine surgery.

There is less agreement as to whether surgery should be considered in cases of degenerative disease. Occasionally, degenerative disease will cause neurologic loss, deformity, and severely painful conditions. The controversy arises when considering surgery on patients with pain that is aggravating but whose condition does not threaten significant deformity or neurologic loss. This is elective surgery and requires careful weighing of the patient's dis-

ability level, pain tolerance, and, most important, the risks of the surgery compared with the danger of the underlying structural abnormality.

Some soul searching needs to be done by the patient and the patient's family or friends. There is major controversy in the media, government, insurance companies, and managed-care organizations as to whether elective spine surgery is necessary. Some of these segments of our society emphatically state that spine surgery is never necessary for back pain alone. Other societies, and countries, are well known for placing patients on disability rather than doing surgery that is expensive and may not be successful. Thus we have a moral controversy. Must we keep every individual at the highest level of function as long as possible, despite the cost? When does surgery become unnecessary and too expensive? Such questions remain to be answered by our society as a whole over a long time. Right now, the individual surgeon and patient need to decide whether surgery will adequately return the patient to significant function.

Dialogue and understanding are essential between the surgeon and the patient. The level of disability needs to be assessed and agreed on by all concerned. Such a disability level needs to be related to structural disease and not psychosocial disease. Obviously, surgery for psychosocial disease is not going to be significantly beneficial.

Are the Goals Realistic?

All individuals concerned about whether or not surgery should be performed should have realistic goals. It is very clear that spine surgery does not always return individuals to full, normal activity. Spine surgery for degenerative disease usually leaves some residual pain and functional limitations, unlike appendectomies or gallbladder and hernia surgery, which may be successful 99% of the time. Spine surgery is one of the least successful of musculoskeletal surgeries.

What is the Level of Function?

The patient's level of function should be assessed. Formal functional capacity evaluations can be done on workers' compensation patients, but in general the patient should self-assess how well he or she is functioning in their daily life compared with a normal person their age. It is relatively easy to look around for individuals of our age bracket and see what normal function appears to be. For an individual to aspire to be in the top 10% or 1% of functioning for a person of the same age is not realistic. Some general guidelines are as follows:

Ages 20 to 30: Heavy work activities including lifting, bending, and rapid movements. Athletics may include racquet sports and contact sports.

Ages 30 to 40: Heavy lifting becomes more difficult. May participate in moderate work activities. No longer engages in contact sports.

Ages 40 to 50: Heavy and moderately heavy work as well as heavy athletics may no longer be possible. May participate in tennis, hiking, swimming, and bicycling.

Ages 50 to 60: After 50 years of age, most individuals do not engage in heavy or moderate labor, or heavy or moderate athletics. Recreational activities of walking, golf, dancing, sailing, and light work are common.

Ages 60 to 70: The average person after 60 years of age is usually retired and does not participate in aerobic athletics.

Given the above guidelines, an individual patient can self-assess. Granted, most of us consider ourselves above average and have great aspirations and desires. That needs to be reality-tested by our family and friends. The physician and surgeon need to help the patient understand that to have surgery in anticipation of higher-than-average function is unrealistic.

The patient who is truly functioning at less than 50% of normal function for age because of back and/or leg pain has a reasonable likelihood of successful improvement with surgery. They are not going to be normal, but an improvement to 70% or 80% of normal function is quite reasonable. An individual who is already functioning at 80% of normal function cannot expect to function at 100% of normal, much less 120% of normal, as many individuals anticipate. It is extremely valuable to have ancillary medical advisors such as psychiatrists, physiatrists, and internal medicine specialists who do not perform surgery, discuss realistic expectations with the patient.

In summary, elective spine surgery should only be contemplated when daily functional activities are significantly below normal, when a very specific diagnosis has been made, and all reasonable conservative measures have been exhausted. The patient should take responsibility for the decision, and not feel that they are being coerced or "talked into" an operation. The surgeon should thoroughly educate the patient and receive his or her truly informed consent. The patient may also be encouraged to obtain a second opinion. A "disinterested" party should help the patient realistically evaluate their level of disability and the anticipated results of surgery.

When to Operate?

It is well understood that in emergencies and with severe conditions of tumor, trauma, and infection, immediate surgery may be necessary. However, decisions regarding surgery for degenerative disease should be much more prolonged and introspective. It is wise to have a multidisciplinary evaluation and second or third opinions prior to doing elective spinal surgery. Some degenerative conditions such as herniated discs are known to improve with time, and most others improve with rehabilitation. The development of strength, endurance, flexibility, and body mechanics takes months. Because time plays such an important role, patients should be given at least 2 or 3 months of evaluation and treatment before surgery. However, waiting too long, in the presence of the psychologic and socioeconomic cascade, can have a negative affect on our outcomes. Also, some neurophysiologic changes may occur with time that can lead to chronic pain and negative surgical results.

Surgical Timing in the Face of Neurologic Deficit

Static neurologic deficit without pain is a frequent and critical issue in spine surgery. To operate on a patient because of a minor neurologic deficit without pain and end up with a patient who still has neurologic deficit and pain may have serious consequences. Surgery can produce additional neurologic injury to a nerve already traumatized by a herniated disc or other condition.

Neurologic deficit that is static has at least a good likelihood of returning to normal. If there is an underlying condition that continues to traumatize an already injured nerve, recovery is much less likely. It is up to the clinician to be sure that the patient is not going to progressively traumatize an already injured nerve. If the patient cannot be relied on to avoid further injury, perhaps surgery is indicated. However, the surgeon should inform the patient that a lack of responsibility on his or her part may result in permanent neurologic deficit and that pain may still be present after surgery.

In the best of all circumstances, static neurologic loss can be monitored daily by the patient and weekly or monthly by the clinician as the neurologic deficit resolves.

Surgical Timing in the Face of Socioeconomic Factors

Nonorganic and nonstructural factors may affect the decision of when to operate (see Chapters 3 and 4). It is well known that individuals who are off work for more than 6 months have less than a 50% likelihood of returning to work. Workers develop bad habits and become so accustomed to being off work that they rarely, if ever, return to work after being off for a year. It is fairly well accepted that surgery should be considered after 3 months of significant disability from back and leg pain. Neurologic loss, scar tissue, and chronic pain are considered by many clinicians to become significant factors after that time.

On Whom to Operate?

What Is the Disability Level?

For elective surgery on degenerative disease of the spine, a critical analysis should be made of the patient's disability level from a structural, psychologic, and socioeconomic standpoint. A patient's physical level of function should be subjectively assessed as described in the previous section and objectively determined by physical examination, objective testing by scans, X-ray studies, and electrodiagnostics.

The patient should be observed in the examining room and in the physical therapy gym or functional capacity evaluation laboratory to determine what his or her true physical capabilities are, aside from the subjective response to pain. The subjective pain should be evaluated through pain drawings, visual-analog scale, psychologic testing, abnormal psychologic responses on physical examination, functional capacity evaluation, and pain provocation and relief tests such as diagnostic blocks and discograms.

The patient's attitude toward his workplace and employer should be investigated as well as the employer's and third-party payor's attitude and experience with the patient (see Chapter 3).

From all of the above disability testing, it is possible to differentiate and apportion the disability between physical structural disease, psychologic pain, and socioeconomic factors. Such factors should be dealt with prior to considering surgery for structural degenerative pain.

What Are the Patient's Expectations?

The patient's expectations need to be correlated with their level of disability to be sure that the expecta-tions are realistic. Patients with severe, chronic, end-stage disease, be it structural or psychosocial, are unlikely to be returned to a very high level of function by surgical intervention. On the other hand, moderate acute conditions, such as a clear-cut herniated disc in a well-trained athlete, can be treated surgically with an expectation of returning the patient to full-scale athletics.

Patients who do heavy labor and have no other form of livelihood who expect to return to heavy labor for 20 years might be better served by a larger operation, perhaps with a fusion if there is any present or anticipated painful instability.

How Severe Is the Disease Process?

Severity implies a greater amount of damage. In structural disease this means greater neurologic involvement and greater deformity or instability. In psychosocial disease the severity increases with the chronicity of the condition and the amount of involvement with drugs, alcohol, litigation, and pain behavior.

As the severity increases the success through surgery decreases. Mild cases of structural disease require minimal surgery with shorter recovery and fewer complications.

What Surgery To Perform?

Spine surgery is one of the most rapidly changing subspecialties of medicine. The number of spine surgeons and the surgical techniques available are nearly doubling every year.

From 1930 to 1960, spinal surgical procedures were virtually limited to laminectomy, discectomy, and fusions without internal fixation. In the 1960s and 1970s, Harrington rod and Knodt rod instrumentation systems were developed. The microscope became available for microdiscectomy and finer neurologic spinal surgery.

In the 1980s and 1990s, there has been a virtual explosion of internal fixation techniques involving the use of bone screws. These internal fixation devices have been used by surgeons attempting to obtain a higher rate of fusion of the spine while holding it in a normal anatomic position (see Chapter 86).

In the 1990s, percutaneous, arthroscopic, and microscopic techniques are advancing in an attempt to remove herniated discs, decompress neurologic structures, and obtain fusions with the least invasive procedures, the shortest hospital stay, and the most rapid return to normal function (see Chapters 73 and 75).

As has been the case in many other surgical fields, we can anticipate that by the year 2000 most spine surgery will be done through scopes. Extraforaminal herniations and foraminal stenosis can be treated through a 1-in. incision lateral to the midline. Then, using a microscope or cylindrical operating scope, the surgeon can channel down to the intertransverse space to directly visualize the lateral herniation or exit zone of the foramen. This, of course, eliminates the problems of entering the intervertebral canal, creating scar tissue, neural tears, nerve injury, and potential instability.

Microscopes, of course, have been used for years to enter the vertebral canal to do a discectomy or foraminotomy. Discectomy is being accomplished more safely with percutaneous arthroscopic techniques. These scopes are passed into the disc via a posterolateral or laparoscopic approach into the body of the disc or intervertebral foramen. They are then passed as closely as possible to the base of the herniation, to laser, shave, or rongeur away as much of the disc as possible without entering the vertebral canal. These procedures can be done as an outpatient and pose comparatively little or no danger to neurologic structures. Best of all, they create no scar tissue within the vertebral canal so that if there is a recurrence, the surgeon is not faced with the troublesome chore of "digging out" a herniated disc from underneath a nerve root that has been encapsulated with scar tissue from previous surgery.

Artificial discs are being developed by many centers (see Chapter 88). These materials can generally be placed within an existing disc that has had a nuclectomy, by any of the above procedures. It is hoped that the artificial disc will restore normal motion after discectomy and avoid the need for fusion.

Fusions are being developed through minimally invasive surgery with better biomechanical constructs, higher fusion rates, and less morbidity (see Chapter 77). From a posterior approach, bone screws can be placed percutaneously. Discectomies and interbody fusions can be accomplished through scopes and can be stimulated by electrical or chemical means (see Chapter 93).

Interbody fusions can be accomplished anteriorly or posteriorly with various synthetic materials, ingrowth material, and threaded cages. These techniques offer better biomechanical stability and alignment, and a higher rate of fusion. Many of them can be placed through microscopic, arthroscopic, or laparoscopic techniques.

Ultimately, if we can identify and limit the structural pain generator to a single source, we will be able to correct the pathology with minimally invasive techniques.

The great value of these new technologies is not just the short recovery time and decreased hospitalization and expense. They obviate the terrible consequences of failed major spine surgery.

Failed open discectomy or fusion occurs as often as 15% of the time. Repeat surgery in such situations fails almost 50% of the time owing to scar tissue, nerve damage, instability, biomechanical disturbances, deconditioning, and psychosocial factors. Minimally invasive surgery, however, can lessen the risk of such troublesome consequences. Although the original minimally invasive technique may not be as successful as an open technique, it can be repeated without traumatizing nerve roots or creating scar tissue, which makes subsequent open surgery more difficult.

Decisions regarding the selection of the appropriate surgical procedure depend on all the factors discussed. The structural diagnosis is probably the most important factor. Posterolateral herniated discs that are contained are amenable to arthroscopic discectomy. Extruded herniations that are fairly well localized are amenable to microscopic discectomy or small laminotomy. Larger herniated discs with more expansive lesions associated with uncinate spurs or stenosis require greater degrees of laminectomy. Instability frequently requires a fusion, and when there is great instability or heavy forces across a segment, internal fixation is frequently necessary. Anterior column disease is usually best approached anteriorly with anterior discectomy or fusion (see Chapter 89). Vague conditions such as internal disc disruption or painful degenerative disc disease, if they are to be operated on at all, usually require discectomy and fusion and still carry a much lower success rate than diagnoses that are better understood.

In choosing a surgical procedure it is important to consider not only the structural diagnosis, but also the patient's level of training. A well-trained individual may tolerate mild to moderate degrees of instability that would otherwise require a fusion in a weak, deconditioned, or obese patient.

The choice of surgical procedure is most difficult in the older patient with degenerative scoliosis and stenosis (see Chapter 91). Decompression is necessary for the stenosis, but it leaves the spine in a considerably weakened condition. The vertebrae are already displaced, and this condition is likely to increase. The patients are elderly, frequently osteoporotic, deconditioned, and may be obese. They frequently cannot tolerate long surgeries encompassing many lumbar segments with great amounts of blood loss.

Outcome studies on surgery procedures are severely lacking in the literature. We have no statistics to verify that any one surgical procedure has benefit over another. Although a fusion may be necessary when there is verifiable instability, we do not know that a fusion added to any of the discectomy or decompression surgeries has any additional benefit in degenerative disease or even herniated disc disease.

Summary

A single type of surgery does not fit all patients. One of the major problems we are having in the current medical economy is "the new surgery flurry," which occurs when a new surgical procedure is developed. There is no panacea for low-back pain. The health-care professional must understand what low-back pain is, and provide the patient with conservative tools to assist him or her in living with that pain. Only occasionally should surgery be performed and then only in very well selected patients who have been extensively screened and conservatively treated and who are willing to take full responsibility for the residual back pain that they are inevitably going to have after back surgery.

Chapter 67

Psychologic Preparation for Surgery

C. Eddie McCoy
Frances A. McManemin
Ramon Cuencas-Zamora

Underlying Concepts

Purpose of Psychologic Evaluation

Complexity of Interdisciplinary Factors

Models and Theories of Pain

Reasons for Referral

Assessment Guidelines for Surgical Candidates

    objective instruments

Preparation for Surgery

    candidacy classifications
    pre- and postsurgical education and
       rehabilitation
    pain drawings and patient profiles
    availability of programs
    outcome predictors

Levels of Treatment

    multidisciplinary behavioral medicine
       models
    chronic pain programs
    work hardening and work conditioning

Behavioral Medicine and Interdisciplinary Cooperation

Patient Responsibility

Underlying Concepts

The assumption that there is a relationship between psychologic factors and outcome after lumbar spine surgery has gained impetus from an increasing number of studies performed during the past three decades.* This chapter will focus on the psychologic issues involved in preparation for surgery, including reassurance and preparation of the patient for the hospital stay (decreased anxiety, reduced drug use, reduction of complications, prompt resumption of activity, and timely discharge), and evaluation of the patient's physical and psychologic readiness for surgery and a long-term positive outcome.[14,20]

While there is less opportunity for psychologic preparation prior to surgery in cases of sudden acute pain requiring emergency intervention, it is extremely important in the evaluation and preparation for surgery of patients with a mixture of chronic and recurrent acute pain. Chronic pain is defined here as pain that has endured from 4 weeks to over 6 months without sufficient underlying physical pathology to explain the severity of the pain reported or the dysfunction observed.[4,5,16,30] An intermixture of acute and chronic pain is often the case when spinal surgeries are undertaken.

Purpose of Psychologic Evaluation

Psychologic preparation for spinal surgery is becoming more popular and can serve a number of useful functions.[28,34] It can be critical in identifying psychosocial and behavioral factors that influence the nature and persistence of chronic pain and that relate to a positive outcome after a surgical intervention. Among the factors that have been identified in our research and clinical practice, as well as in the literature,[8] are the presence or absence of psychopathology which includes affective (emotional processes), cognitive (reasoning and thought processes), behavioral, and personality functioning; use of any addictive substances (e.g., narcotics, benzodiazepines, alcohol, marijuana, and amphetamines); state of the patient's general health; general level of physical conditioning; general functional level; presence or absence of social support; financial and work status; legal status; and language and educational level.

Factors such as beliefs about the etiology of pain and social reinforcement of pain behavior also contribute to the maintenance of pain and dysfunction.

*References 7, 15, 23, 37, and 38

Ignoring these psychologic elements can impede the patient's recovery and interfere with his or her response to rehabilitation. For example, a patient who was first seen 6 years ago and who has had several surgeries during the interim continues to experience disabling pain. He has searched for ways to "get fixed." He has been through extensive training in exercise, aerobic conditioning, biofeedback, functional activities, problem solving, and stress management, but he does not do his exercises or change his lifestyle. He continues to drink, take drugs, smoke, eat a poor diet, and to hurt more than necessary because of his inability to appreciate the role of self-responsibility in the rehabilitation of his back and the reduction of his pain.

Another function of preoperative assessment of psychologic and social stressors has been its effectiveness in predicting surgical outcomes.[28,34] Psychologic preparation for surgery can also aid in identifying specific goals for treatment and vocational rehabilitation. This information aids in the setting of goals for treatment, which result in increased activity levels, decreased intake of medication, improvement of family dynamics, and improvement of stress management and relaxation skills.

Complexity of Interdisciplinary Factors

Although these evaluations can be accomplished from different theoretic perspectives, the utilization of the behavioral medicine model is recommended. This is a multidisciplinary approach to the evaluation and treatment of chronic health problems that works in conjunction with biomedical science when the biomedical model alone is not effective.[6]

The intermingling of somatic and psychogenic factors is one of the most challenging and frustrating aspects of the management of chronic pain and the implementation of successful spinal surgeries.[11,17] For example, the psychologic evaluation cannot give definite information regarding the underlying causes, psychologic or organic, of the pain.[24] The presence of psychologic factors influencing pain and disability does not exclude the possibility of organic pathology, just as the presence of positive physical findings does not necessarily imply the absence of important psychologic influences. To further complicate the issues, the lack of positive physical findings does not indicate that the pain *must* be "psychogenic." This type of thinking perpetuates the outdated conceptual dichotomy between "organic" and "psychogenic," or "functional," pain, an oversimplification that fails to consider current concepts of pain that acknowledge the role of psychologic factors in pain perception, regardless of cause. Additional, it underestimates the complexity of most chronic pain syndromes, in which some mixture of psychologic and organic influences are always found.*

In many cases of chronic pain, the evidence of nociceptive input does not explain the extent of suffering and disability reported, and one must look to other sources of information to understand why a person's pain has continued beyond the normal expected healing time. One alternative in defining the wholeness of chronic pain syndromes would be to create a term that could be used to represent both the organic and psychogenic components. This would not only discourage the ideas of the healthcare provider and the patient that there are essentially two kinds of pain (organic or nonorganic), but could also illustrate that all the factors in the patient's environment can have an influence in the maintenance of chronic pain.

Models and Theories of Pain

Melzac and Wall's[29] proposal of the gate-control theory of pain has provided a scientific model of pain transmission and processing that incorporates cognitive, affective, and sensory processes in explaining the experience of pain. This theory holds that pain perception is a complex interaction of sensory–discriminative, motivational–affective, and cognitive-evaluative components (i.e., the impact on behavior of the intermingling of the person's previous emotional conditioning, his or her ability to process information intellectually, interacting with genetic endowment). This multidimensional concept of pain perception has stimulated researchers as well as clinicians to focus greater attention on psychologic factors thought to influence pain.

With the recognition that traditional medical techniques alone are all too often ineffective in relieving chronic pain[22] and that psychosocial variables influence the persistence of chronic pain problems,[10] there has been increasing utilization of psychologic approaches to the understanding and treatment of chronic pain. This state of affairs has had an increased impact on the clinical management of chronic pain problems, especially with the development and proliferation of the multidisciplinary pain clinic.

Unquestionably one of the most influential approaches has been the operant behavioral model of

*References 4 to 6, 16, 21, 22, 25, 26, and 28.

W.E. Fordyce.[10] He observed that all communication of pain takes place through some form of "pain behavior," such as limping, taking pain pills, grimacing, and verbal report. These behaviors are subject to influence by the consequences (operant conditioning) that follow their occurrence. Operant conditioning is a form of learning in which a behavior becomes more likely to occur as a result of having been reinforced by positive consequences or the removal of aversive consequences. The longer pain persists, the greater are the chances that pain behaviors will come under the control of social environmental contingencies.[3,13] For example, if, when a person limps and grimaces his family shows their concern by rushing to help him lie down and brings water and pain pills, then he is likely to continue limping and grimacing *if* he finds the attention rewarding. Fordyce and his colleagues[12] have demonstrated that modification of such rewarding contingencies can result in a decrease in pain behaviors and dysfunction. In a pain clinic, this approach would consist of ignoring pain behaviors and rewarding desired behaviors such as exercising, walking, and participating constructively in the prescribed program both in the clinic and in the home program.

Another tendency compatible with the concepts of gate-control theory is a growing research and clinical emphasis on cognitive factors that influence pain. Cognitive experiences relevant to pain perception are thought to include focus of attention, beliefs, attributions, expectations, coping strategies, self-statements, images, and problem-solving cognitions.[35] Cognitive theory considers behaviors and emotions as being influenced by the interpretation of an event, rather than solely by characteristics of the event. Thus, an "event" of pain interpreted as signifying ongoing tissue damage or life-threatening illness is likely to produce considerably more suffering and behavioral dysfunction than is one that is viewed as being the result of a minor injury, although the amount of nociceptive input in the two cases may be equivalent. It is important to realize that an evaluation of chronic pain is incomplete if these multidimensional complex interactions are ignored and attention is focused solely on identifying or ruling out organic pathology.[18,36]

Reasons for Referral

Patients suffering chronic pain are usually referred for psychologic evaluation in cases where (1) physical findings or pain generators are not sufficient to explain the pain; (2) the degree of disability or the decline in physical activity greatly exceeds that expected on the basis of physical findings; (3) the patient excessively uses the health-care system or persists in seeking diagnostic tests or treatments when not indicated; (4) addictive behaviors to prescribed medications or alcohol are present; and (5) emotions or stress are affecting pain and physical condition. A psychologic evaluation can be useful in all cases in which pain causes significant impairment in normal functioning or has had a negative impact on interpersonal relationships, or in situations in which a patient is exhibiting signs of significant psychologic distress. Often it is not possible to devote the time required for a thorough psychosocial history in a busy medical office or while doing rounds in the hospital.[21] Consequently, it is advantageous for orthopedists to have contact with a pain clinic or a psychologist who specializes in evaluating patients with both acute and chronic pain. These professionals can also be helpful when communication barriers owing to language or educational deficits are present.

For example, assessment of factors such as recent life distress, substance abuse, educational background, vocational history, psychologic disorders, and family role models of pain or chronic illness can provide worthwhile information helpful in interpreting a patient's current physical complaints and pain behaviors. It is important to recognize that psychologic evaluation alone cannot provide a definitive etiology for a patient's pain. The psychologic evaluation can, however, be quite useful in identifying patients who may be at higher risk for poor surgical outcome because of significant psychologic or behavioral factors. The addition of psychologic evaluation and interventions to the medical/surgical management of chronic pain can be of considerable benefit in clarifying issues and promoting a successful outcome.

Assessment Guidelines for Surgical Candidates

Guidelines for a comprehensive psychologic assessment of a patient with chronic pain or a patient being considered as a surgical candidate are given in the boxes. The upper box opposite outlines the information acquired in the clinical interview, and the lower box lists psychological instruments often used to provide additional information about the interactive impact of psychologic and physiologic functioning.

Based on the information obtained in the psychologic assessment, recommendations can be made about the individual's psychologic preparedness as a surgical candidate.

Components of Clinical Interview

- Identification of presenting problem
- Patient's understanding of problem
- Pain history
- Psychologic history
- Current psychologic status
- Functional limitations
- Family and social relationships
- Cognitive functioning
- Affective status
- Vocational history, status, and plans
- Alcohol and drug history
- Present alcohol and drug use
- Mental status and behavior
- Psychosocial history
- Stress and coping strategies

Psychological Instruments Utilized

- Minnesota Multiphasic Personality Inventory 2—Consists of 567 true–false items. Profile includes 10 clinical scales and three validity scales.
- Dallas Pain Questionnaire—A 16-item visual analog tool that evaluates the effect of chronic pain on patient's everyday life.
- Dallas Pain Drawing—A grid scoring method for the patient's drawing of pain patterns.
- McCoy Incomplete Sentences—Consists of 39 sentence stems reflecting patient's attitudes toward work.

Objective Instruments

The objective instruments utilized in the evaluation are the *Minnesota Multiphasic Personality Inventory-2 (MMPI-2)*, the *Dallas Pain Questionnaire (DPQ)*, the *Dallas Pain Drawing*, and the *McCoy Incomplete Sentences*. The *MMPI-2* provides important information about stress and motivation as well as affective and cognitive functioning. The *DPQ* uses a series of questions about the impact of pain on the activities of daily life, ability to work, leisure and social pursuits, and emotional functioning. Responses are grouped into four subscales and provide a good

Text continues on p. 922.

DALLAS PAIN QUESTIONNAIRE

Name: _____   Date of Birth: _____

Today's Date: _____   Occupation:_____

PLEASE READ: *Mark an "X" along the line from 0 to 100 for each question that tells your doctor how your pain has affected your life. Be sure to mark your own answers. Do not ask someone else to answer the questions for you.*

For example: I feel bad.

Never		Some			Mostly all the time
0%					100%
0	1	2	3	4	5

SECTION I: DAILY ACTIVITIES

1. PAIN AND INTENSITY - to what degree do you rely on pain medications or pain relieving substances for you to be comfortable?

None		Some			All the time
0%					100%
0	1	2	3	4	5

2. PERSONAL CARE - how much does pain interfere with your personal care (getting out of bed, teeth brushing, dressing, etc.)?

None (no pain)		Some		Cannot get out of bed
0%				100%
0	1	2	3	4

3. LIFTING - how much limitation do you notice lifting?

Can lift as I did		Some		Cannot lift anything
0%				100%
0	1	2	3	4	5

Fig. 67-1   *Continued.*

Dallas Pain Questionnaire

4. WALKING - compared to how far you could walk before your injury or back trouble, how much does pain restrict your walking now?

None (can walk the same) 0%			Some			Cannot walk 100%
0	1	2	3	4	5	

5. SITTING - back pain limits my sitting in a chair to:

No pain (same as before) 0%			Some			Cannot sit at all 100%
0	1	2	3	4	5	

6. STANDING - how much does your pain interfere with your tolerance to stand for long periods of time?

None (same as before) 0%			Some			Cannot stand 100%
0	1	2	3	4	5	

7. SLEEPING - how much does your pain interfere with your sleeping?

None (same as before) 0%		Some		Cannot sleep at all 100%
0	1	2	3	4

$$D = \underline{\qquad} \times 3 = \underline{\qquad} \%$$

SECTION II: WORK AND LEISURE

8. SOCIAL LIFE - how much does pain interfere with your social life (dancing, games, going out, eating with friends, etc.)?

None (same as before) 0%			Some			No activities (total loss) 100%
0	1	2	3	4	5	6	7

9. TRAVELING - how much does pain interfere with traveling in a car?

None (same as before) 0%			Some			Cannot travel 100%
0	1	2	3	4	5	6

Fig. 67-1, cont'd
Dallas Pain Questionnaire

10. VOCATIONAL - how much does pain interfere with your job?

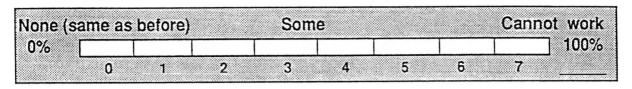

$$W = \underline{\quad} \times 5 = \underline{\quad} \%$$

SECTION III: ANXIETY/DEPRESSION

11. ANXIETY/MOOD - how much control do you feel that you have over the demands made on you?

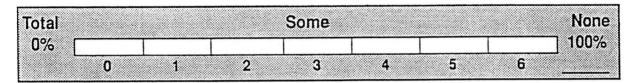

12. EMOTIONAL CONTROL - how much control do you feel you have over your emotions?

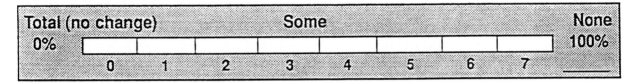

13. DEPRESSION - how depressed have you been since the onset of pain?

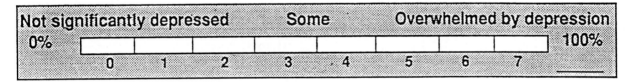

$$A = \underline{\quad} \times 5 = \underline{\quad} \%$$

SECTION IV: SOCIAL INTERESTS

14. INTERPERSONAL RELATIONSHIPS - how much do you think your pain changed your relationship with others?

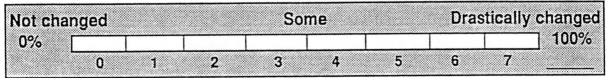

Fig. 67-1, cont'd
Dallas Pain Questionnaire

Continued.

15. SOCIAL SUPPORT - how much support do you need from others to help you during this onset of pain (taking over chores, fixing meals, etc.)?

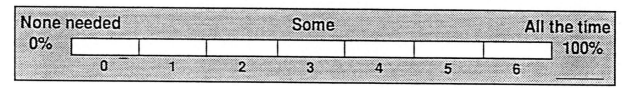

16. PUNISHING RESPONSE - how much do you think others express irritation, frustration, or anger toward you because of your pain?

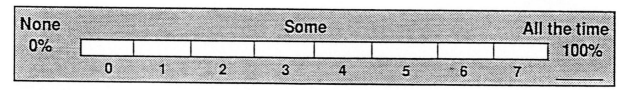

$$S = \_\_ \times 5 = \_\_ \%$$

Fig. 67-1, cont'd
Dallas Pain Questionnaire

overview of the disruption of the individual patient's life by the experience of pain. The resulting scales are Daily Activities (D), Work/Leisure Activities (W), Anxiety/Depression (A), and Social Interests (S). They are expressed in percentages of disruption. The *Dallas Pain Drawing* is a grid that overlays the front and back views of an androgenous human figure. The patient is asked to draw their pain patterns on the human figures. The number of grids having marks in them is counted and then the distortions and/or deviations from physiologically correct pain patterns can be scored.[1] Responses to the *McCoy Sentence Completion* reflects the patient's current attitudes and emotional reactions toward work, daily living, and primary relationships. It also indirectly provides information about the patient's ability to read and communicate.

Preparation for Surgery

Candidacy Classifications

The following classifications were developed at the Dallas Spinal Rehabilitation Center and are based on the individual's psychologic, behavioral, and social functioning.

An individual can be classified as an **excellent** surgical candidate when no significant psychopathology is present as assessed by psychologic evaluation and a clinical interview (see boxes on p 918), the patient is well motivated with no significant social stressors, and the patient has a good understanding of his or her role in the rehabilitation process both before and after surgery.

A **good** classification can be given in the presence of some anxiety if the patient displays good motivation and positive attitudes toward self-responsibility with no significant depression or somatization present. Both the excellent and good candidates will have lifestyles that reflect responsible self care.

A **fair** rating is given when there is evidence of mild psychopathology, such as depression and anxiety or somatization. Anxiety is usually thought of as an emotional state in which the individual is apprehensive and uneasy, without a concrete reason for feelings of dread or distress.[2,33] Depression is usually defined as a mood disorder in which the person feels despondent, pessimistic, sad, and inadequate.[2,33] Relatively positive motivation and attitudes are present in the fair candidate. Often, the fair candidate has a number of lifestyle issues that impair his or her chances of successful surgery. These issues would include significant external stressors, low levels of physical activity, reliance on others to

DALLAS PAIN QUESTIONNAIRE SUMMARY

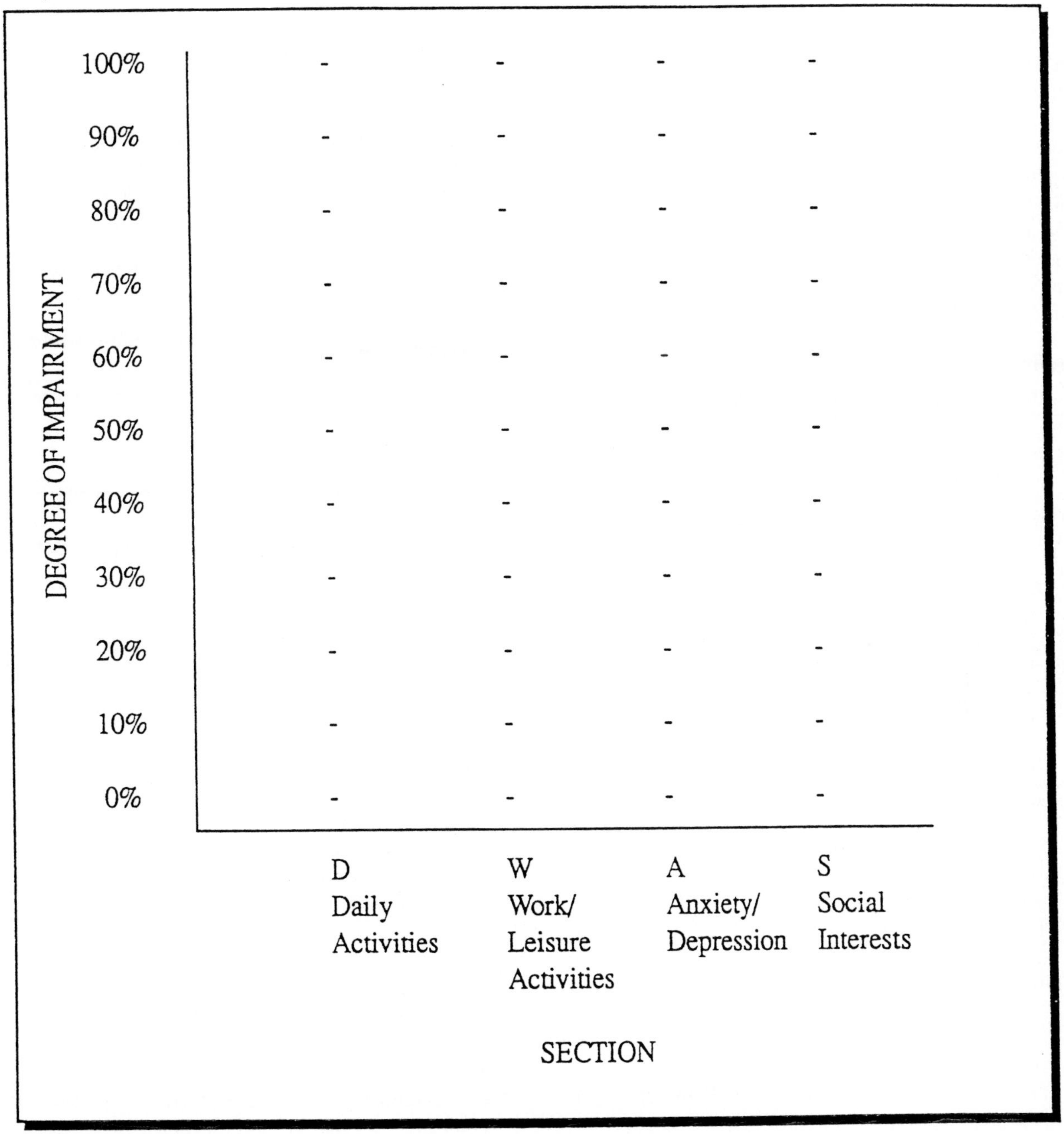
DEGREE OF IMPAIRMENT
100%
90%
80%
70%
60%
50%
40%
30%
20%
10%
0%
D
Daily
Activities
W
Work/
Leisure
Activities
A
Anxiety/
Depression
S
Social
Interests
SECTION

meet needs, poor nutrition, use of alcohol, smoking (tobacco or marijuana), and excessive ingestion of caffeine and/or sugar. The symptoms that might be reported in the physician's clinical evaluation are outlined in the boxed material. The box below and the upper box opposite give the symptoms and the *DSM-III-R* classifications of anxiety, while the lower box opposite and the box on p 925 outline the *DSM-III-R* classifications of mood disorders.

While some positive motivation is often present in the **poor** surgical candidate, psychopathology (moderate to severe depression, high levels of anxiety, and/or intense preoccupation with somatic concerns) is clearly present. Thinking is confused and impulse control is often a problem. There is evidence of seeking external solutions (pills, surgery, "just fix me and I'll be O.K."), and a lack of understanding of the role of self-responsibility in the process of preparation for and recovery from surgery. Usually this patient has excessive and significant social stressors evident in his or her life and experiences signif-

Clinical Symptoms of Anxiety

Motor tension
1. Trembling, twitching, or feeling shaky
2. Muscle tension, aches, or soreness
3. Restlessness
4. Easy fatigability

Autonomic hyperactivity
5. Shortness of breath or smothering sensation
6. Palpitations or accelerated heart rate
7. Sweating, or cold clammy hands
8. Dry mouth
9. Dizziness or lightheadedness
10. Nausea, diarrhea, or other abdominal distress
11. Flushes (hot flashes) or chills
12. Frequent urination
13. Trouble swallowing or "lump in throat"

Vigilance and scanning
14. Feeling keyed up or on edge
15. Exaggerated startle response
16. Difficulty concentrating or "mind going blank" because of anxiety
17. Trouble falling or staying asleep
18. Irritability

From American Psychiatric Association: *Diagnostic and statistical manual of mental disorders,* ed 3, revised. Washington, D.C., 1987, American Psychiatric Association.

DSM-III-R Criterion for Anxiety

300.02 Generalized Anxiety Disorder—Unrealistic or excessive anxiety and worry more days than not.

Other anxiety disorders
Panic disorder
300.21 with Agoraphobia or
300.01 without Agoraphobia
300.22 Agoraphobia without history of panic disorder
300.23 Social phobia
300.29 Obsessive compulsive disorder
300.89 Posttraumatic stress disorder
300.00 Anxiety disorder Not Otherwise Specified (NOS)

From American Psychiatric Association: *Diagnostic and statistical manual of mental disorders,* ed 3, revised. Washington, D.C., 1987, American Psychiatric Association.

Mood Disorders—DSM-III-R Classifications

Bipolar Disorders
296.6x Mixed—both manic and depressed features
296.4x Manic
296.5x Depressed
301.13 Cyclothymia
296.70 Bipolar disorder Not Otherwise Specified (NOS)

Depressive Disorders
Major Depression
296.6x Single episode
296.3x Recurrent

300.40 Dysthymia
311.00 Depressive disorder Not Otherwise Specified (NOS)

Fifth digit x allows coding of current state of disorder: 1 = mild; 2 = moderate; 3 = severe, without psychotic features; 4 = with psychotic features; 5 = in partial remission; 6 = in full remission; 0 = unspecified

From American Psychiatric Association: *Diagnostic and statistical manual of mental disorders,* ed 3, revised. Washington, D.C., 1987, American Psychiatric Association.

Symptoms of Depression

1. Depressed mood or irritable mood
2. Markedly diminished interest or pleasure in activities
3. Significant weight loss or weight gain when not dieting
4. Insomnia or hypersomnia nearly every day
5. Psychomotor agitation or retardation—observable by others
6. Fatigue or loss of energy
7. Feelings of worthlessness or excessive or inappropriate guilt which may be delusional
8. Diminished ability to think or concentrate, or indecisiveness
9. Recurrent thoughts of death, recurrent suicidal ideation without a plan, or a suicide attempt, or a specific plan for committing suicide
10. Lack of reactivity to usually pleasurable stimuli
11. Depression worse in the morning
12. Early morning awakening

From American Psychiatric Association: *Diagnostic and statistical manual of mental disorders*, ed 3, revised. Washington, D.C., 1987, American Psychiatric Association.

icant deficits in his or her ability to cope effectively with almost any difficulty. The lifestyle issues mentioned above are present here as well, usually to a more excessive degree. While they want to get better there is often little motivation to change because these patients find it difficult to conceive that they could initiate effective change or because they simply do not want to make needed lifestyle changes. Patients sometimes say they would rather die than stop smoking or change their diet.

Regardless of test scores, any patient who is emotionally labile, physically debilitated, has significant social stressors, or who has been relying on narcotics, tranquilizers, and/or sleeping pills needs to be given a rating of fair or less. If reliance on medications is part of the daily routine, or suicidal ideations are expressed, the designation of poor needs to be given.

Very poor surgical candidates have extensive psychopathology, while motivation and attitudes are clearly negative. They will, also, have significant social stressors,k poor lifestyle support, and inadequate, as well as destructive means of coping with stress.

They often alienate those who would try to assist or help them. For instance, they often are intense in their efforts to find someone to help them, but reject any suggestions the helper offers. This, combined with the projection of blame, puts them in a double bind that makes improvement almost impossible. Long-term deficits in personality functioning and paranoia have often impaired these patients' ability to act in their own behalf in functional ways. This state of affairs is an absolute indication for avoiding elective surgery. Surgery should be undertaken on these patients only under emergency situations such as acute radiculopathy or neural decompression.

Pre- and Postsurgical Education and Rehabilitation

Each of these patient groups has different needs for preoperative education and pain management, as well as postoperative rehabilitation. **Excellent** candidates will most likely experience successful surgery without extensive education or rehabilitation. They will understand the procedure and will be responsible in following a home program both for preoperative preparation and postoperative recovery if given appropriate instructions.

Good candidates will need to be given careful instructions and follow-up both before and after surgery to allay their anxiety. They are capable of understanding the recommended surgical procedure and its consequences, as well as their role in a home preparation and recovery program, if appropriate education is offered to them before and after surgery. They will not need extensive rehabilitation before surgery unless they are debilitated physically.

Persons who are characterized as **fair** surgical candidates need training to prepare them before surgery is considered. They usually respond well to rehabilitation and education. Their inclusion in a structured pain control/rehabilitation program will considerably improve their chances of a successful surgical outcome. This is accomplished by improving their understanding of physical pathology and of their options in dealing with that difficulty. They have the opportunity to address their psychosocial and lifestyle impairments in a manner that results in a decrease in situational stress and an improvement in depression and anxiety. Equally important is the opportunity to improve strength, flexibility, and endurance through physical and occupational therapies. These measures allow the patient to approach surgery with greatly improved physical and psychologic functioning. Before they are ready to be reconsidered for surgical intervention, the fair surgical candidate should complete a planned pain management/rehabilitation program and 6 to 8 weeks of activity in an independent structured home program that addresses both psychosocial and physical issues.

Patients who are moderately or severely depressed, are anxious, or have been taking narcotics, sleeping pills, or tranquilizers should successfully complete a 4 week multidisciplinary inpatient pain management program or its equivalent, followed by 2 to 4 months of home practice, before a surgical decision is made. A patient who is unable to follow through in a home program is unlikely to be able to do the exercising and self-responsible home care required after surgery.

Poor surgical candidates need extensive education and rehabilitation before surgery can be considered. Their needs are most likely to be met in an inpatient program followed by compliance in a structured home rehabilitation program for 4 to 6 months before being reconsidered for surgery. Their home program should address psychologic, social, and physical issues as well as the development of viable plans for the future. Psychologic debility, physical debility, significant psychosocial stressors, poor coping abilities, or the use of addictive substances are strong indications that a multidisciplinary, inpatient (if available) intervention is needed.

While **very poor** candidates need extensive reeducation and rehabilitation before any surgery should be attempted, they may not have the resources to truly comprehend their need for rehabilitation before surgery is undertaken. As a result, they are quite unlikely to see the need to carry through with a useful home program. Many of these patients may never become even fair surgical candidates. Surgery should only be attempted with them if no other course of action is possible and with the clear understanding that emotional and behavioral factors may interfere with postoperative progress.

Pain Drawings and Patient Profiles

Figures 67-2, 67-3, and 67-4 present the *MMPI-2* profiles, pain drawings, and subscales of the *Dallas Pain Questionnaires* of the three surgical candidates. The 567 true–false questions that comprise the MMPI-2 are examined and grouped into three validity scales (L, F, K) and 10 clinical scales. See box opposite.

These scales provide a profile and summary of information about the patient's current status and con-

cerns about his or her physical and mental health as well as motivation and overall levels of stress, and assist the practitioner in evaluating the interactive nature of these factors. The drawings and profiles of good, fair, and poor patients are often quite dramatic in illustrating the differences between good, fair, and poor surgical candidates.

Description of MMPI-2

L, F, and K are validity scales.

L is called the Lie scale and measures willingness to admit minor social faults. It gives information about social conformity, self-image and self-insight, and denial.

F refers to infrequency and consists of items that are socially unacceptable or have disturbing content. Persons scoring on the low end of this scale are usually conventional and unassuming. Those with elevations are admitting to severe emotional distress and/or psychopathology. Very high scores suggest an invalid profile.

K refers to correction, and the items measure personal resources required to cope with life. Low scores suggest exaggeration of problems or severe emotional distress. Higher scores can result when patients are very confident and in charge or when they are being defensive in their efforts to present themselves as adequate and in control; when in fact their lives are in disarray.

Scales 1 through 10 are the basic clinical scales of the MMPI-2. The information is presented using T scores. A T score of 50 is average; T scores over 65 are in the abnormal range.

Scale 1 is also referred to as the "Hypochondriasis (HS)" scale. This scale consists of items that concern bodily functioning. Many of the items are vague in their content. Persons scoring low on this scale don't have or are denying that they have any physical complaints. Those whose scores are elevated have many physical complaints and concerns. If scores are above 65 physical complaints are often the major focus of the person's life.

Scale 2 is referred to as the "Depression (D)" scale. It consists of items that measure subjective depression, psychomotor slowing and immobilization, physical complaints, mental dullness, and brooding. High scores indicate the presence of depression and low scores indicate those whose affective functioning is within normal limits.

Description of MMPI-2 (continued)

Scale 3 is referred to as "Hysteria (Hy)." It consists of items that indicate whether the individual tends to avoid emotional and social unpleasantness. Those that do may then experience their emotions and stress as somatic complaints. High scorers will often deny psychologic problems and look for concrete solutions to their problems.

Scale 4 is referred to as "Psychopathic Deviate (Pd)." While eight items refer to authority conflicts, the rest of the items deal with family conflicts, denial of social and dependency needs, social alienation, and self-integration. High scorers are often angry, impulsive, in conflict with authority figures in their lives, and are feeling isolated and despondent. High scorers who are not psychopathic are often undergoing stressful transitions in their lives.

Scale 5 is referred to as "Masculinity-Femininity (Mf)." Scores on this reflect traditional versus non-traditional masculine or feminine interests and beliefs, conflicts about sexuality, and interests in aesthetics. Low scores for women suggest feelings of helplessness and dependency, while low scores for men suggest an action-oriented "macho" approach to life. High-scoring males often hold interests in activities usually thought of as feminine and may be experiencing insecurity, helplessness, and conflicts of sexuality. High-scoring females report interest in traditional male patterns, and are often seen as unfriendly, dominating, and aggressive.

Scale 6 is referred to as "Paranoia (Pa)." In addition to paranoia and externalization of blame, this scale contains items related to hypersensitivity, subjectivity, naivete, righteousness, and denial of hostility and distrust. Very high scorers are outright paranoid and may have a thought disorder, while low scorers may be insensitive to others and unaware of other's motives. They may also be denying the presence of paranoid thoughts.

Scale 7 is referred to as "Psychasthenia (Pt)." Items center around the presence of worries, brooding, and rumination. High scorers are seen as anxious and insecure, and may be indecisive. If scores are very high the individual may be compulsive and agitated with feelings of guilt and fear disrupting everyday functioning.

Description of MMPI-2 (continued)

Scale 8 is referred to as "Schizophrenia (Sc)." High scorers are having difficulty with their thinking and feelings. They often feel out of control and unable to take positive action in their own behalf. Extremely high scores are suggestive of severe situational stress. More moderate elevations are seen in those with thought disorders with difficulties in logic concentration, and judgment common.

Scale 9 is referred to as "Hypomania (Ma)." This scale provides information about motivation, physical and emotional activity levels, confidence in social situations, and feelings of self-importance. High scorers are restless, agitated, emotionally labile, and may have racing thoughts. They may also have difficulty delaying gratification and can be impulsive. Manic features appear as scores elevate.

Scale 10 is referred to as "Social Introversion (Si)." This scale provides information about social interests, interpersonal skills, self-consciousness, and feelings of alienation from self or others High scorers are often depressed. They withdraw from social interactions and feel shy and insecure. Low scorers are usually socially extroverted and outgoing.

Availability of Programs

Organized multidisciplinary pain programs are available in many urban areas of the country. These centers will vary in both the philosophy of the treatment approach and the quality of care given. Physicians who disagree with the treatment rationales available to them or who live in areas where an organized multidisciplinary treatment program is not available will need to build a referral network of professionals who are willing to provide needed treatments and interventions that his or her patients require in dealing with acute and/or chronic pain syndromes. Such a network might include a psychologist who is trained to evaluate patients with acute and/or chronic pain; a biofeedback therapist who can provide individual and group therapies; a vocational specialist to evaluate work history and transferable skills and who can help the patient plan for return to active life; a physical therapist to evaluate and provide appropriate training in exercises that will promote increased strength, flexibility, and endurance; and an occupational therapist to evaluate and provide therapeutic services to improve the quality of everyday life and to provide therapies cen-

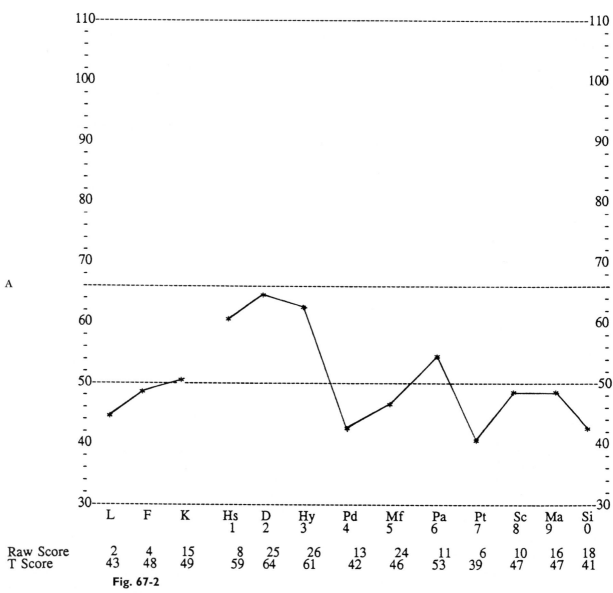

Fig. 67-2

A, MMPI-2 of a "good" surgical patient.

DATE: _____   **NAME:** _____

DALLAS PAIN DRAWING GRID ASSESSMENT
Dr. McCoy/Dallas Spinal Rehabilitation Center, Inc. at Dallas Specialty Hospital
2124 Research Row   Dallas, TX 75235   214/904-6900

Draw the location of your pain on the body outlines and mark how bad it is on the pain line at the bottom of the page.

Percentage of pain in back _____ *90* _____   **Percentage of pain in legs** _____ *10* _____

FRONT   BACK

RIGHT   LEFT   LEFT   RIGHT

B

NO PAIN ┠────────✗────────────────────┨ INTOLERABLE
         MARK YOUR PAIN ESTIMATE   **PAIN**

Fig. 67-2, cont'd   *Continued.*

B, Pain drawing of a "good" surgical patient.

PAIN QUESTIONNAIRE SUMMARY

Good Surgical Candidate

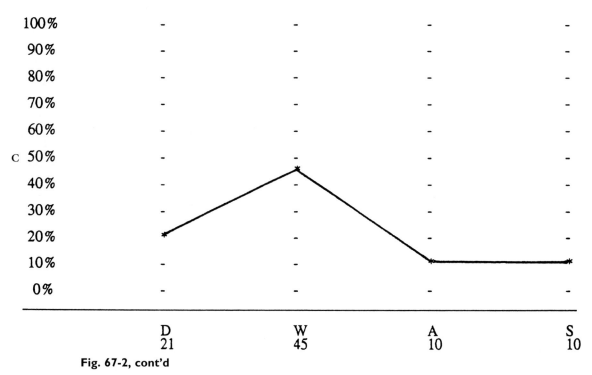

Fig. 67-2, cont'd

C, Dallas Pain Summary of a "good" surgical patient. This 64-year-old patient is a retired engineer with a good support system and no financial stress who wants an improved quality of life. (*D*, daily activities; *W*, work/leisure activities; *A*, anxiety/depression; *S*, social interests.)

tering around functional activities and postural retraining. Some psychologists are able to provide biofeedback, individual and group therapies, and vocational counseling as well as psychologic assessment services. While each of these professionals could provide services within their own private-practice settings, it would be most helpful to the physician and the patients if these efforts could be coordinated through weekly meetings or staffings. Other helpful resources would include a registered dietitian and someone skilled in helping patients with smoking cessation.

Outcome Predictors

There are a multitude of articles in the medical and psychologic literature about chronic pain and outcome predictors for successful surgery.* Recently there has

been some shift in focus on these predictors, with education level coming to the fore as a predictor of importance.[27,31,32] Individuals who are poorly educated do not, as a whole, do as well in dealing with chronic health problems as individuals with higher levels of education. The psychosocial factors that predict poor outcome of surgery also seem to predict the presence of lifestyle disorders such as hepatitis C, cardiovascular disorders, diabetes, hypertension, use of addictive medications, and noncompliance with recommended treatments, which in turn become general medical predictors of poor outcome.[9,27,31,32] Related lifestyle issues include inadequate sleep[19] and nutritional factors such as obesity and diets high in fat, simple sugars, sodium, and caffeine and low in fiber. Other factors less often discussed are the presence of high levels of situational stress associated with financial loss and family disruption.

*References 7, 15, 23, 28, 34, 37, and 38.

MMPI - 2

Fair Surgical Patient

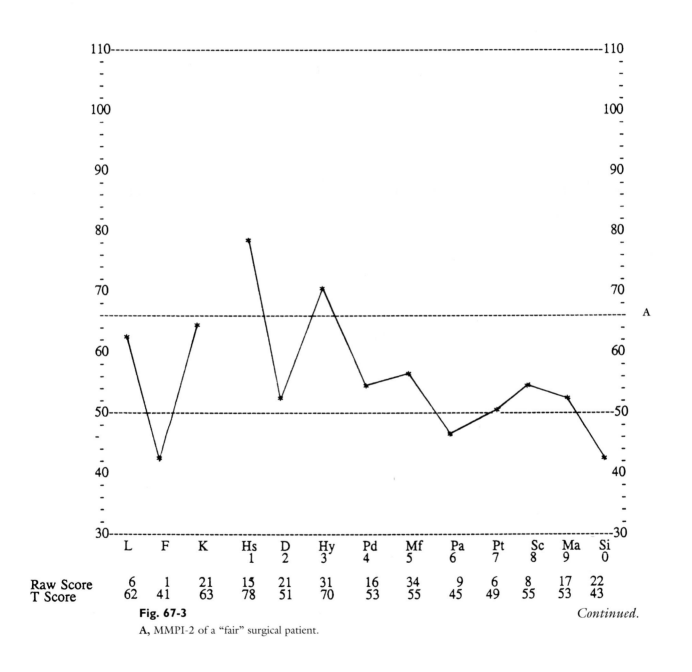

	L	F	K	Hs 1	D 2	Hy 3	Pd 4	Mf 5	Pa 6	Pt 7	Sc 8	Ma 9	Si 0
Raw Score	6	1	21	15	21	31	16	34	9	6	8	17	22
T Score	62	41	63	78	51	70	53	55	45	49	55	53	43

Fig. 67-3   *Continued.*

A, MMPI-2 of a "fair" surgical patient.

DATE: _____   **NAME:** _____

DALLAS PAIN DRAWING GRID ASSESSMENT
Dr. McCoy/Dallas Spinal Rehabilitation Center, Inc. at Dallas Specialty Hospital
2124 Research Row   Dallas, TX 75235   214/904-6900

Draw the location of your pain on the body outlines and mark how bad it is on the pain line at the bottom of the page.

Percentage of pain in back _____*40*_____   **Percentage of pain in legs** _____*60*_____

FRONT   BACK

B

RIGHT   LEFT   LEFT   RIGHT

NO PAIN ├──────────────────────────┤ INTOLERABLE
            MARK YOUR PAIN ESTIMATE   PAIN

Fig. 67-3 cont'd

B, Pain drawing of a "fair" surgical patient.

PAIN QUESTIONNAIRE SUMMARY

Fair Surgical Candidate

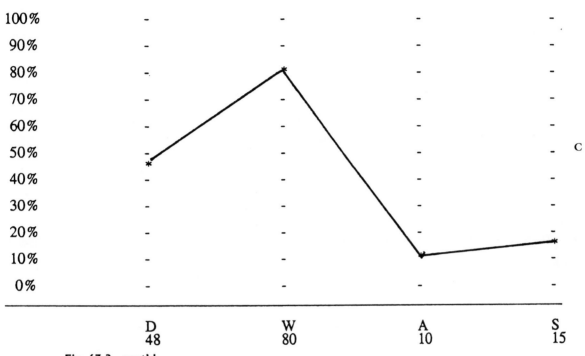

Fig. 67-3, cont'd

C, Dallas Pain Questionnaire Summary of a "fair" surgical patient. This 41-year-old female patient has good support from her husband. She returned to work after 1986, was reinjured in 1987, and is now on Social Security Disability. (*D,* daily activities; *W,* work/leisure activities; *A,* anxiety/depression; *S,* social interests.)

Levels of Treatment

Multidisciplinary Behavioral Medicine Models

The needs of patients with back and neck injuries cannot be met in single-modality intervention programs. The services offered by the Dallas Spinal Rehabilitation Center can be used as a model for a comprehensive multidisciplinary approach to the preparation of patients for surgical intervention, postoperative rehabilitation, and the treatment of chronic pain.

Preoperative Evaluation Program

The Preoperative Evaluation Program (PEP) is a 1-week outpatient program for patients who have physical pathology that the referring physician be-

lieves could be improved with surgical intervention. The multilevel assessment process previously described is used to evaluate psychologic, medical, and physical functioning, and the findings are related to the individual's appropriateness as a surgical candidate. The program seeks to increase understanding of physical problems and options, as well as to improve coping skills and stress-management strategies. Patients are prepared for surgery and their hospital stay through an education process that includes educational groups, videos, and opportunities to ask questions of their surgeons. The importance of self-responsibility and independence is emphasized. Patients are prepared for expected hospital routines such as walking on Day one after surgery and discharge to home with no narcotics for pain. They are taught the exercises to be used both in the hospital and in their independent home rehabilitation and exercise programs. Patients with this preparation show

MMPI - 2

Poor Surgical Patient

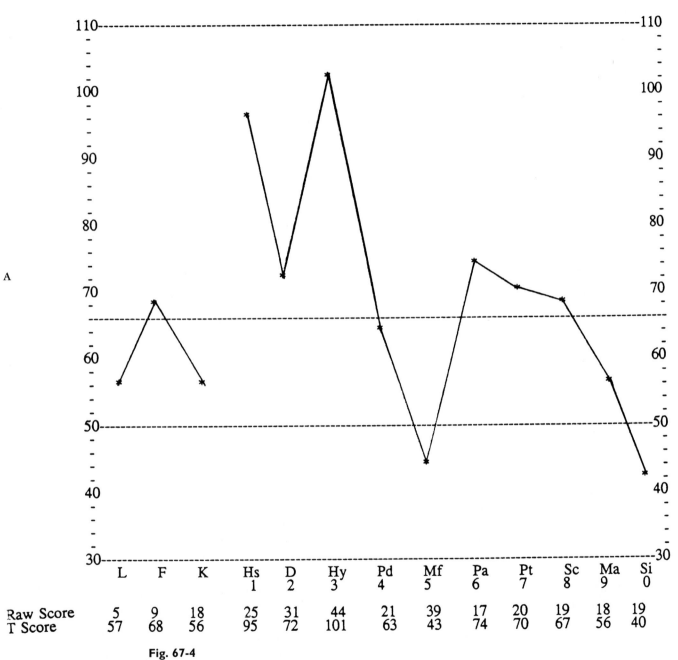

	L	F	K	Hs 1	D 2	Hy 3	Pd 4	Mf 5	Pa 6	Pt 7	Sc 8	Ma 9	Si 0
Raw Score	5	9	18	25	31	44	21	39	17	20	19	18	19
T Score	57	68	56	95	72	101	63	43	74	70	67	56	40

A

Fig. 67-4

A, MMPI-2 of a "poor" surgical patient.

DATE: _____ NAME: _____

DALLAS PAIN DRAWING GRID ASSESSMENT
Dr. McCoy/Dallas Spinal Rehabilitation Center, Inc. at Dallas Specialty Hospital
2124 Research Row   Dallas, TX 75235   214/904-6900

Draw the location of your pain on the body outlines and mark how bad it is on the pain line at the bottom of the page.

Percentage of pain in back ___55___   Percentage of pain in legs ___45___

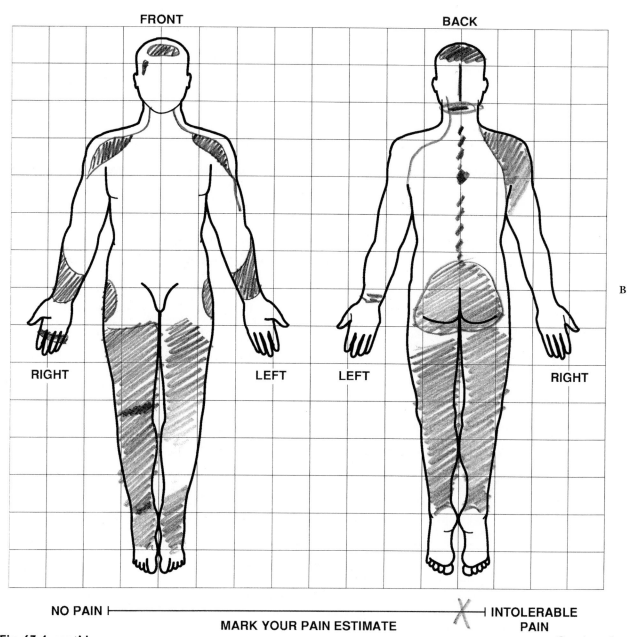

FRONT   BACK

B

RIGHT   LEFT   LEFT   RIGHT

NO PAIN ├─────────────────────────────X─┤ INTOLERABLE
         MARK YOUR PAIN ESTIMATE   PAIN

Fig. 67-4, cont'd

Continued.

B, Pain drawing of a "poor" surgical patient.

PAIN QUESTIONNAIRE SUMMARY

Poor Surgical Candidate

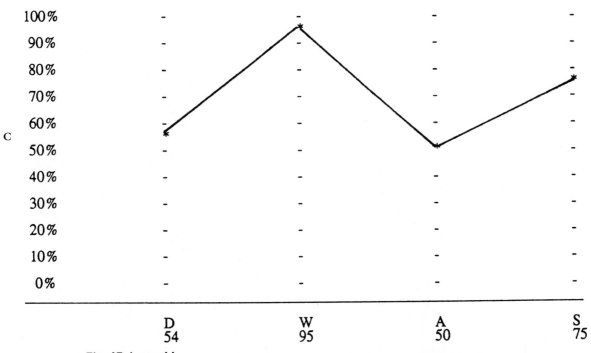

Fig. 67-4, cont'd

C, Dallas Pain Questionnaire Summary of a "poor" surgical patient. This 30-year-old male patient has had two motor vehicle accidents and has been diagnosed with chronic fatigue syndrome. He is taking pain medications and demonstrating lots of pain behavior. (*D*, daily activities; *W*, work/leisure activities; *A*, anxiety/depression; *S*, social interests.)

greater compliance during their hospital stay and after discharge than those who have not had preparatory experiences. Exercises to improve strength, endurance, and flexibility are taught, as are stabilization and neutral spine techniques to improve functional abilities. Each patient is encouraged to formulate future goals and vocational plans.

Factors suggesting good outcome are low to moderate situational stressors, positive motivation and clear goals, absence of significant psychopathology, adequate coping skills, willingness to engage in the exercise program, and overall good health. Factors suggesting poor outcome are severe situational stressors, poor motivation and unclear goals, significant psychopathology, poor physical health, and ongoing legal cases. Approximately 69% of the patients attending the PEP program are offered a surgical option. The remaining patients include those who are

not offered a surgical option because of high levels of psychopathology, physical pathology, mitigating physical problems, or those who elect not to have surgery.

Chronic Pain Programs

Inpatient

The most comprehensive program available is a 4-week inpatient program. This multidisciplinary treatment and evaluation program is for individuals experiencing chronic back or neck pain as a result of injury or progressive degenerative processes. Most patients have underlying physical pathology (>90%) to account, at least in part, for their pain process. This program serves those with severe physical pathology, physical deconditioning, psychologic debility, situational stress, poor coping skills, physical health problems, dependence on medications, and character disorders. Treatment objectives are varied and complex. Assessments and interventions occur at several levels of functioning, including psychologic, social, vocational, functional, physical therapy, occupational therapy, and medical. Educational programs are extensive and seek to assist the patient in understanding what is "wrong" and what options are available. Individual and group interventions address stress-management strategies, coping skills, problem solving, goal setting, motivation, and compliance. Computerized biofeedback equipment is used to both assess and train patients. This training allows patients to utilize information about the electrical activity in their muscles, breathing patterns, and the temperature of their extremities to promote skill in general and specific relaxation strategies, decreasing inappropriate sympathetic nervous system activation, and to improve exercise strategies. Physical and occupational therapies seek to improve strength, endurance, flexibility, and functional abilities as well as proprioceptive, kinesthetic, and sensory awareness. Each patient receives extensive training in stabilization and postural retraining. All therapies and group experiences seek to promote independence in self-monitoring and problem solving. At discharge each patient works with his or her therapist to develop a dynamic home rehabilitation program that serves to build on the gains made while in the program and to develop further a sense of success and self-responsibility.

Outpatient

The 4-week program is also available on an outpatient basis for patients with mild to moderate physical pathology, mild to moderate physical deconditioning, moderate psychologic debility, moderate situational stress, adequate coping skills, no physical health problems, no addictive medications, apparent self-responsibility, and the ability to be cooperative in self-care. Treatment objectives are basically the same as those in the inpatient program.

Work Hardening and Work Conditioning

The work-hardening and work-conditioning programs are structured, goal-oriented treatment programs using rehabilitation techniques and work-simulation tasks to improve the patient's ability to be active. These programs serve those who have reached maximum medical benefit, need to return to active life, need assistance setting constructive goals, use no addictive medications, have no psychologic or sit-

uational problems that would interfere with constructive goal achievement, and need no further medical diagnostic or surgical interventions. The primary objective of the work-hardening program is to improve the patient's ability to return to an active life either in the labor force or in an educational program that will lead to return to work.

Behavioral Medicine and Interdisciplinary Cooperation

These programs are based on a behavioral medicine model that emphasizes a horizontal approach to multidisciplinary interventions rather than the traditional rehabilitation model or the biomedical model. It seeks to integrate disciplines in a manner that approaches patient care from a perspective that recognizes as many of the factors involved in satisfactory outcome as possible. Interdisciplinary cooperation is essential if good outcomes are to be achieved.

Patient Responsibility

A factor that is often not adequately addressed is the need for patient cooperation. The single most essential ingredient to successful outcome is the patient's role in responsible self-care. Traditionally, society teaches us that we can go to the Doctor and soon all will be well. When dealing with chronic illness the situation is reversed[6] and the patient's willingness to comply and make lifestyle changes becomes the most important factor in outcome. This need is perhaps more clear in other chronic illnesses such as diabetes where willingness to comply with dietary change is essential to outcome. This factor is an important ingredient in the need for multidisciplinary intervention programs so that patients can be offered the opportunity to learn about their part in the process of improving the quality of their lives, which is the reason they are willing to have surgery in the first place.

References

1. Achterberg J, Lawlis GF: *Bridges of the bodymind: behavioral approaches to health care,* Champaign, IL, 1980, Institute For Personality and Ability Testing.
2. American Psychiatric Association: *Diagnostic and statistical manual of mental disorders,* ed 3, revised. Washington, D.D., 1987, American Psychiatric Association.
3. Block A, Kremer E, Gaylor M: Behavioral treatment of chronic pain: the spouse as a discrimnative cue for pain behavior, *Pain* 9:243, 1980.

4. Bonica JJ: *Introduction: importance of the problem.* In Aronoff GM, editor: *Evaluation and treatment of chronic pain,* Baltimore, 1992, Williams & Wilkins.

5. Crue BL: *Foreword.* In Aronoff GM, editor: *Evaluation and treatment of chronic pain,* Baltimore, 1992, Williams & Wilkins.

6. Cuencas-Zamora R and others: La medicina conductual: un modelo interdisciplinario en una clinica para el dolor cronico de la columna, *Salud Mental* 14(4):25, 1991.

7. Egbert LD and others: Reduction of post-operative pain by encouragement and instruction of patients, *N Engl J Med* 270:825, 1964.

8. Deyo RA, Diehl AK: Psychosocial predictors of disability in patient with low back pain, *J Rheumatol* 15:1557, 1988.

9. Fischer P, Haley R: *Hepatitis C in the chronic pain patient,* Research in process, 1992.

10. Fordyce WE: *Behavioral methods for chronic pain and illness,* St. Louis, 1976, Mosby.

11. Fordyce WE, Roberts AH, Sternbach RA: The behavioral management of chronic pain: a response to critics, *Pain* 22:113, 1985.

12. Fordyce WE, Shelton JL, Dundore DE: The modification of avoidance learning pain behaviors, *J Behav Med* 5:405, 1982.

13. Fordyce WE, Steger JC: *Chronic pain.* In Pomerleau OF, Brady JP, editors: *Behavioral medicine: theory and practice,* ed 2, Baltimore, 1979, Williams & Wilkins.

14. Frank JD: *Psychotherapy of bodily disease: an overview.* In Garfield CA, editor: *Stress and survival: the emotional realities of life threatening illness,* St. Louis, 1979, Mosby.

15. Freeman C, Calsyn D, Louks J: The use of the Minnesota Multiphasic Personality Inventory with low back patients, *J Clin Psychol* 32:294, 1976.

16. Hayes MA and others: *Alteration in comfort: a nursing challenge.* In Aronoff GM, editor: *Evaluation and treatment of chronic pain,* ed 2, Baltimore, 1992, Williams & Wilkins.

17. Hendler N: *Psychiatric considerations of pain.* In Youmans JR, editor: *Neurological surgery,* ed 3, Philadelphia, 1990, W.B. Saunders.

18. Keefe FJ, Gil KM: Behavioral concepts in the analysis of chronic pain syndromes, *J Consult Clin Psychol* 54:776, 1986.

19. Kellen R: *Sleep patterns and chronic pain.* Thesis, University of North Texas, 1991.

20. Kendall PC, Watson D: Psychological preparation for stressful medical procedures. *Medical psychology: contributions to behavioral medicine,* 1981, Academic Press, p 198.

21. Kinney WW, Brin EN: *Diagnostic evaluation and management of the patient with chronic pain.* In Aronoff GM, editor: *Evaluation and treatment of chronic pain,* Baltimore, 1992, Williams & Wilkins.

22. Linton SJ: A critical review of behavioral treatments for chronic benign pain other than headache, *Br Clin Psychol* 21:321, 1982.

23. Long CJ: The relationship between surgical outcome and MMPI profiles in chronic pain patients, *J Clin Psychol* 37:744, 1981.

24. Love AW, Peck CL: The MMPI and psychological factors in chronic low back pain: a review, *Pain* 28:1, 1987.

25. McCoy CE: *The multidisciplinary team rating as a predictor of success with lumbar fusion on chronic pain patients.* Presentation, North American Spine Society Sixth Annual Meeting, Keystone, CL, July 31-August 3, 1991.

26. McCoy CE: *Pre-operative testing with the Minnesota Multiphasic Personality Inventory as a predictor of success with lumbar fusion on chronic pain patients.* Presentation, North American Spine Society Sixth Annual Meeting, Keystone, CO, July 31-August 3, 1991.

27. McCoy CE, Wolfe C, McGee J: *Educational factors in surgical outcome,* unpublished data, 1992.

28. McCoy CE and others: Patients avoiding surgery: pathology and one year life status follow-up, *Spine* 16:6, 1991.

29. Melzac R, Wall PD: Pain mechanisms: a new theory, *Science* 50:971, 1965.

30. Nachemson AL: Time natural course of low back pain. In White AA, Gordon SL, editors: *Symposium on Idiopathic Low Back Pain,* American Academy of Orthopedic surgeons, 1982, Mosby.

31. Pincus T: Formal education level—a marker for the importance of behavioral variable in the pathogenesis, morbidity, and mortality of most diseases?, *J Rheumatol* 15:10, 1988.

32. Pincus T, Callahan LF, Burkhauser RV: Most chronic diseases are reported more frequently by individuals with fewer than 12 years of formal education in the age 18-64, United States population, *J Chronic Dis* 40:865, 1987.

33. Reber AS: *The Penguin dictionary of psychology,* London, 1985, Viking Penguin.

34. Sorensen LV, Mors O, Skovlund O: A prospective study of the importance of psychological and social factors for the outcome after surgery in patients with slipped lumbar disc operated upon the first time, *Acta Neurochir* 88:119, 1987.

35. Turk DC, Meichenbaum D, Genest M: *Pain and behavioral medicine: a cognitive-behavioral perspective,* New York, 1983, Guilford Press.

36. Turk DC, Rudy TE: Assessment of cognitive factors in chronic pain: a worthwhile enterprise?, *J Consult Clin Psychol* 54:760, 1986.

37. Turner JA, Herron L, Weiner P: Utility of the MMPI pain assessment index in predicting outcome after lumbar surgery, *J Clin Psychol* 42:764, 1986.

38. Wilkinson HA: *The failed back syndrome,* ed 2, New York, 1992, Springer-Verlag.

Chapter 68
Anesthesia in Cervical Spine Surgery
Tracy P. Cotter
Susan L. Goelzer

Preoperative Evaluation

history
physical examination
laboratory evaluation

Intraoperative Management

airway management
induction and maintenance of anesthesia
special considerations
positioning
monitoring

Postoperative Considerations

Summary

Conditions involving the cervical spine affect the anesthetic management of a patient, regardless of the procedure planned. Congenital and acquired abnormalities of the cervical spine can become manifest as a result of intubation and positioning while administering anesthesia for surgery unrelated to the cervical spine. When an injured cervical spine requires operative repair, whether due to disease or trauma, the anesthesiologist faces additional challenges. Each patient must have a thorough preoperative assessment that then guides the anesthesiologist through the intraoperative and postoperative course. Thus, the anesthesiologist aims to protect the patient from injury, to establish conditions that permit the surgeon to reach a prompt and safe conclusion, and to provide physiologic stability, analgesia, loss of awareness, and muscle relaxation when necessary. This chapter will outline the management of the patient with cervical spine diseases, concentrating on the preoperative evaluation and preparation of these patients, the intraoperative management, and possible associated complications.

Preoperative Evaluation

The preoperative evaluation of the patient with cervical spine disease allows the anesthesiologist an opportunity to assess the individual patient's problems and those particular problems associated with the disease. The anesthesiologist is rarely called upon to "clear the cervical spine"; however an appreciation of the anatomy, biomechanics, and disease processes should be a part of his or her clinical repertoire.[4] The acuity, extent, and level of the spinal-cord lesion, as well as the presence of associated conditions, affects the choice of intubation techniques, anesthetic agents, and techniques and monitoring modalities. Communication between the anesthesiologist and surgeon, as well as with pertinent consultants, provides the safest possible outcome for the patient.

History

As always in medicine, evaluation of the patient begins with an adequate history. It is important for the anesthesiologist to be aware of the type and acuity of injury to the cervical spine, the stability of the spine with this injury, and any associated neurologic or cardiovascular impairment, as the anesthetic management of individual patients will change depending on the pathology and associated complications. For example, after a hyperflexion injury the cervical spine is actually more stable in extension. The reverse is true for hyperextension injuries.[45]

Syndromes: Odontoid Hypoplasia

- Down syndrome
- Congenital scoliosis
- Klippel–Feil syndrome
- Neurofibromatosis
- Osteogenesis imperfecta
- Dysproportionate dwarfism
- Morquio syndrome

The ideal time for the patient and the anesthesiologist to meet is several weeks before scheduled surgery. Full evaluation of the patient's medical status may require special laboratory investigations, consultations, and time to assess the response to optimal medical management. Surgery for degenerative joint disease usually suggests an older, possibly more debilitated patient who may need further work-up. Tumors tend to be vascular, setting the stage for rapid blood loss. Infectious cervical spine injuries, such as epidural abscesses, compound management, as the affected patient may be septic and possess the inherent problems of sepsis. Traumatic injuries require immediate attention but the effects on other organ systems should not be forgotten due to the emergent nature of the injury. The actual incidence of cervical spine injury in trauma victims is reportedly 16% to 24%.[6] Seventy percent of trauma victims have multiple injuries, including hemothorax, pneumothorax, blunt abdominal trauma, cardiac tamponade, closed head injuries, and major orthopedic injuries in addition to cervical spine trauma. Hypoplasia of the odontoid process is seen in a number of syndromes (see box above). With these disease processes, hyperextension of the atlantoaxial joint results in subluxation of the atlas anteriorly on the axis with compression of the neural elements. These patients are at risk for traumatic quadraparesis, even with minor trauma.

Many congenital and acquired disorders have been associated with atlantoaxial subluxation (see box on p. 941). Extension of the head may sublux the atlas anteriorly onto the cord with resultant cord compression by the odontoid process. For example, involvement of the cervical spine is a common feature of the inflammatory arthropathies. Radiologic evidence of cervical spine involvement is found in 17% to 86% of patients with rheumatoid arthritis (RA).[22] Atlantoaxial subluxation is the most common radiographic finding in RA, occurring in 25%

Conditions: Axial Subluxation

- Acquired
  Rheumatoid arthritis
  Ankylosing spondylitis
  Still's disease
  Enteropathic arthritis
  Reiter's syndrome
  Psoriatic arthritis
  Traumatic injuries
- Congenital
  Down syndrome
  Mucopolysaccharidoses
  Odontoid anomalies

Mallampati Classification

I: Tonsillar pillars, soft palate, and uvula visualized

II: Tonsillar pillars and soft palate visualized; uvula masked by base of tongue

III: Only soft palate visualized

From Mallampati SR and others: A clinical sign to predict difficult tracheal intubation: a prospective study, *Can Anaesth Soc J* 82:429, 1985.

of patients. All patients with RA presenting for surgery should be evaluated for rheumatoid involvement of the neck. High-risk patients include the elderly, patients with longstanding disease or neck symptoms, patients with subcutaneous nodules, and patients with erosive disease. Lateral cervical spine radiographs should be obtained in the neutral position as well as in flexion and extension. A combination of anterior subluxation with either vertical or subaxial subluxation places the patient at an increased risk for neurologic injury.

Preexisting conditions unrelated to the surgical pathology often dictate anesthetic techniques and monitors. If indicated, these conditions should be fully evaluated by consulting specialists. Congestive heart failure or recent myocardial infarction requires pulmonary artery pressure monitoring and cardiac output monitoring. The sitting position is inadvisable in patients with significant cardiovascular pathology because of depressed cardiac output. Hypertensive patients must have their blood pressure well controlled prior to surgery and their blood pressure monitored closely during the operation with an intraarterial catheter. Patients with chronic obstructive pulmonary disease should be optimized prior to surgery and their baseline lung function documented with pulmonary function testing and arterial blood gases. Neurologic disorders should be well described and systemically evaluated. Any associated sensorimotor deficits must be clearly delineated and well documented preoperatively.

Physical Examination

Physical examination should include evaluation of the airway and cardiopulmonary system, a brief neurologic examination, and a search for sites for vascular access. The airway can be evaluated using numerous techniques. The Mallampati classification offers an easy method to determine the feasibility of tracheal intubation[28] (see box above). The patient's ability to open his or her mouth and, if possible, the range of motion of the cervical spine should be evaluated as well. Although helpful, these techniques do not ensure an uneventful intubation, and adequate alternatives should always be available.

The vital signs should be taken to assess blood pressure and fluid status. The chest should be auscultated to check for murmurs, added heart sounds, wheezing, or rales. New physical findings should always be fully evaluated prior to any elective procedure. Any neurologic findings should be documented preoperatively. Adequate vascular access, including the need for invasive monitoring, should be evaluated preoperatively and discussed with the patient.

During trauma cases, information may be missing owing to a lack of time. The emergent nature of these cases does not always allow for a thorough examination and work-up. The anesthesiologist must be constantly reevaluating these patients as the cases progress. On the other hand, even when the proper studies have been performed, the anesthesiologist must maintain a high level of suspicion. It is well known that a considerable number of cervical spine fractures are missed on initial evaluation in the emergency department.[40] The incidence of missed fractures ranges from 1% to 33% owing to failure to perform an appropriate study or to misinterpretation. These missed injuries are often unstable. The major factor in development of a secondary neurologic injury is failure to immobilize the neck.[38] Therefore, until the patient is awake and a complete examination can be performed, proper immobilization of the cervical spine is essential.

Laboratory Evaluation

Laboratory evaluation should be tailored to the individual patient. Indiscriminate testing is not an effective screening mechanism,[11,36] and should not be used as a substitute for a thorough history and physical.[9] In the appropriate setting, a complete blood count, including platelet count, coagulation studies, electrolyte values, type, and screen, and testing for human immunodeficiency virus (HIV) may be appropriate. Further evaluation, including electrocardiogram, pulmonary function tests, and chest roentgenogram (CXR) are necessary in older patients or those who are deemed at risk. If the need for more complete or invasive studies is necessary, a specialist should be consulted to assist in ordering and interpreting the appropriate evaluations.

After the history has been reviewed and the physical examination performed, the anesthesiologist and surgeon must consult. Estimates of morbidity and mortality, likelihood of benefit, details of the preoperative evaluation and management, planned patient position and surgical approach, special monitors, anticipated complications, need for blood products, and postoperative disposition are reviewed. The patient is given an overview of the events planned for the day of surgery. The patient's decision to proceed with surgery must be fully informed and documented.

Intraoperative Management

Airway Management

In cervical spine surgery specific problems related to the patient's condition are added to the usual difficulties encountered during intubation. The anesthesiologist responsible for securing the airway in this patient population must have a predetermined algorithm for airway management. Anticipation of these difficulties is the most important aspect of airway management. Difficulty in intubation can occur in any patient undergoing general anesthesia, but a careful history, physical examination, and radiologic examination should allow the anesthesiologist to formulate an appropriate plan of action to allow safe control of the airway.[31]

Anesthesiologists are concerned regarding manipulations of the head and neck that are considered safe in the possibly unstable cervical spine. They also need to know what movement is permitted and what might be done to protect the spine and spinal cord during tracheal intubation. For example, after hyperflexion injuries the cervical spine is more stable in extension. The reverse is true for hyperextension injuries. Thus, communication of plans between anesthesiologist and surgeon is important. Ideally, a technique that will provide rapid control of the airway with minimal alteration in the alignment of a possibly unstable cervical spine is desired. Unfortunately, even when the risks are clear, there are no guidelines as to what techniques may be safest. It is up to the individual anesthesiologist's judgment to decide which of many techniques will be best for the individual patient. A review of several techniques, and their benefits and pitfalls, follows.

Control of the airway may be achieved through the use of a mask to deliver gas flow and inhalation anesthetic agents. With proper technique, this will provide a spontaneously ventilating patient who will be properly anesthetized. However, since the airway often needs to be maintained with techniques such as a chin lift or jaw thrust, the unstable cervical spine may be damaged.[1] Also, the use of a mask would interfere with the surgical field owing to the close proximity of the airway and the operative site. Careful bag and mask ventilation is possible during the procedure if proper care is taken; however, it is not appropriate for long-term control of the airway, and alternative methods should be used to secure the airway.

Anesthesiologists are most adept at securing an airway with the use of a laryngoscope to intubate the trachea under direct vision. The laryngoscope helps to align the oral, the pharyngeal, and the laryngeal axes, thus affording the anesthesiologist, in most patients, a clear view of the vocal cords (Fig. 68-1). This method provides rapid airway control, can be performed with or without pharmaceutical intervention, and does not require surgical intervention. Despite its advantages, direct laryngoscopy may not be warranted in the patient with cervical spine disease.

To be effective, direct laryngoscopy requires manipulation of the cervical spine. If the cervical spine is stable and the disease isolated to the lower portions of the cervical spine, direct laryngoscopy is a safe and efficacious manner to control the airway. Although movement is minimal in the lower portion of the cervical spine, atlantoaxial extension is needed to expose the vocal cords adequately during direct laryngoscopy.[5,19,35] Thus, patients with disease at C1-C2, such as those with Down or Morquio's syndrome, osteogenesis imperfecta, rheumatoid arthritis, or achondroplastic dwarfism may be at risk for further injury if direct laryngoscopy is used.[7,10]

If the cervical spine is unstable, the use of direct laryngoscopy is questionable. Historically, it has been believed that direct laryngoscopy is safe with

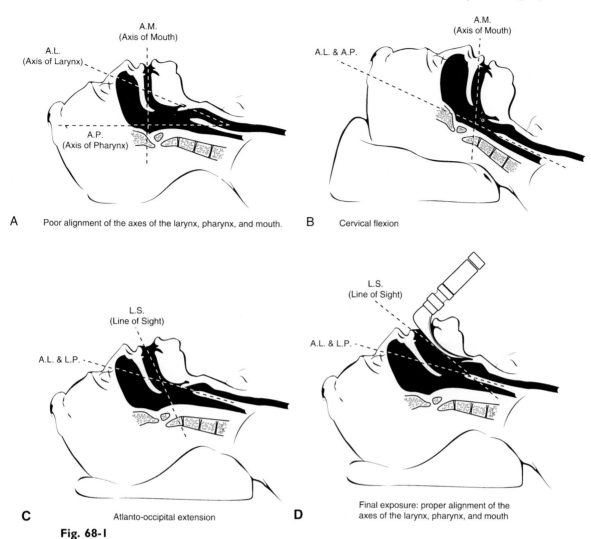

Fig. 68-1

A, Poor alignment of the axes of the larynx, pharynx, and mouth. **B**, Cervical flexion. **C**, Atlantooccipital extension. **D**, Final exposure: proper alignment of the axes of the larynx, pharynx, and mouth. *(Adapted from Finucane BT: Principles of airway management, vol I, Philadelphia, 1988, F.A. Davis, p 127, Figs. 6-3, 6-4, 6-5, 6-6.)*

the use of in-line axial traction during intubation, although no controlled studies have been performed.[3] In both cadaver and human studies, in-line traction has been shown to be less efficacious than previously believed, as neck immobility was not attained.[3,27] There is one case report documenting a sudden worsening of neurologic deficits after traction was applied for spine stabilization.[13] Majernick and associates studied cervical spine involvement during orotracheal intubation with direct visualization in normal controls.[27] Significant movement of the cervical spine was demonstrated and was not reduced with the use of either a soft or hard cervical collar.[29] Axial (longitudinal) traction can be applied manually. A person stands at the head of the patient's bed and places his hands on the patient's mastoid process, applying a traction force of 5 to 10 pounds in the cephalad direction while keeping the mastoid process in line with the axis of the cervical spine. Bivins and colleagues studied the effect of in-line traction during orotracheal intubation in 17 victims of blunt traumatic arrest.[3] In patients with unstable spinal injuries, traction resulted in distraction at the fracture site and up to 4 mm of posterior subluxation. Traction during intubation produced less subluxation than intubation without traction, but the benefit may be negated by the increased distraction at the site of injury. There is no evidence that axial traction increases the severity of injury despite the evidence of distraction at the site of injury.

Any airway maneuver undertaken in a patient with an unstable spinal injury has the potential to do harm. Patients recognized to be at risk and treated with immobilization (tongs, halo, etc.) do not appear to have an increased incidence of neurologic injuries following intubation.

In the patient with an unstable cervical spine when airway control is emergent, after a traumatic injury for example, awake direct laryngoscopy or blind nasotracheal intubation should be performed.[3] Anesthesiologists have long recognized that in a patient with an anticipated difficult intubation, an awake technique, maintaining spontaneous ventilation, is a safe and effective method of securing the airway.[14,15,43] If there is no associated head injury, an awake blind nasal approach has been advocated as a possibly safe technique in patients with cervical spine injury.[8,31] However, this method often requires manipulation of the neck (i.e., flexion and extension), as well as anterior pressure to stabilize the larynx. The failure rate with this technique is 3% to 20%, and the incidence of traumatic intubation is significant.

When the intubation is of an elective nature, fiberoptic intubation should be performed.[37] Fiberoptic intubation is a useful means of intubating the trachea. The technique requires fewer manipulations of the cervical spine to be performed successfully. A fiberoptic instrument, usually a bronchoscope or laryngoscope, can be directed into the trachea via the oral or nasal route without the positional changes in the cervical spine required by direct laryngoscopy.[21] In the elective surgical setting, the patient's airway can be anesthetized topically by any of several methods. Topicalization should not be performed in the patient with a full stomach who is at risk for regurgitation and subsequent aspiration. This technique has been used successfully when extension of the neck is contraindicated or impossible. This technique can be performed on both awake and anesthetized individuals.[32] Proper preparation of the airway, including adequate topicalization and administration of an antisialoagogue, is required for an awake intubation. This technique is difficult to perform in the traumatized airway or in the emergency setting, where topicalization of the larynx is contraindicated and debris and distortion of anatomic landmarks is considerable. Although considerable skill is required to perform fiberoptic intubation, this technique allows intubation to be performed under direct vision and has a success rate close to 100%, and the patient is able to maintain spontaneous ventilation.[37] Rogers and Benumof reviewed the use of fiberoptic bronchoscopy in 25 patients with rheumatoid arthritis, cervical abnormalities, or cervical fusion. All patients were intubated easily in less than 2 minutes with the fiberoptic bronchoscope.[42] Finally, when fiberoptic intubations are performed in the awake patient, neurologic status may be assessed after positioning and prior to induction of anesthesia.

Other methods of airway management include retrograde intubations, transtracheal ventilation, and cricothyroidotomy. Retrograde intubation of the trachea is accomplished by passing a catheter or wire through a needle placed through the cricothyroid membrane.[2,39,41] The catheter is passed cephalad and brought out through the mouth. An endotracheal tube is then placed over the catheter and directed into the trachea using the catheter as a guide. In a recent review, 19 patients with cervical spine injury, maxillofacial trauma, or both were intubated using the retrograde technique. All patients were intubated successfully in less than 5 minutes. Eighty-one percent of these patients had failed intubation using conventional techniques.[41]

Transtracheal ventilation provides oxygenation and ventilation by placing a small (16 gauge) catheter through the cricothyroid membrane and using a jet ventilator to deliver sufficient gas flows. Although effective, it does not protect against aspiration, has a high incidence of barotrauma, and requires specialized equipment.[47] Surgical management of the airway, such as a cricothyroidotomy or tracheostomy, are effective but highly invasive means to control the airway. In an emergency setting with a patient who has an unstable cervical spine, it may be a prudent choice. However, it has a relatively high percentage of complications when performed emergently,[30] and may not always control the airway adequately.[23] In addition, the placement of the cricothyroidotomy and subsequent tracheostomy may interfere with future surgical procedures, particularly anterior approaches to cervical fusion.

Because intraoperative access to the airway is so limited, an endotracheal tube designed to resist obstruction, such as an armored or wire-flexed tube, should be used. Once the endotracheal tube is placed it must be securely fixed in place, as adjustments during the operative procedure are difficult and, oftentimes, dangerous.

Induction and Maintenance of Anesthesia

After reviewing the patient, the appropriate studies, and the proposed operation, the anesthesiologist may select the appropriate induction agents. In elective cases, where no difficulty in intubation is expected, all commonly used induction agents, such as pentathol, etomidate, methohexital, midazolam, or propofol can be used. Propofol may offer some advantages as patients tend to recover from anesthesia faster.[26] If an awake intubation is planned, proper topicalization and sedation with midazolam, narcotics, or propofol should be tailored for the individual patient. In the trauma patient or the patient with hemodynamic instability, ketamine is a useful induction agent.

Succinylcholine is commonly used as a muscle relaxant to facilitate direct laryngoscopy and endotracheal intubation. In patients with neurologic injury, the anesthesiologist should be wary when considering the use of a depolarizing relaxant such as succinylcholine. Perhaps the most important side effect to be aware of with this drug is hyperkalemia.[16] In healthy patients a rise in serum potassium of 0.5 to 1.0 mEq/l does not create a problem. However, in several circumstances, succinylcholine will cause an exaggerated hyperkalemic response and subsequent cardiac arrest. Peak potassium concentrations of 10 to 15 mEq/ml have been reported.[44] There are conditions, then, that are absolute contraindications to succinylcholine. These are listed in the box below. In the acute setting, when fewer then 24 hours have passed since the injury, succinylcholine may be used. However, if more than 24 hours have elapsed, succinylcholine may cause a rapid increase in serum potassium levels and subsequent cardiac arrest. Therefore, succinylcholine should be avoided and such caution should be extended for at least 3 to 6 months after injury to the spinal cord.

Succinylcholine: Contraindications

- Major trauma
- Neurologic disease
- Renal failure
- Severe intraabdominal infection
- Open-eye injury
- Closed-head injury
- Burns
- History of malignant hyperthermia

The intermediate-acting nondepolarizing neuromuscular blocking drugs, atracurium and vecuronium, are alternatively frequently used to facilitate intubation.[34] These agents have minimal side effects, but their onset of action is longer at 90 to 240 seconds and their duration of action is approximately 30 minutes. Therefore, once vecuronium or atracurium is administered it is absolutely necessary to have a foolproof set of plans for maintaining the airway. Also, individual surgeons may prefer that neuromuscular blockade be omitted during surgery, especially when nerve roots are being exposed. The surgeon and anesthesiologist need to communicate prior to surgery to avoid this problem. Finally, longer-acting neuromuscular blockers such as pancuronium, metacurine, pipercuronium, and doxacurium are available, although their prolonged length of action is usually not necessary for these cases.

Maintenance of anesthesia will depend on the condition of the patient and the personal choice of the anesthesiologist. There is not a single "perfect way" to perform an anesthetic for each surgery. Inhalation anesthetics such as halothane, isoflurane, and enflurane provide complete anesthesia and are safe and effective in most patients. Intravenous medications, including propofol, benzodiazepines, and narcotics can deliver complete anesthesia if used appropriately. Alternatively, a balanced technique, using both inhalation and intravenous agents is often useful. In the compromised patient, the anesthetic technique needs to be tailored to the individual. The anesthesiologist must be cognizant of the patient's problems and must attempt to incorporate a technique for each setting.

Emergence from anesthesia should be as smooth as possible, with the patient being free of pain and cognizant enough to perform simple commands (i.e., move his or her legs, etc.). Smooth emergence is best accomplished by titration of anesthetic agents to allow a return to consciousness while maintaining analgesia. Judicious use of narcotics allows a smooth emergence and recovery room phase. Neuromuscular blockade should be reversed and return of normal strength should be documented prior to extubation. After extubation neurologic function should be quickly assessed. If all is in order, the patient can be transferred to the recovery room.

Special Considerations

Spinal Shock

Spinal cord–injured patients may present with neurogenic or spinal shock, hemorrhagic shock, or a combination of both.[33] In either case hypotension and hypothermia are present. The key to the differential diagnosis is the heart rate. In spinal shock the heart rate is usually below 60, slow, and regular, in contrast to the rapid irregular pulse noted in hemorrhagic shock.[12] The bradycardia in spinal shock is secondary to the unopposed parasympathetic effects of the vagus nerve.

In patients with spinal cord injuries above T5 there is a significant risk of marked cardiovascular instability owing to both loss of compensatory vascular reflexes and autonomic dysreflexia.[24] Spinal shock is associated with a decreased peripheral vascular tone and a dilatation of the capacitance vessels secondary to a loss of sympathetic nervous system control. This vasodilatation results in a pooling of blood in the extremities with an inadequate central blood volume. These patients present with a systolic blood pressure of less than 70 mm Hg in addition to a heart rate of less than 60. The use of the Trendelenburg position and/or application of MAST trousers will effectively improve the blood pressure initially. The more specific treatment is cautious volume replacement and the administration of intravenous atropine. Caution must be exercised in the administration of fluid to these patients. They actually may have an adequate blood volume but a problem in the distribution of this volume. That is, they have a relatively low circulating blood volume in relation to their expanded vascular bed. Large increases in volume will result in pulmonary edema. Swan–Ganz catheterization is recommended to assess cardiac function and attain an appropriate volume status.[25] If a blood volume deficit occurs, these patients are unable to maintain cardiac output by sympathetically induced tachycardia or constriction of venous capacitance vessels, nor will blood pressure be maintained by arterial constriction. The heart also will not respond with an increase in contractility. As a result, pulmonary edema is likely to occur with aggressive volume replacement. In the period immediately following the injury, pulmonary edema may occur secondary to lung trauma, volume load, autonomic nervous system imbalance, myocardial contusion, and massive sympathetic stimulation. Loss of compensatory cardiovascular reflexes causes hypotension, especially after rapid position changes. Intermittent positive pressure ventilation will also cause hypotension. Ventilation of the patient should strive to minimize peak and mean airway pressures as much as possible.

Patients with spinal cord injury also will have lost their thermoregulatory ability and will be poikilothermic. They will require passive and active methods of warming (see box following) to avoid significant hypothermia and its complications (see box following). Inability to control the patient's temperature will lead to significant intraoperative problems.

Temperature Maintainence

- Warm room
- Warming lights
- Hyperthermia blanket
- Humidified, warmed (40° C) inspired gases
- Fluid warmers
- Warm peritoneal lavage (43° C)
- Extracorporeal circulation with a heat exchanger

Complications of Hypothermia

- Myocardial depression
- EKG changes
    QT prolongation
    J (Osborn) waves
- Arrhythmias (including ventricular fibrillation)
- Thrombocytopenia
- Decreased calcium mobilization
- Prolonged drug half-lives
- Lactic acidosis

Autonomic Dysreflexia

Autonomic dysreflexia is a sudden, massive sympathetic discharge resulting in severe hypertension with profound bradycardia secondary to intact baroreceptor input.[12] The patient develops abrupt and severe hypertension and bradycardia, pilomotor activity, sweating, dilated pupils, blurred vision, and headache. The blood pressure can rise enough to cause seizures and death. The sympathetic overactivity is initiated by cutaneous or visceral stimuli below the cord lesion. It results from reflex stimulation of the sympathetic neurons in the anterolateral column of the spinal cord below the lesion, which are not under the higher control of the central nervous system. Any lesion at or above T7 may be associated with this condition.

Adequate regional or general anesthesia usually prevents the triggering of this syndrome.[12] Autonomic hyperreflexia can be treated with drugs that block the sympathetic nervous system at either the sympathetic, ganglionic, or peripheral levels. Patients with old spinal cord injuries will often require repeated orthopedic interventions for cervical fusion, osteotomies, debridement of pressure sores, and so on. Although the patient may not require analgesia and anesthesia if the lesion is complete, the patient may still require some form of anesthesia because of the possibility of autonomic dysfunction.

Positioning

Cervical spine surgery can be performed in the supine, prone, lateral, or sitting position with or without the use of Halo traction, tongs, or a Stryker frame. Any of these positions can jeopardize the venous and arterial circulation. Halo traction is often applied to attain reduction and maintain stability of cervical fractures and dislocations. The Halo apparatus is usually applied with local infiltration of lidocaine at each fixation site to all layers of the scalp, including the periosteum. The anterior approach to the cervical spine provides access to the vertebral bodies for spinal fusion, removal of a tumor or disc, and drainage of infection. The posterior approach is used for laminectomy, spinal fusion and decompression. The sitting position is one usually favored by the neurosurgeon.

If the paraplegic patient is to be placed in the prone or sitting position, even greater care than usual must be exercised in making the move. These patients have a decrease in circulating blood volume and absent compensatory mechanisms which, combined with potent anesthetic agents, can result in disastrous falls in blood pressure.

Skin breakdown and subsequent decubiti formation is common in this population. Extreme care must be taken to ensure adequate padding and securing of pressure points, to provide eye protection, and to maintain the patient's head in a fixed position to prevent distortion of the fracture site. Various devices have been designed to support the prone patient and minimize the adverse cardiorespiratory effects of abdominal and consequent inferior vena caval compression. These vary from combinations of pads and pillows to sculptured foam blocks and supporting frames. After each change in position, the position of the endotracheal tube must be rechecked to assure that it has not entered the right mainstem bronchus or been partially withdrawn, especially with flexion and extension of the neck.

The surgical approach to the spine is often through relatively vascular tissues; thus, the blood loss can be large. The anesthesiologist's access to intravenous cannulae is almost as restricted as his or her airway access in these cases. A large bore and securely fastened venous cannula is essential. Short-acting, rapidly metabolized drugs should be used to allow postoperative arousal of the patient for physiologic examination and early extubation. An anesthetic technique allowing rapid but smooth recovery is favorable. At the conclusion of surgery there is often still a relative instability of the cervical spine, and therefore caution must be exercised in handling the patient during extubation. Extreme care must be taken to avoid undue manipulation, coughing, or bucking during extubation. External support can be applied at the conclusion of the procedure to protect the healing vertebrae in the early postoperative period.

Monitoring

The anesthesiologist's responsibilities intraoperatively include providing physiologic homeostasis; providing analgesia, amnesia, and anesthesia; establishing acceptable operating conditions for the surgeon; and protecting the patient from injury. Monitoring devices help us to attain these goals safely. The type of surgery, the positioning of the patient intraoperatively, the patient's underlying medical condition, the surgeon's technique, the anesthesiologist's capabilities, the postoperative facilities available, and the intraoperative monitoring will dictate the type of anesthetic technique.

Cardiorespiratory depression is common in the patient with cervical spine injury and disease. This patient population warrants careful and accurate monitoring. Routinely this would include cardiac and respiratory sounds by esophageal stethoscope, EKG, invasive arterial blood pressure measurement, urine output, temperature, and at times perhaps CVP and/or PAP.

Another useful monitoring modality is somatosensory evoked potentials (SSEPs), particularly in high-risk patients when any clinical examination is severely limited by general anesthesia. Intraoperative monitoring of SSEPs has been used with increasing frequency over the past few years to allow continuous assessment of the functional integrity of the sensory pathways. Somatosensory evoked potentials are noninvasive and have become an important diagnostic method that may also have prognostic value.[18] These evoked potentials are electrical signals of the central nervous system's response to external stimuli. Sensory evoked potentials are recorded by stimulating a peripheral sensory nerve and recording the resultant electric potential at various sites along the sensory pathway to the cerebral cortex. Intraoperative SSEP monitoring has been used during a large number of procedures, including spinal cord decompression and stabilization after acute injury, spinal fusion, resection of spinal cord tumors and cysts, instrumentation correction of scoliosis, correction of cervical spondylosis, and abdominal and thoracic aneurysm repair. Minimal experience has been gained with the use of SSEP monitoring during intraoperative repair of acute spinal cord injury. Most recently, the acute injuries have been less commonly treated by surgical intervention. In addition, complex monitoring is less likely to be available during emergency operations.

Any form of intraoperative monitoring should have clear benefits in comparison with any added risks or costs. Extensive experience with SSEPs has been gained in patients undergoing laminectomy and Harrington Rodding procedures. Of patients undergoing surgical procedures on the spinal cord, 3% to 65% will have intraoperative changes in SSEPs.[17] There is no standard for measuring and evaluating the recorded SSEPs; however, all investigators have described a positive correlation between SSEPs and neurologic findings.[20,46] By convention, a decrease in amplitude of 50% or a 3-msec increase in latency are considered significant changes in waveforms. If these changes reverse spontaneously or are promptly treated by the surgeon or anesthesiologist, the patient will have preserved neurologic function. If these changes in the SSEPs persist intraoperatively, the patient will often have a neurologic deficit postoperatively. However, both false-positive and false-negative results have been reported. In addition, recall that SSEPs to some extent reflect the overall function of the spinal cord but are more accurate at predicting return of dorsal column function than return of motor function.

Many of the drugs used intraoperatively to produce anesthesia, amnesia, and analgesia will influence the intraoperative monitoring of SSEPs. The volatile anesthetics in significant concentrations will cause dose-dependent decreases in amplitude and increases in latency and conduction times. It is possible to use low concentrations of the volatile agents while monitoring SSEPs, avoiding concentrations that obliterate the waveforms. However, since these agents cause significant changes in the waveforms, anesthetic concentrations should not be changed during critical periods of the surgical procedure. Although narcotics also decrease the amplitude of SSEP waveforms, their effects are minimal compared with the volatile anesthetics.[17] Therefore, in my opinion, a narcotic infusion supplemented by a muscle relaxant and a benzodiazepine for amnesia is an ideal anesthetic technique.

Physiologic changes can also result in alterations in the SSEP recordings. Systemic blood pressure, body temperature, and changes in oxygenation will affect the waveforms. Therefore, these parameters should be monitored intraoperatively with interventions available to correct any changes.

Postoperative Considerations

The degree of respiratory compromise depends on the level of the sensory-motor deficit.[12] Patients with injuries at or above C4 suffer respiratory failure because of the lack of diaphragmatic function. Patients with lower lesions may have up to a 70% reduction in forced expiratory volume and in forced vital capacity secondary to the loss of intercostal muscles. The loss of abdominal tone decreases intraabdominal pressure and flattens the hemidiaphragms, reducing the level of maximal tension. Patients with cervical cord injuries are at an increased risk postoperatively for respiratory complications because of their decreased ability to cough and clear secretions, prolonged immobility, and abdominal distension.

Summary

Patients will present to anesthesiologists with potential or actual cervical spine instability for surgery related or unrelated to the cervical spine. The cervical spine abnormality may have resulted from a recent traumatic event or may be chronic, secondary to a congenital abnormality or an acquired disease process. The anesthesiologist should know how to evaluate the cervical spine and estimate the chance of injury. In any patient with a cervical spine abnormality there is a potential for injury during attempts at intubation and while positioning. Very little data are available to guide the anesthesiologist in selecting appropriate airway management techniques. Airway management may need to be directed by the anesthesiologist's skills as well. However, the risks must be identified preoperatively, appropriate assessments must be undertaken, and a plan developed for the safest mode of management intraoperatively and postoperatively.

References

1. Aprahamian C and others: Experimental cervical spine injury model: examination of airway management and splinting techniques, *Ann Emerg Med* 13:584, 1984.
2. Barriot P, Riou B: Retrograde technique for tracheal intubation in trauma patients, *Crit Care Med* 10:712, 1988.

3. Bivins H and others: The effect of axial traction during orotracheal intubation of the trauma victim with an unstable cervical spine, *Ann Emerg Med* 17:25, 1988.

4. Bland JH: *Anatomy and biomechanics. In Disorders of the cervical spine,* Philadelphia, 1987, W.B. Saunders, p 9.

5. Brechner V: Unusual problems in the management of airways. I: Flexion-extension mobility of the cervical vertebrae, *Anesth Analg* 47:362, 1968.

6. Bucholz RW and others: Occult cervical spine injuries in fatal traffic accidents, *J Trauma* 19:768, 1979.

7. Cervical Spine Research Society: *The cervical spine,* Philadelphia, 1983, J.B. Lippincott, p 356.

8. Danzel DF, Thomas DM: Nasotracheal intubations in the emergency department, *Crit Care Med* 8:677, 1980.

9. Delahunt B, Turnbull PRG: How cost effective are routine preoperative investigations?, *N Z Med J* 92:431, 1980.

10. Doolan LA, O'Brien JF: Safe intubation in cervical spine injury, *Anesth Intensive Care* 13:319, 1985.

11. Durbridge TC and others: Evaluation of benefits of screening tests done immediately on admission to hospital, *Clin Chem* 22:968, 1976.

12. Fraser A, Edmonds Seal J: Spinal cord injuries: a review of the problems facing the anesthetist, *Anesthaesia* 37:1084, 1982.

13. Fried L: Cervical spinal cord injury during skeletal traction, *JAMA* 229:181, 1974.

14. Giuffrida JG and others: Prevention of major airway complications during anesthesia by intubation of the concious patient, *Anesth Analg* 39:201, 1960.

15. Gold M, Buechel D: A method of blind nasal intubation for the concious patient, *Anesth Analg* 39:257, 1960.

16. Gronert GA, Theye RA: Pathophysiology of hyperkalemia induced by succinylcholine, *Anesthesiology* 43:89, 1975.

17. Grundy BL: Intraopoerative monitoring of sensory-evoked potentials, *Anesthesiology* 58:72, 1983.

18. Grundy BL, Friedman W: Electrophysiological evaluation of the patient with acute spinal cord injury, *Crit Care Clin* 3:519, 1987.

19. Horton WA, Fahy L, Charters P: Disposition of cervical vertebrae, atlanto-axial joint, hyoid and mandible during x-ray laryngoscopy, *Br J Anaesth* 63:435, 1989.

20. Kaplan BJ and others: Somatosensory evoked potential monitoring of spinal cord ischemia during aortic operations, *Neurosurgery* 19:82, 1986.

21. Keenan MA, Stiles CM, Kaufman RL: Acquired laryngeal deviation associated with cervical spine disease in erosive polyarticular arthritis: use of the fibreoptic bronchoscope in erosive polyarticular arthritis, *Anesthesiology* 58:441, 1983.

22. Komusi T, Munro T, Harth M: Radiologic review: the rheumatoid cervical spine, *Semin Arthritis Rheum* 14:187, 1988.

23. Kress TD, Balasubramanian S: Cricothyroidotomy, *Ann Emerg Med* 11:197, 1982.

24. Lambert DH, Deane RS, Mazuzan JE: Anesthesia and the control of blood pressure in patients with spinal cord injury, *Anesth Analg* 61:344, 1982.

25. Mackenzie CF and others: Assessment of cardiac and respiratory function during surgery on patients with acute quadriplegia, *J Neurosurg* 62:843, 1985.

26. Mackenzie N, Grant IS: Comparison of the new emulsion formulation of propofol with methohexitone and thiopentone for induction of anaesthesia in day cases, *Br J Anaesth* 57:725, 1985.

27. Majernick T and others: Cervical spine movement during orotracheal intubation, *Ann Emerg Med* 15:417, 1986.

28. Mallampati SR and others: A clinical sign to predict difficult tracheal intubation: a prospective study, *Can Anaesth Soc J* 32:429, 1985.

29. McCabe JB, Nolan DJ: Comparison of the effectiveness of different cervical immobilization collars, *Ann Emerg Med* 15:93, 1986.

30. McGill J, Clinton W, Ruiz E: Cricothyroidotomy in the emergency department, *Ann Emerg Med* 11:361, 1982.

31. Meschino A and others: The safety of awake tracheal intubation in cervical spine injury, *Can J Anaesth* 35:S131, 1988.

32. Messeter KH, Pettersson KI: Endotracheal intubation with the fibreoptic bronchoscope, *Anaesthesia* 35:294, 1980.

33. Meyer GA and others: Hemodynamic responses to acute quadriplegia with or without chest trauma, *J Neurosurg* 34:168, 1971.

34. Miller RD and others: Clinical pharmacology of vecuronium and atracurium, *Anesthesiology* 61:444, 1984.

35. Nichol H, Zuck D: Difficult laryngoscopy—the anterior larynx and the atlanto occipital gap, *Br J Anaesth* 55:141, 1983.

36. Olson DM, Kane RL, Proctor PH: A controlled trial of multiphasic screening, *N Engl J Med* 294:925, 1976.

37. Ovassapian A, Dykes M: The role of fibreoptic endoscopy in airway management, *Semin Anesth* 6:93, 1987.

38. Podolsky S and others: Efficacy of cervical spine immobilization methods, *J Trauma* 23:461, 1983.

39. Powell WF, Ozdil T: A translaryngeal guide for tracheal intubation, *Anesth Analg* 46:231, 1967.

40. Reid D and others: Etiology and clinical course of missed spine fractures, *J Trauma* 27:980, 1987.

41. Riou B and others: Retrograde tracheal intubation in trauma patients, *Anesth* 67:A130, 1987.

42. Rogers SN, Benumof JL: New and easy techniques for fibreoptic aided tracheal intubation, *Anesthesiology* 59:569, 1983.

43. Sinclair JR, Mason RA: Ankylosing spondylitis: the case for awake intubation, *Aneasthesia* 39:3, 1984.

44. Tobey RE: Paraplegia, succinylcholine and cardiac arrest, *Anesthesiology* 32:359, 1970.

45. White AA, Southwick WO, Panjabi MM: Clinical instability in the lower cervical spine: a review of past and current concepts, *Spine* 1:15, 1976.

46. York DH and others: Utilization of somatosensory evoked cortical potentials in spinal cord injury: prognostic limitations, *Spine* 8:832, 1983.

47. Zornow M, Thomas T, Scheller M: The efficacy of three different methods of transtracheal ventilation, *Can J Anaesth* 36:624, 1989.

Chapter 69

Positioning the Patient for Lumbar Spine Surgery

W. Bradford DeLong

Charles D. Ray

Access to the Operative Field

Decreased Blood Loss

Anesthesia Access

Radiograph Access

Protection of Peripheral Nerves

Protection of Miscellaneous Pressure Points

Extension Versus Flexion of the Lumbar Spine

Positioning Techniques

    lateral or semilateral

    prone on bolsters

    prone on chest rolls and separate iliac crest supports

    prone on bolsters extending from the chest to the iliac crests

    prone on flat abdominal cradles or frames

    kneeling, "tuck," knee-chest, and prone-sitting positions

    the CeDaR Surgical Platform

    the Andrews frame-platform

Summary

If ideal operative positioning for low-back surgery were available, it would achieve the following benefits:

1. It would provide expandable access to the operative field.

2. It would decrease blood loss.

3. It would provide the anesthesiologist with unrestricted access to the patient's airway and would support the patient's respirations.

4. It would allow unrestricted use of roentgenograms or the C-arm fluoroscope during the operative procedure.

5. It would avoid pressure or traction on peripheral nerves or other susceptible areas, and would avoid rotation of the cervical spine.

6. It would not require expensive paraphernalia.

Access to the Operative Field

The operative position must not restrict the surgeon if he or she decides that the surgical exposure must be developed further as the case proceeds. The incision may have to be extended superiorly or inferiorly, or a unilateral procedure may have to be expanded into a bilateral approach. If an unanticipated spinal fusion becomes necessary, the surgeon will need access to a bone graft donor site.

Some kneeling positions place the surface of the patient's back high off the floor, interfering with the use of the microscope, since some microscope stands will not lift the microscope high enough. Positions that place the patient's back high off the floor may also require the operative team to work standing on a stack of platforms. It is more comfortable for the operating team if the operative position allows them to stand on the floor itself, rather than on platforms.

The ideal operative position would facilitate interlaminal access during the decompressive portion of the procedure by initially placing the curve of the lumbosacral spine in a neutral position, but it would allow the surgeon to restore some degree of lordosis before performing a fusion.

Some operative positions place the lumbosacral spine in a considerable amount of lumbosacral flexion, which can lead to such problems as allowing a periosteal elevator to slip into the spinal canal unexpectedly. This mishap can result in a dural tear at best and neural damage at worst. Excessive flexion can also tighten the paravertebral muscles against the spinous processes, making satisfactory retraction difficult and possibly leading to a postoperative compartment syndrome. If the patient's spine is fused in pelvic flexion, severe lumbosacral biomechanical problems can result postoperatively.

If an orthopedic team is to perform a fusion after a neurosurgical team performs the spinal decompression, it is important for the neurosurgeons to anticipate the needs of the orthopedists. If a bilateral posterolateral fusion is planned, for example, then the initial operative positioning should allow for the wide exposure that will be required later for the fusion. The position chosen should also allow the orthopedists to fuse the spine in an anatomic degree of lumbosacral lordosis.

Decreased Blood Loss

If a patient requires a blood transfusion because of surgical blood loss, he or she is exposed to the risks of transfusion reaction, coagulation problems, hepatitis, or acquired immune deficiency syndrome (AIDS). The use of autologous blood or blood from designated donors can lessen these risks, but it is safest and easiest to use optimal operative positioning to minimize blood loss in the first place.

The key to minimizing intraoperative blood loss is abdominal decompression.* If the patient's position puts pressure on the abdomen, the vena cava will be compressed. This, in turn, will increase the pressure in the spinal venous complex, particularly the epidural veins, making intraspinal operative exposure difficult and bloody. If the patient's abdomen is hanging freely, then the epidural veins will contain blood under relatively low pressure.

In fact, the blood loss difference may be as much as 300% to 400% between the flat abdomen and the free-hanging one. When the abdomen hangs free, hemostasis is rarely a problem. Any bleeding that occurs usually stops promptly with the temporary application of Gelfoam soaked in thrombin. Bipolar coagulation is only occasionally required.

Abdominal compression can lead to problems other than increased intraoperative blood loss. If the vena cava is compressed, cardiac return can be severely compromised and hypotension can occur. This situation can lead the anesthesiologist to think that blood loss has been greater than it actually has been. The patient might then be overtransfused in a futile attempt to correct the hypotension.

A theoretic advantage of optimal abdominal decompression is the lessening of the risk of an intraabdominal vascular catastrophe. It is well known that if an instrument accidentally penetrates the anterior boundary of the disc space, then the aorta, vena cava, or iliac vessels can be lacerated, resulting in an extreme emergency. If the abdomen is well de-

*References 2, 3, 6, 14, and 15.

compressed, the vena cava and iliac veins will be relatively flaccid and the aorta and iliac arteries will not be pushed back against the spinal column. Under these conditions, the vessels stand a better chance of remaining unscathed should they be approached by a disc rongeur, curette, or some other instrument.

An important, unexpected effect of the use of prone-sitting frames is the reduction in arterial pressure. When using a modified Tarlov frame, it was usually important to perform fusions under hypotensive anesthesia; for this procedure an arterial catheter was routinely placed. With the use of the new prone-sitting frames, on the other hand, arterial pressure remains slightly low; thus, hypotensive agents are seldom required. Nonetheless, true hypotension as a surgical complication is not seen. Some patients, on the other hand, have significant fluid loading during the surgery, perhaps related to the dependency of the abdomen and legs. They require subsequent diuresis.

Anesthesia Access

The operative position should support respiration by allowing free excursion of the patient's chest and by permitting free diaphragmatic excursion through satisfactory abdominal decompression. The anesthesiologist must have unrestricted access to the patient's head to deal with any problems that arise from the endotracheal tube and to protect the patient's eyes from pressure.

The anesthesiologist must also have access to intravenous and intraarterial lines. This can be accomplished by abducting the patient's upper extremities on arm boards, allowing the hands to rest beside the head. If a Foley catheter is used, the operative position must allow the nursing staff access to the catheter if any drainage problems arise.

The patient's lower extremities should be gently compressed by elastic stockings, wraps, or compression boots to encourage efficient venous return.

Radiograph Access

Roentgenograms are often needed during spinal surgery. This need cannot always be anticipated, and it is important that the operative position not restrict the placement of the x-ray film cassette or the alignment of the x-ray beam itself.

If lateral x-ray studies are required, a cassette holder can usually be positioned with relative ease. However, various pieces of the frame or holding device can obstruct the x-ray beam if the possible need

for x-ray studies is not kept in mind during positioning of the patient.

Posteroanterior x-ray films can be difficult or impossible to obtain if the patient is positioned in one of the various frames available, because the acute angle of the patient's hips causes the thighs to block placement of the film cassette.

Satisfactory use of C-arm biplane fluoroscopy usually requires the use of a "diving board" extension on the operating table, although some of the frames allow placement of the C-arm tube beneath the prone or kneeling patient for anteroposterior views.

Protection of Peripheral Nerves

The brachial plexus must be protected from traction injuries by avoiding excessive anterior sagging of the shoulders and upper extremities. Similarly, the shoulders should not be forced posteriorly during the procedure. Pads should not press against the axilla during the procedure.

Postoperative ulnar neuropathy can be avoided by paying attention to two points. First, the ulnar nerve should be protected against direct pressure in the ulnar groove at the elbow. This can be done by proper padding and positioning. Second, the ulnar nerve should be protected against a traction injury by avoiding acute flexion of the elbow during surgery.[13] Ulnar neuropathy arising from elbow flexion is less well recognized than neuropathy arising from direct pressure, but both etiologies are important and care should be taken to avoid them.

The common peroneal nerve at the fibular head must be protected from direct pressure, which can occur if the patient's knee migrates laterally against the frame after the operation is underway.

The sciatic nerve must be protected from pressure at the gluteal fold. Such pressure can occur if the patient is sitting back against a frame that allows the lower edge of the gluteal support to press in at the gluteal fold.

The lateral femoral cutaneous nerve can sustain a pressure injury if a pad, sandbag, or frame presses against it during the procedure. This obviously should be avoided, since it can lead to prolonged or permanent dysesthesia of the lateral thigh.

Protection of Miscellaneous Pressure Points

The patient's head must be well supported to avoid accidental pressure over the eyes. Even a few minutes of direct pressure over an eye can cause permanent loss of vision.

If the patient is in a lateral or semiprone position, the neurovascular structures of the axilla must be protected by a roll supporting the upper chest.

If the patient is in a kneeling position, extreme flexion of the hip should be avoided to maintain femoral arterial and venous circulation. A considerable amount of lumbar spine, hip, and knee flexion is obtained in the extreme "tuck" position, for example, and it has been shown that this may produce vascular and nerve compression, particularly in the posterior compartment of the knees. In addition, with prolonged spinal surgical procedures this position has been found to produce permanent changes, albeit rarely, in some of the nerves; for example, the sciatic and peroneal. There may also occur a subsequent massive release of myoglobin (from hypoxic, ischemic damage to the muscles of the lower leg) resulting in acute renal failure.[5] This extreme flexed position may so tighten the posterior paraspinal erector muscles that lateral retraction may be quite difficult.[7,8-10] Additionally, extreme flexion is not tolerable to patients with hip or knee joint disorders, joint destruction, or prosthetic replacements.

Pressure over the anterior superior iliac spines, the knees, the ankles, and the toes should be avoided. If the patient is kneeling, the knees must rest on padding. In general, there should be a distribution of the pressure so that at no place on the skin does the pressure exceed the capillary perfusion pressure; otherwise, burns or necrosis of the skin may occur. Occasional patients will have a short-lived numbness of the forehead, the chin, or at scattered areas around the chest or arms or legs.

There is considerable misunderstanding about the simple physics of cushions and padding. One must remember that the patient's weight applied against the supporting surface (e.g., the operating table, platform, and frame) resulting from gravity remains the same with or without cushions or foam rubber padding. These latter aids simply help to distribute the pressure more evenly around the dependent tissues, and in doing so they prevent pressure points, especially over bony prominences or susceptible structures.

If the patient is extremely obese, or if the procedure will require many hours on the operating table, then the patient should be warned in advance that problems with pressure points, skin "burns," or stiffness of joints may be noticed in the postoperative period.

When the patient is turned supine to prone and back again, the downward upper extremity should be placed along the patient's side to avoid levering the shoulder into a sprain or even a dislocation.

No matter what operative position is used, it is important to minimize the risk of burns associated with the use of electrocoagulation. Burns can occur if the patient's skin comes into contact with metallic parts of the operating table or frame. The patient's skin must be carefully insulated from such contact.

Extension Versus Flexion of the Lumbar Spine

There are reasonable arguments in favor of operative positions that promote increased extension and in favor of those that result in increased flexion. Hyperextension or hyperlordosis (downward swaying of the low back and a free abdomen) may be preferred when the posterior musculature must be relaxed, as in cases when a posterolateral fusion is being performed.

On the other hand, proponents of the hyperflexed position argue that flexion increases the opening of the posterior bony structures to facilitate surgical exposure and decompression. In the case of an ordinary discectomy or decompression of stenosis, hyperextension may force together the posterior structures so closely that posterior interlaminar access can be considerably more difficult.

On balance, however, the relaxation of musculature provided by extension of the lower back is probably more important than achieving moderate additional opening of the posterior interspaces through hyperflexed positions. A well-placed lamina spreader can provide excellent, localized posterior distraction, effectively producing flexion of a specific segment. The rest of the lumbar spine can then remain in its normally lordotic habitus, providing satisfactory muscle relaxation for the exposure.

As noted above, extreme flexion of the lumbar spine leads to tight posterior muscles. Prolonged forceful retraction of the paraspinal muscles can lead to significant muscle atrophy and may lead to a postoperative compartment syndrome. This painful complication occurs with a frequency considerably greater than usually recognized.

Positioning Techniques

The operative position should be safely attainable, requiring a minimum number of operating-room personnel for turning and positioning. The necessary positioning equipment should be readily available at reasonable cost.

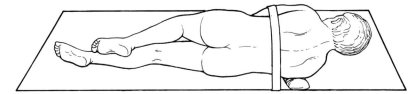

Fig. 69-1

Semilateral position. Abdominal decompression is satisfactory, but the assistant has poor access to the operative site, and it is difficult to perform bilateral procedures in this position. It is important to place an axillary roll under the patient to protect the neurovascular structures.

A number of positioning techniques are available. Many attain the ideal in some respects, but fall short in others.

Lateral or Semilateral

This positioning technique places the patient either on the side in a full lateral position or on the side rolled toward a prone position, in which case the position is called "semilateral" or "semiprone."[1]

The use of either variation—full lateral or semilateral—is generally limited to unilateral discectomy. The pathologic side is placed uppermost. The axillary structures are protected with a roll supporting the chest, and a pillow is placed between the knees. If the patient is in a semilateral position, the uppermost hip and knee are flexed and the uppermost knee brought anterior to the lower knee, providing stability. A wide strap or strip of tape can be placed across the chest to provide further stability, although it should not be severely tightened or respiration will be restricted (Fig. 69-1).

A suction-activated "bean bag" can be used to help stabilize the patient, although x-ray films will be degraded somewhat if the x-ray beam passes through this device.

Advantages of this position include ease of positioning, excellent access to the airway and IV lines, and good support of respiration by providing free excursion of the chest and abdomen. Excellent abdominal decompression is provided, minimizing blood loss. In addition, it is relatively easy to use the operating microscope in this position.

Disadvantages of this position include the lack of flexibility of the surgical exposure. If the exposure must be extended to the opposite side, it is difficult to visualize the downward side of the operative field. Other problems include difficulties in surgical orientation, especially in the semilateral variation. Since the patient is neither fully prone nor fully lateral, he or she is not "square" to the floor of the operating room, and the surgeon can become disoriented in

regard to the location of the lateral and/or anterior aspect of the vertebral body.

Another disadvantage is the restriction of the assistant's ability to see and help with the procedure. The lateral position does not lend itself to use of the assistant's stereoscopic station available on the newer microscopes, because this station is opposite to the surgeon's.

It is also difficult to obtain truly lateral or posteroanterior x-ray films if the patient is not truly lateral or prone.

Prone on Bolsters

If the patient is placed prone, he or she must be supported on bolsters of some sort. Chest rolls are important to maintain adequate chest excursion, but it is unwise to use chest bolsters alone. The abdomen must also be decompressed for the reasons mentioned previously.

Prone on Chest Rolls and Separate Iliac Crest Supports

The patient is placed prone with short chest rolls supporting the chest. The anterior iliac crests are supported separately by padded sandbags or some other firm support. The abdomen is left free between the chest rolls and the iliac crest supports. The operating table can be "broken" (flexed) to bring the lumbosacral spine to a more nearly neutral position. The patient is stabilized by a wide strap secured around the thighs. A footboard can also be used for additional stabilization.

Advantages of this position include some measure of abdominal decompression, which enhances respiratory support. Satisfactory lateral x-ray films can be obtained easily.

Disadvantages include less-than-optimal abdominal decompression, which contributes in some instances to greater blood loss than necessary. Satisfactory posteroanterior x-ray films are difficult to ob-

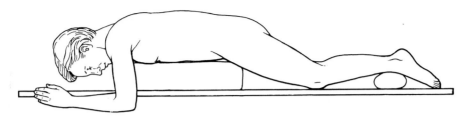

Fig. 69-2

Prone on bolsters. The abdomen cannot be well decompressed in this position, even if separate bolsters are used for the chest and iliac crests.

tain if the operating table is flexed, since the film cassette cannot be positioned for optimal visualization of the entire lumbosacral spine. In this position the lumbosacral lordosis is not neutralized, which may inhibit access to the spinal canal.

Prone on Bolsters Extending from the Chest to the Iliac Crests

This is a variation of the immediately previous technique. Long bolsters are used to support the chest, which are then brought around the lateral aspect of the abdomen and curved back in to support the iliac crests (Fig. 69-2).

The single advantage of this technique over the previous technique is the somewhat increased ease of positioning the patient.

Disadvantages are the same as those of the previous technique, with the added problem of poorer abdominal decompression. It is difficult to position the middle of the long bolsters far enough laterally to avoid abdominal compression.

Prone on Flat Abdominal Cradles or Frames

Several frames place the patient in a prone position by supporting the chest and the anterior iliac crests on pads. These include the Hall, Relton, Basildon (Gardner), Norfolk, Wilson, Kambin, and Cloward frames.

The Hall spinal frame has supporting pads that are adjustable for width but not for height. The pads of the Relton frame adjust for height as well as width. The Basildon (Gardner) frame is similar to the Hall frame, but it provides a horseshoe headrest as part of the device. The Norfolk frame is similar to a Relton frame with a horseshoe headrest.

The Wilson frame consists of a pair of axially parallel, semirigid, upwardly arching cushions that are positioned apart by a crank system. The patient's torso lies cradled in the gap between the cushions in a gentle forward-flexed position. Abdominal pressure is moderately reduced but certainly much less than with the fully pendulous abdominal systems. The gap must be set properly for body width or the patient may sink too deeply between the cushions, or rise too high out of them. The gap is narrowed for smaller patients and widened for larger patients. This frame is lightweight, easily placed, and relatively inexpensive. The Kambin frame is essentially the same as the Wilson frame, but is entirely radiolucent.

The Cloward frame is similar to the Wilson frame in its chest and abdomen section, but has cushion extensions that pass laterally downward and upward so as to cradle nearly the entire body. It includes an attached kneeling cushion. The unit is in two pieces and is applied with the main section and its upper leg component in the form of a stretched Z. The patient lies prone with gentle forward angles at the lumbar area, hips, and thighs. The lower-leg portion attaches at 90° to the main section, on which the flexed knees kneel. This frame, with its distributed cushioning, is particularly applicable to very large patients or those in whom the surgeon feels that widely distributed cushioning is important for intraoperative comfort. The frame comes in three sizes to accommodate most body types.

These frames provide the abdominal decompression necessary to support respiration and minimize blood loss. X-ray access is satisfactory.

Disadvantages include the pressure placed on the anterior iliac crests by the pads in some of the frames, which can lead to skin problems and/or compromise of the lateral femoral cutaneous nerves. This position does not neutralize lumbosacral lordosis, and access to the spinal canal can be less than satisfactory, although the maintenance of lordosis is desirable if a fusion is being performed.

The Hall, Relton, Basildon, and Norfolk frames provide a convenient method of positioning children or small adults and are especially suited for the surgery of scoliosis, where extensive access to the lumbosacral spinal canal is not necessary.

Kneeling, "Tuck," Knee-Chest, and Prone-Sitting Positions

Kneeling, "tuck," knee-chest, or prone-sitting positions have been preferred by many spine surgeons for some years.[3,6,7,11] There are advantages and disadvantages to each position and its associated positioning devices.

Knee-Chest Position Without a Frame

This technique places the patient in a kneeling position on the surface of the operating table. The patient is secured with wide tape or straps. The position provides good abdominal decompression.

However, serious disadvantages exist. The position is difficult to achieve and maintain. Considerable flexion of the hips and knees is necessary to provide stability, and this degree of flexion can lead to compromise of the femoral arterial and/or venous circulation. This degree of flexion can also widen the interlaminar space to a surprising extent, a situation that can lead to accidental interlaminal penetration by a periosteal elevator. This position also tenses the paravertebral muscles against the spinous processes, making retraction of the muscles difficult at times. One should be careful that prolonged forceful retraction of tight paraspinal muscles does not result in a postoperative compartment syndrome, as noted above.

In addition to these disadvantages, posteroanterior x-ray films cannot be obtained because there is no room to position the film cassette anterior to the patient's abdomen. The patient's back is high, and use of the operating microscope is difficult.

Kneeling on the Operating Table, Supported by a Frame

Several frames are available that support the patient in a kneeling position on the surface of the operating table. These include the Hastings frame, the Hicks frame, and the Tarlov seat. The use of these frames has a clear advantage over the simple knee–chest position without a frame. A frame can support the patient in a less extreme kneeling position, protecting circulation to the lower extremities.

Advantages include excellent abdominal decompression, which enhances respiration and minimizes blood loss. The lumbosacral lordotic curve can be neutralized, providing better access to the spinal canal. Frames of this type are fairly simple in design and can be purchased or constructed relatively inexpensively.

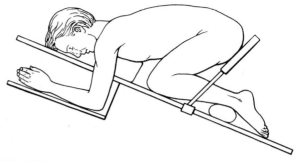

Fig. 69-3

Kneeling on the operating table, supported by a frame. It is difficult to avoid acute flexion of the hips and knees. Flexion of the lumbar region can tighten the paravertebral muscles and make spinal access difficult. It is difficult to place obese or tall patients in this position.

Disadvantages include the difficulty of obtaining satisfactory posteroanterior x-ray films and the difficulty of using the operating microscope when the patient's back is high above the surface of the operating table. If care is not taken, the patient can be positioned in the frame in rather extreme flexion of the hips and knees, leading to circulatory problems in the lower extremities and to the potential for accidental interlaminar penetration when the paravertebral muscles are being stripped from the spinous processes and laminae (Fig. 69-3).

It may be difficult to position and stabilize a particularly tall or obese patient in any of these frames.

Prone-Sitting Attachment Platforms

Frames or platforms are available that attach to the operating table and place the patient in a kneeling or semiseated position. They distribute the patient's weight well between the upper chest and knees, and maintain abdominal decompression. All dependent abdomen frames share the disadvantage of creating lumbar lordosis. Some of the frame designers have attempted to decrease the lordosis by elevating the anterior superior iliac spines with lateral padding, but this does not work very well. The excellent intraspinal venous decompression these frames provide is probably well worth the trade-off of accepting some degree of lumbar lordosis.

The CeDaR Surgical Platform*

The CeDaR Surgical Platform attaches to the operating table and places the patient in a kneeling/sit-

*The platform, cushions, and face-rest units are manufactured by CeDaR Surgical, Inc., 15265 Minnetonka Boulevard, Minnetonka, MN 55345. CeDaR Surgical equipment is available under the brand name, "Raylor™" from Surgical Dynamics, Inc., 2575 Stanwell Drive, Concord California 94520.

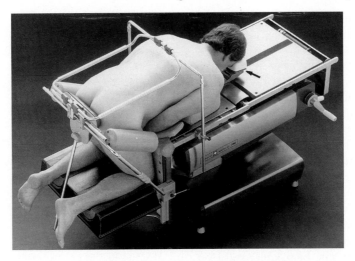

Fig. 69-4

CeDaR kneeling (or prone-sitting) frame. The frame is attached to the footpiece of the operating table.
A posterior yoke holds the seat cushion, to which is attached a removable square-oval retractor ring yoke.
The cephalad end of the ring is attached to a cross yoke, but a chest-rest piece may be used instead, to
support the cephalad end of the ring against the draped chest. An arrow identifies the rocker-shaped face
rest and cushion. Lateral thigh cushions are shown. The kneeling platform locks (handles shown) against
the side rails. Also note the trough-shaped lower leg cushions, the gap at the unsupported patellas, and
a portion of the undermounted elevating stabilizer rod (chromed) beneath the platform. (©C.D. Ray, M.D.)

ting position. Accessory pads and cushions distribute the patient's weight and protect the face (Fig. 69-4).

Chest cushions distribute the weight principally along the upper clavicular and manubrial areas; there is little pressure against the breasts and virtually no pressure on the superior axillary (or lateral subclavicular) areas, which might promote compression of the brachial circulation or nerve plexus.

If the patient's arms are brought overhead or laterally, one must be careful to avoid brachial plexus stretch or compression and shoulder capsule stretch. Alternatively, the arms and hands may be brought downward to pass beneath and anterior to the abdomen. If needed, an additional cushion may be placed on top of the chest cushion to raise the chest farther above the level of the operating table surface, increasing the chest-to-table distance and increasing the angle to which the head and neck will fall forward. Alternatively, the arms may be wrapped in a 1.5-cm foam cushion and placed beneath the pendulous abdomen.

The new knee cushions and lower leg cushions are shaped with a rounded cavity configuration, like troughs, made into the platform of the frame to distribute more evenly the weight applied to the upper tibias, as shown in Fig. 69-4. In addition, there is a gap between the upper portion of these rounded cushions and the operating table; the patellas lie in this gap so that they bear no weight directly. The majority of the weight is therefore distributed along the two tibial plateaus. Further, the lower leg cushion is shaped so that the ankle portion is elevated relative to the knee, as in the normal kneeling position.

The optimal flexion of the hips and knees for patients in this operating table–attached frame is about 60° each. In this way the hip joints and knees are stable; further, sciatic nerve stretch is reduced.

Additional cushions are positioned along the break in the operating table where there is normally a rather prominent edge. Cushions for the buttocks and detachable ones for the thighs are mounted on a large yoke. The yoke is attached to hinges that in turn attach to the platform base; these frame base portions attach to the foot rails of the operating table. The entire unit weighs about 10 kg. Relatively little pressure is applied to the buttocks; this has helped eliminate postoperative sciatic complaints that occur with some of the hyperflexion frames, which may apply significant pressure against the sciatic notches. Incidentally, leaning against one of the lateral thigh cushions is comfortable as a support for the surgeon while operating. The cushioning was therefore developed to optimally accommodate the patient, anesthesia team, and surgeon, an unusual assignment.[11]

Attaching and Adjusting the Platform and Cushions

The foot portion of the standard operating table is placed in the horizontal position and the kneeling platform is slid into place over the side rails and locked at the anticipated correct height, determined by tibial length. The foot portion is then cranked down, perpendicular to the floor. The chest cushion is laid on the table and the surfaces of the platform and chest cushion are covered with a smoothly applied cotton sheet. The retractor ring assembly (shown dorsal to the patient's back in Fig. 69-4) is not yet attached. The anesthetized, intubated, or awake (locally anesthetized) patient is placed on the kneeling platform by a simple bent-knee, roll-over transfer maneuver from the litter. The attached yoke and buttocks cushion are positioned and locked. The lateral thigh cushions are quickly attached and adjusted to accommodate the pelvic width of the patient, and are held in place by a Velcro strap. This entire turning of the patient and positioning generally requires less than 45 seconds, an important element in patient security during this potentially hazardous maneuver.

For some patients it may be necessary to raise or lower the position of the buttocks relative to the chest, thus bringing the dorsal surface of the lumbar spine parallel to the floor. This change may be accomplished in either of two ways. In the first method, the table is pumped up with its hydraulic piston; the stabilizer rod hinge—mounted underneath under the platform—is lowered against the floor. With the side rail locks then loosened, the vertical position of the kneeling platform may be raised or lowered along the side rails of the operating table by pumping the operating table up or down using its hydraulic piston. Alternatively, two persons may hold the yoke base, unlock the foot rail clamps, and manually raise or lower the platform, locking the rail clamps once again into position on the rails. Moving the platform correspondingly changes the buttock elevation relative to the chest (which does not change its height above the operating table surface).

The height of the entire table and patient may then be altered to suit the surgeon's own height. Safety pawls prevent the platform from slipping off the side rails, should the side locks be forgotten.

To prevent any drift of the patient upward on the operating table, when using the CeDaR frame, the hips and knees are bent about 60 degrees (shown in Fig. 69-4). This minor flexion of these joints has nei-

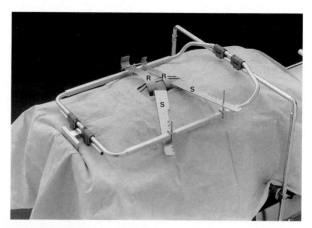

Fig. 69-5

The retractor ring attached at the seat cushion by the steel tongue, locked together with the drapery by a pinch-lock that nondestructively "bites" both drapery and tongue. (R) Raylor malleable retractors and rigid Hibbs-like, notched (S) Sawbill retractors are shown positioned in the wound, being firmly held by ring-attachment devices, mounted to the ring halves. A freely movable mount (not shown) may be attached to the cephalad end of the ring assembly to lie against the draped chest, thus not requiring the cross-thorax yoke (shown). Siderail locks hold the thoracic yoke ends onto the operating table. (©C.D. Ray, M.D.)

ther compromised popliteal venous blood flow nor increased the incidence of deep venous thrombosis. Lateral thigh cushions are then attached and adjusted.

Cushioning the Face

Many patients who have disorders of their lumbar spine also have cervical spine problems. When using an ordinary laminectomy frame in the prone position, the head and neck are usually rather sharply rotated to one side or the other. For the intubated patient, such rotation may present undue lateral pressure against the vocal cords and glottis, as well as an undesirable posture of the neck. If simple forehead cushioning is used, the neck may be hyperextended, as well as rotated. It is not uncommon for some patients to complain of neck or throat difficulties for days or even weeks after such prolonged facial and neck positioning, if their operative procedures have been performed on a standard laminectomy frame (such as the Wilson, Kambin, Cloward, Tarlov, Pronease, CHOP, or others). The cushioned face rest described here[7-11] (indicated by the arrow in Fig. 69-4), used with the prone-sitting frame, obviates abnormal positioning of the head and neck so long as the position of the neck and chest remain in anatomic neutrality.[7] Regular inspection and gentle

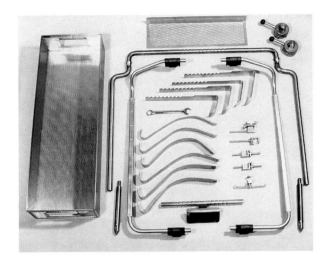

Fig. 69-6

Various mounting, retracting, and positioning devices used with the retractor ring system. A stereotactic unit for laparoscopic use, mounting on the ring side, is not shown. All elements are quickly mounted, demounted, or adjusted by the surgical team. (©C.D. Ray, M.D.)

massage of the face is recommended during lengthy spinal operative procedures to prevent contact "blisters" over bony prominences. Conformal sponge cushions may stretch the skin taught, as the skin is pulled apart by the head weight sinking into the sponge and may thus lead to vascular insufficiency of the tightened skin. Indeed, all cushioning is to be inspected by the surgeon and anesthesiologist just before the operation begins and must be under regular surveillance as the case progresses.

After the patient is brought into the operating room on the stretcher, endotracheal intubation is performed and the face rest is positioned over the patient's face and adjusted for optimal forehead to chin distance. The patient is then turned onto the operating table and positioned on the prone-sitting frame; the face rest is adjusted for elevation of the chin to neutralize almost any curvature of the neck. If the neck is hyperextended, the chest cushion must be raised with additional padding. If not, excessive facial pressure will result. If the neck is hyperflexed, the face rest should be raised by additional padding beneath the unit. The face rest cushions are carefully checked so that supraorbital ridges, eyes, and the lower lip are free from contact or pressure points. Sterile preparation and draping are performed.

Preferably, major components of platform and cushion supports are either x-ray transparent or translucent, permitting intraoperative films to be made or a C-arm to be used. These goals have been variously achieved by the different systems. The orthopedic four-poster CHOP cushion unit provides for film cassettes to be placed beneath the patient, for taking anteroposterior x-ray exposures; intraoperative films or fluoroscopy can be important adjuncts to certain procedures.

Ancillary Attachments that May Be Used with Kneeling Platforms

Following routine preparation and draping of the patient, when using the CeDaR kneeling unit, a steel tongue for attaching a retractor ring unit is pressed deeply into the covering linen into a flat socket, made in the seat (buttocks) cushion casting; a cam lock bites the linen tightly, firmly attaching the tongue to the seat casting and then to the seat-supporting yoke and thus to the operating table.[7] The caudal portion of a squared-oval retractor ring assembly is attached to the stabilized tongue (Fig. 69-4, above the patient, and Fig. 69-5). The upper, cephalad part of the ring attaches to a circular-grooved rod mounted on a plate that simply lies against the sterile drape placed on the patient's upper back. The ring is lightweight and causes no change in respiratory inflation pressure. The retractor "ring" is made in two halves, each of which may be removed separately (if one-sided retraction is needed). The ring will hold a variety of quickly attached retraction blades, rakes, suction, or illumination devices (Fig. 69-6). Using an additional yoke, the system may be applied with any of the currently available patient frame or positioning units, with patients prone or supine.

One of the authors (CDR) has performed decompressions and fusion procedures without surgical assistance using this versatile ring-retractor system. Hibbs-like (Fig. 69-5, "S" for Sawbill), rake, Raylor-like (Fig. 69-5, "R" for Raylor), and special retractors for skin, muscle and even dura may be easily utilized singly or in numbers, as needed (Fig. 69-6). This system, as with all positioning and retracting systems, in addition to its meaningful assistance, provides the requisite safety, effectiveness, and speed for

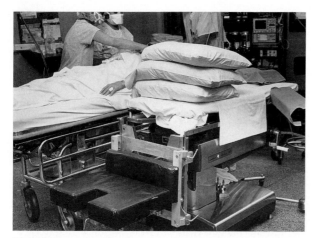

Fig. 69-7

Andrews frame assembly, ready for patient positioning.

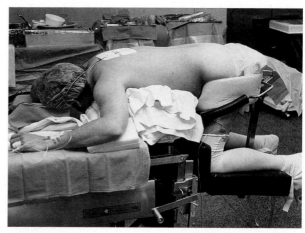

Fig. 69-8

Patient positioned on the Andrews frame. Feet are secured with padded boots that attach to buckles on the undersurface of the horizontal plate. Gluteal plate is adjusted so that the patient sits back slightly against the plate, placing lumbosacral curve in a neutral position. Upper thighs are stabilized by lateral thigh supports and/or wide strap. Three or four pillows support the chest. Elbows are not flexed past 90 degrees, and ulnar grooves are protected from pressure.

the surgical procedure. Retractors are easily released, taken out, or readjusted. This ability to be changed easily prevents the otherwise unending, invariate retraction (especially during long procedures) that may produce excessive muscle injury. In a small, random prospective, unpublished study, one of the authors found that the muscle-injury enzymes (SGOT) in six cases were severalfold elevated and patients had more postoperative deep back pain with the use of a large, crank-type dual bladed, deep retractor (Macelroy), as opposed to an equal number of cases where quickly removable bladed or unilateral pull retractors were used with the present ring system.

The Andrews Frame-Platform*

The Andrews frame uses an assembly that bolts onto the foot section of the operating table. When the foot section is cranked down to a vertical position, the assembly supports a horizontal padded plate on which the patient kneels (Fig. 69-7). The patient's feet are fastened to the horizontal plate by straps attached to padded boots.

The patient's chest rests on pillows or pads placed on the surface of the operating table, and his or her hips are supported by a gluteal plate. Stabilization is completed by using lateral thigh supports and/or a strap around the thighs (Fig. 69-8).

The operative position achieved by the Andrews frame is similar to the Troncelliti position used at Pennsylvania Hospital in Philadelphia by Doctors Richard H. Rothman and Frederick A. Simeone.[4,12]

*The Andrews frame is manufactured and distributed by Orthopedic Systems, Inc., 1897 National Avenue, Hayward, CA 94545.

Advantages of the Andrews frame include the ease of positioning the patient, even one who is obese or tall. Excellent abdominal decompression is achieved, which enhances respiration and minimizes intraoperative blood loss. It is easy to protect pressure points. The lumbosacral lordotic curve can be partially neutralized by allowing the patient to sit back against the gluteal support with the hips and knees in mild flexion, but lordosis can be restored if a lumbosacral fusion is to be done. The patient's back is at a normal level, enhancing use of the operating microscope.

Disadvantages include the difficulty of obtaining posteroanterior x-ray films, because the flexion of the thighs blocks optimal positioning of the film cassette. The frame is more complex than some of the other frames available and is therefore more expensive.

Technique of Positioning in the Andrews Frame-Platform

The use of any specific positioning technique becomes easier as an operating team gains experience with the technique. The following are details of one method of positioning a patient in the Andrews frame.

1. The kneeling plate is attached to the Andrews frame assembly, and the foot of the operating table is cranked down to a 90-degree vertical position, so that the kneeling plate is horizontal.

2. Three or four pillows are placed on the operating table to support the patient's chest.

3. The patient is placed under anesthesia. Intubation is performed while the patient is supine on the gurney.

4. The patient's legs are wrapped. The foot boots are placed on the patient before turning.

5. The gurney is moved down so that the lower margin of the patient's rib cage is adjacent to the vertical foot section of the operating table. This step requires moving the gurney considerably more than the anesthesiologist would generally anticipate, and care must be taken that the breathing circuit tubing has sufficient slack to allow movement of the gurney to this extent.

6. The patient's hips and knees are flexed to 90 degrees before turning.

7. At least four people turn the patient. If the patient is exceptionally tall or obese, more than four people should be used. One person (usually the anesthesiologist) supports the patient's head; one person turns the patient's torso; another person catches the torso; and the fourth person turns the pelvis and flexed lower extremities, easing the knees down onto the horizontal kneeling plate. The foot boots are strapped into the buckles on the kneeling plate.

8. The kneeling plate then is elevated to adjust the height of the patient's pelvis. The gluteal support is put into place, and the patient is moved toward the foot of the operating table so that his or her hips and knees are flexed slightly past 90 degrees. The head of the operating table is elevated slightly so that the patient is sitting back against the gluteal support. The lower edge of the gluteal support must not press into the sciatic nerves at the gluteal folds. The chest pillows are adjusted to achieve maximal abdominal decompression.

9. Arm boards are attached to the center section of the operating table, and the patient's upper extremities are adjusted so the forearms and hands rest beside the head. The shoulders should neither sag too far anteriorly nor be pushed too far posteriorly. The ulnar nerves should be free of pressure at the ulnar grooves. To avoid stretching the ulnar nerves the elbows should not be acutely flexed.

10. If lateral thigh supports are used, they should angle downward toward the floor so they will not impair visualization of the spine on lateral x-ray views (Fig. 69-9). A wide strap is placed around the patient's upper thighs to secure him or her against the gluteal support and to prevent forward sliding during the procedure (see Fig. 69-9).

Variations of the Andrews frame technique include the following:

1. Intubation can be performed while the patient is awake. The patient can then assist in turning him-

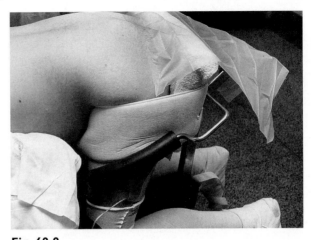

Fig. 69-9

Lateral thigh supports of the Andrews frame are angled inferiorly so they will not interfere with localizing roentgenograms. Note optimal degree of abdominal decompression achieved.

self or herself into a kneeling position on the frame. This may be a useful technique for a particularly obese patient.

2. The foot section of the operating table can be left flat until after the patient is turned. Then the patient's knees can be flexed to 90 degrees and the kneeling plate attached. The foot section is then cranked down 90 degrees to a vertical position, as the patient is gradually moved caudally to the proper position.

The technique of moving the patient from the Andrews frame back onto the gurney includes the following:

1. After the dressing is applied and the drapes are removed, the patient is supported manually while the upper thigh supports and gluteal support are removed.

2. The foot boots are removed. One strap of each boot is unbuckled, and the boot is taken off the patient's foot. The boot then dangles from the kneeling piece by the remaining strap. This minimizes the risk that the boot will be discarded with the disposable operating room debris.

3. The operating table is raised above the level of the gurney.

4. Before turning, the downward arm is moved from the abducted position to a position alongside the patient's torso.

5. The patient's knees and hips are both maintained in 90 degrees of flexion, and the patient is rolled onto the gurney with the knees and hips maintained in flexion. This allows easy turning with minimal lifting by the operating room personnel.

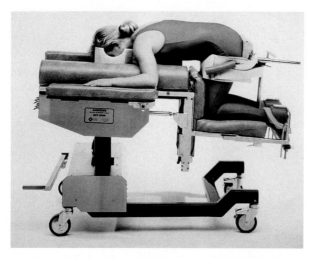

Fig. 69-10

Dedicated Andrews operating table, which places the patient in a prone-kneeling position.

The New Andrews Table

Orthopedic Systems, Inc., manufactures a dedicated Andrews operating table that places the patient in a prone-kneeling position (Fig. 69-10). The technique of positioning the patient on the Andrews table is similar to that described under "Technique of Positioning in the Andrews Frame" above. Rather than using pillows to support the patient's torso, a chest support attached to the table is utilized. Rather than using foot boots to secure the patient's feet, the patient's heels are secured in heel cups.

Any metallic parts of the table that might come in contact with the patient must be covered with padding, to prevent electric burns associated with use of electrocoagulation.

Summary

Each operative position presents advantages and disadvantages. At the very least, the positioning technique chosen should allow the surgeon to extend the operative exposure if necessary. It should provide maximum abdominal decompression to enhance respiration and minimize blood loss. Pressure points and peripheral nerves must be protected. Rotation of the cervical spine should be avoided, or at least minimized.

The position chosen must permit the surgeon to visualize, approach, and perform the procedure with relative comfort, especially when the operating time is long. In today's world, a skin slough, weakened facial muscle, or nerve loss traceable to patient positioning (regardless of the length of the surgical procedure), brings with it the specter of potential legal action if any of these or other effects persist and produce patient discomfort or discontent. In using the CeDaR platform and its ergonomic-oriented cushions, one of the authors (CDR) has noted a definite reduction in postoperative hip, leg, and sciatic complaints, as well as those involving the neck, scalp, and face.

The lumbar hyperextension produced by both the CeDaR surgical frame and the Andrews frame provides the advantage of reducing tension in the paraspinal muscles. This is particularly valuable during posterolateral fusions. If the surgeon requires an increase in the distance between posterior elements (the laminae or dorsal spinous processes) at a given lumbar level, then a simple lamina spreader provides excellent localized posterior distraction (effectively producing flexion of that particular segment).

Both the CeDaR surgical platform and the Andrews frame bring most patients sufficiently close to the operating room floor so that the members of the operating team can stand on the floor itself and do not have to stand on a stack of platforms. This allows the surgeon to operate with less hyperextension of his or her own knees and provides considerably greater comfort for the operating team.

Acknowledgements

Dr. Ray wishes to express his appreciation for the assistance and diligence shown this project by Eugene Dickhudt. Helpful suggestions were made by his associates at the Institute for Low Back Care, especially Matt Garner, PA-C. Five patents have been granted for the major elements of this system, now in wide use. Dr. Ray has indirect royalty rights to this system and associated instrumentation.

References

1. Cannon BW, Ray CD: *The lateral position for lumbar disc surgery* (film), University of Tennessee and Baptist Memorial Hospital, Memphis, TN. Presented at the Annual Meeting of the Southern Neurosurgical Society, Miami, 1959.

2. Cloward RB: *Cloward surgical saddle,* Honolulu, 1984, Surgical Equipment International.

3. Eckert A: Kneeling position for operations on the lumbar spine, especially for protruded intervertebral discs, *Surgery* 25:112, 1949.

4. Finneson BE: *Low back pain,* ed 2. Philadelphia, 1980, J.B. Lippincott.

5. Keim HA, Weinstein JD: Acute renal failure—a complication of spine fusion in the tuck position, *J Bone Joint Surg* 52A:1248, 1970.

6. Orthopaedic Systems, Inc.: Andrews spinal surgery frame (monograph). Hayward, CA, 1992.

7. Ray CD: *Decompressions and the "inaccessible zone."* In Hardy RW Jr, editor: *Lumbar disc disease,* ed 2, New York, 1982, Raven Press, p 123.

8. Ray CD: Head and chin cushioned face-rest for surgery in the prone position, *Anesthesiology* 64:301, 1986.

9. Ray CD: A new kneeling attachment and cushioned face rest for spinal surgery, *Neurosurgery* 20:266, 1987.

10. Ray CD: New techniques for decompression of lumbar spinal stenosis, *Neurosurgery* 10:587, 1982.

11. Ray CD: *Positioning the patient for lumbar decompressions and fusions.* In White AH, Rothman RH, Ray CD, editors: *Lumbar spine surgery: techniques and complications,* St. Louis, 1987, Mosby, p 95.

12. Rothman RH, Simeone FA: *The spine,* ed 2. Philadelphia, 1982, W.B. Saunders.

13. St. John JN: *The elbow flexion test in ulnar entrapment neuropathy.* Paper presented to the Annual Meeting of the Western Neurological Society, Jackson Hole, WY, September, 1982.

14. Tarlov IM: The knee-chest position for lower spinal operations, *J Bone Joint Surg* 49A:1193, 1967.

15. Wayne SJ: The tuck position for lumbar disc surgery, *J Bone Joint Surg* 49A:1195, 1967.

Chapter 70

Perioperative Care of the Spine Patient

George F. Smith

Preoperative Assessment

Preoperative Testing: Rationale and Use

> chest x-ray studies
> electrocardiography
> pregnancy testing
> laboratory studies

Prevention of Common Postoperative Complications

> infection
> thromboembolic disease

Blood Loss and Blood Conservation Techniques

> minimizing blood loss
> restoring lost blood volume

Intraoperative and Anesthetic Considerations

Spinal Surgery in Patients with Specific Illnesses

> cardiac disease
> pulmonary disease
> diabetes
> other endocrine problems
> gastroenterologic disorders
> drug and alcohol abuse

Postoperative Pain Management

Postoperative Rehabilitation and Discharge Planning

The perioperative care of the patient undergoing spine surgery includes preoperative evaluation, intraoperative care, and the postoperative management of pain, medical problems, and surgical complications. Each surgeon must be thoroughly familiar with these aspects of the care of the surgical patient to maximize the opportunity for good outcome.

Preoperative Assessment

The goal of preoperative evaluation is to obtain an accurate assessment of the potential risk of surgical or medical complications. Full assessment includes a history, systemic examination, and any appropriate laboratory studies and consultations. A byproduct of the evaluation is the ability to provide the patient with a chance to give informed consent for a procedure after taking medical factors into consideration. In some circumstances after preoperative evaluation of a patient's condition the surgical decision will need to be changed and tailored to balance the risk:benefit ratio. The factors that need to be included are the type of surgery, anticipated length of time of the surgery, the comorbid medical and psychiatric conditions, current medication use, potential drug interactions, and expected recovery time.

There is great diversity among patients who undergo spine surgery. There are elderly patients with multiple medical problems and collapsing degenerative scoliosis and there are young healthy athletes with acute herniated discs. However, some risks are common to all, including wound infection, reaction to medications, postoperative pain, thromboembolic phenomena, cardiac or pulmonary complications, blood loss, intraoperative positioning, anesthesia, and technical aspects of the procedure. Assessing each individual for his or her relative risks and planning prophylactically to reduce their occurrence will result in reduction of complications, economic savings, and improved patient satisfaction.

Preparing the patient for surgery by a team approach geared toward education and reducing anxiety helps patient and surgeon alike and reduces malpractice claims.[164] At our institution this team consists of a surgeon, an internist specializing in pain management, a psychiatrist, and a nurse-educator. The surgeon gives the patient a complete discussion in lay terms about the proposed procedure, the alternatives to surgery, as well as the possible complications. Then medical and psychiatric evaluations are performed to elucidate and treat any complicating medical or psychologic factors. In conjunction the nurse-educator gives specific instruction to the patient both verbally and by the use of hard copy manuals. Preoperative psychologic evaluation has been shown to be predictive of outcome when either the Minnesota Personality Inventory or a semistructured interview is used.[57] We have shown that preinjury childhood psychologic traumas may inhibit the ability to improve after technically successful surgery.[135,136] Based on an attachment theory model, we have hypothesized that these psychologic traumas inhibit the patient's ability to receive care and nurture. Unfortunately, definitive treatment models for these abnormal psychologic factors to improve outcome have not been studied.

Preoperative medical evaluation has obvious implications to assist in the reduction of complications in patients with comorbid medical problems. In asymptomatic and ostensibly healthy patients, medical consultation has proved to be helpful in patients over the age of 50. In healthy individuals under 50, a screening questionnaire along with blood pressure and hemoglobin determination appear to assess anesthetic risk adequately.[130,174]

The preoperative history and physical examination should focus on risk assessment for intraoperative and postoperative complications (i.e., morbid obesity carries an increased risk of anesthetic difficulty and wound infection). In order to minimize risk, appropriate preoperative studies and consultations should be obtained and a strategy planned to manage comorbid and other potential problems.

Preoperative Testing: Rationale and Use

Chest X-Ray Studies

Routine preoperative chest x-ray studies (CXR) are no longer justified. Abnormalities on CXR increase with age from less than 1% in individuals under the age of 30 to more than 40% in those over 70.[130] Indications for CXR screening have been established for patients undergoing elective noncardiopulmonary surgery and include acute respiratory symptoms, possible metastases, suspected cardiopulmonary disease with no CXR in the past 12 months, and recent immigrants from regions where tuberculosis is endemic and no CXR has been done in the past 12 months.[131]

Electrocardiography

Electrocardiogram (ECG) before surgery is indicated in any patient with a history of cardiovascular disease or in whom cardiac abnormalities are detected during the physical examination. The rate of abnormalities rises with age, and abnormalities include previous myocardial infarction and/or conduction abnormalities.[40] The finding of abnormal ECG in a patient with significant risk factors for coronary disease is an indication for further testing by thallium exercise stress testing or Doppler stress echo to rule out significant coronary disease.

Pregnancy Testing

Robbins notes that any woman who may be pregnant at the time of surgery should have pregnancy testing, except a woman in a monogamous relationship whose partner has undergone sterilization.[130] The incidence of unexpected pregnancy is 1.5% in sexually active premenopausal women who have not undergone surgical sterilization.

Laboratory Studies

Routine testing for laboratory abnormalities in asymptomatic patients has been challenged by multiple studies. Determining the hemoglobin level had positive predictive value for complications in a large series of patients undergoing cholecystectomies.[159] In spinal surgery the predictive value is likely to be higher the more complex the procedure (and therefore the more blood loss anticipated). In addition it is routine to obtain previously donated autologous blood for patients who will undergo instrumented fusions, and the marrow response is variable. In one prospective study at our institution, patients who required homologous blood transfusion had preoperative hemoglobin levels of less than 11 g/dl.[143] It is recommended that if the anticipated blood loss is greater than 1000 ml the hemoglobin should be 12 g/dl or greater prior to surgery.

Urinalysis is needed in all patients undergoing spinal surgery. Specifically, the presence of pyuria is most important. In Turnbull and Buck's study, preoperative pyuria had a positive predictive value of 11% for the development of postoperative urinary tract infection.[159] In patients undergoing spinal surgery this is of particular importance, as many patients are routinely catheterized and there is concern that infection could spread to the spine from the urinary tract through the Batson plexus. It is recommended that if a clean-catch specimen contains greater that five white blood cells in a female patient or three white blood cells in a male, a culture should be taken and the patient treated until the urine is clear and sterile. If pyuria remains after treatment, referral for evaluation of possible subclinical pyelonephritis is recommended.

Preoperative serum creatinine determination is appropriate in patients with spine problems who anticipate undergoing general anesthesia and relative hypotensive anesthesia to reduce blood loss. Creatinine measurement is also recommended in patients taking various nonsteroidal antiinflammatory drugs (NSAIDs), which have the capacity to reduce renal blood flow and glomerular filtration or cause interstitial nephritis. The incidence of newly discovered renal abnormalities has been noted to be 0.2%.[71,159]

Electrolyte disturbances rarely occur except in patients taking diuretics. Mild electrolyte abnormalities did not result in cardiac complications when studied in patients undergoing elective surgery.[159] It should be remembered that hypokalemia, the most common electrolyte disturbance, may be associated with hypomagnesemia, and appropriate treatment requires correction of both abnormalities.

From previous studies it is unclear whether routine preoperative glucose determination is beneficial in patients who are not known to have diabetes. Kaplan found significantly abnormal results in 0.4% of patients.[71] Glucose tolerance is diminished in patients taking diuretics and on corticosteroid therapy. Therefore, testing is prudent in these patients. In diabetic patients this is obviously crucial, and preoperative control will help prevent hyperosmolar states and reduce risk of infection.

There is always concern regarding the state of hemostasis in a patient about to undergo spine surgery because abnormal bleeding may result in an epidural hematoma that could result in both cauda equina compression and increased risk of infection. Tests that assess hemostasis include the prothrombin time (PT), activated partial thromboplastin time (aPTT), bleeding time (BT), and platelet count. In healthy individuals with no prior history of abnormal bleeding only a platelet count is needed.[70] Platelet counts below 100,000 are associated with increased bleeding.[166] In urgently planned surgery (acute cauda equina syndrome), a BT is also appropriate because of the possibility of NSAID use. Treatment for a prolonged BT due to NSAIDs is fresh-frozen plasma and/or desmopressin.[97]

In patients with suspected liver disease (i.e., history of heavy alcohol intake) a PT is indicated to determine if factor VII production is impaired. If the PT is elevated, medical consultation to assess severity is needed.

In a patient with a history of excessive bleeding after tooth extraction, deep bruising, or hemarthrosis, the full battery of tests should be obtained. The most common bleeding abnormality is von Willebrand disease, which is associated with a prolonged BT and possibly prolonged aPTT. The incidence in the general population is estimated to be from 1% to 10% and is associated with blood group O.[132,145] Most forms of this variably expressed disease are able to be treated successfully with fresh-frozen plasma, cryoprecipitate, or desmopressin.[66,98,127] Von Willebrand disease is often serendipitously uncovered when a markedly prolonged BT is found in patients taking NSAIDs.[66,98]

The underlying importance of patients needing to discontinue all NSAIDs prior to spine surgery to prevent bleeding problems is obvious. Aspirin has the most profound effect in that it irreversibly inhibits platelet aggregation for 7 to 10 days (the life span of platelets). We therefore recommend cessation of all NSAIDs for 2 weeks prior to surgery.

Prevention of Common Postoperative Complications

Infection

Infections are a significant cause of morbidity, mortality, and increased cost of care of surgical patients and occur in up to 8% of all surgeries.[50] Nosocomial infections occur as surgical wound infections, urinary tract infections, pneumonia, and bloodstream infections. Infections may also be transmitted from patients to health care personnel.

Wound infection rates for laminectomy/discectomy have been reported to be as high as 3%, with an average of about 1%.[125,146,153] Interestingly, microdiscectomy has a higher rate of infection when compared to standard discectomy (1.4% vs. 0.5%).[153] The incidence of infection after fusions with or without instrumentation has been reported to be up to 6%.[60,91]

Factors that have been shown to affect the surgical wound infection rate are noted in Table 70-1 with their relative weight. The Centers for Disease Control and Prevention (CDC) has adopted guidelines for monitoring and preventing wound infections; these are shown in the box below. Elective spinal surgery has a wound classification of Class I, clean, uncontaminated. These type of wounds carry the lowest infection rates. The overall health and age of the individual are other factors that influence infection rate with an infection rate of 1% in young and healthy patients to 8% in patients at higher risk.[48,50]

Antimicrobial prophylaxis for prevention of surgical wound infections is standard practice. In lumbar spine decompression, Horowitz has demon-

Table 70-1
Factors affecting rate of surgical wound infection

	Relative Increase	Modifiable
Patient Factors		
Age greater than 70	3 times	No
Coexisting medical problems	2 to 3 times	?Yes
Infection at remote site	2 to 3 times	Yes
Immunocompromised	2 times	?Yes
Morbid obesity	2 to 3 times	?Yes
Malnutrition	2 to 3 times	Yes
Anemia	?	Yes
Diabetes	2 times	Yes
Surgical factors		
Emergency surgery	3 to 4 times	No
Length of surgery > 2 hr	3 to 4 times	No
Fusion	4 to 6 times	No
Failure to use antibiotics	2 to 10 times	Yes
Failure to use disinfectant soap shower	2 times	Yes
Failure to report surgeon-specific infection rates to medical staff	2 times	Yes

strated a reduction of infection from 9.3% to 2.4% by the use of both preoperative and postoperative antibiotics.[60] The cephalosporin, cefazolin, has been shown to be the most effective and least expensive prophylactic antibiotic.[5] It has efficacy against the major pathogens in spine surgery, which include aerobic staphylococci, streptococci, and common aerobic gram-negative bacilli. The timing of the initial dose is important. One gram should be administered at least 30 minutes prior to skin incision, with an additional dose if the procedure lasts greater than 4 hours. In patients with a major penicillin or cephalosporin allergy vancomycin should be used. In institutions that have a high incidence of methicillin-resistant *Staphylococcus aureus,* vancomycin may also be a better agent. Vancomycin is given by slow infusion over 60 minutes to reduce the side effects of hypotension and flushing (red neck syndrome).

The recommendation that antibiotics be given postoperatively for 24 to 48 hours is empirical, and there are no data to suggest that treatment beyond

Summary of CDC Recommendations for Prevention of Wound Infections

- Classify and rescore all wound classes at time of surgery.

- Compute class-specific infection rates and report to surgeon.

- Treat and control bacterial infections present prior to surgery.

- Operation site scrubbed with detergent soap, antiseptic solution applied, and patient draped so there is no operator contact with unprepped skin during procedure.

- Tincture of chlorhexidine, iodine, or an iodophor are recommended antiseptics for skin preparation.

- Anyone entering operating room should wear high-efficiency mask fully covering nose and mouth; all hair should be completely covered.

- Scrubbing to the elbows with antiseptic soap should be done by all personnel who will touch the surgical field or sterile instruments.

- Sterile gowns and gloves should be worn. If a puncture occurs, gloves should be changed as soon as safety permits.

- Operator care in handling tissues gently, prevent bleeding, eradicate dead space, and minimize devitalized material in the wound.

- Incisional wounds classified as "dirty" should not be closed primarily.

- If drainage is necessary, a closed suction drain placed through an adjacent stab wound (not the primary incision) should be used.

- Personnel should wash hands before and after taking care of a surgical wound.

- Wound should be inspected if dressings are wet or signs and symptoms of infection are present.

- Increases in wound infection rates should be evaluated.

- Drainage from a wound suspected of being infected should be Gram stained and cultured.

- Prophylactic antimicrobials should be given in operations in which they are expected to significantly reduce infection rates.

Modified from *Guidelines for Prevention of Surgical Wound Infection*, Atlanta, 1985, CDC.

---

this time is superior.[12,55] It has been our practice to limit postoperative antibiotics in nonfusion spine surgery to 16 hours (two doses of cefazolin every 8 hours) postoperatively and to 48 hours in fusion spine surgery. This has resulted in infection rates of 1% for laminectomies and 4% for fusions, in our series of over 1000 cases, which is equal to or lower than in other reported series.[91,143,146,153]

Operating room factors should be optimized to reduce the inoculum into the surgical wound. These include minimizing traffic and keeping the operating room door closed; air flow systems that filter and exchange air at a rate of 25 times per hour; and appropriately fitted suits, head covers, and masks with knee-length shoe covers to reduce shedding of bodily bacteria.[32,128] Two pairs of gloves should be worn, since glove penetration is common in orthopedic procedures.[88]

The surgeon can reduce infections by appropriate handling of tissues. It has been observed at our institution that relaxation of self-retaining retractors every 20 minutes and irrigating tissues with normal saline for 30 seconds result in less muscle necrosis and need for debridement at the end of the procedure.[129] This may contribute to our lower reported infection rate in fusion cases.[143]

Closed suction drains have been used on an empirical basis to reduce hematoma formation.[55] However, data are lacking to prove drains reduce hematoma or infection.

The prevention of pulmonary infection involves minimizing the effects that spine surgery has on normal lung defense mechanisms. Diminished lung defenses are caused by intubation, anesthesia, suppression of cough and deep breathing mechanisms by narcotic analgesics, and pain itself. Hospitalization and antibiotics cause colonization of nosocomial bacteria. Pneumonia has been reported to occur in nearly 1% of discectomies.[134] Kelly et al. have reported depressed pulmonary function and fever to be greater after standard discetomy versus microdiscetomy.[76] The presence of preoperative bronchitis, asthma, or chronic obstructive pulmonary disease (COPD) increases the risk of infection; therefore, preoperative treatment should be maximized prior to surgery. To reduce the risk of postoperative pulmonary complications in smokers, cigarettes must be discontinued 8 weeks prior to surgery.[167] Routine use of incentive spirometry and deep breathing exercises postoperatively reduce the incidence of pulmonary infection.[13]

Urinary tract infections (UTIs) have been reported to occur in up to 10% of patients undergoing discectomy.[134] The occurrence is related to the use of Foley catheterization and preoperative asymptomatic bacteriuria. If an indwelling catheter is used, it should be inserted under aseptic conditions, the drainage system should be kept closed at all times, and the Foley removed as soon as possible. At our institution, bladder catheterization after multilevel decompression or fusion is routine. The catheter is generally removed 48 hours after surgery, usually when patients can stand independently. This practice has resulted in a UTI rate of 3.9%.[143]

Bloodstream infections are noted to be an important cause of morbidity in patients with spine problems.[30] The usual mechanism is from an infected wound, UTI, or pulmonary source. In addition, patients are susceptible to septicemia from indwelling vascular catheters. In complex spine surgeries this may pose a risk, as there is often a need for intravenous access for several days. Arterial or venous lines should be removed as soon as they are no longer essential.

Exposure to blood and sharp instruments during operations with subsequent transmission of bloodborne diseases produces risks to surgeons, healthcare workers, and patients. Protocols for operating room precautions should be established and strictly followed.[67]

Hepatitis and human immunodeficiency virus (HIV) are of highest concern, with rates of infectivity much higher for hepatitis than HIV. Hepatitis B in e antigen–positive circumstances is highly infective.[171] All surgeons and health-care workers who are at potential risk for exposure to blood should receive immunization for hepatitis B, with follow-up antibody response testing.[67] Booster dosing for low levels of antibody is recommended 5 to 7 years after initial immunization. An antibody test for hepatitis C (anti-HCV) has been introduced and is used for screening donated blood. Most cases of non-A, non-B hepatitis are now known to be from the hepatitis C virus.[3] However, a test for the carrier state or vaccine is not available. Particular caution should be exercised to guard against inadvertent contact because of high rates of chronic liver disease after infection from hepatitis C, which has been estimated to be 0.36%.[4,56] Suture needle injuries are thought to be a minimal risk.[7] Surgeons or health-care workers coming in direct contact with HIV-infected blood may choose to use zidovudine (AZT) to modify their risk.[7] Although definitive data are lacking, it is believed that administration within 2 hours of exposure is necessary.[7]

Thromboembolic Disease

Postoperative thromboembolic disease causes significant morbidity and mortality. In several studies evaluating postoperative complications from lumbar decompression, postoperative pulmonary emboli (PE) was the leading cause of death.[102,134,143,146] The incidence of PE has been reported from 0.03% to 1.1%.[72,134,146] Studies specifically evaluating postoperative deep vein thrombosis (DVT) by duplex scanning have shown an occurrence rate of 6% in lumbar discectomies and 14% in lumbar fusion procedures.[36,172]

Patient and surgical factors increasing the risk for thromboembolic disease are listed in the box below. High-risk patients made up 60% of patients in whom DVT developed in Ferree et al.'s study of lumbar procedures.[36]

Modification of risk factors, unfortunately, are limited to discontinuation of estrogen therapy for 6 weeks prior to the procedure, early postoperative mobilization, and limiting operative time in high-risk patients (three or more risk factors).

Prophylactic measures and risk protocols to limit thromboembolic phenomena include the use of medical means (of which heparin, dextran, and warfarin are most studied) and mechanical measures (graded compression stockings [GCS] and external intermittent pneumatic compression boots).[11,19] The use of low-dose heparin or other medical mea-

Factors That Increase the Risk of Thromboembolic Phenomena

Patient Factors	Surgical Factors
Age greater than 40	Procedure greater than 1 hr
Estrogen therapy	General anesthesia
Obesity	Kneeling position
Prior deep venous thrombosis or pulmonary emboli	Spinal distraction
Venous insufficiency	Anterior approach
Malignancy	
Congestive heart failure	
Prolonged postoperative immobilization	
Profound lower-extremity weakness	

sures carry a risk of bleeding that could lead to epidural hematoma. Even though the risk of bleeding in neurosurgical studies have found heparin to be safe, mechanical measures are without bleeding risk and therefore more popular.[6,14]

Thigh-high elastic graded compression stockings have been shown to be effective in reducing the risk of DVT by more than 50% when studied in general surgical patients in randomized, controlled studies.[2,59] No complications have been noted with their use.

External intermittent pneumatic compression (EPC) has been shown to significantly reduce the incidence of DVT in prospective, randomized, controlled studies.[52,120,140,161,176] In a comparison study, EPC was found to be significantly more effective than heparin.[17] Cost effectiveness as compared to other methods has also been demonstrated with EPC.[116] Interestingly, the mechanism of action is likely enhancement of fibrinolysis because effectiveness against lower-extremity DVT has been demonstrated with the use of arm EPC.[81] The combined use of GCS and EPC affords greater prophylaxis in high-risk general surgical patients and in patients with spine problems.[11,37,137] Disadvantages to older devices were due to patient acceptance but newer ones are more comfortable, particularly if a cooling mechanism is used. Their main advantage is simple application and lack of bleeding complications. One report has noted the complications of peroneal neuropathy and lower-leg compartment syndrome associated with EPC in two patients with significant weight loss and cancer.[85]

To be effective, mechanical measures must be applied intraoperatively at the start of the procedure and be worn while the patient is in bed through the hospital stay or until the patient becomes fully ambulatory.[142,160]

In high-risk patients (those with several risk factors and/or prior DVT/PE) the use of subcutaneous heparin with GCS and EPC is warranted. In order for heparin to be effective it must be started preoperatively and continued until discharge.[70,77] In randomized trials there was no increase in wound infection, hematomas, or wound dehiscence. In the author's experience there have been no occurrences of epidural hematoma or excessive bleeding requiring homologous blood transfusion when heparin has been used in those circumstances. The dose is 5000 U given preoperatively and then every 8 hours until discharge.

Blood Loss and Blood Conservation Techniques

The amount of blood lost during spinal surgery depends on the type of surgery and operative technique. Significant blood loss occurs in multilevel posterior spinal fusion procedures. Consideration for blood salvage or transfusion is needed only in procedures in which blood loss is expected to be greater than 1000 ml. Use should be based on effectiveness, risk, and cost. Anemia has not been shown to impair wound healing, increase infection rate, delay bleeding, or lengthen the hospital stay when the hemoglobin is above 7 g/dl.[62] Therefore, old "myths" regarding blood transfusion need to be altered, particularly the 10:30 hemoglobin:hematocrit rule. Even though the risk is low, the use of homologous blood transfusions in elective spinal surgery appears unjustified with current techniques. The obvious exception is life-threatening blood loss. Johnson[62] has noted that 86% of spine surgeons had used homologous blood and that 10% had encountered a post-transfusion disease of hepatitis or HIV. Currently, the risk of hepatitis from screened blood for hepatitis B or C is approximately 1:200. The risk of HIV seroconversion is 1:40,000 to 1:100,000.

Minimizing Blood Loss

Factors that are controllable to reduce the amount of blood loss at the time of surgery are listed in the box below.

Controllable Factors to Reduce Blood Loss during Surgery

1. Desmopressin (DDAVP) given preoperatively at 0.3 μg/kg[65,82]

2. Hypotensive anesthesia with mean arterial pressure at 60 to 80 mm Hg[96,119]

3. Patient positioning to decrease intraabdominal pressure[122]

4. Injection of epinephrine 1:500,000 into the skin and subcutaneous tissues[122]

5. Meticulous control of bleeding points

6. Subperiosteal dissection[106]

7. Use of thrombostatic agents, i.e., topical thrombin preparations

8. Decortication of fusion area after harvesting of donor bone[106]

Desmopressin (DDAVP) has been found to decrease blood loss significantly in spinal fusions with instrumentation for scoliosis or degenerative disc disease in which blood loss exceeded 1000 ml.[65,82] DDAVP was not found to be effective in a randomized, double blind study of two-level laminectomies in which blood loss averaged less than 500 ml.[144] The mechanism of action of DDAVP is release of factor VIII complexes stored in endothelial cells. No increase in thrombosis has been found. Side effects are flushing, transient hypotension, and diminished urine output. We routinely give 0.3 μg/kg (approximately 20 ug) DDAVP at the induction of anesthesia to all healthy patients undergoing multilevel fusion. We have had no directly attributable adverse effects in our 500 cases. The cost is comparable to that of a unit of blood ($300).

Hypotensive anesthesia has been shown in three studies of spinal fusions with instrumentation to reduce blood loss by greater than 50% compared to control groups.[47,96,119] Mean arterial pressures averaged between 60 and 80 mm Hg, and no complications were reported. Caution should be used in patients with cerebrovascular disease, and diminished cardiac output and in the elderly.

Allowing the abdomen to be decompressed by positioning the patient on a Relton or Andrews frame reduces intraabdominal, caval, and epidural venous pressures, which directly reduces oozing during the procedure.[122] The kneeling position used does increase the risk for DVT.

The use of epinephrine 1:500,000 solution injected into the skin and subcutaneous tissues appears to diminish oozing from these tissues.[122] This should not be used in patients with a history of coronary disease or arrhythmias.

Technical aspects of the surgery are extremely important in controlling blood loss. The most obvious is meticulous control of bleeding during the surgery and when the muscle relaxation and hypotension have been reversed. The use of thrombin-soaked Gel-foam (Upjohn, Kalamazoo, MI) for oozing areas may be helpful to ensure clot stability. Milani and Wharton have noted diminished blood loss with a dissection technique that maintains itself in the subperiosteal plane.[106] Also, to reduce oozing from the bony fusion site, decortication of bone should occur as late in the procedure as possible.[106,122]

Restoring Lost Blood Volume

Several techniques that now exist to restore lost blood volume to the patient either intraoperatively or postoperatively are listed in the box opposite.

The use of isovolemic hemodilution to obtain up to four units of whole blood under urgent conditions is simple, safe, and inexpensive (approximately $200).[100] Appropriate patients include those with expected blood loss of greater than 1000 ml or 20% of blood volume who have adequate red-cell mass. The technique involves removing and storing blood in standard blood bags. Volume is then restored with crystalloid and possibly colloid and the stored blood is reinfused during or at the end the procedure. Tissue oxygenation is not impaired when the hematocrit is kept in the 27% to 30% range.[105] This method has also been tolerated in Jehovah's Witnesses who accept it after informed consent, as long as a continuous system exists.[175] No complications have been reported with this technique, but caution is advised in patients with cardiac disease and renal failure as fluid overload is a possibility.[86] Combining the use of induced hypotension and isovolemic hemodilution should be reserved for patients with preoperative American Society of Anesthesiologists class I.

Cell-saver devices for intraoperative autotransfusion have gained great popularity as this device has become more effective and safe.[25,38] This technique returns up to 50% of shed red cells to the circulation. Current systems wash collected red cells and resuspend them in crystalloid for reinfusion. This eliminates debris but also platelets and clotting factors. Therefore, a concern of reduced hemostasis with large amounts of reinfusions is noted and replacement with fresh-frozen plasma may be needed. Additionally, transient hemoglobinuria is common but does not appear to have significant sequelae.[25,38] The cost is significant and its use in procedures in which blood loss is less than 1000 ml is probably not justified.[64] Currently, we recommend its use in multilevel, instrumented fusions or when other methods are not available, such as for Jehovah's Witnesses who accept it.

Postoperative blood salvage and reinfusion from drainage systems is a relatively easy technique, with

Methods to Restore Blood Volume

- Isovolemic hemodilution
- Intraoperative autotransfusion (cell-saver devices)
- Postoperative blood salvage from drainage systems
- Transfusion of stored red blood cells (autologous or homologous blood)

a cost of about $200. Current devices drain shed blood through a filter to remove debris and collect blood into a sterile reservoir that contains an anticoagulant. Collected blood is reinfused using standard peripheral venous access. This technique is limited to blood collected up to 6 hours after the procedure as mild reactions have been reported from blood stored longer.[73] The effectiveness of this technique is variable as it depends on the drainage from the wound, which is a function of the dead space, placement of the drain, and hemostatic control at the end of the procedure. Therefore, this may be most indicated when significant oozing at the end of the procedure has been encountered.

Currently, the most common, effective, safest and comparably inexpensive way of restoring lost blood is by transfusion of predonated autologous blood. This method along with the other aforementioned techniques should entirely replace the use of homologous blood except for extreme medical circumstances. Safe protocols for collection include donating no more than one unit per week while the patient is taking ferrous sulfate 300 mg three times a day.[148]

Different opinions exist in the literature regarding the number of units recommended which in turn depends on the type of procedure. Johnson et al. make the point that they have not needed to transfuse any patient undergoing only decompression and therefore do not recommend predonation in nonfusions.[64] Collatz et al. recommend obtaining one unit for extensive decompressions.[18] Our experience is that there is significant blood loss in multilevel decompressions (particularly in reoperations), and in the elderly, in whom bone is osteoporotic and extensive central and foraminal decompression is needed. In these circumstances we obtain two units of autologous blood. There is agreement that for instrumented fusions it is prudent to obtain two units of autologous blood. For procedures that involve three or more levels, additional units are often needed and obtaining up to four units is appropriate particularly if combined anterior and posterior fusion is planned.

The decision of when and how much to transfuse a patient remains unestablished in nonemergent situations. The subject has not been well studied, particularly for autologous versus homologous blood. The current recommendations are generally too broad.[21,111] Therefore, the decision to transfuse is the physician's judgment. The risks versus benefits of reinfusing autologous blood when acute surgical blood loss has occurred to improve and speed functional recovery and shorten length of hospital stay

are unknown. In a randomized trial Albert et al. noted earlier ambulation and higher reticulocyte counts in patients who received autologous transfusion immediately postoperatively versus later on day 4 after fusion surgery.[1] No difference in nutritional status was noted and all patients received transfusions. Lengths of hospital stay were not compared.

Experience with autologous transfusions at our hospital has proven its safety. In the past 5 years and in over 2000 units reinfused only one incidence of mishap has occurred. This was a technical error in a patient receiving 20 ml of mismatched blood. No reaction or sequelae occurred. We therefore will transfuse all predonated autologous blood in the immediate postoperative period unless fluid overload is a concern. Third space fluid edema will develop in many patients because of intraoperative and postoperative infusions and the concurrence of the syndrome of inappropriate ADH secretion.[101] The use of low-dose furosemide (20 mg) assists in mobilizing this extra fluid safely and seems to result in better patient comfort and less tension on incisions.

The use of the above techniques of blood loss reduction and restoration has limited our use of homologous blood to only two instances in over 1000 consecutive lumbar surgeries (0.2%).[143] It was noted that in both instances the patients had preoperative hematocrits below 34%. Therefore, it appears prudent to delay surgery until the hematocrit is nearly normal; this may reduce the need for homologous blood.

Intraoperative and Anesthetic Considerations

Care of the patient in the operating room is the joint responsibility of surgeon, anesthesiologist, and nursing staff. Proper patient positioning and padding of potential areas of compression are crucial to reduce ischemia to the eyes and peripheral nervous system and to reduce unnecessary blood loss.

The risk of anesthesia depends on preexisting medical conditions (e.g., cardiac disease), the type of anesthesia (general vs. regional), and technical and human factors (machine and operator competency). Overall, anesthetic-induced morbidity and mortality are low, with mortality estimated at 1 per 10,000.[74] The most common cause of mortality is the failure to ventilate adequately. Accurate knowledge of preexisting medical conditions is obviously crucial to modify anesthesia risk. The majority of spinal surgery is performed under general anesthesia, even though there are theoretical advantages to the use of regional (spinal) anesthesia, including diminished postoperative thrombosis, diminished blood loss, and decreased mortality in high-risk patients that have been shown in studies of hip and prostate surgery.[57,107,156,162,165] However, the popularity of general anesthesia persists because of better control of the airway and oxygenation, better hemodynamic control, and better patient comfort for longer cases. Modern general anesthetic risk is quite minimal.

The sources of risk from anesthesia include the stress response to anesthetic drugs and interventions that cause the release of catecholamines. Stress-induced catecholamine release can induce myocardial ischemia and arrhythmias. Inhalational anesthesia causes increased platelet adhesiveness and has a direct depressant effect on myocardium. Higher intraoperative blood pressure and heart rate have been associated with higher rate of myocardial infarction.[5]

The type of general anesthesia may be varied according to the procedure. For example, during scoliosis surgery the use of narcotics are preferred because somatosensory evoked potentials and wake-up tests can be more accurately assessed.[133] In other types of spinal surgery in which spinal cord ischemia is not a consideration, a balanced approach with narcotics and inhalational agents is appropriate. In particular, isoflurane can induce the desired hypotensive effect to reduce intraoperative blood loss.

Important anesthetic drug interactions include the preoperative use of monoamine oxidase inhibitors, which can elicit a malignant hypertension response and should be discontinued 2 weeks prior to surgery. Tricyclic antidepressants can cause ventricular arrhythmias when used with halothane and pancuronium bromide. Lithium carbonate prolongs the neuromuscular blockade by pancuronium and succinylcholine. Cimetidine may result in reduced clearance of lidocaine during regional anesthesia.

Spinal Surgery in Patients with Specific Illnesses

Cardiac Disease

Death due to myocardial infarction is an important cause of mortality in spine surgery. In Deyo et al.'s study it was the leading cause of death in lumbar spine procedures.[30] Determination of those at risk for myocardial ischemia is an important part of the preoperative evaluation. The mere presence of coronary risk factors has not definitively defined which patients are at risk.[20,43,149] The use of dipyridamole thallium imaging has been shown to identify patients at high risk for postoperative cardiac events.[8] When combined with clinical predictors (Q waves on ECG, history of ventricular ectopy, diabetes, age greater than 70, and angina), thallium imaging was highly predictive.[33] The use of stress echocardiography has been reported to be accurate in identifying coronary disease and may be more sensitive than thallium testing.[53,54] We currently use the history of multiple risk factors (smoker, family history of ischemic heart disease, hypertension, hyperlipidemia) for obtaining preoperative noninvasive testing to rule out occult coronary disease. As a result we have had no postoperative myocardial infarctions or cardiac-related deaths in our series of 1000 patients.[143]

Patients should not undergo elective surgery for at least 6 months after a myocardial infarction.[42,149,155] An exception may be patients who have undergone coronary artery bypass grafting who have lower risk.[39] Additionally, patients with a history of congestive heart failure that is well compensated at the time of surgery are at low risk.[43]

Preoperative arrhythmias occur more frequently in patients with known heart disease, and if arrhythmias are noted preoperatively, predict coronary events.[42,163] The presence of significant aortic stenosis in patients undergoing spinal surgery places the patient at high risk for mortality. Treatment with valve replacement is usually recommended prior to elective surgery.

Pulmonary Disease

Smokers have increased risk of atelectasis, pulmonary infections, and respiratory failure even if pulmonary function is normal. Quitting smoking 2 months prior to surgery reduces the risk fourfold.[167] Cessation of smoking for 24 hours prior to surgery lowers the nicotine and carboxyhemoglobin levels and will lower cardiac risk.

COPD and asthma are common conditions in patients undergoing spine surgery. It is important that patients enter the surgery "tuned-up" and that medications be maintained throughout the postoperative period. We will use nebulized bronchodilators for 24 to 48 hours after surgery if a patient is using metered-dose inhaled bronchodilators before surgery. We use corticosteroids perioperatively for asthma patients who have been on steroid therapy recently (within 3 months) or in whom significant wheezing develops despite bronchodilator treatment postoperatively. All patients should be taught deep-breathing exercises and given incentive spirometry to use hourly in the postoperative period to decrease the risk of pulmonary complications.[114,152]

Diabetes

The presence of diabetes in a patient undergoing surgery increases the risks of impaired wound healing, wound infection fivefold, and metabolic disturbances.[24,44] In addition, we have noted a generally less favorable outcome in insulin-dependent diabetics who undergo decompression for radicular symptoms, particularly if peripheral neuropathy is present. A study by Simpson et al. corroborates this finding.[139] They noted that diabetics who undergo lumbar decompression had higher rates of postoperative complications and worse outcomes (particularly if preoperative weakness was present) when compared to nondiabetic controls.

Internal medicine consultation is important for the perioperative treatment of the diabetic patient. Blood glucose levels need to be maintained below 250 mg/dl so that phagocytosis of bacteria by granulocytes is not impaired.[113] Better control of blood glucose results in better wound healing and decreased infection rates.[103,113]

In patients on oral hypoglycemic agents, the use of recombinant insulin by a sliding-scale method is appropriate until a full diet is restored. We have routinely used insulin pumps for younger, type I, insulin-dependent diabetics with excellent control. The key in management of any regimen is frequent monitoring of the blood glucose. Rising insulin requirements in the postoperative period may be an early indication of infection.

Other Endocrine Problems

Another commonly encountered endocrine problem is treated hypothyroidism. Reinstitution of normal doses of thyroid replacement at 24 to 48 hours after surgery is reasonable. Withholding medication until peristalsis is restored does not appear to expose the patient to any undue risk.[169]

It is extremely important to be aware of the patient who has recently been treated with corticosteroids. There is significant risk of decreased adrenal reserve due to suppression of the hypothalamic-pituitary-adrenal axis that can occur with the equivalent of 7.5 mg/day of prednisone for 1 week in the preceding year.[147,150] In patients with spine problems this level may be easily reached with a series of epidural corticosteroid injections. Manifestations of adrenal insufficiency include persistent postoperative hypotension, extreme fatigue, hyperkalemia, nausea, and hyponatremia. Patients who should be given stress doses of corticosteroid include anyone on long-term suppressive therapy and those who have received 2 weeks of suppressive doses within the past 6 months. Coverage should include a preoperative dose of 100 mg of hydrocortisone succinate intravenously and 100 mg every 8 hours for the first 24 hours. The dose can be tapered over the next 72 hours.[75,123,154]

Gastroenterologic Disorders

Patients who have had active peptic ulcer disease and are receiving treatment at the time of surgery and those with a history of gastrointestinal bleeding are at risk for stress gastritis and bleeding ulcers. Treatment with H_2 blockers intravenously is effective in the perioperative period.[177] We had favored ranitidine rather than cimetidine because of its limited drug interactions and lower incidence of disorientation in the elderly.

Diarrhea and constipation are encountered frequently postoperatively. Constipation is most often due to opioid administration. Routine use of stool softeners is recommended. Diarrhea may result from antibiotic therapy, motility changes, or fecal impaction. There may be secretory diarrhea due to intestinal infection by bacteria, viruses, or parasites. Antibiotic-associated colitis may cause diarrhea, which can occur as early as 2 days after the start of antibiotics or as late as 3 weeks after discontinuation of antibiotics. Usually, *Clostridium difficile* is the offending agent, with the diarrhea being due to toxin production. Most episodes are self-limited and do not go on to a full-blown pseudomembranous colitis. Discontinuation of antibiotics and fluid support comprise generally sufficient treatment. If diarrhea persists, gastroenterology consultation is recommended. Treatment usually consists of the use of oral vancomycin or metronidazole.

Occasionally, with anterior lumbar interbody fusion, a severe postoperative ileus is encountered. Invariably, the patient is a significant air-swallower. Decompression with a nasogastric tube to low suction for 48 to 72 hours usually results in prompt relief and allows less tension on the abdominal incision. In addition, we have used trancutaneous electrical nerve stimulation (TENS) applied to the abdomen to stimulate lower tract motility with good result.

Drug and Alcohol Abuse

In an unpublished study funded by the state of California to determine the rate of complications and influencing factors in spine surgery the presence of alcohol- or drug-abuse-related diagnoses were found to be independent risk factors for the occurrence of complications.[9] Other studies of prostate and colon surgeries have noted significantly higher complication rates in alcoholics.[157,158]

A major practical difficulty is screening for the presence of substance abuse prior to surgery. For alcoholism, the use of the CAGE or MAST questionnaires can be helpful.[124] Elevations of the hepatic enzyme γ-glutamyltransferase or the red-cell mean corpuscular volume (MCV) on routine preoperative laboratory tests appear to be confirmatory markers when alcoholism is suspected.[15] However, the problem with screening is that denial is often present. The author has found that asking the patient whether alcohol is used to manage pain is a useful screening question. Alcohol has analgesic properties, and inquiring about its use in the context of a medication appears less threatening.

In 10 to 15 percent of known alcoholics who suddenly become abstinent (such as immediately after surgery) significant alcoholic withdrawal symptoms develop. These may include autonomic dysfunction, hallucinations, and/or seizures.[69,79] Seizures and aspiration add significant morbidity and mortality to what should be low-risk surgical procedures.

Ideally, patients who drink heavily should undergo detoxification before elective surgery. However, the use of benzodiazepines in the postoperative period will usually prevent the alcohol withdrawal syndrome.[29] Another important consideration in alcoholic patients is altered phamacokinetics. In particular, meperidine, which is commonly prescribed for postoperative pain, should be avoided. The half-life of meperidine is doubled with the presence of cirrhosis, and its metabolite normeperidine can cause seizures.[80] Other opioids are cleared more slowly as well, and the use of naloxone may be necessary if inadvertent oversedation occurs to reduce the risk of aspiration. Noninebriated alcoholics also tolerate higher doses of benzodiazepines and may need larger amounts of anesthetics. Alcoholic patients may have abnormal hemostasis due to diminished vitamin K–dependent clotting factors (II, VII, IX, X) and a prothrombin time is indicated for screening.[22] Bleeding may also be increased because of insufficient or abnormal platelets and a bleeding time is also needed to screen for platelet abnormalities.

Other metabolic problems that may be encountered in the alcoholic patient postoperatively include hypoglycemia, ketoacidosis, malnutrition, thiamine deficiency (causing central and peripheral nervous system toxicity), folate deficiency, and hypomagnesemia.

Drug abuse in patients undergoing spine surgery is primarily iatrogenic, with opioids and benzodiazapines being the most frequently overused drugs. The major difficulties in the postoperative period are pain control due to drug tolerance and anxiety states. These problems often lead to prolongation of the hospital stay and significant nursing staff involvement. We recommend discontinuation of these medications for 6 weeks prior to elective surgery to restore suppressed endorphin systems. For management of anxiety postoperatively, lorazepam is effective parenterally and lorazepam or another benzodiazapine, clonazepam (1 mg every 6 hours) are effective orally and are least likely to interfere with early postoperative rehabilitation.

Postoperative Pain Management

All patients who undergo spinal surgery will have the need for postoperative pain management. Therefore, a protocol that includes the prevention and treatment of expected pain is needed. A combined approach of pharmacologic, physical, and psychologic methods works best and is discussed in the box below. Recently, the Department of Health and Hu-

Postoperative Pain Management Techniques

Psychologic measures
  Relaxation techniques, including exercises, music, biofeedback, guided imagery, hypnosis
  Cognitive techniques such as education and instruction
Physical methods
  Ice packs or cooling pads
  TENS
  Mobility exercises, supported bed positioning
Pharmacologic methods
  NSAIDs: for mild to moderate pain (orally administered); exception is ketorolac, which may be administered parenterally
  Antispasmotics: primary site of action is central nervous system, all have sedation as side effect
  Baclofen: oral administration only; dosing flexibility up to 80 mg/day
  Cyclobenzaprine
  Benzodiazepines: lorazepam is preferred because can be given PO, IM, IV, or SL with quick onset and short duration of action (2-4 hours)
  Opioids: administration may be oral, IV, IM, epidural/intrathecal
  Corticosteroids: oral, parenteral, or epidural to relieve nerve-root inflammation; use has questionable scientific support

man Services has recognized undertreatment of postoperative pain as an important health concern and has published an excellent review and practice guidelines on acute pain management.[16]

Multiple studies have demonstrated that postoperative pain is poorly treated in about half the patients.[23,99,151,170] This is due to lack of knowledge of clinical pharmacology (of opioids in particular), poor appreciation of pain intensity and duration, and an exaggerated fear of addiction on the part of physicians and nurses.

From compiled data, Bonica has noted that laminectomy patients are expected to experience moderate to severe pain from the surgical wound and with movement for a duration of 6 days (range, 5 to 9).[7] Sources of pain after spinal surgery include the skin incision, healing muscular tissue with reactive spasm, dural and nerve-root inflammation, bony excision site of vertebae or donor bone site area for fusions, and internal fixation devices interacting with overlying tissues.

Prevention of pain begins with preoperative reduction of anxiety, which is due to patients' fear, uncertainty and impending helplessness. This can be accomplished by informing patients of all aspects of the surgical experience, which will require the use of models, drawings, demonstration of equipment to be used during and after surgery, and possibly hospital tours. Relaxation techniques have been shown to reduce the need for postoperative analgesics and to reduce the length of hospital stay.[35,89] Teaching relaxation training is time-intensive but can be performed by trained staff with physician reinforcement. At our institution, a nurse will spend 30 to 45 minutes counseling patients prior to surgery and then follow them during their hospital stay.

The use of opioids immediately preoperatively can reduce postoperative pain.[78,104] Enhancement of analgesia with local anesthetic blocks performed immediately before surgery has been shown clinically.[104] However, there is reluctance to use epidural local anesthesia.

Intraspinal opioids have been studied as a method to decrease postoperative pain. However, in lumbar fusions Johnson et al. did not find epidural or intrathecal morphine to have an advantage over patient-controlled analgesia (PCA).[63] Concern over late respiratory depression, particularly if supplemental systemic narcotics are used, requires appropriate monitoring.[126] Fentanyl, which is more lipid-soluble than morphine and therefore has less affinity to ascend in the cerebrospinal fluid, appears to be the better choice for intraspinal analgesia because severe respiratory depression has been noted only rarely.[84,93]

Systemic opioids are the mainstay for postoperative pharmacologic pain relief following spine operations. The goal is to obtain adequate therapeutic levels. The most crucial aspect of successful pain management is repeated reevaluation of patient's self-report of pain and the physician's willingness to adapt to individual variability in pain and methods of pain control. It has been demonstrated that poor pain control and patient dissatisfaction is often the result of prescribing opioids on an "as needed" basis.[99,117] Although time-contingent intramuscular injections of opioids is far better, this technique may result in only minimal analgesic concentration for 35% of the dosing interval.[46]

The most convenient and effective method, and the one that patients prefer is the use of patient-controlled analgesia (PCA) devices.[34,45,87] PCA consists of an electronically controlled intravenous infusion with a timing device. The obvious advantage to PCA over other regimens is the minimal time delay between perception of pain and the administration of medication. The patient can, on demand, self-administer a preset amount of analgesic by pressing a button. A "lockout" period (usually 8 to 10 minutes) prevents overadministration. A background infusion or "basal rate" can assist in maintaining blood levels in the analgesic range, although the need for this has been challenged.[118] The author does not recommend the use of basal-rate infusions in the elderly or in anyone with increased risk of respiratory depression (COPD, sleep apnea syndrome). Reassessment of pain levels and appropriate dose adjustments using boluses of medication and dose volume changes will obtain desired analgesia. Other than nursing staff reassessment of pain levels, demands on nursing staff time are reduced. Any parenteral opioid may be used in PCAs. We favor the use of morphine sulfate because of its well-demonstrated analgesic properties, predictable side effect profile, and lack of accumulated metabolites. Meperidine should be used cautiously (for less than 48 hours) if at all because of the potential buildup of a toxic metabolite, normeperidine, which can cause agitation, delirium, and seizures. Hydromorphone (Dilaudid) is the author's second choice with a dose adjustment of about $\frac{1}{4}$ to $\frac{1}{6}$ that of morphine's (0.25 mg vs 1.0 mg). Fig. 70-1 shows a typical PCA order sheet.

Naloxone (Narcan) should be kept at the bedside in case of accidental respiratory depression or overdose. In over 1500 spinal surgeries using PCA, I

1. Medication: _____ morphine _____ mg/ml

   _____ meperidine

   _____ other _____

2. Loading dose (initial bolus): _____ mg

3. Continuous basal rate: _____ mg/hr

4. Dose volume: _____ mg

5. Lockout interval: _____ minutes (usually 8-10)

6. 4 hour maximum dose _____ mg (optional)

7. Additional bolus: _____ mg every _____ minutes prn severe pain

8. Apnea monitor _____ yes   no _____

9. Naloxone (Narcan) 2 ampules taped to PCA machine

10. For oversedation or respiratory depression:

    • hold medication for ____ hours, or until patient is alert

    • decrease basal rate to ____ mg/hr

    • decrease dose volume to ____ mg

    • increase lockout interval to ____ min

    • Administer naloxone 1 to 2 ampules for severe respiratory depression, oversedation, hypotension. If no response call physician stat.

11. For inadequate analgesia:

    check integrity of intravenous line

    bolus of _____ mg

    increase basal rate to _____ mg/hr

    increase dose volume to _____ mg

    decrease lockout time to _____ min

    reassess status in one hour and may repeat.

Fig. 70-1

Sample PCA order sheet.

have seen respiratory depression occur in patients with coexistent sleep apnea syndrome (6 patients) (0.4%). Overmedication has also occurred in 2 patients, whose family members triggered the PCA device. An apnea monitor is recommended in the elderly and in those with respiratory disease.

In the elderly the occurrence of opioid-induced delirium is a not an uncommon side effect. When it occurs, delirium needs to be managed by lowering the dose of medication and supplementation or substitution with ketorolac. Lorazepam is preferred to manage agitation and haloperidol might be used for hallucinations.

PCA is usually needed for about 48 hours after laminectomies and for up to 96 hours after complex fusion surgeries (i.e., combined anterior-posterior fusions). Generally, when patients are taking an oral diet without nausea, parenteral opioids are discontinued and oral narcotics are begun on a time-contingent basis (i.e., hydrocodone or codeine 30 to 60 mg every 4 hours around the clock) allows a smooth transition. In addition, a breakthrough parenteral medication should be available. When changing to an oral narcotic mixed agonist-antagonist opioids (i.e., pentazocine/Talwin) should be avoided because a withdrawal reaction can be precipitated.

Opioid side effects should be anticipated, and contingency orders to manage them should be prepared in advance. Nausea is a frequent side effect, occurring in about 20% of patients. Management with prophylatic antiemetics such as transdermal scopolamine has been demonstrated to be effective in gynecologic surgery.[92] Antiemetics act on receptors in the midbrain and include antihistamines such as diphenhydramine (Benadryl), anticholinergics such as scopolamine, and neuroleptics such as metoclopramide (Reglan) or droperidol.[121] Combinations of the these classes is more effective than any single agent.[109] Pruritus is another common side effect of opioid therapy. The use of diphenhydramine or hydroxyzine (Atarax, Vistaril) appear to be the most efficacious for routine use.

Ketorolac (Toradol), an injectable NSAID, can be used as an analgesic for breakthrough pain or to enhance opioid analgesia with resultant decreased opioid dose.[40,115] Thirty milligrams of ketorolac is approximately equianalgesic to 10 mg of morphine, and there are no significant hemodynamic, respiratory, or CNS side effects.[9,95,110,115] Caution should be exercised in patients with peptic ulcer disease, as reactivation of symptoms and bleeding have been observed. Also, as with other NSAIDs, platelet adherence may be diminished, and theoretically bleeding can occur. Therefore, its use should commence only after postoperative hemostasis has been ensured.

Paravertebral muscle spasm after laminectomy is a very common reaction to surgical dissection. Spasm may occur spontaneously or after turning in bed or getting up and about. It may persist until complete neuromuscular healing has occurred (6 to 8 weeks). Many patients have preoperative muscle spasm as part of their symptom complex. In the postoperative period a combination of ice packs or cooling pads to the wound and antispasmodics gives reasonable relief. Only benzodiazapines are available parenterally, so these are used early in the postoperative period prior to the patient's ability to take oral medicines. We favor the use of the short-acting, flexibly administered lorazepam in a dose range of 1 to 2 mg every 3 to 4 hours. Orally, the use of baclofen appears clinically to be most efficacious.[26]

Systemic or epidural corticosteroids have been used in an attempt to reduce postoperative nerve-root swelling and pain and to shorten the hospital stay. Naylor et al.[112] and Watters et al.[168] had opposite conclusions regarding the efficacy of systemic dexamethasone in prospective, randomized studies. In a nonrandomized trial, Davis and Emmons reported diminished narcotic usage and shorter hospital stay with epidurally administered methylprednisolone.[28] One report notes no benefit from this method and a risk of deep wound infection.[94] It remains unclear what role corticosteroids have in routine postoperative pain management.

Physical measures to alter pain include heat, cold, massage, exercise and TENS. Incisional and deep-tissue cooling techniques appear clinically to be the most efficacious in reducing swelling, pain, and spasm, particularly in posterior lumbar procedures. Existing devices that can supply a comfortable continuous cooled pad can be used without fear of frostbite to the incision. Temperature can be adjusted for comfort and safety, usually to the 42° F to 50° F range. TENS therapy and sham TENS therapy have been shown to reduce significantly subjective pain reports and analgesic use in postoperative patients.[51,61]

Proper positioning and body mechanics can reduce discomfort after spinal surgery. Use of support pillows under the knees while recumbent is beneficial. Patients are taught the "log-roll" turning technique to decrease muscle spasm. Frequent turning assisted by the nursing staff (every 2 hours) in the early postoperative is important for patient comfort. Bed exercises that include mild stretching and isometrics can reduce spasm and reduce deconditioning in the early postoperative period.

Postoperative Rehabilitation and Discharge Planning

Little data exist on the appropriate approach to physical therapy in the postoperative spine patient. There has been a remarkable change in the length of postoperative hospital stay in the past 20 years. Oppel reported in 1977 an average stay of 3 weeks in the hospital.[115a] This contrasts with an average stay of only 3 days for patients undergoing discectomy in California in 1989-1991.[9] The obvious difference is that patients started walking earlier. We currently begin ambulation for all patients on the first postoperative day with a physical therapist and rapidly progress patients to independent ambulation. Patients are taught body mechanics, home exercises, and activities of daily living while in the hospital, with the objective being independent self-care at home. Exercises but no formal physical therapy are prescribed for the first 3 to 4 weeks postoperatively as walking tolerance is increased.

Discharge from the hospital is currently becoming a cost-containment issue in which issues of patient safety and comfort, physician's practice style, and insurance authorization and utilization review must all be considered.

References

1. Albert TJ, Desai D, McIntosh T, et al.: Early versus late replacement of autotransfused blood in elective spinal surgery, *Spine* 18:1071, 1993.

2. Allan A, Williams JT, Bolton JP, LeQuesne LP: The use of graduated compression stockings in the prevention of postoperative deep vein thrombosis, *Br J Surg* 70:172, 1983.

3. Alter MJ, Hadler SC, Judson FN, et al.: Risk factors for acute non-A, non-B hepatitis in the United States and association with hepatitis C virus antibody, *JAMA* 264:2231, 1990.

4. Alter MJ, Margolis HS, Krawczynski K, et al.: The natural history of community-acquired hepatitis C in the United States, *N Engl J Med* 327:1899, 1992.

5. Antimicrobial prophylaxis for surgery, *Med Lett* 23:77, 1981.

6. Barnett HG, Clifford JR, Llewelyn RC. Safety of minidose heparin administratiion for neurosurgical patients, *J Neurosurg* 47:27, 1977.

7. Bonica JJ: *Postoperative pain.* In Bonica JJ, editor: *The management of pain,* Philadelphia, 1990, Lea & Febiger, p 461.

8. Boucher CA, Brewster DC, Darling RC, et al.: Determination of cardiac risk by dypyridamole-thallium imaging before peripheral vascular surgery, *N Engl J Med* 312:389, 1985.

9. California Hospitals Outcomes Project, Office of Statewide Health Planning and Development, Sacramento, CA, David Werdegar MD - director, Harold Luft PhD and Peter Romano MD - principal investigators, September, 1993.

10. Camu F, Van Overberge L, Bullingham R, Lloyd J: Hemodynamic effects of two intravenous doses of ketorolac tromethamine compared with morphine, *Pharmacotherapy* 10:233S, 1990.

11. Caprini JA, Scurr JH, Hasty JH: Role of compression modalities in a prophylactic program for deep vein thrombosis, *Semin Thromb Hemost* 14 (Suppl):77, 1988.

12. Carlson G, Abitibol J, Garfin S: Prevention of complications in surgical management of back pain and sciatica, *Orthop Clin North Am* 22:345, 1991.

13. Celli BR, Rodriquez KS, Snider G: A controlled trial of intermittent positive breathing, incentive spirometry, and deep breathing exercises in preventing pulmonary complications after abdominal surgery, *Am Rev Respir Dis* 130:12, 1984.

14. Cerroto D, Ariano D, Fiacchino F: Deep vein thrombosis and low-dose heparin prophylaxis in neurosurgical patients, *J Neurosurg* 49:378, 1978.

15. Chick J, Kreitman N, Plant M: Mean cell volume and gamma-glutamyl transpeptidase as markers of drinking in working men, *Lancet* 1:1249, 1981

16. Clinical Practice Guidlines: acute pain management: operative or medical procedures and trauma. Washington, DC, February 1992, Department of Health and Human Services.

17. Coe NP, Collins RE, et al.: Prevention of deep vein thrombosis in urological patients: a controlled, randomized trial of low-dose heparin and external pneumatic compression boots, *Surgery* 83:230, 1978.

18. Collatz M, Schwaigler P, Lorenz M, Zindrick M: *Use of autologous blood transfusions in commonly performed spinal procedures.* Poster exhibit at the North American Spine Society meeting, Monterey, CA, August 8-11, 1990.

19. Consensus conference: prevention of venous thrombosis and pulmonary embolism, *JAMA* 256:744, 1986.

20. Cooperman M, Pflug B, Martin E, et al.: Cardiovascular risk factors in parints with peripheral vascular disease, *Surgery* 84:505, 1978.

21. Council of Scientific Affairs: Autologous blood transfusions. *JAMA* 256:2378, 1986.

22. Cowan DH: Effect of alcoholism on hemostasis, *Semin Hematol* 17:131, 1980.

23. Cohen FL: Postsurgical pain relief: patient's status and nurses' medication choices, *Pain* 9:265, 1980.

24. Cruse PJ, Foord R: A five year propsective study of 23,649 surgical wounds, *Arch Surg* 107:206, 1973.

25. Czenscitz TA, Flynn JC: Intraoperative blood salvage in spinal deformity surgery in children, *J Fla Med Assoc* 66:39, 1979.

26. Dapas F, Hartman SF, Martinez L, et al.: Baclofen for the treatment of acute low-back syndrome: a double blind comparison with placebo, *Spine* 10:345, 1985.

27. Davis FM, Laurenson VG: Spinal anaesthesia or general anesthesia for emergency hip surgery in elderly patients, *Anaesth Intens Care* 9:352, 1981.

28. Davis R, Emmons SE: Benefits of epidural methylprednisolone in a unilateral discetomy: a matched controlled study, *J Spinal Disorders* 3:299, 1990.

29. Deutsch JA, Nancy W: Diazepam maintenance of alcohol preference during alcohol withdrawal, *Science* 198:307, 1977.

30. Deyo RA, Cherkin DC, Loeser JD, et al.: Morbidity and mortality in association with operations on the lumbar spine: the influence of age, diagnosis, and procedure, *J Bone Joint Surg* 7A:536, 1992.

31. DiPiro JT, Record KE, Schanzenbach KS, et al.: Antimicrobial prophylaxis in surgery, part 1, *Am J Hosp Pharm* 38:320, 1981.

32. DiPiro JT, Record KE, Schanzenbach KS, et al.: Antimicrobial prophylaxis in surgery, Part 2, *Am J Hosp Pharm* 38:487, 1981.

33. Eagle KA, Coley CM, Newell JB, et al.: Combining clinical and thallium data optimizes preoperative assessment of cardiac risk factors, *Ann Intern Med* 110:859, 1989.

34. Edwards WT: Optimizing opioid treatment of postoperative pain. *J Pain Symptom Manage* 5 (suppl):524, 1990.

35. Egbert LD, et al.: Reduction of postoperative pain by encouragement and instruction of patients: a study of doctor-patient rapport, *N Engl J Med* 270:825, 1964.

36. Ferree BA, Stern PJ, Jolson RS, et al.: Deep venous thrombosis after spinal surgery, *Spine* 18:315, 1993.

37. Ferree BA, Wright A: Deep venous thrombosis following posterior lumbar spinal surgery, *Spine* 18:1079, 1993.

38. Flynn JC, Metzger CR, Czencitz TA: Intraoperative autotransfusion in spinal surgery, *Spine* 7:432, 1982.

39. Foster ED, Davis KB, Carpenter JA, et al.: Risk of noncardiac operations in patients with defined coronary disease: the coronary artery surgery study (CASS) registry experience, *Ann Thorac Surg* 41:42, 1986.

40. Gillies GWA, Kenny RE, Bullingham RE, McArdle CS: The morphine sparing effect of ketorolac tromethamine, *Anaesthesia* 42:727, 1987.

41. Goldberger AL, O'Konski M: Utility of the routine electrocardiogram before surgery and on general hospital admission, *Ann Intern Med* 105:552, 1986.

42. Goldman L, Caldera DL, Nussbaum SR, et al.: Multifactorial index of cardiac risk in noncardiac surgical procedures, *N Engl J Med* 297:845, 1977.

43. Goldman L, Caldera DL, Southwick FS, et al.: Cardiac risk factors and complications in noncardiac surgery, *Medicine* (Baltimore) 57:357, 1978.

44. Goodson WH, Hunt TK: Wound healing and the diabetic patient, *Surg Gynecol Obstet* 149:600, 1979.

45. Graves DA, et al.: Patient-controlled analgesia, *Ann Intern Med* 99:360, 1983.

46. Grossman SA, Sheilder VR: Skills of medical students and house officers in prescribing narcotic medications, *J Med Educ* 60:552, 1985.

47. Grundy B, Nash C, Brown R: Delibrate hypotension for spinal fusion: Prospective randomized study with evoked potential monitoring, *Can Anesth Soc J* 29:453, 1982.

48. Haley RW, Culver DH, Morgan WM, et al.: Identifying patients at high risk of surgical wound infections, a simple multivariate index of patient susceptibility and wound contamination, *Am J Epidemiol* 121:206, 1988.

49. Haley RW, Culver DH, White JW, et al.: The nationwide nosocomial infection rate: a new need for vital statistics, *Am J Epidemiol* 121:159, 1988.

50. Haley RW, Hooton TM, Culver DH, et al.: Nosocomial infections in U.S. hospitals, 1975-1976: estimated frequency by selected characteristics, *Am J Med* 70:947, 1981.

51. Hargreaves A, Lander J: Use of transcutaneous electrical nerve stimulation for postoperative pain, *Nurs Res* 38:159, 1989.

52. Hartman JT, Pugh JL, Smith RD, et al.: Cyclic sequential compression of the lower limb in prevention of deep venous thrombosis, *J Bone Joint Surg* 64A:1059, 1982.

53. Hecht HS, DeBord L, Shaw D, et al.: Digital supine bicycle stress echocardiography: a new technique for evaluating coronary artery disease, *J Am Coll Cardiol* 21:950, 1993.

54. Hecht HS, DeBord L, Shaw R, et al.: Supine bicycle stress echocardiography versus tomographic thallium-201 exercise imaging for the detection of coronary artery disease, *J Am Soc Echocardiogr* 6:177, 1993.

55. Heller JG, Garfin SR: Postoperative infection of the spine, *Semin Spine Surg* 2:268, 1990.

56. Henderson DK, Fahey BJ, Willy M, et al.: Risk for occupational transmission of human immunodeficiency virus type 1 (HIV-1) associated with clinical exposures, *Ann Intern Med* 113:740, 1990.

57. Hendolin H, Mattila MA, Poikolainen E: The effect of lumbar epidural anesthesia on the development of deep vein thrombosis of the legs after open prostatectomy, *Acta Chir Scand* 147:425, 1981.

58. Herron LD, Turner J, Clancy S, Weiner P: The differential utility of the Minnesota Personality Inventory: a predictor of outcome in lumbar laminectomy for disc herniation versus spinal stenosis, *Spine* 10:804, 1985.

59. Holford CP: Graded compression for preventing deep veinous thrombosis, *BMJ* 2:969, 1976.

60. Horwitz NH, Curtin JA: Prophylactic antibiotics and wound infections following laminectomy for lumbar disc herniation: a retrospective study, *J Neurosurg* 43:727, 1975.

61. Jensen JE, Conn RR, Hazelrigg G, Hewett JE: The use of transcutaneous neural stimulation and isodinetic testing in arthroscopic knee surgery, *Am J Sports Med* 13:27, 1985.

62. Johnson RG. Blood loss in spinal surgery: is there a problem? *Spine State Art Rev* 5:1, 1991.

63. Johnson RG, Miller M, Murphy M: Intraspinal narcotic analgesia. A comparison of two methods of postoperative pain relief, *Spine* 14:363, 1989.

64. Johnson RG, Murphy M, Miller M: Fusions and transfusions: An analysis of blood loss and autologous replacement during lumbar fusions, *Spine* 14:358, 1989.

65. Johnson RG, Murphy JM: The role of desmopressin in reducing blood loss during lumbar fusions, *Surg Gynecol Obstet* 171:223, 1990.

66. Johnson RS, Heldt LV, Keaton WM: Diagnosis and treatment of von Willebrand's disease, *J Oral Maxillofac Surg* 45:608, 1987.

67. Joint Working Party of the Hospital Infection Society and the Surgical Infection Study Group: Risks to surgeons and patients from HIV and hepatitis: guidelines on precautions and management of exposure to blood or body fluids, *BMJ* 305:1337, 1992.

68. Kaempfe FA, Lifeso RM, Meiking C: Intermittent pneumatic compression versus coumadin, *Clin Orthop Relat Res* 269:89, 1991.

69. Kaim SC, Klett CJ, Rothfeld B: Treatment of acute alcohol withdrawal states: a comparison of four drugs, *Am J Psych* 125:1640, 1969.

70. Kakkar VV, Spindler J, Flute PT, et al.: Efficacy of low doses of heparin in prevention of deep-vein thrombosis after major surgery: a double-blind trail, *Lancet* 2:101, 1972.

71. Kaplan EB, Sheiner LB, Boechmann AJ, et al.: The usefulness of preoperative laboratory screening, *JAMA* 253:3578, 1985.

72. Kardaun JW, White LR, Shaffer WO: Acute complications in patients with surgical treatment of lumbar herniated disc, *J Spinal Disord* 3:30, 1990.

73. Keating EM, Ritter MA, Fairs PM, et al.: *A system for reinfusion of aspirated whole blood after total hip and knee arthroplasty,* Presented at a meeting of the American Association of Orthopedic Surgeons, Las Vegas, February, 9-11, 1989.

74. Keenan RL, Boyan P: Cardiac arrest due to anesthesia, *JAMA* 253:2373, 1985.

75. Kehlet H: A rational approach to dosage and preparation of glucocorticoid substitution therapy during surgical procedures, *Acta Anaesth Scand* 19:260, 1975.

76. Kelly RE, Dinner MH, Lauyne MH, Andrews DW: The effect of lumbar disc surgery on postoperative pulmonary function and temperature, *Spine* 18:287, 1993.

77. Kiil J, Kiil J, Axelsen F, Anderson D: Prophylaxis against postoperative pulmonary embolism and deep-vein thrombosis by low-dose heparin, *Lancet* 1:1115, 1978.

78. Kiss IE, Kilian M: Does opiate premedication influence post-operative analgesia? A prospective study, *Pain* 48:157, 1992.

79. Klickman L, Herbsman H: Delirium tremens in surgical patients, *Surgery* 64:882, 1969.

80. Klotz V, McHorse TS, Wilkinson GR, et al.: The effect of cirrhosis on disposition and elimination of meperidine in man, *Clin Pharmacol Ther* 16:667, 1974.

81. Knight M, Dawson R: Effect of intermittent compression of the arms on deep venous thrombosis in the legs, *Lancet* 1:1265, 1976.

82. Kobrinsky NL, Letts M, Patel L, et al.: Desmopressin decreases operative blood loss in patients having Harrington rod spinal fusion surgery, *Ann Intern Med* 107:446, 1987.

83. Kobrinsky NL, et al.: Shortening of bleeding time by l-deamino-8-D-arginine vasopressin in various bleeding disorders, *Lancet* 1:1145, 1984.

84. Kreitzer JM, Kirshenbaum LP, Eisenkraft JB: Epidural fentanyl by continuous infusion for relief of postoperative pain, *Clin J Pain* 5:283, 1989.

85. Lachman EA, Rook JL, Tunkel R, Nagler W: Complications associated with intermittent pneumatic compression, *Arch Physiol Med Rehab* 73:482, 1992.

86. Laks H, Pilon RM, Klovekorn WP, et al.: Acute hemodilution: its effect on hemodynamics and oxygen transport, *Ann Surg* 180:103, 1974.

87. Lange MP, Dahn MS, Jacobs LA: Patient-controlled analgesia versus intermittent analgesia dosing, *Heart Lung* 17:495, 1988.

88. Lavernia CJ, Bache H, Godin M: *The incidence of unknown perforations of gloves during routine surgical procedures.* Presented at the Western Orthopedic Association meeting, Anaheim, CA, October, 11-14, 1989.

89. Lawlis FG, Selby D, Hinnant D, McCoy CE: Reduction of postoperative pain parameters by presurgical relaxation instruction for spine pain patients, *Spine* 10:649, 1985.

90. Levinson W: Preoperative evaluation by an interist: are they worthwhile? *West J Med* 141:395, 1984.

91. Lonstein J, Winter R, Moe J, Gaines D: Wound infection with Harrington instrumentation and spinal fusion for scoliosis, *Clin Orthop* 76:272, 1973.

92. Loper KA, Ready B, Dorman BH: Prophylactic transdermal scopalamine patches reduce nausea in postoperative patients receiving epidural morphine, *Anesth Analg* 68:144, 1989.

93. Lortessy A, Magnin C, Viale JP, et al.: Clinical advantages of fentanyl given epidurally for postoperative analgesia, *Anesthesiology* 61:466, 1984.

94. Lowell TD, Errico TJ: *Use of epidural steroids after discectomy may predispose to infection.* Presented at the North American Spine Society meeting, San Diego, October 11-14, 1993.

95. MacDonald FC, Gough KJ, Nicoll RA, Dow RJ: Psychomoter effects of ketorolac in comparison with buprenorphine and diclofenac, *Br J Clin Pharmacol* 28:453, 1989.

96. Malcoln-Smith N, McMaster M: The use of induced hypotension to control bleeding during posterior spinal fusion for scoliosis, *J Bone Joint Surg* 65B:255, 1987.

97. Mannucci PA: Desmopressin for treatment of disorders of hemostasis, *Prog Hemost Thromb* 8:19, 1986.

98. Mannucci PM, Cancione MT, Rota L, Donovan SS: Response of factor VIII/von Willebrand factor to DDAVP in healthy subjects and patients with hemophilia A and von Willebrand's disease, *Br J Haematol* 47:283, 1981.

99. Marks RM, Sachar EJ: Undertreatment of medical inpatients with narcotic analgesics, *Ann Intern Med* 78:173, 1973.

100. Martin E, Hansen E, Peter K: Acute limited normovolemic hemodilution: A method for avoiding homologous transfusion, *World J Surg* 11:53, 1987.

101. Mason RJ, Betz RR, Orzowski JP, Bell GR: The syndrome of inappropiate antidiuretic hormone secretion and its effect of blood indices following spinal fusion, *Spine* 14:722, 1989.

102. Mayfield FH: Complications of laminectomy, *Clin Neurosurg* 23:435, 1976.

103. McMurry JF: Wound healing with diabetes mellitus: better glucose control for better wound healing in diabetics, *Surg Clin North Am* 64:769, 1984.

104. McQuay HJ, Carroll D, Moore RA: Post-operative orthopedic pain—the effect of opiate premedication and local anesthetic blocks, *Pain* 33:291, 1988.

105. Messmer K, Kreimeier V, Intaglietta M: Present state of intentional hemodilution, *Eur Surg Res* 18:254, 1986.

106. Milani JM, Wharton GW: *Blood conservation in lumbar surgery.* Presented at the International Society for the Study of the Lumbar Spine (ISSLS) meeting, Dallas, May 1-3, 1986.

107. Modig J, Borg M, et al.: Thromboembolism after total hip relacement: role of epidural and general anesthesia, *Anesth Analg* 62:174, 1983.

108. Modig J, Malmerj P, Karlstrom G: Effect of epidural versus general anaesthesia on calf blood flow, *Acta Anaesth Scand* 24:305, 1980.

109. Morran C, Smith DC, Anderson DA, McArdle CS: Incidence of nausea and vomiting with cytotoxic chemotherapy: a prospective randomised trial of antiemetics, *BMJ* 1:1323, 1979.

110. Murray AW, Brockway MS, Kenny GN: Comparison of the cardiorespiratory effects of ketorolac and alfentanil during propofol anesthesia, *Br J Anaesth* 63:601, 1989.

111. National Institutes of Health: NIH statement of perioperative red cell transfusion. Nat Inst Health Cons Dev Conf State 7 (4), 1988.

112. Naylor A, Flowers M, Bramley J: The value of dexamethasone in the postoperative treatment of lumbar disc prolapse, *Orthop Clin North Am* 8:3, 1977.

113. Nolan CM, Beaty HN, Bogdade JP: Further characterization of the impaired bactericidal function of granulocytes in patients with poorly controlled diabetes, *Diabetes* 27:889, 1978.

114. O'Donoghue WJ: Prevention and treatment of postoperative atelectasis, *Chest* 87:1, 1985.

115. O'Hara DA, Fragen RJ, Kinzer M, Pemberton D: Ketorolac tromethamine as compared with morphine sulfate for treatment of postoperative pain, *Clin Pharmacol Ther* 41:556, 1987.

115a. Oppel F, Schramm AJ, et al.: Results and complicated course after surgery for lumbar herniation, *Adv in Neuros* 4:36, 1977.

116. Oster G, Tuden RL, Colditz GA: A cost-effective analysis of prophylaxis against deep-vein thrombosis in major orthopedic surgery, *JAMA* 257:203, 1987.

117. Owen H, McMillan V, Rogowski D: Postoperative pain therapy: a survey of patients' expectations and their experiences, *Pain* 41:303, 1990.

118. Parker RK, Holtmann B, White PF: Patient controlled analgesia: Does a concurrent opioid infusion improve pain management after surgery, *JAMA* 266:1947, 1991.

119. Patel N, Patel B, Paskin S, Laufer S. Induced moderate hypotension anesthesia for spinal fusion and Harrington-rod instrumentation, *J Bone Joint Surg* 67A:1384, 1985.

120. Pedegana LR, Burgess EM, Moore AJ, Carpenter ML: Prevention of thromboembolic disease by external pneumatic compression in patients undergoing total hip arthroplasty, *Clin Orthop Relat Res* 128:190, 1978.

121. Peroutka SJ, Snyder SH: Antiemetics: neurotransmitter receptor binding predicts therapeutic actions, *Lancet* 1:658, 1982.

122. Phillips WA, Hensinger RN: Control of blood loss during scoliosis surgery, *Clin Orthop* 229:88, 1988.

123. Plumpton FS, et al.: Corticosteroid treatment and surgery, *Anaesthesia* 24:3, 1969.

124. Porkorny AD, Miller BA, Kaplin HB: The MAST: a shortened version of the Michigan Alcoholism Screening Test, *Am J Psych* 129:118, 1987.

125. Ramirez LF, Thisted R: Complications and demographic characteristics of patients undergoing lumbar discectomy in community hospitals, *Neurosurgery* 25:226, 1989.

126. Rawal N, Wattweil M: Respiratory depression after epidural morphine, an experimental and clinical study, *Anesth Analg* 63:8, 1984.

127. Richardson DW, Robinson AG: Desmopressin, *Ann Intern Med* 103:278, 1985.

128. Ritter MD, Estzen NE, Hart JB, et al.: The surgeons garb, *Clin Orthop* 153:204, 1980.

129. Reynolds J: Personal communication, August 13, 1993, Orthopedic spine surgeon, SpineCare Medical Group, Daly City, CA.

130. Robbins J: *Preoperative evaluation of the healthy patient.* In Stuls J, Dere R, editors: *Practical care of the ambulatory patient,* Philadelphia, 1989, W.B. Saunders Co., p 535.

131. Roberts CJ: The effective use of diagnostic radiology, *J R Coll Phys Lond* 18:62, 1984.

132. Rodeghiero F, Castaman G, Dini E: Epidemiological investigation of the prevalence of von Willebrand's disease, *Blood* 69:454, 1987.

133. Roger MC, editor: *Current practice in anesthesiology,* Philadelphia, 1988, B.C. Decker, p 101.

134. Schepelman F, Greiner L, Pia HW: Complications following operation of herniated lumbar discs, *Adv Neurosurg* 4:52, 1977.

135. Schofferman J, Anderson D, Hines R, et al.: Childhood pyschological trauma correlates with unsuccessful lumbar spine surgery, *Spine* 17:S138, 1992.

136. Schofferman JS, Anderson D, Hines R, Smith GS: *Prospective evaluation of the correlation between childhood psychologic trauma and lumbar surgery outcome.* Presented at the North American Spine Society meeting, San Diego, October 16-18, 1993.

137. Scurr JH, Coleridge-Smith PD, Hasty JH: Regimen for improved effectiveness of intermittent pneumatic compression in deep venous thrombosis prophylaxis, *Surgery* 102:816, 1987.

138. Scurr JH, Ibrahim SZ, Faber RG, LeQuesne LP: The efficacy of graduated compression stocking in the prevention of deep vein thrombosis, *Br J Surg* 64:371, 1977.

139. Simpson JM, Silveri CP, Balderston RA, Simeone FA: *Lumbar spine surgery in patients with diabetes mellitus,* Presented at the International Spine Society meeting, Marseilles, June 11-13, 1993.

140. Skillman JJ, Collins MB, et al.: Prevention of deep vein thrombosis in neurosurgical patients: a controlled, randomized trial of external pneumatic compression boots, *Surgery* 83:354, 1978.

141. Slogoff S, Keats AS: Does perioperative myocardial ischemia lead to myocardial infarction? *Anesthesiology* 62:107, 1985.

142. Smith RC, Elton RA, Orr JD, et al.: Dextran and intermittent pneumatic compression in prevention of postoperative deep vein thrombosis: a multicenter trial, *BMJ* 1:952, 1978.

143. Smith GF, Roos T, Keaney D: *Complications of lumbar spine surgery.* Presented at the North American Spine Society meeting, San Diego, October 14-16, 1993.

144. Smith GF, Schofferman J, et al.: *Preoperative desmopressin (DES) does not decrease perioperative blood loss in two level laminectomy and discetomy,* Poster exhibit at the North American Spine Society meeting, Monterey, CA, August 8-11, 1990.

145. Sorter RF: Antiprostaglandin drugs in von Willebrand's disease, *Am J Obstet Gynecol* 136:696, 1980.

146. Spangfort EV: The lumbar disc herniation, a computer-aided analysis of 2,504 operations, *Acta Orthop Scand* Suppl 142:1, 1972.

147. Spiegel RJ, et al.: Adrenal suppression after short-term coricosteroid therapy, *Lancet* 1:630, 1979.

148. Stanisavljevic S, Walker R, Bartman C: Autologous blood transfusion and total joint arthroplasty, *J Arthroplasty* 1:207, 1986.

149. Steen PA, Tinker JH, Tarlan S: Myocardial reinfarction after anesthesia and surgery, *JAMA* 239:2566, 1978.

150. Streck W, Lockwood D. Pituitary adrenal recovery following short-term suppression with corticosteroids, *Am J Med* 66:910, 1979.

151. Sriwatanakul K, et al.: Analysis of narcotic usage in the treatment of postoperative pain, *JAMA* 215:925, 1983.

152. Stock CM, et al.: Prevention of postoperative pulmonary complications with CPAP, incentive spirometry, and conservative therapy, *Chest* 87:151, 1989.

153. Stolke D, Sollman WP, Seifert V: Intra- and postoperative complications in lumbar disc surgery, *Spine* 14:56, 1989.

154. Symreng T, et al.: Physiological cortisol substitution of long-term steroid treated patients undergoing major surgery, *Br J Anaesth* 53:949, 1981.

155. Tarham S, Moffitt EA, Taylor WF, et al.: Myocardial infarction after general anesthesia, *JAMA* 220:1451, 1972.

156. Thorbun J, Louden JR, Vallance R: Spinal and general anaesthesia in total hip replacement: frequency of deep vein thrombosis, *Br J Anaesth* 52:1117, 1980.

157. Tonnesen H, Schutten BT, Jorgensen BB: Influence of alcohol on morbidity after colonic surgery, *Dis Colon Rectum* 30:549, 1987.

158. Tonnesen H, Shutten BT, Tollund L, et al.: Influence of alcoholism on morbidity after transurethral prostatectomy, *Scand J Urol Nephrol* 12:175, 1988.

159. Turnbull JM, Buck C: The value of preoperative screening investigations in otherwise healthy individuals, *Arch Intern Med* 147:1101, 1987.

160. Turpie AG, Gallus AS, Beattie WS, et al.: Prevention of venous thrombosis and the effectiveness in patients with intracranial disease by intermittent pneumatic compression of the calf, *Neurology* 27:435, 1977.

161. Turpie AG, Gallus AS, Beattie WS, Hirsh J: Prevention of venous thrombosis in patients with intracranial disease by intermittent pneumatic compression of the calf, *Neurology* 27:435, 1977.

162. Valentin N, Lombolt B, et al.: Spinal or general anesthesia for surgery of the fractured hip: a prospective study of mortality in 578 patients, *Br J Anaesth* 58:284, 1986.

163. Varick PE, Davis HS: Cardiac arrythymias during halothane anesthesia, *Anesth Analg* 47:299, 1968.

164. Voshall B: The effects of preoperative teaching on postoperative pain, *Top Clin Nurs* 2:39, 1980.

165. Yeager MP, Glass DD, et al.: Epidural anesthesia and analgesia in high risk surgical patients, *Anesthesiology* 66:729, 1987.

166. Wallerstein RO: Laboratory evaluation of a bleeding patient, *West J Med* 150:51, 1989.

167. Warner MA, et al.: Role of preoperative cessation of smoking and other factors in postoperative complications: a blinded prospective study of coronary bypass patients, *Mayo Clin Proc* 64:609, 1989.

168. Watters WC, Temple AP, Granberry M: The use of dexamethasone in primary lumbar disc surgery: a prospective, randomized, double-blind study, *Spine* 14:440, 1989.

169. Weinberg A, et al.: Outcome of anesthesia and surgery in hypothyroid patients, *Arch Intern Med* 143:893, 1983.

170. Weiss OF, et al.: Attitudes of patients, house staff and nurses toward postoperative analgesic care, *Anesth Analg* 62:70, 1983.

171. Werner BG, Grady GF: Accidental hepatitis B surface antigen positive inoculations: use of e antigen estimate infectivity, *Ann Intern Med* 97:367, 1982.

172. West JL, Anderson LD: Incidence of deep vein thrombosis in major adult spinal surgery, *Spine* 17(8S):S254, 1992.

173. Whang R: Magnesium deficiency: pathogenesis, prevalence, and clinical implications, *Am J Med* 82:24, 1987.

174. Wilson ME, Williams MB, Baskett PJF, et al.: Assessment of fitness for surgical procedures and the variability of anaesthetist judgement, *BMJ* 1:509, 1980.

175. Wong KC, Webster LR, Coleman SS, Deims HK: Hemodilution and induced hypotension for insertions of a Harrington rod in a Jehovah's Witness patient, *Clin Orthop Res* 152:237, 1980.

176. Woolson ST, Watt JM: Intermittent pneumatic compression to prevent proximal deep venous thrombosis during and after total hip replacement, *J Bone Joint Surg* 73A:507, 1991.

177. Zuckerman DO, Shuman R: Therapeutic goals and treatment options for prevention of stress ulcer syndrome, *Am J Med* 83(Suppl 6A):29, 1987.

Chapter 71
Selection of Surgical Treatment by Analysis of Pain Generators
Parviz Kambin

Mechanical Pressure on
the Nerve Roots

Anatomic Status of Perianular
Structures

Hydrostatic Pressure of
the Intervertebral Disc

Postoperative Reduction of
the Disc Height

Degenerative Status of
Intervertebral Disc

Inflammatory Agents and
Pain Syndrome

At present, lumbar discectomy for the treatment of sciatica pain secondary to mechanical pressure on the nerve root is being accomplished by several methods. The open laminotomy[19] procedure has continued to be an acceptable and reliable method of treatment for symptom-producing herniated lumbar discs. Nucleotomy,[22] nucleolysis,[34] or nucleovaporization[4,11] (which is achieved by mechanical tools, chemical means, or laser light) are designed to reduce the nuclear mass. It has been postulated that the core decompression of the nucleus may in turn reduce the size of the protrusion and compression on the nerve root.

Although the outcome of the open discectomy procedure in properly selected patients is somewhat predictable, the efficacy of the nucleotomy technique has been subject to considerable controversy and dispute.[9,22] The above discrepancy in part appears to be due to lack of similarity of preoperative clinical and radiographic findings of the two groups, substandard data-gathering information, and in particular lack of objective clinical evaluation in the latter patient population.

Similar to open laminectomy procedures, the arthroscopic microdiscectomy allows for extraction of posterior and posterolateral fragments and mechanical decompression of the nerve roots through an indirect posterolateral approach.[10,11,16]

The following mechanical, pathologic, anatomic, and biologic conditions may affect the outcome of minimal intervention disc surgery.

Mechanical Pressure on the Nerve Roots

The pathophysiology of pain associated with mechanical pressure or tension on the nerve roots has been the subject of numerous investigations and is well understood. The work of Parke,[26] Delamarter et al.,[5] Olmarker et al.,[23] and Hoyland et al.[8] have clearly demonstrated that the interference with the venous return of the nerve roots seen in association with disc herniation or mechanical foraminal obstruction may be responsible for venous congestion and perineural and intraneural fibrosis. The reduction of oxygen intake in the fibrotic and inflamed nerve root will in turn enhance the clinical manifestation of radicular pain. Rydevik et al.[29] have shown that the mechanical compression of the ganglion may produce intraneural edema associated with abnormal blood supply and pain syndrome.

The classic experimental work of Smyth and Wright[35] has shown that the pull of the nylon loop

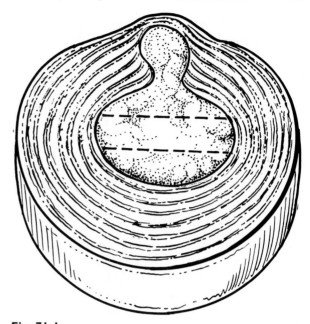

Fig. 71-1

Axial view of schematic drawing of intervertebral disc. Extraction of nucleus from anterior zone must be avoided. Attempt should be made to evacuate posterior zone and remove posterior herniated fragments.

that was passed around the nerve root during the laminectomy procedure reproduced the sciatic pain postoperatively. However, the pull of the dura, ligamentous flavum, and posterior longitudinal ligament caused localized pain and was not associated with radicular complaints. A similar phenomenon also has been demonstrated intraoperatively in the course of the laminectomy procedure under local anesthesia.[17]

In the clinical arena the dramatic relief of sciatica following surgical extraction of a sequestrated fragment has been a thrilling experience for both the patient and the operative surgeon. Any operative technique used for the surgical treatment of a truly symptom-producing herniated disc associated with mechanical pressure on the nerve root must provide the instrumentation and technology to reach and evacuate the posterior and posterolateral corners of the intervertebral disc. A simple core decompression or debulking of a herniated lumbar disc associated with posteriorly lodged collagenized fragment via a straight instrument is doomed to failure.[10,11,13,16] When the straight probe is used and an excess amount of nuclear tissue is removed from the anterior zone (Fig. 71-1) of the intervertebral disc, it may precipitate the posterior expulsion of a subligamentous fragment into the spinal canal. In contrast, a posterior nucleotomy or extraction of nuclear tissue from the posterior zone adjacent to the hernia-tion site may be adequate treatment of small disc herniations.

Anatomic Status of Perianular Structures

The posterolateral approach to the vertebral bodies was described by Craig[3] and Ottolenghi.[24] A simi-lar approach was later utilized for discography and chemonucleolysis. Although the latter approach was extensively used for both diagnosis and treatment purposes, the exact and safe site of entry and anular fenestration was never described or well understood. Extensive cadaveric and radiographic studies con-ducted at the Graduate Hospital in Philadelphia[12,13] led to the identification of a safe zone for fenestra-tion of the anulus and the introduction of the in-struments. The latter also provided the closest access to the posterior zone of the intervertebral disc, thus facilitating the extraction of the posterior and pos-terolateral fragments.

The anterior motor roots and the larger posterior sensory root converge inside the dural sheath, then they may leave the dura separately at the level of the nerve-root foramina. The posterior sensory root continues into the fusiform dorsal-root ganglia. The anterior and posterior roots then join to form the spinal nerve. The dorsal-root ganglia and the ante-rior motor fibers lie posteriorly in the foraminal space. Then they are positioned in the subpedicular notch with branches of lumbar artery, veins, and sinovertebral nerve.[25,27,28]

The spinal nerve then extends distally and later-ally and is positioned anterior to the transverse process of the distal segment. At this junction a triangular zone[11,12] is created that is suitable for safe introduction of instruments for spine surgery through a posterolateral approach. This triangular zone is bordered anteriorly by the spinal nerve, in-feriorly by the proximal plate of the lower vertebrae, and posteriorly by the superior articular process of the distal vertebrae.

The nerve-root complex and the spinal nerves are not fixed. This allows for a certain amount of mo-bility and gliding.[13,28] When a blunt-end instrument is inserted at a 35- to 45-degree angle from a dis-tance of 9 to 10 cm from the midline, it bypasses the spinal nerve before it reaches the anulus. For this reason, it is imperative that the operative surgeon hold the blunt end of the cannulated obturator against the anulus when the access cannula is being

positioned and the anulus fenestration is being car-ried out.

Although L5 radiculopathy is commonly associated with herniation of the intervertebral disc at the L4-L5 level, the L5 root is not subject to insult when the L4-L5 intervertebral disc is instrumented through the posterolateral approach. However, the L4 spinal nerve lies in the path of the inserted instruments.

The posterior longitudinal ligamentum in the lumbar region is detached and mobile at the level of the vertebral bodies. However, its fibers become somewhat interwoven with the superficial layer of the posterior and posterolateral anulus. Parke[25] has shown that the expansion of the posterior longitu-dinal ligament is enriched with sensory nerve fibers supplied by the sinovertebral nerve. This expansion extends laterally over the dorsolateral anulus beyond the nerve-root foramina. Fine filamentous or at times dense fibrous adhesions are found between the ventral dura and posterior longitudinal ligament.[1,18] The latter has prevented us from using a flexible endoscope for epiduroscopy.

The immunohistochemical method has been used to study the status of the innervation of the outer anulus, posterior longitudinal ligament, and facet joints. It has been demonstrated that all the above structures are well innervated.[40,41]

When the posterolateral approach is being used for arthroscopic discectomy, the incision of the an-ulus just outside the foramina may be associated with severe pain. Topical anesthetic or supplemental use of intravenous analgesics prior to anular fenestration may be necessary.

The iliac arteries and veins as well as bowel loops are all positioned anterior to the transverse processes and the intertransverse ligaments. For this reason, great care must be exercised to prevent vertical in-sertion of the needle at the onset of arthroscopic mi-crodiscectomy.

The improper needle positioning at the onset of arthroscopic microdiscectomy will be associated with the wrong placement of the subsequent in-struments and unsatisfactory evacuation of the pos-terior fragments. When the angle of insertion of the needle has not been predetermined by a preopera-tive CT study,[11] it is advisable to insert the needle close to the horizontal line in order to palpate the facet joints; then the operating surgeon, under flu-oroscopy control, is able to withdraw the needle and reinsert it in a more vertical plant until the tip of the needle is properly positioned in the triangular working zone. This maneuver prevents zealous ver-tical introduction of the needle, penetration of the

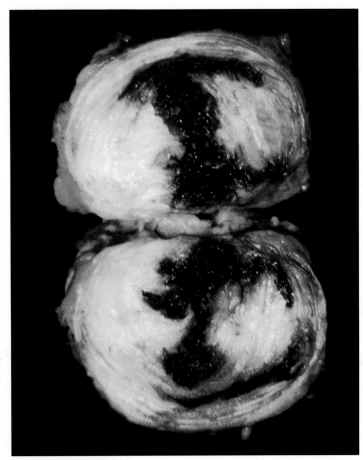

Plate II-1

Cadaveric study following injection of methylene blue into nucleus demonstrates torn, sclerotic, and inverted fibers of anulus, which separate anterior and posterior nuclear tissue by narrow isthmus.

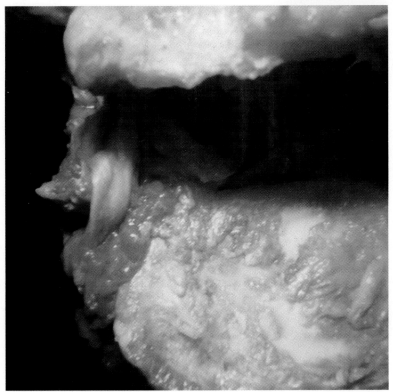

Plate II-2

Cross section of intervertebral disc at L4-L5 in 70-year-old male with slight reduction of height of intervertebral disc, marginal osteophytosis, and symmetrically bulged anulus. Complete derangement and dissication of internal structures of intervertebral disc is demonstrated. Note size and position of spinal nerve. Psoas muscle fibers are seen between anulus and spinal nerve at sight of entry during posterolateral access.

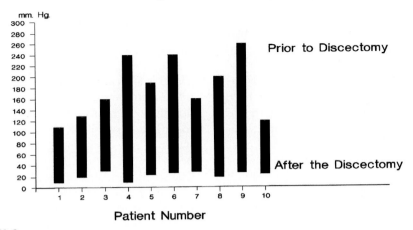

Fig. 71-2

In vivo study demonstrating reduction of intradiscal pressure following anular fenestration and partial nucleotomy *(From Kambin P, Brager M: Percutaneous postlateral discectomy anatomy and mechanism,* J Clin Orthop Relat Res 223:145, 1987.)

intertransverse ligament, and puncture of bowel or vascular structures.

Congenital anomaly of the nerve roots are not uncommon. Hasue et al.[7] reported an incidence of 8.5% abnormal roots in 59 cadavers studied.

Although the presence of extrapedicular communicating nerve fibers is extremely rare, they may interfere with the placement of the instruments for arthroscopic microdiscectomy. The clinical intraoperative expression of severe sciatic pain by the patient and arthroscopic visualization of the entry site are essential for proper protection of the latter. The degenerative changes of the spinal column may be associated with a torn, scarred, or thinned dura sleeve of the nerve roots. The injection of the neurotoxic opaque material during discography or the introduction of chymopapain in an uncontained disc may cause severe neurologic complications due to retrograde migration of the above substances and their contact with the neural tissue.[18]

Hydrostatic Pressure of the Intervertebral Disc

Nachemson's[20,21] classic work has clearly demonstrated the change in hydrostatic pressure of the intervertebral disc in various body positions associated with increase in the bulge of the anulus under load. Tzivian[37] and co-workers also utilized membrane-covered needles to evaluate the intradiscal pressure. The changes in the bulge of the anulus under axial load, flexion and extension also has been reported.[2,38]

Kambin and Brager used slit-tip catheters in an in vivo study to demonstrate the intradiscal pressure prior and following posterolateral anular fenestration and partial nucleotomy in 10 patients.[13] The mean rise of intradiscal pressure with the extension of the trunk with the patient in prone position was 181 mm Hg. Following the anular fenestration with a 5-mm trephine and partial nucleotomy, the pressure was reduced to mean level of 19.4 mm Hg. The finding was statistically significant (Fig. 71-2).

Sakamoto et al.[31] reported the reduction of intradiscal pressure up to 21 months after anular fenestration and mechanical nucleotomy.

It is known that the gelatigenous structure of the nucleus in young individuals behaves hydrostatically.[20,21,38] However, in a clinical arena almost all the disc herniations occur in an already degenerated intervertebral disc associated with dehydration of the nucleus pulposus and thickened, scarred, and partially torn anular fibers. The lasting effect of reduction of hydrostatic pressure of the intervertebral disc and alteration in the bulge of the anulus in the latter patient population by the nucleotomy technique remains highly questionable.

Postoperative Reduction of the Disc Height

The role of the dural ligament in root-compression syndrome has been described by Spencer and his co-workers.[32,33] The dural ligament consists of connective-tissue bands emerging from the ventral and lateral surface of the dura and proximal-root sleeve.

It then extends and joins the fibers of the posterior longitudinal ligament. The above ligament may play a role in pathogenesis of root-compression syndrome, either by tethering the nerve root over the disc protrusion or by applying traction on the fibers of the posterior longitudinal ligament. It has been suggested that the reduction of the height of the intervertebral disc that may occur following chemonucleolysis,[33] laminectomy, discectomy,[6,14] or extensive nucleotomy may be associated with relaxation of the dura ligament and diminishment of the intensity of compression of the nerve root.

Degenerative Status of Intervertebral Disc

For better understanding of the internal structures of intervertebral disc, a cadaveric study of 25 fresh lumbar intervertebral disc was initiated by Kambin et al.[15] A 20-gauge needle was inserted into the center of the intervertebral disc. A mixture of methylene blue and renografin-60 (Squibb Pharmaceutical) was then injected into the center of the intervertebral disc. This step was followed by radiographic examination, dissection, and pathologic evaluation. The disc degeneration was associated with thickened, scarred, and partially torn anular fibers. At times the inverted anular fibers were responsible for compartmentalization of the nuclear space. The expulsion of the collagenized nucleus to the periphery through an isthmus produced by torn inverted annular fibers was not uncommon (see color plate II-1). This finding explains the impotency of nucleotomy techniques for the treatment of posterior and posterolateral herniations. The extraction of the latter can be accomplished only by a direct laminotomy approach or use of deflecting instruments under endoscopic control through an access cannula inserted posterolaterally.

The older specimens showed significant bulging discs with thickened fibrotic anular fibers associated with severely dehydrated and desiccated nucleus (see color plate II-2). It is our belief that the extraction of the nucleus in the latter group will not alter the status of the anular protrusion and its clinical outcome. Most of these individuals presented with signs and symptoms of spinal stenosis that require decompression and at times stabilization.

Inflammatory Agents and Pain Syndrome

There is a growing literature to support the role of inflammatory agents in the production of pain. The dorsal horn of the spinal cord is enriched neuropeptide nerve fibers. Various neuropeptide (substance P and calcitonin gene–related peptide) have been located within the dorsal-root ganglion.[36,39] The level of inflammatory phospholipase A_2 activity in lumbar disc herniation was the subject of an interesting study at the San Francisco Spine Institute and was found to be elevated.[30]

Weinstein[40] has shown that the substance P and VIP (vasoactive intestinal peptide) in the dorsal-root ganglia may be indirectly affected by manipulation of intervertebral disc.

The role of low-frequency vibration in association with changes in the amount of substance P and VIP in the nerve-root ganglia has been reported.[41,42]

The review of this data suggest that the neuropeptide substances from the dorsal-root ganglia are expressed by anular neuroceptors and are seen in association with degenerative process or traumatic event. However, the role of chemical and inflammatory agents in pain production of an already compressed and inflamed nerve root secondary to mechanical compression is not clear and has not been defined.

References

1. Bilkra G: Intradiscal herniated lumbar disc, *J Biomech* 12:453, 1978.
2. Brown T, Hansen RJ, Yorra AJ: Some mechanical tests on the lumbosacral spine with particular reference to the intervertebral disc: a preliminary report, *J Bone Joint Surg* 39A:1135, 1957.
3. Craig F: Vertebral body biopsy, *J Bone Joint Surg* 38A:93, 1956.
4. Davis JK: Laser assisted percutaneous lumbar discectomy: KTP/532 clinical updated in neurosurgery, *Laserscope*, San Jose, CA, 1990.
5. Delamarter RB, Bohlman HH, Dodge LD, Biro C: Experimental lumbar spine stenosis, *J Bone Joint Surg* 72A:110, 1990.
6. Hanley E, Shapiro DE: The development of low back pain after excision of a lumbar disc, *J Bone Joint Surg* 71A:719, 1989.
7. Hasue M, Kikuchi S, Sakuyama Y, Ito T: Anatomic study of the interrelation between lumbosacral nerve roots and their surrounding tissues, *Spine* 8:50, 1983.
8. Hoyland JA, Freemont AJ, Jayson MIV: Intervertebral foramen venous obstruction: a cause of periradicular pain fibrosis, *Spine* 14:538, 1989.

9. Kahanovitz N, Viola K, Goldstein T, Dawson E: *A multi-center analysis of percutaneous discectomy*, Presented at the North American Spine Society meeting, Quebec City, June 29-July 2, 1989.

10. Kambin P: Arthroscopic microdiscectomy, Arthrosc: *J Arthrosc Relat Surg* 8:287, 1992.

11. Kambin P, editor: *Arthroscopic microdiscectomy, minimal intervention in spinal surgery*, Williams & Wilkins, Baltimore, 1990.

12. Kambin P: Percutaneous lumbar discectomy: current practice. *Surg Rounds Orthop* XX:31, 1988.

13. Kambin P, Brager M: Percutaneous posterolateral discectomy anatomy and mechanism, *Clin Orthop Relat Res* 223:145, 1987.

14. Kambin P, Brooks M, Cohen L, Schaffer J: *Comparative incidence of degenerative spondylosis of lumbar spine following discectomy*. Presented at the North American Spine Society meeting, Boston, July 9-11, 1992.

15. Kambin P, Nixon J, Chait A, Schaffer J: Annular protrusion: pathophysiology and roentgenographic appearance, *Spine* 13:671, 1988.

16. Kambin P, Schaffer J: Percutaneous lumbar discectomy—prospective review of 100 patients, *Clin Orthop* 238:24, 1989.

17. Kuslich SD, Ulstrom CL, Michael CJ: The tissue origin of low back pain and sciatica, *Orthop Clin North Am* 22:181, 1991.

18. MacMillan J, Schaffer J, Kambin P: Routes and incidence of lumbar discs with surrounding neural structures, *Spine* 16:167, 1991.

19. Mixter WJ, Barr JS: Rupture of the intervertebral disc with involvement of the spinal canal, *N Engl J Med* 211:210, 1934.

20. Nachemson A: Lumbar intradiscal pressure, *Acta Orthop Scand Suppl* 43:104, 1960.

21. Nachemson A: Disc pressure measurement, *Spine* 6:93, 1981.

22. Onik G, Helms C, Ginsberg L, Hoaglund T, Morris J: Percutaneous lumbar discectomy using a new aspiration probe, *A J R Am J Roentgenol* 144:1137, 1985.

23. Olmarker K, Rydevik B, Holms S: Edema formation in spinal nerve root induced by experimental gaded compression, *Spine* 14:569, 1989.

24. Ottolenghi CE: Vertebral body biopsy, aspiration biopsy, *J Bone Joint Surg* 37A:443, 1955.

25. Parke W: Anatomy of spinal nerve and its surrounding structures, *Semin Orthop* 6:1991.

26. Parke W: The significance of venous return impairment in ischemic radiculopathy and myelopathy, *Orthop Clin North Am* 22:213, 1991.

27. Rauschning W: Normal and pathologic anatomy of the lumbar root canals, *Spine* 12:1008, 1987.

28. Rydevik B, Brown M, Lundberg G: Pathoanatomy and pathophysiology of nerve root compression, *Spine* 9:7, 1984.

29. Rydevik B, Myers RR, Powell HC: Tissue fluid pressure in the dorsal root ganglion, an experimental study on the effects of compression, *Spine* 14:574, 1989.

30. Saal JS, Franson RC, Dobrow R, et al.: High levels of inflammatory phospholipase A_2 activity in lumbar disc herniations, *Spine* 15:674, 1990.

31. Sakamota T, Yamakawa H, Tajima T, Swaumi A: *A study of percutaneous lumbar nucleotomy and lumbar intradiscal pressure*. Presented at the International Symposium on Percutaneous Nucleotomy, Bruxelles, March 17-18, 1989.

32. Spencer DL, Irwin GS, Miller JAA: Anatomy and significance of fixation of the lumbosacral nerve roots in sciatica, *Spine* 8:672, 1983.

33. Spencer DL, Miller JAA, Bertolini JE: The effect of intervertebral disc space narrowing on the contact force between the nerve root and a simulated disc protrusion, *Spine* 9:422, 1984.

34. Smith L: Enzyme dissolution of the intervertebral disc, *Nature* 4887:198, 1963.

35. Smyth MJ, Wright V: Sciatica and the intervertebral disc: an experimental study, *J Bone Joint Surg* 40A:1401, 1958.

36. Takahashi T, Otsuka M: Regional distribution of substance P in the spinal cord and nerve roots of the cat and the effect of dorsal root section, *Brain Res* 87:1, 1975.

37. Tzivian IL, Rayhinstein VH, Motov VF, Ovseychik JG: Results of clinical study of pressure within the intervertebral lumbar discs, *Ortop Travmatol Protez* 6:31, 1971.

38. Virgin WJ: Experimental investigation into the physical properties of the intervertebral disc, *J Bone Joint Surg* 33B:607, 1951.

39. Wall PO, Devor M: Sensory afferent impulses originated from dorsal root ganglion and chronically injured axons: a physiological basis for radicular pain of nerve root compression, *Pain* 17:321, 1983.

40. Weinstein J: Neurogenic and nonneurogenic pain and inflammatory mediators, *Orthop Clin North Am* 22:235, 1991.

41. Weinstein J, Claverie W, Gibson S: The pain of discography, *Spine* 13:1344, 1988.

42. Weinstein J, Pope M, Schmidt R, Seroussi R: Neuropharmacologic effects of vibration on the dorsal horn ganglion: an animal model, *Spine* 13:521, 1988.

Section 2
Minimally Invasive Surgery of the Lumbar Spine

72 Chemonucleolysis

James W. Simmons, Jr.
Eugene J. Nordby

73 Arthroscopic Microdiscectomy

Parviz Kambin

74 Automated Percutaneous Lumbar Discectomy

Gary Onik

75 Microsurgical Discectomy and Spinal Decompression

Bradford DeLong

76 Laser Surgery

Henry Sherk
J.A. Sazy

77 Arthroscopic Lumbar Interbody Fusion

Parviz Kambin

78 Myeloscopic and Endoscopic Herniectomy

Yoshio Ooi
Youkichi Sato
Fujio Mita
Jonathan Schaffer

Chapter 72
Chemonucleolysis

James W. Simmons, Jr.
Eugene J. Nordby

History of Clinical Use

Pharmaceutical and Regulatory History

Biochemistry and Toxicology

    description
    metabolism
    effect on surrounding tissue
    effect on blood vessels
    effect on nerve tissue
    antigenicity

Clinical Trials

Indications

    general criteria
    patient selection
    age considerations

Contraindications

Complications

Operative Technique

Summary and Future Predictions

"If the science of medicine is not to be lowered to the rank of a mere technical profession, it must preoccupy itself with its history"

Emile Littre (1801–1881)

History of Clinical Use

The clinical use of the enzyme chymopapain to dissolve herniated nuclear material chemically was first reported in 1963 by Lyman Smith.[28] He coined the term chemonucleolysis to describe the treatment of intervertebral disc lesions with intradiscal injections of chymopapain.

Decades earlier, in 1941, Jansen and Balls[13] isolated chymopapain from crude papain derived from the latex of the fruit of Carica papaya. In addition to chymopapain, papaya latex contains the enzymes protease, lysozyme, and papain.

Lewis B. Thomas,[36] in 1956, was the first to demonstrate the enzymatic effects of crude papain on the mucoid portion of cartilage. He observed that, within 18 hours after rabbits were injected with a solution of crude papain, their ears drooped. It was noted that "apart from the unusual cosmetic effect" the animals exhibited no evidence of systemic illness or discomfort. Although the structural integrity of the ear cartilage was disrupted, the ears replenished the basophilic chondroid matrix and regained their original shape within 48 hours. Larger doses of injected papain had an impact on joint cartilage, epiphyseal growth plate, and tracheal and bronchial cartilage.

Intrigued by Thomas' article, Smith postulated a possible therapeutic use in chondroplastic tumors. Although chymopapain was found to have no effect on tumors, he found that intradiscal injection in rabbits removed the nucleus pulposus, while leaving the annulus largely intact.[28]

Smith later injected chymopapain into the lumbar intervertebral discs of 22 dogs previously paralyzed because of herniation of the discs; 14 demonstrated a reversal of their paralysis. A postmortem analysis failed to demonstrate any adverse effects attributable to the enzyme. This study laid the foundation for the clinical use of chymopapain.

The initial surgical technique used by Smith in 1963 was the posterolateral approach, in which the needle passes laterally to the dura but within the bony canal and into the center of the disc.[28] The lateral approach for injecting the lumbar discs came into use during a series of studies by Smith and Brown[29] in 1967. This method was rapid and offered less resistance, compared to the resistance of bone, because the needle passed through the soft tissue. This study also confirmed that the use of sodium diatrizoate in discography should be avoided because of its allergenic quality.

In 1971 McNab et al.,[19] reported the results were seen in patients injected with chymopapain. The best results were seen in patients with severe sciatica of short duration associated with marked root tension signs. The worst results were in patients displaying obesity, diabetes, or emotional breakdown.

Pharmaceutical and Regulatory History

After Smith injected the first patient with Discase (chymopapain) in 1963,[28] 75 investigators in the United States and Canada eventually injected about 17,000 patients in the Phase III trial, which ended in July 1975.

A controversial study done at Walter Reed Army Medical Center in 1975[25] triggered the withdrawal of the New Drug Application that had been filed with the Food and Drug Administration (FDA) for use in the treatment of intervertebral disc disease with Discase. This study reported no statistical difference in instance or quality of improvement between the placebo group (49% success rate) and the group tested with Discase (58% success rate). Brown and Daroff[2] criticized the Walter Reed Army Medical Center study because of (1) the early code break,

(2) the lack of inert placebo, (3) the insufficient dose of Discase, and (4) the lack of technical expertise.

Physicians in the United States who had been using the drug with excellent results were disheartened when no progress was made toward an FDA approval. Many patients were referred to Canada for chymopapain. During this time, investigational use of chymopapain continued in Australia and England. A Yugoslavian product (Lekopain) was widely used in the Eastern Bloc countries and to a lesser extent in France and Italy with favorable results.

When no significant progress was made in gaining federal approval for chymopapain, efforts were made to bypass the FDA, and legislation was passed in Illinois, Indiana, and Texas to allow use of chymopapain within each state. Only Texas, however, had a climate conducive to growing papaya fruit, the source of the crude latex required for the manufacture of the finished drug product. As a result, the product Chemolase was developed in Texas and became legal to use in September 1979. A review of 919 patients who underwent chemonucleolysis with Chemolase in Texas between 1981 and 1982 demonstrated a 93% success rate with no deaths.[26]

In 1979, Smith Laboratories developed Chymodiactin, a new formula of chymopapain.[5] In 1981, the results of a randomized double-blind study authorized by the FDA showed composite successful results in 82% of those receiving Chymodiactin and 41% of those who received placebos. No major complications were reported in the 108 patients.[14] In Illinois, a second open study of 1498 patients resulted in a 90% success rate.[18] In this study, however, there were four cases of anaphylactic shock resulting in two fatalities and one case of acute transverse myelitis. An extensive follow-up study failed to establish a causal relationship between chemonucleolysis and acute transverse myelitis.

In November 1982, Chymodiactin received FDA approval and in January 1984, the FDA approved Discase. In the intervening years 6214 doctors attended instructional courses on intradiscal therapy developed by a joint committee of the American Association of Neurological Surgeons (AANS) and the American Academy of Orthopaedic Surgeons (AAOS). In addition, full sets of educational materials on intradiscal therapy were provided to each residency program in neurosurgery and orthopedic surgery.

In spite of the educational effort, Chymopapain administration in more than 120,000 patients resulted in 46 serious neurologic complications, including hemiparesis and paraplegia resulting from in-

trathecal injection. In August 1984, the *FDA Drug Bulletin*[6] recommended modification of chymopapain administration procedures. Smith Laboratories and Baxter Laboratories sold their rights to a larger company, Boots Pharmaceuticals, in part because of the expense in obtaining product liability insurance. Boots Pharmaceuticals discontinued Baxter's Discase and continues to manufacture Chymodiactin.

Biochemistry and Toxicology

Description

Chymopapain, a proteolytic enzyme derived from papaya latex, hydrolyzes the noncollagenous protein that interconnects long-chain mucopolysaccharide. When injected into the nucleus pulposus of the lumbar intervertebral disc, it binds tightly to the mucopolysaccharide protein complex and rapidly hydrolyzes the noncollagenous polypeptides,[8,30] which are responsible for the strong water-binding capacity of the nucleus pulposis.[12,20,21] This liberation of the polysaccharide (GAG) side chains results in loss of their capacity to bind water molecules, which then diffuse out of the cartilaginous matrix of the disc. Depolymerization of the nucleus pulposus lowers the intradiscal pressure and provides relief from the pain.

As manufactured today, Chymodiactin differs from the original formulation by the removal of one protein electrophoretic peak, the omission of sodium bisulfite, which never proved itself as a stabilizer, and the omission of disodium edetate, since no heavy metals should be present in a purified product. In this formulation, Chymodiactin is stable with refrigeration (36° F to 46° F) for up to 3 years.

For more than a quarter of a century, studies have been done on the pharmacology and toxicology of chymopapain[9,10] and a number of clinical trials have been published using chymopapain to accomplish chemonucleolysis.[7,14] Early studies used the weight of the enzyme as the unit of measure, while later work used enzyme activity, which was measured in a variety of ways. As a result, evaluating and comparing the resulting data in any quantitative way is difficult. Standardized interpretation is further complicated by the fact that the enzyme was isolated from a botanical product, which means purity and enzyme activity may have varied with the source and extraction procedure. Because of these uncertainties, a series of three animal studies were done with Chemolase to establish a median lethal dose, identify the pharmacology and toxicology following intradiscal injection, and ascertain the sensitization potential.[27]

Metabolism

The pharmacologic use of chymopapain is contingent on its specific localization. After intradiscal injection, chymopapain or its immunologically reactive fragments diffuse rapidly into the plasma. Chymopapain is absorbed into the blood and is deactivated by the α_2-macroglobulins, a general inhibitor of proteolytic enzymes present in all tissue fluids and sera. After diffusion from the disc, the enzyme remaining bound to the proteoglycan (GAG) and its fragments pass into the circulation and are excreted in the urine, resulting in a moderate increase in urinary acid. Chymopapain is further deactivated by cathepsins and the production of specific antibodies within 7 days.

Effect on Surrounding Tissue

Chymopapain degrades the nucleus pulposus, but the annulus fibrosus remains essentially intact because of its largely collagenous composition. While that allows narrowing of the disc space, in younger tissue reconstitution occurs within a year. Although this indicated that the chondrocyte-mediated synthesis of nuclear proteins is not irrevocably impaired, the phenomenon is dose-related.[1] Doses of enzyme beyond the therapeutic range have no deleterious effect on ligaments, bone, or dura. The margin of safety is reduced, however, should the enzyme enter the subarachnoid space through improper injection. Any variation in placement of the enzyme decreases the desired pharmacologic effect and greatly increases the toxic effect. An intrathecal injection can cause subarachnoid hemorrhage.

Effect on Blood Vessels

Most toxic effects of chymopapain injection result from the proteolysis of glucosaminoglycan in the capillary wall, thereby destroying the endothelial-cell cement (see Chymopapain Toxicology box). Large doses can cause lethal systemic hemorrhage, which is most commonly intrathecal (see Intrathecal Toxicity box). Studies in mice and rats show hemorrhage into the thoracic cavity.[27] The resultant compressive effects of such bleeding can cause paraplegia or death. This catastrophic complication can be prevented in experimental animals by venting the dura with a needle or by opening a flap. If the animal recovers, no residual arachnoiditis is identified. Vessels other than capillaries have a fibrous cover that prevents chymopapain from having any effect on

Chymopapain Toxicology*

1. Mechanism: proteolysis of capillaries, GAG structure
2. Lethality: systemic—from petechial hemorrhage, clots; intrathecal—from cerebrospinal fluid pressure increase
3. Does not affect: sensory or motor nerves (5 mg [2500 units]/kg) dura mater; collagen; heart rate, blood pressure; clotting factors

From Stern IJ: *The biochemistry and toxicology of chymopapain.* In Brown JE, Nordby EJ, Smith L, editors: *Chemonucleolysis,* Thorofare, NJ, 1985, Slack, p 11, with permission.
*Limited by serum inhibition

Intrathecal Toxicity

Mechanism: capillary rupture—cerebrospinal fluid pressure increase via petechial hemorrhage

Cisternal tap controls pressure and prevents death

From Stern IJ: *The biochemistry and toxicology of chymopapain.* In Brown JE, Nordby EJ, Smith L, editors: *Chemonucleolysis,* Thorofare, NJ, 1985, Slack, p 11, with permission.

them.[31] In dogs, there is no measurable effect on heart rate, blood pressure, or clotting factors. The median lethal dose of intravenously administered chymopapain has been found to be 82 mg/kg in mice and 92 mg/kg in rats.[31]

Effect on Nerve Tissue

Because chymopapain does not directly affect sensory and motor nerves or dura mater, it is not neurotoxic. The spinal nerves are not affected by epidural application of chymopapain because they are protected by a fibrous covering. A further margin of safety is provided by the likely inactivation of the enzyme by plasma α_2-macroglobulin.[10,39] Garvin and associates[9] showed that the epidural injection of chymopapain on dogs, even up to a lethal dose, did not penetrate the intact dura. Experiments showing axonal death or intraneural fibrosis are all secondary to interference with the capillary microcirculation exposed to the enzyme.

Antigenicity

As with all foreign proteins, chymopapain can induce antibody production. The potential for anaphylactic reaction is a major complication attributable to the use of chymopapain. About 1% of the world's population has potential for reaction to the pure chymopapain protein because of prior cross-reactive exposure to the antigen through commercial sources of papain, such as meat tenderizers, papaya fruit, beer, toothpaste, digestive aids, cosmetics, contact lens–washing solutions, laboratory reagents, and some treated leathers.[35] Studies have confirmed the high antigenicity for chymopapain that has been reported, further underscoring the care with which the enzyme should be administered.[27]

Sensitivity to chymopapain can be detected prior to injection by skin testing or direct measurement of the patient's antibodies (IgE) by tests such as RAST (radioallergosorbent test) or FAST (fluorescent allergosorbent test). While all procedures can detect sensitivity to chymopapain, it should be noted that anaphylaxis has been reported following epidermal injection for skin test.[15]

Even if all tests for sensitivity have negative results, the highly antigenic property of chymopapain emphasizes the importance of precise placement of the enzyme into the nucleus pulposus in order to benefit from the binding and localization of the enzyme at this site.[27]

Clinical Trials

Chymopapain has undergone rigorous clinical investigation. The early studies of chymopapain in humans suffered from methodologic problems, and the equivocal results generated significant controversy. In the wake of this controversy, new clinical trials were designed to evaluate a new formulation of chymopapain for herniated lumbar intervertebral disc disease in patients with sciatica, taking into consideration a knowledge of previous problems and the elements necessary for well-controlled clinical trials.

The definitive study demonstrating the clinical efficacy of chymopapain was a multicenter, randomized, double-blind, placebo-controlled trial involving 108 patients that was conducted in the United States.[12] At 6 weeks postinjection, Chymodiactin was judged a success in 75% of patients as compared to a 45% success rate for placebo ($p = 0.003$). When measured at 6 months or at the last visit before subsequent surgical intervention, the placebo success rate dropped to 38%, while chymopapain's success rate remained unchanged ($p > 0.001$). When the placebo failures were then treated with chymopapain, 91% responded with partial or total relief of their symptoms. No deaths or serious adverse experiences occurred during this clinical trial.

An open-label, multicenter study of Chymodiactin in 1498 patients confirmed the results of the double-blind study and indicated that, with careful patient selection, success rates ranging from 80% to 90% can be realized. During this open-label trial, two patients died of complications of anaphylaxis, one patient experienced transverse myelitis, and one patient had cauda equina.

Indications

General Criteria

Approximately 80% of patients who experience leg pain from disc displacement will respond favorably to conservative measures, such as bed rest, exercise, anti-inflammatory drugs, body corset, epidural blocks, physical therapy, and traction. Only after all conservative resources have failed should more aggressive treatment be considered.

Chymopapain is indicated in the treatment of unremitting sciatica due to a proven herniated nucleus pulposus that has not responded to adequate conservative management. Because chymopapain acts by changing the water-binding properties of the nucleus mucoprotein, only problems of discogenic origin will benefit from chemonucleolysis. Other causes of sciatica, such as lateral recess stenosis, with not respond.

Chemonucleolysis is contraindicated when profound acute or progressive neurologic changes, particularly the cauda equina syndrome, require adequate neural decompression. Stated simply, the ideal candidate for chemonucleolysis is also the appropriate candidate for elective disc surgery, but the reverse is not always true.

Patient Selection

A series of diagnostic steps will aid the judgment of the surgeon. A complete medical history should be taken that includes the following: allergies, history of symptoms, total duration of back pain, total duration of sciatica, location of sciatica, other significant medical history, and list of medications. In addition, neurologic and muscle testing should include muscle strength testing, deep tendon reflexes, sensation, mechanical tests, sciatic stretch, sitting straight leg raising, and supine straight leg raising.

Neurologic and musculoskeletal assessment, including the evaluation of sensation, muscle strain, and deep tendon reflexes should be well recorded. The mechanical and sciatic stretch test should include sitting and supine straight leg raising, weakness, muscle wasting, and dermatomal dysesthesia. All of these tests and assessments contribute to the clinical diagnosis of radiculopathy, secondary to herniated nucleus pulposus, which must be responsive to chemonucleolysis.

In addition, laboratory studies include routine lumbosacral roentgenographic studies, CT scan, myelography, enhanced CT scan, discography, electromyography, and MRI.

Age Considerations

Age is also a factor when selecting a patient for chemonucleolysis with chymopapain. In adults over age 60, for example, there may be sufficient degeneration to have depleted the mucoprotein in the nucleus pulposus. On the other hand, patients in their early 80s have shown relatively normal hydrated discs on MRI, and theoretically could respond to chymopapain.

There are very few studies of patients under age 20. Sutton has reported results that are 96% satisfactory in 24 patients under the age of 19, as compared to an age-matched cohort previously subjected to open discectomy.[32,34] Lorenz et al.[16] treated 55 adolescents, with 80% successful results.

Contraindications

The major specific contraindications to chemonucleolysis with chymopapain include allergy to papain or papaya (see Contraindications of Chymopapain Injection box). It is widely held that a history of previous chymopapain injection, with its potential for having sensitized the individual, is a clear contraindication. This belief is challenged by Sutton.[33] In a series of 33 reinjections, prior serum testing (Chymofast test) to determine the IgE titer indicated reaction in only 9% of the patients. The last 12 patients in Sutton's series were pretreated with H_1 and H_2 blockers, and there were no allergic reactions.

Pregnancy is a contraindication to treatment with chemonucleolysis. No studies have been done on pregnant women or to determine the effect of chymopapain on fetal development.

The differential diagnosis must not indicate the possibility of spinal cord tumor, metastatic cancer, vertebral osteomyelitis, or disc space infection. X-ray findings should not indicate mechanical insufficiency, spinal stenosis, severe spondylolisthesis, blockage by cervical or thoracic disc as demonstrated

Contraindications of Chymopapain Injection

Absolute
  Allergy to chymopapain
  Cauda equina syndrome—bowel or bladder paresis
  Pregnancy
  Normal discogram

Relative
  Diabetes with peripheral neuropathy
  Spinal stenosis
  Spondylolisthesis, severe
  Old infection of the disc or vertebrae
  Osteoarthritic spur as source of nerve-root pressure
  Extensive osteoarthritis to prevent needle insertion
  Repeat injection of chymopapain
  Allergy to iodine-containing compounds
  Unsuccessful surgery at symptomatic level
  Emotional instability
  Medicolegal cases
  Language barrier

From Nordby EJ: *Diagnosis and patient selection.* In Brown JE, Nordby EJ, Smith L, editors: *Chemonucleolysis,* Thorofare, NJ, 1985, Slack, p 45, with permission.

on myelography, inability to reach disc space via a lateral route, or intrathecal or intravascular flow of contrast dye with discography.

Progressive significant neurologic change such as cauda equina syndrome is a specific contraindication because the response to chymopapain is time-dependent and does not provide the essential prompt relief of neural pressure.

Clearly, the most absolute and obvious contraindication to chemonucleolysis with chymopapain is the finding of a normal disc on discography or MRI.

In addition to these specific contraindications, there are a number of relative contraindications that must be weighed carefully. Osteoarthritis, shown radiographically, may obstruct needle insertion. Since it is possible to rekindle latent infections, history or evidence of old infection of the disc or vertebrae must be considered. Unsuccessful prior open discectomy may inhibit a successful outcome because of the presence of fibrosis. Other relative contraindications include diabetes mellitus, depending on its severity and control, and the presence of neuropathy.

Complications

A review of all "serious" and "unexpected" events reported to the FDA since approval of Chymodiactin (chymopapain for injection) in 1982 covering 121 patients among some 135,000 treated in the United States prior to 1991 has been completed.[23] Included are 7 fatal cases of anaphylaxis, 24 infections, 32 hemorrhagic problems, 32 neurologic complications, and 16 miscellaneous events, with a mortality rate of 0.019%.

Between 1982 and 1989 only 385 anaphylactic reactions occurred among a group of 77,181 patients treated with Chymodiactin, for an incidence of 0.50%. This, however, is misleading because there has been a decrease in frequency over the years, the final year of compilation giving an incidence of only 0.20%.

The anaphylaxis and infections following injection are considered related to chymopapain itself or to the lack of asepsis in its administration. Only 17 (21%) of the 80 hemorrhagic, neurologic, and miscellaneous events can be related to chymopapain or the manner in which it was injected.

Better evaluation of patients in their selection as candidates for injection of chymopapain appears to be the means of eliminating many of the unexpected events.

In spite of the concern for any untoward reactions, a comparison with postoperative discectomy complications shows that neurologic events are 4.7 per 10,000 patients with chemonucleolysis and 29.8 with discectomy or six times less with injection. Infection is 1.8 per 10,000 patients with chymopapain and 30.7 with surgery. Mortality figures are 1.9 per 10,000 patients for chymopapain and 5.9 for laminectomy. Neither of these mortality rates is necessarily related to surgery or chemonucleolysis.

Operative Technique

The chemonucleolysis procedure should be performed in an operating room by a qualified orthopedic surgeon or neurosurgeon. The facilities must be able to supply ample fluoroscopic equipment (radiolucent table, C-arm fluoroscope with image intensifier, equipment to take anteroposterior lateral x-ray films of the lumbar spine during surgery), sterile surgical atmosphere, and presterilized surgical equipment.

The patient is carefully placed on the operating table in a left lateral decubitus position (Fig. 72-1) on a stationary fluoroscopic table and fastened securely to the table with adhesive tape to avoid vary-

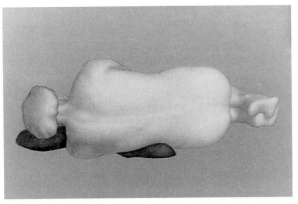

Fig. 72-1

The patient is placed in the left lateral decubitis position with appropriate padding for comfort and padding in the flank to maintain position of the spine in the horizontal position. (Courtesy of Steve Scofield, Boots Pharmaceuticals.)

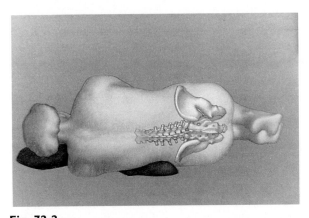

Fig. 72-2

The patient in the left lateral decubitis position with padding and the available landmarks in the appropriate relationship noting in particular the posterior superior iliac spine, iliac crest and the spinus processes. (Courtesy of Steve Scofield, Boots Pharmaceuticals.)

ing from a true lateral position. A portable C-arm fluoroscope is then placed over the stationary table, enabling the surgeon to have biplanar fluoroscopic control. The spine is properly centered and any curvatures of the spine corrected either by inflatable cushion or rolled towel placed in the flank (above the iliac crest) and by the rotating of hips. Proper positioning facilitates easier access to the lumbar disc. Both the lateral and anteroposterior views of the spine are monitored.

The posterior superior iliac spine, iliac crest, and the spinous processes are located (Fig. 72-2) and marked with a marking pen. With a ruler, the area 8 to 10 cm lateral to the tip of the spinous process is marked. This mark is lined up with the intervertebral disc for the point of entrance into the skin. A surgical preparation and drape are done.

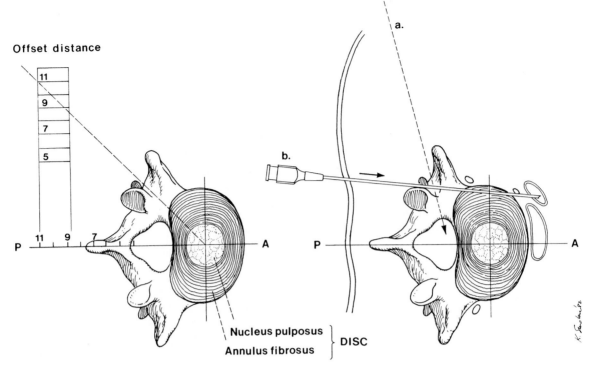

Offset distance

Offset distance is equal
to depth of disc center

Fig. 72-3

Left, triangulation necessary for three dimensional perception of the needle placement. *Right,* the hazards in malplacement of the needle anterior. (Courtesy of Ned Froning, M.D. [deceased].)

There are several technical considerations. First, when the tip of the advancing needles reaches a line adjoining the posterior borders of the vertebral bodies, one should obtain a firm gritty sensation from the anulus. If the tip of the needle passes anterior to this line before the sensation is obtained, the needle will not bisect the disc but will pass anterior and lateral to it (Fig. 72-3). If this occurs, the needle should be inserted at a more acute angle to the sagittal plane. If the angle is to be changed, the needle should first be withdrawn close to the skin surface beyond the lumbodorsal fascia. There may be bony obstructions by the transverse process, the pars interarticularis, or the facet joint. The structures causing bony obstruction can be determined on the lateral roentgenographic projection. Obstruction at the level of the upper half of the vertebral body is probably due to the pars interarticularis. Opposite the disc space, obstruction is probably due to the facet joint. If the transverse process causes obstruction, the site of the needle insertion is moved in a cephalad direction for the L4 intervertebral disc space. If the pars interarticularis or fact joint causes obstruction, the angle of the needle insertion needs to be

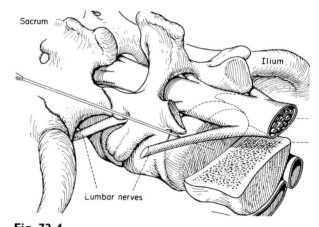

Fig. 72-4

Three dimensional concept of the needle placement. (Courtesy of Ned Froning, M.D. [deceased].)

reduced. However, problems arise if too much attention is paid to the angle of the needle insertion and too little to the overall size and shape of the patient. A clear, three-dimensional mental image of the lower lumbar region is essential (Fig. 72-4). The articulated specimen of the spine in the operating room is helpful.

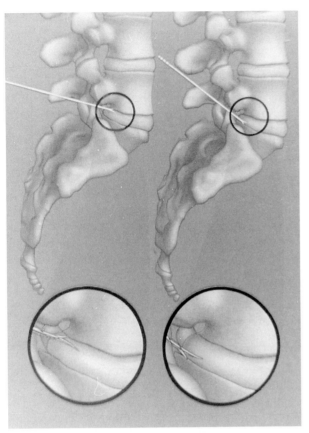

Fig. 72-5

Left, the needle is malpositioned slightly cephalad. *Right*, the needle is malpositioned slightly caudad. (Courtesy of Steve Scofield, Boots Pharmaceuticals.)

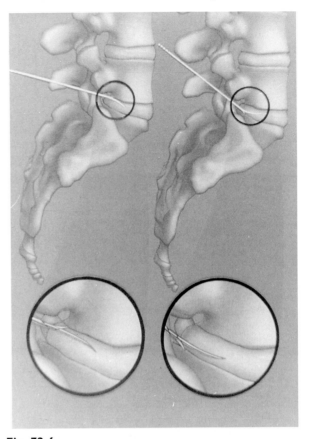

Fig. 72-6

Left, correction of malplacement of the needle cephalad using the bevel position cephalad. *Right*, correction of the needle malpositioned caudad by placing the bevel in the caudad direction. (Courtesy of Steve Scofield, Boots Pharmaceuticals.)

For the L5 intervertebral disc space, the image intensifier is repositioned laterally. The L4 needle may serve as a landmark and guide to the position of the L5 disc space. The L5 needle is inserted at the same angle to the sagittal plane, i.e., 30 degrees, but is directed approximately 45 degrees caudally. This angle is adjusted until the tip of the needle is level and adjacent to the posterior aspect of the vertebral bodies (the L5 disc space). This is of great importance in assessing bony obstruction. Obstruction by the transverse process necessitates reducing the angle of the needle relative to the sagittal plane. There are occasions when a broad transverse process of L5 obstructs this approach. If this occurs, the double-needle technique is used: A 22-gauge needle is placed through an 18-gauge one with the tip of the 18-gauge needle laying just at the level of the inferior of the L5 vertebral body. By curving the distal half inch of the 22-gauge needle with the bevel up, the needle will curve downward and into the L5 intervertebral disc space as it passes out of the tip of the 18-gauge needle (Figs. 72-5 and 72-6). Once

the surgeon has visually verified the correct needle tip placement using the image intensifier, a deionized water-soluble contrast medium is injected. Resistance to flow will give some indication as to the integrity of the disc. The pattern outlined by the dye will give an indication of the morphology and continuity of the anulus.

Lumbar discography is an important step to determine the integrity of the disc before the actual injection of the disc with chymopapain. Inject an adequate amount of dye in the herniated disc to fill the disc. Although an epidural leakage of dye occurs, it is not a contraindication to chemonucleolysis. The procedure should be abandoned in the rare occurrence that contrast material leaks into the subdural or subarachnoid space. A normal disc will have a very high resistance to the flow of the contrast material, a prolapsed disc or herniated disc displaying moderate resistance and a severely degenerated disc demonstrating no resistance. To determine the state of the intervertebral disc in question coordinate the resistance of the flow with the visual monitoring of the dye. Radiograms consisting of anteroposterior and lateral views are taken. Wait at least 10 minutes after injecting the dye for assessment of a possible allergy to the dye.

Chymodiactin is supplied sterile and lyophilized. It is reconstituted with 2.0 ml of sterile water for injection, USP (see insert for directions). Inject 0.2 ml of chymopapain and allow 10 minutes to observe the patient for an anaphylactic response. The remainder of the enzyme (2000 to 4000 pKat units) may be injected if no reaction has occurred within 10 minutes. Inject the enzyme slowly to allow adequate flow and binding of the chymopapain. Slowly remove the needles 3 to 5 minutes after the injection. If no reaction occurs and all vital signs remain stable, the patient may be moved to the recovery room.

Summary and Future Predictions

The first enzyme clinically injected as specific treatment for a disorder in humans, chymopapain, has been shown to provide a procedure that is safe and effective in the short and long term in relieving radiculitis in properly selected patients. More than 160,000 patients in the United States and 300,000 worldwide have been treated with chemonucleolysis.

Studies in rabbits by Williams et al.[38] and Hayashi[11] show that the maximum degradation of the proteoglycans in the nucleus pulposus occurs at a relatively low dose, and in the highest doses the annulus and end plates are digested. Darakjian and Wiltse[4] and others have shown that in a small clinical series, the use of 500 to 700 pKat units per disc have produced successful results. In the future, the optimal dose of chymopapain may prove to be lower than the currently recommended 2000 to 4000 pKats per disc.

There is mounting evidence from France and Spain[3] of the effectiveness of chymopapain in cervical disc herniation. Its acceptance, however, will probably require well-controlled studies with careful patient selection to ensure that the cervical nerve-root compression is not a result of pressure of bony origin, which of course will not respond to chymopapain.

After review of the Soviet employment of chymopapain in the reduction of idiopathic scoliosis in youngsters, there will likely be interest in more studies among this group of candidates. It has been learned that even with the correction obtained, fusion must augment the chemonucleolysis to maintain correction into adulthood.[37]

Another use for chymopapain has been patented. The process, which utilized chymopapain for enzymatic release of stem cells from immunomagnetic microspheres, has received approval for a clinical trial in patients undergoing bone marrow transplantation. The interesting point is that the chymopapain does not harm the fragile cell wall in this procedure.

While many of the former practioners of chemonucleolysis have experimented with automated percutaneous lumbar discectomy, they are now returning to chemonucleolysis. Leon Wiltse reports that chemonucleolysis is "better than percutaneous discectomy . . . and it will enjoy a comeback."[40] John McCulloch said, "automated percutaneous discectomy has been practiced for more than five years in the United States, but over enthusiasm combined with an almost total lack of serious scientific study has virtually destroyed any potential. In my opinion, this procedure does not have a future."[17]

Although not without a history of complications, chemonucleolysis for the excision of a herniated nucleus pulposus is subject to significantly fewer incidents than those recorded for open surgical intervention.[24] No serious complications have occurred in the past 6 years. In the United States, a gradual but persistent return to the use of chymopapain may be attributed to the increased awareness that the most serious neurologic adverse effects have been shown to result from faulty technique and poor patient selection. The only true complication of chemonuleolysis, anaphylaxis, has been controlled with the widespread use of sensitivity screening such as the ChymoFAST test. We conclude that after more than 25 years of clinical use and scientific scrutiny, no other enzyme or percutaneous procedure has withstood the test of time. The research into the optimal dose and uses of chymopapain in other areas continue, and chemonucleolysis has been firmly established as a safe, effective treatment for sciatica as a result of a herniated nucleus pulposus.

References

1. Bradford DS, Oegema TR Jr, Cooper M, et al.: Chymopapain, chemonucleolysis and nucleus pulposus regeneration: biological and biochemical study, *Spine* 9:135, 1984.
2. Brown M, Daroff RB: The double-blind study comparing discase to placebo: an editorial comment, *Spine* 2:33, 1977.
3. Castresana FG, Herrero CV, Horche JBL: *Cervical chemonucleolysis: three years of experience: presentation of 34 cases.* Presented at the International Intradiscal Therapy Society meeting, Nice, France, 1992.

4. Darakjian HE, Wiltse LL: *Low-dose chymopapain as a safe alternative to laminectomy.* Presented at the 3rd annual meeting of the International Intradiscal Therapy Society (IITS), Marbella, Spain, March 7-11, 1990.

5. Data on file, Boots Pharmaceuticals, Inc. Lincolnshire, IL.

6. FDA Drug Bull 14(2), August, 1984.

7. Fraser RD: Chymopapain for the treatment of intervertebral disc herniation: a preliminary report of a double-blind study, *Spine* 7:608, 1982.

8. Garvin PJ, Jennings RB: Long term effects of chymopapain on intervertebral discs of dogs, *Clin Orthop* 9:281, 1973.

9. Garvin PG, et all: Chymopapain: a pharmacologic and toxicologic evaluation in experimental animals, *Clin Orthop* 41:204, 1965.

10. Gesler RM: Pharmacologic properties of chymopapain, *Clin Orthop* 67:47, 1969.

11. Hayashi K: Chymopapain, *J Jpn Orthop Assoc* 65:216, 1991.

12. Hendry NGC: The hydration of the nucleous pulposus and its relation to intervertebral disc degeneration, *J Bone Joint Surg* 40B:132, 1958.

13. Jansen EF, Balls AK: Chymopapain: a new crystalline proteinase from papaya latex, *J Biol Chem* 137:459, 1941.

14. Javid MD, Nordby EJ, Ford LT, et al.: Safety and efficacy of chymopapain (Chymodiactin®) in herniated nucleus pulposus with sciatica: results of a randomized, double-blind study, *JAMA* 249:2489, 1983.

15. Lockey RF, Benedict LM, Turkeltaud PC: Fatalities from immunotherapy (IT) and skin testing (ST), *J Allergy Clin Immunol* 79:660, 1987.

16. Lorenz M, et al.: Chemonucleolysis for herniated nucleus pulposus in adolescents, *J Bone Joint Surg* 67A:1402, 1985.

17. McCulloch JA: *Disorders of the lumbar spine.* Presented at a one-day conference, Nottingham, England, September 20, 1991.

18. McDermott DJ: *Clinical trial results.* In Brown JE, Nordby EJ, Smith L, editors: *Chemonucleolysis,* Thorofare, NJ, 1985, Slack, p 61.

19. McNab I, et al.: Chemonucleolysis, *Can J Surg* 14:280, 1971.

20. Naylor A: The biophysical and biochemical aspects of intervertebral disc herniation and degeneration, *Ann R Coll Surg* 31:91, 1962.

21. Naylor A, Smare DL: Fluid content of the nucleus pulposus as a factor in the disc syndrome, *BMJ* 2:975, 1953.

22. Nordby EJ: *Diagnosis and patient selection.* In Brown JE, Nordby EJ, Smith L, editors: *Chemonucleolysis,* Thorofare, NJ, 1985, Slack, p 45.

23. Nordby EJ, Wright PH, Schofield SR: Safety of chemonucleolysis: adverse effects reported in the USA 1982 to 1989, *Clin Orthop* (293):122-34, August 1993.

24. Ramirez LF, Thisted R: Complications and demographic characteristics of patients undergoing lumbar discectomy in community hospital, *Neurosurgery* 25:266, 1984.

25. Schwetschwenau PR, et al.: Double-blind evaluation of intradiscal chymopapain for herniated lumbar discs, *J Neurosurg* 45:622, 1976.

26. Simmons JW, et al.: Update and review of chemonucleolysis, *Clin Orthop* 183:51, 1964.

27. Simmons JW, Upman PJ, Stavinoha WB: Pharmacologic and toxicologic profile of Chymopapain B (Chemolase), *Drug Chem Toxicol* 7:299, 1984.

28. Smith L, Garvin PJ, Jennings RB, Gesler RM: Enzyme dissolution of the nucleus pulposus, *Nature* 198:1311, 1963.

29. Smith L, Brown J: Treatment of lumbar intervertebral disc lesions by direct injection of chymopapain, *J Bone Joint Surg* 49A:502, 1967.

30. Stern IJ, Smith L: Dissolution of chymopapain in vitro of tissue from normal or prolapsed intervertebral discs, *Clin Orthop* 50:269, 1976.

31. Stern IJ: *The biochemistry and toxicology of chymopapain.* In Brown JE, Nordby EJ, Smith L, editors: *Chemonucleolysis,* Thorofare, NJ, 1985, Slack, p 11.

32. Sutton CJ Jr: Current concepts in chemonucleolysis: International Congress and Symposium Series, *Proc Soc Med Lond* 72:205, 1985.

33. Sutton CJ Jr: Repeat chemonucleolysis, *Clin Orthop* 206:45, 1986.

34. Sutton CJ Jr: *Chemonucleolysis in the management of herniated lumbar discs in the adolescent.* Presented at the International Intradiscal Therapy Society meeting, Fort Lauderdale, FL, March 10, 1988.

35. Tarlo SM, Shaik W, Bell B, et al.: Papain-induced allergic reactions, *Clin Allergy* 8:207, 1978.

36. Thomas LB: Reversible collapse of rabbit ears after intravenous papain, and prevention of recovery by cortisone, *J Exp Med* 104:245, 1956.

37. Vetrile ST, Cherkashov AM: *Chemonucleolysis in the treatment of scoliosis: presentation of 162 cases.* Presented at the International Intradiscal Therapy Society meeting, Houston, TX, April 3-8, 1991.

38. Williams JM, Klester D, Thonar EJMA, Andersson GB: The effects of intradiscal chymopapain on rabbit intervertebral discs, *Proc Orthop Res Soc;* article currently appears in *Spine:* 19(7):747-751, 1994. Keister D, Williams JM, Andersson GBJ, Fugene J-M, Thonar A, McNeill TW: The dose-related effect of intradiscal chymopapain on rabbit intervertebral discs.

39. Wiltse LL: Letter to the editor, *Spine* 2:237, 1977.

40. Wiltse LL, Nordby EJ: Personal communication, December 14, 1992.

Chapter 73
Arthroscopic Microdiscectomy: Lumbar and Thoracic
Parviz Kambin

Introduction

Advantages of Arthroscopic Discectomy

Preoperative Planning

Operative Technique

positioning the patient and the C arm
needle insertion
insertion of the guide wire and cannulated
obturator
insertion of the access cannula and inspection
of the anulus
evacuation of the posterior fragments
biportal arthroscopic microdiscectomy

Postoperative Management

Outcome Analysis

Summary

Arthroscopic Microdiscectomy

Arthroscopic Foraminal Decompression

Endoscopic Thoracic Spine Surgery

Ronald Blackman, George Picetti, III, Kelly
O'Neal
anterior multiple level discectomy for deformity
complications and results
herniated thoracic discs
tumor surgery
summary

The concept of an indirect posterolateral approach to the herniated disc was born by the introduction of chymopapain into clinical use in 1963.[32] At the Graduate Hospital, Philadelphia, mechanical nucleotomy through a posterolateral approach was attempted by the author as early as 1973.[14,18] Hijikata[8,9] also reported on his experience with a nucleotomy technique, which led to the development of the automated nucleotome by Onik et al. in 1985.[23] Friedman[6] used a lateral approach, entering the skin over the iliac crest to access the herniated lumbar discs. However, the latter increased the chance of entrance to the abdominal cavity, and it was later discontinued. Our experimental work in the mid-1970s with nucleotomy technique directed our thought processes toward the development of instrumentations that would allow us to reach the posterior and posterolateral corners of the intervertebral discs. In 1982[18] we submitted our clinical experience with nine patients who were treated by percutaneous posterolateral discectomy under peer review and approval of the Internal Review Board of the Graduate Hospital.

The author's commitment and experience in the development of a safe and effective minimally invasive technique in spinal surgery in the past 15 years has led him to certain beliefs and surgical principles, which have been echoed in his various publications.[14,16,21,30] The close proximity of the spinal nerve and vascular structures require precise placement of the spinal needle on the anulus in the triangular working zone under fluoroscopic control. The patient must be awake to alert the surgeon to any impingement of neural tissues. Since the compression and fenestration of the anulus at the entry point is invariably painful, the arthroscopic visualization of the anulus is necessary in order to rule out neural entrapment. Local anesthesia on the anulus at the point of entry can markedly reduce this pain. Flexible and maneuverable micro instruments are available for manipulation and extraction of posteriorly displaced nucleus.

The technologic advancement leading to the development of a small-caliber 30 and 70-degree scope and deflecting micro instruments in conjunction with the clinical disappointment associated with simple core decompression techniques,[5,11] has led to the development of arthroscopic disc surgery. The latter technique allows for direct visualization and extraction of the posterior and posterolateral herniated fragments. When posterior and posterolateral evacuation of herniated fragments is being attempted, excellent visualization and appropriate fluid management are also required. A satisfactory depth perception is realized only by a biportal approach and triangulation inside the intervertebral disc. Although open operative techniques[1,22] represent a reliable method of treatment of the herniated lumbar disc, it should not be employed for the treatment of small protruded contained disc. The laminectomy should be reserved for extraction of sequestrated fragments or decompression of a stenotic spine.

Lumbar Spine

Advantages of Arthroscopic Discectomy

Minimal interventional surgical techniques are rapidly entering most of the surgical specialties. Nowadays, one would not consider opening a knee joint for meniscus extraction or repair. Endoscopic surgery routinely is being used in urology, gastroenterology, gynecology, and thoracic surgery. The minimal intraoperative injury to the musculoligamentous and osseous structure of the lumbar spine during the course of arthroscopic disc extraction leads to a more rapid recovery and rehabilitation.

A prospective study of 100 patients who were treated either through an access cannula inserted dorsolaterally or by an open laminotomy procedure for herniated lumbar disc has clearly demonstrated a more rapid development of spinal spondylosis and mechanical instability following open operative procedures. These findings were most significant at L4-L5.[17] Panjabi and co-workers[25] have demonstrated the important role of posterior ligamentous structures and the posterior anulus in the preservation of stability of a functional spinal unit following flexion loading. In contrast to the open operative technique the latter structures are not disturbed in the course of the posterolateral approach. The posterolateral approach eliminates the need for entry into the spinal canal; therefore, the complications associated with an open laminectomy procedure—bleeding, scar formation, dural tear, and battered-nerve-root syndrome[28,33]—are not seen following arthroscopic microdiscectomy. The significant role of the neural and perineural venous system in the prevention of venous congestion and neural edema has been the subject of multiple investigations.[3,10,24,26] The injury to the above venous system either by traction on the nerve root or by electrocoagulation may contribute to postlaminectomy pain syndrome.

Furthermore, the herniation of nuclear material through the previously induced anular fenestration associated with recurrence of symptoms is not uncommon.[4,27,31] When a contained intervertebral disc[19] is converted into a noncontained disc by surgical intervention, it invites further expulsion of the nuclear fragment into the spinal canal. Finally, the cost effectiveness of minimal-intervention surgical techniques in spinal surgery has been studied and demonstrated and has proven that the arthroscopic microdiscectomy was more cost effective than open laminectomy procedures, taking into account the occasional necessity of an additional open procedure in failed cases.

Preoperative Planning

The role of conservative therapy in the treatment of lumbar radiculopathy secondary to herniated nucleus pulposus should not be ignored. A great majority of patients do respond to a well-planned treatment consisting of partial bed rest, use of antiinflammatory medications, physical therapy exercise programs, and epidural steroids. Individuals selected for arthroscopic microdiscectomy are a subset of those who are candidates for an open laminectomy procedure. However, when the disc protrusion is associated with stenosis due to degenerative spondylosis and posterior osteophytosis, a simple posterior lateral intradiscal decompression via the arthroscopic technique is doomed to fail. Likewise, at present a large sequestrated displaced herniated fragment is not accessible to the arthroscopic disc extraction technique. The preoperative planning should include vigorous diagnostic work-up in order to exclude the presence of displaced sequestrated fragments or lateral recess or foraminal stenosis.

The inclusion criteria included the failure to respond to conservative therapy, the presence of positive tension signs,[7] neurologic deficit, and positive correlative CT and MRI. The tension signs should be conducted not only in the supine or sitting position, but under the load of weight bearing in flexion and rotation.[12] For the uniportal approach the patient must meet the following criteria: a high-quality MRI must show that the herniation is contained with an intact anular wall, a CT scan with sagittal reformation to visualize the foramina must show that there is no stenosis, and the patient must have unilateral leg pain greater than back pain. The CT scan is essential since MRI has been shown frequently not to visualize stenosis in the foramina. If the patient fits these criteria, he/she should have a 80% to 88% chance for a successful outcome.

In the preoperative phase, the patient should be exposed to at least anteroposterior and lateral roentgenography of the lumbar spine. The latter will provide information regarding the relation of the iliac crest to the surgical site,[14] the height of the intervertebral disc, and the presence or absence of developmental anomalies.

Operative Technique

The minimal-intervention posterolateral approach to the lumbar spine is most frequently achieved through a uniportal approach. The unilateral approach allows intermittent visualization and excision of the nucleus. Arthroscopic microdiscectomy instruments may be used for uniportal or bilateral biportal approaches (Fig. 73-1).

Positioning of the Patient and the C Arm

The operation must be performed with the patient in prone position. This position will provide paramedial access to the intervertebral disc from the left as well as the right side of the lumbar spine. An adjustable radiolucent frame is used to maintain the hips in flexion and to flatten the lumbar lordosis. The frame has two radiolucent bolsters. The distal end of the bolsters are adjusted to provide support under the anterior superior iliac spine. However, the proximal ends of the bolsters are kept apart to provide room for the abdomen and the chest wall (Fig. 73-2). A variety of radiolucent-top operating tables are available. Most operating rooms are equipped with one or two such tables. The extensions used for cardiac pacemaker placement provide good access for the C arm. The fracture table also provides an excellent radiolucent table for arthroscopic microdiscectomy. The distal end of the fracture table, which provides support for the lower extremities, may be used for positioning of the frame and the patient. The fracture table is particularly suitable for minimal-intervention spinal surgery because it is narrower than the operating room tables and does not interfere with the rotation of the C arm from the anteroposterior to the lateral position, or vice versa. The author prefers to position the C arm on the side where the sciatic pain is present while standing on the opposite side of the table at the onset of the operative procedure.

Needle Insertion

For proper evacuation of the herniated fragments from the posterior zone of the intervertebral disc, one should attempt to choose the entry point as far lateral as possible without the risk of entry into the

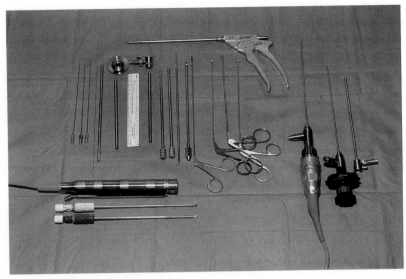

Fig. 73-1

Arthroscopic microdiscectomy instrumentation from left to right: three 18-gauge 6-in.-long spinal needles, guide wire, cannulated obturator, universal access cannula, ruler, second universal access, 3- and 4.5-mm trephines, magnetic retrieval, deflecting tube, three forceps, two discoscopes, and a scope sheath. *Top:* Suction punch forceps. *Bottom:* Disc shavers.

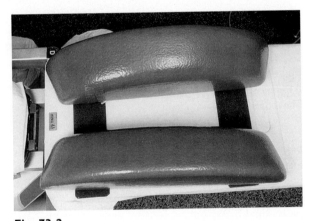

Fig. 73-2

Radiolucent frame with two adjustable bolsters. Proximal ends of bolsters are beveled and kept apart to support chest wall, while distal ends are kept under anterior superior iliac spine.

abdominal cavity. In most individuals, a distance of about 10 cm is adequate. Following the local infiltration of lidocaine solution, an 18-gauge needle 5 to 6 inches in length is inserted at a 35- to 45-degree angle and is directed toward the anulus. When properly positioned, the tip of the needle in the lateral fluoroscopy projection is visualized just posterior to the intervertebral disc, and in the anteroposterior view it is seen in alignment with the middle of the proximal and distal pedicles. Care must be taken to position the C arm properly. Improper po-

sitioning of the C arm at the onset of the procedure will cause distorted images and wrong positioning of the top of the needle. During the needle placement, the C arm is in the lateral position, the tube is then tilted and moved about until the vertebral plates of the segments adjacent to the herniation site are parallel and visualized as a straight line rather than semicircular images.

The tip of the needle should be positioned in the middle of the back wall of the disc as seen on the lateral view. A placement distal to midheight of the anulus as visualized in the lateral fluoroscopy is desirable. When the needle is advanced toward the anulus with a rotary movement, it usually passes through the muscle layers with no resistance. However, one should have no difficulty in feeling resistance when the tip of the needle reaches the anular fibers. A premature insertion of the needle into the anular fibers will mask the exact entry site and should be avoided. When the tip of the needle is properly positioned, before entry into the disc, fluoroscopy should show the tip portion on an anteroposterior view in midpedicular position and on a lateral view at a point on a line going from the back of the superior to the back of the inferior vertebral bodies. When an intraoperative discography is desired, a 22-gauge needle may be inserted into the 18-gauge needle and advanced into the intervertebral disc to an appropriate depth.

Insertion of the Guide Wire and Cannulated Obturator

The guide wire is inserted into the lumen of the 18-gauge needle and advanced to the anular fibers. The needle is then withdrawn. A small skin incision is made, and the cannulated obturator is passed over the guide wire and directed toward the anulus. It is not unusual inadvertently to misdirect the cannulated obturator and bend the wire and find the distal end of the cannula obturator in an unsatisfactory position. It is advisable to review the position of the cannulated obturator via C-arm fluoroscopy in the lateral projection after it has passed the resistance of the fascia to ensure that it is following the exact path of the inserted guide wire (Fig. 73-3). Generous local anesthesia along the path of the dilator prior to insertion will allow the dilator to be inserted in a painless manner. Care must be taken not to anesthetize too deeply or the spinal nerve will be anesthetized. The guide wire should be removed prior to full insertion of the cannulated obturator. It should be noted that the spinal nerve is slightly mobile. The withdrawal of the guide wire will allow the blunt end of the cannulated obturator to bypass the spinal nerve while approaching the anular fibers.

Insertion of the Access Cannula and Inspection of the Anulus

The universal access cannula has an external diameter of 6.4 mm, which provides for an internal working area of 5 mm in diameter. It should be noted that the cannulated obturator has a beveled blunt end that is capable of bypassing the spinal nerve without causing any injury. It is imperative that the operative surgeon hold the cannulated obturator firmly against the anulus with one hand while using his/her opposite hand to introduce the access cannula. When the access cannula is completely inserted, the fluoroscopy view of the surgical site in the lateral projection demonstrates that the round blunt end of the cannulated obturator is well covered by the inserted access cannula. While the access cannula is firmly held against the anulus by the surgeon's hand, a needle test is conducted to be certain that the open end of the access cannula is well centered on the intervertebral disc space. Using the guide wire, poke the four quadrants of the cannula to be certain the patient does not experience a sudden radiating pain, which would indicate that all or part of the spinal nerve is within the opening of the access cannula.

The 30-degree arthroscope provides for a uni-

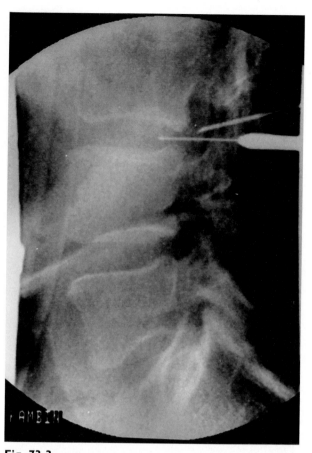

Fig. 73-3

Prior to withdrawal of guide wire, lateral fluoroscopy demonstrates that cannulated obturator is following exact path of inserted guide wire.

portal suction irrigation system and allows the direct visualization of the perianular structures. When the instruments are properly positioned, a loose adipose tissue is usually seen at the site of entry (see color plate III-1). At times a loosely woven fibrous tissue is seen on the surface of the anulus at the entry point. These fibers are thin and do not have the appearance or structure of the spinal nerve (see color plate III-2). When the fatty tissue is extracted, the superficial layer of the anulus fibers and the expansion of the posterior longitudinal ligament is visualized. Although the routine inspection of the spinal nerve is neither necessary nor advisable, a 30-degree video arthroscope may be directed posteriorly and slightly cephalad for the inspection of the spinal nerve and the foramina. However, the fatty tissue that surrounds the spinal nerve may make its visualization somewhat difficult.

Prior to anular fenestration, it is usually necessary to use topical anesthetic or systemic analgesics to reduce the patient's pain and discomfort. The anular fenestration is accomplished first with a 3-mm

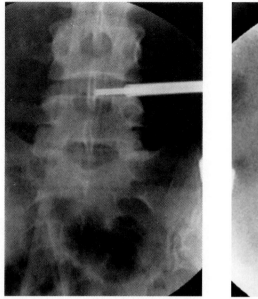
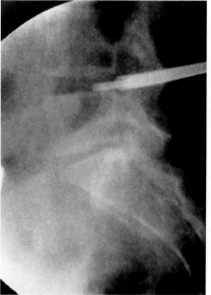

A   B

Fig. 73-4

Anteroposterior and lateral view of inserted trephine into L4-L5 disc space during uniportal discectomy procedure. Note correct position of medial extremity of access cannula on anular fibers, which is in alignment with midpedicular region.

trephine and is then enlarged with the aid of a 5-mm trephine (Fig. 73-4). The design of the instruments does not permit more than 2 cm of penetration of the trephine beyond the medial extremity of the inserted access cannula. While the surgeon is maintaining downward pressure against the access cannula, forceps are used for evacuation of disc material in and around the entry point. Without the fluid adaptor in place, care must be taken not to penetrate through the anulus on the opposite side or anteriorly. Then the access cannula can be advanced into and can engage the anular fibers to prevent the sliding of the cannula into the periannular region.

Evacuation of the Posterior Fragments

Arthroscopic microdiscetomy trimmer blades (4.5 mm) (see color plate III-3) are extremely useful for rapid evacuation of the nuclear material from the posterior zone adjacent to the inner fibers of the posterior anulus. When the trimmer blade is being used, the operating surgeon must make certain that the access cannula is well inserted into the anular fibers. The latter will provide a closed system for effective inflow and outflow of saline solution and is an essential step to protect the spinal nerve at this stage of the operation. It is best to begin with the end-cutting shaver and then use the side-cutting cutter to enlarge the cavity in the nucleus. The cannula can be angled posteriorly, which allows the side-

cutting blade to evacuate more of the nucleus posteriorly. The final evaluation of the nucleus in the posterior position of the disc is performed with manual tools. The defector tube and flexible pituitary rongeur are used when placed through the cannula. The working end of the cannula should be pushed down or anteriorly to allow the instrument better access to the posterior lateral portion of the nucleus. New forceps have been developed that can place the jaws at 110 degrees to the cannula and permit further evacuation of the posterior lateral portion of the nucleus.

Biportal Arthroscopic Microdiscectomy

When a patient has a large central contained herniated disc and has bilateral radicular pain, a biportal approach should be used. When a biportal approach is being used, two straight-punch forceps are first used to develop a communication between the two ports (Fig. 73-5). It should be noted that the biportal approach usually requires deeper penetration of the instruments into the intervertebral disc space. For this reason the sealing fluid adaptor may have to be removed and replaced by a disposable rubber cap, which will allow deeper penetration of the forceps and disc shavers. At this time the 70-degree video arthroscope is inserted from one port and the disc shaver from the opposite side, and under direct visualization the posterior nuclear tissue is resected

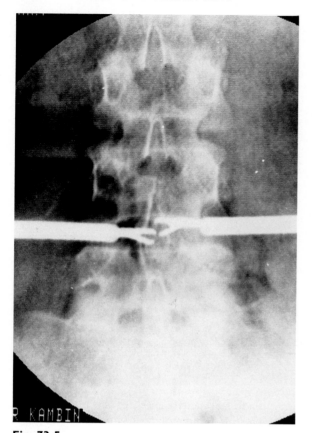

Fig. 73-5

Two manual forceps are used to develop communication between right and left portal in bilateral biportal approach.

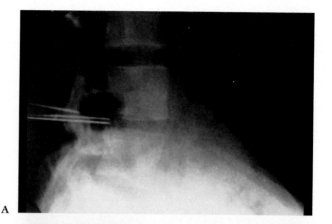

A

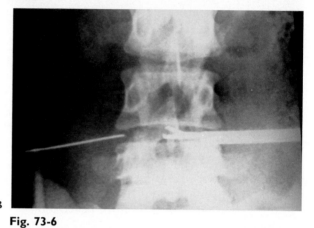

B

Fig. 73-6

Needle positioning in bilateral biportal approach. **A,** In lateral projection tips of needles are seen in alignment with posterior vertebral bodies. Third needle is partially inserted from right side of patient to assist fluoroscopic identification of right and left. **B,** In anteroposterior projection tip of needle is in alignment with line drawn vertically between center of pedicles of proximal and distal segments. Access cannula on opposite side has engaged anular fibers prior to evacuation.

and evacuated. When a bilateral biportal approach is being used, both the right and left needles should be positioned prior to the introduction of the cannulated obturator and the access cannula (Fig. 73-6). It should be noted that when an extraforaminal herniation (far out) (Fig. 73-7) is present, one will have difficulty in positioning the tip of the needle in the midpedicular region (Fig. 73-8).

For a surgeon experienced with spine arthroscopic microdiscectomy, an extruded fragment that is subligamentous may be extracted. As soon as an adequate cavity is created beyond the inner fibers of the posterior anulus and an adequate flow of saline solution is established, the deflecting suction forceps are used to penetrate through the posterior anular fibers in order to facilitate the extraction of subligamentous fragments (see color plate III-4). Since there is no point of reference in the intervertebral disc space to direct the video arthroscope and instruments to the sight of herniation, the entire posterior and posterolateral anulus between the two portals should be probed. However, the visualization of the access cannula from the opposite port

and fluoroscopic visualization of the position of the forceps and the arthroscope in the anteroposterior projection is used as a guide for localization of the herniation site. At the termination of the procedure, the inspection of the spinal nerve may be carried out with the aid of a 30-degree arthroscope (see color plate III-5).

The familiarity with arthroscopic microdiscectomy instrumentation, skill, and biportal approach and triangulation inside the intervertebral disc is essential for percutaneous interbody fusion with or without the use of pedicular fixators. Our removable pedicular fixators and subcutaneous plates have provided a new dimension to the field of spine instrumentation and stabilization (Fig. 73-9). This latter is the subject of a multicenter study in a few highly specialized spine centers.

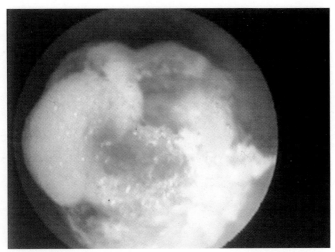

Plate III-1

Arthroscopic view of the anulus at the entry point. Note adipose tissue covering the surface of the anular fibers.

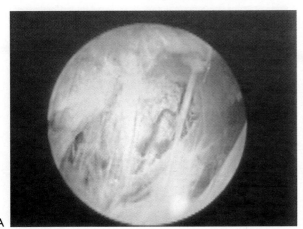

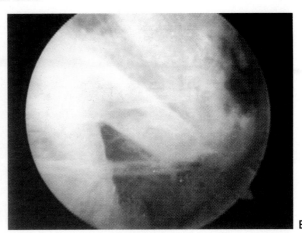

A   B

Plate III-2

A, At times a thin layer of fibrous tissue is seen on the surface of the anulus. These fibers should not be mistaken for the spinal needle. **B,** Magnified view of **A.**

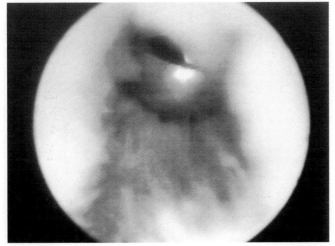

Plate III-3

Biportal arthroscopic view of the trimmer blade while it is being used to create a cavity behind the inner fibers of the posterior anulus.

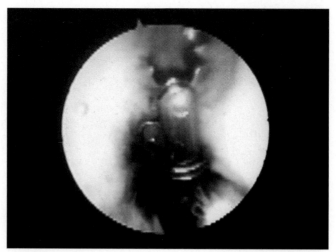

Plate III-4

Deflectable suction forceps are being used under direct arthroscopic visualization from the opposite portal.

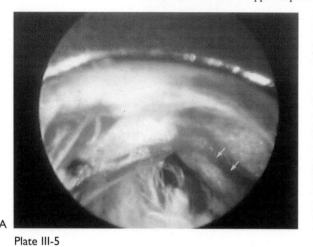

A

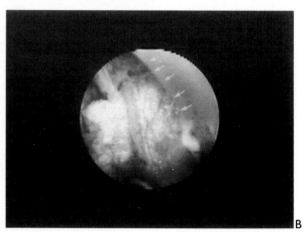

B

Plate III-5

A, Arthroscopic view of the spinal nerve. Note the anular fenestration in the background. **B,** Close-up view of the spinal nerve as shown in **A**.

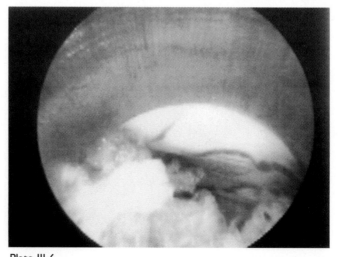

Plate III-6

Arthroscopic visualization of the spinal canal. Magnified nerve root is seen on the top next to the rim of the universal access cannula. The grayish color dura is seen in the background. Foraminal adipose tissue is seen in the foreground.

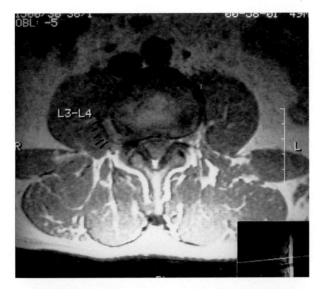

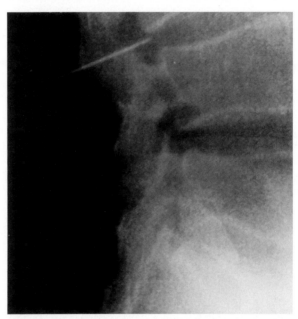

Fig. 73-7

Preoperative MRI study demonstrates extraforaminal herniation at L3-L4 in 34-year-old male with severe anterior thigh pain and depressed patella reflex. *(From Kambin P, Cohen L:* Arthroscopic microdiscectomy vs. nucleotomy techniques. *In Stinson JT, Wiesel SW, editors:* Clinics in sports medicine, *vol 12, no 3, July, 1993, W.B. Saunders Co., p 148.)*

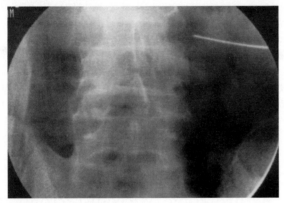

A

Fig. 73-8

Intraoperative fluoroscopy from the patient shown in Fig. 73-7. **A,** In AP projection tip of needle remains away from the pedicle. **B,** In lateral projection tip of needle is seen just posterior to anular fibers. *(From Kambin P, Cohen L:* Arthroscopic microdiscectomy vs. nucleotomy techniques. *In Stinson JT, Wiesel SW, editors:* Clinics in sports medicine, *vol 12, no 3, July, 1993, W.B. Saunders Co., p 146.)*

B

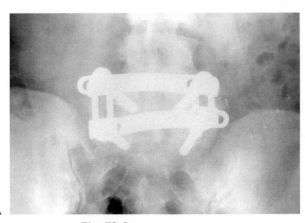

A

B

Fig. 73-9

Anteroposterior- and lateral-view postoperative x-ray films demonstrating removable pedicular fixators with subcutaneous plates and interbody bone grafting.

Postoperative Management

Patients are usually discharged from the hospital on the day of surgery but occasionally are kept overnight for observation and continuation of intravenous antibiotic therapy. Patients usually receive 1 g of cephalosporin intravenously prior to the surgery, followed by three additional doses postoperatively. On discharge, they are instructed to avoid long sitting, lifting, or bending. A great majority of patients express satisfaction and show improvement immediately following their operative procedure. However, as observed after an open discectomy procedure, it is not uncommon for a patient to report some residual pain, numbness, or tingling of the lower extremity. Most of these symptoms subside with the use of antiiflammatory medication and an exercise program. We encourage our patients to participate in swimming exercises as early as 7 days after surgery. The latter is then followed by more rigid exercise program including aqua therapy and isokinetic exercises.

Outcome Analysis

In the past 10 years more than 250 patients with clinical signs and symptoms of disc herniation associated with correlative positive MRI, CT, or myelographic findings have been treated in our institution via a posterolateral approach through a 6.4-mm-outer-diameter access cannula.

Using the pain analog, preoperative and postoperative questionnaires and self-assessment data-gathering in conjunction with preoperative and postoperative findings taking into consideration the patient's ability or inability to return to a functional level, my colleagues and I have reported up to 88% satisfactory results following arthroscopic microdiscectomy.[12,14,21,30]

The complications have been rather minimal. We have reported one incident of instrument breakage, which was withdrawn with the aid of a magnetic rod provided with the instruments. We have had one case of infection detected 10 days postoperatively and treated with prompt culture and sensitivity testing and the use of appropriate antibiotic therapy. Neuropraxia of the peroneal nerve developed in one of our patients as a result of the placement of tight straps around the knee during the operative procedure; the patient is recovering. The psoas hematoma reported in two patients following their surgical procedure has not been observed in our subsequent patient population who have undergone posterolateral discectomy and decompression.

Summary

In 1985 and 1986[16,20] the author reported the minimal invasive posterior evacuation of the herniated lumbar discs for the treatment of disc herniation. The flexible tip forceps, deflector tube, and upbiting forceps were used to reach the posterior corners of the intervertebral disks. Biportal approaches have permitted the extraction of extruded subligamentous herniations.

Our experience with laser disc surgery has been somewhat disappointing. All of the currently used heat-producing lasers are capable of nucleolysis. The attractiveness of blind-laser nucleolysis[2] as well as other nucleotomy techniques[23] appear to be due to its simplicity, quick application, and the fact that it does not require specific skills. It should be noted that the laser does not provide good access to the posterior offending nuclear fragments and that there is an inherent danger associated with the use of a heat-producing laser around the dura and the nerve roots.

Current state of the art in our experience in uniportal use of the laser with a flexible scope does not provide adequate visibility, depth perception, and an appropriate fluid-management system. The latter is necessary for proper visualization and protection of the neural structures during the time of surgery.

Thoracic Spine

Arthroscopic Microdiscectomy

Soft disc herniation of the thoracic spine is not common. However, the paramedial and foraminal herniations may be associated with severe thoracic pain and radiation to the lateral chest wall. A central herniation may cause spastic paraparesis and severe neurological deficit.

Thoracic discs are accessible to the posterolateral arthroscopic approach. As the thoracic nerve root exits the foramina and enters the subcostal grove, it creates ample space in the triangular working zone for insertion of the instruments. Thus, the incidence of thoracic nerve injury via a posterolateral access is less likely than for the lumbar spine.

Due to the size of the vertebral bodies the distance between the anulotomy site and the dura in the thoracic spine is less than in the lumbar spine. This anatomical advantage facilitates the extraction of the posterior herniated fragment through a posterolateral access with relative ease.

The operative technique for posterolateral arthroscopic thoracic discectomy is similar to the previous description for access to the lumbar intervertebral disc with few exceptions. The point of entry is usu-

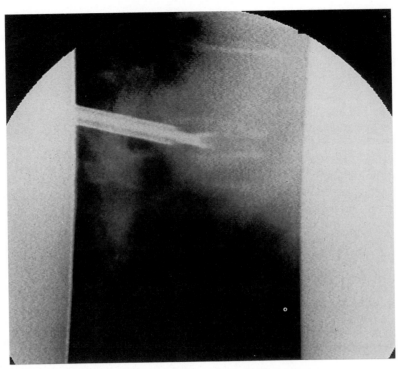

Fig. 73-10

Intra operative fluoroscopic examination demonstrating the position of the access cannula and forceps at T7-T8 intervertebral disc. Note an old compression fracture of T7.

ally about 6 cm from the midline. In order to prevent pleural injury, the proper positioning of the needle tip adjacent to the proximal articular process of the lower thoracic vertebra is essential. The anterior positioning of the instruments increases the chance of pleural penetration. In lateral fluoroscopy, the tip of the needle must be seen in alignment with posterior surface of the vertebra adjacent to the index level.

The arthroscopic inspection of the anulotomy site generally shows less adipose tissue on the surface of the anulus than what is usually observed in the course of arthroscopic examination of the triangular working zone in the lumbar region. Following the fenestration of the anulus, arthroscopic microdiscectomy instruments are used for extraction of herniated disc fragments (Fig. 73-10).

Arthroscopic Foraminal Decompression

The arthroscope, arthroscope irrigation sheet, and cannula assembly permits visualization of perianular and foraminal structures via a uniportal access. In the last five years this author has used a working channel scope (Fig. 73-11) in conjunction with arthroscopic microdiscectomy instruments for perianular and foraminal surgery.[1,29,13]

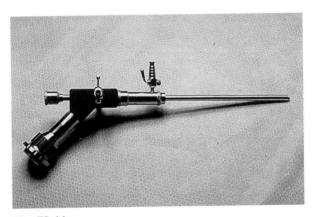

Fig. 73-11

Working channel scope.

It should be noted that most foraminal herniations extend to the extra foraminal region or are part of a paramedial herniated nucleus pulposus. We have used foraminal access for both removal of a foraminal free fragment and for confirmation of adequacy of posterolateral fragmentectomy via an intradiscal approach.

The entry point for foraminal access is usually 10 to 11 cm from the midline. The operating surgeon must avoid vertical insertion of the needle at the onset of the procedure. The articular facets are first palpated with the tip of the inserted needle. The needle is then withdrawn and reinserted in a slightly more vertical angle and positioned into the triangular working zone. This step is followed by insertion of the cannulated obturator and the access cannula.

The working channel scope or 30-degree arthroscope and arthroscope irrigation sheath assembly is passed into the lumen of the univeral access cannula and the anular surface is inspected. At this time the arthroscope, arthroscope irrigation sheath and cannula assembly or working channel scope is medialized and passed under the pars interarticularis for inspection of the nerve root and dura or extraction of a foraminal herniation (see color plate III-6).

Endoscopic Thoracic Spine Surgery

Ronald Blackman, George Picetti, III, Kelly O'Neal

When one watches a thoracic surgeon repair a bleb or do an esophageal myotomy it is obvious that right behind the area where they are working is the spine. All they need to do is pull the lung a little more medial and the view of the spine can be appreciated. Thus was born the endoscopic anterior approach to the thoracic spine.

Our initial decision to explore this technique was prompted by the huge scar on the chest as a result of the open technique. Secondary consideration was the limitation of the open technique to adequately excise discs other than at the apex and one or two adjacent levels. As more discs are involved the ability to see into the disc space becomes difficult.

We also had noticed that in other endoscopic and arthroscopic techniques morbidity and length of hospital stay were significantly decreased and we hoped that the same decrease in morbidity would occur with endoscopic surgery of the thoracic spine.

Three distinct procedures can be identified: anterior multiple level discectomy and release for deformity with and without fusion; surgical excision of herniated thoracic discs; and biopsy and decompression of thoracic spine tumors.

Anterior Multiple Level Discectomy for Deformity

Anterior discectomy over multiple levels has been used in the treatment of scoliosis and kyphosis for more than 30 years. There is no standard as to when this procedure should be carried out but the theory has been that in those kyphotic and scoliotic curves which do not correct well on either extension (for kyphosis) or bending laterally (for scoliosis), then removing the disc may enhance the ability to correct the curve.

This report deals with twenty cases of anterior thoracic spine surgery; usually multiple level discectomy with varying fusion attempts in idiopathic scoliosis, congenital scoliosis and developmental roundback kyphosis. All cases were done anteriorly with an endoscopic technique.

Our techniques were initially developed using anesthetized dogs and pigs. Pigs are difficult to use due to their long trachea and it is difficult to put the lung at rest; dogs on the other hand, have an imperfect mediastinum and producing a pneumothorax on one side produces it on both sides. Despite this, adequate animal trials were performed and the technique was transferred to human cadavers and then to live human subjects. We would suggest that this procedure be initially done in the laboratory. Many hospitals and surgical companies support surgical labs and one can often piggy-back onto the end of a general surgery session of endoscopic cholecystectomy training.

Anesthesia

The success of this procedure depends on proper anesthesia technique. Visualization and performance of surgical technique is improved if the continuous motion of the lung can be eliminated. This goal may be hard to achieve particularly in young children and those with initially poor pulmonary function. Ventilatory function of the lung is the responsibility of the anesthesiologist.

Maintenance of an adequate arterial pO_2 also can be affected by patient positioning. That is, if the patient is in the lateral decubitus position, the "good" lung is usually the down lung and is compressed increasing the ventilatory pressure. Albeit the following techniques are utilized.

The use of a double lumen Carlin type endotracheal tube is used in persons having a large enough trachea to utilize this and get adequate oxygenation. The cut-off is around 45 kg body weight. Often a fiber-optic laryngoscope is needed to visualize and intubate the left main stem bronchus. When the tube is unilaterally clamped, breath sounds on the clamped side should cease. It is important to clamp the tube once or twice prior to the start of the surgical incision to be sure that tube placement is correct.

Gradual decrease in arterial oxygen saturation may occur. There reaches a point where re-oxygenation of the unaerated lung becomes imperative. We have learned that this may be secondary to shifting of the endotracheal tube and can sometimes be rectified by a recheck through the fiber-optic laryngoscope, or just pulling the endotracheal tube up ever so slightly.

In those patients weighing less than 45 kg the trachea may be too small for a double lumen tube or the caliber of the tube is too small to carry adequate ventilation. In those cases intubating only the bronchus of the nonoperative side is the best approach; done with the fiber-optic laryngoscope.

Children 6 years old or less do not tolerate one-lung ventilation well. If the arterial saturation drops it may be necessary to do the procedure with two-lung aeration and deflate the lung adjacent to the surgical work area by light pressure using retractors.

Change of patient position can affect the placement of the endotracheal tube. Initially we flexed the table for better endoscopic visualization opening up the disc spaces. In unflexing, the position of the endotracheal tube dislodged and reintubation was required. It probably is safer to maintain one position once adequate anaesthesia occurs. During the procedure, if a drop in oxygen saturation continues, both lungs can be ventilated by pulling the tube back. A significant drop in arterial oxygen saturation occurred in 4 of our 20 patients and 2 of them were adequately handled in this manner. One 14-year-old with an 80-degree thoracic curve and significant deformity and decreased pulmonary function would not maintain arterial oxygen saturation. This was our first experience with this and the procedure was aborted without trying the above recommendations.

Technique

With the patient in the lateral decubitus position the upper arm is placed in a support at right angles to the body and the shoulders and hips are taped for stability. The skin is marked with the outline of the ribs and scapula and the posterior axillary line is drawn. For scoliosis the initial incision is in line with the posterior axillary line. For kyphosis, the approach is posterior to the posterior axillary line. The intent is to come onto the posterolateral spine to try to avoid working directly towards the spinal cord. The right side is generally a little easier and if one has an option the right side should be chosen. Kyphosis and right thoracic scoliosis fall into this category. Left thoracic curves are more unusual but should be done from the left side.

We prefer to have the surgeon and assistant at the patient's back with a second assistant, if desired, on the side of the patient's abdomen. This keeps the operator working from posterior to anterior away from the spinal cord. Two video cameras are set up so each surgeon and scrub can have a view of the procedure without turning. The endoscope is a 10 mm 45-degree 'scope. For children under 35 kg use 5 mm 45-degree scope. The first port is made 12 mm in length in line with the upper part of the 8th or 9th rib. A finger is inserted to be sure the lung is deflated (if that is the mode) or that the lung is away from the finger at least. An endoscope is inserted through a plastic port for looking around. If the lung is deflated one should be able to see up to the apex of the chest and count the ribs from the first to the twelfth thoracic. The diaphragm limits the inferior exposure, but it's presence and whereabouts is duly noted since remaining ports are made to avoid perforating the diaphragm.

A second and a third incision, 10 to 12 mm in length, are made either up or down from the initial cut, superior to the desired rib. The ports are established and secured with plastic inserts and the spine is usually easily seen. The two other ports are for purposes of retraction and working on the spine. Keeping the desired area of the spine in view a cautery hook is placed on the pleura midway between the head of the rib and the anterior spine overlying a disc space. Normally the disc space has no vessels over it and the pleura can be pulled up by the hook and cauterized in successive movements proximally and distally, leaving the segmental vessels over the body of the vertebra unscathed.

The disc or discs can then be cleaned with a small Kitner sponge. Each disc can be incised with a shortened cautery blade. Removal of disc material can be done in a standard manner of subchondral loosening of the disc attachment by standard Cobb elevator and its' removal by use of rongeurs, angled curettes, and ring curettes. We have tried automatic shavers and burrs and find no advantage in their use. Bleeding of the subchondral bone can be controlled by packing the disc space with Surgicell. Bleeding is magnified through the endoscope and small amounts of blood can obscure the vision. A small stab wound of 5 mm through which a neural type suction tip is inserted may be necessary. Obvious bleeding points can be controlled by cautery forceps. These are standard surgical endoscopic instruments—long forceps with an attachment for the electrocautery. The surgical procedure can then move up or down using either the three initial ports or by making additional ports, the disc space can be approached directly in line of sight.

The goals in kyphosis, idiopathic and neuromuscular scoliosis and congenital scoliosis may be slightly different. In kyphosis the aim is particularly to sever the anterior longitudinal ligament and to remove the anterior part of the disc. The vena cava is immediately adjacent to the anterior longitudinal ligament but the maneuver can be safely performed by lifting up the pleura and gently dissecting between the tissue plane represented by bone/ligament and pleura. A retractor can be placed in this interval or the tissue grasped and an interval created to place a rongeur or angled curette and work from the blind side to the visualized side.

In idiopathic scoliosis the goal is removal of the lateral disc particularly, though as much disc as possible is removed including removal of the anterior longitudinal ligament. The rotation of the spine must be mentally visualized while the disc space immediately adjacent to the head of the rib is cleaned of anulus. Staying anterior to the head of the rib should keep the instruments out of the spinal canal.

In congenital scoliosis the goal is more limited, that is, visualization of the hemivertebra and adjacent disc space and hence the growth plates. This usually looks like a transverse Y and the disc spaces on either side of the Y cleaned and deepened. We have curetted local bone to fill the defect. This should be sufficient to form a fusion. The space is quite small and if pleura is closed over these bone chips healing should, and did, occur.

We now supplement most of the discectomy procedures by filling the defect created with local bone plus Grafton. In lieu of an appropriate delivery system we use the 4 mm tube and cannula from the Craig Bone Biopsy set. The 4 mm tube can be filled with Grafton from its syringe and the tube is then placed into the disc space and its contents expelled by using the solid cannula to push it into the disc space. Ten cc of Grafton is usually sufficient for 5 disc spaces. We do not have to use Grafton, we can use a section of the rib as described in the thoracic herniated disc section for fusion.

Closure of the pleura is difficult and we have experimented with numerous ways. The pleura is often quite thin and readily tears. Simple suture closure takes a long time and risks perforating the lung and vessels. Use of an autosuture appears to offer the best technique for us at this time, though it too is laborious. However, even a few sutures with partial closure may assist in covering open spaces and decrease post-operative bleeding and adhesions.

A chest tube is routinely used to evacuate air and blood for 24 to 48 hours depending on the amount of fluid produced. Normally one of the surgical incisions can be used and chest tube placement into the apex can be done visually through the 'scope.

Complications and Results

Twenty patients underwent the procedure. One patient had the procedure aborted due to inability to maintain her oxygen saturation adequately. This was an early case and we now would not have abandoned the procedure but would use a retractor and aerate the upside lung or reposition the endotracheal tube.

Of the remaining 19 patients, no serious complications arose. In one patient the endotracheal tube dislodged when we changed patient position from acutely flexed in lateral decubitus to normal lateral decubitus position. The patient was turned supine and reintubated. We have stopped flexing the table and feel visualization is not hampered. One other patient with idiopathic scoliosis had rapid loss of arterial oxygen saturation which was cured by repositioning of the endotracheal tube.

Two of the first 3 patients with congenital scoliosis did not tolerate one lung intubation with collapse of the lung on the working side and we performed the procedure with normal lung ventilation. We are using a special rubberized inflatable retractor to push the lung gently away from the working space. The key word is "gently" since both the lung and diaphragm can be easily perforated.

Our second case had a three-stage procedure consisting of anterior thoracolumbar discectomy and fusion followed a week later by anterior thoracic discectomy and one week later by posterior spinal fusion and instrumentation. Her relative correction was excellent. This would seem to be an ideal procedure when both the thoracic and thoracolumbar curve needs to be attacked anteriorly.

Our initial idea was to do an anterior release procedure followed a week later by posterior fusion. However by 72 hours most patients were able to be discharged to await the second procedure. If time permits, we now do the two stages on the same day.

Pulmonary function should not be affected—certainly less so than with an open thoracotomy. We have no scientific means of studying this but have shown pulmonary function (FVC and FEC) not to be any worse. Obviously the relationship between the endoscopic procedure and the actual posterior correction leaves causation to be in doubt but we needed to be sure we were not causing harm.

Blood was likewise difficult to measure scientifically. Each procedure was a little different including lysis of an adhesion which bled but there was no significant acute bleeding and chest tube drainage subjectively appeared little changed from open surgery.

Operative time has gradually decreased from 45 minutes per disc space to 15 minutes per disc space. Setup time appears longer than with open procedures.

Herniated Thoracic Discs

Excision of herniated thoracic discs can be done effectively through the endoscope. The anesthesia and approach is as outlined previously. It is imperative to identify the correct disc level and this is done first by looking into the apex of the chest and counting the ribs. Confirmation by needle placement and x-ray should be done. Long number 18 needles similar to the type used for discography are available. These come in a plastic sleeve. The plastic sleeve is cut 1 cm shorter than the needle and the plastic tube is first placed on the desired disc space and the needle then inserted through the plastic tube into the disc. This ensures a certain amount of safety instead of an open needle waving around in the chest cavity.

The approach is at the posterior margin of the disc. To get there, in the upper chest levels the head of the rib needs to be excised since the head of the rib obscures the posterolateral part of the disc. The rib head and 1 or 2 cm of rib is incised in line with the rib and cleaned subperiosteally. The rib can be cut partially with an osteotome and the cut completed with Kerrison rongeurs. Then the ligaments holding the head of the rib can be incised and the head of the rib removed either in one piece or morselated with a rongeur. The posterolateral and lateral part of the disc is incised as described above and then working laterally the pedicle is identified and the posterior longitudinal ligament can be followed lateral to medial and disc material excised as one goes. A rent in the posterior longitudinal ligament can often be both seen and felt and by focusing the endoscope closer the contents of the disc space can be seen and removed. Looking closely, a tag of disc tissue can be seen at the rent and grasped with a small rongeur removing a much larger free fragment. Fusion can be done if desired as described above.

Tumor Surgery

This area is still in the developmental stage. We have performed biopsies where needle aspirates have been non-diagnostic using the techniques above. In any case where the segmental vessels interfere with the procedure they can be clamped and tied or coagulated. Clips can also be utilized. Once the exposure is done, a plug of bone can be removed in any standard technique and the resulting bleeding can be controlled with thrombin/collagen packing. Tumors tend to bleed and one case required open thoracotomy to adequately control the bleeding.

Decompression of tumors can be performed from the 3rd thoracic to the twelfth but this area remains more experimental. Visualization is excellent and the posterior longitudinal ligament can be cleaned and the cord decompressed but fixation and filling of the defect produced is still to be worked out.

Summary

This approach has been shown to be effective in decreasing morbidity, decreasing hospital stay and successfully performing the desired procedure. Of greatest significance is the substitution of three to five 1 cm scars for the long costal incision. While the adage regarding beauty is appreciated at least to these authors the costal scar is the antithesis of beauty while the small endoscopic scars heal well and are barely visible.

We have no neuroma or neuritic symptoms from the large endoscope between two relatively small ribs and have not had to remove any ribs. This, in itself, may decrease morbidity significantly. The overall correction of the deformity was excellent.

References

1. Dandy WE: Loose cartilage from intervertebral disc simulating tumor of the spinal cord, *Arch Surg* 19:660, 1929.
2. Davis JK: Laser assisted percutaneous lumbar discectomy: KTP/532 clinical updated in neurosurgery, San Jose, CA, 1990, *Laserscope*.
3. Delamarter RB, Bohlman HH, Dodge LD, Biro C: Experimental lumbar spine stenosis, *J Bone Joint Surg* 72A:110, 1990.
4. Epstein JA, Lavine LS, Epstein BS: Recurrent herniation of the lumbar intervertebral disk, *Clin Orthop* 52:169, 1967.
5. Epstein N: Surgically confirmed cauda equina and nerve root injury following percutaneous discectomy at an outside institution: a case report, *J Spine Dis* 3:380, 1990.
6. Friedman WA: Percutaneous discectomy: an alternative to chemonucleolysis, *J Neurosurg* 13:542, 1983.
7. Goddard MD, Reid JD: Movement induced by straight leg raising in the lumbosacral roots, nerves and plexus and the intrapelvic section of sciatic nerve, *J Neuropsychiatry* 28:12, 1965.
8. Hijikata S, Yamagishi M, Nakayama T, et al.: Percutaneous discectomy: a new treatment method for lumbar disk herniation, *J Toden Hosp* 5:5-13, 1975.
9. Hijikata S: Percutaneous nucleotomy: a new concept technique and 12 year experience, *Clin Orthop* 238:9, 1989.

10. Hoyland JA, Freemont AJ, Jayson MIV: Intervertebral foramen venous obstruction: a cause of periradicular pain fibrosis, *Spine* 14:538, 1989.

11. Kahanovitz N, Viola K, Goldstein T, Dawson E: A multi-center analysis of percutaneous discectomy. Presented at the North American Spine Society meeting, Quebec City, June 29-July 2, 1989.

12. Kambin P: Arthroscopic microdiscectomy, *Arthrosc J Arthrosc Relat Surg* 8:287, 1992.

13. Kambin, P: Extra-articular endoscopy of the lumbar spine, instructional course, Arthroscopy Association of North America, San Diego, CA, April 26, 1991

14. Kambin P, editor: *Arthroscopic microdiscectomy: minimal intervention in spinal surgery,* Baltimore, 1990, Williams & Wilkins.

15. Kambin P: Percutaneous lumbar discectomy: current practice, *Surg Found Orthop* 31, 1988.

16. Kambin P, Brager M: Percutaneous posterolateral discectomy anatomy and mechanism, *Clin Orthop* 223:145, 1987.

17. Kambin P, Brooks M, Cohen L, Schaffer J: Comparative incidence of degenerative spondylosis of lumbar spine following discectomy. Presented at the North American Spine Society meeting, Boston, July 9-11, 1992.

18. Kambin P, Gellman H: Percutaneous lateral discectomy of the lumbar spine: a preliminary report, *Clin Orthop,* 174:127, 1983.

19. Kambin P, Nixon J, Chait A, Schaffer J: Anular protrusion: pathophysiology and roentgenographic appearance, *Spine* 13:671, 1988.

20. Kambin P, Sampson S: Posterolateral percutaneous suction-excision of herniated lumbar intervertebral discs: report of interim results, *Clin Orthop* 207:37, 1986.

21. Kambin P, Schaffer J: Percutaneous lumbar discectomy-prospective review of 100 patients, *Clin Orthop* 238:24, 1989.

22. Mixter WJ, Barr JS: Rupture of the intervertebral disc with involvement of the spinal canal, *N Engl J Med* 211:210, 1934.

23. Onik G, Helms C, Ginsberg L, et al.: Percutaneous lumbar discectomy using a new aspiration probe, *AJR Am J Roentgenol* 44:1137, 1985.

24. Olmarker K, Rydevik B, Holms S: Edema formation in spinal nerve root induced by experimental graded compression, *Spine* 14:569, 1989.

25. Panjabi MM, Hausfeld JN, White A: A biomechanical study of the ligamentous stability of the thoracic spine in man, *Acta Orthop Scand* 52:315, 1981.

26. Parke W: The significance of venous return impairment in ischemic radiculopathy and myelopathy, *Orthop Clin North Am* 22:213, 1991.

27. Paus B, Skalpe IO: Recurrence of pain following operation for herniated lumbar disc: fresh herniation or extradural scar tissue, *Int Orthop* 3:113, 1979.

28. Ramirez LF, Thisted R: Complications and demographic characteristics of patients undergoing lumbar diskectomy in community hospitals, *Neurosurgery* 25:226, 1989.

29. Savitz, MH: Same-day microsurgical arthroscopic lateral-approach laser-assisted (SMALL) fluoroscopic discectomy, *J Neurosurg* 80:1039-1045, 1994.

30. Schaffer J, Kambin P: Percutaneous posterolateral lumbar discectomy and compression with 6.9 millimeter cannula: analysis of operative failures and complications, *J Bone Joint Surg* 73A:882, 1991.

31. Shinners BM, Hamby WB: Protruded lumbar intervertebral disc results following surgical and nonsurgical therapy, *J Neurosurg* 6:450, 1949.

32. Smith L: Enzyme dissolution of the intervertebral disc, *Nature* 198, 1963.

33. Stolke D, Sollman WP, Seifert V: Intra- and postoperative complications in lumbar disk surgery, *Spine* 14:56, 1989.

Chapter 74
Automated Percutaneous Lumbar Discectomy
Gary M. Onik

History

Indications

Contraindications

Patient Selection

**Other Treatments Versus Automated
Percutaneous Lumbar Discectomy**

chemonucleolysis
manual discectomy
laser discectomy
laminotomy
open discectomy

Technique

Complications

Results

Future Predictions

History

Automated percutaneous lumbar discectomy (APLD) has now been practiced for 9 years. With more than 50 separate series reported in the literature, a number of conclusions can be drawn about the procedure. The first and most important is that the main goal of the procedure—that of reducing the morbidity associated with disc surgery—has been successfully realized. There is virtually no dispute that APLD is the safest procedure available for treating herniated discs. In all the series reported, comprising over 5000 patients, no instance of a major complication has been reported. The only inherent complication of the procedure appears to be that of a 0.2% discitis rate, three to five times lower than that reported for open discectomy. With over 120,000 procedures performed worldwide, no death has been reported associated with the procedure.

The second conclusion is that despite this safety record, the procedure is markedly underutilized. Since APLD, as well as other intradiscal therapies, requires the selection of patients who have contained herniations rather than free or extruded fragments, it requires the surgeon to expend time and energy to select the correct patient for the procedure. When proper selection is carried out, the success rate for the procedure has consistently been reported in the range of 75% to 85%.[*] When the criteria for selecting patients is ignored, however, the success rate can be less than 50%.[49] Unfortunately, owing to a lack of definitive criteria for patient selection during the introduction of the procedure, many surgeons' initial experience was less than satisfying, with many of them abandoning the procedure during the steep portion of the learning curve, after performing only four or five operations. This fact, coupled with a major financial disincentive to perform the procedure (it was 6 years before National Blue Cross Blue Shield Technology Assessment Committee deemed the procedure nonexperimental and recommended reimbursement for it), stifled the utilization of APLD.

Over the years, much has been learned about the procedure, and clearly defined indications for its use have emerged. With today's major trend to cost containment and the currently ongoing effort to expand the population of patients who are candidates for the procedure to include those with extruded discs, a reemergence of APLD and minimally invasive spine surgery in general is occurring.

[*]References 1 to 5, 7, 8, 10 to 14, 16 to 18, 20 to 27, 29 to 31, 33 to 40, 42, 43, 46 to 48, 53 to 55, 57 to 59, and 61 to 66.

Indications

The success of APLD is dependent on patient selection. Automated percutaneous lumbar nucleotomy was developed to treat patients with contained herniated nucleus pulposus (HNPs)—that is, HNPs that are still confined by the anulus and posterior longitudinal ligament (Fig. 74-1). It is a common misconception that APLD is of value only in patients who have "bulging discs" with vague or equivocal symptoms. A large body of literature on the procedure, however, emphasizes that the procedure is used in the patient with the classic radiographic and clinical findings associated with a focal herniated nucleus pulposus. These patients should have sciatica with leg pain greater than back pain and the classic neurologic findings of wasting, weakness, sensory and reflex changes, and a positive straight-leg raising. These patients should also demonstrate a focal herniated nucleus pulposus on an MRI or CT that is consistent with their clinical picture (Fig. 74-2).

The ability to distinguish between these contained HNPs and extruded (free) fragments falls mainly to radiology, since the only clinical criteria noted to correlate with a poor outcome on APLD has been a cross-positive straight-leg raising.[66] External of those findings, the criteria used to differentiate contained versus noncontained herniations include size, shape, migration, and containment on discography.

Automated percutaneous lumbar discectomy works best on small-to-moderate (less than one third

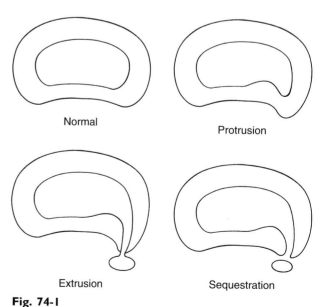

Normal

Protrusion

Extrusion

Sequestration

Fig. 74-1

Varying degrees of nuclear herniation are illustrated. Patients with extrusion and sequestration are not good candidates for APLD.

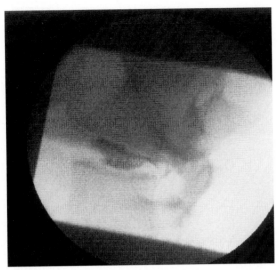

Fig. 74-2

A well-contained herniation seen by discography. Contrast is covering the herniation, and no contrast is noted to flow behind the vertebral bodies, indicating that the anulus is intact.

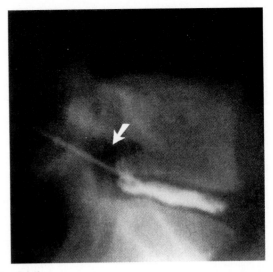

Fig. 74-4

A herniation in which contrast has flowed through a tear in the anulus and has now migrated superiorly (arrow) beyond the disc space. Although there is a tear in the anulus, this disc can be pressurized. Since there is no free flow of contrast into the epidural space, the posterior longitudinal ligament is still intact.

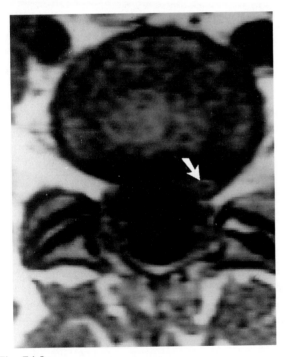

Fig. 74-3

A small focal herniation (arrow) of approximately one third of the thecal sac is shown. This patient is an excellent candidate for APLD.

angulations or irregular shapes are more likely extruded. In addition, intact anular fibers on the sagittal MRI can be evidence for a contained herniation. There can, however, be exceptions to these criteria (Fig. 74-4).

Contraindications

An absolute contraindication to APLD is migration of the disc fragment. Small degrees of migration—that is, 3 mm or less of the herniation—do not preclude the possibility of a good result from APLD. In these cases the epicenter of the herniation is usually still at the disc level. Up until recently this criteria had always been assumed, but never proven by data. In a recently published French study in which 50% of patients had migrated fragments greater than 3 mm, the success rate for APLD was reported at 40%, proving the importance of this criteria.[49]

Patient Selection

It is now clear that the most definitive procedure for selecting patients for APLD is the CT discogram. This procedure demonstrates complete tears of the anulus and posterior longitudinal ligament, indicating those HNPs that are extruded (Fig. 74-5). A CT discogram can also allow assessment of the size of the rent in the anulus that is communicating with the HNP. This is valuable information. When the rent is narrow, giving a mushroom effect to the her-

of the thecal sac) herniated nucleus pulposus (Fig. 74-3). Radiographic literature indicates that herniated discs that comprise 50% or greater of the thecal sac have a 90% chance of being an extruded fragment.[19]

Herniations with smooth obtuse margins are generally contained, while herniations with more acute

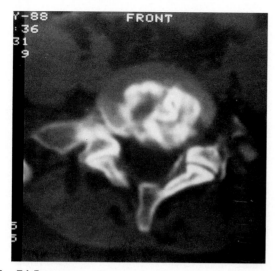

Fig. 74-5

A complete tear of the anulus and the posterior longitudinal ligament. Since contrast flows freely into the epidural space, this disc cannot be pressurized.

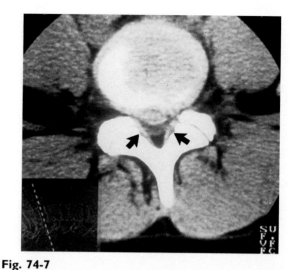

Fig. 74-7

CT scan showing a large herniated nucleus pulposus (arrow) in a teenage girl who injured herself while horseback riding. Although the herniation is large, this patient was treated successfully with APLD.

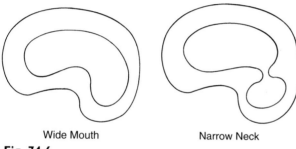

Wide Mouth   Narrow Neck

Fig. 74-6

This illustration shows the appearance of two different anular tears. The wide herniation allows easy retraction of the herniation, making this patient an excellent candidate for APLD. The narrow herniation makes APLD more difficult.

niation, the result of the procedure will be in doubt, with a 50% success rate reported for patients with this finding (Fig. 74-6).[11] When the neck of the HNP is wide with room for transmission of a pressure difference or retraction of the herniation, an excellent success rate of over 80% can be counted on. One of my neurosurgical colleagues now performs CT discography on all candidates for APLD. In his experience, he has an 88% success rate using these selection criteria (Matthew Quigley, personal communication).

Besides the characterization of the herniation on the imaging studies, certain associated radiographic findings should be taken into account when evaluating patients for APLD. Patients with degenerative facet disease should be carefully evaluated prior to APLD. These patients, after the procedure, are more likely to have persistent or possibly worsening of back pain.[38] With this as a consideration, a facet block and/or rhizotomy prior to percutaneous discectomy can help discover what portion of the patient's symptoms are related to the facet arthropathy.

The same considerations should come into play when evaluating patients with spinal stenosis. Patients with congenitally short pedicles may have marked symptomatology due to small herniations. These patients may respond successfully to APLD. Those patients with spinal stenosis and lateral recess stenosis based on facet hypertrophy, however, would be less likely to have a successful result.

Through clinical experience it is now clear there is a certain class of patients who respond particularly well to APLD. These include young patients, patients with far lateral herniations, and patients with previous surgery. Young patients with markedly hydrated discs appear to respond particularly well to APLD. We believe that in these patients, because of the implications of major surgery in this age group, APLD is the procedure of first choice (Fig. 74-7).

Patients with far lateral herniations comprise a group that have a difficult clinical problem. The usual approach to the far lateral herniation often requires significant removal of the facet on the side of the herniation, which could lead to instability. In addition, this can be a technically difficult operation. Automated percutaneous lumbar discectomy is an excellent procedure for the far lateral herniation.[45,60] Since the instrumentation is in extremely close proximity to the herniation or may actually traverse it, results in these patients tend to be immediate and with a high degree of success. Automated percutaneous lumbar discectomy in this patient group may be somewhat more difficult since the nerve is pushed posteriorly by the herniation, closing down the space between the nerve and the anterior surface of the superior articular facet. With maneuvering, however, the nerve can usually be avoided. Any evidence, however, that the herniation has migrated above the disc space should constitute an exclusion for this procedure.

Patients who reherniate after open-back surgery constitute approximately 5% of the population who have that procedure. Unfortunately, patients who are reoperated on with an open discectomy at the same level as previous surgery obtain poor results, as well as being exposed to a very high morbidity owing to the lack of tissue planes caused by the epidural fibrosis.[56] Automated percutaneous lumbar discectomy can be an excellent procedure for this patient population. The route of APLD avoids the epidural space, and therefore APLD in this patient population can be carried out exactly the same way as in other patients. Excellent success rates (as high as 90%) have been reported in this population.[17] The reason for the excellent success rate in this difficult group of patients may be secondary to the fact that the epidural fibrosis decreases the chances of a free fragment occurring. In addition, because of the epidural fibrosis, relatively small changes in the disc pressure may provide greater symptomatic relief. Lastly, this patient population, who has already experienced open discectomy, may be easier to please with any degree of pain relief that avoids a repeat open procedure, being considered by the patient to be a good result. In general, before performing an APLD on this patient population, we obtain a discogram to confirm that a connection between the center of the disc and the HNP exists.

Other Treatments Versus Automated Percutaneous Lumbar Discectomy

Chemonucleolysis

Chemonucleolysis was the first attempt at intradiscal therapy to decrease the morbidity associated with the operative treatment of herniated discs. However, after an initial large patient experience, the use of chymopapain has markedly decreased secondary to the related complications of the procedure. These complications included anaphylaxis, cerebral hemorrhage, seizures, paraplegia, quadriplegia, and a sig-

nificant incidence (30% to 40%) of severe postoperative back spasm associated with the procedure.[9] The spasm results in prolonged hospitalization in some patients with a delayed recuperation period.

Automated percutaneous lumbar discectomy has been compared with chymopapain or chemonucleolysis in at least four different series. Chang compared chemonucleolysis and APLD in 50 patients.[12] In this study, APLD had an 82% success rate versus a 90% success rate for chymopapain; however, APLD had a decreased hospital stay compared with chymopapain, along with an earlier return to function and a quicker return to work. Cooney and associates compared their first 50 chymopapain patients to their experience with their first 50 APLD patients.[14] The APLD patients had an 82% success rate, compared with a 72% success rate for the chymopapain patients. He noted that the major advantage of APLD was the lack of significant back spasm associated with the procedure that he saw in 46% of his chymopapain patients. This resulted in his APLD patients returning to school or work in a markedly reduced time compared with those treated with chymopapain. Based on this experience, in his practice he replaced chemonucleolysis with APLD. These findings were confirmed in a study by Lavignolle and associates, in which 190 patients were studied comparing chemonucleolysis and APLD.[35] In this study, it was found that there was no statistical difference in results between the two procedures at 18 months' follow-up.

The only negative article published comparing chemonucleolysis and APLD was a recent article by Revel and co-workers in which 75 patients in each group were studied.[49] In this study, in which no effort was made to exclude extrusions or migrated free fragments of disc, APLD had a 40% success rate compared with 60% for chemonucleolysis. A low success rate for APLD in this study is not surprising considering that approximately 80% of HNPs in a population will be noncontained and should be excluded from the procedure. The 20% difference in results between the procedures may reflect a patient selection bias or perhaps the ability of chymopapain to flow into the epidural space. The safety implications of this situation, however, can be serious and should not be considered an advantage of chemonucleolysis.

Manual Discectomy

In an effort to improve upon the results of chymopapain, various attempts have been made to non-invasively lower intradiscal pressure by percutaneously removing disc material. In this way the effects of chemonucleolysis, that is, disc decompression, could be accomplished without the hazards of an injectable drug. Manual percutaneous discectomy was the first such procedure. Success rates for this procedure range from 75% to 85%, comparable to chemonucleolysis.[28,52] However, complications such as discitis and major vascular injury have been reported. The technique used in the original manual percutaneous discectomy studies has since been modified by a number of investigators.[32,51] These improvements did not decrease the number of complications associated with manual percutaneous discectomy. When the manual method was compared with APLD, similar success rates were found, but the smaller instrumentation and decreased trauma with APLD resulted in decreased physical therapy needed in the APLD patient with an accelerated return to work over the manual method.[57]

Laser Discectomy

Laser discectomy is the newest entry into the intradiscal therapy arena. While the success rate of the procedure would be expected to be the same as other intradiscal therapies, the lack of inherent safety owing to the spread of heat beyond the confines of the placement of the instrument has already caused injuries to the nerve roots and the bowel.[6,15] Since laser discectomy has no theoretic advantages over mechanical methods of APLD, the use of this technology, except in experimental protocols, does not seem to be justified. For this reason, a laser percutaneous discectomy is considered experimental by almost all third-party payers.

Open Discectomy

There are now two studies that compare laminotomy and APLD. In a series published by Swiecicki, a comparison was made between 100 consecutive laminotomy cases and APLD.[57] In this report, APLD had an equivalent success rate of approximately 80% as compared with a laminotomy. APLD, however, had a markedly shorter hospital stay, return to work, and less need for postoperative physical therapy.

Wilson and associates recently reported a randomized study comparing open discectomy and APLD in patients with a contained HNP.[66] In this study, APLD had a 72% success rate compared with 80% for open discectomy. The authors concluded that due to APLD's low morbidity and early return to function, it was the procedure of choice compared with open discectomy in this patient population.

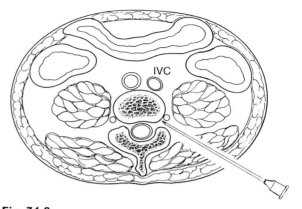

Fig. 74-8

This diagram shows the importance of the posterior vertebral body line.

Technique

The procedure is carried out under local anesthesia, since general anesthesia carries the risk of neural injury. Using sterile technique the patient is placed in either the lateral decubitus or the prone position. The entry point is chosen from a preoperative localization CT scan. By means of this posterolateral approach, an 18-gauge needle is placed down to the disc space. The placement of the trocar (lateral view) should be parallel to and midway between the vertebral body end plates, with the tip of the trocar directed toward the disc center. The point should be touching the posterior vertebral body line when the anulus is felt. If the trocar is anterior to this line and the anulus is felt or if the patient is experiencing any radicular pain, the trocar is withdrawn and redirected. When the anulus is felt and the tip of the trocar is at the posterior vertebral body line, the anteroposterior view is checked to confirm that the tip is not medial to a line connecting the medial aspect of the pedicles, and is therefore not traversing the thecal sac (Fig. 74-8). When the trocar is properly placed, the tip is advanced into the disc center on both the anteroposterior and lateral views. The cannula and dilator are inserted over the trocar. They are then pushed down to the wall of the anulus, and their position is confirmed radiographically in two views. Once placement is confirmed, the dilator is removed, leaving the trocar and cannula in place. The trephine is placed over the trocar and through the cannula. At this point, the fluoroscopic unit is perpendicular to the cannula and trephine, confirming that they are actually against the anulus. After

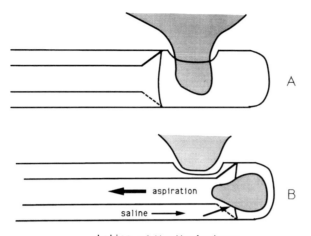

Action of the Nucleotome

Fig. 74-9

This diagram illustrates how the nucleotome applies suction to the central core (**A**). The inner cutting sleeve is pneumatically driven across the side port, guillotining the disc material (**B**). The disc material is then suspended in saline and is aspirated away.

the disc is incised, the trephine and trocar are removed, leaving the cannula in place, and the nucleotome aspiration probe is placed into the disc. The nucleotome position is confirmed and it is turned on to aspirate the disc material (Fig. 74-9). After no more disc material can be removed, the rigid cannula can then be angled to change the position of the nucleotome within the disc. When no further disc material can be removed, the nucleotome is turned off and pulled back into the cannula, and both are removed. The puncture site is covered with a bandage. In most cases, the patient is held for 3 hours and then discharged the same day of surgery.

It has been emphasized in the past that an improperly placed probe could do serious damage to the great vessels or thecal sac.[46] Considering these landmarks, it has been stated in the literature that "injury to these structures is virtually impossible."[5,53] Unfortunately, no technique can eliminate gross error by the operator. There are now two cases reported in the literature of a nucleotome probe being placed erroneously into the thecal sac, resulting in severe nerve injuries. It has been suggested that performance of the procedure under CT guidance could totally eliminate this possibility.[54] It has also been advised that any physician not comfortable with the localization of a needle in two fluoroscopic views should enlist the help of a radiologist to do the procedure or not do the procedure at all.[46] In any case, such injuries are not inherent to the procedure, and should not be considered as a possible complication of a competently performed percutaneous discectomy.

Complications

It is clear from the literature that APLD is the safest procedure that can be performed on patients for a herniated nucleus pulposus. These conclusions can be drawn from over 50 separate articles published, comprising well over 5000 patients.* From this literature, it can be concluded that APLD has fulfilled the most important criteria of a noninvasive procedure: safety. In all these published articles, no major complications were reported. A discitis rate of approximately 0.2%, three to five times lower than that of open discectomy, was the only significant inherent morbidity. In addition to low morbidity, however, the results of the procedure have consistently been reported to be between 75% and 85%. Remarkably, there is yet to be a reported mortality from APLD. It is this safety record that makes APLD the procedure of first choice in patients with contained herniations.[5,23,66]

Results

The first major article published on APLD was a prospective multiinstitutional study by Onik and associates, which consisted of over 500 patients.[44] The prospective inclusion criteria was that of the classic "disc herniation" patient. When the patients met these criteria, a 75% success rate was reported, with failures being due to unrecognized free fragments. Of interest is that only 15% of patients required an open discectomy. If those patients who were successfully treated by a second percutaneous discectomy are included, the success rate increases to 80%.

When the procedure was performed outside the protocol, including patients who were compensation cases or who did not fit the classic symptoms or physical findings of a herniated disc, the success rate of APLD dropped to 50%. Considering the morbidity of the procedure, however, it has been stated that APLD is perhaps a reasonable alternative in this patient population, particularly if all conservative means have failed and the patient is still nonfunctional.[5] This study refuted certain myths that had been associated with APLD, such as the fact that APLD was reserved for a different class of patient, that is, those with bulging discs, who did not fit the classic herniated disc criteria. From the inclusion criteria of this study, it was clear that this was not true and that the classic disc herniation patient was the *best* candidate for this procedure.

*See reference footnote on p 1018.

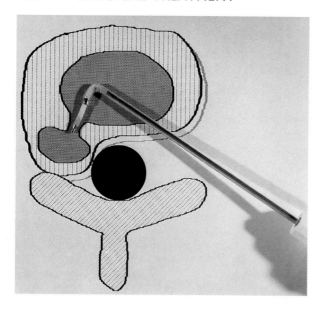

Fig. 74-10

This diagram shows how the curved cannula and nucleotome can be negotiated through the rent in the anulus into the herniation.

Another myth associated with the procedure is that all patients who have APLD would get better anyway with conservative care and that the procedure is just reflecting the natural history of the disease. In the study by Onik, the mean patient symptom duration was 11.5 months, clearly indicating that patients in this study who had APLD were not resolving their symptoms of their own accord. This finding was confirmed by a number of other studies as well.[38,57] In Onik's study, the only major complication was one case of discitis, a rate three to five times less than open or hand discectomy.

The findings of Onik and associates were confirmed by a similar multiinstitutional study carried out by Bocchi and colleagues, in which a 72% success rate was obtained in over 600 patients.[4] Again, the only complication was one case of discitis. The initial results of these multiinstitutional studies are remarkable in that the safety and success of the procedure were confirmed even taking into account the fact that surgeons were all new to the procedure, particularly in regard to patient selection. These studies gave a realistic expectation for the new user of APLD, since it included all the learning curves of the participating physicians.

Since APLD was first used in 1984, long-term results of the procedure are now being published. Schweigel and associates, in a series of 146 patients followed for 2 or more years, reported a 77% success rate with no complications.[53] Ulrich, in a 2-year follow-up, reported a 70% success rate in 45 patients[59]; and Gill, studying 62 patients followed up to 4.5 years, reported a 93% success rate in non-compensation patients, with an overall success rate

of 78%, including compensation patients.[21] Other series have shown a reherniation rate associated with APLD varying from 3% to 5%, with little change in the success rate after 6 months.[38,47]

While all the studies agree that patient selection is critical to the success of APLD, a number of other factors have been shown to be of *little* import in affecting the results. The disc level appears to have no effect on the success rate of APLD, with the L5-S1 level having the same success rate as the L4-L5 level.[5,53] There also appears to be little correlation of the amount of disc material removed in terms of absolute amount; however, virtually all authors suggest removing as much disc material as possible since this might have an effect on the eventual recurrence rate. Clinical experience with APLD confirms the biomechanical studies showing there is little disc-space narrowing associated with the procedure. Follow-up radiographic studies have shown little short-term change in the radiographic picture of the herniation, although definite neurologic improvement in these patients can be shown. This is consistent with the idea of decreased intradiscal pressure, particularly under loading situations, being a major factor in the patient's resolution of symptoms.

Future Predictions

The goal of intradiscal therapy must now be to expand the patient population to include those with extruded or free fragments. While various investigators have tried to obtain disc material from a more posterior position within the disc space, attempts to remove extruded or free fragments of disc consis-

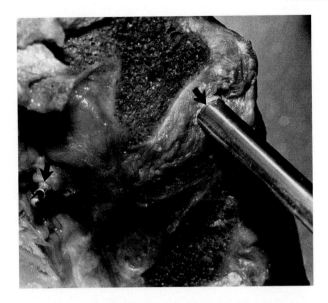

Fig. 74-11

A cadaver spine with a curved nucleotome (arrow) through it. The cannula can be seen entering the disc in relationship to the pedicle, similar to the trajectory of a routine percutaneous discectomy.

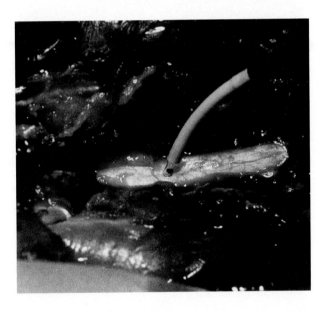

Fig. 74-12

The thecal sac of a dog, exposed by laminectomy. The flat end nucleotome tents the dura, pushing the dura away from the port of the probe. This prevents the nucleotome from sucking the dura up.

tently have been unsuccessful.[41] Requirements for successfully obtaining this result would include the ability to negotiate within the disc, directing an instrument posteriorly that must then be negotiated through the anular rent directly into the herniation. There must be some means of removing the herniation without injuring surrounding structures (Fig. 74-10). While simple in concept, the mechanical requirements needed to accomplish this task are significant. After 3 years in development, a flexible nucleotome that can be negotiated through an anular rent is now available (Fig. 74-11). It is postulated that the blunt end of the instrument and the recessed side port would enable disc material to be removed without injuring the dura, owing to a tent-

ing action by the probe tip (Fig. 74-12). The ultimate success and safety of this approach remain to be determined.

In conclusion, intradiscal therapy appears to be firmly entrenched as an acceptable treatment for contained disc herniations. Of all the methods of intradiscal therapy, APLD has the most clinical experience associated with it and has demonstrated a superior safety record, making it the procedure of choice. It is hoped that continued research and development in this field will expand the patient population suitable for intradiscal therapy and thus decrease the number of patients exposed to the increased risks of open surgical treatment of herniated lumbar discs.

References

1. Benazet JP and others: Treatment of complete lumbar disk herniation by percutaneous discectomy, *Chirurgie (Fr)* 117(1):59, 1991.

2. Blanc C and others: Treatment of herniated lumbar disc by percutaneous nucleotomy with aspiration: preliminary results in 70 cases, *J Neuroradiol* 17(3):182, 1990.

3. Bocchi L, Ferrata P, Passarello F: The Onik method of automated percutaneous lumbar diskectomy (A.P.L.D.): criteria of selection, technique, and evaluation of results, *Ital J Orthop Traumatol* 17(1):5, 1991.

4. Bocchi L and others: La nucleoaspirazione secondo Onik nel trattamento dell'ernia discale lombare analisi multicentrica dei primi risultati su oltre 650 trattamenti, *Riv Neuroradiol* 2(suppl 1):119, 1989.

5. Bonaldi G and others: Percutaneous discectomy using Onik's method: three years' experience, *Neuroradiology* 33:516, 1991.

6. Bonati AO: Arthroscopic lumbar laser discectomy. Toft/Hoogland Course, Munich, November 1991.

7. Bonneville JF and others: CT of the lumbar intervertebral disc space after automated percutaneous nucleotomy: comparison with chemonucleolysis, *Rachis* 1(2):113, 1989.

8. Capanna AH, Capanna DM: *Correlations of amount of disk removed by percutaneous lumbar diskectomy and clinical results.* In Mayer HM, Brock M, editors: *Percutaneous lumbar diskectomy,* Berlin, 1989, Springer-Verlag.

9. Carter H and others: Post-nucleolysis low-back pain: influence of early ambulation. Toft/Hoogland Course, Munich, November 1991.

10. Cartolari R, Davidovits P, Gagliardelli M: *Automated percutaneous lumbar diskectomy (APLD).* In Mayer HM, Brock M, editors: *Percutaneous lumbar diskectomy,* Berlin, 1989, Springer-Verlag.

11. Castro WHM and others: Restriction of indication for automated percutaneous lumbar discectomy based on computed tomographic discography, *Spine* 17(10):1239, 1992.

12. Chang SK: Chemonucleolysis vs percutaneous automated nucleotome in lumbar disc surgery, *Konruk University School of Medicine Academic Journal* 34(2):43, 1990.

13. Chen SC, Chatterjl S, Solanki R: Automated percutaneous lumbar discectomy: experience in a district hospital, *Orthop Prod News,* February 1992, p 28.

14. Cooney FD: *Comparison of chemonucleolysis with chymopapain to percutaneous automated diskectomy: a surgeon's first 50 cases of each.* In Mayer HM, Brock M, editors: *Percutaneous lumbar diskectomy,* Berlin, 1989, Springer-Verlag.

15. Cooney FD: Comparison of the early results of laser lumbar decompression to chemonucleolysis and automated percutaneous lumbar discectomy. Toft/Hoogland Course. Munich, November 1991.

16. Corkill G, Kimple J, Corkill R: *Automated percutaneous nucleotomy by pain scale.* In Mayer HM, Brock M, editors: *Percutaneous lumbar diskectomy,* Berlin, 1989, Springer-Verlag.

17. Davis GW, Onik GM, Helms CA: Automated percutaneous discectomy, *Spine* 16(3):359, 1991.

18. Dei-Anang K, Weigand H, Mader U: Is the percutaneous disectomy an alternative to chemonucleolysis? *Radiologe* 30:70, 1990.

19. Edwards W, Orme T, Orr-Edwards B: CT discography: prognostic value in the selection of patients for chemonucleolysis, *Spine* 12:792, 1987.

20. Flynn LM and others: Arthroscopically-assisted lateral percutaneous lumbar disckectomy using the Onik Nucleotome, *J Neurol Orthop Med Surg* 9(1):45, 1988.

21. Gill K, Blumenthal SL: Clinical experience with automated percutaneous diskectomy—the nucleotome system, *Orthopedics* 14(7):757, 1991.

22. Gobin P and others: Percutaneous automated lumbar nucleotomy, *J Neuroradiol* 16:203, 1989.

23. Gobin P and others: Percutaneous automated lumbar nucleotomy; *J Radiol* 71(6–7):401, 1990.

24. Goldstein TB, Mink JH, Dawson EG: Early experience with automated percutaneous lumbar discectomy in the treatment of lumbar disk herniations, *Clin Orthop* 238:77, 1989.

25. Gomez-Castresana F, Vazquez Herrero C, Baltes Horche JL: Cervical chemonucleolysis: three years of experience. Toft/Hoogland Course, Munich, November 1991.

26. Hammon W: Percutaneous lumbar nucleotomy, *Neurosurgery* 24(4):635, 1989.

27. Hidalgo Ovejero AM and others: Resultados iniciales de la nucleotomia percutanea automatizada en el tratamiento de las hernias discales, *Rev Ortop Traum* 35(6):428, 1991.

28. Hijikata S: Percutaneous nucleotomy: a new concept technique and 12 years' experience, *Clin Orthop* 238:9, 1989.

29. Jacchia GE, D'Arienzo M, Pavolini B: Results in the first 100 cases of lumbar disc herniation treated with percutaneous discectomy, *J Bone Joint Surg [Br]* 74-B(suppl 1):51, 1992.

30. Jacobson S: Lumbar percutaneous diskectomy, *Bull Hosp Jt Dis Orthop Inst* 48(1):67, 1988.

31. Kahanovitz N and others: A multicenter analysis of percutaneous discectomy, *Spine* 15(7):713, 1990.

32. Kambin P, Schaffer JL: Percutaneous lumbar discectomy: review of 100 patients and current practice, *Clin Orthop* 238:24, 1989.

33. Kaps H, Cotta H: *Early results of automated percutaneous lumbar diskectomy.* In Mayer HM, Brock M, editors: *Percutaneous lumbar diskectomy,* Berlin, 1989, Springer-Verlag.

34. Kovac D: Significance of automatic endoscopic percutaneous diskectomy in the treatment of lumbar disc herniation, *Lijec Vjesn* 113:158, 1991.

35. Lavignolle B, Castagnera L, Grenier N: Comparative study of nucleolysis versus percutaneous nucleotomy versus automated discectomy in treatment of herniated disc, *Nucleotomie Percutanee Manuelle Et Nucleoaspiration* 287.

36. Lesion F and others: La Nucleotomie percutanee automatisee en pathologie discal lombaire, *J Chir (Paris)* 126:185, 1989.

37. Lisai P and others: Percutaneous nucleotomy: the indications and limits. *Arch Putti Chir Organi Mov* 38(2):311, 1990.

38. Luft C and others: Automated percutaneous lumbar discectomy (APLD)—method and 1-year follow-up, *European Radiology* 2:292, 1992.

39. Magalhaes ACA, Weigand H, Barros Filho TE: Herniated lumbar disc: automated percutaneous discectomy, *Rev Hosp Clin Fac Med S Paulo* 44(6):285, 1989.

40. Maroon JC, Allen RC: A retrospective study of 1,054 APLD cases: a twenty-month clinical follow-up at 35 US centers, *J Neurol Orthop Med Surg* 10(4):L335, 1989.

41. Mayer HM, Brock M: Percutaneous endoscopic discectomy: surgical technique and preliminary results compared to microsurgical discectomy, *J Neurosurg* 78:216, 1993.

42. Moison JJF and others: Results of a multicentric study of 297 cases automated percutaneous discectomy. Toft/Hoogland Course, Munich, November 1991.

43. Morris JM: Percutaneous discectomy, *West J Med* 155(2):172, 1991.

44. Onik GM, Helms CA: Automated percutaneous lumbar diskectomy, *Am J Roentgenol* 156:531, 1991.

45. Onik G, Maroon J, Shang Y: Far-lateral disc herniation: treatment by automated percutaneous diskectomy, *AJNR* 11:865, 1990.

46. Onik GM and others: Automated percutaneous discectomy: a prospective multi-institutional study, *Neurosurgery* 26(2):228, 1990.

47. Phelip X, Troussier B, Chirossel JP: La nucleotomie percutanee automatisee dans le traitement des hernies discales lombaires, *La Presse Medicale* 21(34):1604, 1992.

48. Pitto E, Fabbri D, Pitto RP: Clinical experience with automated percutaneous diskectomy, *Arch Putti Chir Organi Mov* 38(2):321, 1990.

49. Revel M and others: Automated percutaneous lumbar discectomy versus chemonucleolysis in the treatment of sciatica, a randomized multicenter trial, *Spine* 18(1):1, 1993.

50. Rezaian SM, Silver ML: *Percutaneous diskectomy—personal observations of 27 cases.* In Mayer HM, Brock M, editors: *Percutaneous lumbar diskectomy*, Berlin, 1989, Springer-Verlag.

51. Schaffer JL, Kambin P: Percutaneous posterolateral lumbar discectomy and decompression with a 6.9-millimeter cannula, *J Bone Joint Surg [Am]* 73-A(6):822, 1991.

52. Schreiber A, Suezawa Y: Transdiscoscopic percutaneous nucleotomy in disk herniation, *Orthop Rev* 15(1):75, 1986.

53. Schweigel J: *Automated percutaneous discectomy: comparison with chymopapain.* In *Automated percutaneous discectomy*, San Francisco, 1988, Radiology Research and Education Foundation.

54. Seibel RMM, Gronemeyer DHW, Sorensen RAL: Percutaneous nucleotomy with CT and fluoroscopic guidance, *JVIR* 3:571, 1992.

55. Solini A, Paschero B, Ruggieri N: Automated percutaneous diskectomy according to the Onik method: conclusive considerations, *Ital J Orthop Traumatol* 17(2):225, 1991.

56. Stolke D, Sollmann WP, Seifert V: Intra- and postoperative complications in lumbar disc surgery, *Spine* 14:56, 1989.

57. Swiecicki M: *Results of percutaneous lumbar diskectomy compared to laminectomy and chemonucleolysis.* In Mayer HM, Brock M, editors: *Percutaneous lumbar diskectomy*, Berlin, 1989, Springer-Verlag.

58. Troussier B and others: La nucleotomie percutanee automatisee: technique, indications et resultats. A propos de 50 patients, *Rhumatologie* 42(9):307, 1990.

59. Ulrich HW: Automated percutaneous diskectomy: indication, technique and results after 2 years, *Z Orthop (Germany)* 130(1)45, 1992.

60. Vanneroy F and others: A new deal with far lateral lumbar disk herniations (FLHD) automated percutaneous discectomy, *European Radiology* 1(Suppl): S163, 1992.

61. Vanneroy F and others: Percutaneous automated nucleotomy in the treatment of foraminal and extra-foraminal lumbar disk herniation: review of 18 cases, *Rachis* 3(4):323, 1991.

62. Vogel KE, Leclercq TA: Percutaneous lumbar disc excision: experience with sixty cases and review of the literature, *J La State Med Soc* 143:25, 1991.

63. Vogl G and others: Neuroradiologic treatment possibilities of intervertebral disk displacement, *Wien Klin Wochenschr (Austria)* 104(8):243, 1992.

64. Weigand H: Perkutane Nukleotomie—Eine nichtoperative, perkutane Behandlungsmethode des lumbalen Bandscheibenvorfalls, *Jahrbuch der Radiologie* 169–176, 1991.

65. Weigand H, Weissner B: Percutaneous nucleotomy: a new interventional radiological technique for lumbar disk removal, *Ann Radiol* 32(1):34, 1989.

66. Wilson LF, Mulholland RC: Automated percutaneous discectomy versus surgery: a prospective randomised study of treatment for lumbar disc protrusions. Presented at the Third Annual Meeting of the European Spine Society, Cambridge, September 3, 1992.

Chapter 75
Microsurgical Discectomy and Spinal Decompression
W. Bradford DeLong

History and Current Trends

Indications

Microsurgical Techniques Compared with "Standard" Techniques

    advantages of the operating microscope
    disadvantages of the operating microscope
    the principles of spinal surgery

The Technique of Microsurgical Spinal Surgery

    preoperative evaluation and preparation
    intraoperative medications
    operative positioning
    the operating microscope
    instruments
    intraoperative roentgenograms
    operative technique

Variations

    local anesthesia
    outpatient microsurgery
    the lateral position
    preserving the ligamentum flavum
    bilateral decompression for spinal stenosis
    limited disc removal versus curettage of
        the disc space

Potential Complications

    inexperience using the microscope
    postoperative neurologic deficit
    retained disc fragments
    cerebrospinal fluid leaks
    postoperative infection
    mistaken level of surgery
    perforation of the great vessels

Results

Predictions for the Future

History and Current Trends

Yasargil demonstrated that the operating microscope contributes greatly to the success of neurosurgical procedures.[28] Stereoscopic magnification combined with intense coaxial lighting along the surgeon's line of vision increases the ease and accuracy of surgical dissection.

Williams advocated use of the operating microscope for lumbar discectomies.[25] Now many neurologic and orthopedic surgeons use the microscope during lumbar spinal surgery, but there is considerable confusion regarding the definition of terms such as "microsurgical discectomy."

Williams rigidly defines the term *microlumbar discectomy*. He applies it specifically to a procedure that includes "no laminectomy, no facet trauma, no scalpel incisions in the anulus fibrosus, and no curettement of the intervertebral tissue."[24] Williams preserves all fat and healthy disc tissue, and permits no electrocoagulation of any kind within the spinal canal. Williams applies the term *microlumbar discectomy* to the treatment of soft virgin disc herniations in the absence of spinal stenosis or other bony spinal pathology.

Other terms remain less well defined. The term *microsurgical discectomy* is currently applied not only to the specific procedure defined by Williams, but also to more extensive procedures, which can include laminotomy or partial laminectomy, medial facetectomy, foraminotomy of the intervertebral canal, and curettage of the interspace.

It would probably be best if the term *microlumbar discectomy* were used to define the specific limited discectomy defined by Williams, without bone removal and without curettage of the interspace. The term *microsurgical discectomy* can be applied to a discectomy that includes a limited partial laminectomy (a so-called "laminotomy"), and may or may not include curettage of the interspace. If the nerve root needs to be decompressed in the subarticular lateral recess or in the intervertebral canal (the so-called "neural foramen"), then the appropriate procedural term would be "microsurgical spinal decompression." If a discectomy also is required, then the appropriate term would be "microsurgical discectomy and spinal decompression."

Indications

The indications for microsurgical spinal procedures are the same as the indications for "standard" discectomies or operations for spinal stenosis. Microsurgical spinal procedures are performed primarily to relieve leg pain. The patient may or may not have back pain as well. Very few, if any, individuals with back pain alone will experience a satisfactory result with discectomy or lateral spinal decompression.

Microsurgical Techniques Compared with "Standard" Techniques

Advantages of the Operating Microscope

There is controversy concerning whether the operating microscope is necessary for performing lumbar spinal surgery, or whether it even offers an advantage. The results in the literature, summarized below, suggest that patients who have undergone microsurgical disc excisions leave the hospital sooner and return to full activity sooner than do patients who have had a "standard" laminectomy.

Use of the microscope probably offers several specific advantages. Magnification allows the surgeon better appreciation of the anatomy. A nerve root distorted and flattened by a disc fragment anterior to it can be recognized before it is accidentally incised by the surgeon, who may think it is part of the compressed anulus. The epidural veins can be recognized and preserved, to maintain venous drainage of the nerve root. Tissue planes between a nerve root and an adherent disc fragment can be more easily developed if magnification is available. If a dural tear occurs, it can be repaired more accurately under magnification.

The newer microscope stands offer a balanced microscope secured by electromagnetic locks that allow the surgeon to "float" the microscope into position by touching a button or by pressing a mouthswitch and moving the microscope with his or her teeth and mouth (Fig. 75-1). These systems have greatly improved the ease of maneuvering the microscope, and give the surgeon as much freedom as he or she normally has when wearing loupes* and a headlight.

The magnification afforded by the microscope is stereoscopic, because the system of prisms within the

---

*"Loupes", technically, are single lenses fit into eyeglasses, worn to magnify a field of work. A jeweler would generally wear a set of loupes. The term *surgical telescopes* can be used to indicate a sophisticated set of multiple lenses fit into a barrel attached to each lens of a pair of eyeglasses. The use of multiple lenses allows considerable choice in regard to power of magnification and depth and width of field. (Designs-for-Vision, 760 Koehler Ave., Ronkonkoma, NY 11779.)

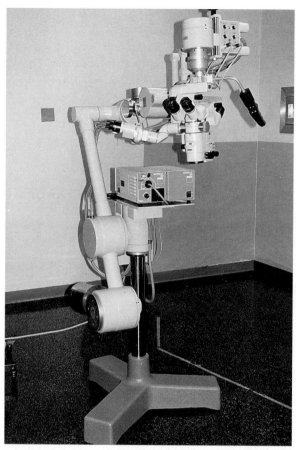

Fig. 75-1

The Zeiss Varioskop operating microscope on the Contraves electromagnetic stand. The stand is balanced, and allows the surgeon to "float" the microscope into position easily.

microscope "compresses" the surgeon's interpupillary distance. The objective lenses are closer together than the surgeon's pupils (Fig. 75-2). The lenses of surgical telescopes are only slightly closer together than the surgeon's pupils, and do not allow stereoscopic vision within deep operative fields.

The light projected by the microscope is very intense and is more nearly coaxial with the surgeon's line of vision than the light from most headlights (Fig. 75-2).

Current optical accessories for the microscope include a truly binocular viewing station for the assistant surgeon, and attachments for video observation and recording of the procedure. Therefore, the assistant surgeon can participate in the procedure to a much greater extent than he or she can during procedures in which the surgeon's head blocks the view (Fig. 75-3). Other members of the operating team can also participate more effectively when they can follow the procedure on a video monitor. Improved observation and recording of the procedure is especially important in teaching situations.

The microscope, with its stereoscopic magnification and intense coaxial lighting, allows the surgeon to work effectively in a narrow, deep operative field. Therefore, he or she can use a smaller incision and limit soft-tissue trauma. The shorter incision protects the paravertebral muscles from extensive denervation, decreases blood loss, and is more cosmetic, thus increasing patient acceptance of the operative procedure.

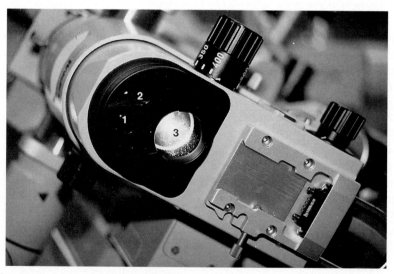

Fig. 75-2

The objectives are closer together than the surgeon's interpupillary distance, allowing true stereoscopic viewing in deep, narrow operative fields. The intense light is projected fiberoptically so that it is nearly coaxial with the surgeon's view. 1 and 2 = objective lenses; 3 = coaxial light.

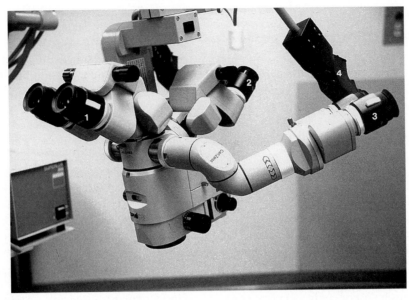

Fig. 75-3

Optical accessories allow true stereoscopic viewing by the assistant surgeon. The binocular observation tube gives a third observer a good view of the operative field, but since it attaches to only one port of the beam splitter, it provides only a "pseudostereoscopic" image, which is somewhat flatter than the assistant's and surgeon's views. 1 = surgeon's stereoscopic station; 2 = assistant's stereoscopic station; 3 = observer's "pseudostereoscopic" station; 4 = motorized hand controls for changing zoom magnification setting, focus, and microscope position.

Disadvantages of the Operating Microscope

The main disadvantage of the operating microscope is the time and practice the surgeon must devote to learning its use. The surgeon should become thoroughly familiar with the microscope before using it in surgery, either during residency or fellowship, or by attending one of the many postgraduate courses in spinal microsurgical techniques. At the very least, the surgeon should practice using the microscope in a laboratory or "after hours" in the operating suite, referring to books and training videos.[8,18,28]

The Principles of Spinal Surgery

There is really nothing magical about the use of the microscope. It simply provides a way of seeing the operative field better, though the remarkable increase in hand–eye coordination that occurs when the surgeon works under magnification sometimes seems almost magical.[8] The microscope allows reconstructive surgeons to perform freehand anastomoses of blood vessels smaller in diameter than the wire of a paper clip, using needles finer than a human hair and suture material only three times the diameter of a red blood cell.

However, the surgeon who is inexperienced in the use of the microscope may become so involved with his or her attempts to manipulate the instrument that he or she forgets the basic principles of spinal surgery.

Fager, in a critique of microsurgical techniques applied to lumbar disc surgery, has summarized these principles.[11] First, the exposure must accomplish decompression of the neural elements before attempting to deal with the lesion itself. Following this principle avoids damage to the nerve roots or cauda equina during removal of the lesion or as an effect of postoperative edema. Second, the neural elements must be satisfactorily released longitudinally. If a nerve root or the cauda equina remains restricted cephalad or caudad to the lesion, neurologic damage may occur during excision of the lesion. If the bony removal is not extended adequately cephalad or caudad, disc fragments that have migrated may be missed. Third, the lesion should be approached laterally to minimize retraction on the nerve root or cauda equina and to allow better visualization and preservation of the epidural veins.

These principles can easily be followed during microsurgical spinal procedures, as long as the surgeon is comfortable with the microscope and does not get distracted and frustrated by maneuvering it inadequately during the procedure.

The Technique of Microsurgical Spinal Surgery

Following is this author's technique for performing microsurgical lumbar discectomy, decompression of lateral spinal stenosis, or a combination of the two.

Preoperative Evaluation and Preparation

A patient who is a candidate for spinal surgery will have failed to respond to a program of conservative therapy. The best surgical candidates will have more leg pain than back pain. A patient who has only back pain is probably not a candidate for discectomy or lateral spinal decompression alone.

Because of the precision of the microsurgical approach, it is very important to define exactly the pathology involved, using preoperative imaging studies of good quality. The exact location of extruded or sequestered disc fragments must be demonstrated, and the degree of subarticular lateral recess stenosis or intervertebral canal stenosis must be defined. Usually an MRI scan will suffice, but if the patient has significant disc resorption and narrowing at the involved level, then a CT scan may also be necessary to study the lateral region of the spinal canal and define the degree of stenosis present.

Epstein points out the importance of using CT scanning preoperatively to identify Type I–IV posterior vertebral limbus fractures.[10] Dealing with these lesions surgically generally requires more extensive bone removal than excising a simple disc herniation, and preoperative planning is important.

If the patient has had previous spinal surgery, then an intravenously enhanced MRI scan will be helpful in distinguishing a recurrent disc herniation from postoperative fibrous tissue. A myelogram followed by an enhanced CT scan may also be necessary.

It is unusual for an individual undergoing a microsurgical procedure to require a blood transfusion. However, most of our patients wish to reduce the chance they might receive a transfusion from an unknown donor to the lowest level. Therefore, most of them provide a unit of packed red cells for their surgery through autodonation or through the use of a designated donor.

Fibrin adhesive is prepared from the donated blood, for use in sealing a dural tear, should one occur.[16,22]

We routinely use prophylactic intraoperative and postoperative antibiotics, usually one of the cephalosporin preparations.

Intraoperative Medications

Before making the incision, the skin and paravertebral muscle attachments are infiltrated with 0.5% lidocaine containing 1:200,000 epinephrine.

In the spinal canal, hemostasis is secured by the temporary application of Gelfoam (absorbable gelatin sponge, USP) soaked in thrombin, USP (1000 Units/ml).

Before closure, 0.25% plain Marcaine without preservatives is instilled into the disc space, the exposed epidural space, and the attachments of the interspinous and supraspinous ligaments.

Antibiotic irrigation is used throughout the case, usually Bacitracin (50,000 Units/500 ml).

Operative Positioning

The patient is placed in a modified knee–chest position on one of the operative frames available, usually the Andrews frame (Fig. 75-4).* This provides optimal abdominal decompression and prevents the great vessels from being compressed against the anterior aspect of the vertebral column, probably protecting them from injury.

The Operating Microscope

The Zeiss operating microscope is the "gold standard" of intraoperative magnification.† Most operating suites have at least the Zeiss OPMi I model, which has manual magnification settings of 6×, 10×, 16×, 25×, and 40×.

The actual magnification achieved is somewhat less than the settings indicate and depends on the selected combination of oculars (e.g., 12.5×, 16×, or 20×), objective (e.g., 200 mm, 250 mm, 300 mm, 350 mm, or 400 mm), and binocular tube length (125 mm or 160 mm).[18,28]

To achieve the full magnification indicated on the settings of the Zeiss OPMi I microscope, one would have to use 20× oculars, a 200-mm objective, and a 160-mm binocular tube length, but this is not a satisfactory configuration for spinal surgery. The use of 16× oculars, a 300-mm objective, and a 160-mm binocular gives actual magnifications of one half the indicated settings—3× at a setting of 6×, 5× at a setting of 10×, and 8× at a setting of 16×.

---

*Andrews frame available from Orthopedic Systems Inc, 1897 National Ave., Hayward, CA 94545.
†Carl Zeiss Inc, 1 Zeiss Dr., Thornwood, NY 10594.

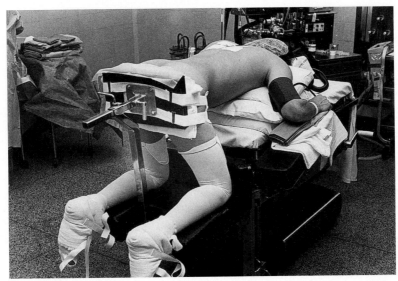

Fig. 75-4

The patient on the Andrews frame in the modified knee–chest position.

For disc surgery, a 300-, 350-, or 400-mm objective can be used. The 300-mm lens attenuates the illumination less and provides a brighter field, but the 400-mm objective provides greater clearance for the manipulation of the instruments. I prefer the 300-mm lens, but some surgeons use the 350-mm option as a reasonable compromise. Either 12.5×, 16×, or 20× high-eyepoint oculars can be used. It is important to use high-eyepoint oculars because they provide a wider field of view than the standard oculars. They can also be used with eyeglasses if the surgeon must wear them. An angled binocular should be used for lumbar spinal surgery. The binocular tube comes in focal lengths of 160 mm and 125 mm. The 160-mm option provides higher magnification, but it is longer and puts the surgeon farther from the surgical field. I prefer the shorter 125-mm binocular.

Therefore, if I am using the OPMi I model, I use it with 16× high-eyepoint oculars, an angled 125-mm binocular, and the 300-mm objective. This combination gives actual magnification of 2.5× at a setting of 6×, 4× at a setting of 10×, 6× at a setting of 16×, 10× at a setting of 25×, and 16× at a setting of 40×. At a setting of 16× (6× actual magnification), the field of vision is 33-mm wide.[18,28]

There are several other Zeiss models available more sophisticated than the OPMi I. The OPMi II model has a power zoom magnification changer, which gives a range of actual magnification similar to the manual settings on the OPMi I. The new Varioskop model has motorized zoom and focus controls, which allow continuous variation of the focal length of the objective to allow for changes in the depth of the operative field. For instance, the surgeon can place the microscope as close as 200 mm or as far away as 400 mm without having to change the objective lens.

As noted above, accessories are available that allow two surgeons to view the operative field with true stereoscopic vision. This greatly enhances the ability of the assistant to participate in the operation and enhances the teaching value of the operating microscope.

The surgery will become unduly difficult if the microscope and the stand are not configured properly. The Contraves stand is electromagnetically controlled and can be balanced, which improves the maneuverability of the microscope to a remarkable degree. It is expensive, but in this age of diagnosis-related groups (DRGs), it is a cost-effective piece of equipment, because it decreases surgical time. However, many hospitals do not yet have one available.

If the Contraves stand is not available, a tall 1900-mm stationary stand should be used. The more common 1600-mm stand is too short for spinal cases. The 1900-mm stand should be fitted with extra extension arms, and the microscope should be suspended from the extension arm by a fitting that allows the microscope to rotate in an oblique plane.

Superior lighting increases the accuracy of surgical dissection. If the operating microscope is used, then internal fiberoptic lighting with a halogen or xenon light source can provide brilliant coaxial illumination. If surgical telescopes are used, then a fiberoptic headlight can be used to illuminate the

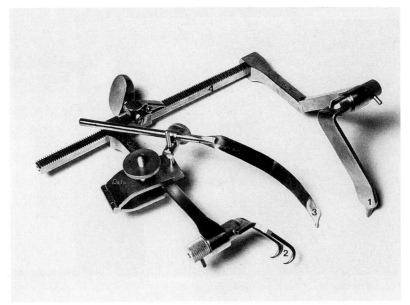

Fig. 75-5

The modified Taylor-type blade and opposing hook attached to a Haverfield–Scoville retractor frame. The Cloward self-retaining nerve root retractor is clamped in position. 1 = Taylor-type retractor blade; 2 = opposing hook; 3 = Cloward self-retaining nerve root retractor; 4 = Haverfield–Scoville retractor frame.

surgical field in near-coaxial fashion. However, if surgical telescopes and a headlight are used instead of the operating microscope, the surgeon's comfort is decreased because of the weight of the devices and because of the head and neck position required to maintain focus and illumination.

Instruments

It is important to use self-retaining retractors. To retract the paravertebral muscles, we use a narrow custom-made Taylor-type blade that attaches to the Scoville–Haverfield retractor. Countertraction is provided by a small double hook attached to the other side of the Scoville–Haverfield retractor (Fig. 75-5). Alternatives are a regular Taylor retractor that has been cut to a narrow width (1.5 cm),[5] the Williams microdiscectomy retractor,[18] or the McCulloch retractor system. The nerve root can be retained medially by a Cloward self-retaining nerve root retractor, which is clamped to the Scoville–Haverfield retractor (Fig. 75-5).[*]

[*]The Williams microdiscectomy retractor, the Scoville–Haverfield retractor frame, and the Cloward self-retraining nerve-root retractor are available from Codman & Shurtleff, New Bedford Industrial Park, New Bedford, MA 02745. The Taylor-type retractor blades and double-hook retractors were obtained on special order from Codman & Shurtleff. The McCulloch retractor system is available from Baxter V. Mueller, Lake Cook 2-2, 1425 Lake Cook., Rd., Deerfield, IL 60015.

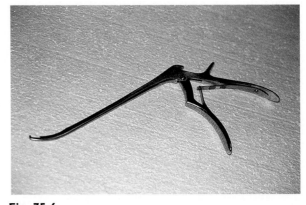

Fig. 75-6

The curved Link–Beatty rongeur, ueeful for relieving intervertebral canal stenosis by allowing resection of the anterior aspect of the superior articular process of the inferior vertebra.

Electrocoagulation within the spinal canal should be avoided. Williams emphasizes the importance of this.[24] Crock[7] points out the importance of relieving obstruction to the venous drainage of the nerve roots in operations for spinal stenosis. He emphasizes that great care should be taken to protect the arteries and veins associated with the nerve roots; he also avoids the use of diathermy within the spinal canal. He almost always arrests bleeding within the spinal canal only with the application of Gelfoam.[7]

If the surgeon feels compelled to use electrocoagulation within the spinal canal, then bipolar coagulation is essential, to minimize the spread of the coagulating current to sensitive neural tissue.

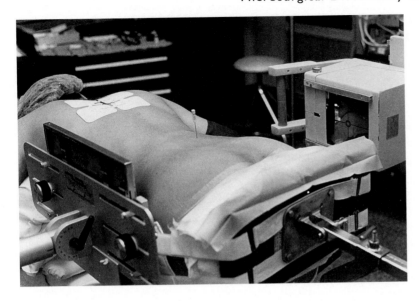

Fig. 75-7

The lateral localizing portable x-ray.

A standard angled Kerrison rongeur, a straight chisel, and/or a high-speed drill is used for bone removal. If the anterior aspect of the superior articular process must be resected to accomplish a foraminotomy of the intervertebral canal, then a curved Link–Beatty rongeur is used (Fig. 75-6).[4]* Standard discectomy instruments are used for nerve-root mobilization and disc excision.

Intraoperative Roentgenograms

When utilizing a small incision for microsurgical spinal surgery, it is essential to use localizing x-ray films to confirm the level being approached (Fig. 75-7).

The first localizing lateral x-ray film is taken before making the skin incision. It can be obtained either before or after the skin is prepared. The location of the involved interspace is estimated, and the skin over this point is prepared if full preparation has not yet been done. An 18- or 19-gauge spinal needle is used as a marker, with the stylet in place. A smaller needle may be difficult to visualize on the portable x-ray films.

The needle is inserted beside the spinous process at the involved level and on the side of the disc herniation. It is advanced until it contacts the lamina or facet. Care is taken not to penetrate the interlaminar space to avoid damage to the nerve root and to avoid creating a troublesome cerebrospinal fluid leak.

The intervertebral space at L5-S1 lies directly anterior to the superior portion of the interlaminar space, but at L4-L5 it lies anterior and superior to

*The curved Link–Beatty rongeur is available from Link America, 321 Palmer Rd., Denville, NJ 07834, or from Elekta Instruments, 8 Executive Park West, Atlanta, GA 30329.

the inferior margin of the L4 lamina. At L3-L4 the intervertebral space lies approximately anterior to the junction of the lower and middle thirds of the lamina. Keep these relationships in mind when placing the marking needle, since the surgical incision should be centered over the involved disc space rather than over the interlaminar space.

The marking needle is inserted perpendicular to the floor so that its relationship to the involved disc space can be easily determined on the portable x-ray film (Fig. 75-8). If the needle is angled superiorly or inferiorly, it is easy to become disoriented once the skin incision has been made.

If the portable x-ray film shows that the needle is properly placed at the involved level, the site of the tip of the needle is marked by using a tuberculin syringe to inject 0.1 ml of indigo carmine through the needle. (Use indigo carmine, not methylene blue. Methylene blue is neurotoxic and has no place in the operating room when there is even the slightest chance it might be accidentally injected into the cerebrospinal fluid.)

The anatomic level of the involved disc space usually can be located by reference to surface anatomy. Preoperative x-ray films or CT scans will demonstrate the relationship of the intercristal line to the involved disc space. Usually it runs near the L4-L5 interspace. The posterior superior iliac spine is at the level of the S2 spinous process. If the patient is obese or if a transitional vertebra is present, it may be helpful to insert a marking needle at each of two levels. After the roentgenogram is taken, the desired one is chosen for the indigo carmine injection.

After the lamina over the involved interspace has been marked with the indigo carmine, the needle is

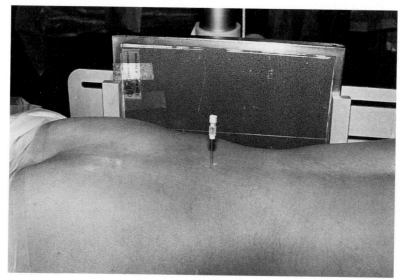

Fig. 75-8

The needle used to localize the interspace on the portable x-ray machine is inserted perpendicular to the floor. This helps the surgeon maintain orientation to the intended interspace during the operative approach.

removed. Residual dye within the needle will leave a small blue dot at the site of the needle puncture to distinguish it from other skin markings.

If there is any doubt whatsoever about the level being approached after the self-retaining paravertebral muscle retractor has been placed, then a second localizing lateral x-ray film is taken. A clamp or other metallic marker is placed on the interlaminar soft tissue to confirm the correct level. If the expected pathology is not encountered within the spinal canal, a roentgenogram should be taken to confirm the level being approached.

If the L5-S1 interspace cannot be defined on the films, the x-ray procedure must be repeated with better alignment and penetration. If the patient has a transitional vertebra or if the intrasacral interspaces are well developed, it is easy to be misled by the localizing portable x-ray film. In these cases the intraoperative x-ray films must be closely correlated with the preoperative x-ray and imaging studies.

Operative Technique

Preparation

Under general anesthesia, the patient is positioned on the Andrews frame. The localizing x-ray film is taken. Skin preparation is done and the site of the incision marked with a sterile marking pen, 1 to 1.5 inches long and centered over the involved intervertebral space. The operative field is draped, using an iodophor coated plastic adhesive sheet to cover

the skin. I prefer to stand on the side of the operating table opposite the involved nerve root because this makes it easier to decompress the subarticular lateral recess and intervertebral canal.

Exposure

Lidocaine (0.5%) with epinephrine is injected before making the incision. A small amount of subcutaneous fat is removed to facilitate visualization into the depths of the operative field. It is placed in Depo-Medrol and used as a free fat graft in the epidural space at the conclusion of the operation.

The lumbodorsal fascia is incised 1 cm lateral to the midline to preserve the supraspinous and interspinous ligaments. This preserves spinal stability and reduces postoperative pain.[2] The paravertebral muscles are mobilized subperiosteally and retracted laterally by the assistant with a Meyerding retractor.

Soft tissues are swept off the laminae, the ligamentum flavum, and the facet capsule. This portion of the dissection is done by the feel of the instruments, taking care not to penetrate the interlaminar space accidentally. The tooth of the modified microsurgical Taylor blade is engaged by the lateral edge of the pars interarticularis or by the lateral edge of the facet. The double hook of the retractor is placed opposite the blade and engages the supraspinous ligament. The blade and hook are then attached to the Haverfield–Scoville retractor, and the retractor is opened.

Bone Removal

At this point, the operating microscope is brought in. If the localizing indigo carmine is not obvious or if there is any doubt whatsoever about the interspace being approached, a second localizing x-ray film is obtained at this time.

Remaining soft tissue is excised from the ligamentum flavum and from the facet capsule. The lateral aspect of the pars interarticularis is identified. Enough of the pars is preserved to avoid sacrificing the inferior articular process. The inferior rim of the lamina above, the superior rim of the lamina below, and the medial edge of the inferior articular process are excised with an angled Kerrison rongeur, a straight chisel, or a high-speed drill using a 2-mm steel burr or a matchhead-shaped burr.* The medial edge of the superior articular process is scored with a straight chisel to create a stress riser, and then removed with a 2- or 3-mm angled Kerrison rongeur or the high-speed drill (Fig. 75-9).

The ligamentum flavum is picked up with vascular forceps and excised with a #15 blade or a #67 Beaver blade.† The epidural fat and veins are separated from the anterior aspect of the remaining ligamentum flavum with a blunt dissector. The angled Kerrison rongeur is used to resect remaining fragments of the ligamentum flavum and the superior ridge of bone to which the ligament attaches, being careful to avoid damaging the epidural veins.

Any free (sequestered) disc fragments that may have migrated away from the interspace should have been identified on the preoperative imaging studies. The laminar resection may have to be extended superiorly or inferiorly to reach them.

Epidural fat is preserved, and the epidural veins are visualized and protected. They are not coagulated. Bleeding from them can usually be arrested by the temporary application of Gelfoam soaked in thrombin.

The dural sheath of the nerve root is visualized. The bone removal is extended laterally far enough to expose the posterior anulus well beyond the lateral margin of the dura. The medial shelving edge of the superior articular process is resected back to the medial edge of the pedicle of the inferior verte-

bra, to make sure that any subarticular stenosis has been relieved and that the nerve root and epidural veins have been well decompressed (Fig. 75-9, E).

If the preoperative imaging studies or intraoperative exploration demonstrates the presence of a narrow intervertebral canal ("neural foramen"), the anterior aspect of the superior articular process of the vertebra below is removed with the Link–Beatty rongeur.[4] If an uncinate spur arising from the posterior aspect of the vertebral body is compromising the foramen, it must be removed with the chisel, down-biting curettes, the high-speed drill, or angled bone tamps.

Exposed cancellous bone is coated with bone wax to discourage future spur formation and to decrease irritation of the adjacent nerve root.

If the patient's symptoms are secondary to disc resorption and subarticular or intervertebral canal stenosis, these steps may complete the operation, since disc excision may not be necessary. The anterior aspect of the spinal canal should be explored to make sure that a disc fragment or uncinate spur is not compromising the nerve root from the ventral direction.

Disc Excision

If all the bone removal can be accomplished before the herniated disc is excised, there is less likelihood of increasing nerve root compression during medial mobilization. If a large disc herniation compromises the bone removal, it should be excised when encountered and the bone work finished later on. However, it is important not to compromise the nerve root by trying to drag a large herniated disc fragment out through an inadequate bony opening. Sometimes the surgeon has to work back and forth between bone removal and piecemeal excision of large herniated disc fragments.

If a sequestered disc fragment or a portion of an extruded disc is evident in the epidural space, it is removed before mobilization of the nerve root. The nerve root then is gently mobilized medially and held in place with the Cloward self-retaining nerve-root retractor. If the herniated portion of the disc is contained by thinned out anulus and/or the posterior longitudinal ligament, these structures are perforated with a small dissector, such as a Penfield #4.

A small stab incision (with a pointed #67 Beaver blade) may be required to facilitate entry into the anulus, but a large incision or wide resection of the posterior anulus is avoided. Often, herniated disc material will extrude through the opening at that point and can be removed by grasping it with the

---

*If it is available, I prefer the Midas Rex drill with the AM attachment and #8 matchhead-shaped burr, from The Midas Rex Company, 2929 Race St., Fort Worth, Texas 76111. The Anspach drill with the "Blue" attachment and #8 matchhead-shaped burr is an alternative, available from the Anspach Company, 1349 South Killian Dr., Lake Park, FL 33403.
†Beaver blades available from the Beaver Company, 411 Waverley Oak, Waltham, MA 02154.

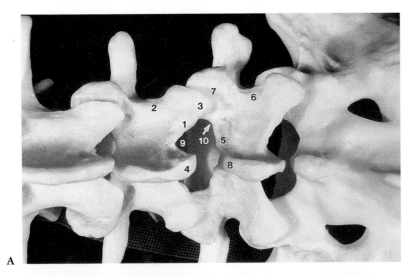

A

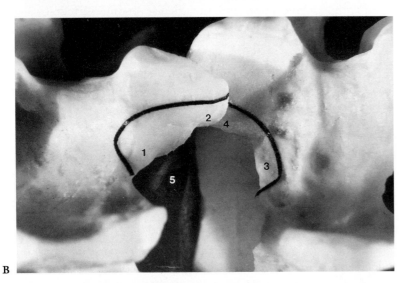

B

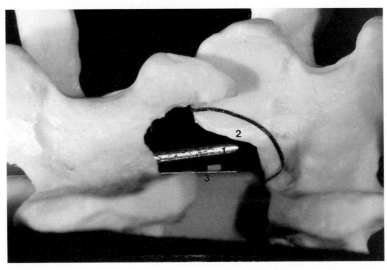

C

Fig. 75-9

A. A model of the lumbar spine, demonstrating the surgeon's orientation to the L4-L5 level. The approach is made through a short paramedian incision in the lumbodorsal fascia. The supraspinous and interspinous ligaments are preserved; 1 = inferior edge of L4 lamina; 2 = L4 pars interarticularis; 3 = L4 inferior articular process; 4 = L4 spinous process; 5 = superior edge of L5 lamina; 6 = L5 pars interarticularis; 7 = L5 superior articular process; 8 = L5 spinous process; 9 = L4-L5 intervertebral disc; 10 (arrow) = subarticular region medial to L5 pedicle.

B. The L4-L5 level, marked to indicate the intended bone resection. 1 = inferior edge of L4 lamina; 2 = medial edge of L4 inferior articular process; 3 = superior edge of L5 lamina; 4 = medial edge of L5 superior articular process, partially hidden anterior to the inferior articular process of L4; 5 = L4-L5 intervertebral disc.

C. The inferior edge of the L4 lamina and the medial edge of the L4 inferior articular process have been resected with the high-speed drill. The nerve root passes anterior to the medial shelving edge of the L5 superior articular process. 1 = L5 nerve root; 2 = medial edge of the L5 superior articular process; 3 = dural sac.

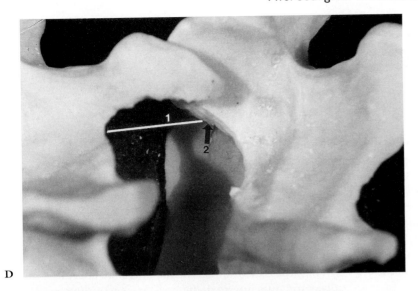

D

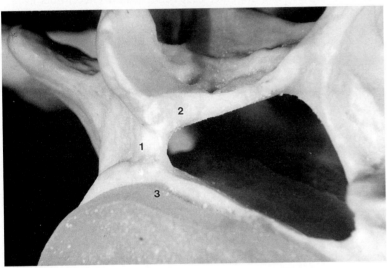

E

Fig. 75-9, cont'd

D. The high-speed drill has been used to complete the bone resection. If more severe subarticular stenosis is present, more of the superior edge of the L5 lamina and more of the medial edge of the L5 superior articular process will have to be removed than is indicated here. 1 = course of L5 nerve root; 2 (arrow) = medial edge of L5 pedicle.

E. Oblique view of the opened subarticular lateral recess superior and medial to the L5 pedicle. The L5 nerve root and its accompanying epidural vessels have been decompressed. 1 = pedicle of L5, 2 = resected medial edge of L5 superior articular process; 3 = L4-L5 intervertebral disc.

disc rongeur. The opening then is gradually dilated until a disc rongeur can be inserted into the interspace itself.

Removal of degenerated material from within the disc space is generally confined to the ipsilateral posterior disc quadrant, although obvious loose and/or degenerated material is removed even if it lies in the anterior quadrant or across the midline. Cup curettes, ring curettes, down-biting Epstein curettes, and disc rongeurs are used, but no intentional attempt is made to remove the cartilaginous end plates. Firm anular material is not removed unless it projects posteriorly into the spinal canal or unless it is associated with a posterior limbus fracture that must be widely resected.[10] The instruments are kept away from the anterior boundary of the interspace to minimize the risk of damage to the aorta, vena cava, or iliac vessels.

If the disc has herniated into the axilla of the involved nerve root, it may have to be initially approached medial to the nerve root. No initial attempt is made to retract the nerve medially in these cases. Once the root has been decompressed by the removal of the herniated material, it can then be moved medially so the interspace itself can be approached lateral to the root.

Extruded or sequestered disc fragments may be adherent to the dura of the nerve root or to the dural sac itself and may have to be sharply dissected away from the root or dura with a #67 or #64 Beaver blade. Use of the operating microscope increases the accuracy of this dissection and lessens the chance of a cerebrospinal fluid leak.

After the degenerated disc material has been removed, the epidural space is very thoroughly searched for any additional disc material that may have migrated away from the interspace. Care is taken that additional disc material is not hidden between the posterior cortex of the vertebral body and the posterior longitudinal ligament superior or inferior to the interspace.

Closure

Before closure, 0.25% plain Marcaine without preservatives is instilled into the interspace and the exposed epidural space. It is also injected into the attachments of the supraspinous and interspinous ligaments. The free fat graft is gently laid over the exposed dura and nerve root. There is no need to suture the muscles. The lumbodorsal fascia, subcutaneous tissue, and skin are closed according to the surgeon's preference. I use synthetic absorbable sutures to close the fascia and subcutaneous tissue and a subcuticular suture of the same material to close the skin.

Postoperative Management

Usually, little or no narcotic medication is required. The patient begins ambulation the day of surgery or the next day. The day after surgery, gentle midrange therapeutic exercises are started in both flexion and extension. The patient leaves the hospital when he or she is ambulating comfortably and independently, usually on the first or second postoperative day.

The therapeutic exercise program is developed further after discharge. Walking and swimming are encouraged. The program of spinal education is continued. I encourage the patient to become involved in a formal conditioning program using low-impact aerobic exercises and supervised weight training with the goal of making spinal exercise and general fitness lifelong habits.

Variations

Local Anesthesia

Some surgeons perform microsurgical lumbar procedures under local anesthesia, supplemented with intravenous sedation.[15] If needed, light spinal anesthesia can be administered through a #30 needle inserted through the dura exposed in the operative field.

Outpatient Microsurgery

Some surgeons are performing microsurgical lumbar procedures as outpatient procedures through the same-day surgery facility of their hospital or surgicenter.

The Lateral Position

Some surgeons prefer placing the patient in a lateral position, with the affected side up. This accomplishes abdominal decompression and prevents epidural venous engorgement. It is also relatively easy to position the patient in the lateral position. However, we believe the lateral position has several disadvantages. It is very difficult to extend the operation to the down side of the spine. This might become necessary to remove a large central disc fragment or spur that resists excision from one side alone.

The other disadvantage of the lateral position involves the difficulty that the assistant encounters in trying to see and reach into the operative field. This position does not allow the assistant to take advantage of the binocular stereoscopic station available on the newer microscopes, which is located opposite the surgeon.

Preserving the Ligamentum Flavum

Some surgeons believe that the ligamentum flavum should be preserved to decrease postoperative epidural fibrosis. They resect the medial edges of the inferior and superior articular processes, lateral to the attachment of the ligamentum flavum, then retract the ligamentum medially along with the nerve root. We have been concerned that in some cases hypertrophy of the ligamentum flavum may be difficult to recognize, and the mass of the ligament in the epidural space may compromise the nerve root or the epidural veins. We prefer to resect the ligamentum flavum and the cephalad bony ridge to which it attaches, to decompress the nerve roots and epidural veins as much as possible.

Bilateral Decompression for Spinal Stenosis

Crock[7] believes strongly that bilateral decompression should be carried out when disc resorption has resulted in subarticular lateral recess stenosis, even though the leg pain may be unilateral. He feels that further disc resorption will result in compromise of the contralateral nerve root and epidural veins in a significant percentage of cases. This problem can be prevented by proceeding with a bilateral decompression initially.

Crock preserves the spinous processes and central ligaments to maintain spinal stability, and approaches the spinal canal through two paramedian incisions in the lumbodorsal fascia, one on each side of the midline. At present, Crock does not advocate use of the operating microscope for spinal surgery, especially for bilateral procedures, but the rationale for the bilateral approach applies to microsurgical procedures as well as to standard spinal procedures.[7]

Limited Disc Removal versus Curettage of the Disc Space

Williams advocates simple removal of the herniated disc fragment without curettage of the interspace. He reports a 4.1% incidence of true recurrence of the herniated disc at the site of the initial microlumbar discectomy.[26] Most reports in the literature document rates varying from 1% to 5% for recurrence of disc herniation at the same level and same side as the initial procedure, whether the interspace is curetted or not.[*] An exception is Rogers's report, which notes a 21% recurrence rate in 33 patients in whom the interspace was not curetted versus a 0% rate in 35 patients in whom ". . . as much of the intervertebral disc as possible was removed. . . ."[21] A recent report of the recurrence of disc herniation in standard discectomies notes a similar incidence whether the interspace is curetted or not.[3]

Potential Complications

Kardaun and co-workers studied 3289 patients with surgically treated lumbar disc herniation and found an overall complication rate of 3.7%.[14] In this epidemiologic study, no distinction was made between patients treated with microsurgical techniques and those treated with standard techniques. This study probably could not identify the incidence of cerebrospinal fluid leaks created and repaired at surgery. Transient postoperative neurologic deficits would probably have been missed if they did not appear on the discharge ICD codes.

The complication rates reported in the various series that studied microsurgical procedures range from 2.2% to 22% for the microsurgical procedures, and from 3% to 33.4% for the standard procedures.[†] These include such complications as exploring an unintended level, dural tears, hemorrhage severe enough to require transfusion, superficial wound infections, disc-space infections, aseptic discitis, new postoperative neurologic deficits, hematomas of the wound, epidural hematomas, damage to retroperi-

toneal structures including the great vessels or ureter, gastrointestinal problems such as gastritis or hemorrhage, and cardiovascular problems including thrombophlebitis and pulmonary embolism.

These complications can occur with any sort of disc surgery, microsurgical or standard. None is specifically associated with the use of microsurgical techniques, nor can any of them necessarily be avoided specifically with the use of microsurgical techniques. However, some of them may be associated with inexperience or inadequate training in using the operating microscope.

Inexperience Using the Microscope

When intraspinal surgery is performed, the principles of intraspinal surgery must be followed, whether the surgeon is using microsurgical or standard techniques.[11] If they are not followed, the incidence of complications will be higher. A surgeon trying to use the microscope without sufficient training and experience will tend to become distracted by the problems of maintaining maneuverability of the microscope and alignment with the operative field. He or she will also tend to leave the microscope on lower magnification, neglecting the accuracy of dissection afforded by the higher magnifications.

Postoperative Neurologic Deficit

Unfamiliarity with the microscope can lead to a greater incidence of postoperative neurologic deficits from attempts to extract large disc fragments through inadequate bony openings and from failure to identify accurately the degree of bony resection required to deal with subarticular and intervertebral canal stenosis.

Retained Disc Fragments

Sequestered disc fragments may be missed if their exact location has not been determined by close examination of the preoperative imaging studies.

Cerebrospinal Fluid Leaks

Most of the microsurgical series report an incidence of intraoperative dural tears of 2% to 6%, which is a range similar to that reported in other series dealing with standard discectomy.[9] Rogers reported an incidence of 16% in patients undergoing microsurgical disc excisions.[21]

*References 6, 9, 12, 18, 26, and 27.
†References 1, 6, 9, 13, 17 to 19, 21, 23, 26, 27, and 29.

The inexperienced spinal microsurgeon may have more than his or her share of cerebrospinal fluid leaks because insufficient bony resection does not allow adequate mobilization of the nerve root, and because the inexperienced surgeon tends to use too-low a magnification setting when trying to separate epidural adhesions with sharp dissection.

Most surgeons will occasionally create a cerebrospinal fluid leak during intraspinal dissection when operating on patients who have had previous surgery. It is important to learn the techniques of suturing and knot tying under the microscope so that these leaks can be repaired.[8] 7-0 Prolene suture works well and is fairly easy to handle under magnification. A microsurgical needle holder, preferably bayonet-shaped, should be used.

If there is a ragged opening in the dura, it can be repaired by cutting lyophilized dura into an oversized patch, placing a traction suture in its center, and inserting it through the defect into the subarachnoid space. The pressure of the cerebrospinal fluid will tend to hold the patch against the edges of the dural defect. The patch should then be sutured to the edge of the dural defect.[24]

A sutured dural leak should be coated with fibrin adhesive, if available.[22] Dural leaks that are anteriorly located may not be accessible for suturing. They can still usually be sealed by placing a free fat graft over them and coating the fat and surrounding dura with fibrin adhesive. Laws, in a discussion of Shaffrey and associates, suggests delivering the fibrin glue to the region of the dural leak by holding a thrombin-soaked piece of Gelfoam next to the dural leak and infiltrating the Gelfoam with the cryoprecipitated fibrinogen using a single syringe and a fine needle.[16] This technique avoids the problem of having to manipulate two syringes simultaneously in a small operative field.

Postoperative Infection

If the microscope is carefully covered with a sterile plastic drape and if sterile technique is followed, the incidence of postoperative infections should not be any higher than that of standard spinal procedures.

Mistaken Level of Surgery

The surgeon must take steps to identify carefully the spinal level involved with the pathology. It is all too easy to be off by one level when operating through a small incision. The most common error involves operating one level higher than the intended level.[18]

Preoperative x-ray films should be obtained, with a spinal needle in place as described above, and indigo carmine injected for intraoperative identification of the level. If there is any doubt about the level once the lamina and facet capsule are exposed, or if the expected pathology is not encountered inside the spinal canal, another x-ray film should be taken.

Perforation of the Great Vessels

Damage to the aortic, vena cava, or iliac vessels can occur when either microsurgical procedures or standard procedures are used to remove disc material from the interspace. The operating microscope offers the advantage of direct vision into the interspace during disc removal, and its use probably lessens the chance that the anterior boundaries of the interspace will be penetrated.

Results

To the best of my knowledge, there have been no randomized, prospective, controlled studies comparing the results of spinal procedures performed with microsurgical techniques and the results of procedures performed with standard techniques. Several studies have made retrospective, uncontrolled comparisons, and these suggest that patients who have undergone microsurgical procedures may leave the hospital sooner and return to work faster than those who have had standard spinal procedures.[6,13,23,27]

These studies also suggest that the incidence of recurrent disc herniation at the same level and side and the incidence of complications are similar whether spinal procedures are performed with microsurgical or standard techniques.

Proponents of microsurgical spinal procedures generally claim superior results for their techniques, compared with standard techniques, but these claims cannot be supported statistically by any study done thus far. Some of the claims seem too good to be true. Reported satisfactory results range from 76.3% to 98.8%, depending upon whether the surgeon is reporting results as "good/excellent," "satisfactory," "able to return to work," or some other standard.

Williams reports surgical "cures," which he defines as "a patient who is economically productive, if he or she so desires, physically comfortable without addictive medication, and free from sciatic pain." He reports a total 15-year surgical "cure" rate of 98.8%, including patients who ultimately benefitted from reoperation.[26]

McCulloch is more stringent in his criteria for success. He groups his results into "satisfactory" and "unsatisfactory." A "satisfactory" result is a patient who has either complete relief of symptoms or only mild discomfort with the ability to participate in all activities and not requiring medications or bracing. He reports 84.0% satisfactory results in 100 patients without previous surgery and without lateral zone stenosis undergoing microdiscectomy for a herniated disc.[18]

Pappas and co-workers studied 654 patients who underwent microsurgical spinal procedures over a 4.5-year period.[19] They emphasize the importance of using a standardized ordinal rating scale to determine results more nearly objectively and to allow better comparison of results among different studies. They report their results in terms of Prolo's Functional-Economic Outcome Rating Scale, which allows scores of 2 (worst) through 10 (best)[20] (Table 75-1). They consider Functional-Economic Ratings of 8, 9, or 10 as "good," and 76.3% of their patients fell into this range. Prolo and associates considered scores of 9 and 10 as "excellent," and scores of 7 and 8 as "good."[20] Postoperative scores of 7 through 10 were achieved in 85.5% of the patients studied by Pappas and colleagues.[19]

Most of the results of microsurgical spinal procedures reported in the literature thus far are not clear. Comparison among different series is impossible. Prolo and Pappas and their associates are correct: An objective, standardized rating system must be applied to the analysis of surgical results. Prolo himself devised his scale for the study of patients who had undergone posterior lumbar interbody fusion, but his system is well suited to the study of other procedures as well.

Balagura studied the effects of keeping lumbar spinal incisions small and off the midline.[2] He compared days to discharge and postoperative narcotic medication in two groups of 10 patients each. Both groups had a lumbar herniated disc removed by the same surgeon, who used 3.5× surgical telescopes in all cases. In one group, the disc was approached through an 8- to 10-cm midline skin incision with incision and reflection of the supraspinous and interspinous ligaments. In the other group, the approach was through a 4-cm midline skin incision and a 4-cm paramedian incision in the lumbodorsal fascia. The ligaments were left intact. The bone removal and dissection within the spinal canal were the same in both groups. Fiberoptic illumination was used to aid visualization through the small incision.

Table 75-1
Prolo functional-economic outcome rating scale*

ECONOMIC STATUS

E1	Complete invalid
E2	No gainful occupation (including ability to do housework or continue retirement activities)
E3	Able to work but not at previous occupation
E4	Working at previous occupation on part-time or limited status
E5	Able to work at previous occupation with no restrictions of any kind

FUNCTIONAL STATUS

F1	Total incapacity (or worse than before operation)
F2	Mild to moderate level of low-back pain and/or sciatica (or pain same as before operation but able to perform all daily tasks of living)
F3	Low level of pain and able to perform all activities except sports
F4	No pain, but patient has had one or more recurrences of low-back pain or sciatica
F5	Complete recovery, no recurrent episodes of low-back pain, able to perform all previous sports activities

The patient is scored according to the numbers associated with each of the two scales. For example, a patient who fell into E3 and F4 would score a "7." A patient in E4 and F5 would score a "9." The lowest possible score is a "2" (E1 plus F1).

*From Prolo DJ, Oklund SA, Butcher M: Toward uniformity in evaluating results of lumbar spine operations: a paradigm applied to posterior lumbar interbody fusions, *Spine* 11:601, 1986.

The "mean postoperative days in the hospital" for the patients who had their ligaments incised and reflected was 6 days, and each patient used a mean total of 1200 mg of Demerol. Patients with the short paramedian fascial incision were discharged in 2.5 days and used 150 mg of Demerol each. Balagura believes that a shorter and more comfortable postoperative stay can be achieved without using the operating microscope, provided that the incision is kept small and midline ligamentous dissection is avoided. He does not believe that intraspinal microsurgical techniques *per se* are responsible for shorter hospital stays.[2]

Balagura is probably correct. If a surgeon follows the principles of spinal surgery and removes enough bone to decompress the neural elements without destabilizing the spine, and if he or she is gentle but thorough with the intraspinal dissection and avoids coagulation of the epidural vessels, then good results will follow. If the surgeon also keeps the incision small and keeps the midline ligaments intact, then the results will probably be even better.

The point is this: Once a surgeon has become familiar with the operating microscope, it is easier and physically more comfortable to work through a small incision with the microscope than it is to use surgical telescopes and a headlight. The study of microsurgical technique simply familiarizes the surgeon with instruments designed to be used in small spaces and gives him or her the ability to suture dural tears more accurately should the need arise. Hand–eye coordination also improves as magnification increases, and it is easier to achieve higher magnification with the microscope than it is with surgical telescopes.

Predictions for the Future

The use of microsurgical techniques in spinal surgery will probably become increasingly widespread as improvements in instrumentation and the operating microscope continue. Further improvements in the operating microscope will probably make it smaller and even more maneuverable than it is now.

However, with the further improvement of arthroscopic instrumentation, arthroscopic microsurgical and laser techniques will probably largely replace open surgical techniques for the treatment of most herniated discs. Right now, arthroscopic and/or laser disc decompression is being used for the treatment of contained disc herniations, but current instrumentation is not well suited to the removal of a disc fragment that has extruded into the spinal canal, especially if a portion of the fragment has migrated cephalad or caudad from the level of the interspace.

Soon, arthroscopic instruments will probably be available that will allow the surgeon to visualize the epidural space from a unilateral approach. The instruments will then allow the surgeon to move extruded disc fragments from the epidural space into the interspace, where they can be vaporized with the laser. Right now, this can sometimes be done with a biportal arthroscopic approach, but a biportal approach is considerably more traumatic than a unilateral approach and may not offer any advantage over an open microsurgical approach.

Open microsurgical techniques will probably be necessary for some time to come for the removal of disc fragments that have become sequestered within the spinal canal away from the interspace, for the treatment of lateral zone stenosis, and for the treatment of disc herniations associated with disc resorption in which the interspace is too narrow to admit an arthroscope.

References

1. Abernathey CD, Yasargil MG: *Results in microsurgery.* In Williams RW, McCulloch JA, Young PH, editors: *Microsurgery of the lumbar spine,* Rockville, MD, 1990, Aspen, p 223.
2. Balagura S: Lumbar discectomy through a small incision, *Neurosurgery* 11:784, 1982.
3. Balderston RA and others: The treatment of lumbar disc herniation: simple fragment excision versus disc space curettage, *J Spinal Dis* 4:22, 1991.
4. Beatty RA: Foraminotomy rongeur, *Spine* 16:1388, 1991.
5. Bell WO, Lavyne MH: Retractor for lumbar microdiscectomy: technical note, *Neurosurgery* 14:69, 1984.
6. Caspar W: *Results in microsurgery.* In Williams RW, McCulloch JA, Young PH, editors: *Microsurgery of the lumbar spine,* Rockville, MD, 1990, Aspen, p 227.
7. Crock HV: *A short practice of spinal surgery,* ed 2. Wien-New York, 1993, Springer-Verlag, pp 23, 28, 32, 138.
8. DeLong WB: *The inner limits: basic microsuturing technique.* Videotape. 20 minutes. 1975. Sponsored by The Ethicon Suture Company, US Route 22, Somerville, MD 08876. Available from W. Bradford DeLong, MD; One Shrader St., 4th floor; San Francisco, CA 94117.
9. Ebeling U, Reichenberg W, Reulen H-J: Results of microsurgery lumbar discectomy: review of 485 patients, *Acta Neurochirurgica* 81:45, 1986.
10. Epstein NE: Lumbar surgery for 56 limbus fractures emphasizing noncalcified type III lesions, *Spine* 17:1489, 1992.
11. Fager CA: *Microsurgical intervention for lumbar disc disease: a critique.* In Williams RW, McCulloch JA, Young PH, editors: *Microsurgery of the Lumbar Spine,* Rockville, MD, 1990, Aspen, p 249.
12. Goald HJ: Microlumbar discectomy: follow-up of 477 patients, *J Microsurg* 2:95, 1980.
13. Hudgins RW: The role of microdiscectomy, *Orthop Clin North Am* 14:589, 1983.
14. Kardaun JW, White LR, Shaffer WO: Acute complications in patients with surgical treatment of lumbar herniated disc, *J Spinal Dis* 3:30, 1990.
15. Kuslich SD: *Microsurgical lumbar nerve root decompression utilizing progressive local anesthesia.* In Williams RW, McCulloch JA, Young PH, editors: *Microsurgery of the lumbar spine,* Rockville, MD, 1990, Aspen, p 139.

16. Laws ER Jr: Discussing Shaffrey CI, Spotnitz WD, Shaffrey ME, Jane JA: Neurosurgical applications of fibrin glue: augmentation of dural closure in 134 patients, *Neurosurgery* 26:207, 1990.

17. Maroon JC, Abla A: Microlumbar discectomy, *Clin Neurosurg* 33:407, 1985.

18. McCulloch JA: *Principles of microsurgery for lumbar disc disease,* New York, 1989, Raven Press.

19. Pappas CTE, Harrington T, Sonntag VKH: Outcome analysis in 654 surgically treated lumbar disc herniations, *Neurosurgery* 30:862, 1992.

20. Prolo DJ, Oklund SA, Butcher M: Toward uniformity in evaluating results of lumbar spine operations: a paradigm applied to posterior lumbar interbody fusions, *Spine* 11:601, 1986.

21. Rogers LA: Experience with limited versus extensive disc removal in patients undergoing microsurgical operations for ruptured lumbar discs, *Neurosurgery* 22:82, 1988.

22. Shaffrey CI and others: Neurosurgical applications of fibrin glue: augmentation of dural closure in 134 patients, *Neurosurgery* 26:207, 1990.

23. Silvers HR: Microsurgical versus standard lumbar discectomy, *Neurosurgery* 22:837, 1988.

24. Williams RW: *Final thoughts and conclusions.* In Williams RW, McCulloch JA, Young PH, editors: *Microsurgery of the lumbar spine,* Rockville, MD, 1990, Aspen, p 263.

25. Williams RW: Microlumbar discectomy: a conservative surgical approach to the virgin herniated lumbar disc, *Spine* 3:175, 1978.

26. Williams RW: *Results in lumbar microsurgery.* In Williams RW, McCulloch JA, Young PH, editors: *Microsurgery of the lumbar spine,* Rockville, MD, 1990, Aspen, p 211.

27. Wilson DH, Harbaugh R: Microsurgical and standard removal of the protruded lumbar disc: a comparative study, *Neurosurgery* 8:422, 1981.

28. Yasargil MG: *Microsurgery applied to neurosurgery,* New York, 1969, Academic Press.

29. Young PH: *Microsurgery of the lumbar spine: a 4-year experience.* In Williams RW, McCulloch JA, Young PH, editors: *Microsurgery of the lumbar spine,* Rockville, MD, 1990, Aspen, p 215.

Chapter 76
Laser Surgery

John A. Sazy
Henry H. Sherk

Surgical Lasers

    infrared lasers
    visible-light lasers
    ultraviolet lasers

The Evolution of Minimally Invasive Discectomy

Experimental Basis for Laser Discectomy

Clinical Application of Laser Discectomy

Technique of Percutaneous Laser Discectomy

Summary

Recent advances in technology have fostered the growth and application of minimally invasive surgical techniques throughout a wide range of surgical procedures. Fiberoptics, and the miniaturization of delivery systems, for example, have allowed surgeons to deliver laser energy to sites deep within the body in a percutaneous manner for cutting, sculpting, and ablating. These techniques permit access to areas of the body that would otherwise require a major open surgical procedure.

Percutaneous discectomy has already been extensively developed using mechanical debridement with suction and cutting devices and chemical dissolution with chymopapain or collagenase. The delivery of laser energy to the disc is a logical extension of these techniques; this chapter will review our experience in this regard. Laser energy is created by focusing light emitted from a lasing medium that has been excited by an external power source. The laser beam emitted is monochromatic (of one wavelenghth), coherent (nondivergent), and collimated (light waves in phase). These properties permit the laser to be precisely used based on the power level (watts), pulse mode (joules/time), and wavelength (μm) of the specific laser. Laser energy must be absorbed by tissue to be effective at creating various desired surgical results. Currently, the infrared, visible-light, and ultraviolet lasers have clinical application in surgery.

Surgical Lasers

Infrared Lasers

Infrared lasers are categorized as far-infrared, mid-infrared, and near-infrared. The far-infrared laser is a CO_2 laser having a wavelength of 10.6 μm, which is highly absorbed by water. CO_2 lasers have excellent ablative capabilities with minimal heat diffusion into surrounding tissues. CO_2 lasers are delivered to the tissues via a waveguide, and are not fiberoptic capable. This quality makes their clinical use less adaptable in many surgical procedures. The mid- and near-infrared laser energy can be delivered to the operative site through small cannulas or needles by an optical fiber. These lasers include the 2.1-μm Holmium:YAG, and the 1.06-μm, 1.32-μm, and 1.44-μm Nd:YAG lasers. The 2.1-μm Holmium:YAG laser is less well absorbed by water than the CO_2 laser; however, its ablation threshold as defined by the amount of energy required to begin ablating tissue produces a high ablation yield with minimal thermal diffusion. Near-infrared lasers are poorly absorbed by water and produce a less effective ablation ratio and yield. These lasers have high ablation ratios, with more heat diffusion into surrounding tissues. Near-infrared lasers are not absorbed by the white avascular tissue of menisci, articular cartilage, or nucleus pulposus, and therefore have little effect on these tissues. Near-infrared lasers can be made more effective by the addition of pigment to the target tissue, providing a chromophore, thus allowing the tissue to absorb the laser energy. The fiber tip can be adapted to absorb the laser energy, creating a thermal probe that can then ablate tissue in a contact mode. Various materials, including sapphire crystals and ceramic tips, are used to convert laser energy to thermal energy; however, near-infrared lasers are not effective for intradiscal ablation.

Visible-Light Lasers

Visible-light lasers are poorly absorbed by water, and therefore have high ablation thresholds. Chromophore is essential for these lasers to have ablative activity in tissues containing water. Pigments such as hemoglobin or melanin lower the ablation threshold for water-rich tissue. Both near-infrared and visible-light lasers tend to diffuse into white avascular tissue with significant heat diffusion, until the temperature reaches 100° C, producing vaporization and usually a char-lined crater. The pigment of the char then absorbs the visible light and lowers the ablation threshold, allowing for further enlargement of the tissue defect.

Ultraviolet Lasers

Protein bonds within collagen molecules absorb the laser energy, causing a photochemical decomposition of the peptide bond and subsequent tissue ablation. The products of decomposition are removed as a gas. Ultraviolet lasers are more powerful than infrared and visible-light lasers, and have lower ablation thresholds per joule of energy. These properties also permit the use of these lasers at lower energy levels owing to the strength of the laser fiber emitting the beam. They ablate tissue at much lower rates at these energy levels, making their clinical use ineffective at this time.

The Evolution of Minimally Invasive Discectomy

Middleton and Teacher[14] in 1911 were among the first to recognize intervertebral nuclear material in the spinal canal as a cause for neurologic deficit. Complete laminectomies were performed and the tissue removed using the transdural approach of Oppenheim and Krause.[18] Surgeons at this time were operating under the assumption that these spinal masses were tumors. In 1939, Love[11] successfully removed disc material from the spinal canal with a less destructive hemilaminectomy. This technique is currently widely used for disc excision.

The concept of minimizing tissue destruction through less open approaches was furthered by Williams,[23] who in 1976 performed a large series of microdiscectomies. This procedure was performed on 530 patients who had positive straight-leg raising, motor deficit, and failed conservative management. Eighty-six percent of his patients had myelographic evidence of herniation. He reported that 91% of his patients had a satisfactory result, returning to an economically productive lifestyle without need of analgesic medication. Williams states the benefits of the procedure as being the elimination of surgical trauma to the lamina and facets, preservation of all extradural fat, blunt rather than sharp entrance to the annulus, and preservation of healthy nonherniated disc material. Microdiscectomy continues to be a frequently used approach in the treatment of disc herniation.

Hijikata[8,9] was the first to report on percutaneaous microdiscectomy in 1975. He reported the results of 136 patients who had undergone this procedure over a 12-year period. The procedure was performed on patients who had positive physical findings of straight-leg raising, radiculopathy, motor weakness, back pain, and failed conservative treatment. The patients' results were rated according to the Modified Japanese Orthopedic Association's score for low-back pain. Patients with bulging and protruding discs were included in the study. Patients with extruded discs were excluded. Dr. Hijikata's technique involved the percutaneous insertion of a 5-mm suction cannula into the annulus with removal of 1 to 3 grams of disc material. This technique is performed under fluoroscopic control. Guide tubes are used to direct suction cannulas, and cutting rongeurs. Dr. Hijikata reported that 72% of his patients had good to excellent results, while 28% failed to benefit from this treatment modality. He also reported that patients with degenerated discs who had referred pain on discography also benefitted from percutaneous microdiscectomy.

This technique has been refined with the addition of specially designed rongeurs and motorized cutting tools by Onik and associates.[17] Further advancement of this technique involves the addition of a second portal that permits the insertion of an endosope, allowing direct visualization of the disc space while debriding nuclear material. These more refined techniques require larger bore cannulas for the specially designed instrumentation, which decreases miniaturization and has the potential for increased morbidity.

The enzymatic digestion of nuclear material by percutaneous injection of chymopapain was once a popular method of discectomy. The enzyme chymopapain would interact with the peptidoglycan of the nucleus pulposus, thereby sparing the annulus. Reports of neurologic injury and anaphylaxis have prompted second thoughts regarding this technique of discectomy.

Experimental Basis for Laser Discectomy

The intervertebral disc is composed of the annulus fibrosus and nucleus pulposus. The annulus is primarily Type I collagen at the periphery. The collagen structure becomes Type II near the central portions of the annulus. The nucleus pulposus is composed of a highly hydrated proteoglycan that has a gel-like quality. The annulus is composed of approximately 60% to 70% water, a proportion that remains constant throughout life. The nucleus pulposus is 90% water in the infant; it declines to 80% in young adults, becoming approximately 70% water with further aging.[16] It stands to reason that the most effective laser for ablation of disc material would be one absorbed by water.

Lane and associates[10] studied the ablative properties of the CO_2 (10.6-μm wavelength), argon, Nd:YAG (1.32-μm wavelength), and Holmium:YAG (2.1-μm wavelength) lasers. Cummings and associates[6] studied the Nd:YAG (1.44-μm wavelength) on the ablation of thawed fresh-frozen human intervertebral discs. Effectiveness of disc ablation was demonstrated to be a function of water absorption of the laser studied. The lasers with the highest water absorption were most effective at ablating disc material, without producing large regions of thermal necrosis and heat transmission to the vertebral end plates or posterior longitudinal ligament. The lasers that are poorly absorbed by water did not effectively ablate disc material, and had a much larger region of thermal necrosis and heat transmission (Fig. 76-1). Lane and associates[10] also demonstrated that even though the CO_2 laser is highly absorbed by water, and effective at ablating tissue, the waveguide delivery system may have been responsible for the increased intradiscal temperatures and moderate thermal necrosis (Table 76-1). This data demon-

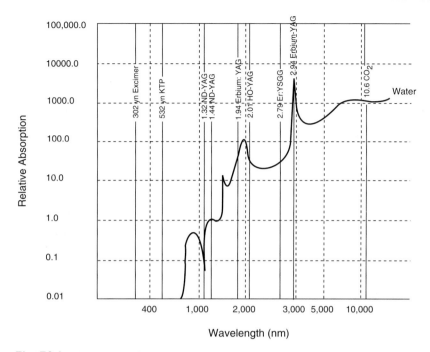

Fig. 76-1

Absorption spectra versus wavelength of various lasers. *(From Lane GJ et al:* An experimental comparison of CO_2, Argon, Nd:YAG and Ho:YAG Laser Ablation of Intervertebral Discs. *In Sherk H, editor,* Laser Discectomy; Spine State of the Art Reviews, *vol 7, no 1, 1993. Hanley & Belfus, Inc., Philadelphia.)*

Table 76-1

Laser ablation and temperature measurements on human intervertebral areas

	CO_2	Argon	1.32 Nd:YAG	1.44 Nd:YAG	2.01 Ho:YAG
Energy imparted (J)	1200	1200	1200	1200	1200
Size of defect (l × w × h) (cm)	1.3 × 1.2 × 0.6	1.1 × 0.4 × 0.2	1.7 × 1.0 × 0.4	3.0 × 2.0 × 0.45	2.5 × 1.6 × 0.6
Approximate volume ablated (cm^3)	0.936	0.88	0.68	2.7	2.4
Temperature change (°C)					
I.D.	16	14	40	*	10
P.L.L.	3	2	7	*	1
Vertebral end plate	4	3	8	*	4
Thermal necrosis	Moderate	Moderate	Large	Minimal	Minimal

* No data available.

(From Sherk HH: *Results of percutaneous lumbar discectomy with lasers.* In Sherk H, editor, *Laser Discectomy; Spine State of the Art Reviews,* vol 7, no 1, 1993. Hanley & Belfus, Inc., Philadelphia.).

strate that suitably sized defects are produced in the nucleus pulposus without significant temperature elevation in surrounding structures by lasers that are both highly absorbed by water and have fiberoptic delivery capability. Canine studies were conducted by Gropper and colleagues,[7] who compared the radiographic and histologic effects of a CO_2 laser and mechanical anterior discectomy. They found that the disc could be easily, safely, quickly, and more com-

pletely ablated, compared with mechanical anterior cervical discectomy. Choy and associates[3] also studied the effects of percutaneous laser disc decompression in canines, and concluded that there were no deleterious effects in canines sacrificed at 2 weeks.

Decompression of the disc by removing the contents of the disc is the goal of discectomy. The effectiveness of disc ablation in decompressing the disc has been studied by several investigators. Choy and

Altman[2] introduced 1000 joules of 1.32-μm Nd:YAG energy via a 400-μm quartz fiber into the L5-S1 interspace of cadaveric human spines. They found that the intradiscal pressures fell to 55.6% of the pre-lased value while the disc space was under a constant load. Prodoehl and colleagues[19] studied the effects of human cadaveric disc decompression by imparting 1200 joules of 2.1-μm Holmium:YAG laser energy into the L4-L5 disc space. Five fresh human specimens were studied by taking four pressure measurements pre- and post-lasing. Their data demonstrated a significant drop in post-lasing disc pressure at all four vertical load measurements. These investigations provided the necessary data demonstrating that laser discectomy is safe, that significant disc ablation can be created, and that significant decompression of the disc space occurs with ablation of the central portion of the disc. These experiments laid the ground work for clinical trials.

Clinical Application of Laser Discectomy

Choy and associates,[3,4] after studying the effects of Nd:YAG (1.32-μm wavelength) percutaneous discectomy on cadaver and animal models, were the first to begin clinical application in 1986. Their initial work demonstrated that 9 of 12 patients had immediate relief of symptoms, with 5 having recurrence of their symptoms at a later time. These authors used an Nd:YAG laser with a 1.32-μm wavelength imparting 1200 joules of energy to the disc. In a follow-up investigation using Macnab criteria,[12] Choy and associates,[5] in a prospective uncontrolled study, reported that 261 of 333 patients (78.4%) had a good to fair response, and 72 of 333 (21.6%) had a poor response to lumbar laser discectomy. Eleven patients had repeat laser discectomy, with seven (64%) having benefitted from the second procedure. Patients who did not respond to this treatment had open discectomy. Patients were included on the basis of MRI or CT scan evidence of a contained disc herniation, radicular symptoms corresponding to the level of the herniation, failure to respond to conservative therapy for at least 3 months, absence of degenerative or deforming spinal conditions, electromyelogram, no pending litigation, no previous disc surgery, no hemorrhagic diathesis, cardiac clearance, and informed consent. The KTP/532 (0.532-μm wavelength) laser was the first to be approved by the FDA for clinical application in laser discectomy. This laser can be used in conjunction with the chromophore indigo carmine (indigotindisulfinate

sodium), which is used to stain the disc material to enhance the absorption of the laser energy, which lowers the laser ablation threshold.

Yeung,[24] in a prospective uncontrolled study, reported good to excellent results in 840 of 1000 (84%) patients undergoing laser disc decompression with the 0.532-μm KTP laser. Their patients received 1250 joules of laser energy, as previous work had established this as the amount of energy needed to lower the intradiscal pressure by 50%. Patients were considered candidates for the procedure if they had a contained disc herniation confirmed by MRI or CT scan, no dye leak with discography either at time of work-up or surgery, clinical findings of leg pain greater than back pain, positive straight-leg raising on examination, or neurologic findings of decreased reflexes or motor strength, and, lastly, failure to respond to conservative treatments.

Rhodes and colleagues,[20] in a prospective uncontrolled study, reported on the results of 25 patients undergoing lumbar laser discectomy with a 2.1-μm Holmium:YAG laser. The laser was set at 1.5 W/pulse at 10 Hz, with 5 J of laser energy delivered to the nucleus with 5-second intervals between delivery of laser energy to the nucleus. A total of 1200 J of laser energy was imparted to the nucleus in each patient. These patients ranged from 24 to 60 years in age, and had symptoms of low-back pain, sciatica, and MRI evaluation demonstrating a prolapsed or extruded intervertebral lumbar disc. All patients had failed at least 10 weeks of conservative therapy, and had no evidence of degenerative or deforming spinal disease. Twenty of the 25 patients reported a 20% or better improvement of their symptoms on the Dallas Pain Questionnaire. One patient underwent open laminectomy-discectomy for an extruded disc. Twenty-three patients had resolution of abnormal physical findings, and 15 of 21 employed individuals returned to work after their procedure.

Sherk and colleagues[22] performed an expanded prospective, nonrandomized, controlled study with 47 patients in the laser treatment group, and 21 patients in the control group, who did not receive percutaneous laser discectomy. A 2.1-μm Holmium:YAG laser was used, set at 1.7 W/pulse at 10 Hz. Thirty to 50 joules of laser energy were delivered to the disc with 5-second intervals between each delivery. A total of 1200 to 1500 J was delivered to the disc of each patient. Patients were followed up 1 week after the procedure, at which time they completed a Dallas Pain Questionnaire. The patients were also evaluated on their ability to return to work. Patients who remained symptomatic continued conservative treat-

Table 76-2

Analysis of differences between laser treatment and control groups

Variable	Mean (S.D.) of Treatment Group	Mean (S.D.) of Control Group	p Value
Age (yr)	41.3 (11.9)	36.5 (7.5)	0.045*
Sex	60% male	52% male	0.541
Follow-up (mo)	6.9 (4.9)	5.3 (4.3)	0.159
Compensation/litigation	55% yes	76% yes	0.105
Smoker	43% yes	43% yes	0.963
Level	72% L4-L5	90% L4-L5	0.769
Preoperative duration of symptoms (mo)	29.8 (35.3)	32.2 (31.7)	0.800

*Statistically significant difference as judged by *t*-test.
(From Sherk HH: *Results of percutaneous lumbar discectomy with lasers.* In Sherk H, editor, *Laser Discectomy; Spine State of the Art Reviews*, vol 7, no 1, 1993. Hanley & Belfus, Inc., Philadelphia.).

Table 76-3

Analysis of change in pain questionnaire

Variable	Mean (S.D.) of Treatment Group	Mean (S.D.) of Control Group	p Value
DPQ	17.3 (24.3)	15.3 (16.9)	0.702
DPQ categorical	0.44 (0.88)	0.52 (0.75)	0.700
Signs	45.7 (22.1)	18.1 (27.5)	0.000*

*Statistically significant difference as judged by *t*-test.
(From Sherk HH: *Results of percutaneous lumbar discectomy with lasers.* In Sherk H, editor, *Laser Discectomy; Spine State of the Art Reviews*, vol 7, no 1, 1993. Hanley & Belfus, Inc., Philadelphia.).

ment. Forty-seven patients were in the laser treatment group; 21 were in the control group. Patients refused randomization; therefore, their decision for or against percutaneous laser discectomy placed them in the treatment or control group. The only significant difference between groups was their age, with older patients opting for percutaneous laser discectomy (Table 76-2). There appeared to be no significant differences in the Dallas Pain Questionnaire results, whereas physical findings were believed to be significantly different between the treatment and control groups (Table 76-3). Significant findings involved sex, compensation/litigation, and preoperative duration of symptoms. Women experienced more relief from their symptoms than men. Patients with pending litigation or compensation did not experience relief from their symptoms after percutaneous laser discectomy (Table 76-4).

Technique of Percutaneous Laser Discectomy

Lumbar laser discectomy is performed using a percutaneous approach. The patient is positioned in either a lateral decubitus (pain side up) or prone position. Image intensification with fluoroscopy is used to obtain anteroposterior and lateral views of the spine. The procedure is performed under sterile conditions, and can be performed in a radiology suite or operating room. The point of entry when the patient is in the lateral decubitis position is 7 to 8 centimeters, and when in the prone position 10 centimeters, from the midline (Fig. 76-2.). The painful or symptomatic side is chosen as the entry site. Lidocaine is injected into the subcutaneous tissues at 45° to the coronal plane down to the level of the annulus with a 16-gauge needle. If leg pain is encountered, the needle can be redirected. The position of the needle is continuously confirmed in the sagittal and coronal planes with fluoroscopy during needle localization of the target disc. Once the disc is entered, the stylet is withdrawn and a 400-μm laser fiber is inserted into the disc through the needle. Placement is confirmed with fluoroscopy. The tip of the laser fiber is observed to be equidistant in the center of the disc space in both the coronal and sagittal planes. The laser is then activated. When 1.32-μm Nd:YAG laser discectomy is performed, the laser is calibrated for 20- to 23-watt output at the tip of the laser fiber. The laser is activated in 1-second pulses with 1-second pauses until 1000 to 1850 joules has been delivered to the disc space.[5]

Table 76-4

Multiple regression analysis of the effect on outcome of laser treatment

Variable	Regression Coefficient	Standard Error	p Value
Dependent variable: DPQ			
Sex	11.92	2.85	0.0001
Compensation/litigation	−8.17	4.80	0.0936
Preoperative duration of symptoms	0.156	0.09	0.0740
Dependent variable: DPQ categorical			
Sex	0.237	0.087	0.0081
Preoperative duration of symptoms	0.005	0.003	0.0992
Dependent variable: signs			
Treatment	25.22	2.09	0.0000
Preoperative duration of symptoms	4.17	0.08	0.0387

(From Sherk HH: *Results of percutaneous lumbar discectomy with lasers.* In Sherk H, editor, Laser Discectomy; *Spine State of the Art Reviews,* vol 7, no 1, 1993. Hanley & Belfus, Inc., Philadelphia.).

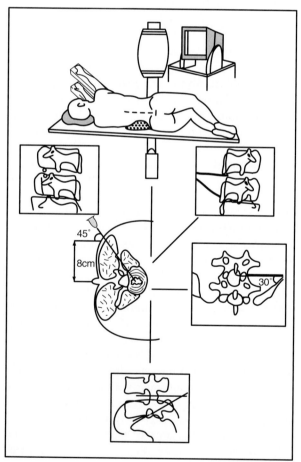

Fig. 76-2

Lateral positioning of the patient, demonstrating needle placement and fluoroscopic images confirming needle position. *(From Siebert W: Percutaneous laser disc decompression: the European experience. In Sherk H, editor, Laser Diccetomy; Spine State of the Art Reviews, vol 7, no 1, 1993. Hanley & Belfus, Inc., Philadelphia.)*

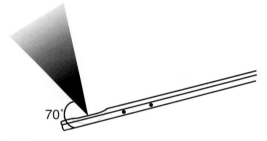

Fig. 76-3

Spine Stat probe illustrating the blunt tip diverting laser energy 70°. *(From Yeung AT: Consideration for the use of the KTP laser for disc decompression and ablation. In Sherk H, editor, Laser Diccetomy; Spine State of the Art Reviews, vol 7, no 1, 1993. Hanley & Belfus, Inc., Philadelphia.)*

KTP/532 laser discectomy involves a similar localization procedure and the introduction of a 1.8-mm "SpineStat" probe that optically diverts the laser energy 70°, resulting in a vaporization zone 60° to 80° from the axis of the fiber owing to the 20° beam divergence (Figs. 76-3 and 76-4). A total of 1250 to 1875 joules of energy can be delivered with this system.

The 2.1-μm Holmium:YAG laser involves the same disc localization procedure, with the patient in the prone position. Once the 400-μm fiber is confirmed to be centrally located in the disc by coronal and sagittal fluoroscopy, the laser is activated using a 1.5-J pulse at a repetition rate of 10 Hz, delivering not more than 15 J of energy to the nucleus at one time. There is a 5-second pause after every 15 J of laser energy imparted to the nucleus. This process is repeated until a total of 1200 J of energy is delivered to the nucleus. Next, a flexible guidewire is

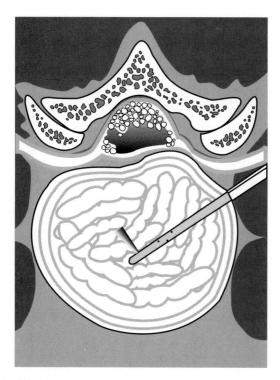

Fig. 76-4

Spine Stat probe in the disc space delivering laser energy to the nucleus pulposus. *(From Yeung AT: Consideration for the use of the KTP laser for disc decompression and ablation. In Sherk H, editor, Laser Discectomy; Spine State of the Art Reviews, vol 7, no 1, 1993. Hanley & Belfus, Inc., Philadelphia.)*

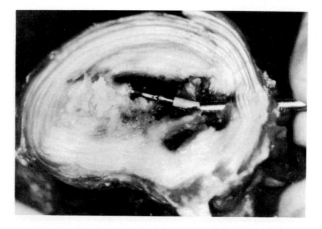

Fig. 76-5

Transaxial view of a lumbar disc with the flexible endoscope and laser fiber in the disc space after obliteration of the nucleus pulposis.

placed into the 16-gauge needle, and the needle removed. A 2-mm cannula with an inner trephine sleeve is then introduced into the disc over the guidewire. An adjustable stop on the cannula is then positioned against the patient's skin to stabilize the cannula. The trephine is advanced into the disc space over the flexible guidewire. The cannula is advanced through the annulus into the disc over the trephine and guidewire. The trephine and guidewire are then removed, leaving the cannula in the disc space. The 1.7-mm endoscope is then advanced through the cannula into the disc space (Fig. 76-5). The endoscope is a triaxial device that contains channels for the laser fiber, illumination fiber, image fiber, and flush lumen. The endoscope is focused, and flushed prior to being used. The endoscope has a flexible tip that permits deflection in a 90° arc of motion, which is controlled from the handpiece. Direct visualization of disc ablation is made possible by this system, and is initiated when disc material is encountered upon entry of the disc. Ablation of the disc is begun by delivering 1.5-J pulse at 15 Hz in 15- to 20-joule increments with 5-second pauses between energy delivery. Irrigation of the disc is accomplished

with this system, which also increases the amount of laser energy required for ablation to approximately 10,000 to 15,000 joules. Once the disc is ablated the instruments are removed and the patient returned to the recovery room. Patients are routinely discharged home several hours after the procedure.

Summary

The prolapsed or extruded disc and its role in the etiology of back and leg pain remains a subject for investigation. Mixter and Barr[15] were first to describe the decompression of lumbar nerve roots and the resolution of sciatica by removing herniated disc material. Their work laid the foundation, and provided a conceptual framework for discectomy in the treatment of herniated disc material. Laminectomy with discectomy became the standard treatment of symptomatic herniated discs. Love[11] popularized a less destructive hemilaminectomy technique in 1939. In 1978 Williams[23] helped popularize a microdiscectomy technique that avoided dissection of the posterior elements and preserved the epidural fat, thereby reducing adhesion formation. Hijikata[8,9] reported on a percutaneous technique of disc decompression using cannulas, suction, and rongeurs. This technique has been advanced by Onik and associates,[17] and other investigators introducing various cutting tools aiding the decompression. Choy introduced percutaneous laser decompression, which has been advanced by others, and has produced similar results to all other less-invasive forms of discectomy. The goal of all these techniques is the removal of disc material. The mechanism by which the disc produces symptoms may be severalfold. Chemical irritation, and initiation of a chemical-mediated inflammatory response from the acidic glycosaminoglycan of the nucleus pulposus,[13] mechanical compression from a herniated disc producing ischemia of the involved nerve root,[21] and disruption of the innervation of the annulus fibrosus[1,25] are all current theories of pain resulting from disc herniation. Removing disc tissue addresses all these proposed mechanisms. It stands to reason that the least invasive means of accomplishing this result would be the most beneficial for the patient. Currently, laser discectomy is the least invasive means by which discectomy can be performed. Experimentally reliable defects in the nucleus pulposus with decompression of the disc space can be reproduced in the clinical population. Currently, controlled studies on the efficacy of laser discectomy are, however, inconclusive.[22] Most but not all patients experience relief from their symptoms after laser discectomy. Further prospective, randomized, controlled, and blinded studies may help to determine the patient profile that might benefit from this procedure.

References

1. Bogduk N, Tynan W, Wilson AS: The nerve supply to the human intervertebral discs; *J Anat* 132:39, 1981.
2. Choy DSJ, Altman P: Fall of intradiscal pressure with laser ablation; *Spine State Art Rev* 7(1)11–16:, 1993.
3. Choy DSJ, Case R, Fielding W: Percutaneous laser ablation of lumbar discs: a preliminary report of in vitro and in vivo experience in animals and four human patients (abstract 323). Thirty-third Annual Meeting of the Orthopaedic Research Society, San Francisco, January 1987.
4. Choy DSJ, Case RB, Fielding W: Percutaneous nucleolysis of lumbar disc, *N Engl J Med* 317:771, 1987.
5. Choy DSJ and others: Percutaneous laser decompression: a new theraputic modality. *Spine* 17(8):949, 1992.
6. Cummings RS and others: Laser ablation of intervertebral discs using the Nd:YAG 1.44 μm laser, *Spine State Art Rev* 7(1):37, 1993.
7. Gropper GR, Robertson JH, McClellan G: Comparative histological and radiographic effects of CO_2 laser versus standard surgical anterior cervical discectomy in the dog, *Neurosurgery* 14:42, 1984.
8. Hijikata S: Percutaneous nucleotomy: a new concept technique and 12 years experience, *CORR* 238:24, 1989.
9. Hijikata S, Yamagishi M, Nakayama T: Percutaneous discectomy: a new treatment method for lumbar disc herniation, *J Toden Hosp* 5, 1975.
10. Lane GT and others: An experimental comparison of CO_2, argon, Nd:YAG, and Ho:YAG laser ablation of intervertebral discs, *Spine State Art Rev* 7:1, 1993.
11. Love GJ: Removal of protruded intervertebral disc without laminectomy, *Mayo Clin Proc* 14:800, 1939.
12. MacNab I: Negative disc exploration: an analysis of the causes of nerve root involvement in sixty-eight patients; *J Bone Joint Surg* 53A:891, 1971.
13. McCurron RF and others: The inflammatory effect of nucleus pulposus: a possible element in the pathogenesis of low-back pain, *Spine* 12:760, 1987.
14. Middleton GS, Teacher JH: Injury of the spinal cord due to rupture of an intervertebral disc during muscular effort, *Glasgow Med J* 76:1, 1911.
15. Mixter WJ, Barr JS: Rupture of the intervertebral disc with involvement of the spinal canal, *N Engl J Med* 211:210, 1934.
16. Oegema RT: Biochemistry of the intervertebral disc, *Clin Sports Med* 12(3):419, 1993.
17. Onik GM, Morris J, Helms C: Percutaneous lumbar discectomy using an aspiration probe: initial patient experience, *Radiology* 162:129, 1987.
18. Oppenheim H, Krause F: Veber einklemmung bzw. Strangulation der cauda equina, *Deutssche Med Wochnchr* 35:697, 1909.
19. Prodoehl JA and others: The effect of lasers on intervertebral disc pressures, *Spine State Art Rev* 7:17, 1993.
20. Rhodes A and others: Clinical use of the 2.1 micron holmium:YAG laser and percutaneous discectomy, *Spine State Art Rev* 7:49, 1993.
21. Rydevik D and others: Nutrition of the spinal nerve roots: the role of diffusion from the cerebrospinal fluid. Transactions of the 30th Orthopedic Research Society Meeting 9:276, 1984.
22. Sherk HH and others: Results of percutaneous laser discectomy with lasers, *Spine State Art Rev* 7:141, 1993.
23. Williams RW: Microlumbar discectomy: a conservative approach to the virgin herniated lumbar disc, *Spine* 3:175, 1978.
24. Yeung AT: Considerations for use of the KTP laser for disc decompression and ablation, *Spine State Art Rev* 7:67, 1993.
25. Yoshizawa H and others: The neuropathology of intervertebral discs removed for low back pain, *J Pathol* 132:95, 1980.

Chapter 77
Arthroscopic Lumbar Interbody Fusion
Parviz Kambin

Indications

Limitations of Arthroscopic Lumbar Fusion

Instruments

      pedicular jig
      cannulated obturator
      access cannula
      bolts
      extension bar

Operative Technique

Potential Use of Bone Substitutes and Bone Morphogenetic Protein for Arthroscopic Spine Fusion

Potential Use of Titanium Cage in Minimally Invasive Arthroscopic Lumbar Fusion

Mechanical instability of lumbar segments and the need for surgical stabilization of the vertebral column have attracted the interest of surgeons for decades.

Albee[1] reported in 1911 on the use of tibial bone graft to obtain stabilization for patients with Pott's disease involving the spinal column. In 1912, Hibbs[12] reported on posterior fusion of the lumbar segments affected by tuberculosis.

Posterolateral fusion[37,40] is an acceptable means of stabilization of the lumbar motion segments and is still popular today.

Posterior interbody fusion, advocated by Cloward,[4] has continued to provide a satisfactory method of approach for spinal stabilization.

Whether it is accomplished anteriorly,[6,9,34] posteriorly,[4,7,39] or posterolaterally[16,17,19-22,24] under arthroscopic control, broad surface contact of vertebral bodies and adequate blood supply at the fusion site have contributed to the success and popularity of interbody fusion.

The contribution of Harrington and Tullos[11] to the development of lag screws along with the enormous contribution of other spine surgeons[25,32,33,35] has been a giant step toward the maintenance of reduction and stabilization of the lumbar motion segments.

Recent advancements in arthroscopic disc surgery[18] and an understanding of safe dorsolateral access to the intervertebral disc have lead to the development of instrumentation for percutaneous interbody fusion and utilization of fixators through a minimally invasive operative technique.

Percutaneous insertion of bolts eliminates the need for wide exposure and injury to myoligamentous structures, thus promoting early mobility and restoration of function. The pedicular jig assists in the precise positioning of the guide pins and bolts under fluoroscopic control. Subcutaneously positioned plates, washers, and nuts can be readily accessed and extracted within a few months pending satisfactory arthrodesis. This procedure may become necessary for further MRI or CT studies on patients who have remained symptomatic.

Experience with percutaneous interbody fusion without instrumentation has been somewhat disappointing.[21,22] This view is also shared with other investigators.[24] Reduction of the height of the intervertebral disc, absorption of the bone chips, and mechanical difficulty leading to inadequate intraoperative decortication of the vertebral plates have been common causes of failure.

The concept of the use of percutaneous pedicular fixators was first introduced by Magerl.[26,27] External fixators were used for stabilization of fractures involving the thoracic and lumbar spine. However, the bulk of external fixators are somewhat cumbersome and generate certain physiologic and physical limitations. Furthermore, the concern for development of pin-track infection has limited its wide utilization.

Leu and Schreiber[24] have used external fixators after percutaneous posterolateral interbody fusion with satisfactory results. These authors use long screws and insert them through a stab skin incision into the pedicle under fluoroscopic control. Shortcomings of this operative technique include the inability of the surgeon to examine the medullary canal of the pedicles to rule out cortical penetration, and to change the position, diameter, or length of the screws if deemed necessary. When the screws are positioned through an access cannula placed over the pedicles, the above difficulties are eliminated. Other problems with this technique include the cumbersome and inconvenient nature of the external fixators and the potential for development of pin-track infection.

Indications

Restabilization of lumbar motion segments is indicated when there is demonstrable objective evidence of instability that can be correlated with patients presenting signs and symptoms.

Instability can be described as the loss of integrity of one or more supportive structures of the spinal unit associated with abnormal translation of the vertebrae, or deformation of the spine that is not present under physiologic conditions, thus potentially compromising the spinal canal and its neural content.

The functional spinal unit includes the adjacent two lumbar segments, the intervertebral disc facet joints, and the spinal ligaments.

Instability of the lumbar segment motion may occur following trauma associated with fracture dislocation or may be seen in conjunction with degenerative changes of the spinal column. The incidence of degenerative spondylolisthesis and the reduction of the height of the intervertebral disc following laminotomy and discectomy or decompressive procedures is not uncommon.

The developmental anomaly of the spine, destructive tumors, and infections are also capable of causing symptoms associated with spinal instability.

The inclusion criteria for arthroscopic lumbar fusion are similar to the generally accepted indications for spine arthrodesis. However, at this stage of its development, arthroscopic lumbar fusion aug-

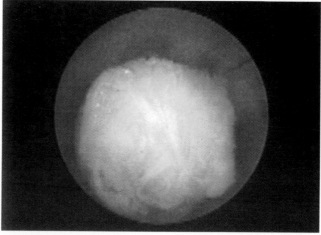

Plate IV-1

Arthroscopic visualization of the anular fibrosis at the site of entry. Note thick fibrous bands on the surface of the anulus and the absence of nerve entrapment.

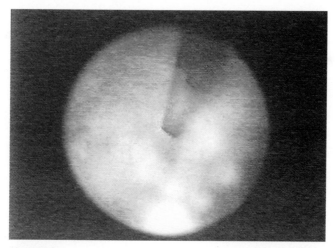

Plate IV-2

Nd:YAG 1064 nm laser being used for the vaporization of nuclear debris.

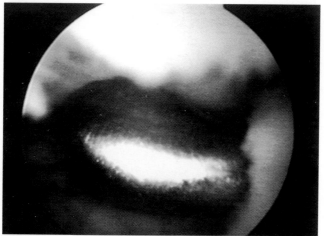

Plate IV-3

Arthroscopic view demonstrates the use of a long-handled curved curette to remove cartilaginous plate of the vertebral bodies at the fusion site.

mented by bolts and removable subcutaneous plates must be confined to a single motion segment and certainly should not be extended beyond two adjacent intervertebral discs.

The diagnosis of lumbar instability and need for surgical stabilization of degenerative or postdecompressive instability of the lumbar spine has been the subject of much controversy. However, when the condition is properly diagnosed, arthroscopic lumbar fusion can be substituted for conventional methods of lumbar segmental stabilization.

The forward and backward translation of one lumbar segment against another, visualized in the lateral erect flexion and extension roentgenogram,[13,23,30] provides valuable information for the diagnosis of lumbar instability. When severe pain is present, analgesics and at times epidural blocks may be used prior to the above diagnostic study.

Multiple recurrent disc herniations in a short time span may call for surgical stabilization of the involved spinal unit. Individuals with failed back syndrome who have had multiple decompressive spine surgeries may benefit in particular from arthroscopic lumbar fusion. Since intraoperative impingement or stimulation of scar tissue in these individuals does not produce pain, it has been postulated that the scar tissue is capable of producing pain by causing tension and traction on immobile but well innervated posterior longitudinal ligamentum and neural structures with movement and activity.

Discography is commonly used for diagnosis of internal disc disruption syndrome associated with disabling back pain. The pattern of distribution of the injected opaque substance when visualized in postinjection CT study, in conjunction with reproduction of the patient's symptoms, is used as a diagnostic tool for appropriate selection of the site of arthrodesis.

It has been suggested that the pain reproduction following discography may be secondary to the presence of the defect at the site of attachment of outer anular fibers to the vertebral plates.[10] These outer anular defects are likely due to mechanical stress and failures, independent of radial or concentric tears or clefts that are seen in the course of degeneration of the intervertebral disc. The granulation tissue and nerve ingrowth at the site of the defect of outer anular fibers has been demonstrated in cadaveric studies.[31] Since the intervertebral disc in this group of patients is the prime source of pain, anterior discectomy and fusion or 360-degree arthrodesis have been advocated in their treatment.[34] Arthroscopic disc extraction and fusion with percutaneous pedicular fixation certainly will reduce the morbidity associated with an anterior retroperitoneal approach.

When intractable back pain is associated with degenerative changes involving a single spinal unit as evidenced by the presence of traction spurs combined with MRI documentation of dehydration and global bulging of the intervertebral disc and satisfactory response to facet blocks, the arthroscopic lumbar fusion and stabilization may be used as an alternative method to arthrodesis.

Bolts and subcutaneous plating may be used for stabilization of unstable fractures of the lumbar spine.[26,27] If bone grafting is deemed necessary, the cancellous bone may be introduced via an access cannula positioned percutaneously in the pedicles of the involved segment.

Temporary stabilization of the lumbar motion segment for diagnosis and determination of the necessity of fusion may be achieved via percutaneous pedicular fixation and subcutaneous plating.

Symptomatic spondylolisthesis secondary to pars defect may be treated with arthroscopic lumbar fusion augmented by subcutaneous fixators. When decompression of pars interarticularis is deemed necessary, it is accomplished through a separate small posteromedial incision under magnification.

Bolts and subcutaneous plating may also be used in conjunction with an open posteromedial decompressive procedure. This author has used the above fixators following laminotomy and decompression of neural elements and posterolateral intertransverse fusion.

Limitations of Arthroscopic Lumbar Fusion

When considerable narrowing and reduction of the height of the intervertebral disc has taken place, certain difficulties associated with the placement of the access cannulas and decortication of the vertebral plates may be encountered.

The deformities of the spine are usually associated with distorted anatomy of pedicles and neural structures, which demand wide exposure and visualization of the surgical site.

Infections and tumors of the spine commonly require extensive debridement and block resection along with bone grafting and even prosthetic replacement and are considered unsuitable conditions for arthroscopic lumbar arthrodesis.

Individuals who have had failed open interbody fusion may not be good candidates for arthroscopic lumbar fusion.

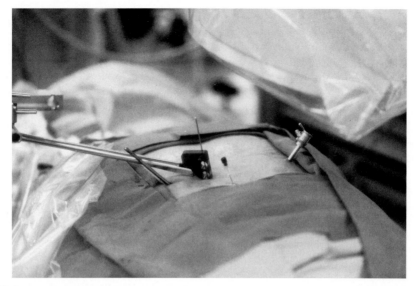

Fig. 77-1

The pedicular jig is being used for localization of the pedicle under C-arm fluoroscopy and insertion of the guide pin.

Instruments

Pedicular Jig

The appropriate positioning of the screws even during an open operative procedure is at times difficult. Weinstein and associates reported a 21% failure rate and unacceptable positioning in eight fresh cadaveric specimens.[38]

The pedicular jig (Fig. 77-1) allows for precise positioning of the guide pin in the center of the pedicle, which in turn accommodates proper positioning of the cannulated bolt.

The jig has a 36-in. handle and can be maneuvered by the surgeon outside the operating field, minimizing radiation exposure. A specially designed universal clamp allows the surgeon to maneuver the tip of the pedicular jig in all directions until the correct position is obtained. A locking mechanism is attached to freeze the jig in any given position.

Cannulated Obturator

The cannulated obturator (Figs. 77-2 and 77-3) is 12 cm in length and 9 mm in diameter. Its blunt extremity allows separation of the muscle fibers without undue injury to myoligamentous structures.

Access Cannula

The access cannula (Figs. 77-2 and 77-3) has an inner diameter of 10 mm, which slides with ease over the inserted cannulated obturator. It provides access to the pedicle and a path for the insertion of the pedicular taps, bolts, extension bars, and various wrenches.

Bolts

The bolts are cannulated. Several bolts in various lengths and diameters are available. The proximal extremity of the bolts above the cancellous threads are cylindrical, thus keeping the hex of the bolt above the posterolateral bone graft. This facilitates the engagement of the wrench and extraction of the bolt without interfering with the posterolateral bone mass.

Extension Bar

Two kinds of extension bars (Fig. 77-2)—straight and offset—are available in varying lengths. The extension bars are screwed clockwise to the threaded proximal extremity of the bolts, allowing for attachment and linkage via plates and nuts above the deep fascia layer at the lumbar region.

The offset extension bars are particularly useful when multiple segments are instrumented. Rotation of the extension bars facilitates alignment of the bolts prior to the placement of subcutaneous plates.

The offset extension bar is also useful when arthrodesis of L5-S1 is attempted. The bolts may have a tendency to converge, particularly when they are extended to a level above the fascia. The offset extension provides adequate space between the proximal extremity of the extension bars and facilitates the placement of subcutaneous plates.

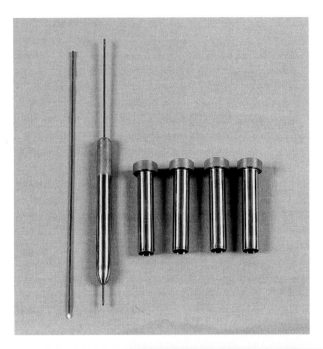

Fig. 77-2
Left to right: guide pin, cannulated obturator, four access cannulas.

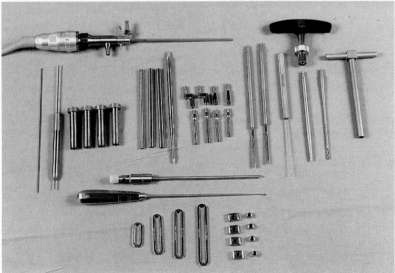

Fig. 77-3
Top: videodiscoscope: second row, left to right: guide pin, cannulated obturator, four access cannulas, various cannulas for access to the intervertebral disc, bolts with straight and offset extension bars, two screw taps, flexible sound, torque wrench, cannulated drill, bolt wrench, bone reamer, long-handled curette, plates, washers, and nuts.

Washers and nuts are beveled in order to minimize soft-tissue irritation.

Operative Technique

The patient is positioned prone on a radiolucent bolster and operating room table. The operative site is prepped and draped in routine fashion. Prophylactic antibiotic is administered prior to surgery and followed postoperatively for six additional doses. A bilateral biportal approach to the intervertebral disc is established, prior to localization of the site of introduction of bolts with the aid of the pedicular jig. The concern of injuring the spinal nerve while introducing instruments through the posterolateral approach is well founded. However, in skilled hands it is unlikely. As the spinal nerve departs the foramina, it descends distally, anteriorly, and laterally. It is then positioned safely anterior to the transverse process of the lower lumbar segment. The descent of the spinal nerve in the above fashion creates a triangular working zone[18] suitable to accommodate the inserted instruments. The triangular working zone is bordered by the spinal nerve, proximal plate, and proximal articular process of the lower segment.

Great care should be exercised when placing the instruments within the sacrospinalis, quadratus lumborum, and psoas major muscles. A far lateral approach increases the chance of entry to the abdominal and peritoneal cavity. The iliac arteries and vein are located anteriorly and are usually not in the path of the instruments. It should be noted that deep penetration or perianular slippage of the access cannula can cause injury to these structures. To provide

added safety, the design of the instruments does not permit more than 2 cm penetration into the intervertebral disc.

The point of entry varies from 8 to 10 cm from the midline. In thin individuals a distance of 8 to 9 cm may be adequate. Obese patients require a further distance from the midline.

Both right and left needles should be properly positioned at the onset of the operation. Otherwise the instruments positioned on the opposite side may interfere with proper fluoroscopic visualization of the tip of the needle being inserted. Two 18-gauge needles, 6 in. in length, are introduced dorsolaterally on an angle of approximately 35 to 45 degrees from the horizontal plan. The angle of the introduction and the entry site may be predetermined by a prone preoperative CT scan study (Fig. 77-4).

The position of the tip of the needle is first visualized with the C-arm in the lateral projection. The point of the needle should be just posterior to the edge of the intervertebral disc or slightly anterior to it (Fig. 77-5). Since there is ample space in the lower half of the triangular working zone, it is more desirable to position the needle closer to the inferior vertebral plate than to the plate of the upper segment. The C-arm is then turned into the anteroposterior (AP) position. In this position the tip of the needle should be visualized at the midpart of the pedicle or slightly lateral to it (Fig. 77-6). If a preoperative discography is requested, the surgeon

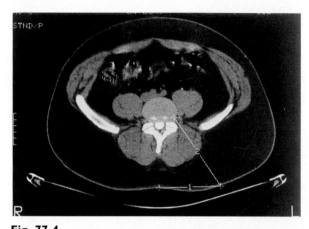

Fig. 77-4

Preoperative CT study in prone position confirms safe passage of the instruments through the muscle layers from a distance of 11 cm from the midline.

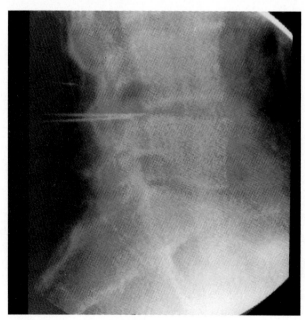

Fig. 77-5

Intraoperative lateral fluoroscopic examination shows proper positioning of the needle tip on the anular fibers.

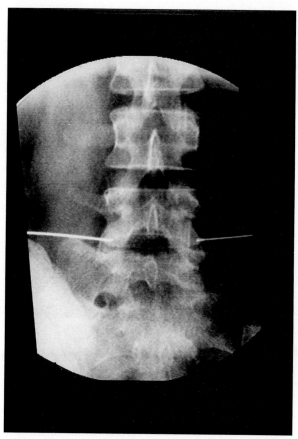

Fig. 77-6

Anteroposterior fluoroscopy during surgery, showing acceptable position of the tip of the needle, which is in alignment with the midpart of the pedicles of the adjacent segments.

may introduce a 22-gauge needle inside the lumen of the 18-gauge needle, and pass it into the center of the intervertebral disc for the above study. If discography is not conducted, the stylet of the needle is replaced by a 9-in. long Kirschner wire and the needle is then withdrawn. When intraoperative discography is not required, an 0.45 blunt tip Kirschner wire may be substituted for the 18-gauge needle and positioned on the anulus as described above.

At this time a cannulated trocar is introduced over the Kirschner wire (Fig. 77-7), thus allowing precise placement of the cannulated obturator on the anulus within the triangular working zone.

The universal access cannula is then placed over the cannulated obturator and directed toward the anulus with a rotary movement. Prior to full insertion of the access cannula, the surgeon must make certain that the blunt end of the cannulated obturator is well fitted and held against the anular fibers. The blunt extremity of the cannulated obturator has a tendency to push the spinal nerve aside, allowing the access cannula to reach the surface of the anulus.

When the access cannulas are properly positioned, AP fluoroscopy of the distal extremity shows the cannulas in alignment with the midportion of the pedicle (Figs. 77-8 and 77-9).

The arthroscopic inspection of the anulus is now carried out. Invariably one observes a loose adipose tissue on the surface of the anulus. To visualize the anular surface and rule out nerve root entrapment,

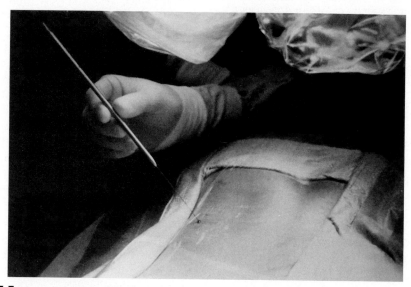

Fig. 77-7

The cannulated obturator is being inserted over the previously positioned guide wire, thus minimizing the incidence of soft-tissue injury and development of hematomas.

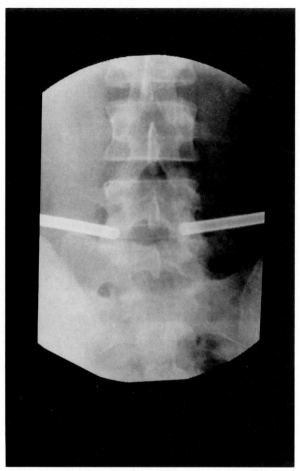

Fig. 77-8

Intraoperative anteroposterior fluoroscopy demonstrating the bilateral biportal approach to the L4-L5 intervertebral disc. Note the proper positioning of the distal extremities of the access cannulas, which are in alignment with the line drawn at the midpart of the pedicles or slightly lateral to them.

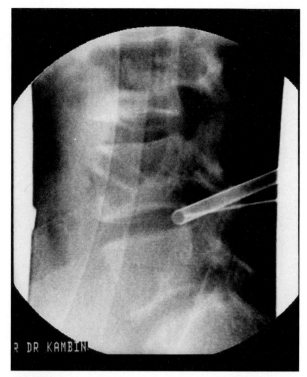

Fig. 77-9

Lateral x-ray film showing the proper positioning of one access cannula and the needle that has been placed on the anulus from the opposite side.

the fatty tissue is removed with pituitary forceps or crushed and rubbed off with a cottonoid held by pituitary forceps. The absence of spinal nerve entrapment can then be unequivocally confirmed (see color plate IV-1).

At this time needle testing is conducted to make certain that the distal opening of the access cannula is well positioned on the anulus fibers. The strength and durability of the access cannulas allows a certain mobility of the inserted sheaths through the paraspinal muscles. While holding the access cannula firmly against the anulus, the surgeon first uses a small and than a larger trephine circular cutter to penetrate the anular fibers. The large trephine may be left in the intervertebral disc as a guide while the access cannula is pushed into the anular fibers with a firm rotary and downward movement.

These steps are repeated to create another portal from the opposite side (see Fig. 77-8).

For adequate disc extraction and access to the vertebral plates, two access cannulas, larger in diameter, are customarily telescoped over the universal cannulas.

Oval-shaped access cannulas provide a working space of 6 × 8 mm and may be used to gain wider access to the intervertebral disc. A specially designed auxiliary jig, which is inserted next to the cannulated obturator, is used for placement of the oval cannula.

Nuclear tissue is extracted with the aid of manual and aggressive trimmer blades. The laser has been found to be a useful adjunct to the above instruments by enabling rapid nucleolysis and removal of fine nuclear debris that can be left in the intervertebral disc space (see color plate IV-2). Most of the commonly used and available lasers in the operating room, including Nd:YAG 1064 nm, KTP 532 nm, and Holmium:YAG may be used.

A meticulous extraction of the cartilaginous plate of the vertebral bodies is accomplished with the aid of power-driven reamers and a curved curette (see color plate IV-3).

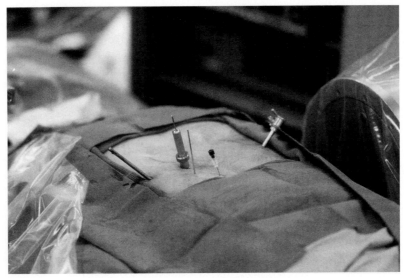

Fig. 77-10

Cannulated obturator and access cannula are placed over the previously positioned guide pin in the pedicle of the fourth lumbar vertebra. Note the two intervertebral disc cannulas inserted dorsolaterally. The needle is used for administration of spinal anesthesia during the surgery.

The pedicular jig is attached to the operating room table. The 6-in. guide pin is inserted into the radiolucent tip of the pedicular jig. The C-arm is draped and positioned for AP fluoroscopic examination. It should be noted that the tube is tilted 20 degrees lateral from the pedicle that is being instrumented. The handle and the entire length of the pedicular jig is manipulated through the universal clamp until the guide pin is viewed as a radiographic dot positioned slightly above the center of the pedicle. At this time the jig is locked into place by turning the appropriate knob on top of the universal clamp.

The guide pin is then hammered into the pedicle. At times a hand or power drill must be used to penetrate the cortical bone at the entry site.

An incision approximately 1.5 cm long is made adjacent to the guide pin with a #11 knife blade, following the path of the guide pin, and the deep fascia is incised. This permits the passage of the blunt end of the cannulated obturator.

The cannulated obturator is now placed over the guide pin and is passed through the fascia and the muscle layer with a slow twisting movement until it reaches the bony structures at the entry site.

At this time the pedicular access cannula is placed over the cannulated obturator and driven through the fascia and paravertebral muscle fibers until resistance is felt (Fig. 77-10). With the use of the cannulated drill, the cortical bone is penetrated at the entry site prior to the use of the pedicular bolt taps.

The C-arm is turned to the lateral position and the direction of the guide pin in the pedicle and the vertebral body are visualized. One should make certain that the C-arm is properly positioned and the vertebral plates of the segments adjacent to the fusion site are viewed parallel to one another. If the position of the guide pin is incorrect, it may be withdrawn and reinserted into the medullary canal of the pedicle in a more acceptable position.

The medullary canal of the pedicle is taped in preparation for insertion of the bolt.

A flexible sound may be used to examine the medullary canal of the pedicle and to make certain that the cortex of the pedicle has not been violated.

A number of bolts varying in length and diameter should be available. A bolt appropriate in length and diameter is chosen and placed over the guide pin to be driven through the medullary canal of the pedicle and into the vertebral body of the segment adjacent to the site of fusion. The position of the bolt is inspected via a lateral fluoroscopic examination (Fig. 77-11).

An extension bar is then chosen and attached to the proximal extremity of the bolt, allowing extension to the level above the deep fascia of the lumbar spine. A special wrench is used to immobilize the bolt while the extension bar is inserted with a hex screwdriver. When more than two segments are fused or when L5-S1 stabilization is performed, the offset extension bar may be used. This allows for correct alignment of the bolts in preparation for the in-

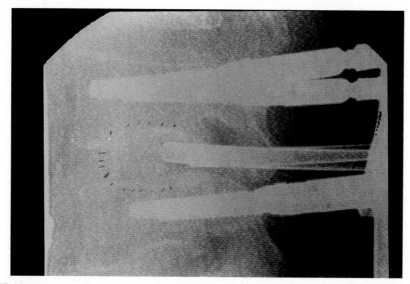

Fig. 77-11

Intraoperative lateral fluoroscopic examination demonstrates four bolts and extension bars in place. Two access cannulas are used for decortication of the vertebral plates and impaction of bone grafts.

sertion of subcutaneous plates. The access cannulas are removed following the insertion of the bolts. The subcutaneous plates are then passed under the skin through the incision that was made previously for the introduction of the access cannulas. The plates are attached to the extension bars with beveled washers and nuts. The hex screwdrivers may be placed in the proximal extremity of the extension bar to provide compression or distraction prior to placement and tightening of the washers and nuts.

The wounds are irrigated. The subcutaneous tissue is closed with interrupted absorbable sutures; subcutaneous sutures are used for skin closure.

Autogenous bone graft is harvested through a small incision placed over the posterior superior iliac spine. Sufficient cancellous and cortical bone is extracted and packed between the vertebral bodies at the fusion site through the previously positioned cannulas into the intervertebral disc (see Fig. 77-11).

Although nucleotomy, along with insertion of access cannulas into the intervertebral disc, can be performed under local anesthesia, the harvesting of bone from the pelvis and the introduction of the pedicular bolts requires general or spinal anesthesia.

Spinal anesthesia is provided by the surgeon. A 22-gauge spinal needle is inserted into the subarachnoid space two or three levels above the fusion site (see Fig. 77-10).

If the surgeon has acquired skill with arthroscopic microdiscectomy and is able to visualize the perianular structures, he or she may proceed with general anesthesia for the entire operative procedure.

Potential Use of Bone Substitutes and Bone Morphogenetic Protein for Arthroscopic Spine Fusion

Orthopedic surgeons generally favor an autogenous bone graft over allografts and synthetic material. However, the absorption of bone chips placed between the vertebral bodies in the course of arthroscopic interbody fusion may result in nonunion and an unfavorable outcome.[22]

In addition, the harvesting of bone from the ilium requires a separate incision. This procedure both is time-consuming and increases postoperative morbidity and the chance of development of postoperative infection. Numerous synthetically prepared bone substitutes have been used on animals and in clinical studies. These materials include hydroxyapatite, tricalcium phosphate, collagen type I, demineralized bone matrix, growth factors, biopolymers, matrix proteins, and ceramic.

The hydroxyapatite from coral and tricalcium phosphate, when used as bone substitutes, lack osteoinductive capabilities and mechanical strength.[3,5] However, they are biocompatible and bond readily with the recipient's bone. Mooney and Selby and associates reported a high rate of nonunion in clinical use of hydroxyapatite compared with autogenous bone grafts.[29,34]

It has been demonstrated that bone induced by demineralized bone matrix can achieve 35% torsional strength of normal bone together with an increased capacity to deform under load.[2,8,36] Hopp and co-workers[14] reported a favorable outcome pertaining to mechanical strength and rate of union when osteoinductive demineralized bone matrix and hydroxyapatite demineralized bone matrix composite were used as graft substitutes in rabbits.

There are many convincing laboratory and clinical studies on the bone-inductive capacities of bone morphogenetic protein when used in conjunction with synthetic osteoconductive material or fresh bone marrow.[15,28,36,41]

Future availability and experience with osteoconductive or osteoinductive material used in conjunction with autogenous bone will certainly enhance the incidence of development of solid arthrodesis and the level of interest in minimally invasive arthroscopic lumbar fusion.

Potential Use of Titanium Cage in Minimally Invasive Arthroscopic Lumbar Fusion

Ongoing research into the development of an expandable cage that can be placed between the vertebral plates will add another dimension to minimally invasive arthroscopic lumbar fusion. Currently, a clinical study on the efficacy and feasibility of the use of a BAK titanium cage placed between the vertebral bodies through an anterior laparoscopic approach is being conducted by Yuan and co-workers.[42] This procedure may prove to be an acceptable operative technique in the field of minimally invasive spine surgery.

References

1. Albee FH: Transplantation of a portion of the tibia into the spine for Pott's disease: a preliminary report, *JAMA* 57:855, 1911.
2. Bolander ME, Balian G: The use of demineralized bone marrow in the repair of segmental defects, *J Bone Joint Surg (Am)* 68:1264, 1986.
3. Bucholz RW, Carlton A, Hommes RE: Hydroxyapatite and tricalcium phosphate bone graft substitutes, *Orthop Clin North Am* 18:323, 1987.
4. Cloward RB: The treatment of ruptured lumbar disc by vertebral body fusion: indications, operative technique, after care, *J Neurosurg* 10:154, 1953.
5. Cook SD and others: Hydroxyapatite-coated titanium for orthopedic implant applications, *Clin Ortho* 232:225, 1988.
6. Crock HV: Anterior lumbar interbody fusion: indication for its use and notes on surgical technique, *Clin Orthop* 165:157, 1981.
7. Dommisse GF: Lumbo-sacral interbody spinal fusion, *J Bone Joint Surg* 41:87, 1959.
8. Einhorn TA and others: The healing of segmental bone defects induced by demineralized bone matrix: a radiographic and biomechanical study, *J Bone Joint Surg* 66:277, 1984.
9. Fang HSY, Ong GB, Hodgson AR: Anterior spinal fusion: the operative approaches, *Clin Orthop* 35:16, 1964.
10. Fraser RD, Osti OL, Vernon-Roberts B: Intervertebral disc degeneration, *Eur Spin J* 1:205, 1993.
11. Harrington PR, Tullos HS: Reduction of severe spondylolisthesis in children, *South Med Assoc* 62:1, 1969.
12. Hibbs RA: An operation for Potts disease of the spine, *JAMA* 59:433, 1912.
13. Hirsch C, Lewin T: Lumbosacral synovial joints in flexion-extension, *Acta Orthop Scand* 39:303, 1968.
14. Hopp SG, Dahners LE, Gilbert JA: A study of the mechanical strength of long bone defects treated with various bone autograft substitutes: an experimental investigation in the rabbit, *J Orthop Res* 7:579, 1989.
15. Johnson EE, Urist MR, Fineman GAM: Distal metaphyseal tibial nonunion: deformity and bone loss treated by open reduction, internal fixation, and human bone morphogenetic protein (HBMP), *Clin Orthop* 250:234, 1990.
16. Kambin P: Arthroscopic lumbar fusion with pedicular bolts and removable subcutaneous plates, ISMISS Scientific Exhibit, AAOS Meeting, San Francisco, CA, February 18-22, 1993.
17. Kambin P: Arthroscopic lumbar fusion with pedicular bolts and subcutaneous plates, ISMISS Scientific Exhibit, AAOS Meeting, Washington, D.C., February 20-25, 1992.
18. Kambin P: Arthroscopic microdiscectomy, *Arthroscopy J Arthroscopic Rel Surg* 8(3):287, 1992.
19. Kambin P: Percutaneous segmental stabilization in situ and with pedicular screws and subcutaneous fixators, Symposium, The Graduate Hospital, Philadelphia, November 1, 1991.
20. Kambin P: Posterolateral approach to the lumbar intervertebral discs: from nucleotomy to segmental stabilization, International Symposium on Percutaneous Intervertebral Surgery with Discoscopy, Zurich, Switzerland, June, 1991.
21. Kambin P: *Posterolateral percutaneous lumbar interbody fusion, arthroscopic microdiscectomy, minimal intervention in spinal surgery,* Baltimore, 1991, Williams & Wilkins, p 117.
22. Kambin P, Schaffer JL: Poster exhibit, Arthroscopic lumbar fusion augmented with removable pedicular fixators and subcutaneous plates, Advanced course on pedicular fixation of the lumbar spine and other advanced techniques, Scoliosis Research Society and NASS, Orlando, FL, May 13-15, 1993.
23. Knuttson F: The instability associated with disc degeneration in the lumbar spine, *Acta Radiol* 25:593, 1944.
24. Leu HJ, Schreiber A: *Percutaneous lumbar restabilization, arthroscopic microdiscectomy, minimal intervention in spinal surgery,* Baltimore, MD, 1991, Williams & Wilkins, p 123.

25. Luque ER: The anatomic basis and development of segmental spinal instrumentation, *Spine* 7:256, 1982.

26. Magerl FP: *External skeletal fixation of the lower thoracic and the lumbar spine,* In Uhthoff HK, Stahl E, editors: *Current concepts of external fixation of fractures,* New York, 1982, Springer-Verlag.

27. Magerl FP: Stabilization of the lower thoracic and lumbar spine with external skeletal fixation, *Clin Orthop* 189:125, 1984.

28. Mahy PR, Urist MR: Experimental heterotopic bone formation induced by bone morphogenetic protein and recombination human interleukin-1B, *Clin Orthop* 237:286, 1988.

29. Mooney V, Derian C: *Synthetic bone graft lumbar spine surgery techniques and complications.* White A, Rothman RH, Ray CD, editors. St. Louis, 1987, Mosby, p 471.

30. Pennal GF and others: Motion studies of the lumbar spine, *J Bone Joint Surg* 54B:442, 1972.

31. Rauschning W: Pathoanatomy of central and lateral stenosis, *The lumbar spine: State of the Art,* IV Instructional Course, International Society for the Study of the Lumbar Spine, Rome, June 13-14, 1993.

32. Roy-Camille R: Osteosynthese du rachis dorsal, lombaire et lombo-sacre par plaques metalliques visees dans les pedicules vertebraux et les apophyses articulaires, *Pres Med* 78:1447, 1970.

33. Roy-Camille R and others: *Early treatment of spinal injuries.* In MacKibbin B, editor: *Recent advances in orthopaedics number three,* Dublin, 1979, Churchill Livingstone, p 57.

34. Selby DK and others: *Anterior lumbar fusion.* In White AH, editor: *Lumbar spine surgery,* St. Louis, 1987, Mosby, p 383.

35. Steffee AD, Biscup RS, Sitkowski DJ: Segmental spine plates with pedicle screw fixation: a new internal fixation device for disorders of the lumbar and thoracolumbar spine, *Clin Orthop* 203:45, 1986.

36. Urist MR, Strates BS: Bone formation in implants of partially and wholly demineralized bone matrix, including observations on acetone-fixed intra and extracellular proteins, *Clin Orthop* 71:271, 1970.

37. Watkins MB: Posterolateral fusion of the lumbar and lumbosacral spine, *J Bone Joint Surg* 34A:1014, 1953.

38. Weinstein JN and others: Spinal pedicle fixation: reliability and validity, Third Annual Meeting, NASS, July 1988.

39. Wiltberger R: Intervertebral body fusion by the use of posterior bone dowel, *Clinical Orthopedics,* 35:69, 1964.

40. Wiltse LL and others: The paraspinal sacrospinalis-splitting approach to the lumbar spine, *J Bone Joint Surg* 50A:919, 1968.

41. Yasko AW and others: Comparison of biological and synthetic carriers of recombinant human BMP (rhBMP-21): induced bone formation. Orthopaedic Research Society, 38th Annual Meeting, Washington, D.C., Feb. 17-20, 1992.

42. Yuan HA and others: Preliminary report on laparoscopic L5-S1 anterior discectomy and fusion using BAK cage, SICOT/ISMISS Congress, Seoul, Korea, September 3, 1993.

Chapter 78
Myeloscopy and Endoscopic Nucleotomy

Yoshio Ooi
Youkichi Satoh
Fujio Mita
Jonathan L. Schaffer

Historical Aspects

Myeloscopic Technique

equipment
examination
normal findings
pathologic findings
summary

Endoscopic Nucleotomy

equipment
examination

Summary

Historical Aspects

A myeloscope is a small-caliber endoscope designed to view the intrathecal and epidural spaces. The history of myeloscopy dates back to Dr. Michael Burman's work in 1931, at the Hospital for Joint Diseases in New York, when he attempted to view the cauda equina of cadavers by the use of an arthroscope.[1] Burman was unable to enter the intrathecal space because of the size of the endoscope.

Elias Stern, from Sydenham Hospital, New York, and staff surgeon of the Clinic for the Relief of Intractable Pain, reported the possibility of endoscopic examination of the intrathecal space in the *Medical Record* in 1936.[25] He examined living subjects, but did not describe the number of cases or elaborate on his findings which he recorded in handwritten sketches. Stern called the endoscope a spinaloscope.[25] He speculated that the ultimate observation of this human cavity would be by endoscopic methods. In 1938, J. Lawrence Pool, at the Neurological Institute of New York at Columbia Presbyterian Hospital, developed a hot-lamp system specifically designed for intrathecal observation.[21] He observed the cauda equina and the accompanying vessels. Dr. Pool examined more than 400 patients in the following years, published at least three papers, and made valuable observations regarding arachnoiditis and spinal tumors.[21-23] His handdrawn sketches were precise in detail, even though his endoscope was not comparable to the present cold-light system. Dr. Pool, who later became the Chairman of the Department of Neurological Surgery at Columbia Presbyterian Hospital, should be honored as the initial investigator of myeloscopy in humans. He discontinued his study of myeloscopy after 1942, possibly due to technical problems.

In 1966, the senior author independently performed the first intrathecal observation of a patient diagnosed with intervertebral disc herniation with spondylolisthesis (Fig. 78-1).[13] Documentation of the pathology was recorded and the patient subsequently underwent an open procedure.[13] The endoscope was the type used in the ENT clinic, with an outer diameter of 5.6 mm (Fig. 78-2). After this initial case, several cases of low-back pathology were then studied and photographed, including patients with spinal cord injuries and spina bifida. The author then was able to spend a number of months working under Dr. H.A. Rusk at the Institute of Rehabilitation Medicine at New York University in 1967 and also was able to interact with Dr. Pool, then Chairman of Neurosurgery at Columbia University. On his return to Japan in 1969, his work in myeloscopy continued.

Progress in medical technology, especially in the field of lens polishing and glass-fiber engineering, has led to the use of small-diameter, cold-light systems. Thus, the outer diameter of the myeloscope has decreased from 5.6 mm in 1966 to 2.8 mm in 1972, down to 1.7 mm in 1977, and finally to 0.8 mm in 1987 (Fig. 78-3). In 1991, the thinner fiberglass optics became available so that endoscopes with a 0.35-mm outer diameter now had resolution sufficient for operative procedures. In 1981, the second author reported the investigation of the movement of the L4 and L5 nerve roots while testing straight leg raising in a living subject.[14] Nerve-root

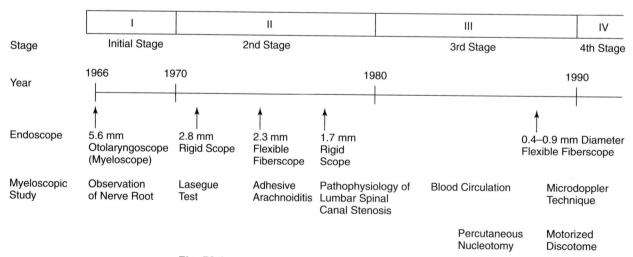

Fig. 78-1

Historical timeline of myeloscopic development by authors.

movement caudally, anteriorly, and laterally was visualized through the myeloscope.

The introduction of integrated video systems facilitated the visualization of the vasculature within the cauda equina. Further work on chronic arachnoiditis began in 1981.[10] Following the suggestions of Drs. Leon Wiltse and Ian MacNab, Dr. S. Dohring, an orthopedic surgeon from the University of Dusseldorf, joined our laboratory to investigate the clinical use of myeloscopy. He performed myeloscopic and histologic investigations of artificially induced arachnoiditis in monkeys.[2] The cauda equina of monkeys are ideally suited for observation. Chronic aseptic adhesive arachnoiditis was induced by the injection of proteolytic enzymes. Intrathecal collagenase produced drastic changes in the vessels of the cauda equina.[2] In our laboratory, research turned toward the clarification of the pathophysiologic mechanism of intermittent claudication in lumbar spinal canal stenosis. It had been postulated that the disturbance of either extradural or intradural venous blood return leads to vasocongestion and is associated with the gradual onset of neurogenic claudication.[12] However, the etiology still remains unclear. J.A. Epstein's excellent study found that approximately 50% of patients with lumbar spinal canal stenosis had chronic aseptic adhesive arachnoiditis.[3] In that investigation it was suggested that constriction of the dural sac and obstruction of cerebrospinal

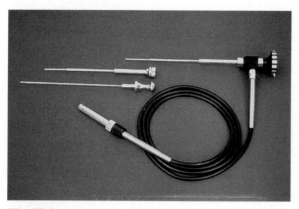

Fig. 78-2

Rigid-type myeloscope and its attachments used in 1966. Outer diameter was 5.6 mm.

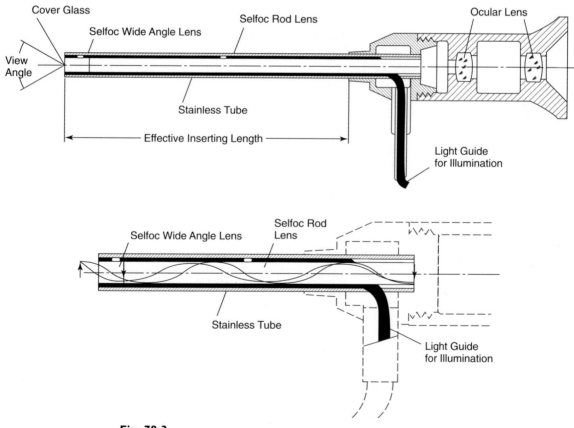

Fig. 78-3

Schematic of myeloscope currently being used, with diameter of 1.7 mm.

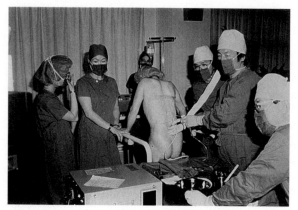

Fig. 78-4

Myeloscopic observation while patient walks on treadmill.

fluid flow may have precipitated the aseptic adhesive arachnoiditis changes. Mita inserted the 1.7-mm diameter myeloscope into a patient with lumbar spinal canal stenosis and put the patient on a treadmill[12] (Fig. 78-4). Intermittent claudication appeared within a few minutes of treadmill use. He then compared the pretreadmill and posttreadmill myeloscopic findings. Engorgement of the accompanying blood vessels in the cauda equina was observed, as well as dilation of the venous plexus in the extradural space (color plate V-1). Differentiating between the vein and the artery within the cauda equina was quite impossible through the myeloscope, but theoretically it is mostly venous return that should have been obstructed. Patients with herniated nucleus pulposus served as controls and did not show any stagnation of flow within the blood vessels of the cauda equina. Whether an increase or decrease of blood flow in cauda equina vessels is present in patients with spinal stenosis is yet another interesting question that remained unanswered. In order to evaluate blood flow within the accompanying vessels, a specially designed micro-Doppler sensor (F502575, Primtec Company) was inserted through the trochar together with a myeloscope; however, the technique was difficult because we were unable to attach the sensor satisfactorily on the roots in the cauda equina. In 1991, a successful result was obtained and reported at the International Society for the Study of Lumbar Spine meeting (Boston, 1991).

It would be interesting to observe myeloscopically the effects of vasodilating or vasoconstricting agents on this exercise-related vasocongestion. Such work is currently under way at our laboratory. Porter and Hibbert[24] did report some beneficial clinical effect with calcitonin on patients with lumbar spinal canal stenosis. Considerable improvement in walking tolerance was noted in 11 of 41 patients with a diagnosis of neurogenic claudication who were treated with calcitonin. We have initiated studies demonstrating significant effect with intravenous calcitonin, nicardipine, and adrenaline on blood flow within cauda equina vessels. In other work, the authors continued their in vivo, endoscopic disc studies. These were presented to the symposium at the annual meeting of the International Society of Radiology in Brussels in 1981.

In 1975, Dr. Hijikata took myeloscopy a step further and developed the percutaneous nucleotomy by successfully inserting the punch forceps into an intervertebral disc and removing degenerated nucleus pulposus material.[4] He performed the procedure percutaneously through a posterolateral approach. Concurrently, Dr. Parviz Kambin independently initiated his work on the posterolateral percutaneous lumbar discectomy technique for removal of the herniated fragment comprising a nerve root and has now reported on two prospective series of patients.[5-7] Dr. Gary Onik developed the automated nucleotome for debulking the center of a nucleus pulposus.[8] In 1987, Ooi and Mita introduced a single puncture technique for endoscopic herniectomy by use of a working cannula[11] (Fig. 78-5 & color plate V-2). The technology of flexible myeloscopy is improving rapidly, leading to a promising future.

Myeloscopic Technique

Equipment

There are a number of myeloscopes now available.[9,15,16,17,18,19] These vary according to outer diameter; flexible or rigid construction; lateral, oblique, or direct view systems; and glass fiber systems. Medical instrument companies, including Olympus Camera Company, Machida Medical Instrument Company, and Shinko Medical Instrument Company have supplied us with excellent-quality endoscopes. The authors use a specially adapted Olympus camera with Kodak ASA400 film and the Sony videotelevision system. The length of fiberoptics should be greater than 15 cm to reach the entire lumbar intraspinal canal satisfactorily. The authors use fiberoptics that have been custom-manufactured (Asahi Kohgaku Company). Color discrepancy with Selfoc fiberoptics is minimal, and resolution is inadequate for the operative visualization. Additional supplies required for the procedure are surgical knife, local anesthetic, suturing set, drapes, and skin disinfectant such as that used for routine surgical preparation.

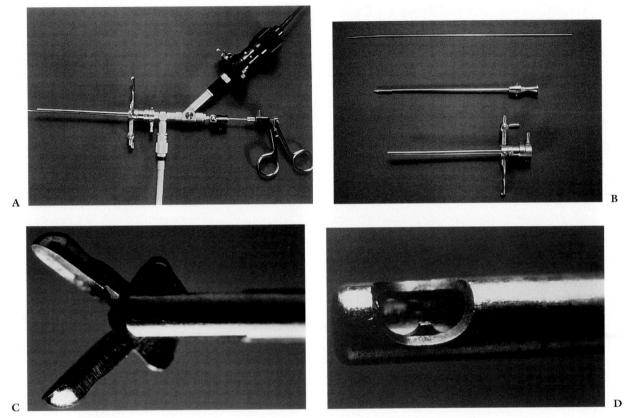

Fig. 78-5

Myeloscope and attachments for arthroscopic nucleotomy. **A,** Double-hole rigid scope and forceps with camera and light source attached. **B,** Guide wire, trochar, and scope sheath. **C,** Forceps. **D,** Discotome.

Examination

The patient is asked to lie on the operating table in the lateral decubitus position. After infiltration with local anesthesia, an incision less than 0.5 cm is made in the midline. A trochar needle is inserted into the intraspinal canal at the level of L4-L5 or L5-S1 using technique one would use for a spinal tap procedure. The trochar needle is replaced with the myeloscope in order to observe the extradural space and structures. The myeloscope should be connected to a video system, which allows for viewing on the monitor and for concurrent video recording (Fig. 78-6). After viewing and identifying the epidural space, the trochar needle is reinserted and the dura mater is punctured to permit the entry into the intrathecal space. The myeloscope is placed intrathecally and the cauda equina and their accompanying blood vessels are observed.[18] Flushing with normal physiologic saline clears the endoscopic view if bleeding obstructs or hinders the view. Dexamethasone (2 mg) in the epidural space has been used occasionally, as it may be beneficial after the myeloscopy. The total examination time is usually around 30 minutes,

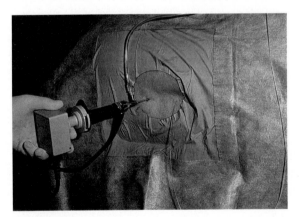

Fig. 78-6

Myeloscope connected to camera.

depending on the aim of the investigation. To prevent postexamination headache, possibly due to the loss of cerebrospinal fluid during the examination, 500 ml of normal saline is administered intravenously. After the myeloscopy, all patients are asked to lie in bed for 3 or more hours, maintaining a head-down position. Patients may stay one or two nights in the hospital or may go home during the examination day.

After washing out the endoscope with a large amount of sterile water, it is immersed in concentrated chlorhexidine gluconate for 15 minutes. However, because of the possible risk of viral infection, we perform viral serologic studies on each patient before examination. After myeloscopy, the endoscopes are routinely disinfected with a 24-hour ethylene oxide gas protocol.

Normal Findings

The cauda equina with its accompanying vessels has a normal appearance that is a slightly pale, bluish white color with reddened vessels (color plate V-3). The diameter of one cauda equina nerve root is approximately 5 to 10 times greater than its accompanying vessel. The appearance of the normal cauda equina is somewhat obscured with the nearly transparent arachnoid membrane. The color of the dura mater is pale white and semitransparent in the young adult, whereas in the elderly, it is thick and white. Observation of the accompanying vessels improves with experience. The Y-shaped branch vessels often found at the sites of kinking are helpful landmarks, especially during observation of nerve-root movement, such as during a straight leg raising test. Maneuvers such as the straight leg raise should be done in the lateral decubitus position, as would be done when performing a lumbar puncture, with an assistant slowly moving the patient's leg while the main observer records and investigates. It is interesting to note not only the movement of the cauda equina, but also the dynamic blood flow within the cauda equina. Occasionally, it is possible to demonstrate the cessation of blood flow or even a reversal of the flow during the straight leg raising test.

In elderly patients, the nerve roots often show a folded redundant pattern. The structures that can be observed by the use of the myeloscope include the supraspinal and interspinal ligaments, the ligamentum flavum, the epidural space, the nerve roots, the intrathecal cauda equina, the anterior and posterior longitudinal ligaments, and the disc material.

Pathologic Findings

Over 700 cases of myeloscopy have been accumulated in the authors' clinic.[9,12,13,14,15,16,17,18,19] Among these series, some examples of pathologic conditions have been demonstrated (color plate V-4). Chronic aseptic adhesive arachnoiditis is seen in many patients who do not have many subjective or objective findings. Patients who have undergone back surgery demonstrated widely varying degrees of arachnoiditis. This led the authors to suspect that predispositions or familial tendencies for scar tissue formation or minor collagen abnormalities may play a role in the development of arachnoiditis.

Summary

Myeloscopy is a helpful diagnostic technique with minimum risk, as only one patient had stigmata of an infection and was successfully treated. In the over 800 cases performed to date, only one patient had a temporary cerebrospinal fluid leak. The procedure is easy to perform and almost no complications have been noted. Continued experience with this procedure will permit development of diagnostic and potentially therapeutic procedures.

Endoscopic Nucleotomy

Equipment

The endoscopic nucleotomy apparatus consists of a double-holed trochar, an endoscope, forceps, an electric shaver for hernia mass removal, and a light source. The trochars are oval, with outer diameters of 3.9×2.3 mm and 4.4×2.8 mm and internal diameters of 3.7×2.1 mm and 4.2×2.6 mm, respectively.

Examination

The patient is placed on the operating table in the prone position. Before the skin incision, local anesthesia, typically 1% lidocaine, is injected into the superficial tissues. Preoperative administration of an intravenous narcotic is also helpful for the patient. We have also used general anesthesia for added safety in over 75% of our cases. The posterolateral approach, as described by Carlos Ottolenghi[20] is routinely used, but this approach is often modified. The trochar hole for the endoscope should be aligned so that it is always placed in the lateral position, and the forceps side should be medial.

At this time, the transpinal canal approach has not been adopted, but it could become possible because the diameter of the whole trochar is getting smaller. The basic idea of percutaneous nucleotomy is not the removal of protruded nucleus pulposus, but rather the decreasing of intradiscal pressure.[4,11] It is therefore reasonable to think that, based on our experience, the posterolateral approach is safe. However, this procedure has inherent limitations. Pro-

Plate V-1

Flow changes in blood vessels of the cauda equinae in a patient with lumbar spinal canal stenosis.

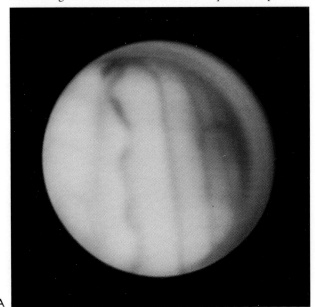

A

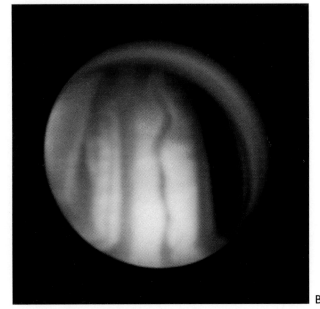

B

A, Before walking.

B, After walking on a treadmill.

Plate V-2

Intraoperative visualization of intradiscal instrument placement.

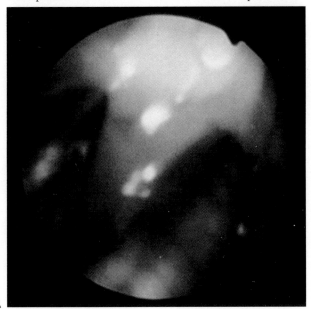

A

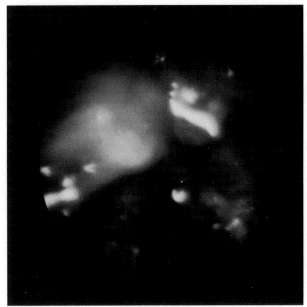

B

A, Arthroscopic visualization of the forceps.

B, Arthroscopic visualization of the discotome.

Plate V-3

Myeloscopic visualization of normal anatomy.

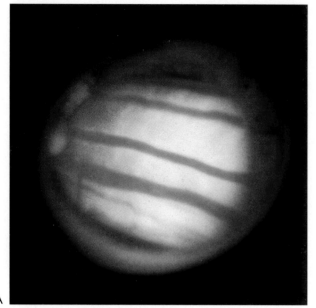

A, Cauda equina, normal.

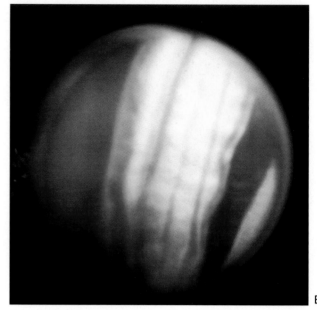

B, Cauda equina, standing.

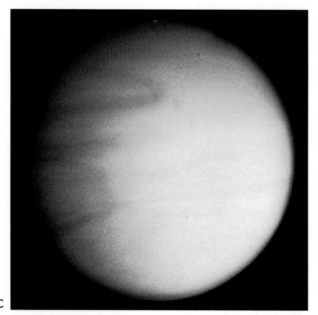

C, Surface of the dura.

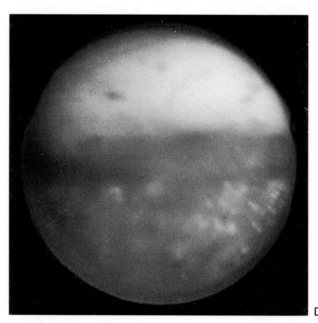

D, Dura and epidural fat tissue.

Plate V-4
Myeloscopic visualization of the pathological findings in chronic aseptic arachnoiditis.

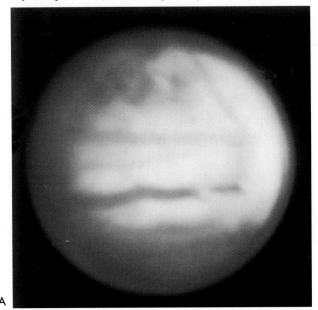

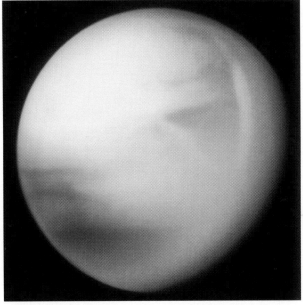

A, Discoloration of the cauda equina.

B, Hypertrophied dural sac.

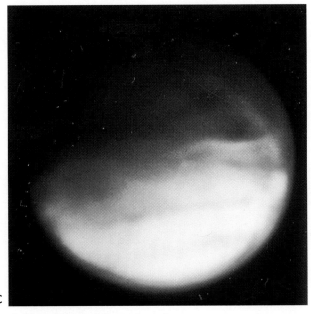

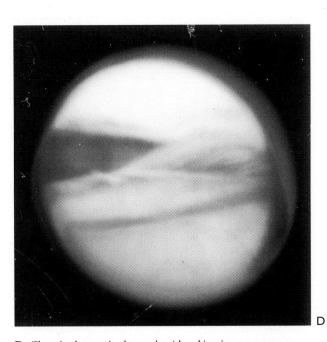

C, Matted fibers of the cauda equina.

D, Chronic changes in the arachnoid making its appearance cloudy and white as opposed to the normal transparent appearance.

lapsed or sequestered disc material cannot be removed. Also, if disc material has adhered to the nerve root, then there will probably be no improvement after percutaneous nucleotomy procedure, and open surgery would then be indicated in such cases.

Summary

These procedures can now be visualized through the accompanying endoscope. The technique of percutaneous herniectomy is safe and simple. Future developments will include laser applications and the transpinal canal approach.

We sincerely appreciate the editorial efforts of Steven H. Richeimer, M.D.

References

1. Burman MS: Myeloscopy or the direct visualization of the spinal canal and its contents, *J Bone Joint Surg* 13A:695, 1931.
2. Dohring S, Ooi Y, Schulitz KP, Satoh Y: Myeloscopic findings in the region of the lower lumbar spinal column, *Beitr Orthop Traumatol* 31:120, 1984.
3. Epstein JA, Epstein BS, Lavine LS, et al.: Obliterative arachnoiditis complicating lumbar spinal stenosis, *J Neurosurg* 48:252, 1978.
4. Hijikata S: A method of percutaneous nucleus extraction: a new therapy modality of intervertebral disc herniation, *J Toden Hosp* 5:39, 1975.
5. Kambin P: Arthroscopic microdiscectomy, *Arthroscopy* 8:287, 1992.
6. Kambin P: Posterolateral percutaneous lumbar discectomy and decompression: arthroscopic microdiscectomy. In Kambin P, editor: *Arthroscopic microdiscectomy, minimal intervention in spinal surgery*, Baltimore, 1991, Urban & Schwarzenberg, p 67.
7. Kambin P, Schaffer JL: Percutaneous lumbar discectomy: review of 100 patients and current practice, *Clin Orthop* 238:24, 1989.
8. Onik G, Helms CA, Ginsburg L, Hoaglund FT, Morris J: Percutaneous lumbar diskectomy using a new aspiration probe, *AJR Am J Roentgenol* 144:1137, 1985.
9. Ooi Y: Myeloscopy (in Japanese), *Orthop Trauma Surg* 24:659, 1981.
10. Ooi Y: Myeloscopy, diagnosis to adhesive arachnoiditis (in Japanese), *Clin Orthop* 22:130, 1987.
11. Ooi Y, Mita F: Endoscopic percutaneous nucleotomy to lumbar disc hernia (in Japanese), *Med Book Orthop* 18:81, 1989.
12. Ooi Y, Mita F, Satoh Y: Myeloscopic study on lumbar spinal canal stenosis with special reference to intermittent claudication, *Spine* 15:544, 1990.
13. Ooi Y, Morisaki N: Intrathecal lumbar endoscope (1st report) (in Japanese), *Clin Orthop Surg* 4:295, 1969.
14. Ooi Y, Satoh Y, Inoue K, et al.: Myeloscopy, with special reference to blood flow changes in the cauda equina during Lasegue's test, *Int Orthop* 4:307, 1981.
15. Ooi Y, Satoh Y, Morisaki N: Myeloscopy: a preliminary report, *J Jpn Orthop Assoc* 47:619, 1973.
16. Ooi Y, Satoh Y, Morisaki N: Myeloscopy (in Japanese), *Orthop Surg* 24:181, 1973.
17. Ooi Y, Satoh Y, Morisaki N: Myeloscopy (in Japanese), *Igaku Ayumi* 81:209, 1972.
18. Ooi Y, Satoh Y, Morisaki N: Myeloscopy: possibility of observing lumbar intrathecal space by use of an endoscope, *Endoscopy* 5:90, 1973.
19. Ooi Y, Satoh Y, Sugawara S, et al.: Myeloscopy, *Int Orthop* 1:107, 1977.
20. Ottolenghi CE: Diagnosis of orthopaedic lesions by aspiration biopsy, *J Bone Joint Surg* 37A:443, 1955.
21. Pool JL: Direct visualization of dorsal nerve roots of the cauda equina by means of a myeloscope, *Arch Neurol Psychiatry* 39:1308, 1938.
22. Pool JL: Myeloscopy: diagnostic inspection of the cauda equina by means of an endoscope (myeloscope), *Bull Neurol Inst* N Y 7:178, 1938.
23. Pool JL: Myeloscopy: intraspinal endoscopy, *Surgery* 11:169, 1942.
24. Porter RW, Hibbert C: Calcitonin treatment for neurogenic claudication, *Spine* 8:585, 1983.
25. Stern EL: The spinascope: a new instrument for visualizing the spinal canal and its contents, *Med Rec* 143:31, 1936.

Section 3

Open Surgery of the Lumbar Spine

79 The Controversy of "Large Versus Small": The Present Role of Minimally Invasive Surgery of the Spine

Charles V. Burton

80 Lumbar Spinal Stenosis: Reliable Methods of Decompression

Charles D. Ray

81 Posterior Lumbar Interbody Fusion: Biomechanical Selection for Fusions

James W. Simmons, Jr.
John N. McMillin

82 Anterior Approach for Lumbar Fusions and Associated Morbidity

Robert J. Henderson

83 Anterior Lumbar Interbody Fusion and Combined Anteroposterior Fusion

Richard M. Salib

84 Results of Anterior Interbody Fusion

Robert G. Watkins

85 Anatomic Strategies of Internal Fixation

R. Charles Ray

86 Instrumented Posterior Lumbar Surgery

John H. Peloza
David K. Selby

87 The Vermont Spinal Fixator for Posterior Application to Short Segments of the Thoracic, Lumbar, or Lumbosacral Spine

Martin H. Krag
Bruce D. Beynnon

88 Posterior Lumbar Interbody Fusions by Implanted Threaded Titanium Cages

Charles D. Ray

89 Anterior Lumbar Instrumentation and Fusion

John D. Schlegel
Rand L. Schleusener
Hansen A. Yuan

90 Lumbar Pathoanatomy: Soft- and Hard-Tissue Decompression

Charles D. Ray

91 Degenerative Spondylolisthesis

Paul J. Slosar
James B. Reynolds

92 Spondylolisthesis: Isthmic Congenital, Traumatic, and Post-Surgical

James B. Reynolds

93 The Use of Electrical Stimulation for Spinal Fusion

Kevin Finnesey

Chapter 79

The Controversy of "Large Versus Small": The Present Role of Minimally Invasive Surgery of the Spine

Charles V. Burton

Introduction

Chemonucleolysis by Chymopapain (Chymodiactin)

Invasive Spine Care

The Procedure "Report Card"

  chymopapain
  automated percutaneous lumbar
    discectomy
  arthroscopic microsurgical discectomy,
    uniportal
  arthroscopic microsurgical discectomy,
    biportal
  primary laser discectomy
  anterior laparoscopic microdiscectomy
  arthroscopic microsurgical fusion
  laminectomy
  microsurgical discectomy
  microdiscectomy
  intracapsular lateral decompression
  paraspinal (paralateral) decompression
  fusion

Conclusion

"The execution of the laws is more important than the making of them."

Thomas Jefferson

Introduction

In the field of health care, information serves as the basis for our "laws." Similar to Jefferson's legislative process, the manner in which information is interpreted and applied is more important than the information itself. Because medicine has always been more of an art than a science there now exists an unwieldy plethora of information and opinion to sort through. Only recently has there been a focus of attention and effort on the need to delineate and define information and to begin to document outcomes.

Productive change in medicine requires the prudent interpretation of, and the appropriate application of, information. This represents a great deal more than just data capture. It is not an infrequent phenomenon to have incorrect conclusions drawn from basic facts. The successful conclusion of the process of improving health-care delivery also requires something which, at times, seems to be a rare commodity, "common sense."

In no area of medical practice is there a greater need for productive change than in the field of spinal care. If low-back problems alone do not represent the largest expenditure of health-care dollars in the United States, they certainly represent the area of most inefficient application of resources, and, after the common cold, the leading cause of missed work.[8,10,11]

Appropriate use of information is a primary means by which the challenge of low-back pain (LBP) can be effectively addressed. Of concern in this regard, however, has been the concerted effort by some to consider certain types of information as being sacrosanct.

Randomized, double-blind, controlled, and prospective (RDCP) studies represent the highest order of well-defined information. Such studies also represent the smallest segment of information presently available in spine care (Fig. 79-1) and, despite their high value, are likely to continue to represent only a minuscule portion of the information on which we can base effective change in the immediate future.

Unfortunately, RDCP studies have become a "temple of worship" for some who neglect to subject such studies to critical review of methodology and substance before creating medical "laws" based on invalid conclusions. This has been particularly true in regard to invasive therapy for spinal care (see Invasive Spine Care box on p. 1078). It is interesting to observe that invasive therapy (as opposed to noninvasive conservative care) has represented one of the few areas in spinal therapy in which private funding has been consistently available in the past for research study. Even so there have been few valid RDCP studies performed. Even when excellent data is available the U.S. experience with chemonucleolysis by chymopapain serves as an instructional guide as to "how not to proceed" following the completion of a valid research study.

Chemonucleolysis by Chymopapain (Chymodiactin)

On May 13, 1983, the *Journal of the American Medical Association* contained the report of an RDCP study on chymopapain for the treatment of herniated lumbar disc.[12] The success rate, at 6 months, for those patients receiving enzyme (rather than placebo) was 82%, and for those initially receiving placebo and then the enzyme was 91%. On the basis of this information the U.S. Food and Drug Administration approved chymopapain (chymodiactin) for routine use in the United States. The chymodiactin study was initiated and financially supported by Smith Laboratories of Northbrook, IL. This effort represented one of the most expensive and meticulous RDCP studies ever carried out in the field of

Spine Care Information

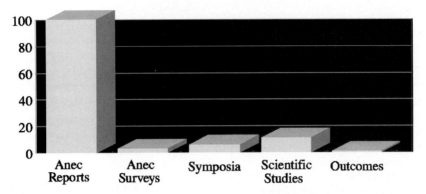

Fig. 79-1

The relative amount of different information in spine care is shown. Anecdotal information represents, by far, the largest category.

spine care and demonstrated dramatic efficacy for this minimally invasive procedure. Today, Smith Laboratories no longer exists and chymopapain is only infrequently used in the U.S. How can this be? The reasons for this sad situation should cause us all to reflect carefully upon the appropriate collection and interpretation of information and the use of "common sense" in extending information into the arena of patient care.

As one of the investigators in the chymodiactin study, this author (often identified as "and others" when the JAMA article is referenced), has had adequate opportunity to study the situation. All the study clinician participants were surgeons who used, as a primary focus of their attention, sciatica and neurologic status rather than LBP or segmental dysfunction. Only minimal attention was directed to the observation that intradiscal injection of any substance has the potential to be a direct infusion into the venous vascular tree or that the rapid decrease in discal volume could serve as a means of increasing LBP. Following the FDA approval, based on the observation that 91% of those receiving enzyme had successful results, over 6,000 orthopedists and neurosurgeons participated in a 1 day "dry lab training course," following which they were considered to be "qualified" to perform the procedure by the hospitals in which they practiced. Many of these surgeons had no previous experience with special spine procedures or even the use of biplane fluoroscopy. Chymopapain failure in the U.S. has really been a reflection of the complications associated with the delivery of this enzyme rather than the efficacy of the procedure itself. Although the research was an

RDCP study, and done well, the criteria were limited. Chemonucleolysis lost credibility because of problems related to its implementation rather than its value as demonstrated by scientific study.

Reason dictates that all credible information needs to be used for the purpose of good decision making. Not all information has equal value. Why not rate information according to its quality, in the same way the financial markets rate bonds? The challenge today is to best utilize available information resources until such time as more meaningful and valid scientific study and outcomes data are available.

Invasive Spine Care

The present spectrum of invasive spine care is reviewed in the box on the next page. Unfortunately, in today's world, the application of these procedures is often neither a medical nor a well-informed decision. This choice may now be made by a third-party payor and not infrequently on the basis of proprietary information not available to the public[1] or the treating physician. The patient liabilities produced by this are reflected in the Blue Cross Blue Shield of Minnesota coverage guidelines for medications, procedures, and services judged by them to be "investigative" and thus not reimbursable[21](the box on the next page). If these guidelines were strictly applied to the field of invasive spine care now, the only procedure that would appear to qualify for BC/BS coverage in Minnesota *might* be chemonucleolysis with chymodiactin.

In 1987, 250,000 discectomies (1990 average direct cost $13,000; total cost, including indirect,

$26,000) and 115,000 fusions (1990 average direct cost range $23,000 to $30,000; total cost, including indirect, $46,000 to $60,000) were performed

Invasive Spine Care

1. Special procedures (i.e., injections and blocks)
2. Minimally invasive procedures
   Chemonucleolysis
       Chymopapain (CHY)
       Collagenase
   Automated percutaneous lumbar discectomy (APLD)
   Arthroscopic microsurgical discectomy, uniportal (AMD UNI)
   Arthroscopic microsurgical discectomy, biportal (AMD BI)
   Primary laser discectomy (PLD)
   Anterior laparoscopic microdiscectomy (ALM)
   Arthroscopic microsurgical fusion (AMF)
3. Surgery
   Laminectomy (LAM)
   Microsurgical discectomy (MSD)
   Microdiscectomy (MD)
   Intracapsular lateral decompression (INTCP)
   Paraspinal (paralateral) decompression (PARA)
   Fusion (FUS)

Blue Cross Blue Shield of Minnesota Medications, Procedures and Services Considered Investigative
Criteria Used to Evaluate New Technology (January, 1993)

1. The technology must have final approval from the appropriate government regulatory bodies.
2. The scientific evidence must permit conclusions concerning the effect of the technology on health outcomes.
3. The technology must improve the net health outcome.
4. The technology must be as beneficial as any established alternatives.
5. The improvement must be attainable outside the investigational settings.

in the United States. The average failure rate of discectomy was 8% and fusion was 15%.[17,20] In 1981 the most common reason (57.5% of all cases) for the "failed back surgery syndrome" was the presence of lateral spinal stenosis.[9] In 1992 lateral spinal stenosis still remains the most common reason for this problem.[2] It is clear that a great deal needs to be done in improving the efficacy and cost of spinal surgery. Minimally invasive procedures, with their associated decreased operative time and shortened hospital stay, can certainly decrease cost. It still remains to be demonstrated that they can also provide a higher level of safety and efficacy.

The Procedure "Report Card"

As a practical means of attempting to respond to the need to use presently available data on a rational and productive basis, I suggest that attention be focused on the development of procedure "report cards" based on expanded criteria (in the following box).

Criteria to Compare Invasive Spine Care Procedures

1. Patient safety
   The relative morbidity and mortality risks to the patient.
2. Efficacy
   The relative likelihood of a good patient result.
3. Cost
   Includes the relative direct costs of surgery and hospitalization.
4. Surgical control
   The relative amount of surgical control allowed by the nature of the procedure.
5. Potential for abuse
   The relative ease with which the procedure can be used unnecessarily.
6. Long-term liability
   Does performance of the procedure create additional long-term problems for the patient?
7. Scientific documentation
   References the amount of scientific information collected over time.
8. Outcomes data
   The amount of outcome data presently available for review.

In this effort consideration is given to areas such as the abuse potential of procedures and also potential associated patient liabilities.

Each procedure has been rated in the multiple criteria using an 8-point scale from −4 to +4 (Fig. 79-2). At this time each category is being given equal rating. This is certainly something that can be modified in the future as experience accumulates. The first "report cards" are summarized in Tables 79-1 (minimally invasive) and 79-2 (invasive) along with a final "grade." These ratings reflect those initiated by myself and then reviewed by a panel of experienced spine surgeons. It should be clear that this effort represents, at this time, only the beginning of a format designed to reflect the best of anecdotal information arrived at by consensus. The meaning and value of an effort such as this will be seen by using the format for more widespread consensus surveys and symposia developed specifically to survey these criteria.

Consensus is not possible without a consistency of understanding of the procedures being identified.

Report Card Rating System

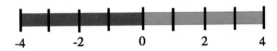

Fig. 79-2
The rating schema used in developing the surgical report card.

Table 79-1

Criteria to compare minimally invasive spine care procedures*

				Procedure			
Criteria	CHY	APLD	AMD UNI	AMD BI	PLD	ALM	AMF
1. Patient safety	3	4	3	3	4	1	3
2. Procedure efficacy	3	1	2	3	1	3	2
3. Procedure cost	−1	−2	−2	−2	−2	−2	−3
4. Surgical control	1	1	2	2	1	3	2
5. Abuse potential	−4	−4	−1	−1	−4	−1	−1
6. Long-term liability	?	?	?	?	?	?	?
7. Scientific documentation	3	1	3	2	1	?	?
8. Outcomes data	1	1	1	1	?	?	?
Report Card Grade	**6**	**2**	**8**	**8**	**1**	**4**	**3**

*See the Invasive Spine Care box on p. 1078 for procedure abbreviations.

Table 79-2

Criteria to compare invasive spine care procedures*

			Procedure		
Criteria	LAM	MSD	MD	INTCP	PARA	FUS
1. Patient safety	3	3	3	3	3	3
2. Procedure efficacy	4	4	3	4	4	3
3. Procedure cost	−3	−3	−3	−3	−3	−4
4. Surgical control	4	4	3	4	3	4
5. Abuse potential	−3	−3	−4	−2	−2	−4
6. Long-term liability	?	?	?	?	?	−3
7. Scientific documentation	3	3	3	3	3	3
8. Outcomes data	2	2	1	1	1	2
Report Card Grade	**10**	**10**	**6**	**10**	**9**	**4**

*See the Invasive Spine Care box on p. 1078 for procedure abbreviations.

At this time such consistency does not exist, but illustrated glossaries are now available for reference purposes.[6]

It is surprising to find that "report cards," which are such a common part of our educational experience, are not regularly applied in the evaluation of health care, although some are now being published by health maintenance organizations.[24] This eminently reasonable approach using groups of relevant and appropriate criteria needs to be a greater part of professional information provided to physicians as well as the public.*

Chymopapain

Chemonucleolysis with chymopapain (CHY) (Fig. 79-3) has been used sufficiently, and internationally, for a long enough time to document its reasonable value. Unfortunately, very little data are available to assess the long-term liabilities of interspace collapse and increased plasticity of the vertebral motion segment. Low-dose therapy, using 25% of normal dose, has been reported by Wiltse and Darakjian and may represent a means of moderating these changes. Chemonucleolysis appears to be of particular value in underdeveloped countries where basic spine surgery, as well as more sophisticated technology, is unavailable.

Automated Percutaneous Lumbar Discectomy

Despite high grades for patient safety, the net APLD grade is low because of the high abuse factor. This procedure can be performed by practitioners of many disciplines and is often used when other noninvasive and effective means of therapy would be more appropriate (Fig. 79-4). It remains to be demonstrated that partial debulking of a disc alone produces significant benefit in the long term.

Arthroscopic Microsurgical Discectomy, Uniportal

This procedure best represents the emerging minimally invasive technology as competition to laminectomy (Fig. 79-5). Arthroscopic microsurgical discectomy allows the surgeon a reasonable degree of operative control. At the present time clinical efficacy seems directly related to the skill and experience of the operator. Given its safety and decreased cost, AMD shows real potential.

*References 4, 6, 7, 13 to 16, 18, 19, 22, and 23.

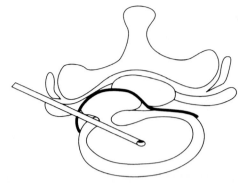

Fig. 79-3
Intradiscal needle placement for chemonucleolysis. A large contained disc herniation is depicted. (*From Burton CV: Recent surgical developments, In Kirkaldy-Willis WH, Burton CV, editors Managing low back pain, vol 3, New York, 1992, Churchill-Livingstone, p 382.*)

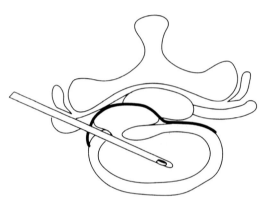

Fig. 79-4
An automated suction/cutting cannula for disc debulking. (*From Burton CV: Recent surgical developments. In Kirkaldy-Willis WH, Burton CV, editors: Managing low back pain, vol 3, 1992, Churchill-Livingstone, p 382.*)

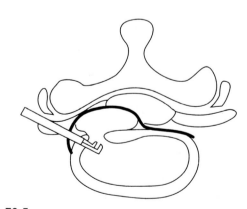

Fig. 79-5
Miniaturized surgical instruments are alternated with endoscopic visualization. (*From Burton CV: Recent surgical developments. In Kirkaldy-Willis WH, Burton CV, editors: Managing low back pain, vol 3, New York, 1992, Churchill-Livingstone, p 382.*)

Arthroscopic Microsurgical Discectomy, Biportal

Arthroscopic microsurgical discectomy as a biportal procedure (Fig. 79-6) is more invasive but also may be more effective. The data is not available to judge this now.

Primary Laser Discectomy

At this point in time PLD (Fig. 79-7) is a very controversial subject. Laser seems to be an orphan looking for a home with invasive spine care. Because abuse and cost are high and because most cases being treated with this modality would probably do as well (if not better) with noninvasive means, there is no compelling reason to provide a "passing grade" for PLD at this time.

Anterior Laparoscopic Microdiscectomy

The transabdominal approach to the disc space is logical and potentially valuable. Risk factors for this approach are simply not yet well appreciated and would depend, to a high degree, on operator experience. Laparoscopic technology is rapidly advancing. It is increasing direct medical costs but dramatically reducing indirect costs, which include time lost from work. In the future ALM may have an important link to minimally invasive fusion and the implantation of artificial discs.

Arthroscopic Microsurgical Fusion

As technical tour-de-force, AMF may open many doors for innovative thinking but will have to demonstrate impressive cost savings and improved safety in order to replace standard fusion techniques. Spinal arthroscopes seen to be almost "Lilliputian" when compared with those presently in use in orthopedic joint surgery, general surgery, and obstetrics/gynecology.

Laminectomy

Laminectomy continues to be the "gold standard." The surgical dictum relating to the importance of adequate exposure is still valid.

Microsurgical Discectomy

Defined as the addition of magnification and illumination to laminectomy by the inclusion of loupes, operating telescopes, or operating microscopes. Microsurgical discectomy appears to have a positive ef-

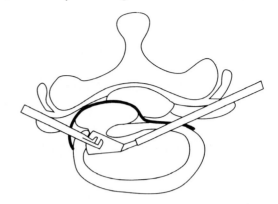

Fig. 79-6
Continual endoscopic monitoring is possible with the biportal technique. *(From Burton CV: Recent surgical developments. In Kirkaldy-Willis WH, Burton CV, editors: Managing low back pain, vol 3, New York, 1992, Churchill-Livingstone, p 382.)*

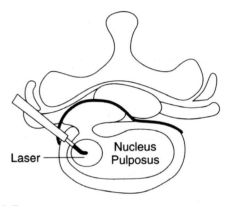

Fig. 79-7
A small laser is inserted into the disc. Small endoscopes are often part of the system. *(From Burton CV: Recent surgical developments. In Kirkaldy-Willis WH, Burton CV, editors: Managing low back pain, vol 3, New York, 1992, Churchill-Livingstone, p 382.)*

fect on efficacy. Most probably MSD should have the highest grade of all spine surgery procedures.

Microdiscectomy

Microdiscectomy, meaning a microsurgical procedure performed through the smallest possible surgical opening, is an excellent procedure for some patients. It has been subject to criticism because the surgeon is not always able to visualize adequately spinal recess stenosis, lateral stenosis and other pathology because of the limited operative field.

Intracapsular Lateral Decompression

This is a medial approach designed to preserve the lateral portion of the facet joint and also to decompress the foraminal and extraforaminal zones while also avoiding direct contact with the exiting neurovascular bundle. It also allows surgical access from the central to the extraforaminal zones.

Paraspinal (Paralateral) Decompression

This is a highly efficacious procedure for approaching spinal pathology presenting in the foraminal and extraforaminal zones. The appropriate application of these approaches requires the surgeon to define accurately the nature and site of the lesion prior to surgery. This can usually be achieved by sophisticated spinal imaging.

Fusion

With today's impressive modern spinal instrumentation (essentially all of which, according to the FDA, is still "investigational") solid fusion and good clinical results are possible, even in smokers. The grade for fusion would be higher if the postfusion spinal liabilities (stress on instrumentation, adjacent motion segments, and the spine in general) could be diminished and consistent agreement achieved as to who constitutes a good candidate for this procedure. Postfusion spine health daily maintenance programs, which include stabilization exercises and intermittent, controlled, antigravitational unloading, may prevent many of these problems related to increased spine stress from fusion.

Conclusion

Surgeons have made great strides in improving results and decreasing the risks of invasive spine therapy. There continues to be room for even greater effort in this direction, as well as in reducing cost. Basic procedures, such as laminectomy, continue to be of high value and the mainstay of clinical practice.

Despite the attention focused on the cost of invasive procedures, the real cost savings will be realized only through the implementation of prevention as a specific discipline, effective nonoperative care, posttherapy low-back health-care maintenance programs, and the implementation of common-sense measures designed to potentiate life expectancy and quality of the spine itself (eugonomics) (see the following box).[3,5]

The mandate from big business and government is clear. We need to continue to advance health care by all of our talents and, at the same time, also search for cost-saving techniques. The latter is, most certainly, an example of "smaller being better."

The Comprehensive Field of Spine Care

1. Prevention
2. Therapy
   Noninvasive
   Invasive
      Special procedures
      Minimally invasive procedures
      Traditional surgery
3. Health maintenance
4. Eugonomics*

*The science of modifying and potentiating "normal" body structure and function through the process of intentional design.

Meanwhile, we all must deal with significant integrity lapses in the health-care system. Much of this is typified by efforts of third-party payers to avoid providing their contractual financial responsibilities to subscribers by any means possible. It is also characterized by behavior designed to obfuscate what is "reasonable and necessary" in providing medical care to those in need of such. In some states, third-party payers work cooperatively with the medical profession, the public, industry, and government. In others, they have adopted, and continue to maintain, adversarial relationships in which all parties lose. This is "dysfunctional behavior," and it must change.

The author would like to express his sincere appreciation to Drs. Charles Ray, Leon Wiltse, David Selby, David Fardon, James Weinstein, and David Radosevitch for their kind advice and editorial assistance.

References

1. Blue Cross Blue Shield of Minnesota, Provider letter, Kim Quesnel, R.N., Chairperson, Medical Policy Committee, January, 1993.
2. Burton CV: Causes of failure of surgery on the lumbar spine, *Mt. Sinai J Med* 58(2):183, 1991.
3. Burton CV: How can athletes potentiate their spines for the future?: eugonomics—the next step beyond ergonomics, *Spine State Art Rev* 4(2):297, 1990.
4. Burton CV: *Neurosurgery, past, present, and future.* In Kirkaldy-Willis WH, Burton CV, editors: *Managing low back pain,* vol 3, New York, 1992, Churchill-Livingstone.
5. Burton CV: Preparing the back for the age 100, *J Back Musculoskel Rehab* 1:49, 1991.
6. Burton CV: *Recent surgical developments.* In Kirkaldy-Willis WH, Burton CV, editors: *Managing low back pain,* vol 3, New York, 1992, Churchill-Livingstone.

7. Burton CV: Surgical discectomy 1991: status report, *Semin Orthop* 6:92, 1991.

8. Burton CV, Cassidy JD: *Economics, epidemiology, and risk factors.* In Kirkaldy-Willis KW, Burton CV, editors: *Managing low back pain,* vol 3, New York, 1992, Churchill Livingstone.

9. Burton CV and others: Causes of failure of surgery on the lumbar spine, *Clin Orthop* 157:191, 1981.

10. Frymoyer JW: *Epidemiology.* In Frymoyer JW, Gordon SL, editors: *Perspectives low back pain,* St. Louis, 1990, Mosby.

11. Frymoyer JW: An overview of the incidences and costs of low back pain, *Orthop Clin North Am* 22:263, 1991.

12. Javid MJ and others: Safety and efficacy of chymopapain (chymodiactin) in herniated nucleus pulposus with sciatica, *JAMA* 249(18):2489, 1983.

13. Kambin P, Gellman H. Percutaneous lateral discectomy of the lumbar spine: a preliminary report, *Clin Orthop* 174:127, 1983.

14. Kirkaldy-Willis W, Burton CV, Heithoff KB: Lateral spinal nerve entrapment, *Pain* March/April:93, 1990.

15. Obenchain TG: Laparoscopic lumbar discectomy: case report, *J Lap Surg* 1:145, 1991.

16. Onik G and others: Percutaneous lumbar discectomy using a new aspiration probe, *Am J Roentgenol* 144:1127, 1985.

17. Ray CD: *The artificial disc: introduction, history and socioeconomics.* In Weinstein J, editor: *Clinical efficacy and outcome in the diagnosis and treatment of low back pain,* New York, 1991, Raven Press.

18. Ray CD: *Decompressions and the "inaccessible zone."* In Hardy RW, editor: *Lumbar disc disease,* ed 2, New York, 1993, Raven Press.

19. Ray CD: *Far lateral decompressions for stenosis: the paralateral approach to the lumbar spine.* In White AH, Rothman RH, Ray CD, editors: *Lumbar spine surgery: techniques and complications,* St. Louis, 1987, Mosby.

20. U.S. Department of Health and Human Services, National Center for Health Statistics, Vital and Health Statistics: *Detailed diagnoses and procedures,* National Hospital Discharge Survey 1986, 1987, vols 127, 128, Series 13, 1988, 1989.

21. Wilson KS, Christiansen TA: Secret proprietary standards of care, *Minn Med* 73:19, 1990.

22. Wiltse LL: Personal communication, March 10, 1993.

23. Wiltse LL, Spencer CW: New uses and refinements of the paraspinal approach to the lumbar spine, *Spine* 13:696, 1988.

24. Winslow R: Report card on quality and efficacy of HMOs may provide a model for others, *Wall St J,* March 9, 1993, p B1.

Chapter 80

Lumbar Spinal Stenoses: Reliable Methods of Decompression

Charles D. Ray

Anatomy and Variations of Stenoses

Indications and Patient Selection for Surgical Decompression

decompressions for central stenosis
decompressions for subarticular stenosis
methods of decompression for lateral and
far-out stenosis

Anatomy and Variations of Stenoses

Central stenosis is often referred to simply as "spinal stenosis." This latter designation is, of course, an error because central stenosis is a specific anatomic diagnosis, besides being a far less common source of compression or irritation than lateral spinal, or foraminal, stenosis* (Fig. 80-1). In most cases of lumbar spinal stenosis, anatomic pathology can be accurately diagnosed only through the use of CT or MRI scans; sometimes both are required.† Myelography has a high error rate in identifying stenosis located at or distal to the ganglion, and is not used in

*References 1, 2, 5, 7, 9, 10, 15, 18, 20, 25, 33, 35, and 36.
†References 3, 4, 12, 14, 21-24, and 34.

the work-up unless severe central stenosis is suspected.[13,38]

We recognize four types of spinal stenosis, namely (1) central stenosis, (2) subarticular or lateral recess stenosis, (3) lateral or foraminal stenosis, and (4) extraforaminal stenosis (which has been called "far-out" stenosis).[12,14] Ray also recognized three forms of lateral foraminal stenosis: cephalocaudal or "up-down" stenosis; anterior-posterior, or "front-back" stenosis; and combined or "pin-hole" stenosis[12,27,28] (Fig. 80-2). In a review of 9484 routine CT scans for all indications, taken over a 1-year period (1987-1988) and documented by Heithoff and Ray, 71% of all the scans were of the lumbar spine.[11] That is, 71% of all the patients who came for a CT scan for any purpose were studied for a symptomatic lumbar spine problem. A structural diagnosis of some form

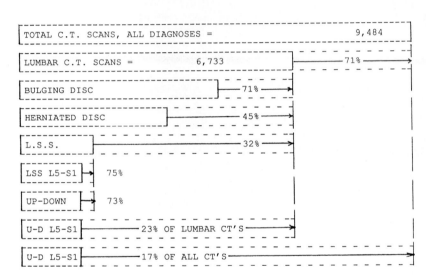

Fig. 80-1

Approximate incident of up-down lateral stenosis at the lumbosacral junction (L5-S1).

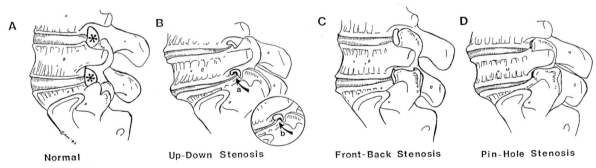

Normal   Up-Down Stenosis   Front-Back Stenosis   Pin-Hole Stenosis

Fig. 80-2

Diagram showing left lateral foraminae at the L4-L5 and L5-S1 lumbar levels. **A,** The normal foraminal configurations *(asterisks)*. **B (a),** The most common form of lateral spinal (foraminal) stenosis, in which an uncinate spur on L5 forms the inferior (caudal) wall of a gutter or valley through which the ganglion passes laterally. Since the ganglion and emerging spinal nerve are tethered to the inferior aspect of the pedicle and deep in the valley between both the uncinate spur and the pedicle, the emerging ganglion becomes tightly compressed between them. **B (b),** A variant in a case of spondylolisthesis in which the anterior slippage of L5 on S1 buckles the anulus, thus forming a part of the inferior wall of the gutter or valley. **C,** The lateral stenosis formed between the ventral aspect of the facet joint and the dorsum of the vertebral body. **D,** A combined or pin-hole stenosis. Note the drop in vertebral body height, occurring with progressive degeneration (including lateral or circumferential spur formation.) *Copyright 1993 Charles D. Ray, Ltd., reprinted by permission.*

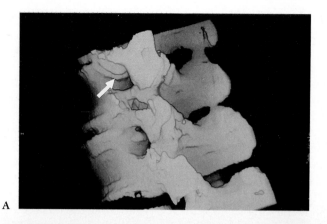

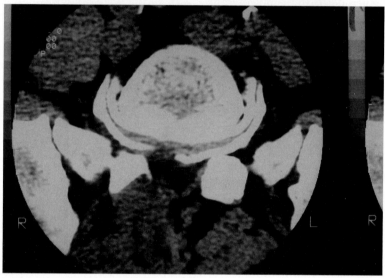

Fig. 80-3

A, Three-dimensional reconstruction of lumbar segments L3 through S1 from a routine CT scan. The film shows the uncinate spur on the lateral margin of the end plate of L5 *(white arrow)*. The valley or gutter where the ganglion lies is immediately cephalad to the spur and caudad to the pedicle. **B,** CT scan "slice" passing through the two spur ridges (L5 and S1) such that these spur ridges resemble parallel "tram tracks." The more medial of these tracks is the L5 ridge. Anulus tissue lies in between the tracks. This finding is pathognomonic of up-down lateral foraminal stenosis. *Copyright 1993 Charles D. Ray, Ltd., reprinted by permission.*

of "stenosis" was made in 32% of these lumbar scans. Of these having a "stenosis" diagnosis, 75% of the lesions occurred at the lumbosacral level. Up-down stenosis is by far the most common, comprising 72% of those patients who had a diagnosis of lateral spinal stenosis at the lumbosacral level.[28,29,31] Thus, percent of "stenosis" designated cases had one principal lesion, namely, unilateral or bilateral L5-S1 uncinate spur formation.

These observations clearly indicate that up-down lateral foraminal stenosis arising as an entrapment by an uncinate spur is by far the most common non–soft-tissue diagnosis in a spine-focused practice dealing with lumbar degenerative disc disease. Further, L5-

S1 uncinate spurs producing lateral foraminal stenosis comprised 23% of all cases having lumbar CT scans and 17% of all cases having CT scans for any reason, as shown in Fig. 80-1. Lateral spinal stenosis is a common problem among symptomatic lumbar spine cases, although the absolute incidence of such stenoses in the general population is unknown.

The uncinate spurs, responsible for the clear majority of cases of lateral stenosis, develop along the inferior lateral margin of the L5 vertebral disc (in a position equal to that in the cervical spine) and produce an entrapment of the emerging ganglion in a deep valley between this spur and the inferior aspect of the superior pedicle[12,30,32] (Figs. 80-2 to 80-4).

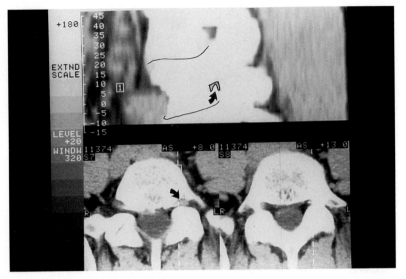

Fig. 80-4

Combined sagittal reconstruction (retouched for clarity) and transaxial views from a routine CT scan in a case of L5-S1 up-down foraminal stenosis. The uncinate spur and the associated entrapped ganglion are indicated on the two images by the curved arrows. *Copyright 1993 Charles D. Ray, Ltd., reprinted by permission.*

The front-back form of stenosis occurs as a result of hypertrophy of the facet joint, which produces an entrapment in an anteroposterior (AP) fashion, squeezing the emerging ganglion against the dorsum of the vertebral body. This occurs slightly less than one quarter as frequently as the up-down variety. The combined or pin-hole stenosis (a combination of the above lesions) is seen one sixth as often as the up-down type.[11,27,28]

The relative occurrence of each general type of stenoses (central, recess, foraminal, or extraforaminal) was reviewed among a more recent cohort of 287 cases, again by Heithoff and Ray.[11] These cases, having lumbar stenosis of any type, showed central stenosis to be present in 25% and recess stenosis (central recess or subarticular) in 23% of them. Those diagnosed as having lateral stenosis comprised 47% of the cohort, while far-out stenosis was seen in 5%. Again, lateral or foraminal stenosis proved to be the most common diagnosis involving stenosis (again, about 75% of these being the up-down type). Generally, lateral stenosis is often clinically quite significant when it is rated as "moderate to severe," but clinical significance of central stenosis is usually found only when it is diagnosed as "severe" or "extreme."[10,12] Thus, symptomatic central stenosis occurs even less often than one might expect, if one compares anatomic interpretations of scan reports alone.

Indications and Patient Selection for Surgical Decompression

An important clinical element of this symptomatic problem is the presence of neurogenic claudication that begins after walking short distances.[1,17,23,36,37] This problem is often the major sign for both central and lateral stenosis and may become progressively more restrictive to the patient, either slowly or somewhat precipitously. Precipitous clinical changes are usually related to a fresh soft-tissue lesion, e.g., a herniated fragment into an already tight canal, or a traction injury to the nerve or ganglion, which is held very tightly between the uncinate spur on the inferior aspect and the pedicle in the superior. In the past, it was commonly thought that the tip of the superior facet might impinge on the ganglion, pressing it against the pedicle above, but this condition is rarely seen and probably does not account for clinical stenotic problems. (If the compromise of the ganglion from the superior tip of the superior facet were a genuine problem, patients with lateral stenosis would develop acute root signs during hyperextension of the segment; they seldom do and even then, the ganglionic compression is most likely the result of buckling of the facet capsule and subjacent ligamentum flavum.) From a clinical point of view, the findings in lateral stenosis are otherwise rather sparse. Most patients have a basically negative neurologic examination but may sometimes show denervation potentials on an electromyogram (EMG). If this latter condition exists, it is further evidence that decompression may not help; that is, the changes may not be reversible. Without doubt, however, lateral stenosis may well lead to a progressively disabling neurogenic problem commonly associated with claudication symptoms in the leg or low back.

Proper planning for surgery is necessarily based on good scanning images for decisions regarding lesion location, approach, landmarks, and the retention of sufficient posterior and lateral bony anatomy to prevent the development or worsening of segmental instability.[19,26,28,37]

To reach an essential decision on where and how to operate, a detailed transaxial CT scan using 3-mm slices at the stenosing level or a parasagittal MRI study must be obtained. In addition, diagnostic root injections using a very small volume (0.2 ml) of a dilute local anesthetic (0.25% bupivacaine containing a corticosteroid, e.g., 0.5 ml Celestone Soluspan) should be performed to identify further the specific, entrapped nerve and to obtain some indication of prognosis and outcome from decompression of that specific nerve (Fig. 80-5). The local anesthetic in this small quantity will give the patient both motor and sensory changes in the exact dermatome of the injected root, lasting approximately 4 hours. During this time, the patient is encouraged to be as active as possible in order to test the certainty of pain relief in its "usual" clinical distribution. The corticosteroid (approximately 0.5 ml of Celestone Soluspan) should give the patient prolonged improvement, lasting perhaps over a matter of days or weeks. Patients having symptoms for longer than 1 year who obtained excellent, very short-lived (only hours) temporary relief from such injections are suspect as to the probable clinical outcome of their decompression. That is, if the stenosis has been present for a long time, there may very well be permanent changes within the ganglion or postganglionic nerve that will not be reversed by decompression. The corticosteroid prolongation of relief is a reasonable indication that the patient may have a good, permanent outcome from a decompression.[6]

The spinal surgeon must understand the exact anatomy and surgical approaches to these various stenosing lesions, not only to properly address the stenosis but also to spare adjacent, normal bony anatomy as far as possible. Generally speaking, rather little bone needs resecting to treat properly any of the stenoses. In the course of surgical decompression, the preservation of stability is important to prevent further instability at the involved segment. This

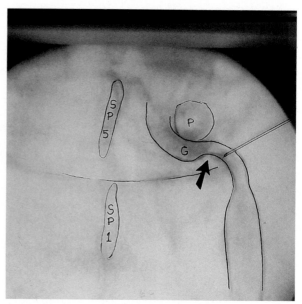

Fig. 80-5

Retouched AP fluoroscopic x-ray view following the injection of contrast dye in a routine spinal nerve (or nerve sleeve) injection. Note the uncinate spur on L5 (arrow) producing an "hour-glass" constriction causing swelling of the emerging spinal nerve. **SP**-5 is the spinous process of L5; **SP**-1, of S1. **G** is the ganglion and **P** is the pedicle of L5. The nerve sleeve forms an arc as it passes dorsolaterally over the lateral margin of the tram-track disc bars, to the right of the arrow. *Copyright 1993 Charles D. Ray, Ltd., reprinted by permission.*

has been well documented in the surgical literature.* Of course, if the disc space is essentially collapsed, with or without symptoms, the likelihood of worsening the segmental instability is extremely low and decompressions may, with safety, be more radical.

Decompressions for Central Stenosis

Clinically significant central stenosis is most commonly of the hypertrophic degenerative type, produced by a confluence of thickened ligamentum flavum and overgrown facet joints narrowing inwardly on the central canal, usually to the exclusion of the midline retrodural fat pad. In decompressing this condition it is essential to remove the ligamentum, particularly its cephalad bony attachment. This prominent ridge (the tightest part of the central canal) is normally part of the ventral aspect of the neural arch (Fig. 80-6). Since the ligamentum originates from this ridge and the underside of the lamina, hypertrophy of the ligamentum in response to

*References 9, 16, 18, 19, 27, and 29.

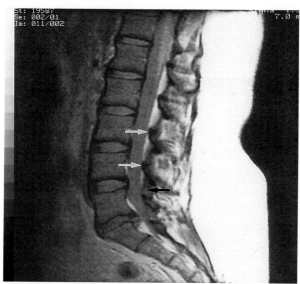

Fig. 80-6

Midsagittal MRI scan (loss of signal and degeneration also shown at the L5-S1 disc space) showing the normally narrowest portions of the central canal *(white arrows),* the ventrally protruding ridges across the center of the lamina. The ligamentum flavum *(black arrow)* originates on these ridges, passing under the laminas caudally to insert onto the dorsum of the laminas at each level below. Hypertrophy of the ligamentum flavum is, together with degenerative slip of the segment, the principal cause of acquired central stenosis. In congenital central stenosis, this ridge and the thick lamina form a napkin-ring around the central canal, especially in association with short pedicles. *Copyright 1993 Charles D. Ray, Ltd., reprinted by permission.*

excessive pull at an unstable segment will simultaneously lead to thickening of the bony origins and insertions. From this ridge the ligamentum descends, covering the posterior dura, while it attaches all the way down to its insertion as a flattened plane along the dorsum of the inferior lamina. Clearly the overdevelopment of the ligamentum occurs due to use-hypertrophy—that is, in the attempt to help stabilize the progressively degenerating segment. Thus, all associated ligaments thicken. Of course there are lateral reflections of the ligamentum, but they play a minor role in central narrowing; however, thickening of the lateral reflections are common in both lytic and degenerative spondylolisthesis and contribute to the soft-tissue component of lateral stenosis. If one carefully examines thin (3-mm) slices of a CT scan of central stenosis, one will see the narrowest area of the canal at the afflicted spinal level, immediately at the midpoint of the pedicle. Removing the thickened ligament from this area, the cephalad anchor or origin of the ligamentum, and downward (caudally) is the key to a good decompression.

The procedure can take a destructive approach, with complete removal of the posterior neural arch via bilateral total laminectomies, but the final cutting of the narrow arch can be hazardous as well.[9,18,20,28,36] Preferably, as advocated here, one should take a simpler approach, which requires a moderate bilateral inferior laminotomy at the segment, followed by bilateral resection of the entire central and dorsal ligamentum ventrally attached beneath the arch. This cutting and scraping away of the ligamentum uses small (#000 size) and larger (#3 and Scoville) straight and up-cutting, curved curettes. When the ligamentum is quite gone, each side of the central canal, in turn, may be carefully undercut using 4-mm wide, 30° bent-tip osteotomes (actually small, tapered chisel-edged ones), peeling away the ventral, traversing, bony fibers of the neural arch. As each layer is split away with chisel and mallet (sometimes angled across from the opposite side, passing under the base of the dorsal spinous process), a small curette further cleans the bone fragments. This cut-chip-and-clean method is aided by careful use of Kerrison punches (2-, 3-, and 4-mm wide) cutting as parallel to the central canal as possible, until the arch is decompressed. This method works very well for the common degenerative central stenosis but often cannot serve in the very unusual cases with congenital narrowing (where the pedicles are short and the bony arch is too narrow and too tough); further, hypertrophy of the ligament plays a relatively lesser role, in bony central stenosis.

The question of predecompression or postdecompression segmental instability is another matter. In most cases one need only perform the central decompression, without fusion. Further, in many older patients the bone is already soft and the facets are virtually fragmented, giving a potential fusion a questionable outcome. Fortunately, if back pain is the lesser component of the syndrome, the quasi-stable patient usually does well without fusion.

Patients who present with acute signs of central compression (such as severe claudication or cauda equina syndrome) almost always have a soft-tissue lesion (herniated disc) that has triggered off the clinical problem in the presence of a longer-standing central stenotic segment.

In rare cases, the posterior neural arch can be cut off completely using a high-speed drill or a careful bilateral resection utilizing wide (3-mm) curved-tip osteotomes, which may be used to split each side of the spinous process away from the arch and yet not penetrate through the arch and on to the dura.[31] The base or attachment of the cut spinous process may then simply be "popped off" using medium curettes. From then on, the central canal may be lat-

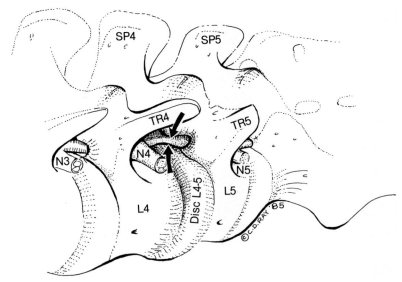

Fig. 80-7

Subarticular stenosis. Semitransverse view from high on left side. Indicated are L4 and L5 vertebral bodies, and their respective dorsal spinous processes *(SP4, SP5)* and transverse processes *(TR4, TR5)*. Superior medial lamina of L5 overhangs herniated nucleus pulposus (at disc L4 to L5) catching traversing L5 nerve root in a squeeze *(arrows)*. In most cases definitive treatment is removal of laminar overhang, leaving disc anulus undisturbed and intact.

erally decompressed using osteotomes and a Kerrison punch aided by small curettes.

One must remember that central stenosis is seldom a clinical problem unless it is rated as severe or very severe. The presence of a small amount of fat dorsal to the dura near the central portion of the neural arch does not of itself mean that central stenosis is not present or is not clinically significant.

Decompressions for Subarticular Stenosis

Subarticular stenosis, or spinal recess stenosis, occurs primarily at the superior lateral margins of the lamina beneath which the root passes.[8,28] Subarticular stenosis just above the disc margin is usually related to a congenitally narrowed lateral recess and is not significant (unless the traversing root is swollen owing to trouble at the next cephalic disc space). Thus, the most common anatomy of this disorder occurs just distal to the point where the axilla of the root has permitted the root sleeve to part from the central spinal sac and the root then passes beneath the cephalad edge of the lamina (Fig. 80-7). Here, the slight bulging of a disc may compress the preganglionic root against a low, overhanging dorsal lamina. This will produce a form of "stand-up" disc, meaning that this compromise in a tight lateral re-

cess particularly occurs when the patient bears weight on the disc space and it bulges circumferentially or especially posteriorly.

In decompressing this lesion for ultimately safe passage of the root, one must "raise the bridge" dorsally by resecting part of the superior lamina. It is often not necessary to tamper with the disc itself (like "lowering the river" for the boat/root to pass under), since bulging of the disc can no longer trap the traversing root against the bony "bridge" of the resected superior lamina. When passing significantly caudal along the lamina, and especially if extending the decompression laterally, one must be extremely careful not to tear the dura of the sleeve or the central dura. This is an extremely tight region and, in my experience, the decompressions are best performed with small osteotomes, which allow one to crack the medial bone dorsally and medially away from the traversing root. Fortunately, it is seldom necessary to decompress the root along its entire course medial to the pedicle, even though it may seem a bit tight.

In cases of congenital narrowing, the nerve in the lateral recess is in a remarkably tight space, resembling the brim of an inverted Mexican sombrero, on transaxial CT slices throughout its course medial to the pedicle; here it may be necessary to remove more of the lateral aspect of the central canal, medial to the pedicle. Again, small, sharp tools suffice, particularly small, narrow chisels.

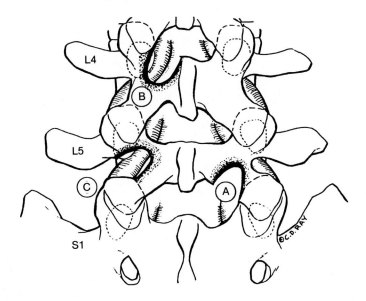

Fig. 80-8

Typical laminotomies and their primary applications. **A,** Inferior laminotomy (most common, for removal of herniated nucleus pulposus). **B,** Superior laminotomy (used in decompressions for subarticular stenosis but useful in certain cases of lateral stenosis to achieve good access to inferior medial aspect of pedicle). **C,** Lateral laminotomy (used for lateral stenoses and offending lateral osteophytes). I refer to this as a midline paramedial approach. After exposure is made to osteophyte, a bone impactor is usually used in decompression.

Methods of Decompression for Lateral and Far-Out Stenosis

Three somewhat unusual but highly effective surgical approaches have been designed to direct the attack on stenosing spurs: (1) a lateral laminotomy in which part of the lateral pars is removed to gain access to the spur; (2) a transverse midline approach which entails the approach to cut the spur by undercutting the facet and crossing beneath the spinous process from the opposite side; and (3) a paralateral approach in which one enters the skin about 15 cm lateral to the midline, then medially traverses through the paraspinal muscles to the lesion. These surgical techniques differ quite considerably from the usual laminectomy or facetectomy methods and are used, as indicated, in patients of all ages. These procedures are very often performed, with the patient lightly sedated, under epidural block and local analgesia. This latter recipe permits a close interaction between the surgeon and the patient, who may help guide the surgeon to localize, decompress, and yet protect the irritable portion (always the most highly stenosed part) of the nerve or ganglion. I have used one or more of these methods in perhaps 500 cases over the past 8 years.[27] A brief anecdotal follow-up survey indicates that approximately 75% of these cases had 50% or more lasting improvement over their preoperative pain.

Lateral Laminotomy

A lateral laminotomy (also referenced in the chapter on lumbar soft- and hard-tissue decompressions) is a variation of the standard laminotomy, but it is begun from the lateral aspect of the lamina, essentially in the region of the pars interarticularis[27,30] (Fig. 80-8). After coagulating the lateral segmental arterial branch, a part of the neurovascular bundle arising from the posterior primary division, the lateral laminotomy is performed either with a small osteotome, a small curette and punch, or a high-speed turbine drill. Usually, the lateral lamina in this region is too thick to be easily removed with a Kerrison punch. Therefore, the posterior aspect of this portion of the lamina is thinned out so that the punch can then be passed beneath it to cut the lateral lamina. However, one must be careful in passing any instrument inside the foramen, ventral to the lamina, so as not to injure further the entrapped ganglion. A small probe may be passed from lateral to medial through the foramen to determine its tightness. Displacing the ganglion to approach the stenosing uncinate spur may be something of a challenge. Once the lateral laminotomy has been widely performed (sparing the pars from potential fracture by avoiding excessive bone removal), the ganglion should be fully decompressed and rather freely movable.

The Technique of Impaction

Used in concert with a number of approaches to the osteophytes, disc bars, or end-plate irregularities, the technique of impacting bone may be extremely helpful at times (Figs. 80-9 and 80-10). Using a variety of shaped impaction tools, bony prominences may be driven inward into the softer cancellous portions, broken, and fragmented or simply flattened. Other instrumentation may be very important in the overall procedure for decompressions of stenotic lesions, including small curved osteotomes and a variety of

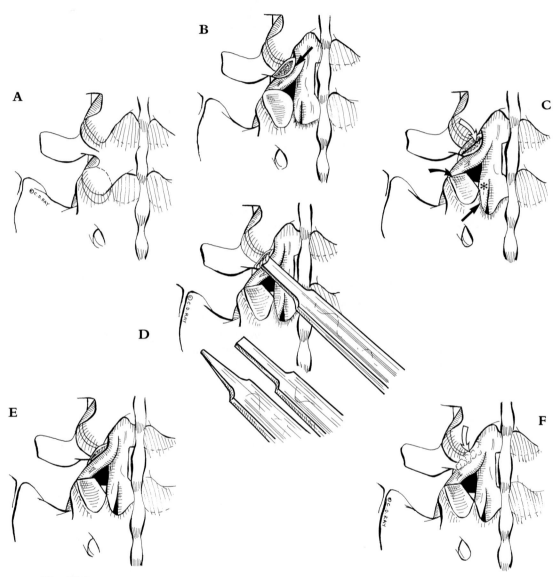

Fig. 80-9

Impaction for decompression of inferior pedicle. **A,** Exposure of left sided L4-L5 and L5-S1 is diagramed. **B,** Full left hemi-laminectomy has been performed, showing tight situation of L5 nerve as it passes around its pedicle *(arrow),* somewhat as a rope would pass around a pulley. Exposures are usually not this extensive. Disc space should have been found to be quite stable so that total facetectomy will not destabilize the segment. **C,** Tip of the superior facet *(curved black arrow)* at S1 has been cut. Inferior pedicle *(open white arrow)* has been cut across (slotted) with an osteotome. S1 root passing over L5-S1 disc margin is indicated by asterisk. (If subarticular stenosis of L5-S1 were present, the location of an appropriate decompression is indicated by the straight black arrow.) **D,** Impactor, shaped to fit inferior curve of pedicle, is tapped with nylon mallet, aiming upward and laterally, driving cortical portion of pedicle away from root, allowing it to relax. Root is carefully protected from possible pinching by impactor as it is struck. Two other types of impactors are also shown. **E,** Root is now relaxed as it passes around impacted pedicle. If need be, more of the pedicle can be resected and impacted. Exposure is often sufficient to permit exploration and impaction of possible disc spur or bar at L5-S1 level. **F,** Small fat graft has been placed between impacted pedicle and L5 root/ganglion.

quite small, neurosurgical-type curettes. I have found that high-powered air drills have limited use in the tight confines of the foramen and introduce a significant element of danger to both the patient and the operator.

The Transverse Approach

The transverse approach is the most interesting, sometimes difficult, but most satisfactory means for removal of a stenosing uncinate spur. This technique requires a midline exposure, approaching the spur from the opposite side, passing across, beneath the inferior margin of the spinous process at a very low angle[27] (Fig. 80-11). Most of the patients on whom I have operated with this technique received a combination of epidural and local block analgesia. The safety provided (when dissecting around the ganglion in a very tight situation) by this analgesic combination is often of considerable value. That is, the patient, although highly sedated, is still capable of responding to an acute irritation or compression of

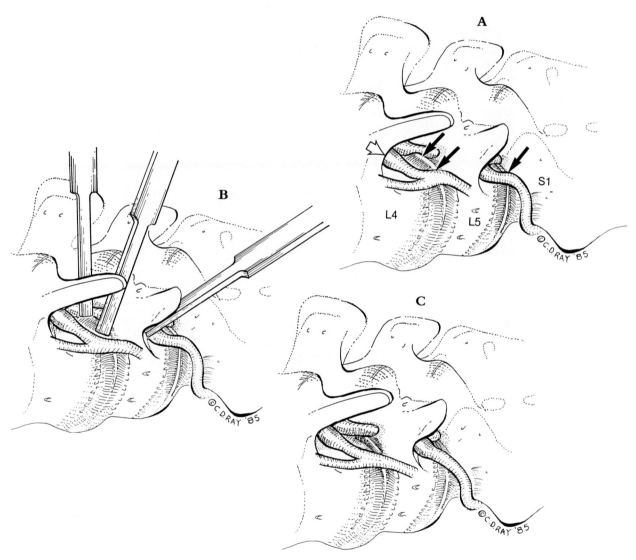

Fig. 80-10

Lateral approach to impaction of pedicles and disc bars or spurs. Shown are left side of vertebral bodies at the L4, L5, and S1 levels. **A,** Tight pedicle situation, as shown in Fig. 80-9, is indicated by open arrow at L4. Similar compression is located at L5 but not indicated with an arrow. Disc bars and spurs are indicated by solid arrows, covered with anular fibers so that they appear as smooth mounds elevating spinal nerves L4 and L5. **B,** Impactors being used to decompress nerves by driving spur or bar into the vertebral body. Impaction of inferior aspect of pedicle of L5 is shown; this has already been done at L4 in this diagram. A footed impactor is particularly useful for impacting spurs beneath the dura, ventral to a ganglion or a spur inside a foramen. **C,** Postimpaction situation showing relaxed position of L4 and L5 nerves as they now pass over impacted bony ridges, caudad to impacted pedicles.

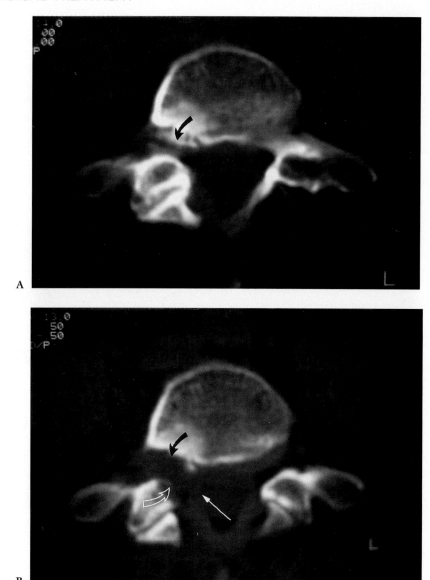

Fig. 80-11

Transaxial CT scans of patient with tram-track uncinate spurs at right L5-S1; **A,** preoperative *(arrow)* and **B,** postoperative *(arrow)* transverse midline decompression. Part of the ventral facet *(open white arrow)* has been resected. The cutting off of the spur was approached along the path shown by the long white arrow, beneath the spinous process from the opposite side. *Copyright 1993 Charles D. Ray, Ltd., reprinted by permission.*

the nerve, should this occur during the procedure. This responsiveness may also set the limits to which the ganglion can be maneuvered during exposure or undercutting. Thus, when removing the base of the spur with an osteotome or when leveraging in order to fracture the inferior lip of the deep valley (that is, the uncinate spur itself), one may obtain immediate information from the drowsing patient who will suddenly awaken and complain of acute disturbance in the leg. It is well known that the portion of a nerve or ganglion, or even the dura, for that matter, that

has been irritated, inflamed, or compressed by a lesion is considerably more sensitive to mechanical (or electrical) stimulation than other portions of that nerve or ganglion. Thus, one can probe along the nerve or ganglion and determine exactly where the most sensitive area lies, thus locating the apex of the stenosing lesion, hard or soft.

The transverse approach for subarticular decompression of laterally stenosing uncinate spurs is shown in a series of illustrations (Fig. 80-12). Assuming that the spur is on the right side, at L5-S1, for example,

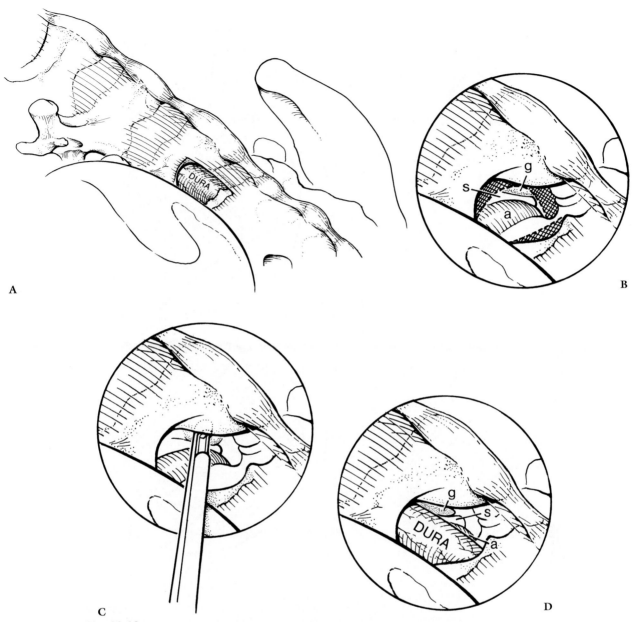

Fig. 80-12

Transverse midline approach for removal of an uncinate spur on the right side at L5.

A, Following a midline incision from L2 through S2, the paraspinal muscles have been widely retracted using very deep Gelpi retractors; the ligamentum flavum and two thirds of the most ventral interspinous ligament are resected. The view shows the anatomic orientation of the approach, via a low (more ventral) pathway from the left side. The ligamentum flavum is removed bilaterally along with the ventral two thirds of the interspinous ligament. The dura is exposed.

B, Bilateral standard laminotomies are performed (in the drawing the dura has been removed for illustrative purposes only). The laminotomy opening is enlarged in all directions by punching bone out along the dashed lines, undercutting the opposite-side superior facet, reaching across from the left side beneath the interspinous ligament but dorsal to the dura and also removing bone form the left and right laminas (all the cross-hatched areas), providing further access to the anulus (*a*), the uncinate spur (*s*), and the entrapped ganglion (*g*).

C, A Kerrison punch crosses the midline, passing under the interspinous ligament at a low angle, to remove small ventral portions of the right superior facet and capsule.

D, With the dura again drawn in position, one can see the uncinate spur (*s*), the badly compressed emerging ganglion lying in the narrow "valley" between the ridge of the spur and the cephalad pedicle (*g*), the lateral anulus (*a*), and the pedicles of L5 and S1.

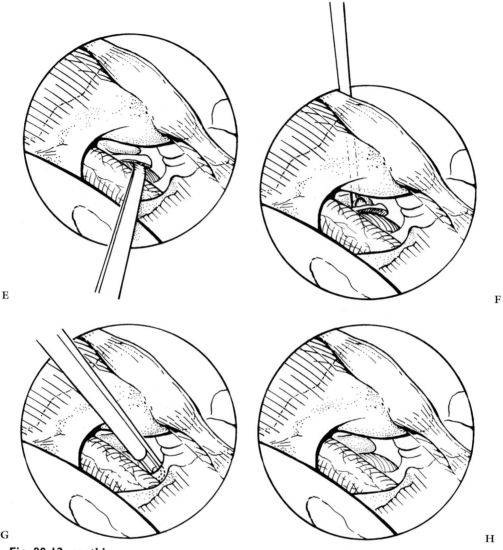

E

F

G

H

Fig. 80-12, cont'd

E, A small osteotome with a down-cutting curve at the tip cuts the base of the spur at its attachment to the vertebral end plate. The dura is again shown in its natural position.

F, A small neurosurgical curette, leveraged against the laminotomy of the right side, breaks the spur at its base, caudally away from the ganglion, with caution not to compress the ganglion itself. The remnant base of the removed uncinate spur may be curetted or impacted away.

G, The punch may now be used to remove remnant lateral portions of the broad-based spur, cutting around the superior aspect of the pedicle.

H, The freed ganglion is now movable; it descends away from the pedicle, filling the space just occupied by the spur, and passes dorsally over the lateral anulus (often resected in part). Fragmented remains of the spur may be further resected, curetted, or impacted, to provide a smooth bed for the emerging ganglion. At no time should the ganglion be battered, stretched, compressed, or in any way injured. It will normally swell considerably on being released from its entrapment and should be freely movable; if not, a lateral extension of the spur (bar) may need resection, perhaps via a more lateral approach such as a lateral laminotomy. *Copyright 1993 Charles D. Ray, Ltd., reprinted by permission.*

a standard inferior laminotomy is performed bilaterally at L5. The more ventral portion of the interspinous ligament is removed as well as the ventral and more cephalad aspect of the attachment of the ligamentum flavum to the lamina on the right side.

Crossing over from the left side at a very low angle, the ventrolateral aspect of the lamina and the foramen are resected, largely with small osteotomes, punches, and curettes. The most ventral portions of that facet joint are partly undercut in a similar manner, removing some of the soft-tissue component of the stenosis (ventral facet capsule) and providing greater space for visualization of the spur.

The most important anatomic detail to remember here is that the uncinate spur arises from the inferior lateral aspect of the given vertebra and entraps the ganglion in a deep valley between that spur and the inferior aspect of the pedicle of the same vertebra. Therefore, either limited or excessive removal of the superior facet will not solve the problem, as the ganglion remains tight within the deep valley between the spur and the pedicle. The inferior aspect of the spur as it is attached to the disc plate is amputated with a small osteotome and then broken away with a small curette placed between the ganglion and the spur. One must be careful not to leverage the curette against the ganglion. That is, the final curetting must be performed so that the ganglion is not squeezed against the pedicle. Once the spur has been broken free and removed and the base of the spur cleaned out by further curettage, the ganglion should now be freely movable. The upper foramen may then be explored with a ball-tipped probe for adequacy of decompression. Small, angled, or upcutting curettes also may be used to open further the deep valley and to help in the removal of the usually present lateral disc bar.

Starting near the superior base of the pedicle of S1 and progressing cephalad, coagulating large and small veins located in the axilla of the root, one exposes the inferior base of the uncinate spur (essentially the end-plate margin of L5). In the process of exposing the lateral aspect of the posterior vertebral body of L5, the spur can be seen rising rather sharply close (cephalad) to the pedicle of S1 (Fig. 80-12, D). The base of the spur and attached anulus are cut using a small, long, narrow (2-4 mm) osteotome and then removed using a small curette. Cutting the spur in the "right spot" is a bit like cutting a diamond in the correct location (Fig. 80-12, E). Generally speaking, since these spurs are not a true portion of the vertebral body but are only attached to its end-plate marginal cortical bone, they will fracture away in a caudal direction using a small (#00 or #1) neurocurette. The curette is leveraged against the remnant laminar margin in the right-sided L5 laminotomy; one must guard against any direct application of leveraging force against the ganglion (Fig. 80-12F). Amputating the base of the spur in this fashion and further resecting its base with a curette will remove not only the hard attachment of the spur to the marginal end plate but also its attachments to the superior aspect of the anulus. Now, if needed, the dissection may proceed laterally out the foramen. A small or medium Kerrison punch may be used to reach around the caudal pedicle to remove lateral elements of the uncinate spur, as shown in Fig. 80-12, G. Remember that the postganglionic nerve must rise dorsally, lateral to the displacing disc bar (as the nerve traverses laterally out of the deep valley), and then ventrally as it proceeds downward and ventral to the ala. Here again, there may be some form of entrapment needing to be relieved (the "far-out" stenosis). Out this far, laterally through the foramen, one will usually encounter some small arterial bleeders and small branches of the posterior primary that enter into the lateral aspect of the facet joint.

There is a point beyond which lateral dissection from the midline approach is neither safe nor practical—namely, if the spur proceeds laterally out the foraminal zone, beyond the margin of the S1 pedicle (as determined in advance by the CT or MRI scans). During the procedure, one should also decide whether this portion of the spur is likely to be truly entrapping the postganglionic nerve, being confirmed by exploring the foramen and comparing the observed anatomy with the scan images (best seen on sagittal MRI slices). That is, one should know where the postganglionic nerve rises over a lateral disc bar before the nerve descends to become part of the lumbosacral plexus, and whether this rise (or displacement) is significant. Thus, if this spur or bar (as well as those that may constitute a "far-out" stenosis) are too far lateral to be successfully approached from the midline, one must elect either to resect most of the facet joint and continue the lateral decompression or to abandon the midline approach and perform the further decompression via a lateral laminotomy. The decision here being a trade-off relating to ultimate stability of the segment, that is, retaining a major portion of the facet joint, versus a wider, more aggressive removal of bone for decompression of the nerve.

The Paralateral Approach

This technique was described also in the chapter on lumbar hard- and soft-tissue decompression. In this procedure, the approach to the target is taken through a skin incision placed approximately 12 to 16 cm (Fig. 80-13) lateral to the midline and the dissection traverses in the septum between the spinal erector muscles (longissimus and iliocostalis) to reach the lateral aspect of the target space[27-30] (Fig. 80-14). Decompressions by this approach are not

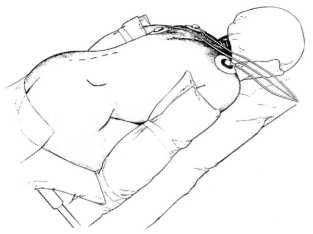

Fig. 80-13

A patient positioned on a prone-sitting frame. The incision for a paralateral approach is indicated by the curving incision placed quite lateral to the midline, just above the iliac crest (for an L3 to L5 approach). *Copyright 1993 Charles D. Ray, Ltd., reprinted by permission.*

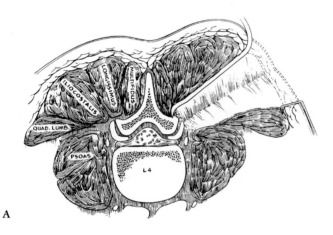

A

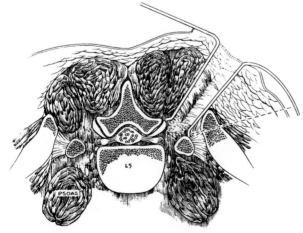

B

Fig. 80-14

Paralateral approaches through the muscle septa at the L4-L5 (**A**) and L5-S1 (**B**) lumbar levels. As indicated, one may need to resect a portion of the posterior superior iliac spine to facilitate a low-angle approach at L5-S1. *Copyright 1993 Charles D. Ray, Ltd., reprinted by permission.*

difficult at L4-L5 and above; however, when performed at the L5-S1 level the method is considerably more difficult. This is owing to the high-rising medial edge of the iliac crest, which may prevent reaching the L5-S1 foramen at a sufficiently lateral, flat angle to permit good decompression of the spur. Therefore, a portion of the superior posterior ilium may have to be removed. A modification of the approach at this level uses a somewhat more posterolateral, closer path, taking out the dorsal aspect of the medial sacral ala and from there then working toward the spur, using a path rather similar to a lateral laminotomy. One must remember that the paralateral approach does not permit visualization of lesions or structures that are medial to the pedicle.

Once having arrived at the spur either paralaterally or via the previously discussed lateral laminotomy, one may use impaction instruments to fracture and depress the spur or lateral bony disc bar. If the spur is thus morcelized, all the bone fragments must be carefully removed to prevent subsequent irritation of the ganglion by a retained piece.

References

1. Arnold CC and others: Lumbar spinal stenosis and nerve root entrapment syndromes: definition and classification, *Clin Orthop* 115:4, 1976.
2. Burton CV and others: Computed tomographic scanning and the lumbar spine. Part II: Clinical considerations, *Spine* 4:356, 1979.
3. Burton CV and others: Causes of failure of surgery on the lumbar spine, *Clin Orthop* 157:191, 1981.
4. Crenshaw C and others: The use of nuclear magnetic resonance in the diagnosis of lateral canal entrapment, *J Bone Joint Surg (Br)* 66:711, 1984.
5. Crock HV: Isolated lumbar disc resorption as a cause of nerve root canal stenosis, *Clin Orthop* 115:109, 1976.
6. Derby R and others: Steroid response and duration of radicular pain as a predictor of surgical outcome, *North Am Spine Soc Proc Ann Meet,* Aug 1, Keystone, CO, 1991.
7. Epstein BS, Epstein JA, Jones MD: Lumbar spinal stenosis, *Radiol Clin North Am* 15:227, 1977.
8. Epstein JA and others: Sciatica caused by nerve root entrapment in the lateral recess: the superior facet syndrome, *J Neurosurg* 36:484, 1972.
9. Getty CJM: Lumbar spinal stenosis: the clinical spectrum and the results of operation, *J Bone Joint Surg* 62B:481, 1980.
10. Heithoff KB: *Pathogenesis and high-resolution computed tomographic scanning of direct bony impingement syndromes of the lumbar spine.* In Genant HK, Chafez N, Helms CA, editors: *Spine update 1982,* San Francisco, 1982, Department of Radiology, University of California.
11. Heithoff KB, Ray CD: Lumbar spinal stenoses in a sample of 9,800 scans, Presented at Institute for Low Back Care Symposium, Minneapolis, April, 1990.

12. Heithoff KB, Ray CD: *Principles of the computed tomographic assessment of lateral spinal stenosis.* In Genant HK and others, editors: *Spine update 1984,* San Francisco, 1984, Radiology Research and Education Foundation.

13. Heithoff KB and others: *Computed tomography versus myelography.* In Genant HK, editor: *Spine update 1987,* San Francisco, 1987, Radiology Research and Education Foundation.

14. Heithoff KB and others: *CT and MRI of lateral entrapment syndromes.* In Genant HK, editor: *Spine update 1987,* San Francisco, 1987, Radiology Research and Education Foundation.

15. Helms CA: CT of the lumbar spine—stenosis and arthrosis, *Comput Radiol* 6:359, 1982.

16. Herkowitz HN, Garfin SR: Decompressive surgery for spinal stenosis, *Semin Spine Surg* 1:163, 1989.

17. Herkowitz HN, Kurz LT: Degenerative lumbar spondylolisthesis with spinal stenosis, *J Bone Joint Surg* 73A:802, 1991.

18. Hopp E, editor: *Spine: state of the Art Reviews—Stenosis,* Philadelphia, 1987, Hanley & Belfus.

19. Johnson K-E, Willner S, Johnsson K: Postoperative instability after decompression for lumbar spinal stenosis, *Spine* 11:107, 1986.

20. Katz JN and others: The outcome of decompressive laminectomy for degenerative lumbar stenosis, *J Bone Joint Surg* 73A:809.

21. Kirkaldy-Willis WH and others: Lumbar spinal nerve lateral entrapment, *Clin Orthop* 169:171, 1982.

22. Kirkaldy-Willis WH and others: Lumbar spinal stenosis, *Clin Orthop* 99:30, 1974.

23. Kirkaldy-Willis WH and others: Pathology and pathogenesis of lumbar spondylosis and stenosis, *Spine* 3:319, 1978.

24. Kornberg M, Rechtine GR: Quantitative assessment of the fifth lumbar spinal canal by computed tomography in symptomatic L4-L5 disc disease, *Spine* 10:328, 1985.

25. Onel D, Sari H, Doenmez C: Lumbar spinal stenosis: clinical/radiologic therapeutic evaluation in 145 patients, *Spine* 18:291, 1993.

26. Rauschning W: Normal and pathologic anatomy of the lumbar root canals, *Spine* 12:1008, 1987.

27. Ray CD: *Decompressions and the "inaccessible zone."* In Hardy RW Jr, editor: *Lumbar disc disease,* ed 2, 1992 New York, Raven Press.

28. Ray CD: *Extensive lumbar decompression: patient selection and results.* In White AH, Rothman RH, Ray CD, editors: *Lumbar spine surgery: techniques and complications,* St. Louis, 1987, Mosby.

29. Ray CD: *Lateral spinal decompression using the paralateral approach.* In Watkins RG, Collis JS Jr, editors: *Lumbar discectomy and laminectomy,* Rockville, MD, 1987, Aspen.

30. Ray CD: *Methods of resection of bone spurs, osteophytes and bony encroachment.* In White AH, Rothman RH, Ray CD, editors: *Lumbar spine surgery: techniques and complications,* St. Louis, 1987, Mosby.

31. Ray CD: New techniques for decompression of lumbar spinal stenosis, *Neurosurgery* 10:587, 1982.

32. Ray CD: Transfacet decompression and dowel fixation: a new technique for lumbar lateral spinal stenosis, *Acta Neurochir* 43:48-54, 1988.

33. Simeon FA, Rothman RH: Clinical usefulness of CT scanning in the diagnosis and treatment of lumbar spine disease, *Radiol Clin North Am* 21:197, 1983.

34. Verbiest H: *Lumbar spine stenosis.* In Youmans JR, editor: Neurological surgery, vol 5, ed 3, Philadelphia, 1990, W.B. Saunders, p 2805.

35. Verbiest H: The significance and principles of computerized axial tomography in idiopathic developmental stenosis of the bony lumbar vertebral canal, *Spine* 4:369, 1979.

36. Weinstein PR: Diagnosis and management of lumbar spinal stenosis, *Clin Neurosurg* 30:677, 1983.

37. Wiltse LL, Kirkaldy-Willis WH, McIvor GWD: The treatment of spinal stenosis, *Clin Orthop* 115:83, 1976.

38. Wiltse LL and others: Alar transverse process impingement of the L5 spinal nerve: the far out syndrome, *Spine* 9:31, 1984.

Chapter 81

Posterior Lumbar Interbody Fusion: Biomechanical Selection for Fusions

James W. Simmons, Jr.
John N. McMillin

Indications

Clinical Advantages

Comparative Options

Technique

Complications

Results with Posterior Lumbar
    Interbody Fusion—Literature
    Review

Predictions

"There is nothing either good or bad but thinking makes it so."

William Shakespeare

In 1911, Hibbs and Albee first described an inter-laminar fusion of the lumbar spine that became the standard fusion technique.[31] Mercer,[57] in 1936, was apparently the first to suggest that "the ideal operation for fusing the spine would be an interbody fusion, but the surgical difficulties encountered in performing such a feat would make the operation technically impossible." Posterior interbody fusion after lumbar disc removal was first reported by Jaslow[36] in 1946. It is Ralph Cloward, however, who is undoubtedly the "father" of posterior lumbar interbody fusion (PLIF). In 1947 the Cloward[11] report, "The Treatment of Ruptured Lumbar Disc by Intervertebral Fusion—Report of 100 Cases" was read at the Harvey Cushing Society meeting at Hot Springs, Virginia. With the exception of Cloward's own publications,[8,9,12] there was little early enthusiasm for PLIF.

After Cloward, most of the initial enthusiasm was outside the United States. Crock,[14,15] of Australia, indicated that theoretically the ideal operation for isolated disc resorption (localized spondylosis) was PLIF, allowing bilateral nerve-root canal decompression. James and Nisbet[35] of New Zealand used intervertebral fusion in patients with spondylolisthesis, as well as prolapsed discs. They reported the use of tibial grafts for body-to-body fusion, stating "posterior intervertebral body-to-body fusion is a neater operation." LeVay[44] reported that PLIF is favored by neurosurgeons in England. In Germany, Junghanns and Schmorl[38] advocated Cloward's concept of the PLIF. Junghanns[37] believed that unstable lumbar segments should not only be fused but distracted as well. "In the lumbar spine this could only be achieved posteriorly by removing disc tissue, eliminating the cartilaginous endplate, unfolding (distraction) of the disc space, and positioning of the osseous packs." The use of spinal fusions was then extended by the application to anterior interbody fusion methods by Hodgson.[32]

There were several isolated reports of the PLIF procedure in the United States prior to 1980. Wiltberger[92,93] favored PLIF, evacuating the disc material and using a unilateral approach to insert dowel grafts into the intervertebral disc space. Christoferson[7] reported 92% good results placing lamina in the intervertebral disc space after discectomy. There was increased usage and innovation in the United States during the late 1970s and early 1980s. Lin[45,48] modified Cloward's technique, and his continuing interest culminated in the formation of the first Posterior Lumbar Interbody Fusion Workshop and Symposium in 1981.[46] Ma[51] and Collis[13] both introduced new instruments and reported on the use of allograft bone. Simmons[77] reported on the use of autograft chips obtained at the time of laminectomy.

Current trends that will probably increase the general acceptance of PLIF include improved posterior spinal fixation, particularly bone screw devices and the wider use of allograft bone. Roy-Camille[65,66] first developed the concept of using bone screws with plate fixation. Magerl[53] and Olerud and coworkers[60,61] had important roles in the development of pedicle fixation. Steffee[81] is probably responsible for the wide popularity of this technique in the United States. In 1988 he reported on the use of pedicle fixation in combination with PLIF.[82] The use of pedicle fixation with PLIF achieves immediate three-column spinal stability. This allows wider decompression, prevents graft dislodgement, and improves fusion rate.[74,82] Biomechanically, the construct is load-sharing[74,94] and protects the graft while maintaining disc height and interpedicular distance. A side benefit of immediate stability is quicker patient mobilization, shorter hospitalization, and no brace requirement. Improved instrumentation in conjunction with the advantages of pedicle fixation will lead to more widespread use of PLIF.

Another trend that may affect the general use and acceptance of PLIF is the use of bone allografts in orthopedic surgery.[55] Use of allografts avoids the complications associated with iliac crest autografts. Allografts, when used for interbody fusions, appear to have a consistent, acceptable fusion rate.[82] This may be the result of the compression forces across the graft or of the presence of osteoprogenitor cells in the subchondral plate. The risk of disease (autoimmune deficiency syndrome, or AIDS) transmission is still somewhat controversial, although no human immunovirus (HIV) transmission has been reported with processed bone.[70]

Indications

Junghanns and Schmorl[38] were the first to describe the lumbar intervertebral disc as being only a part of the motor segment or motion segment ("bewegungssegment"). The motion segment consists of the intervertebral disc, foramina, facet joints, interlaminar space, ligamentum flavum, spinous processes, and the adjoining ligaments. Junghanns' concept was that with a change in the disc space, there is also an associated change in all of the motion segment. When a lumbar disc is degenerative or surgically removed, the intervertebral space will settle, and the narrowing is followed by sequential changes of the motion segment as a whole. In addition to disc herniation, there would be posterior vertebral spur formation, facet subluxation with hypertrophy, and ligamentum flavum hypertrophy and invagination. The size of the intervertebral foramen is further reduced by the coverage of ligamentum flavum extending laterally as it covers the facet joint to its lateral limit. Various combinations result in neural compression at different sections of the spinal segment. Spinal stenosis, either central, subarticular, or foraminal, may occur following simple discectomy. These phenomena also are described by Kirkaldy-Willis,[40] Farfan,[19,20] Crock,[14] Finnison,[22] and Cauthen.[4]

In addition to these mechanical effects, more is being learned about the chemical etiology of low-back and sciatic pain.[26] The apparent leakage of intradiscal breakdown products—proteoglycans—appears to figure prominently in the pain generation process. The roles of PLA-2,[67] substance-P,[88,89] and serotonin have yet to be fully defined. However, this line of investigation may have an increasing role in any procedure emphasizing "total disc displacement."[13]

The essential indicator for a PLIF procedure is low-back pain with or without sciatica as a result of abnormalities of the "motion segment"[64] or "functional spinal unit."[91] Key to this issue is localization of the pain-producing source. MRI scanning is proving to be a valuable initial screen,[72,80,86] especially in patients who do not present with a clear, single-root, unilateral syndrome. Clinical findings and experience, as described by O'Brien,[18,59] and torsion and compression testing, as described by Farfan,[19,21] may be useful adjuncts to the standard neurologic examination. Probably most important, however, is the use of provocative tests to localize pain. Awake discography has been most helpful,[1,75,80,87] with facet and nerve-root blocks occasionally necessary.

Some researchers propose definitive indications for PLIF. In recommending the procedure for the chronic symptomatic degenerated disc, Collis[13] describes several indications, including lumbar pain with or without sciatica, a degenerated disc with or without a protrusion, or a midline disc protrusion. Such factors as "discectomy syndrome" following lumbar laminectomy or a recurrent soft-tissue protrusion as well as spondylolisthesis, grade I or grade II, or reverse spondylolisthesis are also signs that the PLIF procedure is needed. Any combination of the preceding seven conditions also may serve as indication for the procedure.

Keim[39] has listed 10 factors as indications for lumbar spine fusions. Unstable joint complex associated with a long history of low-back pain, spondylolisthesis with or without spondylolysis, as well as congenital anomaly, transitional transverse process, or spondylolysis without spondylolisthesis may signal a need for a lumbar spine fusion. Additional indications include localized lateral spinal stenosis or degenerative spondylosis at one level, facet resection from previous surgery, or a history of heavy labor or sports activity associated with simple disc herniation (with or without degenerative change). Bilateral disc herniation, massive midline herniation, and previous disc surgery at that level may indicate the need for lumbar spine fusion. Finally, Keim lists reconstruction for failed back surgery syndrome (FBSS), including pseudoarthroses from lateral fusion, and bilaterally extruded discs in obese patients that prevent rapid postoperative settling of the disc space as indications for lumbar spine fusion. In addition, the indications described by Cloward[12] have not changed after 45 years of experience—that is, "the treatment of low-back pain with or without sciatica due to lumbar disc disease."

Our indications for the PLIF include a combination of pathophysiology, musculoskeletal function, and significantly impaired lifestyle requirements. Specific indications include spinal stenosis, segmental instability, discogenic disease, and the postlaminectomy syndrome. Spinal stenosis, particularly subarticular or foraminal, may require partial or complete facetectomy, destabilizing the functional spinal unit. Segmental instability may be difficult to define radiographically.[16,27,30,42,63,73,83,84] Primary sagittal or rotational instability, as well as secondary signs[3] such as the vacuum gas sign, MacNab traction spur,[52] spondylolisthesis,[62] retrolisthesis,[25] and previous total laminectomy[2] may be helpful in determining the need for fusion. Discogenic disease not responding to job or activity modification covers a broad spectrum of disease processes, from dysfunction to stabilization as defined by Kirkaldy-Willis,[41,42] and probably includes intractable disc pain of chemical origin.[67] The use of MRI and awake discography is particularly helpful in defining this indication. Postlaminectomy syndrome includes a combination of segmental instability with epidural fibrosis.[69] In the postoperative spine, radiographic instability may be difficult to define, but epidural scar tissue exacerbated by clinical instability will be apparent.

Clinical Advantages

Lin[47] lists six clinical advantages of the PLIF procedure. First, the normal anatomic relationship between the motion segment and the neural structures is restored, with the narrow disc space returning to normal anatomic alignment. Second, further degenerative processes of the fused motion segment are arrested with successful PLIF. However, this increases the range of motion of the adjoining vertebral disc spaces, possibly enhancing their degenerative processes. Third, recurrent lumbar disc herniation is prevented at the level where the total discectomy was needed for PLIF. Fourth, the lack of motion after a successful PLIF prevents mechanical pulling of the nerve root by the surrounding scar tissue. Thus, PLIF prevents painful nerve-root irritation from postoperative perineural adhesions. Fifth, all neural compression from structures other than the disc is relieved by wide laminotomy in PLIF, especially in cases of lateral spinal stenosis. Sixth, stress and motion from an abnormal motion segment result in a tropism of the facets. The motion is arrested by stabilization; thus PLIF prevents recurrence of tropism or lateral spinal stenosis.

Cauthen[4] lists several clinical advantages of the PLIF procedure. The procedure reconstitutes the normal anatomic relationship between the motion segment and the neural structures. The narrow disc space and the motion segment are restored to normal anatomic alignment. Successful PLIF also arrests further degenerative processes of the fused motion segment. However, because of an increased range of motion of the adjoining vertebral disc spaces, their degenerative processes can be enhanced by PLIF. The total discectomy needed for PLIF prevents recurrent lumbar disc herniation at that level. Posterior lumbar interbody fusion prevents painful nerve irritation from postoperative perineural adhesions. Lack of motion after a successful PLIF prevents mechanical pulling of the nerve by the surrounding scar tissue. Wide laminotomy in PLIF relieves all neural compression, especially in cases of lateral spinal stenosis. And finally, Cauthen points out that PLIF restores a constant relationship between all the components of a motion segment. It also prevents tropism of the facet.

According to Cautilli,[5] the PLIF procedure has several advantages. A wide area of bone surface is provided, and there is an adequate blood supply through the cancellous portion of the vertebral body once the cortical plate has been removed. In addition, the fusion is proximate to the center of motion and compression forces.

The procedure allows for complete visualization of the area of nerve-root compression while providing complete access for removal of the areas of compression centrally (anteriorly and posteriorly), as well as laterally, at the foraminal trough. Finally, the procedure preserves interbody distance so there will be no ensuing disc space collapse and possible lateral stenosis as a sequela of disc excision.

Evans[17] has presented a biomechanical model supporting the clinical advantages already noted. His flagpole concept presents a rationale for performing PLIF rather than a less demanding procedure. In this concept, the central graft placement represents the flagpole while the facets, remaining anulus anteriorly, and posterior ligamentous restraints represent surrounding guy wires. Only this combination achieves balance of both compression and torsional forces. The intervertebral graft placement, including the lateral disc space, optimizes the load-bearing capacity of the vertebral segment and simultaneously produces stability. Necessary to achieving this model is total posterior disc excision while maintaining or reconstructing the posterior restraints. After significant facetectomy or sacrifice of posterior ligaments, use of interpedicular fixation may reestablish the construct.

In addition to the flagpole model, the more routine orthopedic concept of load sharing is relevant to the discussion. The use of interbody cortical-cancellous grafts in conjunction with interpedicular fixation is a load-sharing construct. This protects both graft and screw from failure and favorably affects fusion success.

Comparative Options

The PLIF procedure is technically demanding; however, to the trained spinal surgeon it allows dynamic decompression of the nerve root by restoring and maintaining disc space height. In addition, the posterior approach is familiar and allows wide decompression. Decompression to the pedicle permits total disc excision, epidural veins can be cauterized with less risk, and neural elements are more easily identified. Allograft bone for total disc replacement (TDR) decreases blood loss and surgical time and avoids the morbidity associated with iliac crest bone harvesting. The exposure necessary to perform the PLIF allows direct visualization of the medial border of the pedicle, simplifying screw insertion for pedicle fixation devices. The inherent stability provided by PLIF in combination with pedicle fixation allows quick patient mobilization with decreased discomfort and less external support.

In comparison, the anterior LIF also achieves TDR, with dynamic decompression by restoration or maintenance of disc space height while avoiding the neural canal.[6,14,24,28,34,68] However, the exposure is less familiar to most spine surgeons and carries the risks of exposing the retroperitoneal area and inducing vascular injury[14,29] and retrograde ejaculation[23,24] with possible sterility. In addition, fixation, although evolving, is less readily available for ALIF. Probably most important, however, is the inability to manage significant posterior pathology from the anterior approach.[6,34] Free-fragment herniations and significant stenosis are contraindications to this approach. This makes preoperative evaluation all the more important and allows little possibility for intraoperative correction for missed posterior pathology.

The lateral intertransverse fusion is currently the most popular alternative with spine surgeons. It uses the familiar posterior approach and allows decompression as necessary. This might allow for less neural manipulation than the PLIF: however, it is unclear whether that results in less epidural scar formation.[94] The lateral intertransverse fusion does not achieve TDR or restore disc space height without placing unnecessary tension on the pedicle fixation system. This is in contradistinction to the load-sharing construct of the PLIF with pedicle fixation.[56,94] It is still to be clarified whether retained nuclear substance after solid intertransverse fusion plays a role in continued pain. Finally, intertransverse fusions require autogenous iliac crest graft to maximize fusion potential.

The final option is the simultaneous combined anterior and posterior fusion (SCAPF) described by Kozak and O'Brien[43] and Linson and Williams.[50] As originally described, this combines a standard ALIF with a posterior intertransverse fusion and instrumentation, although pedicle fixation could by easily substituted. This approach does achieve TDR with immediate stability. However, if posterior decompression is required, this becomes an extensive procedure with the combined risks of anterior and posterior spinal surgery.

"Change is not made without inconvenience, even from worse to better."

Richard Hooker

Technique

The PLIF procedure is quite technical and requires meticulous attention to detail, starting with positioning the patient. The knee-chest positioning table has been very useful both for abdominal dependency and C-arm positioning. In addition, it allows control over lumbar lordosis prior to plate application. Hypotensive anesthesia,[54] cell saver, and autologous blood should be routine considerations, especially in multiple level or repeat surgery. Prophylactic antibiotics are administered preoperatively and are continued 48 hours postoperatively. Antiembolus stockings with sequential gradient pumps are used intraoperatively.

A standard midline approach with electrocautery from dermis to spinous process is used to control bleeding from the outset. Electrocautery and periosteal elevators are used to expose the posterior elements subperiosteally to the base of the transverse process. If pedicle fixation is to be used, exposure should extend 1.5 levels above and 1 level below, while sparing the uninvolved level facet capsules.

Wide laminectomy with Kerrisons and osteotomes is performed (Fig. 81-1). Bilateral partial facetectomy, exposing nerve roots to the pedicle or further laterally if indicated by preoperative studies or intraoperative findings, is performed (Fig. 81-2). Bipolar cautery is used in the epidural fat and veins to expose the disc bilaterally. Total discectomy in-

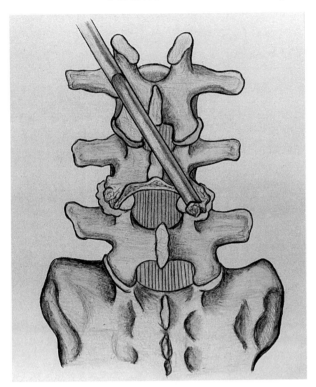

Fig. 81-1
The posterior elements are debrided of exostosis and hypertrophic bone, including the medial and lateral facets of the spinal canal.

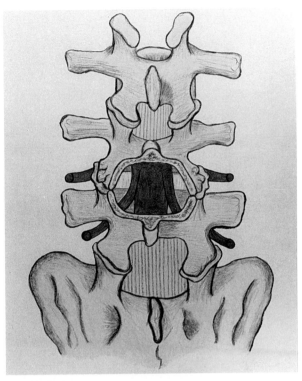

Fig. 81-2
A wide exposure out to the pedicles is necessary to expose the nerve roots and insert the graft. An adequate amount of the apophyseal joint remains for posterior stability.

cluding lateral disc, midline anulus, and posterior longitudinal ligament is performed. Osteotomes, pituitary rongeurs, Scoville curettes, and a posterior longitudinal ligament resector are all useful (Figs. 81-3 and 81-4).

End-plate preparation is critical to secure graft fit and incorporation (Figs. 81-5 and 81-6). Disc space depth and width are then determined (Fig. 81-7). An appropriate disc spacer is placed unilaterally (Fig. 81-8). An appropriately sized and contoured iliac crest bone plug is then impacted on the contralateral side. Graft may be bicortical or tricortical, allograft or autograft (Fig. 81-9). If allograft is used, local autogenous chips can be impacted anterior to the graft, creating a composite graft. The spacer is then removed (Fig. 81-10) and a second bone plug is inserted (Fig. 81-11). Puka chisels (Fig. 81-12) are used to position the grafts, and a third plug or autogenous chips may be placed in the remaining space (Figs. 81-13 and 81-14).

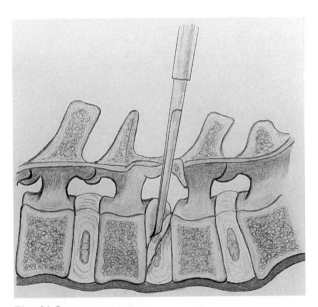

Fig. 81-3
The cartilaginous end plate is separated from the bony end plate.

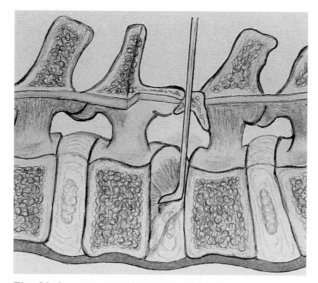

Fig. 81-4

Removal of the disc, particularly the lateral most portions of the disc, with a reverse Scofield curette.

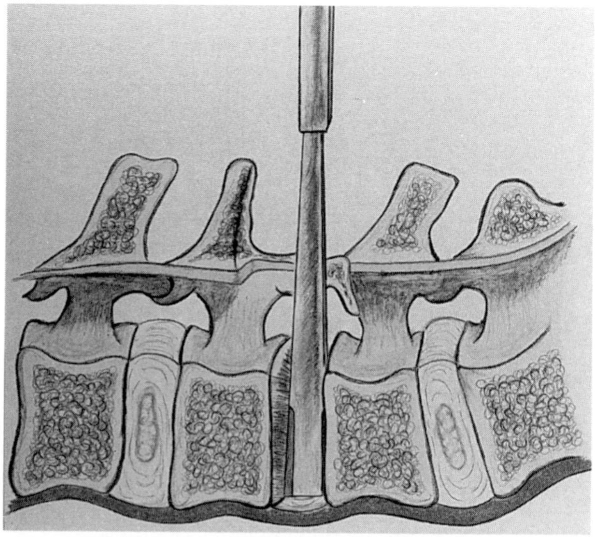

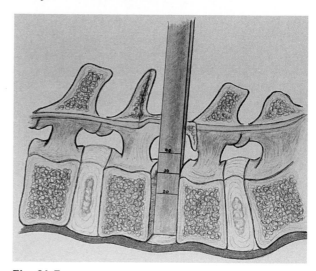

Fig. 81-5

The disc space is fashioned to receive bone plugs. Here the Collis shapers is demonstrated.

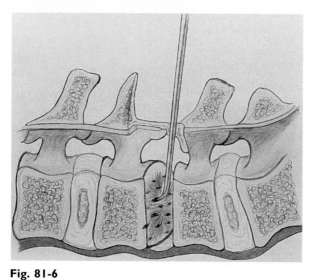

Fig. 81-6

Adequate bleeding of the end plate for vascularization is necessary. A Cloward punch can be used to fracture the bony end plate.

Fig. 81-7

The disc space is measured with spanners as demonstrated.

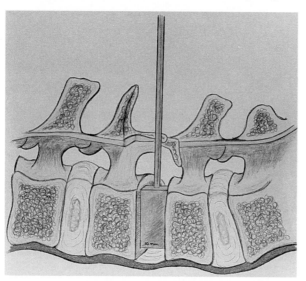

Fig. 81-8

A spacer in the disc space maintains distraction for placement of the opposite bone plug.

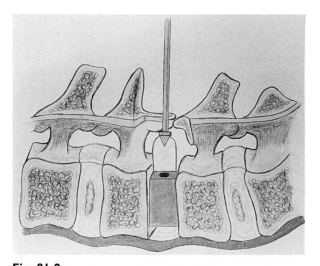

Fig. 81-9

Allograft bone plug is inserted on the opposite side using a holding device.

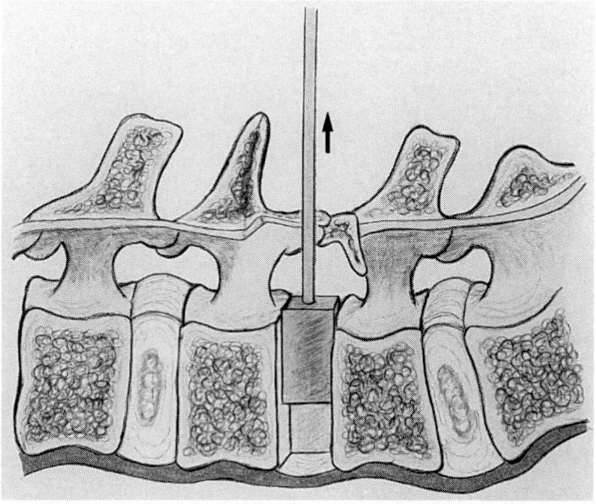

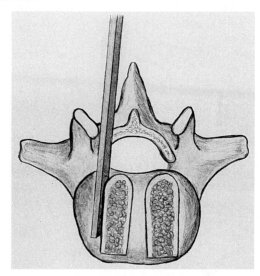

Fig. 81-10

The spacer is removed with the bone plug inserted on the opposite side.

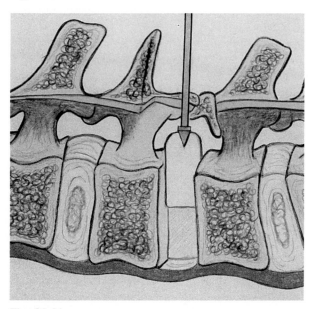

Fig. 81-11

A second bone plug is inserted after removal of the spacer.

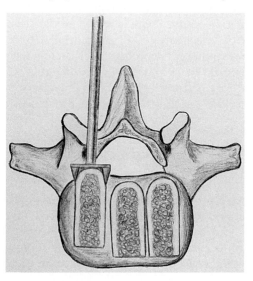

Fig. 81-12

Puka chisels are used to "walk" the bone plug medially.

Fig. 81-13

A third or fourth bone plug can be inserted to fill the disc space. The plugs are impacted slightly below the posterior rim of the vertebral body.

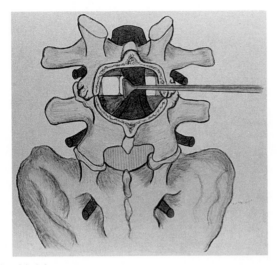

Fig. 81-14

The bone plugs fill the intervertebral disc space, maintaining disc space height.

After graft impaction, the nerve roots are inspected for any residual impingement, a fat graft is placed between the dura and the graft, posterior to the dura. A layered watertight closure over suction drainage is performed.

If pedicle fixation is used, the screws may be placed prior to discectomy or after graft placement. Prior to plate placement, normal lordosis should be restored, locking in the grafts.

Complications

Posterior lumbar interbody fusion is major spine surgery and requires a thorough understanding of the spine and neuroanatomy involved. A complete understanding of bone and fusion physiology also is necessary. The risks of PLIF include all the same risks of any posterior spine surgery: blood loss, epidural bleeding, intraabdominal vascular injury, instability, infection, arachnoiditis, and dural tears.

Complications specific to PLIF include nerve root injury, pseudoarthrosis, graft resorption, epidural scarring, graft retropulsion, and adjacent level degeneration. All of these either present a special problem or have been particularly implicated in PLIF. Nerve root injury should be avoided by careful decompression and retraction. Lateral disc exposure with ample facetectomy protects both exiting and traversing roots at the time of graft impaction. Anesthetic paralysis should be avoided, and if lower extremity movement occurs during graft impaction, roots should be inspected.

Epidural scar has been implicated as particularly troublesome with PLIF. Hemostasis, gentle retraction, and fat grafting may help. The stability provided with PLIF and pedicle fixation prevents excessive neural traction by epidural scar.

Pseudoarthrosis can be minimized by adequate end-plate preparation, good carpentry or graft fit, and complete disc space packing with low-antigenicity allograft,[79] autograft, or composite graft. Complete excision of nucleus and posterior anulus is essential. If a pseudoarthrosis still occurs, it can be managed by external pulsed electromagnetic fields[58,78] or supplemental lateral intertransverse fusion. Similarly, graft resorption can be prevented by use of high-quality, low-antigenicity allograft or composite grafting.[79] Maintenance of stability without overcompression with the fixation device is important as well.

Graft retropulsion is specific to PLIF, but it is avoidable by end-plate shaping, graft sizing, and countersinking. The routine use of pedicle fixation should nearly eliminate this complication.

Adjacent-level degeneration is an increasingly discussed complication.[90] It can best be minimized by appropriate preoperative examinations. Awake discography should help predict and decrease this risk. Technically, it is important to spare the facets adjacent to the fused segment.

Results with Posterior Lumbar Interbody Fusion— Literature Review

Evaluating published results of the PLIF procedure is difficult. Many reports are technique-oriented, while those reporting clinical results do so in a wide variety of ways. Different gauges of fusion and clinical and functional success are used, as are a variety of graft types. Table 81-1 represents an attempt to summarize results, with some editorial license. A grade of "excellent/good" can generally be regarded as representing no neurologic deficits, minimal or no requirement for pain medication, and return to work. Lin's[49] "satisfactory" grade approximates the "excellent/good" rating offered by other investigators.

Predictions

Posterior lumbar interbody fusion often has been criticized for being too fraught with complications to warrant general use. Like many procedures, it has been criticized most by those using it least. If due caution is exercised by a trained spine surgeon, the procedure can be accomplished with an acceptable

Table 81-1
Literature review of PLIF results

Author	Patients (#)	Fusion (%)	Clinical Results (% excellent/good)
Cloward[10]			
(1981)	97	86	98
Collisi[13] (1985)	50	94	88
Lin[49] (1983)	465	88	82 (satisfactory)
Ma[51] (1985)	100	74	74
Christoferson[7]			
(1975)	418	10	95
Wiltberger[93]			
(1964)	46	87	70
Hutter[33] (1985)	142	91	78
Simmons[76,77]			
(1980, 1985)	113	91 (stable)	54
Steffee[82] (1988)	36	100	92
Schecter[71]			
(1991)	25	95	89
Stonecipher[85]			
(1989)	35	100	NR*

*Not reported.

complication rate. Recent advances make the procedure even more attractive. Pedicle fixation and PLIF are two procedures meant for each other. The routine use of bone screw devices will improve fusion rates, prevent graft dislodgement and resorption, and allow sufficiently wide decompression to make graft impaction less risky. At the same time, the rigid stability provided by the two in combination will allow quick patient mobilization with decreased hospitalization. The use of low-antigenicity allografts will decrease patient morbidity. Future studies will verify the safest way to procure and process bone, but to date no HIV transmission has been shown with processed bone. Until prosthetic disc replacement is a reality, PLIF best addresses and corrects the pathology of the diseased motion segment.

References

1. Antti-Poika I and others: Clinical relevance of discography combined with CT scanning: a study of 100 patients, *J Bone Joint Surg [Br]* 72:480, 1990.
2. Bradford DS: Spinal instability: orthopaedic prospective and prevention, *Clin Neurosurg* 27:591, 1980.
3. Bradford DS, Gotfried Y: Lumbar spine osteolysis: an entity caused by spinal instability, *Spine* 11(10):1013, 1986.
4. Cauthen JC: *Lumbar spine surgery: indications, techniques, failures and alternatives,* Baltimore, 1983, Williams and Wilkins.
5. Cautilli RA: *Theoretical superiority of PLIF.* In Lin PM, editor: *Posterior lumbar interbody fusion,* Springfield, IL, 1982, Charles C Thomas.
6. Chow SP and others: Anterior spinal fusion for deranged lumbar intervertebral disc, *Spine* 5(5):452, 1980.
7. Christoferson LA, Selland B: Intervertebral bone implants following excision of protruded lumbar discs, *J Neurosurg* 42:401, 1975.
8. Cloward RB: Lesions of the intervertebral discs and their treatment by interbody fusion methods, *Clin Orthop* 27:51, 1963.
9. Cloward RB: Posterior lumbar interbody fusion updated, *Clin Orthop* 193:16, 1985.
10. Cloward RB: Spondylolisthesis: treatment by laminectomy and posterior interbody fusion: Review of 100 cases, *Clin Orthop* 154:74, 1981.
11. Cloward RB: The treatment of ruptured lumbar discs by intervertebral fusion: a report of 100 cases. Read at the Meeting of the Harvey Cushing Society, Hot Springs, VA, November 15, 1947.
12. Cloward RB: The treatment of ruptured lumbar intervertebral discs by vertebral body fusion: indications, operative technique, after care, *J Neurosurg* 10:154, 1953.
13. Collis JS: Total disc replacement: a modified posterior lumbar interbody fusion: Report of 750 cases, *Clin Orthop* 193:64, 1985.
14. Crock HV: Anterior lumbar interbody fusion: indication for its use and notes on surgical technique, *Clin Orthop* 165:157, 1982.
15. Crock HV: *Practice of spinal surgery,* p 1, Vienna, 1983, Springer-Verlag.
16. Dupuis PR and others: Radiologic diagnosis of degenerative lumbar spinal instability, *Spine* 10(3):262, 1985.
17. Evans JH: Biomechanics of lumbar fusion, *Clin Orthop* 193:38, 1985.
18. Fairbanks JCT, O'Brien JP: Engineering aspects of the spine, *Eng Med* 7:135, 1980.
19. Farfan HF: *Mechanical disorders of the low back,* Philadelphia, 1973, Lea & Febiger.
20. Farfan HF: Muscular mechanism of the lumbar spine and the position of power and efficiency, *Orthop Clin North Am* 6:135, 1975.
21. Farfan HF: The use of mechanical etiology to determine the efficacy of active intervention in single joint lumbar intervertebral joint problems: surgery and chemonucleolysis compared, a prospective study, *Spine* 10(4):350, 1985.
22. Finnison BE: *Low back pain,* Philadelphia, 1973, J.B. Lippincott.
23. Flynn JC, Price CT: Sexual complications of anterior fusion of the lumbar spine, *Spine* 9(5):489, 1984.
24. Freebody D: Anterior transperitoneal lumbar fusion, *J Bone Joint Surg* 74(B):211, 1965.
25. Frymoyer JW, Selby DK: Segmental instability: rationale for treatment, *Spine* 10(3):280, 1985.

26. Garfin SR, Rydevik BL, Brown RA: Compressive neuropathy of spinal nerve roots: a mechanical or biological problem?, *Spine* 16(2):162, 1991.

27. Gertzbein SD and others: Centrode patterns and segmental instability in degenerative disc disease, *Spine* 10(3):257, 1985.

28. Goldner JL and others: Anterior disc excision and interbody spinal fusion for chronic low back pain, *Orthop Clin North Am* 183:22, 1984.

29. Harmon PH: Anterior extraperitoneal lumbar disc excision and vertebral body fusion. II. Operative technic including observations upon variations in the left common iliac veins and their connections, *Clin Orthop,* 18:185, 1960.

30. Hayes MA and others: Roentgenographic evaluation of lumbar spine flexion-extensions in asymptomatic individuals, *Spine* 14(3):327, 1989.

31. Hibbs RA, Albee FH: An operation for progressive spinal deformities, *NY State J Med* 93:1013, 1911.

32. Hodgson AR, Stock FE: Anterior spinal fusion: a preliminary communication of the radical treatment of Pott's disease and Pott's paraplegia, *Br J Surg* 44:266, 1956.

33. Hutter CG: Spinal stenosis and posterior lumbar interbody fusion, *Clin Orthop* 193:103, 1985.

34. Inoue SI and others: Anterior discectomy and interbody fusion for lumbar disc herniations, *Clin Orthop* 183:22, 1984.

35. James A, Nisbet NW: Posterior intervertebral fusion of lumbar spine: preliminary report of a new operation, *J Bone Joint Surg [Br]* 35(2):181, 1953.

36. Jaslow IA: Intercorporal bone graft in spinal fusion after disc removal, *Surg Gynecol Obstet* 82:215, 1946.

37. Junghanns H: Spondylolisthesis Ohne Spalt im Zwischengelenkstueck (pseudospondylolisthesis), *Arch Orthop Unfallchirurgie* 29:118, 1931.

38. Junghanns H, Schmorl G: *The human spine in health and disease,* ed 2, New York, 1971, Grune & Stratton.

39. Keim HA: Indications for spine fusions and techniques, *Clin Neurosurg* 25:266, 1977.

40. Kirkaldy-Willis WH: *Managing low back pain,* New York, 1983, Churchill Livingstone.

41. Kirkaldy-Willis WH, Farfan HF: Instability of the lumbar spine, *Clin Orthop* 165:110, 1982.

42. Knutsson F: The instability associated with disc degeneration in the lumbar spine, *Acta Radiologica* 25:593, 1944.

43. Kozak JA, O'Brien JP: Simultaneous combined anterior and posterior fusion: An independent analysis of a treatment for the low back pain patients, *Spine* 15(4):322, 1990.

44. LeVay D: A survey of surgical management of lumbar disc prolapse in the United Kingdom and Eire, *Lancet* 1:1211, 1967.

45. Lin PM: *Current techniques in operative neurosurgery,* New York, 1977, Grune & Stratton.

46. Lin PM: First Temple PLIF Workshop, Nazareth Hospital, Philadelphia, April 4 and 5, 1981.

47. Lin PM: *Introduction of PLIF, biomechanical principles and indications,* Springfield, IL, 1982, Charles C Thomas.

48. Lin PM: A technical modification of Cloward's posterior lumbar interbody fusion, *Neurosurgery* 1(2):124, 1977.

49. Lin PM, Cautilli RA, Joyce MF: Posterior lumbar interbody fusion, *Clin Orthop* 180:154, 1983.

50. Linson MA, Williams H: Anterior and combined anterior-posterior fusion for lumbar disc pain: a preliminary study, *Spine* 16(2):143, 1991.

51. Ma GW: Posterior lumbar interbody fusion with specialized instruments, *Clin Orthop* 193:57, 1985.

52. MacNab I: The traction spur: an indication of segmental instability, *J Bone Joint Surg [Am]* 53:663, 1971.

53. Magerl FP: Stabilization of the lower thoracic and lumbar spine with external skeletal fixation, *Clin Orthop* 189:125, 1984.

54. Malcolm-Smith NA, McMaster MJ: The use of induced hypotension to control bleeding during posterior fusion for scoliosis, *J Bone Joint Surg [Br]* 65:255, 1983.

55. Mankin HJ and others: Current status of allografting for bone tumors, *Orthop* 15(10):1147, 1992.

56. Matsuzaki H, Tokuhashi Y: Problems and solutions of pedicle screw plate fixation of lumbar spine, *Spine* 15(11):1159, 1990.

57. Mercer W: Spondylolisthesis with a description of a new method of operative treatment and notes of ten cases, *Edinburgh Med JNS* 43:545, 1936.

58. Mooney V: A randomized double blind prospective study of the efficacy of pulsed electromagnetic fields for interbody lumbar fusions, *Spine* 15(7):708, 1990.

59. O'Brien JP: Anterior spinal tenderness in low back pain syndrome, *Spine* 4(1):85, 1979.

60. Olerud S, Hamburg M: External fixation as a test for instability after spinal fusion L4-S1: a case report. *Orthop* 9:547, 1986.

61. Olerud S, Karlstrom G, Sjostrom L: Transpedicular fixation of thoracolumbar vertebral fractures, *Clin Orthop* 227:44, 1988.

62. Penning L and others: Instability in lumbar spondylolysthesis: a radiographic study of several concepts, *Am J Roentgenol* 134:293, 1980.

63. Posner I and others: A biomechanical analysis of the clinical stability of the lumbar and lumbrosacral spine, *Spine* 7(4):374, 1982.

64. Rolander SD: *Motion of the lumbar spine with special reference to the stabilizing effect of posterior fusion,* Gothenburg, Sweden, 1966, Tryckeri.

65. Roy-Camille R, Demeulenaere C: Osteosynthese du rachis dorsal, lombaire et lombo-sacre par plaque metalliques vissees dans les pedicules vertebraux et les apophyses articularies, *Presse Med* 78:1447, 1970.

66. Roy-Camille R, Roy-Camille M, Demeulenaere C: Fixation par plaques des metastases vertebrales dorso-lombaires, *Nouv Presse Med* 1:2463, 1972.

67. Saal JS and others: High levels of inflammatory phospholipase A-2 activity in lumbar disc herniation, *Spine* 15(7):674, 1990.

68. Sacks S: Anterior interbody fusion of the lumbar spine, *J Bone Joint Surg [Br]* 47:211, 1965.

69. Sano S and others: Unstable lumbar spine without hypermobility in postlaminectomy cases: mechanisms of symptoms and effect of spinal fusion with and without spinal instrumentation, *Spine* 15(11):1190, 1990.

70. Scarborough NL: Current procedures for bone banking allograft human bone, *Orthop* 15(10):1161, 1992.

71. Schecter NA, France MP, Lee CK: Painful internal disc derangements of the lumbarsacral spine: discographic diagnosis in treatment by posterior lumbar interbody fusion, *Orthop* 14(4):447, 1991.

72. Schiebler ML and others: In vivo and ex vivo magnetic resonance imaging evaluation of early disc degeneration with histopathologic correlation, *Spine* 16(6):635, 1991.

73. Schuerman H: Roentgenologic studies of the origin and development of juvenile kyphosis, together with some investigations concerning the vertebral epiphyses in man and in animals, *Acta Orthop Scand* 5:161, 1934.

74. Shirado O and others: Biomechanical evaluation of methods of posterior stabilization of the spine and posterior lumbar interbody arthrodesis for lumbosacral isthmic spondylolisthesis, *J Bone Joint Surg [Am]* 73(4):518, 1991.

75. Simmons EH, Segil CM: An evaluation of discography in the localization of symptomatic levels in discogenic disease of the spine, *Clin Orthop* 108:57, 1975.

76. Simmons JW: Posterior interbody fusions: Presented at the Seventh Annual Meeting of the International Society for the Study of the Lumbar Spine, New Orleans, 1980 (abstract).

77. Simmons JW: Posterior lumbar interbody fusion with posterior elements as chip grafts, *Clin Orthop* 193:85, 1985.

78. Simmons JW: Treatment of failed posterior lumbar interbody fusion (PLIF) of the spine with pulsing electromagnetic fields, *Clin Orthop* 193:127, 1985.

79. Simmons JW and others: The antigenicity of homologous goat bone prepared by two methods. Presented at the Mid-American Orthopaedic Association Meeting, Point Clear, AL, March 29, 1990.

80. Simmons JW and others: Awake discography: a comparison study with magnetic resonance imaging, *Spine* 16(6S):S216, 1991.

81. Steffee AD, Biscup RS, Sitkowski DJ: Segmental spine plates with pedicle screw fixation: a new internal fixation device for disorders of lumbar and thoracolumbar spine, *Clin Orthop* 203:45, 1986.

82. Steffee AD, Sitkowski DJ: Posterior lumbar interbody fusion and plates, *Clin Orthop* 227:99, 1988.

83. Stokes IA, Frymoyer JW: Segmental motion and instability, *Spine* 12(7):688, 1987.

84. Stokes IA and others: Assessment of patients with low back pain by biplanar radiographic measurement of intervertebral motion, *Spine* 6(3):233, 1981.

85. Stonecipher T, Wright S: Posterior lumbar interbody fusion with facet-screw fixation, *Spine* 14(4):468, 1989.

86. Tretti M and others: Disc degeneration in magnetic resonance imaging: a comparative biochemical, histologic and radiologic study in cadaver spines, *Spine* 16(6):629, 1991.

87. Walsh TR and others: Lumbar discography in normal subjects: a controlled prospective study, *J Bone Joint Surg [Am]* 72:1081, 1990.

88. Weinstein J: Mechanisms of spinal pain: the dorsal root ganglion and its role as a mediator of low back pain, *Spine* 11(10):999, 1986.

89. Weinstein J and others: The effects of low frequency vibration on dorsal root ganglion substance-P, *J Neuro Orthop* 4:24, 1987.

90. Wetzel, FT, LaRocca H: The failed posterior lumbar interbody fusion, *Spine* 16(7):839, 1991.

91. White AA, Panjabi M: *Clinical biomechanics of the spine*, Philadelphia, 1978, J.B. Lippincott.

92. Wiltberger BR: The dowel intervertebral body fusion as used in lumbar-disc surgery, *J Bone Joint Surg [Am]* 39(2):284, 1957.

93. Wiltberger BR: Intervertebral body fusion by the use of posterior bone dowel, *Clin Orthop* 35:69, 1964.

94. Yashiro K and others: The Steffee variable screw placement system using different methods of bone grafting, *Spine* 16(11):1329, 1991.

Chapter 82

Anterior Approach for Lumbar Fusions and Associated Morbidity

Robert J. Henderson

Indications

Choice of Exposure

Team Approach

Contraindications

Surgical Technique

  anterior abdominal wall exposure
  retroperitoneal exposure
  vertebral disc exposure
  disc excision
  graft-site preparation
  graft placement

Bone Grafts

Potential Complications

  blood loss
  other vascular complications
  impotence
  retrograde ejaculation
  sympathetic causalgia, or reflex sympathetic
      syndrome
  postsympathectomy syndrome
  serum sickness syndrome
  inguinal pain
  interbody graft displacement
  psoas abscess

Summary

Indications

The past 10 to 15 years have seen a significant expansion and utilization of the indications for performing interbody fusions, particularly anterior lumbar interbody fusions. These indications have included anterior interbody fusions (1) as a remedial stabilizing procedure for prior failed posterior fusion[6]; (2) as a mechanism for "load sharing" when using internal fixation posteriorly, or in providing additional stabilization for a posterior fusion to heal; (3) in ablating or extirpating an identified "pain generator" as with discogenic pain[1]; (4) in reestablishing disc space height in a cascading spine; or (5) as the final solution in preventing recurrent disc herniations.*

Over the past 5 years it has become increasingly apparent that anterior lumbar fusions enhance the success of posterior fusions and help alleviate symptoms. It is theorized that spinal segment stability is initially provided by the "wedging" effect of the anterior bone graft. This initial stability accelerates and improves the success of the posterior fusion. Then the long-term stability of the posterior fusion enhances the slower incorporation of the anterior fusion into a solid mass.

It is well known that a "stand-alone" anterior or posterior fusion does not necessarily immobilize the entire motion segment.[15] The successes of the properly performed anterior-posterior fusion that addresses all identified pain generators will lead to increased use of anterior fusions in properly selected patients.

Choice of Exposure

The safest, most expedient, bloodless exposure of the anterior lumbar spine is through an extraperitoneal approach. The easiest to learn is the paramedian approach, mobilizing the rectus muscle laterally from the midline and incising the posterior rectus sheath near its lateral border (Figs. 82-1 to 82-3). This allows the peritoneum to be dissected free easily from the overlying transversus muscle. The paramedian approach provides maximum exposure and versatility to handle complications, and the appropriate interspaces are easily identified. The problem with the paramedian approach is that it has a well-established record of developing incisional hernias because of the poorly developed integrity of the posterior rectus sheath that occurs in approximately 5% of the population. Good surgical technique minimizes hernia occurrences in this approach, but they

*References 1, 2, 4, 6, 9, 11, 12, and 14.

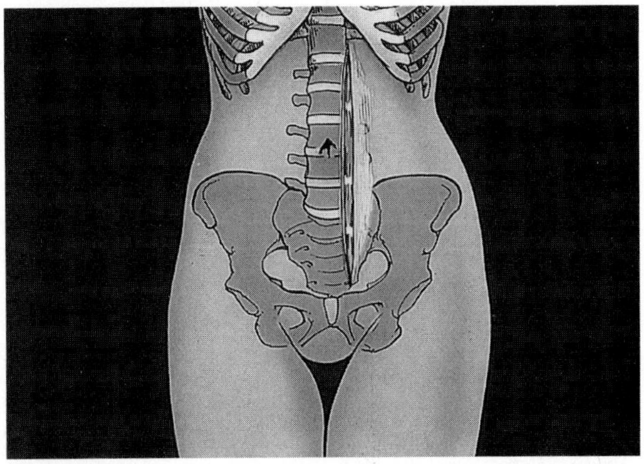

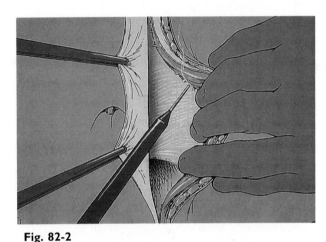

Fig. 82-1
Paramedian approach two fingerbreadths lateral to midline. *(© MediVisuals, Inc., Dallas, TX.)*

Fig. 82-2
Mobilizing rectus from midline out laterally, taking great care to avoid damage to epigastric vessels lying on undersurface of rectus muscle. *(© MediVisuals, Inc., Dallas, TX.)*

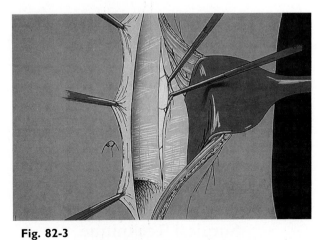

Fig. 82-3
Incising underlying posterior rectus sheath near its lateral border down to peritoneum. Sometimes, particularly when more cephalad, this involves incising through transversus muscle prior to reaching peritoneum. *(© MediVisuals, Inc., Dallas, TX.)*

will occur with an incidence of at least 5%. The use of an abdominal binder for the first 6 weeks postoperatively may help minimize the problem.

The oblique approach is one of the original approaches to the lumbar spine and is excellent when extensive exposure is needed for complete multilevel vertebrectomies, etc. The most significant problem with this approach is the incidence of eventration and hernias that occur due to inadvertent, accidental, or necessary transection of one or more of the motor nerves that supply the oblique musculature. Also, the exposure to the spine is from a lateral direction, which increases the possibility for damage from dissection or traction on the exiting nerve roots, which are hidden in the paraspinous musculature.

The transverse approach to the anterior lumbar spine has proved to be expedient, safe, and bloodless and in most cases does not lead to hernias.

Team Approach

The use of a team approach with two sets of skilled hands will keep one out of potentially life-threatening situations. The approach does have a learning curve. It is important that the surgeon creating the exposure be experienced in vascular surgery and in working in the retroperitoneal area. This experience gives one the skills to minimize dissection and achieve the surgical objectives without unnecessarily destroying structures.[15] The people holding retractors are also very important and play an integral part in minimizing potential complications.

Severe vascular complications, including exsanguination, and limb loss can occur when surgeons are just beginning to do anterior surgery on the spine.

Contraindications

Unless the surgeon is experienced and the longer instruments are available to accomplish this procedure, the anterior approaches to the lumbar spine should not be used in the following situations: (1) prior radiation to the abdomen; (2) retroperitoneal dissections (radical lymph node dissections); (3) a history of iliofemoral deep venous thrombosis; (4) bacterial discitis; (5) aortic bypass grafts; (6) prior anterior lumbar fusions and (7) significantly obese patients.

Surgical Technique

The key to developing good surgical technique in this procedure is the ability to identify and dissect in the proper tissue planes. This will result in an almost bloodless and extremely expeditious procedure with a minimum of morbidity and more than adequate exposure.

Approach to the anterior lumbar spine is important in effecting the ease, efficiency, and effectiveness of the spinal fusion procedure itself and in many cases the end result.[5,8,9,13] Therefore, due deliberation must be given to the type of exposure to be attempted and the appropriate level of the skin at which to initiate the approach. It is important to delineate the anatomic relationship between the highest interspace to be fused with the superior iliac crest on the ipsilateral side (Fig. 82-4). This is done by evaluating the anterior-posterior lumbar x-ray films. Usually the transverse incision overlying the left rectus muscles will be just below the umbilicus when exposing for the L4-L5, or L4-L5 and L5-S1 levels, and approximately midway between the umbilicus and symphysis pubis when exposing the L5-S1 level only (Fig. 82-5). Individuals who require more than two sequential levels, or skip levels to be fused, or who are more than moderately obese, or who require a fusion above the L3-L4 level need to have a paramedian vertical incision approach.[15]

Anterior Abdominal Wall Exposure

After incising the skin and subcutaneous tissues on a transverse plane overlying the left rectus muscle, dissection is carried down to the anterior rectus sheath and hemostasis is obtained with electrocautery. The anterior rectus sheath is incised transversely (Fig. 82-6) and extended caudally on the medial side and cephalad on the lateral side (Fig. 82-7). The rectus muscle is then freed hemostatically

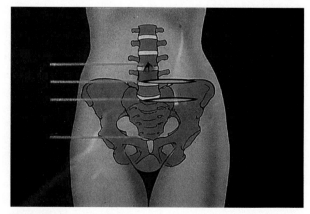

Fig. 82-4

Relationship of lower lumbar interspaces to bony landmarks. *(© MediVisuals, Inc., Dallas, TX.)*

with electrocautery from the anterior rectus sheath (Fig. 82-8) and mobilized medially, exposing the neurovascular bundles. Usually there are one or two of these bundles that need to be divided between hemoclips to facilitate exposure (Fig. 82-9). They provide motor innervation to the rectus muscle, but as long as more than two contiguous bundles are not sacrificed, crossover innervation will prevent denervation and eventual eventration of the muscle.

Retroperitoneal Exposure

The posterior rectus is then incised on a vertical plane near the lateral border of the rectus sheath down to the peritoneum (Fig. 82-10). This is to en-

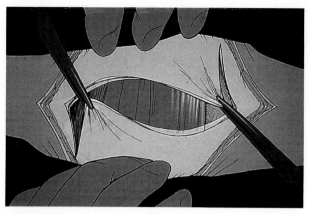

Fig. 82-7

Extending incision in anterior rectus sheath cephalad at lateral margin and caudally at medial margin. (© MediVisuals, Inc., Dallas, TX.)

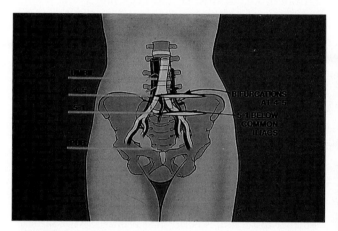

Fig. 82-5

Relationship of lower lumbar interspaces to vascular structures. Incision should be made at level of most cephalad disc to be operated on. (© MediVisuals, Inc., Dallas, TX.)

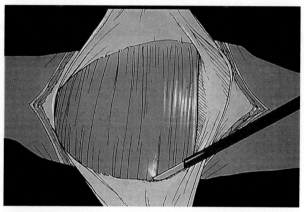

Fig. 82-8

Freeing of muscle from anterior sheath to facilitate mobilizing rectus muscle medially. (© MediVisuals, Inc., Dallas, TX.)

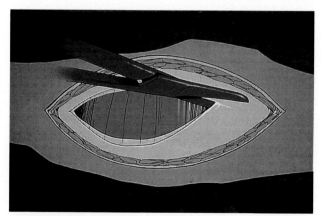

Fig. 82-6

Incision transversely across anterior rectus sheath. (© MediVisuals, Inc., Dallas, TX.)

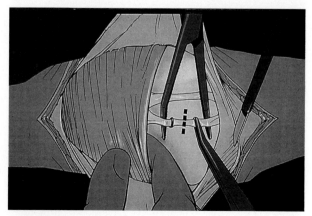

Fig. 82-9

Division of neurovascular bundles in front of posterior rectus sheath. (© MediVisuals, Inc., Dallas, TX.)

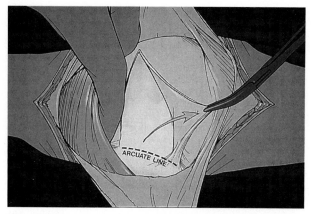

Fig. 82-10

Incision of posterior rectus sheath near its lateral border down to peritoneum. (© MediVisuals, Inc., Dallas, TX.)

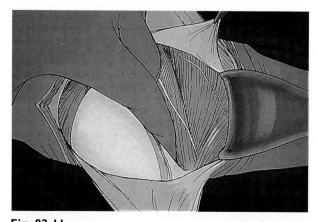

Fig. 82-11

Blunt finger dissection into extraperitoneal space and back into retroperitoneum. Spreading with fingers and pulling sac up and medially across midline not even touching genitofemoral, ilioinguinal nerves. (© MediVisuals, Inc., Dallas, TX.)

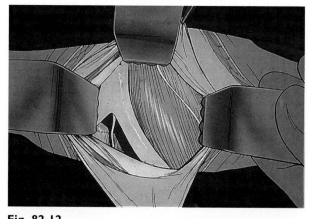

Fig. 82-12

Exposure of iliac vessels allowing ureter to remain with peritoneal sac. (© MediVisuals, Inc., Dallas, TX.)

sure a distinct separation between the peritoneum and the posterior rectus sheath, which as the surgeon moves medially becomes one contiguous layer. It is also very helpful when making this incision to use a fresh scalpel blade so that a minimum of pressure is needed to incise through the fascia. Blunt finger dissection is then used to free and mobilize the peritoneal sac over the psoas musculature and across the midline, to the right, along with the left ureter. When done correctly this maneuver need not disturb the ilioinguinal or genitofemoral nerves, which should be left lying in situ (Fig. 82-11). As the iliac vessels are exposed, they are left in situ (Fig. 82-12). Palpation with the fingertips will allow one to discern the location of the intervertebral spaces. One should continue to dissect over these interspaces because they are avascular. All of the dissection in the retroperitoneum thus far has been finger dissection only. Occasionally, the exposure may not be adequate, appears too difficult to maintain, or reveals the angulation of the L5-S1 space to be too oblique, or because of the size of the patient, the lower interspace may not be available to exposure. In those circumstances, using the T incision by caudal extension of the skin, subcutaneous, and anterior rectus fascia, along the same plane as the original division of the anterior sheath at the medial border (Fig. 82-13, *A* and *B*), will overcome these obstacles.

At this point, right-angled, blunt-tipped retractors (Hibbs) of an appropriate length (4, 6, 8, or 10 in.) (Fig. 82-14) are inserted to allow direct visualization. Further dissection is performed primarily with Kitner dissector pads (Fig. 82-15) directly over the palpable, avascular, intervertebral space. Levels are determined by counting up from the palpable L5-S1 sacral promontory. Confirm these levels with a cross-table lateral x-ray film using a metal probe placed within the interspace. Dissection of the lower lumbar intervertebral spaces is facilitated by having the patient in a hyperextended position. This is accomplished by positioning the patient over a retractable kidney rest built into the operating table that can be repositioned intraoperatively (Fig. 82-16).

Vertebral Disc Exposure

When exposing the L5-S1 interspace, the bifurcation of the iliac vessels is mobilized cephalad and to the right and left. Presacral vessels are divided between hemoclips to facilitate and maximize exposure. Only blunt dissection is used, sweeping from the midline laterally to avoid inadvertently injuring the branches of the sympathetic nerve plexus (Fig. 82-17).

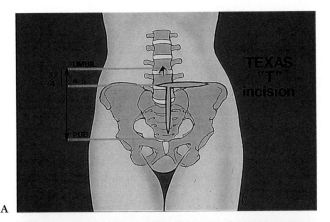

A

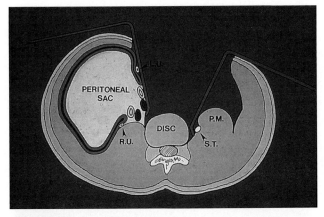

B

Fig. 82-13

A and **B**, Texas T provides additional exposure and room to maneuver and is gained by extending incision caudally, creating flap that is rolled out laterally to side and down. (© MediVisuals, Inc., Dallas, TX.)

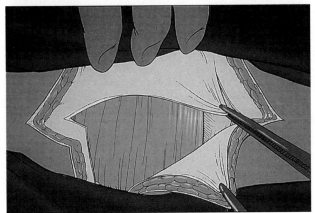

Fig. 82-14

Peritoneal sac rolled anteriorly and across midline and held aside with right-angled modified Hibbs retractors. (© MediVisuals, Inc., Dallas, TX.)

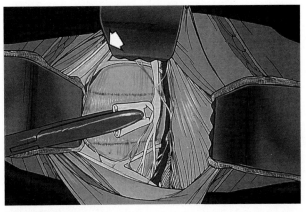

Fig. 82-15

Blunt dissection over avascular interspace representing L4-L5, with distal aorta and proximal iliac vessels retracted to right and sympathetic chain beginning to fimbriate over L5 vertebral body. (© MediVisuals, Inc., Dallas, TX.)

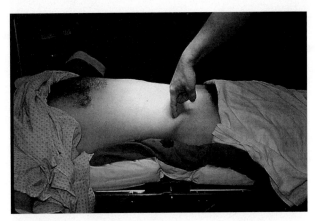

Fig. 82-16

Patient positioned correctly over kidney rest for L4-L5 and/or L5-S1 interbody fusion. (© MediVisuals, Inc., Dallas, TX.)

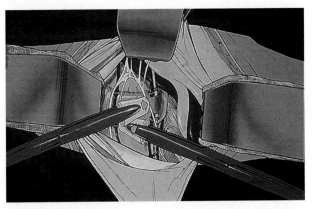

Fig. 82-17

Dividing presacral vessels with appropriately sized hemoclips. Careful blunt dissection of fimbriated sympathetic nerves beneath bifurcation iliac vessels at L5-S1. (© MediVisuals, Inc., Dallas, TX.)

Exposure of the L4-L5 interspace is also done by blunt dissection, mobilizing the distal aorta and the left common iliac vessels to the right (see Fig. 82-15). The sympathetic trunk is usually intact at this level and can be easily moved to the left as shown in Fig. 82-18. It is sometimes necessary to divide small

branches off of the left common iliac vessels to augment satisfactory exposure. Occasionally, the ascending lumbar vein, the first major branch off the common iliac vein, will need to be transected after first securing it with double ligatures on each side. Additional exposure can be obtained by dividing the prevertebral transverse vessels, usually crossing the midportion of the vertebral bodies beginning with L4.

After obtaining exposure of the interspace across the midline and above and below the vertebral end plates, it is important to maintain exposure in such a way as to protect the major vessels from accidental injury from the dissection instruments being used. Proper exposure to the anterior spine makes the actual discectomy and interbody fusion technique relatively straightforward.

Using the modified Crock dowel technique[1] further enhances the efficiency, reproducibility, and graft placement precision of the anterior lumbar fusion.

Disc Excision

Use electrocautery to dissect the anterior longitudinal ligament and annulus away from the end plates in a hemostatic fashion (Fig. 82-19, *A*) while identifying the "gray line" that denotes the end plates on either side of the interspace and remaining aware of the sympathetic chain and iliac vessels. The disc can then be separated away from the end plates with the periosteal elevator, following the concavity of the end plate posteriorly (Fig. 82-19, *B*). The annulus is incised with a no. 11 scalpel medially and laterally. The disc is then grasped with a Kocher clamp and dissected free of its remaining attachments with the periosteal elevator or sometimes pulled out piecemeal with a pituitary rongeur (Figs. 82-20 to

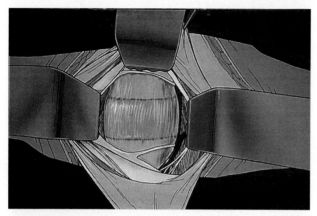

Fig. 82-18

Retraction of sympathetic trunk, Note "gray line" on edges of interspace. (© *MediVisuals, Inc., Dallas, TX.*)

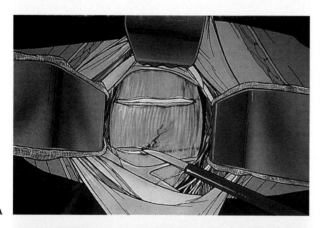

A

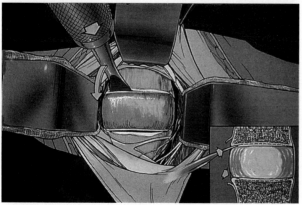

B

Fig. 82-19

A, Subperiosteal exposure. **B,** Separating disc and end plate from subchondral bone. (© *MediVisuals, Inc., Dallas, TX.*)

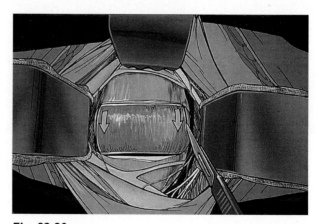

Fig. 82-20

Incising anulus medially and laterally. (© *MediVisuals, Inc., Dallas, TX.*)

82-22). The interspace is further cleared of remaining disc material and end plate down to subchondral bone using the Crock curette (Fig. 82-23) and/or the Oswestry curette (Fig. 82-24). Both of these instruments allow definitive control of the posterior dissection back to the posterior margin of the interspace while allowing leverage to be applied in a controlled fashion to remove the cartilaginous end plate.

Graft-Site Preparation

At this point, with a "cleaned out" interspace, the depth is measured (Fig. 82-25). If necessary, any osteophytes on the anterior lip are resected to allow the "starter" chisel to create the initial cut (Fig. 82-26) to seat the teeth of the cutting reamer. It is important that the starting cut be of sufficient depth to prevent the reamer from "jumping" and damag-

ing the adjacent neurologic or vascular structures. The dowel cutters come in four graduated sizes so that an appropriate size cut can be made that incises through the end plate to a width at least as wide as

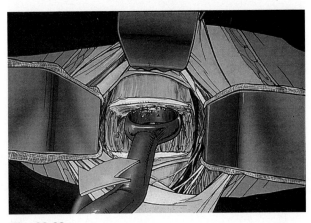

Fig. 82-23
Crock curette may be used to clean down to subchondral bleeding bone. (© MediVisuals, Inc., Dallas, TX.)

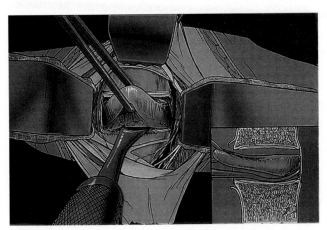

Fig. 82-21
Dissecting disc free and removing en bloc. (© MediVisuals, Inc., Dallas, TX.)

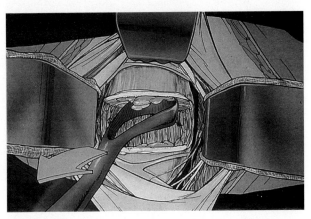

Fig. 82-24
Oswestry curette. (© MediVisuals, Inc., Dallas, TX.)

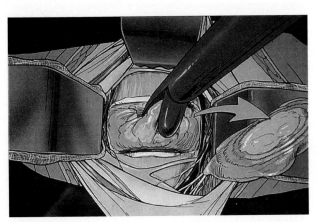

Fig. 82-22
Dissecting disc piecemeal with rongeur. (© MediVisuals, Inc., Dallas, TX.)

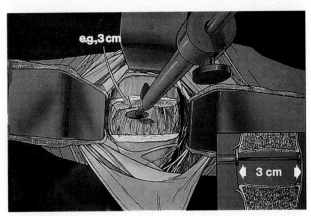

Fig. 82-25
Determining depth of interspace. (© MediVisuals, Inc., Dallas, TX.)

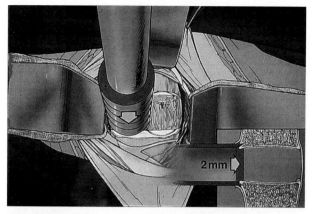

Fig. 82-26

Starter chisel allows dowel cutter to be seated firmly. (© MediVisuals, Inc., Dallas, TX.)

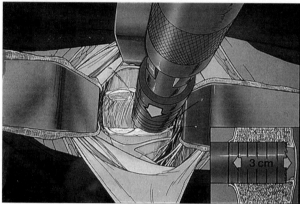

Fig. 82-27

Dowel cutter. Note remaining posterior rim of bone left in situ. (© MediVisuals, Inc., Dallas, TX.)

the dowel graft to be inserted. Be sure to allow for the concavity of the interspace when making the cuts. Remember, the deeper the cut into the vertebral body the weaker the bone structure, so choosing the appropriate size cutter can be a significant decision.

The dowel cutter is used to ream a circular cut across the intervertebral space. It is imperative at this point that adequate lighting is used. A headlamp and some form of magnification is also very beneficial. Having previously cleaned out the interspace, it is possible to visualize the depth of the cut as well as monitor the depth by watching the graduated lines on the cutter. The depth of the cut should be such that it leaves a 3- to 5-mm shelf posteriorly for the graft to abut, preventing posterior extrusion (Fig. 82-27). The cutter can be turned on a Hudson brace, T-ratchet handles, or on a powered drill.

The core evacuator gouge is helpful in removing the cut bone without damaging or enlarging the cut surfaces of the vertebral bodies (Fig. 82-28). With the widened interspace, additional soft tissue can be removed from the posterior interspace. Great care should be taken to avoid disrupting the epidural vessels.

Graft Placement

Figure 82-29 demonstrates the site prepared for seating of the grafts. Again, note that there is bleeding bone on the cut surfaces, the interspace is well cleaned out, and there is a buttress of bone between the graft and the dura. With the kidney rest still further elevated, the next-larger-size dowel grafts are inserted and tapped home (Fig. 82-30). The kidney rest is let down and the grafts checked for stability.

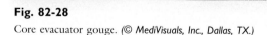

Fig. 82-28

Core evacuator gouge. (© MediVisuals, Inc., Dallas, TX.)

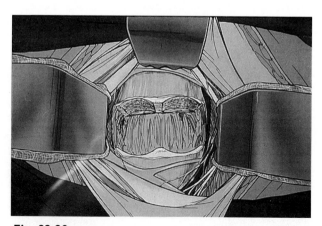

Fig. 82-29

Prepared beds with symmetrical cuts into subchondral bone. (© MediVisuals, Inc., Dallas, TX.)

Rough or protruding edges should be smoothed with a rongeur.

Place a piece of Surgicel over the grafted interspace. This will provide hemostasis and help prevent infection, which may result from the surgical violation of the lymphatic drainage that serves the lower intestinal tract (Fig. 82-31).

Closure of this approach is anatomic, in reverse order of the exposure technique, and done in individual layers with running absorbable suture: posterior rectus sheath, anterior rectus sheath, Scarpa's fascia, and skin (Figs. 82-32 to 82-35).

Bone Grafts

Tricortical iliac crest is available as fresh donor from the patient, but creates a full-thickness defect in the crest, with its attendant morbidity.[2] These grafts heal very quickly. When obtained from a bone bank, the fusion rate seems to be no different from the autogenous grafts but does take longer. Obviously there is no morbidity associated with its harvesting and al-

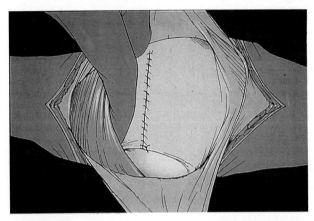

Fig. 82-32
Closing posterior rectus sheath. (© MediVisuals, Inc., Dallas, TX.)

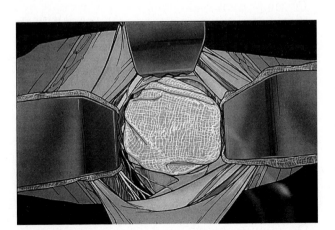

Fig. 82-30
Dowel grafts inserted against posterior ledge. (© MediVisuals, Inc., Dallas, TX.)

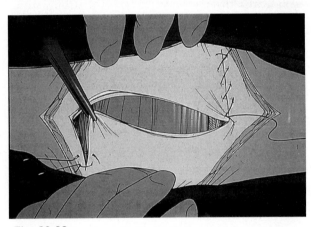

Fig. 82-33
Closing anterior rectus sheath. (© MediVisuals, Inc., Dallas, TX.)

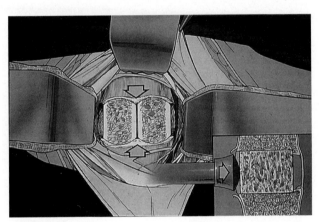

Fig. 82-31
Surgicel used for hemostasis and antibacterial properties. (© MediVisuals, Inc., Dallas, TX.)

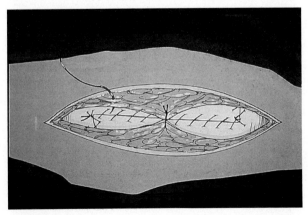

Fig. 82-34
Closing Scarpa's fascia. (© MediVisuals, Inc., Dallas, TX.)

lows the patient's crests to be used for posterior fusion or other future needs. Collapse of these grafts is not seen when used in conjunction with a posterior fusion, particularly with the added load sharing of internal fixation. Once healed they provide a large surface area of contiguous bone across the interspace.

Patellar dowel grafts are dense cancellous bone that provides the needed early structural strength but avoids the extracortical bone, which takes much longer to incorporate into the fusion mass.

Femoral dowel grafts, although readily available and structurally very strong, have proven to be brittle and to fracture easily. They also may dislocate from their intended position because they do not "grip" the vertebrae with their smooth cortical surface.

Femoral ring grafts have gained a lot of acceptance since the technique of filling the cancellous core with autogenous cancellous bone. This allows earlier and more successful development of bone fusion across the interspace because of strong structural support from the cortical ring. Several cases have shown that femoral rings, when used above and below a vertebral body, have led to a fracture of the intervening vertebral body. Femoral ring grafts do not lend themselves to the dowel-cutting technique and therefore do not have the reproducible precision of fitting the prepared interspace.

Interference screws, usually made of titanium, are being used successfully with the larger cortical grafts to prevent "backout" of the femoral rings or dowels.

Potential Complications

Blood Loss

Blood loss can be minimized by using electrocoagulation on the anterior longitudinal ligament and hemoclips (titanium) for dividing vessels and repairing venous tears. It is important to use the appropriate size hemoclips to maintain patency of the repair and to be assured that the hemoclip will maintain a secure grip on the tissue. Considerable blood can be lost from the cut surface of the vertebral bodies. This can be treated with hypotensive anesthesia, expedient insertion of bone plugs, and the use of the cell saver. Packing the interspace with a gauze sponge is usually sufficient to "stem the tide" until the graft is prepared. Epidural venous bleeding is best addressed by using Gelfoam at the back of the interspace prior to inserting the bone plugs.

A tear in the iliac venous system can result in massive blood loss very quickly. The exposure should be

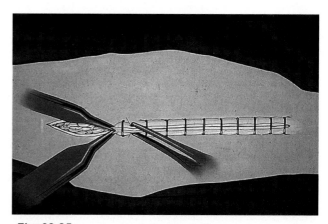

Fig. 82-35
Closing skin (© MediVisuals, Inc., Dallas, TX.)

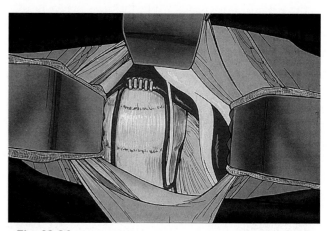

Fig. 82-36
Sequential application of appropriately sized hemoclips to repair venous tears. (© MediVisuals, Inc., Dallas, TX.)

maintained and the bleeding controlled by direct pressure with Kitners, retractors, or sponge stick. Obtain proximal and distal control by pressure over the vessel and then, in a sequential, tangential fashion, begin the repair with hemoclips (Fig. 82-36). Attempting to mobilize to cross clamp the vessels will lead to additional blood loss and increased morbidity from stripping the lymphatics and sympathetic nerves off the iliac vessels and the presacral area. This leads to problems with retrograde ejaculation, sympathetic causalgias, postsympathectomy syndrome, possible lymphedema, and neuralgias of the genitofemoral and ilioinguinal nerves.

Other Vascular Complications

Occlusion or thrombosis of the iliac artery may also occur. An arteriosclerotic plaque may fracture, creating a clot. If the intimal lining of the artery is in-

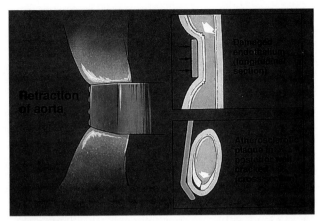

Fig. 82-37

Pathophysiology of thrombus formation. (© MediVisuals, Inc., Dallas, TX.)

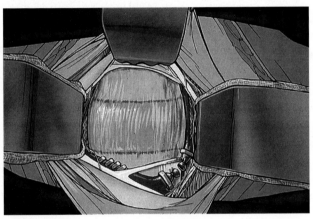

Fig. 82-38

Division of ascending lumbar vein. (© MediVisuals, Inc., Dallas, TX.)

jured, a platelet aggregate may be created, leading to a complete thrombosis (Fig. 82-37). The use of hand-held retractors can help minimize these thrombotic complications. It is imperative that these situations be recognized "on the table" and be addressed immediately. After removing the drapes, or before, evaluate the integrity of the pedal pulses and check for symmetry of temperature. If in doubt, consider the effects of possible anesthetic-induced hypotension and use Doppler to determine if there is adequate blood flow to both lower extremities. Usually femoral arteriotomy, balloon thrombectomy, or often balloon angioplasty (dilatation) is all that is necessary to correct compromised lumens if recognized and dealt with expeditiously.

The ascending lumbar vein is the first branch off the left common iliac vein. It is sometimes necessary to divide this vein to facilitate exposure. This vein is very short for its diameter and if avulsed will retract into the psoas muscle and bleed if not securely ligated prior to division. A ligature and a hemoclip should be used if this vessel is divided (Fig. 82-38).

The renal vein can be easily missed, cut into, or avulsed at the L2-L3 level when it has been stretched or compressed empty of blood. The renal artery is sometimes atherosclerotic and can be avulsed or occlude when excessive tension is applied to facilitate exposure. Many times intraoperative hemorrhage will not be the presenting sign, but postoperative hypotension may be. This may be secondary to delayed bleeding into the retroperitoneal space during the early postanesthetic period after "normotension" and intravascular volume are restored.

Often the prevertebral vessels, both arteries and veins, do not need to be divided for exposure, but when mobilizing the distal aortic vessels to the right it sometimes becomes advantageous to sacrifice these vessels for additional exposure. The veins can be easily divided between hemoclips. The arteries require three hemoclips: two on the proximal or aortic side, one on the distal side.

During the dissection, the ureter should be kept with peritoneal structures to preserve its blood supply. If it is stripped free, an ischemic segment may become somewhat fibrotic and/or stenotic over a period of weeks or months. It has also been found that an obstruction can occur from scarring in the retroperitoneal area due to an infection, if it takes a prolonged time to resolve a retroperitoneal hematoma, and/or if there is a propensity for idiopathic retroperitoneal fibrosis. If there is free blood or a clot being metabolized in the retroperitoneal space, there is the possibility of diapedesis into the urinary collecting system, resulting in hematuria. This normally clears within a few days. It is not a worrisome sign unless dissection was in the upper lumbar region involving the kidneys directly.

Impotence

The inability to obtain a penile erection is a potential problem only if dissection is carried out into the sacral plexus below the sacral promontory. Stay out of this area, as it will only cause bleeding and denervation. It does not facilitate exposure to "free up" this area. The top of the first sacral vertebral body should be the caudal end of the exposure.

Retrograde Ejaculation

This results from a violation of the sympathetic nervous system that lies as a trunk along the anterior lateral edges of the vertebral bodies and fimbriates at the L4, or more commonly the L5, level and passes either behind or on top of the common iliac vessels. Therefore, one must limit the dissection surrounding the iliac vessels.

Retrograde ejaculation is a potential and eventually unavoidable complication of dissection along the anterior spine. When it occurs, this presents a problem of insemination, not fertility or sensation. A simple and reliable solution to achieve fertilization after a retrograde ejaculation is to empty the bladder first, achieve ejaculation (into the bladder), again empty the bladder, draw up the semen in a syringe and deposit it into the vaginal vault.

Sympathetic Causalgia, or Reflex Sympathetic Syndrome

This syndrome is manifested by a cold, extremely sensitive extremity. This condition when it persists, results in atrophy of the distal musculature due to disuse. It can occur if the sympathetic trunk is damaged by traction, compression, or partial laceration. The syndrome can also arise in an extremity following a period of ischemia, which may occur when retracting the iliac vessels for prolonged periods without intermittently releasing the pressure to allow additional flow of oxygenated blood into the lower extremity. It will not occur when the sympathetic trunk has been severed completely, but then there is the possibility of postsympathectomy syndrome.

Postsympathectomy Syndrome

Postsympathectomy syndrome can be miserable and debilitating and is manifested primarily by dependent edema and pain in a warm extremity after the sympathetic trunk has been severed or severely damaged. Treatment includes elevating the involved extremity and applying custom-fitted compressive hose. Over time the symptoms may resolve. This is not a "nice" syndrome. The surgeon should take special precautions to protect the sympathetic nerves and think carefully before intentionally performing a sympathectomy.

In a less overt form, postsympathectomy syndrome presents only with unilateral warming of the affected extremity. This is usually self-limited and resolves in 6 to 12 weeks. In a smaller percentage of patients it is permanent. It is interesting that most patients wonder why the unaffected extremity is so cool, when in reality its temperature is normal.

A sympathectomy effect is frequently achieved by removing the pain generator (i.e., herniated nucleus pulposus, discogenic pain, foraminal stenosis, etc.)

that is stimulating the dorsal root ganglion and subsequently the sympathetic trunk via its connection through the gray rami communicans. The benefits of sympathectomy are achieved without the potential detrimental side effects of mechanically dividing the sympathetic chain. Frequently, patients come to the operating room with their socks on to keep their chronically cold feet warm; they awake from surgery with their "pain generators" removed, their sympathetic chains intact, and their feet warm.

Serum Sickness Syndrome

Acute and subacute postoperative problems may arise that are peculiar to patients who have undergone anterior lumbar fusion. Serum sickness syndrome is a problem that is manifested by recurrent spiking temperature curves usually beginning 24 hours after surgery and ranging from above 101.5°F to 103°F to 104°F. It is always associated with profuse sweating (soaking clothes and bed linens) and a general feeling of malaise and almost flulike symptoms, but without the nausea. When this persists into or past the third postoperative day it should be treated with a single intramuscular injection of methylprednisolone, 50 mg. Within a few hours the signs and symptoms of the syndrome should resolve. It is thought that the serum sickness syndrome results from an immune response to retained foreign protein in the allografted bone.

Inguinal Pain

Burning or discomfort can present in the first few weeks postoperatively as a result of the irritation and inflammation, and sometimes scarring, that occurs on the left side of the retroperitoneum in the area of previous dissection. This is more likely to present transiently if a hematoma or seroma developed in the retroperitoneum and is being metabolized and phagocytized and results from irritation of the genitofemoral and ileoinguinal nerves that are lying on top of the psoas muscle.

Interbody Graft Displacement

Interbody graft displacement can result in an almost immediate return of preoperative symptoms. It is important to order plain films when a person has a sudden recurrence of symptoms after a symptom-free period. If this occurs in the first 3 weeks postoperatively one may reenter through the same approach with relative ease. Later than this, tissue planes have fused together and tissues are friable, making dissection tedious. There is also the possibility of injuring both vascular and nerve structures. An extruded relatively asymptomatic graft should be left in situ if not discovered prior to 3 weeks postoperatively. If discovered later, the longer the wait prior to reentering this same area the better.

Psoas Abscess

My colleagues and I have had experience with two patients in whom psoas abscesses developed in the late postoperative period. One was 6 months post-operation, the other almost 2 years. Both had successful fusions. It is believed that the infection is a secondary blood-borne "seeding," usually from the gastrointestinal tract. The patient has increased pain, usually in the low back, lists to the affected side, and sometimes has fever and an elevated white-cell count. The diagnosis should be confirmed by CT or MRI scan. The treatment is usually open drainage, but could be done through directed needle drainage, with or without catheter placement, depending on the size of the abscess. To prevent this occurrence from being more frequent or arising in the early postoperative course, the patient should follow a simple preoperative bowel preparation regimen, including a Fleets enema the night prior to surgery. Prophylactic antibiotics that cover the gram-negative spectrum should be prescribed both preoperatively and postoperatively. The patient should not leave the hospital until he/she has had a bowel movement. If the patient has not had a movement by the third postoperative day, despite being on routine postoperative stool softeners (bulking agents), the bowels should be evacuated on the fourth day by whatever means necessary.

Summary

The pitfalls, complications, and morbidity of exposures to the anterior lumbar spine can be minimized with the development of a team approach. That team must not be passive observers, but must be actively aware of the goals to be achieved during the procedure. Efficient and careful surgical technique is important. Knowledge of what the operative goals are and when they are achieved usually results in a safe procedure. Having the appropriate, sharp instruments minimizes tissue damage and helps initiate healing. And finally, proper patient selection, as always, is the best key to obtaining a good outcome.

References

1. Crock HV: Anterior lumbar interbody fusions, indication for its use and notes on surgical technique, *Clin Orthop* 165, 1981.
2. Crock HV: Practice of spinal surgery, New York, 1983, Springer-Verlag.
3. Crock HV: Observations on the management of failed spinal operations, *J Bone Joint Surg* 58B:193, 1976.
4. Crock HV: Traumatic disc injury. In Vinken, Bruyn editors: Handbook of clinical neurology, Amsterdam, 1976, North-Holland Publishing Co.
5. Freebody D: Anterior transperitoneal lumbar fusion, *J Bone Joint Surg* 53B:617, 1971.
6. Goldner JL et al.: Anterior disc excision and interbody spinal fusion for chronic low back pain, *Orthop Clin North Am* 2:543, 1971.
7. Harmon PH: Anterior excision and verteral body fusion operation for intervertebral disk syndromes of the lower lumbar spine: three- to five-year results in 244 cases, *Clin Orthop* 26:107, 1963.
8. Hodgson AR, Stock FE: Anterior spinal fusion: the operative approach and pathological findings in 412 patients with Pott's disease of the spine, *Br J Surg* 48:172, 1960.
9. Hodgson AR, Wong SK: A description of a technic and evaluation of results in anterior spinal fusion for deranged intervertebral disc and spondylolisthesis, *Clin Orthop* 56:133, 1968.
10. Humphries AW, et al.: Anterior interbody fusion of lumbar vertebrae: a surgical technique, *Surg Clin North Am* 41:1685, 1961.
11. Johnson PM: Internal disc disruption, *J Arkansas Med Soc* 81:425, 1985.
12. Kirkaldy-Willis WH, et al.: Surgical approaches to the anterior elements of the spine: indications and techniques, *Can J Surg* 9:294, 1966.
13. Land JE Jr, Moore ES Jr: Transperitoneal approach to the intervertebral disc in the lumbar area, *Ann Surg* 127:537, 1948.
14. Sacks S: Anterior interbody fusion of the lumbar spine: indications and results in 200 cases, *Clin Orthop* 44:136, 1966.
15. Selby DK, Henderson RJ: Anterior lumbar fusion. In White, Rothman, Ray, editors: Lumbar spine surgery, St. Louis, 1987, Mosby, p 383.
16. Stauffer RN, Coventry MB: Anterior interbody lumbar spine fusion, *J Bone Joint Surg* 54A:756, 1972.

Chapter 83

Anterior Lumbar Interbody Fusion and Combined Anteroposterior Fusion

Richard M. Salib

Introduction

Biomechanics of Anterior Lumbar
  Interbody Fusion

Risks Specific to Anterior Lumbar
  Interbody Fusion

Advantages of Anterior Lumbar
  Interbody Fusion

The Role of Anterior Lumbar
  Interbody Fusion

Anterior Fusion Versus Combined
  Anteroposterior Fusion

  indications for anterior fusion
  indications for simultaneous combined
    anteroposterior fusion

Surgical Techniques

  tricortical iliac blocks
  fibular graft
  femoral cortical-cancellous composite
    allograft

Summary

Introduction

Anterior lumbar interbody fusion (ALIF) was first reported by Barber in 1933 as a technique to stabilize spondylolisthesis. Acceptance of the technique as a valuable procedure with reasonable risks has been slow. Much of the concern over the technique of ALIF has been related to the inconsistent rate of arthrodesis reported—56% to 99%[3,8-10,22,23]; and to the perception that the surgical technique has a high complication rate.[3] This technique is certainly not a procedure that is in the armamentarium of every orthopedic surgeon or neurosurgeon performing spine surgery. However, those surgeons who dedicate their practice to the spine or who have a predominance of spine surgery in their practice should learn the skills necessary to safely perform ALIF, because the technique has distinct advantages under certain situations (discussed later).

Biomechanics of Anterior Lumbar Interbody Fusion

Anterior lumbar interbody fusion increases the stiffness of the lumbar spine by 80%. There is a shift in the center of rotation of the remaining lumbar spine cephalad and anteriorly when L5-S1 is fused.[14] It can be presumed that the same would occur if L4-L5 and L5-S1 are fused. In a bilateral lateral (transverse process) fusion, the center of rotation is shifted cephalad only, and in a posterior fusion, the center of rotation is shifted cephalad and posteriorly. The shift in the center of rotation cephalad is greater with the bilateral lateral fusion than it is with an anterior interbody fusion or posterior fusion. The center of rotation of the lumbar spine has not been established for fusions combining the anterior and posterior columns.

All types of fusion result in increased motion at adjacent motion segments.[14] This may occur equally at the first and second levels above the fusion, at only the second level above the fusion, or at only the first level above the fusion. Stress to the anterior and posterior columns of the motion segment immediately cephalad to the fused segment is shifted anteriorly after an anterior interbody fusion, placing more stress on the disc. A posterior fusion places more of the stress on the facet joints, and a pure lateral fusion, with no extension of fusion dorsally, distributes the stress more equally between the disc and the facet joint.

The biomechanics of obtaining solid interbody fusion are not completely understood, but I have found that the rate of arthrodesis increases with the increased immobilization of the motion segment at the time of surgery.[21] The degree of immobilization is affected by the degree of distraction and the size of the anterior interbody graft and the degree of stability provided by posterior structures or fixation devices. Tsuji and colleagues demonstrated a statistically significant increase in the rate of fusion using autologous tricortical iliac graft when a ceramic block was placed posteriorly between the spinous process.[26] They hypothesized that this occurred because of a more evenly distributed compressive force on the graft's vertebral interface when the interspinous process block was used. The block also decreased the motion at the level of fusion. The fusion rate in their series went from 79% when the interspinous process block was not used to 98.9% when it was used. The increased rate of fusion has been observed with increased stability provided by a posterior fixation device in other types of fusion as well; therefore, it is not surprising that Tsuji and colleagues observed this increased fusion rate.[26] What is not known is how much fixation is needed to optimize the fusion rate of the various techniques of fusion. Tsuji's results parallel my own experience with anterior interbody fusions in that posterior stabilization significantly increases the rate of arthrodesis of the anterior graft. I have observed an 82% fusion rate without posterior fixation, compared with 98% with posterior pedicle fixation in a series of patients having anteroposterior fusion.[21]

Risks Specific to Anterior Lumbar Interbody Fusion

1. Damage to the nerve roots of the cauda equina resulting from posterior placement of the interbody graft or fracture of the posterior cortical margin of the vertebral body during graft insertion.
2. Injury to the superior hypogastric (sympathetic) plexus with the resultant loss of ejaculation in 0.42% of male patients, according to Flynn.[6] In one fourth of those with retrograde ejaculation the problem reverts to normal with time. The true incidence of sexual dysfunction is not known, owing to a lack of adequate documentation in all published series.
3. Impotency related to damage to the parasympa

thetic network in the presacral region occurring in 0.44%, according to Flynn.[6] This in general should not be a problem unless the exposure inadvertently is extended below the sacral promontory.

4. Injury to the vascular structures in the retroperitoneal space immediately overlying the vertebral column. The inferior vena cava and the iliac veins are very fragile and difficult to repair. Injury to the abdominal aorta or iliac arteries are more rare and more easily repaired.

5. Potential increase of pulmonary embolism or deep-vein thrombosis associated with retraction of the left iliac vein when operating on the L5-S1 or L4-L5 level.

6. Abdominal wall hernia or partial paralysis of the rectus abdominis muscle. This can be avoided with proper technique. (No more than one neurovascular bundle to the rectus abdominis muscle should be sacrificed.)

7. Reflex sympathetic dystrophy involving the left lower extremity.

Advantages of Anterior Lumbar Interbody Fusion

1. Biomechanically, anterior interbody fusion increases the axial stiffness by 80%. Bilateral lateral fusion increases stiffness by 40%, and dorsal fusion by 10%.[22]

2. Immobilizes the anterior column (disc) of the spine more effectively than posterolateral or posterior fusion.

3. Allows restoration, or at least maintenance, of normal lumbar lordosis by hyperextending the patient during the surgical procedure. Many patients in whom lumbar fusion is performed have a decreased lumbar lordosis before the surgical procedure.

4. Avoids violation of the spinal canal and its nerve roots, thus reducing the formation of scar tissue in the epidural and perineural regions of the spinal canal.

5. Offers some degree of immediate stabilization of the motion segments and restores the vertical height of the disc space, alleviating both bone and soft-tissue compression of nerve roots within the foramen and, to some degree, in the spinal canal. (A marked increase in the vertical height of the disc space is not advised in patients with adhesive arachnoiditis, because stretch on the nerve roots

may increase the pain of the tethered nerve roots.) The restoration of vertical height is more likely to be maintained when internal fixation is used.[21]

The Role of Anterior Lumbar Interbody Fusion

The advantage of completely replacing the disc with an interbody graft would clearly suggest that painful disc derangement would be the ideal indication for performance of an anterior interbody fusion. However, there has been no controlled study to determine whether or not it is necessary to actually remove the disc in situations where the disc seems to be the principal pain generator. In other words, it is not known whether the disc tissue itself has to be removed to eliminate the pain most effectively or whether simply immobilizing the disc by posterolateral fusion may provide similar results.

The principal role of ALIF today is in the salvage of difficult problems in spine surgery, such as pseudarthrosis, but if an acceptable rate of fusion (90%) can be obtained, the technique can be used whenever a fusion is indicated. In most situations more consistent results are achieved by combining anterior fusion with posterolateral fusion and/or posterior instrumentation.

Anterior Fusion Versus Combined Anteroposterior Fusion

The number of surgeons performing anterior lumbar spine fusion has clearly increased during the 1980s; however, most surgeons are using the technique of a combined anteroposterolateral fusion rather than only an anterior fusion. The primary reason for this is related to the difficulty in obtaining a high rate of fusion with an anterior fusion alone, as well as the increased experience and knowledge concerning the types of cases in which posterolateral fusion alone does not provide a high rate of fusion. Examples of situations in which the risk of pseudarthrosis by performing a posterolateral fusion (PLF) alone is particularly high are

1. Repairing a pseudarthrosis of a previously attempted posterolateral fusion.[12,13]

2. A patient with a history of cigarette smoking.

3. Multilevel fusions, particularly beyond two levels.[11,19]

4. Diabetes mellitus or other metabolic bone disorders.[22]

A combination of anteroposterior fusion (APF) has yielded a significantly higher success rate than ALIF or PLF alone in these more difficult cases. As a primary procedure, APF is gaining acceptance because it provides the highest percentage of fusions, and it appears that the clinical outcome of a spinal fusion is better if the patient can obtain solid fusion on the first attempt and is not required to undergo multiple attempts at fusion at the same level.[11,19]

Indications for Anterior Fusion

Most surgeons have found that anterior fusion at the L5-S1 motion segment is more likely to fuse than at the L4-L5 level. Repair of a pseudarthrosis of a PLF at one level is another indication for ALIF. Repair of pseudarthrosis posteriorly by performing a PLF results in a 49% to 60% fusion rate when a PLF with bone screw fixation is used.[13,14] Pettine and Salib[21] have documented a 91% fusion rate in repairing pseudarthroses by performing an anterior fusion without using any internal fixation. The addition of posterior instrumentation and posterolateral graft increased the fusion rate to 98%. There was no statistical difference between the anterior fusion and combined anteroposterolateral fusion.[16]

Mooney reported a 93.5% fusion rate with one-level anterior fusions, 88.9% with two-level anterior fusions, and 88.9% with smoking patients when a pulsed electromagnetic field (PEMF) device was used in the postoperative period.[18] More experience with PEMF is necessary before it can be recommended as being cost effective or superior or equal to the results of combined APF in obtaining a solid arthrodesis.

Indications for Simultaneous Combined Anteroposterior Fusion

When anterior and posterior fusion were first used as a means of salvaging the most difficult types of spinal conditions, it was believed by many practitioners that performing both surgical procedures at the same time would lead to higher complication rates and problems for the patient. However, all reports that have directly compared the complication rate and the cost of performing (1) an APF under two separate anesthetics 5 to 10 days apart, with (2) the simultaneously performed anterior and posterior procedures under the same anesthetic, have concluded that the complication rate, the cost, and the overall outcome of the procedure are superior when the procedures are performed under the same anesthetic.[11,20,25]

Circumstances under which I believe that the combined APF approach is valuable to obtaining a high rate of arthrodesis are

1. Repairing the pseudarthrosis of a previous PLF.

2. Fusion of more than two levels.

3. A patient who has had multiple previous laminectomies, particularly if there has been complete removal or the posterior elements and/or very small transverse processes.

Cigarette smoking by the patient is a relative indication for combined APF. Although the use of internal fixation alone in performing a PLF clearly improves the rate of fusion in patients who smoke, the addition of the anterior fusion allows the surgeon to achieve the rate of fusion which he or she would customarily see in performing a PLF in nonsmokers. Therefore, although it is not an absolute indication that a patient who smokes have an APF, one should certainly evaluate one's success rate in patients who smoke; if a low fusion rate is identified, the addition of the anterior fusion to the PLF will clearly result in a higher success rate.

Surgical Techniques

The surgical approach described by Henderson is recommended and will not be reviewed in this portion of the book. Several surgical techniques have evolved in performing ALIF. The literature contains no data to show that one technique is superior to the other. There are merely different methods, which have evolved over time. One controversial topic is whether autologous bone or allograft bone should be used. The results with autologous bone range from a 50% to an 98.9% fusion rate. In studies in which autologous bone and allograft bone have been used in the same series, no difference has been seen in the rate of fusion between the allograft bone and autologous bone for interbody fusion.[18] I have used allograft bone in all my ALIF procedures and have had a high fusion rate,[21,24] but I have not compared this to autologous bone. The success of allograft bone used in interbody fusions is difficult to explain, particularly since its use for PLFs has not been successful. Two possible explanations may be (1) in an interbody fusion, the graft is under compressive load, and (2) the bone marrow and bone precursor cells existent within the vertebral body may seep into the allograft, thus creating a more suitable environment for the replacement of the allograft bone.

Surgical Technique using Tricortical Iliac Blocks

Multiple tricortical blocks have been the most common surgical technique used for anterior interbody fusions.

Once the spine has been exposed anteriorly and the great vessels safely retracted, the anterior longitudinal ligament and the anulus are excised. The nucleus and the inner portion of the anulus, as well as the cartilaginous end plate, are removed by using a combination of rongeur or curettes. Angle curettes can be very helpful in reaching the end-plate surfaces, which are difficult to see. I have also found that, particularly at the L5-S1 level, it is extremely helpful to place the patient in Trendelenburg position, which allows better visualization of the L5 end plate. Once the cartilaginous end plate is completely removed, the cortical surface of the bone is either scarified or removed, exposing bleeding cancellous bone. It is not known whether the removal of the cortical bone leads to a higher or lower fusion rate. There are advocates of both techniques, but if the cortex is removed, care should be taken to remove as little of the cancellous bone as possible to minimize the risk of getting into the softer portion of the cancellous bone. Preparing the end plates so that they are parallel to one another makes it easier to shape the tricortical graft to fit the interspace accurately. The key to success of any anterior interbody fusion is good carpentry. It is important to leave the posterior annulus intact to avoid inadvertent placement of the graft into the spinal canal. Two or three tricortical grafts are then tightly impacted into the disc space. Care should be taken so that the cancellous portion of the graft maintains flush contact with the vertebral end plates and that none of the grafts loosen as the others are impacted. The grafts should fill the entire prepared interspace. Lee and associates have demonstrated a need to cover 30% or more of the vertebral end plate.[15]

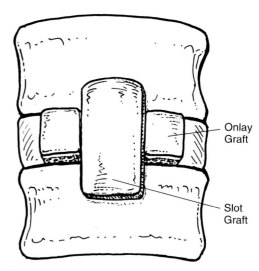

Fig. 83-1

Tricortical slot graft described by Barber[1]

Barber has described a variation on the technique of tricortical grafting in which the center tricortical graft is taller, acting as a slot graft (Fig. 83-1).[1] It is not known whether this technique has any advantages over the previously described technique.

Crock[4,5,6,9] has described another variation on the use of tricortical iliac bone in which autologous bone graft is cut from the ilium using cylinder dowel cutters. Dowel cavities are created with appropriate drills. They are slightly smaller than the cylinder dowel obtained from the iliac crest. Two dowels are then impacted into the disc space in a manner similar to the tricortical iliac block (Fig. 83-2). The potential advantage of this technique is a simplified method of carpentry, ensuring good contact of the tricortical graft with the vertebral end plates. Theoretically, there is the potential for improved stability in the rotational plane because of the round shape of the grafts, but this has not been demonstrated, nor has there been any direct comparison of the fusion rate of this technique with the standard tricortical technique.

Fibular Graft

Raney[29] and Watkins[30] have advocated the use of autologous fibular graft after repairing the interspace in the usual manner with parallel surfaces of bleeding subchondral bone. Practically speaking, this technique is limited to one level because of the amount

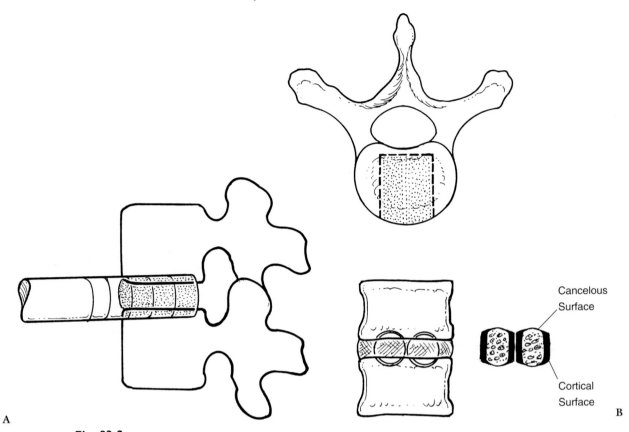

A   B

Fig. 83-2
Lower lumbar dowel cavities. **A,** The use of a dowel cutting instrument in the lumbar spine. **B,** The anteroposterior orientation of two dowel cavities in the lower lumbar area.

of fibula available from one leg. I do not know of anyone who has reported a series in which allograft fibular was used; therefore, it is not yet known whether allograft fibular would work as successfully as autologous fibula. The technique is tedious, and it is difficult to get all of the grafts to fit tightly. Incorporation of the graft will clearly be slower. Flynn has shown that it takes the average iliac crest graft approximately 2.5 years to incorporate, and the fibular graft 5.2 years to incorporate.[5]

Femoral Cortical-Cancellous Composite Allograft

The substitution of the femoral cortical-cancellous composite allograft for a tricortical graft in ALIF was first performed by Salib[28] and Brown in the same month, totally independent of one another. This technique for performing ALIF has gained wide ac-

ceptance in the United States, for at least three reasons: (1) the short supply of allograft tricortical iliac bone; (2) the fact that only a single graft is necessary to fill the interspace; and (3) this type of allograft is biomechanically stronger than two tricortical grafts, and therefore less likely to collapse.

The exposure and the preparation of the end plates is essentially the same technique used for tricortical iliac grafts. Once the cartilaginous end plates are removed, the vertebral end plates must be made parallel, with removal of as little cancellous bone as possible. Intervertebral spacers are available from a variety of companies to ensure that the end plates are parallel and the space is uniform from side to side and front to back. Distraction of the interspace is accomplished by maximum elevation of the kidney rest and extension of the table just prior to graft insertion. The typical prepared area is 30 mm across and 28 to 32 mm deep, varying with the vertebral size. A femoral diaphysis, which has been precut in

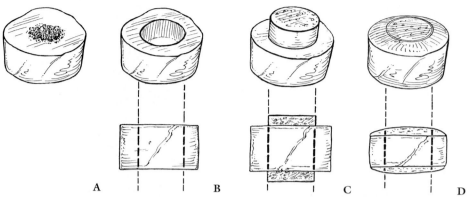

Fig. 83-3

Preparation of a composite graft from a femoral diaphyseal ring and a cancellous dowel. **A,** The average medullary canal of the femoral diaphyseal ring is too small to accept the required dowel. **B,** Ream the femoral ring to 16-18 mm in diameter. **C,** A pre-cut cancellous dowel at least 3-4 mm longer than the height of the femoral ring is driven into the femoral ring. **D,** Using a burr, bevel the graft as shown leaving the central portion 2-3 mm higher than the periphery. The height of the periphery should be the same as the space prepared. *(Modified from: Salib RM, Graber J: Femoral cortical ring plus cancellous dowel: an alternative in anterior lumbar interbody fusion. Osteotech, Inc., Shrewsbury, NJ, 1990.)*

2-mm increments of height, is selected to be from 0 to 4 mm taller than the created space. It is important to select the largest diameter graft that will fill the space prepared. The typical graft can be shaped with a burr into an oval shape, usually longer from left to right than anterior to posterior. The medullary canal of the femoral diaphyseal graft should be filled with a large amount of cancellous graft (Fig. 83-3). I have used allograft for this, but it certainly would be possible to obtain autologous bone if your preference is to use autologous cancellous graft. The minimum diameter of the cancellous graft (the minimum inside diameter of the femoral diaphysis) should be 16 mm, but is usually 18 mm. In most cases, it is necessary to ream the inner diameter of the femoral ring with a burr to obtain this size. The cancellous portion of the graft is allowed to protrude 1 mm beyond the surface of the cortex to ensure good contact between the cancellous portion of the graft and the vertebral end plates. I have recently been using femoral grafts that are between 2 and 4 mm larger than the disc space repaired, rather than exactly the same size. I then use a burr to dome both the superior and inferior surfaces of the composite graft so that the femoral cortex is the same size as the disc prepared, but the cancellous portion is 2 to 4 mm taller than the space prepared. I do not have enough experience with this modification of my technique to know whether it will result in any improved fusion rate, but it does provide

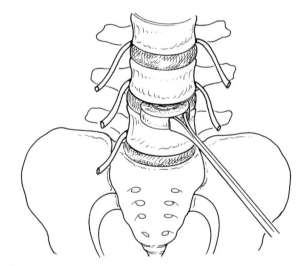

Fig. 83-4

Technique for implanting a composite graft for anterior lumbar interbody fusion. *(Modified from: Salib RM, Graber J: Femoral cortical ring plus cancellous dowel: an alternative in anterior lumbar interbody fusion. Osteotech, Inc., Shrewsbury, NJ, 1990.)*

for a tighter fit and better immobilization of the disc space and should decrease any chance of a graft displacing anteriorly. This modification was suggested by Dr. Casey Lee, who has shown that this shape appears to be more optimal than having a flat surface in contact with the vertebral end plate. Dislodgement of the graft has only occurred in cases of spondylolisthesis in which I have had no posterior fixation. Therefore, I do not see anterior displacement of the graft as a significant problem as long as the graft is put in tightly. There is the potential for improved resistance to sheer stress in rotation by doming both the graft surfaces that contact the vertebral body. Once the graft is impacted into the disc space (Fig. 83-4), the anterior cortex of the femoral allograft should rest flush with the anterior surface of the vertebral body to provide better weight-bearing lines and to minimize the chance of subsidence into the vertebral body.

This technique, in my hands, has provided a higher rate of fusion than I was able to achieve using tricortical iliac grafts. One of the problems with tricortical iliac grafts is the variation and the strength of the graft. With the femoral allograft, the compression strength is clearly not an issue. Morales and associates have demonstrated that the average femoral diaphyseal allograft can resist 15,000 pounds of compression. My experience with tricortical grafts is that if failure occurs, it usually occurs because the graft collapses and there is an area that has not been completely revascularized in the center portion of the graft. This revascularization process clearly takes a long time. This type of collapse has never been observed with the femoral allograft, but there is another problem that is seen from time to time with the femoral allograft, related to subsidence into the vertebral body. This has occurred in cases where too much of the vertebral end plate has been removed, the host is osteoporotic, or when a graft was used that did not immobilize the motion segment well enough.

Pettine,[21] reporting on the first 101 fusions using femoral allograft in my patients, reported a 98% fusion rate when internal fixation was used and an 82% fusion rate when internal fixation was not used. However, there was no statistical difference in these two groups ($p = 0.58$). Nearly all the patients who did not heal in the "no posterior fixation" group were smokers.

Posterior fixation is strongly encouraged when more than one segment is fused, regardless of the specific surgical technique used. The distraction achieved at the time of surgery will only be maintained when internal fixation is used with the femoral allograft. This cannot be said for tricortical iliac graft; however, it is important to realize that permanent distraction of the interspace is only necessary or desirable when foraminal stenosis is a concern.

Summary

In summary, anterior fusion and, more so, anterior posterior fusion of the lumbar spine is a valuable and sometimes necessary technique to salvage some of the most difficult spinal problems. There are some additional risks, but the risk of the fusion failing with other techniques must also be considered.

References

1. Barber B: *Anterior lumbar interbody fusion: step-by-step procedure and pitfalls,* In *Lumbar Spine Surgery: Techniques and Complications* St. Louis, 1987, Mosby, p 368.

2. Crock HV: Anterior lumbar interbody fusion: indications for its use and notes on surgical technique, *Clin Orthop* 165:157, 1982.

3. Crock HV: Observations on the management of failed spinal operations, *J Bone Joint Surg* 58B:193, 1976.

4. Crock HV: A short practice of spinal surgery, ed 2, Wien, 1993, Springer Verlag.

5. Flynn JC, Hogue MA: Anterior fusion of the lumbar spine: End result study with long term followup, *J Bone Joint Surg* 61A:1143, 1979.

6. Flynn JC, Price CT: Sexual complications of anterior fusion of the lumbar spine, *Spine* 9:489, 1984.

7. Fujimaki A and others: The results of 150 anterior lumbar interbody fusion operations performed by two surgeons in Australia, *Clin Orthop* 165:164, 1982.

8. Harmon PH: Anterior excision and vertebral body fusion operation for intervertebral disc syndromes of the lower lumbar spine: three to five year results in 244 cases, *Clin Orthop* 26:107, 1963.

9. Harmon PH: Anterior lumbar disc excision and fusion. I. Study of the long term results, various grafting materials, *Clin Orthop* 18:169, 1960.

10. Harmon PH: Anterior lumbar disc excision and fusion. II. Operative technique including observation upon variations in the left common iliac veins, *Clin Orthop* 18:185, 1960.

11. Kozak JA, O'Brien JP: Simultaneous combined anterior and posterior fusion: an independent analysis of a treatment for the disabled low-back pain patient, *Spine* 15:322, 1990.

12. Lauerman WC and others: Management of pseudarthrosis after arthrodesis of the spine for idiopathic scoliosis, *J Bone Joint Surg* 73A:222, 1991.

13. Lauerman WC and others: Results of lumbar pseudarthrosis repair, *J Spinal Dis* 5:149, 1992.

14. Lee CK, Langrana NA: Lumbosacral spinal fusion: a biomechanical study, *Spine* 9:574, 1984.

15. Lee CK and others: NASS general session, 1992.

16. Linson MA, Williams H: Anterior and combined anteroposterior fusion for lumbar disc pain: a preliminary study, *Spine* 16(27):143, 1991.

17. McAfee PC and others: The biomechanical and histomorphometric properties of anterior lumbar fusions: a canine model, *J Spinal Dis* 1(2):101, 1988.

18. Mooney V: A randomized double-blind prospective study of the efficacy of pulsed electromagnetic fields for interbody lumbar fusions, *Spine* 15:708, 1990.

19. Morales: A comparison of tricortical graft and femoral graft compressive strength NASS 1991

20. O'Brien JP and others: Simultaneous combined anterior and posterior fusion: a surgical solution for failed spinal surgery with a brief review of the first 150 patients, *Clin Orthop* 203:191, 1986.

21. Pettine KA, Salib RM: Anterior lumbar interbody fusion using femoral-cancellous allograft, NASS meeting, 1991.

22. Raney FL, Adams JE: Anterior lumbar disc excision and interbody fusion used as a salvage procedure, *J Bone Joint Surg* 47B:211, 1965.

23. Sacks S: Anterior interbody fusion of the lumbar spine, *J Bone Joint Surg* 47B:211, 1965.

24. Salib RM, Pettine KA: Wiltse pedicle screw and rod fixation results, NASS meeting, 1991.

25. Shufflebarger HL and others: Anterior and posterior spinal fusion: staged versus same-day surgery, *Spine* 16:930, 1991.

26. Tsuji H and others: Ceramic interspinous block (CISB) assisted anterior interbody fusion, *J Spinal Dis* 3(1):77, 1990.

27. Watkins: Personal communication

28. Zdeblick TA, Ducker TB: The use of freeze-dried allograft bone for anterior cervical fusions, *Spine* 16:726, 1991.

Chapter 84

Results of Anterior Interbody Fusion

Robert G. Watkins

Proper Review of Results

Proper Diagnostic Studies

Indications for Anterior Lumbar Surgery

    determining the need for fusion
    importance of accurate diagnosis

Preoperative Evaluation

    procedure for discography

Morbidity Criteria

There are numerous problems in evaluating fusion studies in general, particularly anterior lumbar fusion studies. Numerous methods have been used for spinal fusion. The anterior lumbar fusion appears to be, theoretically, an ideal method of stopping motion in any neuromotion segment. Because of a lack of understanding of the technique, the popularity of the operation has never matched similar operations such as the anterior cervical fusion. In the past, studies of the results of anterior lumbar fusions have varied from very high fusion rates to low fusion rates, from very high clinical success rates to low clinical success rates.

There are several problems in evaluating these papers, as well as those of other fusion methods. Prospective studies comparing fusion to nonfusion patients is quite difficult. Most studies making this comparison use patients who are being decompressed for radicular symptoms and in whom outcome depends primarily on the adequacy of the decompression, not the fusion. A better comparison would probably be between fusion patients and patients not treated, or treated nonsurgically.

Proper Review of Results

Several measures can be used in a proper review of the results of a specific operation without double-blind prospective comparisons:

1. Proper assessment of the preoperative morbidity

2. Establishing a diagnosis

3. Standardization of operative technique

4. Proper assessment of a postoperative morbidity

5. Determination of structural result such as fusion

Clinical morbidity should be determined by a scale encompassing function, pain, and occupation. In a modern society with a high unemployment rate, return to prior occupation after back surgery is hardly the sole criteria for improvement of human pain and suffering. The functional activities of the patients, their ability to become active community ambulators as opposed to bedridden patients, the ability to avoid narcotic medications, and a change from constant pain to intermittent pain may be more than enough justification for a specific operation. It is very important to know how sick are these patients who are proposed for fusion. Patients who have had a mild problem for a short time will often get well with no treatment, good nonoperative treatment, or with a safer operation. Fusion permanently changes spinal biomechanics. There is added stress and strain at adjacent levels. An unfused healed disc is better than a fused one. It is important that fusion patients have significant morbidity to warrant the operation.

The best way to judge this consistently is to use a standardized evaluation of morbidity. A proper morbidity scale should be evaluated preoperatively and at proper postoperative intervals. Documentation should be made in a standard—preferably numerical—form of the patient's pain, function, and occupational status. Subjective evaluation by the surgeon and sometimes by the patient is often inaccurate. Too often these evaluations are more a reflection of their expectations of clinical results rather than the true clinical result.

Finally, an independent reviewer is preferred when reviewing a surgeon's work.[9,10] A truly independent review is difficult to obtain. Anyone reviewing clinical material with sufficient knowledge to understand it may have some inherent biases with regard to its results.

Proper Diagnostic Studies

Proper diagnostic studies are at the heart of any review of surgical results. Without understanding the diagnosis for which the operation was performed, very little information can be determined from the results of the operation. Most fusion studies have used a great variety of methods for determining which levels to fuse: the presence of spondylolisthesis, hypermobility on motion films, hypomobility on motion films, and the presence of radiographic changes on plain x-ray films, myelograms, discograms, electromyograms (EMGs), clinical examinations, CT scanning, and different combinations of these tests. To compare one fusion study that uses myelographic changes as its indication for fusion to one that uses motion studies for its indication for fusion is quite difficult. There must be a consistent diagnosis and consistent diagnostic testing criteria to compare clinical results.

As for anterior interbody fusion, it is imperative that the surgical approach be standardized and done by the most skilled hands available for this type of surgery. There are certain inherent complications in an anterior approach to the spine, and every effort should be made to standardize the technique in the approach to keep these complications to a minimum.[32] In addition to the approach, grafting technique is a consideration. There are a number of grafting techniques available, from the dowel method[4,5,10] to fibular grafts, to tricorticate iliac crest grafts,[17,19] and autograft. For evaluation of a series of cases it is best to have the same grafting technique in all the cases. Having a great mixture of grafting techniques and bone graft used will introduce many factors into the clinical study.

Different reviewers often have a marked difference in opinion concerning what constitutes a fusion.[6] Plain radiographic evaluation of possible postoperative fusion is difficult indeed. CT scanning techniques have improved this method and may be a future source of determination of fusion. Bone scanning techniques offer a very gross evaluation of the activity of a fusion. Motion studies are probably the best method of determining stability but fall short of defining what type of tissue is present in the fusion area. Evaluation of fusion results should be a combination of radiographic appearance, as well as motion studies. Specifically, vigorous flexion/extension films with documentation of the amount of motion at a prior fusion levels should be the test to use. The margin for error in doing this measurement is not well defined.

Indications for Anterior Lumbar Surgery

Any fusion operation should proceed with the basic understanding that abnormal motion is present in the area of the spine to be fused. The spine is a multiunit, biomechanical structure in which each disc and its two facet joints combine with adjacent levels to produce a combined motion. The disc and its two facet joints, the nerves innervating that area, and the muscles and ligaments attached to that area are considered one neuromotion segment. The mechanical forces present in a neuromotion segment are a complex variety of coupled motions, for example, flexion, extension, rotation, shear, compression, and tension. A neuromotion segment is a living viscoelastic structure that responds with creep, hysteresis, stress strain, injury, and permanent deformity. The biomechanical changes in a neuromotion segment are continually evolving in response to prior stimuli. The neuromotion segment is richly innervated with sensory fibers and can respond to noxious stimuli with intense pain. Disc herniations, disc-space infections, acute annular tears, fractures, and other pathologic conditions can totally immobilize the patient with pain. It is most difficult to determine how much motion is abnormal, what type of motion is abnormal, and how much stress is needed to produce pain through an abnormal motion.

In making the decision to stop motion surgically in a neuromotion segment, one must be concerned with documenting abnormal motion and pain production from that neuromotion segment. Motion x-ray films in flexion/extension films can be of benefit, but they are hindered by the fact that the abnormal motion present may in no way be reflected as hypermobility. Very often the most inflamed, painful disc is splinted and will be moving less than an adjacent, normal disc whose hypermobility is a reflection of the pathology at the abnormal level. Flexion/extension films reflect only certain aspects of the motion present in a neuromotion segment. The best use of flexion/extension films is probably in degenerative spondylolisthesis. The operative care of degenerative spondylolisthesis is usually conducted for radicular disease and involves a decompression. The flexion/extension film is an indicator of future radicular disease due to progressive olisthesis. Flexion/extension films are a less reliable indicator of fusion for back pain in degenerative spondylolisthesis. In cervical spine disease, fusing either the stiff or the hypermobile segment for neck pain may lead to diagnostic error.

The fact that the cases in which union was achieved often do not match the cases in which the greatest clinical successes were achieved has led investigators to the skeptical opinion that fusion was not the causative factor in the patient's clinical outcome and therefore should not be a worthy therapeutic method. An anterior lumbar fusion operation may not produce a total ablation of all motion at that neuromotion segment. A pseudoarthrosis may produce a sufficient ablation of the noxious motion at that neuromotion segment and thereby produce an excellent clinical result. A pseudoarthrosis may have eliminated all the shear forces through an intervertebral disc but not eliminated 3 to 5 degrees of flexion on a vigorous flexion/extension film. Despite this possibility, any fusion operation should be designed and conducted to achieve solid bony union with no motion present in the neuromotion segment. Consistent inability to obtain solid union requires that the surgical technique and procedures be reevaluated.

A prerequisite for anterior lumbar fusion is that the pathologic condition can be affected by an operation on the anterior column of the spine. As a general rule, spinal column pain, discogenic pain, and axial pain are more likely to respond to anterior interbody fusion than posterior column pain, radicular pain, and leg pain. The latter is treated commonly by a decompressive operation of the posterior column. An ideal would be one procedure for both anterior and posterior disease. One example is anterior cervical fusion, which is indicated for and has the best results in cervical radiculopathy. Another is the posterior lumbar interbody fusion. Anterior lumbar fusions have been shown to produce significant improvement in radicular symptoms. Stopping motion in a neuromotion segment does decrease nerve-root irritation from a lesion adjacent to the nerve root, but it is important to choose the most efficient and effective method of dealing with a specific pathologic situation. A large primary space-occupying lesion, such as disc herniation or free fragment, is best removed posteriorly, whereas a nerve root scarred to a disc that is moving abnormally may best be handled with an anterior interbody fusion. Anterior lumbar fusion may or may not be the most effective method of dealing with radicular pain, depending on the cause of the radicular pain.

Determining the Need for Fusion

The first step in determining the need for anterior lumbar fusion is to determine the need for fusion. With the acknowledged difficulties in documenting the type of abnormal motion present in a neuromotion segment, clinical decision making is often on an empirical basis using indirect criteria. Criteria for fusion at the time of an initial disc herniation include a long history of mechanical back pain before the herniation and radiographic signs of abnormal mechanical stress at the disc space, such as hypermobility or traction spurs. The predictive value of the height of the disc space is questioned because the higher the disc space the greater the chance for hypermobility and instability. Yet the narrowing of early degeneration in a disc may indicate abnormal mechanical stress on an intervertebral disc and result in severe back pain but less overall motion. Relative indications for primary fusion include a massive central herniation in which the anulus is totally insufficient for any hope of normal biomechanics in that disc in the near future.

Disc herniation with spondylolysis or spondylolisthesis is an indication for fusion. Rehorniation in cases other than a reextruded fragment within the first 6 weeks is a reasonable indication that the disc has undergone sufficient damage that prophylactic fusion will improve the overall clinical result.

Age is an important consideration. Young patients are more likely to have instability from an injury or disc herniation but are more likely to heal. Fusions in young people are more likely to produce degenerative change at adjacent levels because they are under higher activity loads for longer periods of time. The young to midportion of life is the most economically productive time; thus, people are less able

to endure a long disability. Immediate fusion that ensures stability, although it may be prophylactic in nature, is often preferred over two potential periods of disability and convalescence. As patients near retirement they are usually less willing to undergo a procedure with a high complication rate just because the procedure offers hope of total perfection when successful. Physiologically, the older the patient, the less likely a fusion is needed. Neuromotion segments stiffen naturally. If symptoms are the result of spinal stenosis, the segment is usually stable. The prime time for fusion for disc disease appears to be ages 35 to 55. A clinician must be very selective in using these relative criteria for the choice of fusion in any specific patient.

Importance of Accurate Diagnosis

Diagnostic accuracy is a key to successful surgical results in most medical conditions, and spinal fusions are no exception. Obviously, if the wrong level is fused a poor clinical result can be expected. Motion studies are limited by a lack of understanding of abnormal motion in a neuromotion segment. Static studies of the spinal column are limited by our knowledge of which structural abnormalities cause pain under what biomechanical conditions. Myelographic and CT scan changes may not be the source of a patient's pain. Discography is a test commonly used to determine candidates for fusion.[11,21] Discography offers the ability to evaluate the structural integrity of the intervertebral disc through the morphologic changes seen on the discogram. Also, it allows a symptomologic reproduction of pain. The discogram reproduces the patient's pain by introducing noxious stimuli into an inflamed, irritated, or injured area. The injection of the needle, the pressure of the fluid introduced, or the chemical irritation of the fluid introduced will usually reproduce pain from an injured, symptomatic intervertebral disc. The clinician may also block the disc with local anesthetic, hopefully relieving the patient's pain.

There are difficulties encountered in interpreting discography, just as there are with other diagnostic tests. Some patients are too emotionally distraught to participate in pain-reproduction studies. Their tests will be inaccurate. Often patients with a long history of pain are too suggestible and subjectively involved in their pain to report pain reproduction accurately. When conducted accurately, discography offers the potential for identifying which neuromotion segment is responsible for the patient's pain. Further evidence can be achieved by ablation of that pain with local anesthetic. It improves the chances of an operation designed to stop motion in that neuromotion segment, relieving the patient's pain. Multilevel discography has the additional benefit of allowing evaluation of levels adjacent to that proposed for fusion. Patients with multilevel symptomatic degenerative disc disease are less likely to improve from an isolated-level fusion. Multilevel positive discography is a relative contraindication to an isolated-level interbody fusion. Multilevel discography has demonstrated cases in which the most obviously degenerated spondylolisthetic level was not the source of the patient's pain, while an adjacent, normal-appearing radiographic level was. There will be cases in which symptomatic discs on discography may not be the source of the patient's pain either.

Preoperative Evaluation

Preoperative evaluation of a patient with back pain must include some method to eliminate intrathecal tumors and high lumbar disc herniations as a source of the pain. Myelograms, contrast CT scans and/or MRI are important in this area.

Discography is a test for discogenic disease.[21] Myelograms and CT scans are a better test for radicular disease. Often the two disease processes may be present in the same patient, but they may not be. Discography should not be the diagnostic procedure of choice for a predominantly radicular clinical problem. An evaluation of potential fusion patients should pinpoint as accurately as possible the neuromotion segment or segments responsible for a patient's pain. Diagnostic accuracy is imperative in anterior fusions, and discography should be an integral part of the diagnostic work-up. Very little information can be confirmed at surgery, therefore complete reliance is on preoperative tests.

The discograms are performed under direct fluoroscopic guidance in the radiology department. The discogram need not be a terrifying ordeal for the patient. In a cooperative patient a three-level discogram could be completed in approximately 30 minutes.

Procedure for Discography

The patient is premedicated before coming to radiology, but not sedated too much to respond. A modified lateral approach is used rather than a midline approach. First and most important, the dural sac is avoided. This reduces the incidence of headaches and other side effects so frequently encountered during myelography. Second, any epidural extravasation would imply anular and ligamentous disruption and

must not be confused with potential leakage of contrast through the needle tract. In patients with clinical radicular pain, the approach used is the side opposite to their leg pain, to avoid any confusion that might occur if the lumbar nerve is encountered with the needle. The patients are placed in the prone semioblique position with a bolster under the abdomen in an effort to open up the disc spaces. After sterile preparation, local anesthesia is employed so the patient is awake and can relate any pain response on disc injection. Using fluoroscopy, exact measurements on needle placement are not needed. The procedure can be performed in the surgical suites with a mobile C-arm fluoroscopic unit. The patient is in an oblique position so that the "Scotty dog" appearance of the posterior arch is visible. After local anesthesia with lidocaine, an 18-gauge spinal needle is inserted down to the midpoint of the disc until contact with the anulus fibrosus is achieved. At certain levels it is necessary to angle the C-arm or fluoroscopic x-ray tube so that the disc space is seen in profile. If a nerve is accidentally encountered by the needle, the patient relates this to the radiologist, who subsequently repositions the needle.

There are a variety of discogram needles ranging from 3- and 3/4-in. spinal needles to 8-in. needles for obese patients. A skinny 22- or 23-gauge Chiba needle (20 cm in length) is passed through the 18-gauge needle after the stylet has been removed. The patient may feel some discomfort as the anulus is punctured. The 22-gauge needle can be manipulated by forming a curve 2 to 3 cm from its tip. This is usually necessary for the L5-S1 level, but it is generally not required for other levels. By turning the beveled needle in either direction, the needle tip can be deflected in the direction away from the bevel. Using such maneuvers, the Chiba needle is advanced until its tip is within the center of the disc space. This is confirmed with the patient either turning onto the side or stomach or by rotating the C-arm so that the disc and needle are visualized in two planes. Once the position of the needle is centrally located within the disc, contrast material is carefully injected while monitoring the flow of contrast and the patient's pain response.

With a normal disc, between 0.5 and 1 ml can be injected, whereupon there is resistance to further injection. Herniated or degenerated discs may accommodate up to 4 or 5 ml with little or no resistance. Injection should be stopped with either increased resistance to injection, frank anular rupture with extravasation of contrast, or reproduction of the patient's clinical pain. Finally, before the removal of the needle intradiscal lidocaine or bupivacaine was injected for symptomatic relief and to avoid confusing pain responses at different levels.

With this technique, there is little morbidity and discomfort to the patient. The complication rate is quite low.

Morbidity Criteria

Patients proposed for anterior lumbar fusion should have sufficient morbidity to justify an operation with potential complications that produces a spine with different biomechanics. The complication rate with anterior lumbar fusion in some reviews approaches 20%. The inherent risk of vascular complications is rarely present in posterior approaches. Careful assessment of the patient's morbidity may determine that the potential hope of success with the operation warrants the potential complications. The more disabled patients are before surgery, the more they will notice the improvement and the more tolerant they will be of complications and a failure to improve. Combining morbidity ratings with time of pain and disability offers a reasonable indication of severity of the symptoms. Not only can one establish criteria for fusion in one's own patient, but one can also have an objective assessment of clinical results.

To fuse a disc—especially in the midportion of the lumbar spine—produces unusual biomechanics. This unusual situation may be a marked improvement over the painful abnormalities present before surgery, but any realistic expectations after anterior interbody fusions would take into account that mechanics are different. There are increased stresses at adjacent levels. Patients who have suffered an injury to an intervertebral disc at one level are more likely to suffer an injury at another level. Even with normal discography at adjacent levels, degenerative changes are more likely to occur in people who have had other degenerated levels, although the chance of suffering a second totally incapacitating disabling injury will be much less. Pain from degenerative disc disease and disc injury is a ubiquitous problem. Only a fraction of patients suffering this type of pain should ever require spinal fusion.

An additional indication for fusion is a failure of nonsurgical treatment. Properly conducted nonsurgical treatment results in a very high success rate in treating patients with discogenic problems. Only after proper nonsurgical treatment methods will one have an accurate assessment of the true role of the operation in the patient's improvement. The clinician will also significantly increase the overall patient

success rate by conducting these aggressive nonsurgical treatment methods.

If it is accepted that abnormal motion is present and fusion is indicated, the method of fusion is considered immediately. The posterior approach to the spin offers a great variety of surgical procedures. There is the ability to decompress the neurologic structures and achieve stabilization after that decompression. Methods include posterior and posterolateral fusion; decompression, laminectomy, and foraminotomy with lateral fusion; decompression, lateral fusion, and internal fixation; and posterior lumbar interbody fusion. Each of these posterior methods has been conducted with good results by numerous clinicians. A brief review of specifics and difficulties with these procedures includes:

1. *Posterior and posterolateral fusion.*[30] Success with posterior and posterolateral fusion for relieving back pain alone has not been accepted as sufficient to warrant the procedure except in cases of spondylolisthesis. The amount of residual motion in the disc space after a solid posterior and posterolateral fusion may be sufficient to allow continued anular pain because of flexibility of the posterior fusion mass. The paraspinous approach does offer good exposure of the area to be fused and the ability to avoid the scarred midline area.

2. *Decompression with posterolateral fusion.* The procedure allows a maximum decompression and attempts to compensate for instability by fusing the remaining posterior elements. Decompression removes a significant portion of bone available for fusion. This may compromise the union rate and produce a greater chance of instability. There is a greater chance of pain due to motion under a solid fusion because it decreases the bulk of the fusion mass.

3. *Decompression, posterolateral fusion, and internal fixation.* Internal fixation may or may not improve fusion rates, probably depending on the method of internal fixation. The techniques of internal fixation of the lumbar spine are varied and continually under revision and, hopefully, improvement. Multilevel fixation and bone-screw fixation have great promise but will follow the same evolution of successes and failures as internal fixation in other orthopedic conditions. A successful interbody fusion offers a good chance of complete immobilization of a neuromotion segment. At least it should have a greater chance of having a profound effect on the motion of a neuromotion segment than a posterior fusion.

4. *Posterior lumbar interbody fusions* offer the opportunity for total decompression in addition to fu-

sion.[3,20] This operation is technically demanding. The usual indication for posterior lumbar interbody fusion is a postlaminectomy syndrome patient with back and radicular pain. Postlaminectomy patients are the most difficult ones on whom to perform additional back surgery because of the dural scarring; they will have the highest neurologic complication rate. Posterior lumbar interbody exposure of articular surfaces to be fused is not as good as the anterior exposure. The carpentry is less precise compared to the anterior exposure. The exposure itself causes intense scarring, and when fusion is unsuccessful it may contribute to postoperative pain.

5. *Anterior lumbar interbody fusion.* Anterior interbody fusion offers the ability to avoid prior areas of neurologic scarrings as in postlaminectomy cases and to avoid prior posterior column infected areas. It offers excellent disc exposure and the ability to use skill and precision in the carpentry of the fusion technique under direct visualization. Approaching the spine through a transperitoneal or retroperitoneal approach is similar to numerous transperitoneal and retroperitoneal operations for other conditions. The disadvantages are that decompression of neurologic structures is usually done in an indirect manner by stopping motion. Although direct removal of tissue from the posterior anulus and spinal canal through the disc space is possible, it is technically difficult. There is an approximate 10% complication rate that must be considered with the choice of an anterior lumbar fusion. Anterior lumbar fusion should be considered a one-time operation. Repeat approaches to the anterior lumbar spine have a high vascular complication rate. Biomechanical considerations of the effects of anterior resection of the anulus and anterior longitudinal ligament are unknown.

Several past published reports (Table 84-1) stand out. An overall view of experience with anterior lumbar fusion demonstrates varying success with the procedure. The best results were with one surgeon doing all the cases.* This allowed an accumulation of experience that improves results. Retrospective reviews of a number of surgeons at one institution does not show as good results.[1,7,29] Most of the cases with fewer numbers have less than ideal results.[1,7,28] Using the same grafting technique helps to compare results, but there is variance of technique between and within studies.[8,12,33]

Among the many contributions in this area, several studies offer specific information. Chow and as-

*References 2, 8, 9, 18, 22, and 28.

Table 84-1
Results of past studies

First Author	Union, %	Clinical Success, %
Calandruccio[1]	32	56
Chow[2]	63	89
Flynn[7]	67	52
Freebody[8]	85	91
Fujimaki[10]	96	76
Goldner[11]	81	82
Harmon[12]	83,99	
Harmon[14]		100
Harmon[15]	83	95
Harmon[16]	95,85	79
Hodgson[17]	83	96
Hoover[18]	70	70
Humphries[19]	78	70
Nisbet	42	74
Raney[22]	83	63
Raney[23]	81	76
Ragstad[24]	81.6	82.2
Sacks[25]	72	88
Sacks[27]		88
Sijbrandij[28]	61	
Stauffer[29]	56,64	56
Taylor	44	

sociates,[2] in relating the Hong Kong experience, reviewed 97 patients, most of whom had back and leg pain from disc disease. Using strict radiographic criteria for union of their corticocancellous autogenous iliac plugs, they showed a marked disparity between one- and two-level fusion rates—85% to 45%. There was a 95% relief of sciatica and a 32% complication rate.

Freebody's work[8,9] was standardized by technique and surgeon and was reviewed independently. The fusion rate was 92.4% with disc lesions of a lower rate with spondylolisthesis of 84.3%. The clinical success was excellent, 90%.

Goldner et al.'s review[11] has a wealth of information. Discography was used effectively, and other diagnostic methods were discussed. The diagnostic categories were defined and the technique—iliac corticocancellous plugs—explained. There was 78% relief of back pain and 85% relief of leg pain. There was an 83% overall fusion rate that decreased with multilevels.

Harmon's diagnostic criteria[12-16] are difficult to understand. He uses Panto-paque myelogram and motion studies; 244 of 650 cases were reviewed, meaning a great number of cases were not included. Those included had a strangely low complication rate of 1%, and great results of a clinical success rate of 90% and union rate of 95%.

Raney[22,23] had an 81% union rate and 76% clinical success rate using a combination of fibula and iliac crest. There is an extensive list of complications and methods to avoid them.

Ragstad et al.[24] showed a lower union rate with spondylolisthesis of 76.9% compared to an overall rate in all cases of 87.0%. There was no correlation between the 82.2% who had good success and age, duration of symptoms, duration of disability, or union.

Sacks[25-27] has published extensively on anterior lumbar fusions. Using broad indications, a mixture of autologous and allogenous graft and occasional internal fixation, he had an 88% clinical success.

Stauffer and Coventry[29] found a low 36% clinical success rate and advised use only when posterior fusion could not be done. The fusion rate was 56% and thought to be increased by a spica cast after surgery. There were no consistent diagnostic criteria or standard technique among the seven surgeons who tried the procedure over an 8-year period. This study may be a better example of the ineffectiveness of anterior lumbar interbody fusion as an occasional operation rather than an indictment of faulty mechanics resulting from the anterior approach.

Flynn and Hogue[7] had a union rate of 56% and clinical success of 52%. There was no correlation between union and clinical success. They presented retrograde ejaculation to be a transitory, overrated complication.

In a review of severe failed back patients in whom was performed an anterior lumbar fusion using a single midline strut with cancellous packing, the union rate was 77% and the clinical success rate was 90%.[33]

A composite of papers of this kind shows what type of results can be expected. It allows one to choose some factors responsible for success.

1. Experience
2. Good grafting technique
3. Safe approaches

In a retrospective review of anterior lumbar fusions I reviewed the results of another surgeon.[32] An attempt was made to evaluate all cases done within

Morbidity Ratings

Pain

1. No pain to mild pain, minimal discomfort with activity
2. Moderate pain, may take nonnarcotic medication
3. Constant low-grade or severe intermittent pain, intermittent narcotic use, may interfere with sleep
4. Constant severe pain, regular narcotic use, minimal to no relief of pain

Function

1. No impairment
2. Impairment of function
3. Inaffective community ambulator
4. Inaffective household ambulator

Occupation

1. Full-time
2. Part-time
3. Changed jobs
4. Unemployment

Table 84-2

Preoperative morbidity review of total cases

	Pain		Function		Occupation	
Scale 1	0	0%	3	3.5%	9	11%
Scale 2	7	8.5%	16	19.5%	14	17%
Scale 3	16	19.5%	24	29%	16	20%
Scale 4	59	72%	39	48%	43	52%
TOTAL	82		82		82	

the certain period of time. There was good clinical chart data on 82 patients; 60 were seen in follow-up.

The preoperative and postoperative morbidity was assessed by comparison of three categories of pain, function, and occupation (see box). The severity of preoperative morbidity is critical in justifying the operation (Table 84-2). The patients had 85 months with preoperative back pain and averaged 32 months of preoperative disability. Using the rating scales (Tables 84-3 to 84-5), the patients showed an average disability of 3.37, with 1 being minimum dis-

Table 84-3

Preoperative and postoperative pain ratings of patients available for review

Scale	Preoperative		Postoperative	
1	0	0%	26	43%
2	6	10%	25	42%
3	13	22%	3	5%
4	41	68%	6	10%
TOTAL	60		60	

Table 84-4

Preoperative and postoperative function ratings of patients available for review

Scale	Preoperative		Postoperative	
1	3	5%	22	37%
2	12	20%	24	40%
3	19	32%	10	17%
4	26	43%	4	6%
TOTAL	60		60	

Table 84-5

Preoperative and postoperative occupation ratings of patients available for review

Scale	Preoperative		Postoperative	
1	8	13%	22	42%
2	8	13%	6	12%
3	10	17%	9	17%
4	34	57%	15	29%
TOTAL	60		52	

ability and 4 being the maximum. A 4 rating would be unable to work, bedridden, or on narcotics because of spinal pain. Of all the patients, 53% were work compensation cases, most were laborers or housewives, and 49% had at least one prior laminectomy.

The diagnosis for these patients was segmental instability. To condense the diagnostic criteria the patients had a history of mechanical and/or radicular pain with activity; 80% had positive straight leg rais-

ings. Surgical decisions were based predominantly on multilevel discography. All patients had discography, and 60% had myelography, an important adjunctive test. Discography showed abnormal configuration, reproduced the patient's symptoms, and usually allowed symptom blocking with local anesthesia at each level to be fused.

The technique was the transperitoneal approach, iliac crest (autogenous and allogenous) tricorticate plugs after disc space distraction and chiseling of the endplate.

The postoperative clinical improvement was dramatic—91% improved, 6% remained the same, and 3% worsened (Table 84-6). The morbidity ratings fell from 3.37 to 2.03; 41% improved their occupational rating.

The union rate was determined by flexion/extension films and radiographic appearance; 2 degrees of motion was labeled a nonunion. The union rate was 60%. Although it is significantly low, it had no correlation with clinical improvement. A significant number of fibrous unions and nonunions showed clinical improvement.

Postlaminectomy patients showed improvement equal to primary surgical patients. This may be an indication that anterior lumbar fusion is a reasonable choice for postlaminectomy patients because most other operative methods would have a lower success rate compared to primary surgery. Also, when worker's compensation cases with morbidity ratings of 3 to 4 in every category were reviewed as a separate group, they had an excellent recovery rate, indicating that anterior lumbar fusion has a role as a salvage operation for difficult patients (Table 84-7).

What are the indications for anterior lumbar interbody fusion? The ideal case is a patient who has had multiple operations, who is totally disabled with back and with leg pain. Discography is positive at one level (L4-L5) only, without spondylolisthesis. In discussing indications an assumption is made that the patient has sufficient morbidity and failure to respond to nonsurgical care to warrant an operation. It is best that the problem be confined to one or two levels with normal adjacent levels confirmed by discography. Relative indications include:

1. Primary large central disc herniation
2. Anular tear and segmental instability of an intervertebral disc
3. Primary disc herniation with a long history of disabling back pain
4. Postlaminectomy syndrome resulting from segmental instability
5. In combination with a posterior fusion and instrumentation for instability or deformity

Table 84-6

Clinical improvement

	Number	Percent
Improved	55	91
Same	4	6
Worse	1	3

Table 84-7

Postoperative clinical success rate in severely disabled patients (rating 3 and 4)

	Pain	Function	Occupation
GENERAL POPULATION			
Asymptomatic	40%	19%	22%
Improved	47%	44%	19%
Same	11%	6%	27%
Worse	2%	0%	2%
SEVERELY DISABLED WORKER'S COMPENSATION CASES			
Asymptomatic	22%	20%	9%
Improved	61%	73%	36%
Same	12%	7%	46%
Worse	5%	0%	9%

6. In combination with anterior instrumentation in lumbar scoliosis

Special circumstances in which anterior lumbar fusion has distinct advantages over other methods include:

1. More back pain than leg pain
2. Scar around nerve and posterior elements
3. Posterior pseudarthrosis
4. Prior posterior infection
5. Disc space infection

When choosing anterior lumbar fusion as treatment for a lumbar spine problem, a surgeon should be comfortable with not only the technique of the operation but also the philosophy of the operation. Being well trained and knowledgeable concerning anterior lumbar fusions requires a reasonable number of cases to become proficient. Most surgeons performing this operation come in three groupings.

1. The surgeon who rejects entirely interbody fusion as a treatment for disc damage producing back pain regardless of the amount of pain and any concomitant conditions such as sciatica. These surgeons may use anterior lumbar fusion for lumbar scoliosis, disc-space infection, and fractures only.

2. The second group of anterior lumbar surgeons consists of those who reserve the operation for the most difficult of lumbar spine disc problems. This includes circumferential fusions for certain types of lumbar instabilities such as spondylolisthesis, posterior pseudarthrosis, posterior infection, kyphotic deformities, and failed surgery cases with predominantly back pain.

3. The third category of surgeons includes the most frequent users of anterior lumbar fusion. They would use anterior lumbar fusion, in addition to the indications outlined above, for primary disc herniations, postlaminectomy syndrome, an anular tear of the intervertebral disc with back pain only, and degenerative spondylolisthesis. These surgeons believe in the use of discography and anterior lumbar fusion as surgical treatment for incapacitating pain from the anulus of the intervertebral disc. It becomes a primary surgical procedure.

Some parameters of application for anterior lumbar fusion have been presented, but its exact role in the operative care of the lumbar spine may ultimately be an individual clinical-patient decision.

References

1. Calandruccio RA, Benton BF: Anterior lumbar fusion, *Clin Orthop* 35:63, 1964.
2. Chow SP, et al.: Anterior spinal fusion for deranged lumbar intervertebral discs, *Spine* 5:452, 1980.
3. Cloward RB: Spondylolisthesis: treatment by laminectomy and posterior interbody fusion: review of 100 cases, *Clin Orthop* 154:74, 1981.
4. Crock HV: Observations on the management of failed spinal operations, *J Bone Joint Surg* 58B:193, 1976.
5. Crock HV: Anterior lumbar interbody fusion: indications for its use and notes on surgical technique, *Clin Orthop* 165:157, 1982.
6. DePalma AF, Rothman RH: The nature of pseudoarthrosis, *Clin Orthop* 59:113, 1968.
7. Flynn JC, Hogue MA: Anterior fusion of the lumbar spine, *J Bone Joint Surg* 61A:114B, 1979.
8. Freebody D: Treatment of spondylolisthesis by anterior fusion via the transperitoneal route, *J Bone Joint Surg* 46B:788, 1964.
9. Freebody D, et al.: Anterior transperitoneal lumbar fusion, *J Bone Joint Surg* 53B:617, 1971.
10. Fujimaki A, et al.: The results of 150 anterior lumbar interbody fusion operations performed by two surgeons in Australia, *Clin Orthop* 165:164, 1982.
11. Goldner JL, et al.: Anterior disc excision and interbody spinal fusion for chronic low back pain, *Orthop Clin North Am* 2:543, 1971.

12. Harmon PH: Experiences with anterior interbody spinal fusion, *J Bone Joint Surg* 41A:562, 1959.

13. Harmon PH: Operative technique and some ten year end results from abdominal disc excision and vertebral body fusions in the lumbar spine, *J Bone Joint Surg* 41A:1355, 1959.

14. Harmon PH: Anterior lumbar disc excision and fusion. I. Study of the long term results, various grafting materials, *Clin Orthop* 18:196, 1960.

15. Harmon PH: Anterior lumbar disc excision and fusion. II. Operative technique including observation upon variations in the left common iliac veins, *Clin Orthop* 18:185, 1960.

16. Harmon PH: Anterior excision and vertebral body fusion operation for intervertebral disc syndromes of the lower lumbar spine: three to five year results in 244 cases, *Clin Orthop* 26:107, 1963.

17. Hodgson AR, Wong SK: A description of a technique and evaluation of results in anterior spinal fusion for deranted intervertebral disc and spondylolisthesis, *Clin Orthop* 56:133, 1968.

18. Hoover NW: Indications for fusion at the time of removal of intervertebral disc, *J Bone Joint Surg* 50A:189, 1968.

19. Humphries AW, et al.: Anterior interbody fusion of the lumbar vertebrae: a surgical technique, *Surg Clin North Am* 41:1685, 1961.

20. Hutter CG: General orthopedics: posterior intervertebral body fusion, 25 year study, *Clin Orthop* 179:86, 1983.

21. Kingston S, Watkins RG: *Principles and techniques of spine surgery*, Baltimore, 1986, Aspen Systems.

22. Raney FL Jr, Adams JE: Anterior lumbar disc excision and interbody fusion used as a salvage procedure (proceedings of the Western Orthopedic Association), *J Bone Joint Surg* 45A:667, 1963.

23. Raney FL Jr: Anterior lumbar interbody fusion, *Spinal Disorders* 162, 1977.

24. Ragstad TS, et al: *Acta Orthop Scand* 53:561, 1982.

25. Sacks S: Anterior interbody fusion of the lumbar spine, *J Bone Joint Surg* 47B:211, 1965.

26. Sacks S: Experiences with posterior, anterior and posterolateral spine fusions, *J West Pacific Orthop Assoc* 6(1):187, 1969.

27. Sacks S: Anterior spinal surgery in Ballarat (proceedings of the Australian Orthopedic Association), *J Bone Joint Surg* 52B:392, 1970.

28. Sijbrandij S: The value of anterior interbody vertebral fusion in the treatment of lumbosacral insufficiency, with special reference to spondylolisthesis, *Arch Chir Neeland* 14:37, 1962.

29. Stauffer RG, Coventry MD: Anterior interbody lumbar spine fusion, *J Bone Joint Surg* 54A(4):756, 1972.

30. Watkins MB: Posterolateral bone grafting for fusion of the lumbar and lumbosacral spine, *J Bone Joint Surg* 41A:388, 1959.

31. Watkins RG: *Surgical approaches to the spine*, New York, 1983, Springer-Verlag.

32. Watkins RG: Anterior interbody fusion: a clinical review. Presented at the American Academy of Orthopedic Surgeons meeting, Las Vegas (Submitted for publication).

33. Watkins RG, et al.: Comparisons of preoperative and postoperative MMPI data in chronic back patients treated by anterior lumbar fusion, *Spine*, 1985 (In press).

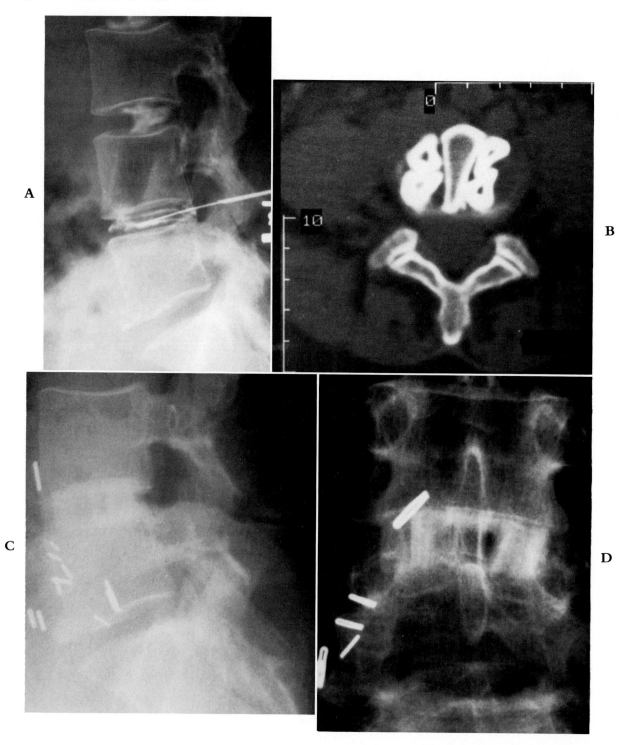

Fig. 84-1

A, 39-year-old woman who had 10-year history of recurring episodes of mechanical axial back pain. With childbirth and delivery patient developed excruciatingly severe back pain that predominantly confined her to bed rest for 6 months before evaluation. Patient had severe mechanical back pain that increased on coughing, sneezing, and straining. There was no radiculitis or radiculopathy. Myelogram and CT scan (not shown) had no evidence of intracanal lesion. Preoperative discography demonstrated normal levels at L2-L3, L3-L4, L5-S1, and symptomatic abnormal discography at L4-L5. L4-L5 disc was blocked with local anesthetic, producing significant relief in patient's symptoms. **B,** Postoperative CT scan showing 4 fibula and 1 iliac crest graft. **C** and **D,** At follow-up, patient is totally asymptomatic with no motion present in disc space.

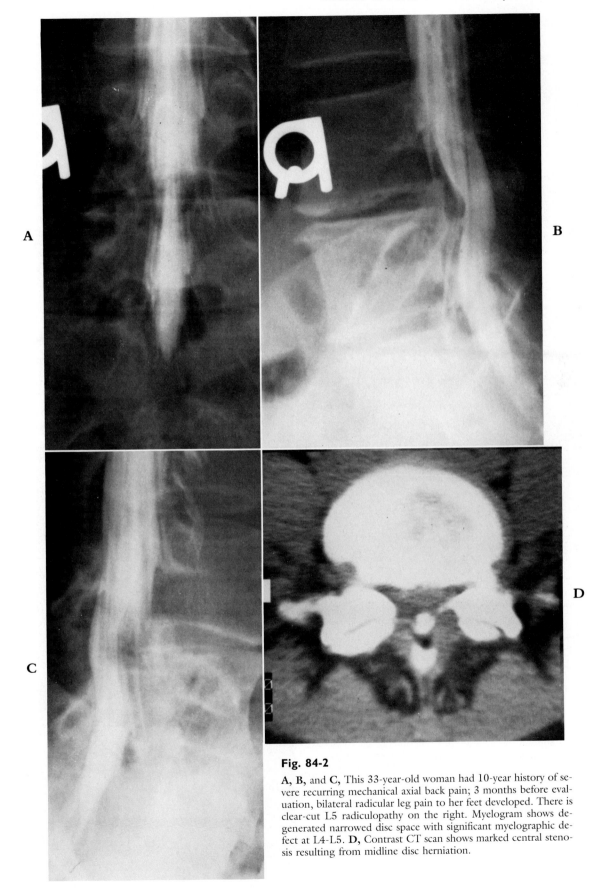

Fig. 84-2

A, B, and **C,** This 33-year-old woman had 10-year history of severe recurring mechanical axial back pain; 3 months before evaluation, bilateral radicular leg pain to her feet developed. There is clear-cut L5 radiculopathy on the right. Myelogram shows degenerated narrowed disc space with significant myelographic defect at L4-L5. **D,** Contrast CT scan shows marked central stenosis resulting from midline disc herniation.

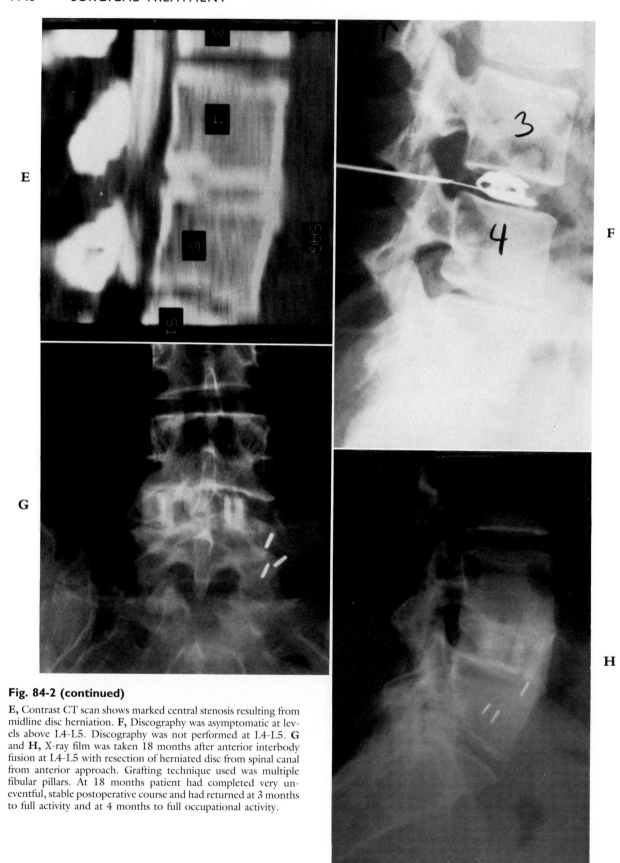

Fig. 84-2 (continued)

E, Contrast CT scan shows marked central stenosis resulting from midline disc herniation. F, Discography was asymptomatic at levels above L4-L5. Discography was not performed at L4-L5. G and H, X-ray film was taken 18 months after anterior interbody fusion at L4-L5 with resection of herniated disc from spinal canal from anterior approach. Grafting technique used was multiple fibular pillars. At 18 months patient had completed very uneventful, stable postoperative course and had returned at 3 months to full activity and at 4 months to full occupational activity.

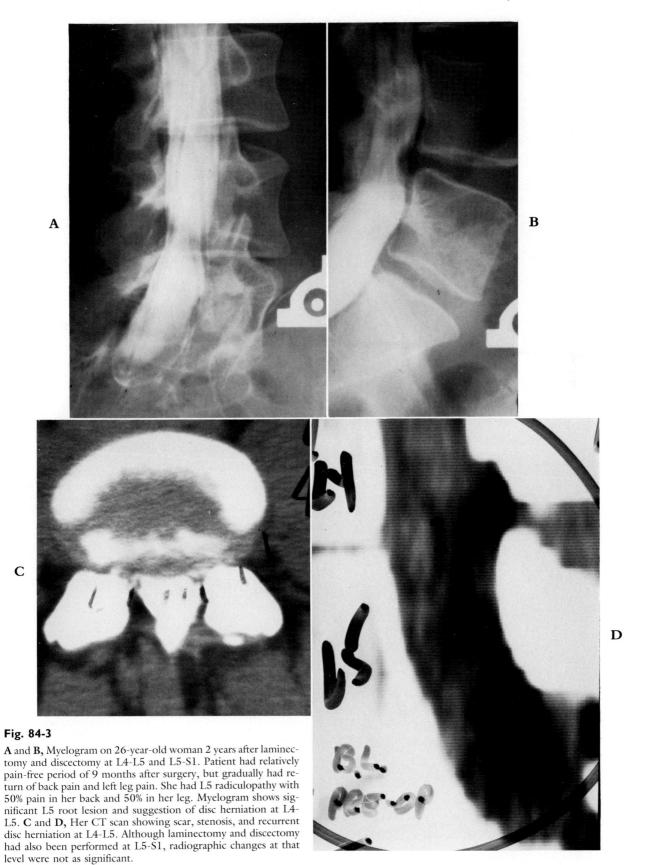

Fig. 84-3

A and **B,** Myelogram on 26-year-old woman 2 years after laminectomy and discectomy at L4-L5 and L5-S1. Patient had relatively
pain-free period of 9 months after surgery, but gradually had return of back pain and left leg pain. She had L5 radiculopathy with
50% pain in her back and 50% in her leg. Myelogram shows significant L5 root lesion and suggestion of disc herniation at L4-
L5. **C** and **D,** Her CT scan showing scar, stenosis, and recurrent
disc herniation at L4-L5. Although laminectomy and discectomy
had also been performed at L5-S1, radiographic changes at that
level were not as significant.

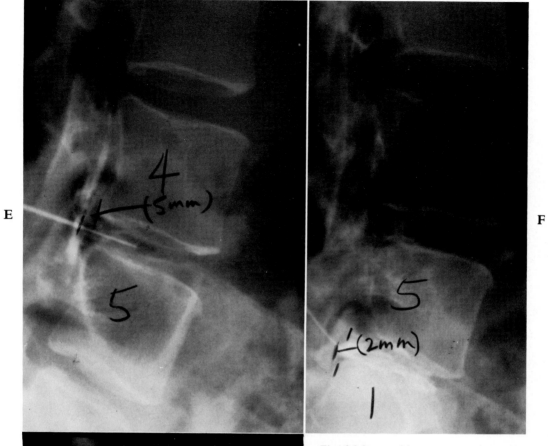

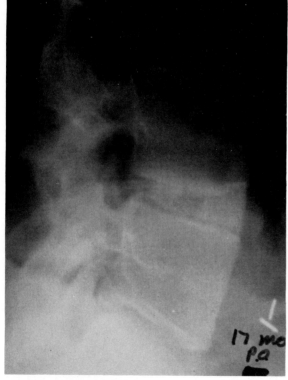

Fig. 84-3, cont'd

E and **F,** Discography at L2-L3 and L3-L4 were negative. Discography at L4-L5 reproduced patient's pain exactly and allowed for partial ablation of pain with local anesthetic injection. L5-S1 disc was asymptomatic on discography. **G,** X-ray film was done 17 months after anterior interbody fusion using fibular graft. Patient is totally asymptomatic, has returned to work, and is working in body reconditioning program. It was elected not to fuse L5-S1 level because patient had minimal symptoms from that area, had clear-cut myelographic, CT scan, discographic lesion at L4-L5 that matched her clinical symptoms.

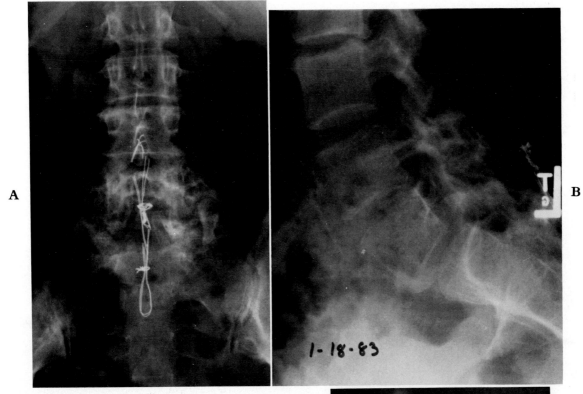

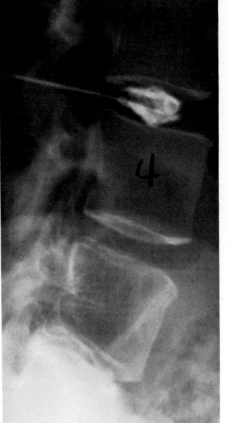

Fig. 84-4

This 41-year-old woman had history of three prior spine operations, the last a posterior and posterolateral fusion at L4 to S1.
She was pain-free approximately 6 months and then developed
severe back and radiating leg pain. Her pain was with forward
bending and had a reproducible mechanical component. Discography could not be performed because of size of posterior fusion
mass, but motion was measured through center of fusion mass,
indicating pseudarthrosis. **C,** Discography at level above fusion
mass proved to be negative. There is narrowing of L2-L3 disc
space. This was asymptomatic on discography.

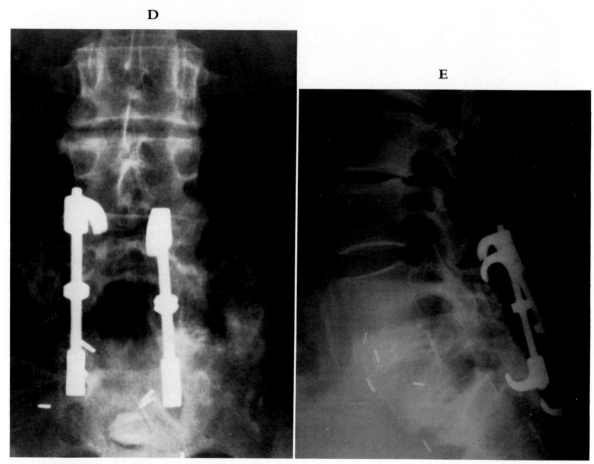

Fig. 84-4 (continued)

D and **E,** Patient underwent two-stage anterior and posterior fusion, first stage being posterior pseudarthrosis resection, regrafting and Knodt rod internal instrumentation. Bony bed posteriorly for re-grafting was very poor. Second stage was two-level anterior lumbar fusion. Patient has had marked symptomatic improvement but is still unable to work 2 years after surgery. Poor quality of bone posteriorly was believed to be totally inadequate for posterior refusion.

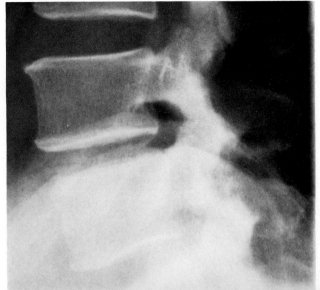

A

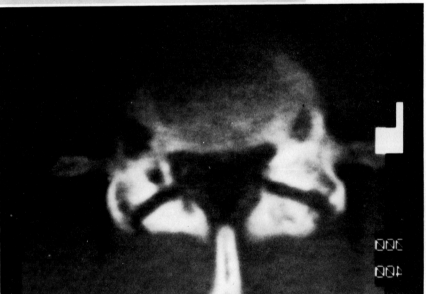

B

Fig. 84-5

A, This 46-year-old man had history of 6 months of back and leg pain before evaluation by orthopedic surgeon. Based on positive myelogram and CT scan for disc herniation, patient underwent chemonucleolysis. **B,** CT scan taken 30 days after surgery reveals evidence of infection. Patient had normal sedimentation rate and was afebrile, but he had extreme back pain with drop foot on left. Based on this CT scan he underwent major posterior decompression and debridement. Postoperative cultures were negative, but they showed intense red granulation tissue. **C,** CT scan done 11 months after laminectomy shows that total facetectomy and laminectomy had been carried out. Patient had return of significant back and leg pain after 3-month pain-free interval.

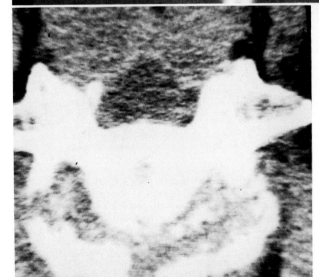

C

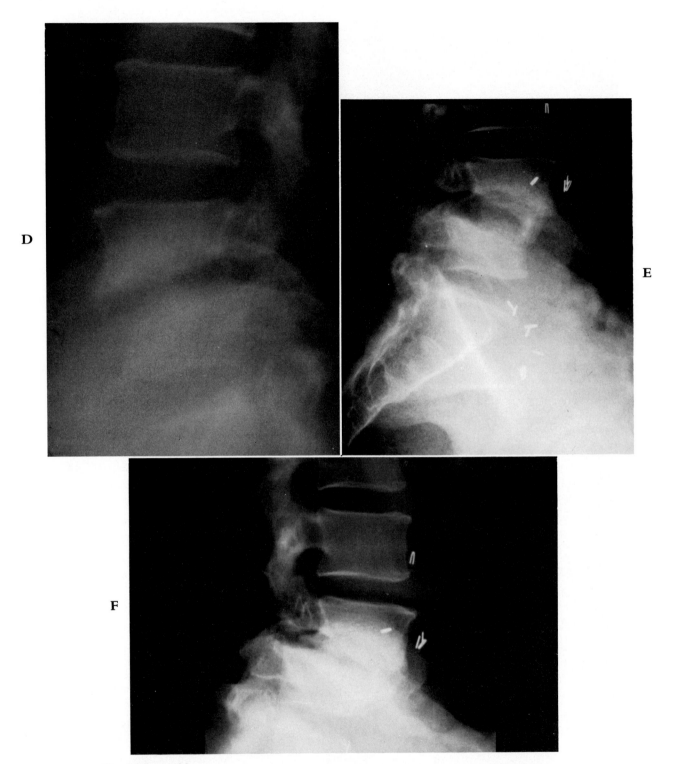

Fig. 84-5 cont'd

D, Patient's x-ray film, demonstrating what appears to be an infection; 11 months after surgery the patient had a Craig needle biopsy, revealed no evidence of infection or reactive bone. Cultures were negative. Sedimentation rate was 28. At this point patient has excruciating back pain, is unable to ambulate, and is unrelieved by narcotic medication. **E,** Immediate postsurgical films demonstrate satisfactory disc space distraction and graft in place. Anterior fusion was carried out after anterior debridement revealed no evidence of infection on Gram's stain or frozen section. There was excellent bleeding and clean bone for grafting surface. Autogenous iliac crest was used. **F,** Graft collapse and suggestions of early fusion 8 months after surgery. Patient is asymptomatic.

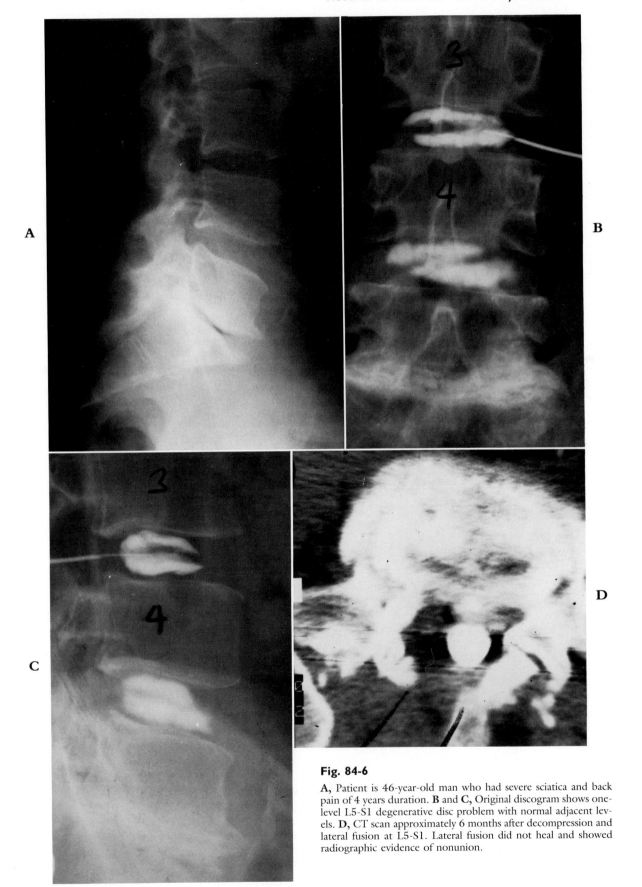

Fig. 84-6

A, Patient is 46-year-old man who had severe sciatica and back pain of 4 years duration. **B** and **C,** Original discogram shows one-level L5-S1 degenerative disc problem with normal adjacent levels. **D,** CT scan approximately 6 months after decompression and lateral fusion at L5-S1. Lateral fusion did not heal and showed radiographic evidence of nonunion.

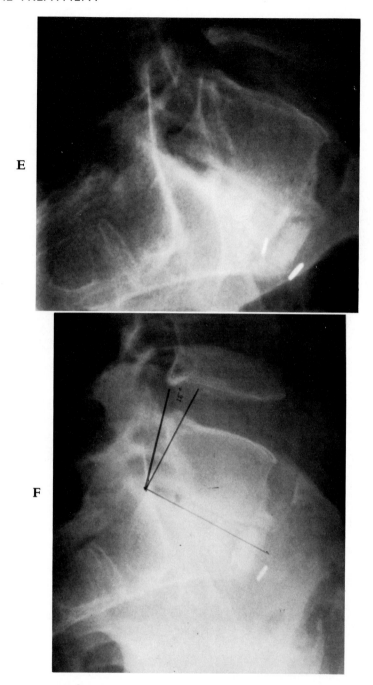

Fig. 84-6, cont'd

E, Immediate postsurgical anterior lumbar fusion demonstrating distraction of disc space. F, Follow-up film showing progression of satisfactory union with no motion on flexion/extension films. There is improvement in symptomatology at 16 months after surgery.

Chapter 85
Anatomic Strategies of Internal Fixation
R. Charles Ray

Spinous Process

Lamina

    hooks

    sublaminar wires

Facet-Joint Fixation

Pedicle Fixation

Vertebral Bodies

Disc Space

Lumbosacral-Junction Fixation

Future Trends

The concept of rigid bony fixation to secure proper anatomic alignment and hold it while bony union occurs while simultaneously allowing adjacent segment motion is one that is well accepted in the treatment of extremity fractures. The acceptance of these principles by the spinal surgery community has been slow for several reasons.

First of all, there has been a lack of adequately controlled studies documenting the efficacy of internal fixation in achieving successful arthrodesis. Spine fusion rates without internal fixation have been quoted anywhere from 56% to 90%[56] successful, and fusion rates with internal fixation have shown a similar spread. Only recently have prospective studies such as Zdeblick's[61] shown an improvement in, not only healing rates, but also clinical satisfaction with rigid internal fixation.

The second reason for poor acceptance of internal fixation in the lumbar spine has been the poor tools and techniques we have had for accomplishing our goals. The development of adequate fixation implants has been stymied by government bureaucracy as well as by the difficulty of the task itself. Unlike other parts of the body, the spine often presents us with poor quality of bone for fixation, leading to instrumentation failure at the bone-implant junction. Our techniques of transverse process fusions are a holdover from Brittain,[11] an engineer by training, who developed extraarticular fusion techniques to avoid opening of septic tuberculous joints. Current lumbar spine fusion techniques often leave the surrounding muscles denervated and devascularized. A femoral rodding technique that routinely left the quadriceps a noncontractile mass of scar tissue would never be accepted as a reasonable form of treatment, but such results are accepted in the lumbar spine. This is all complicated by the difficulty even in assessing whether the fusion has successfully united the segments the surgeon was attempting to fuse.[12] We have been slow to appreciate the three-column significance of the spine, trying to accomplish everything from one column or another. The importance of load sharing between the posterior implants and anterior structures has become obvious with the more rigid posterior implants, which fail more dramatically than their weaker predecessors, which merely loosened allowing the spine to sag into malalignment.

We also have been slow in sorting out the issues in back pain as a clinical phenomenon. When the spine is realigned, painful joints are solidly fused, nerve-root pressure has been relieved, but the patient still complains bitterly of pain, is this a problem with our fixation, with our fusion strategy, or with one of the myriad other problems that beset our patients that has nothing to do with the spine itself?

To get a broad view of internal fixation strategies, the bone-implant junctions from an anatomic standpoint will be examined. The current choices of materials and how the current systems have been put together will be reviewed. Third, what is needed for the implant system of the future will be summarized.

Spinous Process

The spinous process was the first structure used for internal fixation in the spine. Hadra[26] of Galveston used a figure-eight silver wire in 1891 in the treatment of a cervical fracture. Albee[1] popularized the interspinous process fusion originally described in 1911. Since he used a tibial graft held in place by sutures, this construct was of questionable significance as far as internal fixation is concerned. In 1931 Gibson[25] used a tibial graft that blocked extension by fitting snugly between the bases of the spinous processes. The "clothespin" graft, as it has been called, was recognized to restore facet alignment, reduce lumbar lordosis, and open intervertebral foramina. It had the added advantage of not using metal. The Wilson[60] plate described in 1952 used metal on one side of the spinous process for stability and bone graft bolted to the other side for the fusion mass.

The simplest construct for spinous process fixation remains the tension band wire, either in the form of a simple loop placed through holes or around the ends of the spinous process as a whole. Converting this to a figure-eight changes little in the properties of the fixation. This construct, which restricts flexion only, tends to cut through bone with the same principle used to make cheese cutters. With the current emphasis on adequate decompression, the spinous process is seldom left totally intact. The bone quality is mostly cancellous with a very thin cortical shell and hence is a poor choice in the lumbar spine in terms of relative strength for a fixation device.

The area of the junction of the spinous process with the lamina has been proposed as an alternative to sublaminar wiring. Drummond et al.[21] have developed a fixation technique using the relatively strong bone in the junctional area of the spinous process and the lamina. The forces on the cortex are dissipated by using a washer buttress for the wire. This increases pull-out strength by 40% over the wire alone. This technique is used with doubled rods for multiple level fixation as a safer alternative than sublaminar wiring.

Lamina

The lamina historically has been the most commonly used area of lumbar fixation before the recent popularization of pedicle fixation. It can be thinned and partially resected for decompression while still maintaining adequate strength for fixation. Laminar fixation takes the form of hooks or wires.

Hooks

All systems designed for thoracic and lumbar instrumentation include a various assortment of hook shapes and sizes based on the original design of Harrington.[27] They have been modified to improve fit along anatomic lines and minimize intrusion into the canal. Building on Harrington's ideas with his threaded rod, Cotrel et al.[20] perfected the concept of placing hooks anywhere along an anatomically contoured rod while providing both distraction and/or compression at different levels in the same rod. Prior to this, distraction instrumentation in the lumbar area, such as Harrington or Knodt rods,

while opening intervertebral foramina, tended to reduce the normal lumbar lordosis and produce a "flat back" syndrome.[9,45,59]

With distraction instrumentation, even if the rod is bent into lordosis, distraction on the posterior elements produces a kyphosis at the top level of the instrumented segment. This can be prevented by reversing the top hook to capture the top segment in a "claw" configuration (Fig. 85-1). This can be done with either two hooks on the same lamina or two adjacent levels. Roach et al.[47] have shown that a claw across two levels is nearly the same strength as a claw across one. Since the length of the lamina is limited, a claw can also be constructed with the opposing hooks on two different rods if the rods are rigidly linked together.

Sublaminar Wires

Luque[39] was the first to popularize an entire system based on sublaminar wires. This allowed for correction of scoliotic and some kyphotic deformities, except spondylolisthesis reduction. While being a rea-

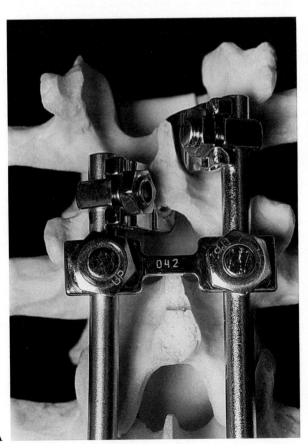
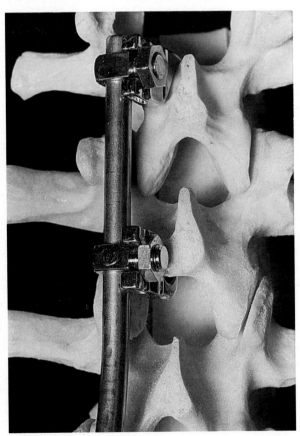

A   B

Fig. 85-1
Hooks. **A,** Single-level claw with two rods and cross link. **B,** Two-level claw with one rod.

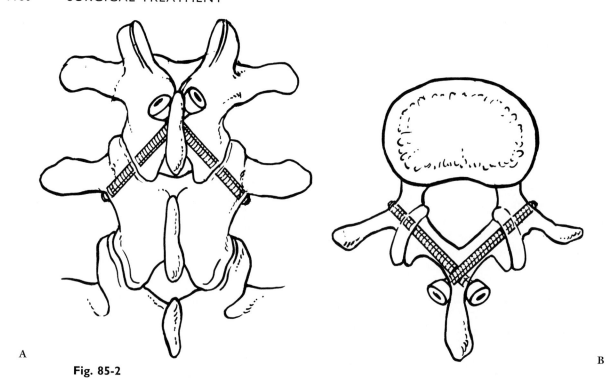

A   B

Fig. 85-2

Mangerl's facet joint fixation. *(From Magerl F: Stabilization of the lower thoracic and lumbar spine with external skeletal fixation,* Clin Orthop *189:128, 1984.)*

sonable fracture and scoliosis system, it had several problems in the lumbar spine. First, sublaminar wire fixation to the sacrum is difficult because of the small or absent lamina and often requires wiring into the body of the lateral mass or ala. Second, the junction between the wire, rod, and lamina is not a rigid construct and allows some motion to persist in short segment constructs, especially with axial compression and rotation.[4] With the advent of multistrand[55] titanium and stainless steel cables that are stronger and more fatigue-resistant than single-strand stainless steel wires, some renewed interest is being shown in this type of fixation. The titanium cable overcomes the poor fatigue strength of single-strand titanium wire. The flexible cable is probably safer to handle in the patient as well.

Facet-Joint Fixation

Since the spine moves at the disc and facet joints and since facet-joint degeneration like other arthritic joints in the body seems to be a common cause of back pain, it seems reasonable to approach the treatment of back pain by fixating and fusing the arthritic joints themselves. In 1948 King[33] described a method of facet-joint fixation using short screws directly across the facet. Boucher[8] modified this pro-

cedure using longer screws in a more oblique direction toward the junction of the pedicle and the transverse process. Magerl[40] further modified the technique into a translaminar, transfacet-into-upper-pedicle-type path by starting the screw on the contralateral side of the spinous process (Fig. 85-2). This technique does require additional small incisions to accommodate the oblique path of the drill and screwdriver but should avoid the possibility of nerve-root injury. Two such cases described by Boucher were thought by him to be due to improper screw placement. Proper screw direction is aided by an end-point aiming guide. This technique, while not the strongest available, does require less metallic bulk under the paraspinal muscles than any pedicle-fixation system. Renewed interest in minimal invasive technique for fusions has led to a renewed interest in this concept.

Pedicle Fixation

Pedicular fixation has a varied history of contributors. Roy-Camille[49] is generally considered to be the father of this technique. Schoellner[53] described the reduction of a spondylolisthetic slip with a dual threaded screw attached to a plate. Louis[37,38] described a simple lumbosacral plate with multiple

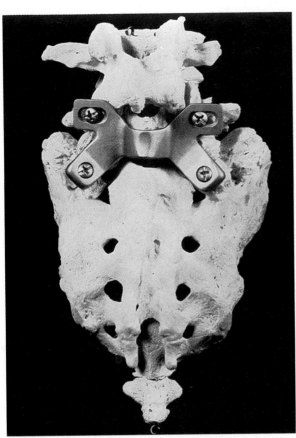

Fig. 85-3

Louis plate and bone-screw fixation. *(From Louis R: Fusion of the lumbar and sacral spine by internal fixation with screw plates, Clin Orthop 203:18, 1986.)*

screws that attached to one or two lumbar levels bilaterally (Fig. 85-3). The first American to design and implant a pedicle screw was Harrington, who used it for spondylolisthesis reduction in 1965.[28] The concept of pedicular fixation is an attractive one. The pedicles are seldom involved in decompressive resection. The quality of bone varies from nearly all cortical in the young patient, to a thin cortical tube in the elderly but is usually the strongest area in a particular vertebra. Steffee et al.,[57] who have done a great deal to popularize this technique (Fig. 85-4), have described the pedicle as the "force nucleus," where all the posterior forces can be transmitted anteriorly to the vertebral body. Zindrick et al.[63] have studied the anatomic morphology of the pedicles. The important lesson is that the cross-sectional diameter varies between individuals and between levels in the same individual. Likewise, the longitudinal axis of the pedicle and the angle it makes medially with the floor of the canal varies in a fairly consistent manner at different lumbar levels. This becomes important when an instrumentation system does not allow for these differences, forcing the screws to be placed more to accommodate the instrumentation than the patient. Inserting a screw into any particular pedicle is not difficult. Getting screws that have been inserted into multiple pedicles each with a differing axis to line up with a straight plate can be difficult to say the least (Fig. 85-5). The angles of the pedicle-body alignment and the cross-sectional size of the pedicles can all be determined by preoperative CT scans[7] and should enter into preoperative planning of the fixation.

Just as long bones undergo certain changes with age, the pedicle undergoes similar changes. There is a gradual enlargement resulting from periosteal new bone formation with thinning of the cortex and enlargement of the medullary canal accompanied by loss of trabecular bone centrally. The studies of Zindrick et al.[35,64] showing the relative pullout strengths of differing screw designs demonstrate that it is important to fill up the pedicle with the largest screw possible and that variations on pitch, thread design and other factors are of secondary importance. Krag et al.,[34] however, showed that a screw inserted 50% of the way into the vertebral body had only 75% of the strength of one inserted to an 80% depth. Triangulation of the screws between the two sides of one level and linking the two longitudinal connectors can also increase the overall stability.[15] Ruland et al.[51] showed that pullout strength of individual screws are only as strong as the bone immediately surrounding the screw, but if the screws are first rigidly connected together, pullout is resisted by all the bone between the screws (Fig. 85-6).

Pedicular fixation usually takes the form of screws attached to some other connecting device such as a longitudinal plate or rod. The increased rigidity afforded by segmental fixation at every level is attractive. How rigid the fixation system becomes depends on both the rigidity with which the screws and longitudinal members are connected and the rigidity of the connection of the longitudinal members to each other. With rigid cross connections the system obtains resistance to torsional forces as well as flexion and side bending.[30] Any pedicle-fixation system must allow for variations in the medial/lateral angle between the screws and the connecting member, for varying distances between the screws and the connecting member, and for differing sagittal angles between adjacent levels to allow for differing lordotic curves. Each system accommodates these requirements in a somewhat different manner. Because of the cantilever of the screw off the plate/rod, how much distraction across the disc space they can maintain is unclear and may be limited by the quality of the bone at the bone-im-

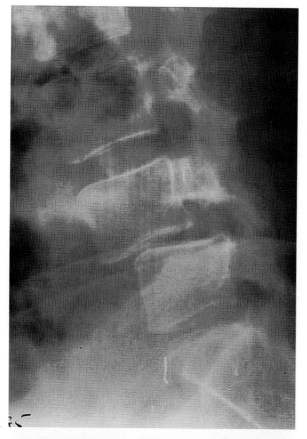

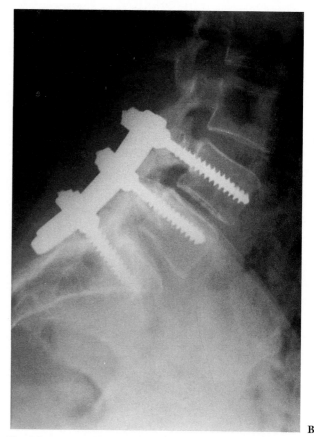

Fig. 85-4

A 56-year old female with progressive degenerative spondylolisthesis treated with Steffee instrumentation.

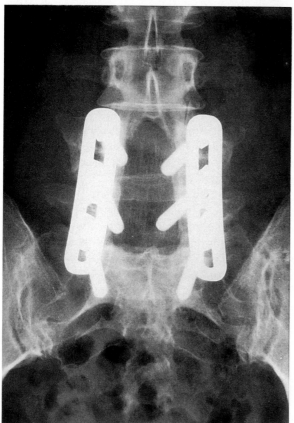

plant junction.[42] This same cantilever loading may lead to late fatigue failure screw breakage even in the presence of a solid posterior fusion due to the micromotion left across the disc space.[18,43] Without solid anterior column support, short-segment pedicle fixation is not always successful in maintaining alignment. Any discussion of the strength of a system has to specify not only the strength of the parts but also the quality of bone for the implant and the number of bony attachment points sharing the load. The ideal pedicle screw system will be addressed later in the future trends section.

Vertebral Bodies

In 1969 Dwyer et al.[23] introduced the concept of a tension band fixation applied to the vertebral body on the convexity of the scoliotic curve. This device used a flexible cable attached to a staple-screw device at each level.

The next advance on the Dwyer apparatus was made by Zielke and Berthet[62] by modifying the screw-staple arrangement and substituting a semi-flexible threaded rod and nuts for the flexible cable. This allowed a more controlled determination of lordosis and allowed a greater correction of rotational deformity.

Zielke's device was strengthened by Kaneda et al.[31] for use as a fracture device (Fig. 85-7). Two rigid rods were used to connect two screws placed in a trapezoidal configuration at the segment above and below the fracture. Rotational stresses were opposed by linking the two rods with two connecting plates. This system was later modified to allow treatment of scoliosis by multisegment instrumentation.

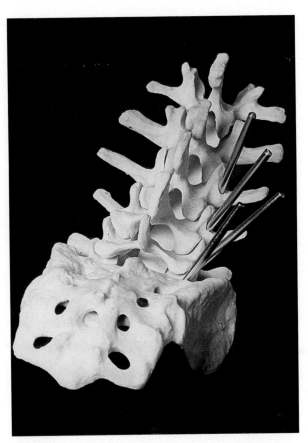

Fig. 85-5

Central axis of pedicle is different at each level. Spinal instrumentation must somehow, in its design, take this into consideration.

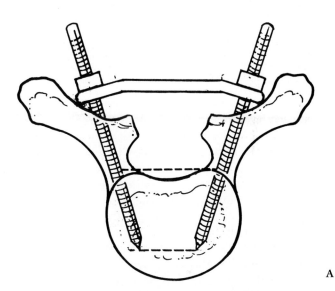

A

Fig. 85-6

Strength of fixation of single bone screw is determined by amount of bone within screw threads. If large reduction forces are applied in attempt to correct spondylolisthesis or scoliosis, the screw tends to loosen, pull out, or even fracture the pedicle. With triangulated connection between pedicles, however, strength of fixation is determined not only by amount of bone within bone screw, but also by area of bone within trapezoid formed by screws. *(Ruland CM, et al.: Triangulation of pedicular instrumentation: a biomechanical analysis, Spine 16:S272, 1991.)*

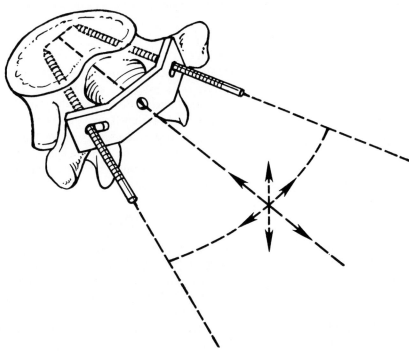

B

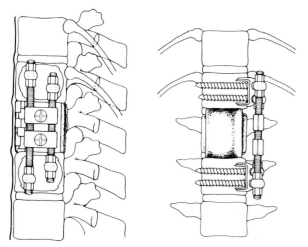

Fig. 85-7

Kaneda device for thoracolumbar fractures. *Note:* Bicortical purchase of screws and reconstruction of anterior column by bone graft. *(From Acromed Technical Brochure, ed 2, Cleveland, Ohio 1990.)*

Compression or distraction forces could be adjusted at each level to select the lordosis desired.

A somewhat different approach for scoliosis is used by the Texas Scottish Rite Hospital (TSRH[58]) group using a single smooth rod. Rotational and scoliotic deformities are corrected simultaneously with rod rotation similar to the principle used posteriorly for thoracic scoliosis reduction by Cotrel-Dubousset (CD) and TSRH systems.

Because of the bulk of these rod-screw systems in the lumbar spine, there have been a number of plate systems developed that try to retain the best parts of the rod systems yet reduce the overall profile. Experience with these systems is limited so far.

All anterior types of fixation for the lumbar spine suffer from two basic drawbacks. First, instrumentation to L5 can be difficult, and to the sacrum essentially impossible. Second, the risk, however low, exists of retrograde ejaculation in males with anterior sacral dissection. Certain other risks with this approach to the spine include renal failure secondary to retroperitoneal fibrosis; direct trauma to the iliac veins, spleen, or ureters; and in the past late postoperative arterial damage caused by erosive pressure of the metal on arterial vessels if implanted in contact with them.[22] The latter can be avoided by placement of the instrumentation on the lateral side of the vertebrae away from arterial vessels. All current anterior systems are designed with this factor in mind. This becomes particularly important when dealing with fracture reconstruction. Since the instrumentation sits on the lateral aspect of the vertebral body with the screws cantilevered to the opposite side, it is critical to provide contralateral support

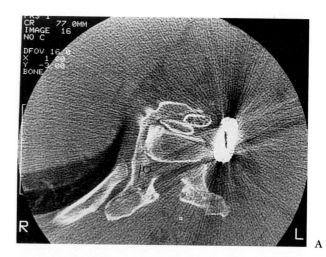

A

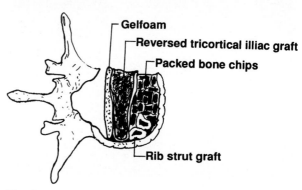

- Gelfoam
- Reversed tricortical illiac graft
- Packed bone chips
- Rib strut graft

B

Fig. 85-8

A, Well-reconstructed anterior column with tricortical iliac crest graft with tricortical portion placed on contralateral side of instrumentation supplemented with two rib grafts. **B,** Success of anterior instrumentation depends in large part on adequate reconstitution of anterior columns with bone grafting. This is especially important on contralateral side of instrumentation.

with the bone graft that reconstitutes the vertebral body (Fig. 85-8).

The vertebral body, featuring a cortical shell and cancellous bony core, requires a fairly large screw thread for fixation. Forces on the proximal cortical shell can be distributed by a washer or staple device,[5] although Ashman's studies suggest a washer does not contribute significantly to fixation, while a staple does. The best screw fixation is achieved by engaging the far cortex with the screw.

Disc Space

Blocking motion by fixation of the area where motion occurs around the axis of rotation has long been an attractive idea. The disc is the site of primarily compressive loading that stimulates bone healing. The vertebral end plates form a large well-vascularized area for graft incorporation. The materials used for fixation of this area have included bone,[17] sin-

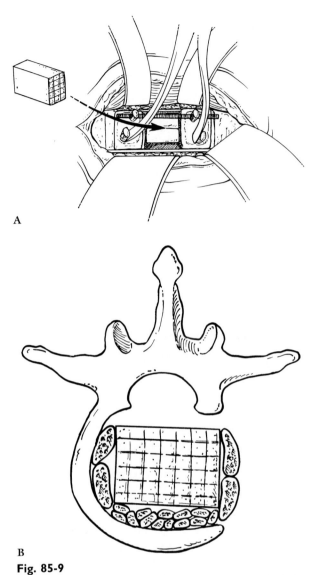

Fig. 85-9

A, Anterior column reconstruction can be performed using methylmethacralate, titanium mesh blocks or, as shown here, ceramic spacers. **B,** Whether biologic or inert materials are used, principles of anterior column reconstruction remain same. If long-term survival is expected, some bone grafting material should be added to inert spacers. *(From Kaneda K, et al.: The treatment of osteoporotic-posttraumatic vertebral collapse using the Kaneda device and a bioactive ceramic vertebral prosthesis, Spine 17 (Suppl 8):296, 1992.)*

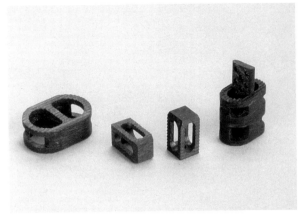

Fig. 85-10

Various carbon fiber cages have been designed to allow immediate structural strength as well as long-term bony ingrowth by filling interior spaces with bone graft. *(Courtesy AcroMed® Corp., Cleveland, Ohio.)*

tered titanium blocks,[16] ceramics[32] (Fig. 85-9), and cages of carbon fiber[10] (Fig. 85-10) or titanium.[6,13] The treatment of discogenic pain by attempting to stop disc motion at sites other than the disc has always seemed peculiar to this author. Rolander[48] has shown how some disc motion occurs even with rigid fixation of all the posterior elements as a result of the viscoelastic behavior of bone.

Resection of the cortical end plate, although sometimes desirable, weakens the supporting structure for the implant. Substituting a cancellous bone bed for the original cortical plate greatly enhances the bony incorporation of the fusion, but the strength of the bone in resisting impaction of the grafts diminishes rapidly with the distance from the end plate.

This has led numerous authors to suggest distributing the forces as widely as possible by "filling up the interspace" with graft material (Fig. 85-11). When an interbody fusion is done through a posterior approach as advocated by Cloward,[17] fixation achieved anteriorly by the bone plugs is best supplemented by some sort of posterior neutralization fixation across either the pedicle, lamina, or spinous process to help prevent posterior dislocation or loosening of the bone plugs.[54] Interbody fusions done from a posterior approach are probably the most technically demanding of the fixation techniques and are associated with some of the potentially greatest risks, including nerve-root impingement by displaced plugs, nerve-root injury by excessive manipulation or stretch, and excessive scar formation.

The use of posterior instrumentation after either an anterior or posterior interbody fusion relieves the bone plugs of the dual task of acting as graft mate-

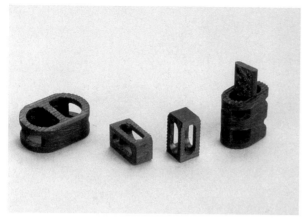

Fig. 85-11

Lin's interbody fusion technique. *(From Lin PM, editor: Posterior lumbar interbody fusion, Springfield, IL, 1982, Charles C Thomas, Publisher.)*

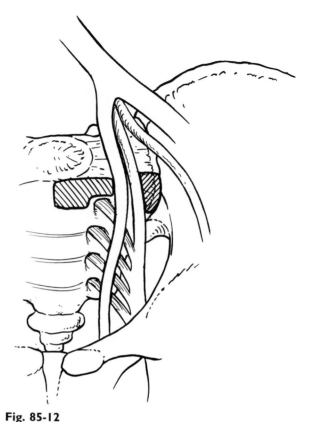

Fig. 85-12

Anteroposterior sacrum: safe zones for screw placement. *(From Mirkovic JJ, et al.: Anatomic consideration for sacral screw placement, Spine 16:S293, 1991.)*

rial and stabilization by doing a much better job of the latter. Difficulties in obtaining donor bone of sufficient quantity and size have led to the division of the mechanical support and osteoinductive functions. Titanium and carbon-fiber cage implants have been developed to hold bone graft chips that provide the osteoinductive and osteoconductive structure. These have been used as single disc space spacers or entire vertebral body substitutes for corpectomy cases.

Lumbosacral-Junction Fixation

Lumbosacral-junction fixation has long been the unmet challenge of spinal instrumentation systems. The forces in this area are the greatest encountered anywhere in the spine.[36,41] The body of the sacrum is difficult to reach through an anterior approach. Work in this area is associated with its own unique potential hazards, usually vascular. The lamina is sometimes absent posteriorly and is often thin when compared to the lamina of the adjacent segments. The relative canal size at the sacrum is often small, allowing a lesser degree of safety for hooks that protrude into the canal itself. Failure of laminar fixation in the sacrum can result in catastrophic sacral nerve-root injury. The safest areas for fixation are the ala and pedicle regions. The alar area, representing an enlargement of the transverse processes, presents an option for fixation not found in other areas of the lumbar spine. Since the ala sit so far laterally, contouring rods to the lamina more medially over short segments has been difficult, and pedicle fixation has in general supplanted this option. Options for pedicle fixation include single or doubled screws, screw plus hook or intrasacral rod,[29] plates with multiple

screws, or techniques that cross the unfused sacroiliac joint.

Single sacral screws are usually medially directed near the superomedial corner of the S1 pedicle. The strongest bone of the sacrum is found in this region. However, the cancellous bone of this area is much thinner than in a corresponding area of a lumbar vertebra and may be nearly totally replaced with fat. Fixation often requires engaging the far cortex of the sacrum either anteriorly near the midline, laterally near the sacroiliac joint, or in the end plate of S1. Anatomic strategies for sacral screw placement have been studied by a number of authors.[3,24,44] Not only must the strength of the bone be considered but also the vital structures adjacent to the anterior cortex where the screws will penetrate. Fortunately, there are two relatively "safe areas" as described by Mirkovic et al. (Fig. 85-12).[44] These are directly anterior to the midsacral body and laterally in the region of the sacroiliac joint.

If a second sacral screw is used next to the first, it is placed slightly caudal to the medially directed first sacral screw and is directed laterally.

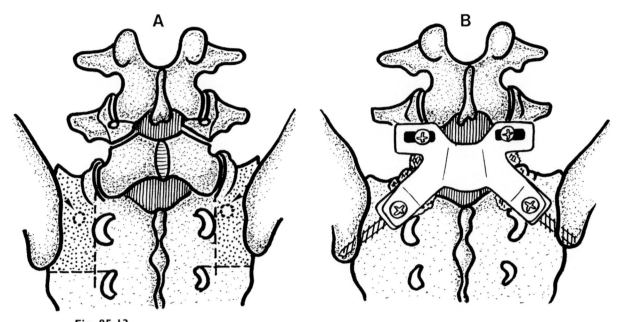

Fig. 85-13

Diagram showing positioning of L5-S1 lumbosacral plate after laying bare L5-S1 posterior intervertebral joints, zone of osteolysis, and interposition of bone fragments taken from spinous processes and laminae.

Sacral-plate fixation was described by Louis in 1976[37,38] (Fig. 85-13). His plate had bilateral sacral screws into the sacrum with L5 bone screws in the same plate. These screws were not rigidly fixed to the plate. Variations in the distance between the pedicle of L5 and the sacrum were accommodated by varying the placement of the sacral screws. This system did allow for some flexibility in variations of the interpedicular distance of L5 but not in accompanying multiple-level fixation. The unilateral plates of Roy-Camille et al.[50] allowed for multiple screw fixation into the sacrum as well as multiple-level fixation. Asher and Strippgen[3] built on the principles of Louis, but their "Isola" plate required cutting holes in the ilium to accommodate the screw direction (Fig. 85-14). They described a nonrigid fixation using a malleable plate and cancellous screws. The design was never perfected for clinical use. Variations in interpedicular distances of the sacrum can be solved by making unilateral plates that are connected to each other via rigidly connecting longitudinal rods. The Chopin[19] block uses two screws, one directed medially and slightly cephalad and a second directed straight laterally (Fig. 85-15). The Tacoma sacral plate[46] has both two- and three-screw versions (Fig. 85-16). Both versions feature a medially directed S1 bone screw. Since the primary mode of failure is with a flexion-bending moment, the second screw of both versions of the plate is directed obliquely caudally and laterally to increase the lever

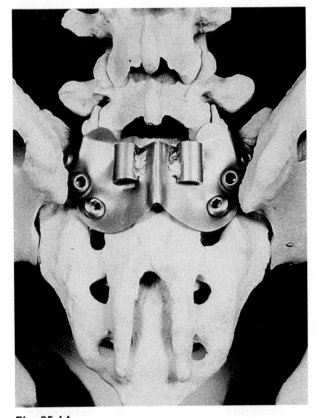

Fig. 85-14

Isola sacral implant prototype. *(From Asher MA, Strippgen WE: Anthropometric studies of the human sacrum relating to dorsal transsacral implant designs, Clin Orthop 203:61, 1986.)*

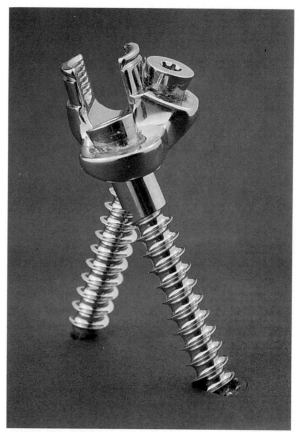

Fig. 85-15

Chopin block for sacral fixation for use with CC-D System *(Courtesy Sofamor/Danek, Memphis, Tennessee.)*

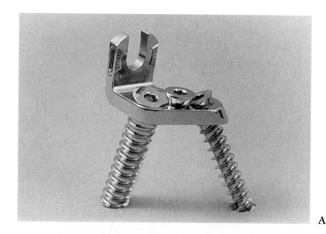

A

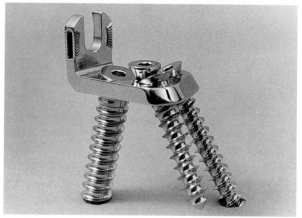

B

Fig. 85-16

Tacoma sacral plate. **A,** Two-screw Tacoma sacral plate with variable angle goalposts for TSRH instrumentation. **B,** Three-screw Tacoma sacral plate with variable-angle goalposts for TSRH instrumentation.

arm resisting this force. The three-screw plate uses the same two screws and adds a third laterally directed screw. Since Camp et al.[14] have shown that sacral screws tend to fail by first coming together before pulling out, it is important to note that the screws in both the Chopin and Tacoma plates lock rigidly with the plate to prevent this type of failure.

Some of these problems have been avoided with bypassing the sacrum and fixating to the ilium. The Galveston technique of attaching Luque rods to the pelvis described by Allen and Ferguson[2] is, by far, the strongest lumbosacral junction fixation available (Fig. 85-17). This, however, poses the additional problem of the fixation crossing the unfused sacroiliac joint, which has led to some cases of symptomatic sacroiliitis and the need for subsequent rod removal. If adequate fixation to the sacrum using plates with multiple screws can be achieved without this risk, it seems reasonable to do so.

Future Trends

It seems to this author that internal fixation in the future will allow two different trends. The first is a refinement of our present techniques. The second parallels the current trend toward minimally invasive techniques.

The future system will hopefully solve the current shortcomings of today's hardware. There are seven major problem areas that have not been adequately solved by any lumbar system on the market today. These can be viewed as the requirements for any system of the future. (1) The system must be user-friendly for the average spine surgeon who can adequately place a screw through the pedicle and the vertebral body. (2) The two pedicle screws at each level must be rigidly connected to each other before attachment to the longitudinal rod or plate. (3) The system must allow for variation in the bone-screw

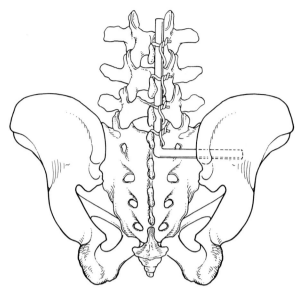

Fig. 85-17
Galveston technique for pelvic fixation. Rod is inserted intraosseously into ilium starting near posterior inferior iliac spine and passing close to sciatic notch. Rod is contoured down to sacral lamina to minimize prominence subcutaneously. *(From Allen BL, Ferguson RL: The Galveston technique for L-rod instrumentation of the scoliotic spine, Spine 7:282, 1982.)*

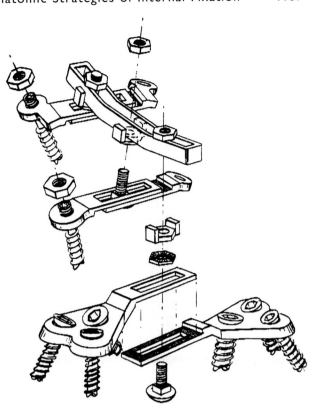

Fig. 85-18
Component parts of Tacoma Monorail System. Top plate is of offset designed to minimize interference with superiormost facet joint. Bottom plate incorporates multiple screw technology for maximum purchase in sacrum. Middle plate is for intermediate levels.

axis at different lumbar levels. It must also allow for variations in the screw distances between the right and left sides for the plate fixation mentioned before. It must also allow for differing screw axes between one level and the next to accommodate the appropriate sagittal alignment. (4) The system must have an adequate way to avoid disruption of the facet joint of the first unfused segment. (5) The system must allow for reduction of spondylolisthesis and degenerative scoliosis. (6) The bulk of the system must be minimized as much as possible and moved to the midline between the paraspinal muscles instead of over the area of the fusion graft. (7) Finally, the system must allow for further diagnostic tests. Whether an implant-material change from stainless steel to titanium or carbon fiber will solve this problem remains to be seen.[52]

One system currently under development attempts to address all these issues. As can be seen from Fig. 85-18, the screws can be inserted into the best position in each pedicle without concern for the position of the screw at the next level. The two screws at each level are then rigidly linked together with a device that accommodates for variations in interscrew distance and difference between the insertion axis between the two sides, if any (Fig. 85-19). This connecting plate has a different shape at the superior most level to avoid damage to the next facet joint. The sacral plate takes advantage of the current

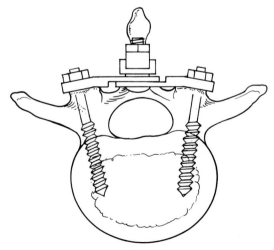

Fig. 85-19
With plates of differing angles, two different bone-screw angles can be accommodated at same level and varied at each level as necessary.

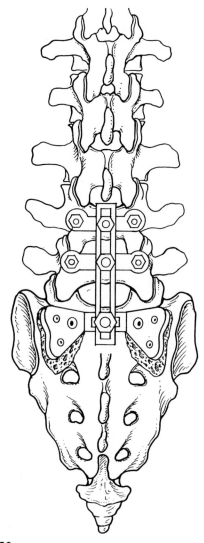

Fig. 85-20

Three-level instrumentation using Tacoma Monorail System showing three types of plate design.

rigid, multiscrew technology (Fig. 85-20). The longitudinal plate can be contoured for the desired lordosis and provides a rigid platform for correction of both the flexion and translational aspects of the spondylolisthesis deformity. The greatest bulk of the implant is in the midline, where the spinous processes normally form an attachment for the paraspinal muscles. Whether this implant made in titanium will allow for better visualization on MRI is theoretical at this point but it seems that it would have a better chance than others.

As far as minimalistic invasive techniques are concerned, these can be divided into three types, percutaneous, subfascial and translaminar. The percuta-

neous techniques of the AO group such as the fixator external are troubled by both the real problems of secondary infection control and the physical and emotional problems such devices represent, i.e., special mattresses, chair comfort, clothes fit, etc.

The conversion of this type of device to a subcutaneous or subfascial level is limited by the lack of subcutaneous fat in this area in the average male and many female patients.

This leaves further development of techniques such as transfacet joint screw fixation, which do not require longitudinal connectors. Similar techniques can be developed for anterior laparoscopic fusion techniques for the vertebral body as well.

References

1. Albee FH: Transplantation of a portion of the tibia into the spine for Pott's disease: A preliminary report, *JAMA* 57:885, 1911.
2. Allen BL, Ferguson RL: The Galveston technique for L-rod instrumentation of the scoliotic spine, *Spine* 7:276, 1982.
3. Asher MA, Strippgen WE: Anthropometric studies of the human sacrum relating to dorsal transsacral implant designs, *Clin Orthop* 203:58, 1986.
4. Ashman RB, et al.: Mechanical testing of spinal instrumentation, *Clin Orthop* 117:113, 1988.
5. Ashman RB, et al.: *TSRH universal spinal instrumentation.* Dallas, TX, 1993, Hundley & Assoc.
6. Bagby GW: Arthrodesis by the distraction-compression method using a stainless steel implant. *Orthopedics* 11:931, 1988.
7. Banta CJ, et al.: Measurement of effective pedicle diameter in the human spine, *Orthopedics* 12:939, 1989.
8. Boucher HH: A method of spinal fusion, *J Bone Joint Surg* 41B:248, 1959.
9. Bradford DS: Instrumentation of the lumbar spine: an overview, *Clin Orthop* 230:185, 1986.
10. Brantigan JW, Steffee AD, Geiger JM: A carbon fiber implant to aid interbody lumbar fusion: mechanical testing, *Spine* 16:277, 1991.
11. Brittain HA: *Architectural principles in arthrodesis,* ed 2, Edinburgh, 1952, E. & S. Livingstone, Ltd.
12. Brodsky AE, Kovalsky ES, Khalil MA: Correlation of radiographic assessment of lumbar spine fusions with surgical exploration, *Spine* 16(6s):261, 1991.
13. Butts SD, et al.: Biomechanical analysis of a new method for spinal interbody fixation, *Adv Bioeng Ref*, 1978.
14. Camp JF, et al.: Immediate complications of Cotrel-Dubousset instrumentation to the sacro-pelvis: a clinical and biomechanical study, *Spine* 15:932, 1990.
15. Carson WL, et al.: Internal forces and moments in transpedicular spine instrumentation: the effect of pedicle screw angle and transfixation—the 4R-4Bar linkage concept, *Spine* 15:893, 1990.

16. Chow SP, et al.: The use of porous titanium implant in anterior spinal fusion: a preliminary report, *J West Pac Orthop Assoc* 16:2, 1979.

17. Cloward RB: The treatment of ruptured lumbar intervertebral discs by vertebral body fusion: indications, operative technique, after care, *J Neurosurg* 10:154, 1953.

18. Coe JD, et al.: Influence of bone mineral density on the fixation of thoracolumbar implants: a comparative study of transpedicular screws, laminar hooks, and spinous process wires, *Spine* 15:902, 1990.

19. Cotrel Y: *Compact Cotrel-Dubousset instrumentation (CC-D)*, Presented at the 8th International Congress on Coutrel-Dubousset Instrumentation, Montpellier France, 1991.

20. Cotrel Y, Dubousset J, Guillaumat M: New universal instrumentation in spinal surgery, *Clin Orthop* 227:10, 1988.

21. Drummond D, et al.: Interspinous process segmental spinal instrumentation, *J Pediatr Orthop* 4:397, 1984.

22. Dunn HK: Anterior stabilization of thoracolumbar injuries, *Clin Orthop* 189:116, 1984.

23. Dwyer AF, et al.: An anterior approach to scoliosis: A preliminary report, *Clin Orthop* 62:192, 1969.

24. Esses SI, et al.: Surgical anatomy of the sacrum: A guide for rational screw fixation, *Spine* 16:283, 1992.

25. Gibson A: A modified technique for spinal fusion, *Surg Gynecol Obstet* 53:365, 1931.

26. Hadra BE: Wiring of the vertebrae as a means of immobilization in fracture and Pott's disease, *Times Reg* 22:423, 1891.

27. Harrington PR: Surgical instrumentation for management of scoliosis, *J Bone Joint Surg* 42A:1448, 1960.

28. Harrington PR, Tullos HS: Reduction of severe Spondylolisthesis in children, *South Med J* 62:1, 1969.

29. Jackson RP, Ebelke DK, McManus AC: *The sacroiliac buttress and new methods for correction with CD pedicle instrumentation.* Presented at the 8th International Congress on Cotrel-Dubousset Instrumentation, 1991.

30. Johnston CE II, Ashman RB, Corin JD: Mechanical effects of cross-linking rods in Cotrel-Dubousset instrumentation, *Orthop Trans* 11:96, 1987.

31. Kaneda K, Abumi K, Fujiya K: Burst fractures with neurologic deficits of the thoraco-lumbar spine. Results of anterior decompression and stabilization with anterior instrumentation, *Spine* 9:788, 1984.

32. Kaneda K, et al.: The treatment of osteoporotic—posttraumatic vertebral collapse using the Kaneda device and a bioactive ceramic vertebral prosthesis, *Spine* 17(858):295, 1992.

33. King D: Internal fixation for lumbosacral fusion, *Am J Surg* 66:357, 1948.

34. Krag MH, et al.: Depth of insertion of transpedicular vertebral screws into human vertebrae: Effect upon screw-vertebra interface strength, *J Spine Disord* 1:287, 1988.

35. Krag MH, *Biomechanics of transpedicle spinal fixation.* In: Weinstein JN, Weisel S, eds. *The lumbar spine.* Philadelphia: WB Saunders, 1990; 916

36. Krag MH, et al.: Screw fixation in the human sacrum. An in vitro study of the biomechanics of fixation, *Spine* 17:S196, 1992.

37. Louis R: Fusion of the lumbar and sacral spine by internal fixation with screw plates, *Clin Orthop* 203:18, 1986.

38. Louis R, Maresca C: Les arthrodeses stables de la charniere lombo-sacree (70 cas), *Rev Chir Orthop* 62 (Suppl II):70, 1976.

39. Luque E: The anatomic basis and development of segmental spinal instrumentation, *Spine* 7:256, 1982.

40. Magerl FP: Stabilization of the lower thoracic and lumbar spine with external skeletal fixation, *Clin Orthop* 189:125, 1984.

41. McAfee PC, et al.: Biomechanical analysis of lumbosacral fixation, *Spine* 17(Suppl 8):S235, 1992.

42. McAfee PC, Weiland DJ, Carlow JJ: Survivorship analysis of pedicle spinal instrumentation, *Spine,* 16:422, 1991.

43. McAfee PC, Werner FW, Glisson RR: A biomechanical analysis of spinal instrumentation systems in thoracolumbar fractures: A comparison of traditional Harrington distraction instrumentation with segmental spinal instrumentation, *Spine* 10:204, 1985.

44. Mirkovic JJ, et al.: Anatomic consideration for sacral screw placement, *Spine* 16:289, 1991.

45. Moe JH, Denis F: The iatrogenic loss of lumbar lordosis, *Proc Scoliosis Res Soc,* 1976.

46. Ray RC, Asher RB: *Biomechanical comparison of a new sacral fixation method.* Presented at the 25th annual meeting of the Scoliosis Research Society, Minneapolis, September 24–27, 1991.

47. Roach JW, Ashman RB, Allard RN: The strength of a posterior element claw at one verses two spinal levels, *J Spinal Disord* 3:259, 1990.

48. Rolander SD: *Motion of the lumbar spine with special reference to the stabilizing effect of posterior fusion,* Doctoral thesis, Gothenburg, Sweden, 1966, University of Gothenburg.

49. Roy-Camille R, Roy-Camille M, Demeulenacre C: Osteosynthese du rachis dorsal, lomaire et lombosacre par plaques metalliques vissees dans les pedicules vertebraux et les apophyses articulaires, *Presse Med* 78:1447, 1970.

50. Roy-Camille R, Saillant G, Mazel C: Internal fixation of the lumbar spine with pedicle screw plating, *J Clin Orthop* 203:7, 1986.

51. Ruland CM, et al.: Triangulation of pedicular instrumentation: A biomechanical analysis, *Spine* 16:270, 1991.

52. Rupp R, et al.: Magnetic resonance imaging evaluation of the spine with metal implants: general safety and superior imaging with titanium, *Spine* 18:379, 1993.

53. Schoellner O: Ein neues verfahren zur resposition und fixation bei spondylolisthesis, *Orthop Prax* 4:270, 1975.

54. Shirado O, et al.: Biomechanical evaluation of methods of posterior stabilization of the spine and posterior lumbar interbody arthrodesis for lumbosacral isthmic spondylolisthesis: a calf-spine model, *J Bone Joint Surg* 73A:518, 1991.

55. Songer MN, et al.: The use of sublaminar cables to replace Luque wires, *Spine* 16(8s):418, 1991.

56. Stauffer R, Coventry M: Anterior interbody lumbar spine fusion, *J Bone Joint Surg* 54A:756, 1972.

57. Steffee AD, Biscup RS, Sitkowski DJ: Segmental spine plates with pedicle screw fixation: a new internal fixation device for disorders of the lumbar and thoracolumbar spine, *Clin Orthop* 203:45, 1986.

58. Turi M, Johnston CE II, Richards BS: Anterior correction of idiopathic scoliosis using TSRH instrumentation, *Spine* 18:417, 1993.

59. White AH, Zucherman JF, Hsu K: Lumbosacral fusions with Harrington rods and intersegmental wiring, *Clin Orthop* 230:185, 1986.

60. Wilson PD, Straub LR: *Lumbosacral fusion with metallic-plate fixation*, AAOS Inst Crs Lectures, vol 9, Ann Arbor, 1952, JW Edwards, p 53.

61. Zdeblick TA: *A prospective, randomized study of lumbar fusion*. Presented at the AAOs meeting, Washington, DC, February 20–25, 1992.

62. Zielke K, Berthet XX: Ventrale derottionsspondylodese-Vorlanfiger bericht uber 58 falle, *Veitr Orthop Traumatol* 25:85, 1978.

63. Zindrick MR, et al.: Analysis of the morphometric characteristics of the thoracic and lumbar pedicles, *Spine* 12:160, 1987.

64. Zindrick MR, Wiltse LL, et al.: Biomechanical study of interpedicular screw fixation in the lumbosacral spine, *Clin Orthop* 203:99, 1986.

Chapter 86
Instrumented Posterior Lumbar Surgery

John H. Peloza

David K. Selby

Internal Fixation
Types of Instrumentation

   nontranspedicular screw fixation
   transpedicular screw fixation

Complications

   neural injury
   vascular injury
   instrumentation failure
   pseudarthrosis
   infection
   miscellaneous complications

Transpedicular Internal Fixation
   Design

   screw plate
   screw bolting

Other Issues Related to Transpedicular
   Screw Systems

   screw placement
   depth of the screw penetration
   cross linking

The Wiltse System

   components
   advantages
   modifications
   mechanical testing
   indications
   contraindications
   surgical technique
   clinical results

Although there are many techniques for spinal fusion for which successful outcomes are reported, the primary dilemma for the spine surgeon is to determine for what patients and under what conditions spinal arthrodesis should be performed. The broad indications for fusion by category include degenerative disc disease, trauma, neoplasm, infection, inflammation, and congenital, idiopathic, and acquired deformity of the spine. The common denominator for all these conditions is pain. Spinal pain may originate from mechanical, inflammatory, or neurochemical sources.[10,56,72,73] The exact mechanisms for spinal pain are not clearly understood, but vertebral motion does play an important role. The purpose of spinal fusions is to eliminate pathologic motion or mechanical insufficiency at the involved spinal segments. In cases of deformity, primary or secondary to the aforementioned pathologic processes, fusion maintains correction or prevents progression of the deformity. The most effective and consistent way to obtain spinal fusion is through the use of internal fixation.

The purpose of this chapter is to discuss internal fixation in general, and transpedicular fixation specifically. The advantages, disadvantages, biomechanics, indications, contraindications, and particular issues of transpedicular internal fixation will be reviewed. A specific discussion of the Wiltse system, including surgical technique and clinical results will end with discussion.

Internal Fixation

Internal fixation of the lumbar spine is a major advance in surgical treatment of the spine. The improvement of internal fixation systems has made it possible to treat successfully almost any condition of the spine. But, without successful arthrodesis, all internal fixation systems eventually fail. Therefore, choosing a fixation system appropriate to the patient's pathology is important. Load sharing between the internal fixation and the anterior column reduces stress and increases the longevity of the internal fixation. Exacting surgical technique is required when

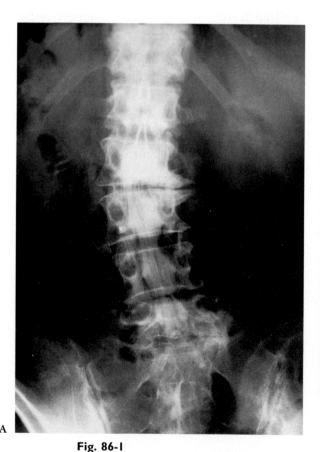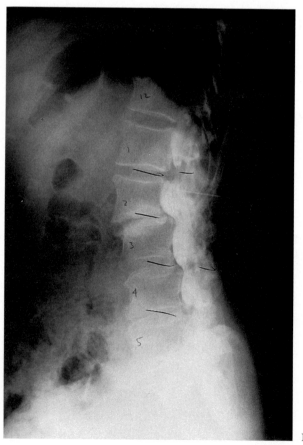

A   B

Fig. 86-1

A, Anteroposterior, and **B,** lateral lumbar spine, degenerative scoliosis, status post decompression and fusion with pseudarthrosis and spinal stenosis.

preparing the graft bed, selecting and preparing the graft material, influencing local and systemic factors to enhance fusion, and implanting the internal fixation properly.

Internal fixation has many purposes, among them to correct deformity and maintain the correction until fusion is complete. Without internal fixation, deformity cannot be corrected and fusion rates are lower. Fusion rates for noninstrumented cases range from 60% to 80%. In multilevel fusions without instrumentation, pseudarthrosis is more frequent* (Fig. 86-1). Even if fusion occurs without instrumentation, spinal alignment may be lost, especially in cases with instability—e.g., spondylolisthesis, scoliosis, trauma, neoplasm, and iatrogenic conditions.

Another potential benefit of internal fixation may be improved rehabilitation. By providing immediate stabilization of the motion segments, patients can increase the pace and intensity of exercise. For most situations, internal fixation precludes the need for bed rest, cumbersome external bracing, or electrical stimulation.

Types of Instrumentation

Nontranspedicular Screw Fixation

There are two main types of instrumentation in the lumbar spine: Nontranspedicular screw fixation and transpedicular screw fixation. Nontranspedicular screw fixation systems include hook/rod (Fig. 86-2), sublaminar wire/rod constructs, facet joint screws, or spinous process plates. All these systems require posterior elements (i.e., lamina) for the purchase of either a hook, wire, screw, or plate. In cases of prior laminectomy or concomitant decompression, normal segments must be included in the fusion construct in order to obtain purchase.[58] This is obtained at the expense of normal adjacent motion segments and has adverse mechanical consequences.

The rigidity of nontranspedicular fixation is less than that of transpedicular screw fixation. Fixation

*References 15, 16, 36, 52, 58, 67, and 79.

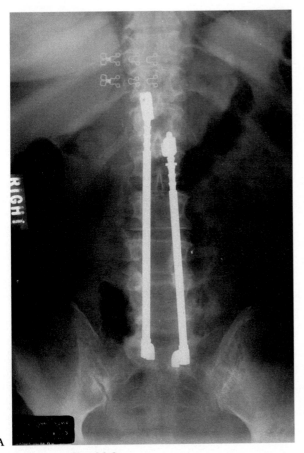
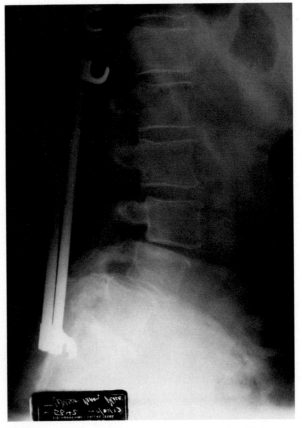

A   B

Fig. 86-2

A and **B,** Preoperative anteroposterior and lateral lumbar spine, degenerative spondylolisthesis, status post decompression, fusion and Harrington rod instrumentation with pseudarthrosis.

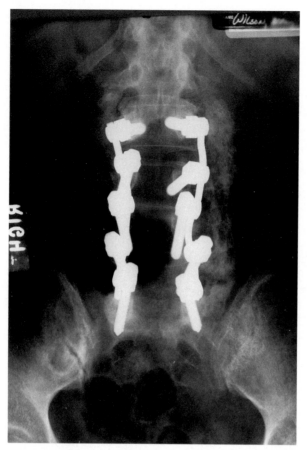

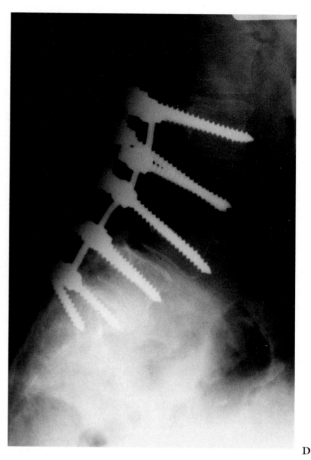

C

D

Fig. 86-2, cont'd

C and **D,** Anteroposterior and lateral lumbar spine, status post radical decompression, instrumentation, and fusion.

to lamina, particularly at the sacrum, is inferior.[23] The hook/rod systems depend on distraction and ligamentotaxis, which decreases lumbar lordosis with adverse biomechanical consequences. Their ability to resist flexion, extension, torsion, and especially axial loading varies depending on the system, but the non-transpedicular fixation systems are all inferior to transpedicular screw systems.[1,8,9,23]

Transpedicular Screw Fixation

A major advance in lumbar spine implants is transpedicular screw fixation (Fig. 86-3). Bone screws resist loads of any type at the strongest part of the vertebra. They do not rely on distraction, compression, or ligamentotaxis for rigidity. Bone screw systems do not depend on posterior elements for fixation; therefore, they are the implant of choice for patients with a previous laminectomy or with concomitant decompression with total laminectomy and/or facetectomy (Fig. 86-4). Fusion is limited to

the pathologic segments, thereby preserving normal adjacent levels. The linking members of the construct (i.e., plates or rods) can be contoured to restore physiologic alignment. In addition, excellent fixation is achieved at the sacrum. Bone screw systems are superior in their ability to resist three-dimensional loads on the spine, but are even better in torsion, angular moments, and axial loading.*

Complications

The use of bone screw fixation systems has a number of potential complications associated with it, including nerve injury, vascular injury, hardware failure, pseudarthrosis, loss of correction, infection, and adjacent facet joint injury. Spine surgeons need to be familiar with these complications, their avoidance, and their treatment.

*References 1, 9, 23, 26, 27, 29, 37, 59, and 80.

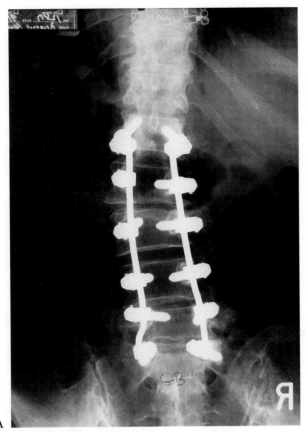

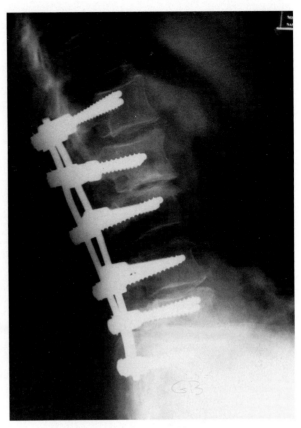

Fig. 86-3

A, Anteroposterior, and **B,** lateral status post radical decompression, fusion and Wiltse instrumentation, early postoperative.

Neural Injury

Injury to neural structures results from a number of sources. Malposition of a drill bit, pin, awl, curette, tap, or screw can directly or indirectly involve the nerve root, or spinal cord at a level higher than L1. Roy-Camille et al.[53] reported a 10% and Louis[46] a 1.3% incidence of malpositioned screws causing nerve injury in their early series. Weinstein et al.[71] demonstrated a 21% incidence of screw malposition in their experimental study, although significant improvement was noted toward the end of the study, which was attributed to a practice effect.

Screw penetration at the medial and inferior wall of the pedicle may injure the exiting nerve root because of its juxtaposition to the pedicle wall. Screw penetration in an excessively upward direction may injure the nerve root, exiting at the foramen above. In addition to direct nerve injury, dural tears are a possibility. Indirect nerve injury may occur if a tap or screw expands, fractures, or cuts out of the pedi-

cle. This situation is more likely in an osteoporotic bone and when forces of distraction or compression are placed on the screw. All these problems are increased by preexisting stenosis, deformity, or listhesis.

Instrument malposition may be avoided by having a thorough knowledge of pedicle anatomy. Krag[39,40] and Zindrick[83] and their colleagues described pedicle morphology in the transverse, coronal, and sagittal planes, as well as the cortical diameter and shapes of the pedicle at different vertebral levels. A preoperative imaging study may reveal anatomic abnormalities. With experience, this complication is reduced drastically and reported rates of clinical neurologic injury in the lumbar spine are low.[17]

Vascular Injury

Vascular injury may be catastrophic, but fortunately its incidence is very low. At or above L4, penetration of the anterior cortex can injure the aorta or vena cava. At L5, the common iliac vessels are suf-

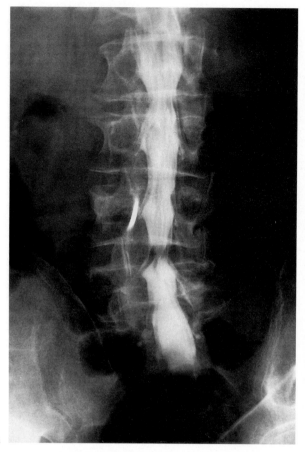

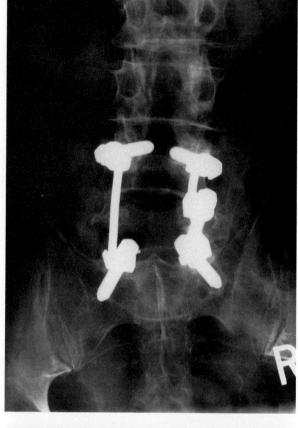

A

B

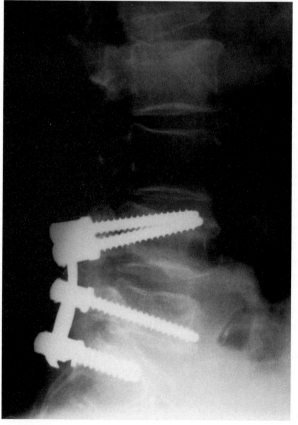

C

Fig. 86-4

A, Anteroposterior, lumbar spine, spinal stenosis. **B** and **C,** Status post decompression with transverse process fusion and Wiltse internal fixation. Left L5 pedicle was skipped in order to make rod bend more easily, but still maintain segmental fixation with pedicle screw in L5 pedicle on right. This obviated need for cross link.

ficiently lateral so that anterior penetration is less likely to injure them. The most worrisome area is the sacrum. The common iliacs bifurcate at the sacral ala into the internal and external iliac vessels. Anterior cortical penetration at the ala may injure these vessels. In addition, penetration at the S1 and S2 vertebrae can damage the L5 and S1 roots, respectively.

These complications can be easily avoided. Purchase to the anterior cortex with a screw is rarely needed, because an 80% depth of penetration provides adequate strength of fixation in most cases.[37-39] At the sacrum, anterior medial screw direction through the S1 pedicle, or posterolateral orientation to the sacral ala are both safe and provide similar strength of fixation.[6,7,80] If anterior cortical purchase is desired, then proper drilling and tapping aided by fluoroscopy can be used.

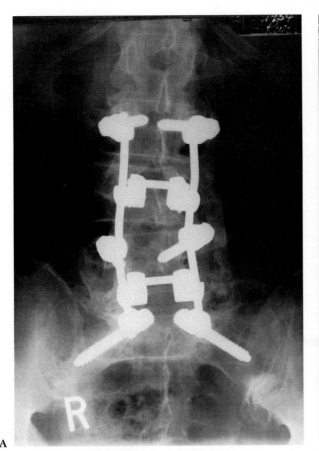
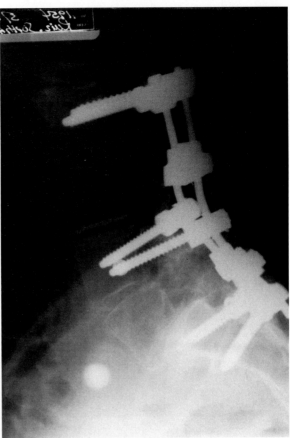

Fig. 86-5

A, Anteroposterior, and **B,** lateral lumbar spine, degenerative scoliosis, status post decompression, fusion, and instrumentation. Instrumentation is with cross links. Cross links were used to decrease operative time by using fewer bone screws, which would also make rod bend more easily. This patient was elderly, with multiple medical problems, and it was quite advantageous to decrease operative time.

Instrumentation Failure

Instrumentation failure was a frequent problem in early series, but is less so now. Screw failure is associated with metal stress fatigue. Roy-Camille et al.[53] reported a 25% failure rate in acute lumbar fractures; Louis[46] reported 8 of 401 patients with broken screws and another 6 patients with loose screws. The AO tibial dynamic compression plate attached to the spine by bone screws had a screw breakage rate of 6.5%.[3] Steffee[62] had a 6.7% screw failure rate with the VSP system, which decreased substantially after modifications of the instrumentation. Most of these failures were the result of poor screw and linkage system design. Luque's report noted only one broken and one loose screw in 57 patients utilizing a semirigid screw and plate system.[48]

Loss of fixation can be caused by screw malposition, pedicle fracture, or hardware failure, but the most important factor is bone quality. Osteoporosis should raise a red flag because it might be a contraindication to transpedicular screw fixation. Bone quality may be even more important than screw design.[16,82] In osteoporotic bone, anterior cortical purchase, as well as end-plate penetration increases screw pull-out strength. Augmenting bone fixation with pressurized polymethylmethacrylate can increase screw pull-out strength to 96%.[80] However, polymethylmethacrylate is dangerous because it might leak into the vertebral canal or anteriorly into the retroperitoneum. If postoperative infection occurs, treatment and removal of hardware is much more difficult because it usually requires radical excision of the bone and cement.[82]

Other fixation techniques that are useful in poor bone are cross links (Figs. 86-5 and 86-6) and screw/bolt fixation systems. These techniques provide a purchase that is not solely dependent on the screw pull-out strength. Cross links reduce internal forces and movements that occur within a

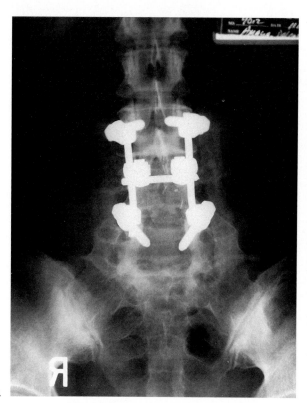
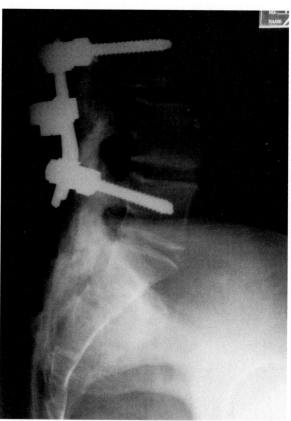

Fig. 86-6

A, Anteroposterior, and **B,** lateral lumbar spine, status post anterior interbody fusions, decompression, and posterior transverse process fusion with internal fixation and repair of a previous pseudarthrosis. This case uses cross links for skipped pedicles at L4.

construct.[14,39,54] Screws with a large major diameter have greater pull-out strength, and cortical purchase is stronger than cancellous purchase.[80] Thus, the largest screw that can be implanted through the pedicle with cortical and end-plate penetration, using a screw/bolt design and cross links, more or less bone cement can be used in cases of poor bone. The addition of an anterior column construct (i.e., interbody fusion graft) will also decrease bending and axial forces at the screw and bone, resulting in a fixation that is more load-sharing. Postoperative bracing limits gross spinal range of motion and reduces applied moments onto instrumented segments but does not limit axial load transfer.

In order to avoid hardware failure or loss of fixation, surgeons must understand the patient's pathology and the strengths and weaknesses of various internal fixation systems. Then, they must select a fixation and fusion construct that can withstand the forces to be applied to it.

Pseudarthrosis

The main reason to use internal fixation is to improve the fusion rate, particularly at the lumbosacral junction. There are many different transpedicular screw systems. Most reports about screw systems are difficult to compare because they describe particular screw systems for a variety of spine pathologies. However, bone screw systems are shown to improve fusion results. Roy-Camille[53] reported a 0% pseudarthrosis rate with his screw plate system. Louise[46] reported a 2.6% nonunion rate in acute fractures with only posterior fusion and fixation, but had 100% union with combined anterior/posterior fusion and fixation. Dick,[20] using his "fixateur interne," reported a 1.6% pseudarthrosis rate, while Aebi et al.[3,4] had a 6.7% nonunion rate with the same system. Krag and colleagues[42] developed the Vermont spinal fixator, and they report a 9% to 10% nonunion rate for initial VSF implantation depending on the indications for surgery.

Early series with plate screw systems include the AO tibial dynamic compression plate and the first Steffee VSP systems. The AO series had a 72% fusion rate.[49,65] Steffee et al.[62] reported a 4.1% pseudarthrosis rate. West,[75,76] Whitecloud,[77] and Zucherman[85] and their colleagues reported pseudarthrosis rates ranging from 11% to 18%, with pseudarthrosis repair yielding the poorest result. Heim and Luque[31] developed a semirigid screw plate system, and the multicenter study group outcome revealed a 7% pseudarthrosis rate in 220 patients.

More recent studies now confirm higher fusion rates with transpedicular internal fixation. Lorenz et al.[47] showed prospectively a fusion rate of 100% in the instrumented group versus 58.6% in the noninstrumented group. Steffee and Brantigan[64] also prospectively confirmed higher fusion rates—93% overall; 91.6% failed back, 96.8% spondylolisthesis—with instrumented fusion of three levels or less. A prospective, randomized study by Zdeblick[79] found solid fusions in 95% of the cases that used rigid internal fixation but only 77% solid fusions with the use of semirigid fixation and 65% solid fusions without fixation.

There are many other transpedicular systems, including the Wiltse, Cotrel-Dubousset, ISOLA, Texas Scottish Rite, Danek, and Zielke systems. Fusion results using pedicle instrumentation have been reported both retrospectively[18,33] and prospectively[43,64,79] to be higher in instrumented groups than in noninstrumented groups.[24,34,44,78,79]

Factors responsible for pseudarthrosis include local and systemic conditions, the graft material's ability to stimulate a healing process, surgical preparation of the graft site, and the biomechanics of the graft/internal fixation construct. These factors must all be optimized in order to obtain a solid fusion. If pseudarthrosis occurs, internal fixation constructs that work in compression are more successful than fixation constructs in distraction.[28] Load-sharing constructs or circumferential fusion constructs are also very effective.[57]

Infection

Unfortunately, the risk of injection increases with internal fixation. A larger dissection is required to implant screw fixation. This condition creates more dead space and increases operating time. The hardware itself is also a nidus for infection. Roy-Camille[53] and Steffee[62] and their colleagues reported a 6% incidence of infection in their respective series. Zucherman et al.[84] noted a 5.2% deep wound infection rate.

Other authors have reported infection rates from 0% to 5%.[18,31,47] By using strict antiseptic techniques, perioperative antibiotics, careful handling of the soft tissues, decreased operating room traffic and equipment, and by working with a high degree of dexterity, the infection rate can be reduced.

Miscellaneous Complications

Damage to the adjacent facet joints is another complication that can happen at the time of surgery (i.e., injury to the facet at the time of implantation) or later (i.e., degeneration of the adjacent segments due to increased stress). Because of the relationship between the pedicle and the facet joint, the facet may be compromised while inserting the screw. Even if the joint is not damaged, there may be mechanical compromise because the hardware abuts the facet. This problem can be eliminated by directing a superior screw in a cephalad and lateral-to-medial orientation.[39,74] Late degeneration of the adjacent segment may occur with any fixation system and is probably due to forces from a healed fusion being transferred to the mobile segment and not to the fixation, per se.[43]

Hardware that extends above the facet joints occasionally seems to cause pain. The pain may be caused by the friction between the muscles and the metal, resulting in an inflamed bursa. There may also be skin problems due to pressure, particularly in thin patients and patients requiring postoperative braces.[28] If the hardware causes symptoms, it can be easily removed after the fusion is solid.

Although there are significant theoretical complications with transpedicular internal fixation, the actual problems in clinical practice are few. Davne and Myers[17] studied 486 patients over a 5-year period. Their overall neurologic complication rate was 1.1%, with no neural injuries in the last 333 cases. The infection rate was 2.6% (0.6% deep wound). The hardware failure rate was 4.3%. They showed that, in the hands of experienced spine surgeons, transpedicular screw internal fixation is safe, with very low morbidity.

Transpedicular Internal Fixation Design

There are two major types of transpedicular screw designs: a screw plate construct and a screw bolt construct. They differ in their mechanism of attachment to the screw and in the screw loading mechanism each system employs.

Screw Plate

The screw plate, secured between the pedicle (i.e., the bone) and a nut on the distal end of the screw, is attached to the bone by tightening the screw. The predominant loads are an axial load (P) and a bending moment (M)(Fig. 86-7). The axial load applies a shear force on the screw that is resisted by the transverse force distributed along the screw to the bone interface.[39] The bending moment applies a tensile force to the screw (F)—i.e., a claw-hammer effect. The tensile force is resisted by a longitudinal distributed shear force at the bone screw interface (f). The moment is maximized at the ends of the construct because the moment arm (d) is longest at the ends. The pull-out forces (F) tend to extract the screw from the bone, which loosens the plate connection. When this happens, the plate can no longer resist axial load or the bending moment. If any bone resorption or compression occurs under the plate, the same condition is reproduced. This will tend to toggle the screw in the plate and change the loading on the screw from tensile (F) to cantilever bending. This mechanism is responsible for the high screw breakage rate seen with these systems.

In order to solve this problem, a system was designed to attach the screw rigidly perpendicular to the plate.[62] If the screw is not perpendicular to the plate, the screw shaft will bend as the distal nut is tightened,[80] or the screw will not sit securely against the plate. Either situation will increase the shear stress on the screw and tend to cause screw failure.[39] During surgery, it is difficult to have every screw aligned perpendicular to the plate, especially when performing multilevel fusions and in deformity cases.

The newest modification of the Steffee system has addressed the problem by using angled and different height spacers between the plate and the bone in order to ensure a proper fit. The Danek system has addressed this problem by designing full-length, scalloped, open-slot plates. Bone screw orientation may be optimal without plate design limiting screw position. These plates allow 15 degrees of medial lateral and 30 degrees of craniocaudad angulation without applying increased stress on the screws.[31]

Screw Bolting

Dominant loads applied to the screw in a screw bolting system are similar in axial load, but very different in bending moment to those applied to the screw in a screw plating system (Fig. 86-8). An axial load (P) applies a shear force to the screw that is resisted

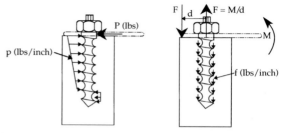

Fig. 86-7

Reactions at bone-screw interface due to applied loads in bone screw plating system. **A**, Reaction to axial load. **B**, Reaction to moment. *(Courtesy of Advanced Spine Fixation Systems, Inc., Cypress, CA.)*

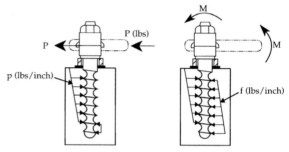

Fig. 86-8

Reactions at bone-screw interface due to applied loads in bone screw bolting system. **A**, Reaction to axial load. **B**, Reaction to moment. *(Courtesy of Advanced Spine Fixation Systems, Inc., Cypress, CA.)*

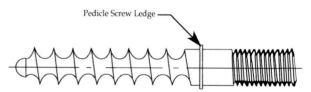

Fig. 86-9

Bone screw showing integral ledge on screw used with screw bolting system. *(Courtesy of Advanced Spine Fixation Systems, Inc., Cypress, CA.)*

by a transverse distributed force along the screw-bone interface. The difference in the screw bolt system is that the bending moment (M) transfers load directly by bending rather than by tension. The bending moment is resisted by a transverse force along the screw-bone interface. Thus, no tensile force is produced to pull out the screw. The integral ledge on the screw (Fig. 86-9) isolates the load to the screw and not to the vertebral body, thereby eliminating the prying mechanism (i.e., the claw-hammer effect) that exists in a plate system. Because the bending moment is transferred directly to the

$$\sigma_t = \frac{M}{\frac{D}{2}\left(\frac{\pi D^2}{4}\right)} = \frac{8M}{\pi D^3}$$

$$\sigma_b = \frac{MD}{2\left(\frac{\pi D^4}{64}\right)} = \frac{32M}{\pi D^3}$$

Fig. 86-10

Stresses on screws. **A,** σt is tensile stress for screw plate system. **B,** $\sigma\beta$ is bending stress of screw bolt system. *(Courtesy of Advanced Spine Fixation Systems, Inc., Cypress, CA.)*

screw and tensile force pull-out is eliminated, the possibility of rod loosening because of extraction (i.e., screw pull-out) is much less.

In a screw bolt system, the screw must resist higher bending loads than in a screw plate system. The bending stress ($\sigma\beta$) on the screw in a screw bolt system is four times greater than the tensile stress ($\sigma\tau$) on the screw in a screw plate system (Fig. 86-10). Even so, the tensile load on a screw in a screw plate system is resisted by the shear strength of the vertebral body, the weakest element in an instrumented spinal segment. Bending moment on the screw is resisted by the strength of the screw. The screw is designed to minimize bending stress with a margin of safety so that there is no risk of pull-out from the screw or screw breakage.

In a screw bolt system, the screw must resist most of the applied load. The inner diameter (i.e., the solid core) of the screw is the most important factor in bending and fatigue strength. The major diameter, which includes the threads, does not significantly affect the strength, stiffness, or fatigue life of the screw, but it does affect pull-out strength. The optimal screw design is a full radius thread with cancellous-type pitch and large inner diameter.[6,39] Large-inner-diameter screws produce little loss in pull-out strength, because they are not under tensile load, and a large gain in bending strength.

Other Issues Related to Transpedicular Screw Systems

Screw Placement

Screws may be placed straight ahead, inward, or up-and-in. Pedicle morphology determines their placement. Screw orientation may be altered by changing the starting hole. To protect the normal adjacent facet, the safest method for placing screws is up-and-in or lateral placement.[74] An up-and-in approach is

also easier, requiring less dissection to implant. The oblique orientation, i.e, the lateral, and up-and-in placement, allows for a longer screw, which increases bone implant purchase and a three-dimensional locking effect (toenailing or delta configuration), which resists lateral shifting. This locking effect lessens the need for a cross linking to longitudinal members to increase construct rigidity.[39]

In the sacrum of S1, screws can be positioned in two directions—posterolateral to anteromedial (i.e., in the sacral promontory) or anteromedial to posterolateral (i.e., in the sacral ala). Zindrick et al.,[80] found that the pull-out strength of the screws is greater if angulated into the sacral ala. Asher and Strippgen[7] found a medial orientation into the sacral promontory to be stronger. The difference in pull-out strength is small, and clinically there is no advantage to either technique. However, the screws should not be implanted straight ahead because anterior cortical penetration might injure the vessels or lower sacral plexus, especially the L5 root, and fixation is weaker.[80]

Depth of the Screw Penetration

There is a linear relationship between the strength of screw purchase and the percentage of vertebral body penetration. The strongest screw purchase occurs when the anterior cortex is engaged.[80] Significant strength is achieved at 80% penetration.[37-39] Clinically, 80% penetration is adequate for most situations, especially when using screw bolt systems. That percent penetration eliminates the potential complications of neurovascular injuries that are due to anterior cortical penetration. Anterior cortical penetration is probably optimal in cases of osteoporosis, reduction of deformity—where bone implant stress is greater—and in screw plate systems that fail by screw pull-out.

Cross Linking (See Figs. 86-5 and 86-6)

Cross links were initially used to increase overall construct rigidity in scoliosis cases. They do increase torsional rigidity,[39] but do not increase any other element of stiffness. Cross links can decrease stress on smaller screws, but the effect is less important as the screw diameter increases more than 5 mm. Cross linking does not reduce screw stress if the screws are oriented out of the sagittal plane (i.e., greater than 30 degrees).[39] Cross linking can prevent lateral shifting of the implant, but is not necessary if screw orientation is out of the sagittal plane (i.e., toenailing).[39] If the construct permits screw orientation

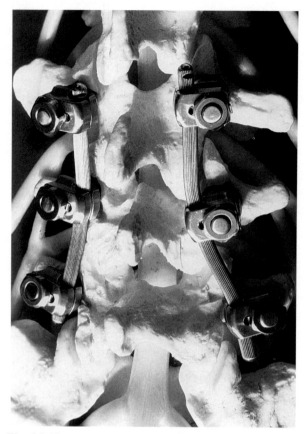

Fig. 86-11

Two-level Wiltse construct implanted into spine model.

medial to the sagittal plane and uses large-diameter screws, and the bone quality is good, cross linking is not necessary. If torsional instability (i.e., trauma or tumor) is a concern or if there is screw orientation of less than 30 degrees from the sagittal plane, poor bone quality, lack of load sharing in the construct, or pedicle levels must be skipped within the construct, then cross linking can increase construct rigidity.

In conclusion, transpedicular screw systems provide superior stability as compared with non-transpedicular screw systems. The improved rigidity of the transpedicular screw systems is due to the fixation of the screw into the vertebral pedicle. This construct controls three-dimensional motion and can resist linear forces and moments about the vertebrae. Bone screws do not rely on ligamentotaxis and can be used over fewer spine segments without the need for posterior elements.

Complications are possible, but are usually related to surgical technique. Device-related complications have decreased because screw system designs have improved. Construct rigidity is decreased by poor bone screw purchase, especially in cases of osteo-

porosis, but this problem can be overcome. Nevertheless, poor bone quality is a relative contraindication for transpedicular screw use.

Internal fixation should be used in a load-sharing manner. Implant survival will be enhanced if forces are shared between the metal and the biologic tissues. If fusion is not achieved, the fixation devices will most likely fail.

The Wiltse System

The Wiltse spinal internal fixation system (see Fig. 86-3) is a transpedicular screw system for the lumbar and lower thoracic spine. It is a screw/bolt (rod) design that is semirigid and is intended to conform to the spine rather than have the spine conform to the internal fixation (Fig. 86-11) (also see Fig. 86-4). The unique component that allows this construct is a saddle/clamp assembly that attaches to the screw. The screw is placed in an optimal position and a malleable rod is contoured to fit into the saddle clamp. A very thorough description of the system and the technical details of its use have been reported by Arnold.[6]

Components

Screws

The screws are made of 316 L Vacuum Melt stainless steel. A screw has an integral ledge (Fig. 86-12) to isolate loads to the screw and a flat edge so the saddle clamp orientation may be adjusted and rotation may be prevented. The screws are manufactured in diameters of 5.0, 5.8, 6.5, 7.0, and 7.5 mm and lengths from 35 to 60 mm. The screws have a full-radius cancellous thread with a large inner diameter to resist bending moments. In addition, the top of the screws are blunt so that inadvertent anterior cortex penetration will not injure anterior soft-tissue structures.

Rods

The rods are made of 316 LVM stainless steel and are 4.4 mm in diameter. The rods are serrated and available in lengths from 65 to 304 mm. The rods are the weak link in the construct and will fail before the screw does.

Saddle Clamp

The saddle clamp assembly connects the rod to the screw. The assembly comes in a single or double con-

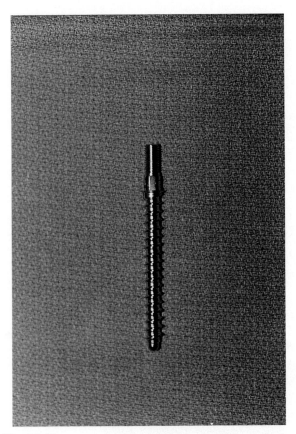

Fig. 86-12
Wiltse transpedicular screw.

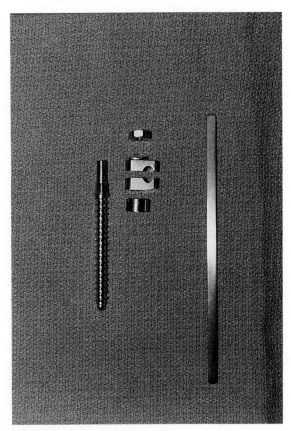

Fig. 86-13
Left-to-right: Wiltse screw, upper and lower saddles with apertures. *Top:* hex-head screw. *Bottom:* Spacer. *Right:* Wiltse serrated rod.

figuration to allow single or double rod constructs. The saddles are also manufactured in offsets from 15 to 45 degrees to preserve the integrity of the facet joints adjacent to the fusion/instrumentation construct. Each of the two saddles in the assembly has a concave aperture (Fig. 86-13). When the two saddles are clamped together they secure the rod at 90 degrees to the center line of the screw (Fig. 86-14). As the nut is tightened, the saddle clamp assembly and rod connect directly to the screw and not the vertebra. The screw does not bend, nor is the pedicle damaged during the tightening process. Spacers ranging in size from 2 to 10 mm placed between the integral ledge and the screw threads stop the screw from further advancement into the pedicel (Fig. 86-15). This placement prevents facet impingement, allows easier rod contouring, and increases the space available for the bone graft. Mid and end cross link saddle clamps are also available to increase torsional rigidity or allow the surgeon to skip pedicles, if necessary.

Advantages

Advantages of the Wiltse system are its screw/bolt design, its relative ease of insertion, its low profile, and its versatility. Because the screws are placed in an optimal position in the pedicle and the rod is contoured to fit the saddle clamp assembly, the Wiltse system is one of the easiest systems to implant. The ease of insertion decreases operative time and potential infection rates. The system is also low profile, which reduces bursa formation around the hardware. The ductile rod allows application in cases of deformity (see Fig. 86-5). The ability to change the system from semirigid to rigid is useful in patients with severe instability, for example, in those who have reconstruction after trauma, tumor, or infection.

Modifications

Two modifications of the Wiltse system were devised by the senior author of this paper. The Selby I

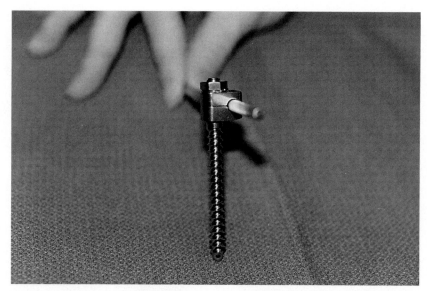

Fig. 86-14

Saddle clamp assembled with rod.

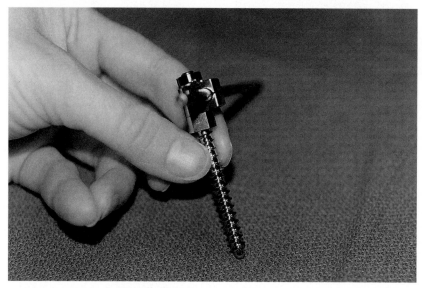

Fig. 86-15

Saddle clamp assembly, including spacer.

(Fig. 86-16) system uses sublaminar wires attached to a bent rod and secured to the sacrum with two sacral bone screws. The Selby II (Fig. 86-17) system uses two laminar hooks connected to a modified Knott rod and secured to the sacrum with two sacral bone hooks. These systems use fewer bone screws, decrease risk to neural structures, and significantly reduce operative time because they are so easy to insert. They are significantly less rigid than bone screw systems—especially in relation to axial load and torsion—require posterior elements, rely on distraction and ligamentotaxis, and are unable to reduce deformity. The Selby systems should only be used in degenerative cases with an interbody graft construct for load sharing. The Selby II system should not be used if more than two levels are included in the fusion, because it will often decrease lumbar lordosis (flat back).

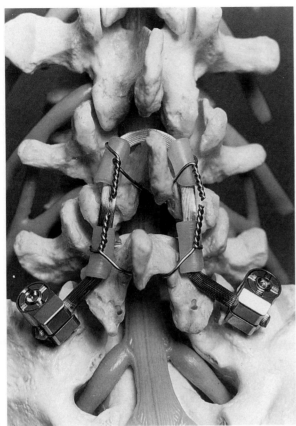

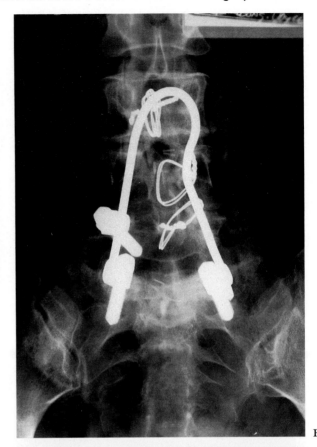

Fig. 86-16

A, Selby I construct implanted on a model representative of the human spine. **B, C,** Selby I construct implanted after decompression and 360 fusion.

Mechanical Testing

Mechanical testing to establish cyclical fatigue failure was conducted. Cyclic testing is more predictive of the long-term in vivo life of an implant than simple strength or stiffness testing. A one-level construct was tested to 10 million cycles, representing a 7-year lifetime. All Wiltse components meet mechanical testing specifications established by the FDA.[2,6]

The Wiltse system was also compared to a Luque rod/sublaminar wire construct and a Harrington rod construct. These systems were tested in intact spines, after partial laminectomy, after total laminectomy, and after facetectomy in cadaveric lumbosacral spines. The Wiltse system was 200% more rigid in flexion, extension, and lateral bending than other systems.[2,6] Panjabi et al.,[50] tested five bone screw systems and facet screw fixation for multidirectional stability. The double- and single-rod Wiltse, the Steffee, Cotrel-Dubosset, and AO systems were evaluated. The most stable system was the Wiltse double-rod system, followed by the Wiltse single-rod and the Steffee plate systems.

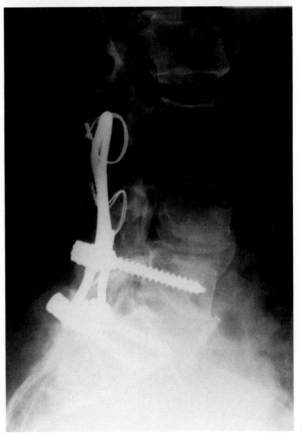

C

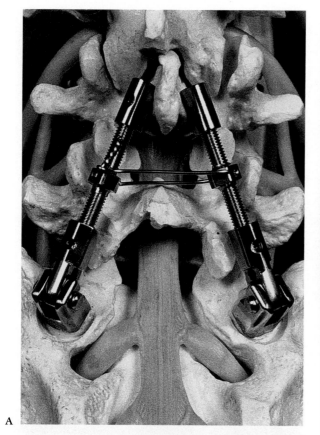

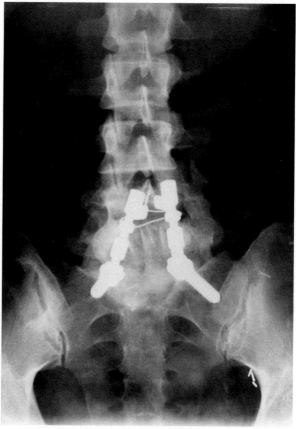

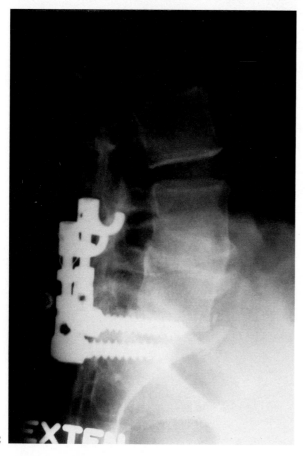

Fig. 86-17

A, Selby II fixation in spine model. **B** and **C,** Selby II fixation status post 360 fusion and decompression.

Indications

Trauma
  Fractures, fracture/dislocation
  Discoligamentous lesion
  Internal disc disruption (Fig. 86-18)
Tumor (reconstruction)
  Posterior
  Combined with anterior reconstructive construct
Deformity
  Degenerative lumbar scoliosis (see Figs. 86-1, 86-3, and 86-5)
  Flat back syndrome (status post osteotomy)
  Spondylolisthesis (Fig. 86-19)
Degenerative
  Spinal stenosis (status post destabilizing decompression) (See Fig. 86-4)
  Fusion for current herniated nucleus pulposus
  Iatrogenic instability
  Degenerative spondylolisthesis (see Fig. 86-11)
Pseudarthrosis
Multilevel fusions

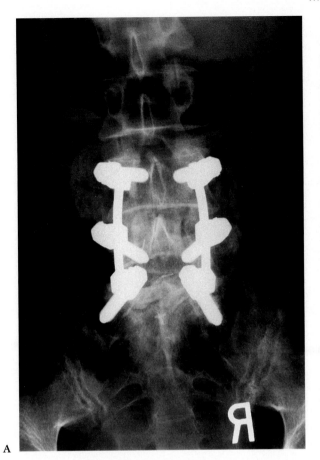

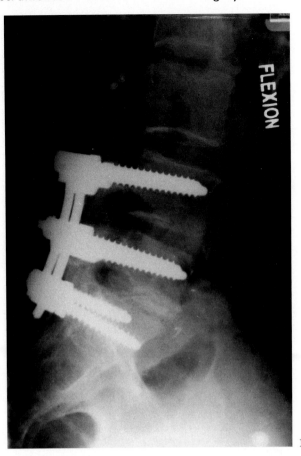

Fig. 86-18

A and B, Postoperative anteroposterior and lateral 360 fusion with Wiltse instrumentation for internal disc disruption.

Anterior (see Fig. 86-18)
Posterior (see Fig. 86-5)
Inflammation
    Seropositive, e.g., rheumatoid arthritis
    Seronegative, e.g., anklosing spondylitis
Infection
    Resolved
    Instability
    Status Post reconstruction, e.g., tuberculosis
Smoker/nicotine use
Contraindications
    Active infection*
    Osteoporosis*

Surgical Technique

Exposure

Two main types of exposure can be performed in the lumbar spine: midline and paraspinal. The mid-

*May use internal fixation in these cases depending on the particular case.

line approach is used when a central decompression is to be performed. The midline approach is also preferred cranial to L3 even if a decompression is not performed. If a decompression is not required, then a paraspinal approach,[78] particularly below L3 in obese or heavily muscled patients is preferred. This approach requires less dissection and tissue trauma and gives the surgeon a direct view to the pedicles and bony surfaces. Alternatively, a lateral stab wound can be made to direct screws medially when a midline approach is used.

Screw Insertion

There are many techniques to localize the pedicle and insert a screw.* Intraoperative fluoroscopy has been advocated by most authors. The American Association of Orthopaedic Surgeons (AAOS) recommends direct visualization of the medial and inferior pedicle wall, which requires limited decompression.[5]

*References 5, 20, 32, 39, 40, 46, 48, 62, and 74.

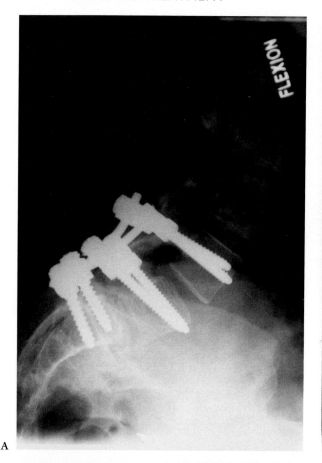

A

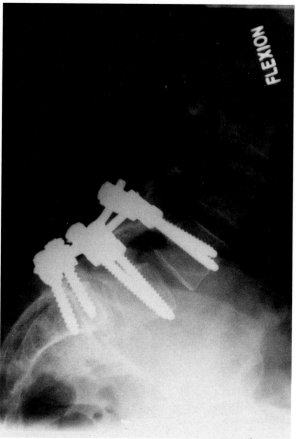

B

Fig. 86-19

A, Grade I spondylolisthesis. **B** and **C,** Anteroposterior and lateral lumbar x-ray films, status post decompression, fusion, and internal fixation.

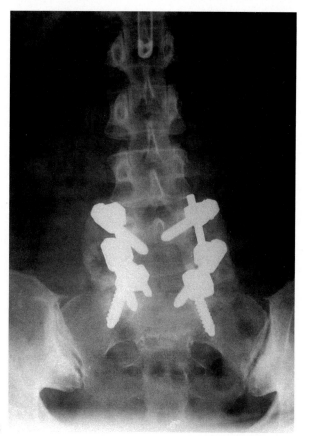

C

We feel that fluoroscopy is cumbersome and unnecessary and that direct visualization is time consuming and not required, but surgeons should use whatever technique they are most comfortable with. Descriptions of either technique are well described elsewhere.

The landmarks for the pedicle starting point are completely visualized after the exposure. The transverse process is seen from the lateral tip to its junction with the outer surface of the superior articular process. A line bisecting the superior and inferior edges of the transverse process intersects with the outside edge of the superior process. This marks the starting point. At S1, the starting point is similar, but the screw can be directed medially into the sacral promontory or laterally into the sacral ala. At S2, the starting point is slightly medial and caudal to a point midway between the first and second sacral foramen. The screw is best directed laterally at S2. Prior to beginning a surgery, a preoperative imaging study should be obtained to account for any variability in

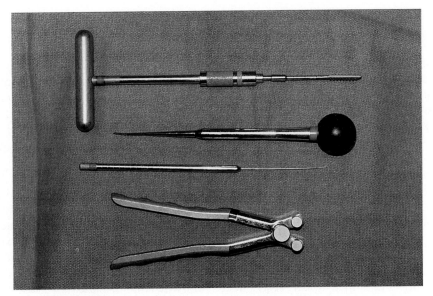

Fig. 86-20

Top-to-bottom: Pedicle tap, pedicle awl, pedicle feeler, hand-held bender.

normal anatomy. The starting point is then decorticated with a high-speed burr.

After the starting point is made, the pedicle is entered with a blunt-tipped, curved awl (Fig. 86-20) that enters the medullary cavity of the pedicle. As standard procedure, the alignment of the awl and pedicle is checked with plain cross-table lateral radiography. This entry into the pedicle gives us our orientation for the insertion of all subsequent instruments into the pedicle. The pedicle is then tapped with an appropriately sized tap for the selected screw. The tap is 15% smaller than the screw, which enhances screw purchase and reduces the chance of expanding or fracturing the pedicle.[6] The tap has a blunt tip and threads so that inadvertent anterior or pedicular cortical penetration does not injure the soft tissues. Only the pedicle is tapped when anterior cortical penetration is not desired. Once the pedicle has been tapped, it is checked with a pedicle sound or probe. The probing is done in a 3, 6, 9, and 12 o'clock orientation to ensure a bone margin around the pedicle. If a decompression has been performed, direct visualization of the pedicle wall and sounding of the pedicle will ensure proper positioning.

At this point, the screw is inserted. Prior to inserting the screw, appropriately sized spacers are selected in order to allow space for the bone graft on the transverse process. In addition, the spacers allow the bottom saddles of the construct to clear the adjacent facet joints, thus avoiding any damage to them. More importantly, by varying spacer height,

the rod can be contoured much more easily. The anterior/posterior rod bend plane can be reduced or eliminated, thus changing a three-dimensional bend into a two-dimensional medial/lateral and craniocaudal bend. If there is no deformity, proper screw orientation within the pedicle can reduce or eliminate the medial/lateral and craniocaudal incongruities into a single plane. With skilled placement of screws and appropriately sized spacers, a complex three-dimensional contouring problem can be changed into a slightly bent or even a straight rod. In deformity cases, the rod needs to be bent considerably in only one plane.

Instrumentation Assembly

At this point, the bottom saddles are applied to the screws. The saddles must be flush with the integral ledge and flat edge of the screw shank. The flat shank prevents the lower saddle from rotating on the screw. The orientation of the screw/saddle can be manipulated to make rod contouring easier. There are offset saddles available to protect the facet joints adjacent to the fusion.

Prior to assembling the fixation construct, the fusion is performed to maximize bone decortication and fill the graft bed with as much bone as possible. The bone is decorticated along the transverse process, superior articular process, and pars interarticularis with a high-speed burr. Then, cancellous bone strips are placed over and between the transverse processes much like the overlapping technique of brick masonry. Smaller pieces of bone are packed into any gaps.

Once the bottom saddles are in place, a rod is selected and contoured. First, an appropriate rod length is determined. The rods come in multiple lengths and can be cut with a bolt cutter for proper fit. If good screw orientation has been performed and appropriate spacer selection has been made, the rod can be contoured freehand with a hand-held bender. If this is not possible, an aluminum rod may be used as a template for a more accurate fit. An aluminum rod, which bends easily, is placed over the bottom saddles, and a perfect fit is constructed. The template is then placed in a C-clamp bending vise, or for more difficult bends, a major support rod bending system. The stainless steel rod is then contoured to match the aluminum template precisely. This shaping is performed with several bending tools that come with the system.

Fusion

When the final contour of the rod has been shaped, it is placed on the bottom saddles. The top saddles are placed on the screws over the rods and locked in place with a nut. The nut is tightened with a wrench while a counter torque is applied with the crow's-foot wrench on the top saddle to prevent pedicle injury, rotation of the screw/saddle, and adverse loading of the screw. Once the final assembly is completed, the nuts are locked into place by crimping the lock washer located on the top saddle. The rods and inner aperture of the saddles are serrated to prevent rotation of the rods in the saddles.

A cross-link assembly can be used at this time. The system has midline and end cross-link constructs. The mid cross link is applied after the main construct is secured. The end cross links are applied at the time of the main rod assembly.

After the entire assembly is completed, final details are addressed. Any remaining bone graft is placed in the graft bed around the fixation. Throughout the operation, the wound is frequently irrigated in order to dilute any bacterial contamination and to keep soft tissues moist. Large suction drains are placed over the fusion bed, and the wound is closed in anatomic layers.

Clinical Results

The Wiltse system has been in clinical use since 1985. The results have been recorded by a national

multicenter study and independent studies. These studies document the efficacy and safety of the Wiltse system.

The earliest review of the Wiltse system was from the Wiltse Spinal Institute by Horowitch et al.[32] This study reflected the earliest experience with this system, and the findings led to improvement in the design and implantation techniques. The patient population included a variety of surgical pathologies, including previous surgical failures, pseudarthrosis, multilevel fusions, deformity, etc. The overall fusion rate was 68%, with clinical improvement in 70% and no improvement or worsening symptoms in 30%. The complications included 4 infections, 2 neurologic injuries and 11 hardware failures in 99 patients.

Other early studies showed better results. Guyer et al.[30] reported a 71% fusion rate at 1-year follow-up with 90% of patients reporting improvement in pain—52% greatly improved, 26% improved, 13% slightly improved. Complications in 222 patients included 4 hardware failures, 7 dural tears, and 1 superficial infection. They reported no neurologic injury or deep wound infection. Capen et al, in a retrospective study of 105 patients, reported an overall fusion rate of 85% in a mixed population. Complications included 5 hardware failures, all associated with pseudarthrosis, 6 transient neurologic deficits, and 20 hardware removals. There were 2 deep and 3 superficial wound infections, with 30 patients requiring drainage of a seroma. Blumenthal and Gill[11] reported their experience with the Wiltse system in 476 patients. Their overall fusion rate was 91%, with an overall complication rate of 6%. They had 15 hardware failures and 2 neurologic deficits (0.4%). Their infection rate was 2%, with 3 superficial and 5 deep wound infections. In addition, they had to drain 2 seromas.

Salib et al.[57] reported the first prospective series using the Wiltse system for spinal fusion. The overall fusion rate was 93%. The type of surgical procedure influenced the fusion rate. The fusion rate for a posterior lumbar interbody fusion/posterolateral fusion was only 58%, while the posterolateral fusion alone was 95% and the combined anterior lumbar/posterolateral fusion procedure (360) was 100%. Repair of a preoperative pseudarthrosis had a lower fusion rate of 88%.

The clinical outcome was measured based on the preoperative diagnosis and surgical procedure. Patients with disc disruption syndrome had 100% satisfactory results, while degenerative disc disease, spondylolisthesis, segmental instability, and pseudarthrosis had 82%, 93%, 82%, and 70% satisfactory results, respectively. Patients who had a combined anterior/posterior fusion had an 80% satisfactory result, while the posterolateral and PLIF procedure produced 76% and 75% satisfactory result, respectively.

The complications were infrequent. Hardware failure occurred with one screw and one rod (0.28%) breakage. There were 12 nerve root injuries, of which 8 were transient. Four patients underwent surgical reexploration—2 screws were cut out of the pedicle, and symptoms resolved with screw removal. Two neurologic deficits were not related to the hardware. There was one superficial (0.9%) and 2 deep (1.8%) wound infections.

The Phase III limb of the national multicenter study[2] is now complete. Only degenerative diseases—degenerative disc disease, degenerative spondylolisthesis, spinal stenosis—were included in the study protocol of 206 patients. Forty-six percent of the patients had prior surgery and 50% were smokers. Fifty-two percent had a posterior transverse process fusion, 37% had a transverse process/posterior lumbar interbody fusion, and 18% had an Anterior Lumbar Interbody Fusion/Transverse Process Fusion. The overall fusion rate was 95% and the Transverse Process Fusion/Posterior Lumbar Interbody Fusion procedure was responsible for 10 of the 15 nonunions. Seven patients were smokers, and 3 nonunions were multilevel fusions. Pain assessment shows pain to be eliminated or greatly reduced in 55% of patients, while 34% reported improvement in their pain. Functionally, patients able to perform moderate or normal activity increased from 14% preoperatively to 78% postoperatively. Ninety-one percent of the patients with successful fusion showed improvement in pain as compared with 62% with nonunions. Similarly, postoperative function improved in 81% of successful fusions as compared with 38% of nonunions.

The complication rate was low. Hardware failure occurred, with 6 broken screws out of 967 implanted (0.62%) and 13 broken rods of the 415 implanted (3.1%). There were 5 wound infections, 13 seromas, and 1 hematoma. There were 7 dural leaks unrelated to the hardware and no neurologic injuries or deficits secondary to the hardware.

The Wiltse system is a semirigid, transpedicular internal fixation system designed to obtain fusion primarily for degenerative disease of the lumbar spine. It is easy to implant, versatile, safe, and efficacious. This device is a valuable tool in the armamentarium of the spine surgeon.

References

1. Abumi K, Panjabi MM, Duranceau JS: Biomechanical evaluation of spinal fixation devices. Part III. Stability provided by six spinal fixation devices and interbody bone graft, *Spine* 14:1249, 1989.
2. Advanced Spine Fixation Systems, Incorporated, 11730 Seaboard Circle, Stanton, California 90680.
3. Aebi M, Etter C, Kehl, T et al.: Stabilization of the lower thoracic and lumbar spine with the internal spinal skeletal fixation system: indications, techniques, and first results of treatment, *Spine* 12:544, 1987.
4. Aebi M, Etter C, Kehl T, et al.: The internal skeletal fixation system: a new treatment of thoracolumbar fractures and spine disorders, *Clin Orthop* 227:30, 1988.
5. American Academy of Orthopaedic Surgeons, Summer Institute in San Diego, California, 1988.
6. Arnold DM: *The Wiltse system of internal fixation*. In Arnold DM, Lonstein JE, editors: *Pedicle fixation of the lumbar spine*, Spine State of the Art Reviews, vol. 61, no. 1, Philadelphia, 1992, Hanley & Belfus, Inc., p. 55.
7. Asher MA, Strippgen WE: Anthropometric studies of the human sacrum relating to dorsal transsacral implant designs (abstract), *Clin Orthop Relat Res* 203:58, 1986.
8. Ashman RB, Bechtold JE, Edwards T, et al.: In-vitro spine implant mechanical testing protocol, *J Spinal Disord* 2:274, 1989.
9. Ashman RB, Galpin RD, Corin JD, Johnston CE: Biomechanical analysis of pedicle screw instrumentation systems in a corpectomy model (abstract), *Spine* 14:1398, 1989.
10. Badalamente MA, Dee R, Ghillani R, et al.: Mechanical stimulation of dorsal root ganglia induces increased production of substance P: a mechanism for pain following nerve root compromise, *Spine* 12:552, 1987.
11. Blumenthal SL, Gill K: *Complications of pedicle screw fixation*. Presented at the annual meeting of the International Society for the Study of Lumbar Spine, Hamburg, Germany, 1991.
12. Boucher HH: A method of spinal fusion, *J Bone Joint Surg* 41B:248, 1959.
13. Brodsky AE, Hendricks RL, Khalil MA, et al.: Segmental ("floating") lumbar spine fusions, *Spine* 14:447, 1989.
14. Chopin D, Matta J: *Selective study of the treatment in idiopathic scoliosis double major curves using traditional CD constructs and combined pedicle fixation with cross plates* (abstract). Presented at the International Congress of CD Instrumentation, 1991.
15. Cleveland M, Bosworth DM, Thompson FR: Pseudarthrosis in the lumbosacral spine, *J Bone Joint Surg* 40A:91, 1948.
16. Coe JD, Warden KE, Herzig MA, McAfee PC: Influence of bone mineral density on the fixation of thoracolumbar implants: a comparative study of transpedicular screws, laminar hooks, and spinous process wires, *Spine* 15:902, 1990.

17. Davne SH, Myers DL: Complications of lumbar spinal fusions with the transpedicular instrumentations, *Spine* 17:S184, 1992.

18. Dean SM, Hall BB, Johnson RG: Analysis of posterolateral lumbar fusion and VSP pedicle screw and plate fixation. In *Proceedings of the 57th Annual Meeting of the Academy of Orthopaedic Surgeons,* 1990.

19. DePalma AF, Rothman RH: The nature of pseudarthrosis, *Clin Orthop* 59:113, 1968.

20. Dick W: The "fixateur interne" as a versatile implant for spine surgery, *Spine* 12:882, 1987.

21. Drummond DW, Guadagni J, Keene JS, et al.: Interspinous process segmental spinal instrumentation, *J Pediatr Orthop* 4:397, 1984.

22. Edwards CC: Presented at the Spinal Fixation Study group, Baltimore, 1987.

23. Ferguson RL, Tencer AF, Woodard P, Allen BL Jr: Biomechanical comparisons of spinal fracture models and stabilizing effects of posterior instrumentations. *Spine* 13:453, 1988.

24. Frymoyer JW, Hanley EN, Howe J, et al.: A comparison of radiographic findings in fusion and nonfusion patients ten or more years following lumbar disc surgery, *Spine* 4:435, 1979.

25. Frymoyer JW: The role of spine fusion, *Spine* 5:284, 1981.

26. Gaines RW, Carson WL, Satterlee CC: Groh GI: Improving quality of spinal internal fixation: evolution toward ideal immobilization. A biomechanical study (abstract), *Proc Scoliosis Res Soc*, 1986.

27. Gelpin RD, Corin J, Ashman R, Johnston CE: *Biomechanical testing of pedicle screw instrumentation in a burst fracture model.* Presented at the 22nd annual meeting of the Scoliosis Research Society, Vancouver, British Columbia, September 1987.

28. Georgis T, Rydevik B, Weinstein JN, Garfin SR: *Complications of pedicle screw fixation.* In Garfin SR, editor: *Complications of spine surgery,* Baltimore, 1989, Williams & Wilkins.

29. Gurr KR, McAfee PC, Shih CM: Biomechanical analysis of anterior and posterior instrumentation systems after corpectomy: a calf-spine model, *J Bone Joint Surg* 70A:1182, 1988.

30. Guyer RD, Hochschuler SH, Stith WJ, et al: Initial results and complications of pedicle screw fixation. Poster exhibit at the annual meeting of the North American Spine Society, Monterey, CA, 1990.

31. Heim SE, Luque ER: *Danek plate and screw system.* In Arnold DM, Lonstein JE, et al, editors: *Pedicle fixation of the lumbar spine.* Spine State of the Art Reviews, vol. 6, no. 1, Philadelphia, 1992, Hanley and Belfus, Inc., p. 201.

32. Horowitch A, Peek RD, Thomas JC, et al.: The Wiltse pedicle screw fixation system: early clinical results, *Spine* 14:461, 1989.

33. Kabins MB, Weinstein JN, Spratt KF, et al.: Isolated L4-L5 fusions using the variable screw placement system: unilateral versus bilateral, *J Spinal Disord* 5:39, 1992.

34. Kelly RP: Intertransverse fusion of the low back, *Trans South Surg Assoc* 74:193, 1963.

35. Kim SS, Denis F, Lonstein JE, Winter RB: Factors affecting fusion rate in adult spondylolisthesis, *Spine* 15:9, 1990.

36. King D: Internal fixation for lumbosacral fusion, *J Bone Joint Surg* 30A:560, 1948.

37. Krag MH, Beynnon BD, Pope MH, et al.: An internal fixator for posterior application to short segments of the thoracic, lumbar, or lumbosacral spine, design, and testing, *Clin Orthop* 203:75, 1986.

38. Krag MH, Breynnon BD, DeCoster TA, Pope MH: Depth of insertion of transpedicular vertebral screws into human vertebrae: effect upon screw-vertebrae interface strength, *J Spinal Disord* 1:287, 1988.

39. Krag MH: *Spinal fusion: overview of options and posterior internal fixation devices.* In Frymoyer JW, editor: *The adult spine: principles and practice.* New York, 1991, Raven Press.

40. Krag MH, Weaver DL, Breynnon BD, Haugh LD: Morphometry of the thoracic and lumbar spine related to transpedicular screw placement for surgical and spinal fixation, *Spine* 13:27, 1988.

41. Krag MN, Beynnon SD, Pope MN, et al.: An internal fixator for posterior application to short segments of the thoracic lumbar or lumbosacral spine: design and testing, *Clin Orthop* 203:75, 1986.

42. Krag MN: *Vermont spinal fixator.* In Arnold DM, Lonstein JE, et al., editors: *Pedicle fixation of the lumbar spine,* Spine State of the Art Reviews, vol. 6, no. 2, Philadelphia, 1992, Hanley & Belfus, Inc., p. 121.

43. Lee CK: Accelerated degeneration of the segment adjacent to a lumbar fusion, *Spine* 13:375, 1988.

44. Lehmann TR, Spratt KF, Tozzi JE, et al.: Long-term follow-up of lower lumbar fusion patients, *Spine* 12:97, 1987.

45. Lenke LG, Birdwell KH, Bladus C, et al.: *Results of in-situ fusion for isthmic spondylolisthesis.* Presented at the annual meeting of the scoliosis research society, Minneapolis, MN, September 27, 1991.

46. Louis R: Fusion of the lumbar and sacral spine by internal fixation with screw plates, *Clin Orthop* 203:18, 1986.

47. Lorenz M, Zindrick M, Schwaegler P, et al.: A comparison of single level fusions with and without hardware, *Spine* 16:S455, 1991.

48. Luque ER: *Semirigid interpedicular fixation in correction of instability of the low back.* Presented at the North American Spine Society meeting, 1990.

49. Muller ME, Allgower M, Schneider R, et al.: *Techniques recommended by the AO group, in 1979 Manual of Internal Fixation,* Berlin, 1979, Springer-Verlag.

50. Panjabi MM, Tammamoto I, Oxland T, et al.: *Biomechanical comparison of the stability provided by four pedicle screw systems and facet screw fixation.* Presented at the annual meeting of the Scoliosis Research Society, Amsterdam, The Netherlands, September 17-22, 1989.

51. Panjabi MM, Abumi K, Duranceau J, Crisco JJ: Biomechanical evaluation of spinal fixation devices: part II. Stability provided by eight internal fixation devices, *Spine* 13:1135.

52. Ranson N, LaRocca S, Thalgott J: *Comparative results of three posterolateral lumbosacral arthrodesis techniques: no instrumentation, sublaminar wiring and A.O. intrapedicular screw and plate fixation.* Presented at the annual meeting of the American Academy of Orthopaedic Surgeons, New Orleans, February 1990.

53. Roy-Camille R, Saillant G, Mazel C: Internal fixation of the lumbar spine with pedicle screw plating, *Clin Orthop* 203:7, 1986.

54. Ruland CM, McAfee PC, Wardem KE, Cunningham BW: Triangulation of pedicular instrumentation: a biomechanical analysis, *Spine* 16:S270, 1991.

55. Rutkow IM: Orthopaedic operation in The United States, 1979-1983, *J Bone Joint Surg* 68A:716, 1986.

56. Saal JS, Franson RC, Dobrow R, et al.: High levels of inflammatory phospholipase A2 activity in lumbar disc herniations, *Spine* 15:674, 1990.

57. Salib R, Pettine K, Akins W: *Prospective evaluation of lumbar fusions utilizing Wiltse pedicle screw fixation.* Presented at the annual meeting of the North American Spine Society, Keystone, CO, 1991.

58. Selby D: Internal fixation with Knodt's rods, *Clin Orthop* 203:179, 1986.

59. Shirado O, Zbeblick TA, Ward KE, McAfee PC: *Biomechanical evaluation of posterior spine stabilization methods for lumbosacral isthmic spondylolisthesis.* Presented at the 52nd annual meeting of the American Academy of Orthopaedic Surgeons, New Orleans, February 1990.

60. Soshi S, Shiba R, Kondo H, Murati K: An experimental study of transpedicular screw fixation in relation to osteoporosis in the lumbar spine, *Spine* 16:1335, 1991.

61. Stauffer RN, Coventry MB: Posterolateral lumbar spine fusion, *J Bone Joint Surg* 54A:1195, 1972.

62. Steffee A, Biscup R, Sitkowski D: Segmental spine plates with pedicle screw fixation, *Clin Orthop* 227:82, 1988.

63. Steffee AD, Sitkowski D: Reduction and stabilization of Grade IV spondylolisthesis, *Clin Orthop* 227:82, 1988.

64. Steffee AD, Brantigan JW: *The VSP fixation system—report of a prospective study of 250 patients enrolled in FDA clinical trials.* Presented at the North American Spine Society meeting, 1992.

65. Thalgott JS, LaRocca H, Aebi M, et al.: Reconstruction of the lumbar spine using AO DCP plate internal fixation, *Spine* 14:91, 1989.

66. Thompson WA, Gristina AG, Healy WA: Lumbosacral spine fusion: a method of bilateral posterolateral fusion combined with Hibb's fusion, *J Bone Joint Surg* 56A:1643, 1974.

67. Thompson WAL, Ralston EL: Pseudarthrosis following spine fusion, *J Bone Joint Surg* 31A:400, 1949.

68. Truchley G, Thompson WAL: Posterior lateral fusion of the lumbosacral spine, *J Bone Joint Surg* 44A:505, 1962.

69. Truchly G, Thompson WAL: Posterior lateral fusions: 14 years experience with a salvage procedure for failures of spine fusion, *J Bone Joint Surg* 52A:826, 1970.

70. Watkins MB: Posterior lateral fusion in pseudarthrosis and posterior element defects of the lumbosacral spine, *Clin Orthop* 35:80, 1964.

71. Weinstein JN, Spratt KF, Spengler D, et al.: Spinal pedicle fixation: Reliability and validity of roentgenogram-based assessment and surgical factors on successful screw placement, *Spine* 13:1012, 1988.

72. Weinstein JN, Claverie W, Gibson S: The pain of discography, *Spine* 13:1344, 1988.

73. Weinstein JN, Pope MH, Schmidt R, Seroussi R: Neuropharmacologic effects of vibration on the dorsal root ganglion, an animal model, *Spine* 13:521, 1988.

74. Weinstein JN: Kabins MB: *The evolution and efficacy of pedicle fixation of the spine.* In Stauffer RN, editor: *Advances in operative orthopaedics,* vol. 1, St. Louis, 1993, Mosby.

75. West JL, Bradford DS, Ogilvie JW: *Complications of Steffee plate pedicle screw fixation.* Presented at the North American Spine Society meeting, 1989.

76. West JL, Bradford DS, Ogilvie JW: *Steffee Instrumentation: two-year results.* Presented at the 23rd annual meeting of the Scoliosis Research Society.

77. Whitecloud TS III, Skalley TC, Morgan EL, et al.: *Radiographic measurement of pedicle screw penetration.* Presented at the North American Spine Society meeting, 1989.

78. Wiltse LL, Bateman JG, Hutchinson RH, et al.: The paraspinal sacrospinalis splitting approach to the lumbar spine, *J Bone Joint Surg* 50A:919, 1968.

79. Zdeblick TA: A prospective, randomized study of lumbar fusion, *Spine* 18:983, 1993.

80. Zindrick MR, Wiltse LL, Widell EH, et al.: A biomechanical study of intrapedicular screw fixation in the lumbar spine, *Clin Orthop* 203:99, 1986.

81. Zindrick MR, Lorenz MA, Knight GW, et al.: *The effect of methylmethacrylate augmentation upon pedicle screw fixation.* Presented at the International Society for the Study of the Lumbar Spine meeting, Dallas, TX, June 1987.

82. Zindrick MR: The role of transpedicular fixation systems for the stabilization of the lumbar spine, *Orthop Clin North Am* 22:333, 1991.

83. Zindrick MR, Wiltse LL, Doornik A, et al.: Analysis of the morphometric characteristics of the thoracic and lumbar pedicles; *Spine* 12:160, 1987.

84. Zucherman J, Hsu K, White A, et al.: Early results of spinal fusion using variable spine plating systems, *Spine* 5:570, 1988.

Chapter 87

The Vermont Spinal Fixator for Posterior Application to Short Segments of the Thoracic, Lumbar, or Lumbosacral Spine

Martin H. Krag

Bruce D. Beynnon

Design Objectives

   minimal length of spinal involvement
   three-dimensional adjustability
   three-dimensional positional control
   spinal-canal avoidance
   use of safest surgical approach

Design Issues

   in vivo loads
   vertebral morphometry
   bone-screw design
   articulating clamp
   depth of screw penetration into vertebra
   screw placement

Methods

   vertebral morphometry
   bone-screw design
   articulating clamp
   depth of screw penetration into vertebra
   screw placement

Results

   vertebral morphometry
   bone-screw design
   articulating clamp
   depth of screw penetration into vertebra
   screw placement
   current design

Discussion

   vertebral morphometry
   bone-screw design
   articulating clamp
   depth of screw penetration into vertebra
   screw placement
   in vivo loads

Clinical Experience

Summary

The Vermont Spinal Fixator (VSF), intended for application to "short-segment" spinal defects such as disc degeneration, fracture, spondylolisthesis or tumor, has undergone extensive biomechanical testing and clinical use, beginning in the mid-1980s. Its major characteristics are (1) three-dimensional adjustability, which allows anatomically and biomechanically optimal screw placement (without having to align screws to holes or slots in a plate) and also easy reduction of fracture/dislocations or spondylolisthesis; (2) three-dimensional fixation that prevents loss of alignment, even without anterior intervertebral body load sharing; (3) compact, simple design with very few parts to reduce "fiddle factor," to allow as short as single motion-segment instrumentation, and to reduce adjacent soft-tissue irritation; and (4) use of bone screws for attachment, which eliminates deliberate encroachment into the spinal canal (e.g., Luque wires or Harrington hooks) and allows much more secure fixation than do hooks, even to the sacrum or to laminectomized vertebrae.

Extensive investigations for the VSF have included study of the following issues: (1) CT-measured pedicle morphometry to define allowable screw diameters and lengths; (2) effect of pitch, minor diameter, and tooth profile on screw pull-out strength; (3) static and fatigue strength of a compact, three-dimensionally adjustable, strong, articulating clamp; (4) the relationship between screw depth of penetration into the vertebra and screw-bone interface strength; and (5) biomechanical comparison between sacral screws placed anteromedially (into the promontory) and anterolaterally (into the ala). In addition, clinical experience with the VSF is summarized.

Major advances have been made in the field of spinal surgery in recent years.* Important contributions to these advances have come from the application of biomechanics to spine problems† and from the growing variety of spinal implants that have become available.‡

An important group of spinal implants is comprised of devices that attach to the posterior aspect of the spine by means of screws placed through the pedicle into the vertebral body. One of these implants is the Vermont Spinal Fixator (VSF), the concept for which was formed in 1981, based on exposure by the

author to the Roy-Camille plate and screw system and to the external fixator work of Magerl and Schläpfer.[106-109,152,153] The basic idea was to "internalize an external fixator." At that time, almost all the basic morphometric and biomechanical issues remained to be resolved. Presented here is the rationale for the VSF design, the results of anatomical and biomechanical investigations relevant to it, and a summary of clinical experience with it.

Design Objectives

Minimal Length of Spinal Involvement

When fusion is indicated for single-level instability, only two vertebrae in principle need to be incorporated in the fusion mass. Even in the case of instability from a severely comminuted fracture, only three vertebrae need to be fused. From a mechanical viewpoint, a short fusion is not strengthened by adding to its length (a one-foot length of chain is as strong in tension as a three-foot length of chain). From a biologic viewpoint, unnecessary disruption of normal tissue should certainly be avoided.

Despite this, five, six, or even seven vertebrae are typically involved when using Harrington distraction rods, the most commonly used implant for dealing with instability, used either in their standard configuration,* or with modifications.† This is related to the history of Harrington rods,[66] which were devised for management of long-segment deformities, such as scoliosis, and then subsequently applied to short-segment problems (instability, spondylolisthesis, fracture).

Since the mechanical characteristics of short-segment problems are quite different, an implant specifically designed for such problems would probably function better. Placement of Harrington hooks more closely together than five vertebrae fails to achieve adequate stabilization. This same dependency on five or more segments occurs with posterior plates and screws, such as Williams,[174,179] Wilson,[64,101,180] or Roy-Camille.[68,103,143,145] One method of decreasing the fusion length is the "rod long, fuse short" technique,[4,24,71,72] in which the rods are removed after the graft is solid. Not only does this involve a second operation, but early evidence[76,77] suggests that facet arthrosis may become a problem at the levels temporarily immobilized but not grafted.

*References 15, 57, 69, 70, 134, and 160.
†References 7, 19, 23, 41, 43, 44, 58, 61, 73, 74, 79, 81, 84, 98, 100, 102, 111, 113, 116, 121, 124, 125, 136, 141, 152, 153, 156, 157, 161, 167, 168, 171, 172, 176, 177, 181, 182, and 185.
‡References 6, 14, 17, 21, 42, 59, 62, 78, 103, 104, 108, 109, 117, 128, 132, 133, 137, 140, 143, 145, 148, 158, 159, 166, and 170.

*References 1, 4, 24, 25, 33, 35, 39, 51, 52, 63, 65, 74, 75, 112, 114, 129, 150, 155, 163, 174, 178, and 183.
†References 13, 18, 20, 34, 41, 45, 46, 48, 50, 53, 56, 73, 80, 117, 122, 154, 162, 164, 165, and 182.

Three-Dimensional Adjustability

Three-dimensional adjustability means that the longitudinal linking element (e.g., rod or plate) is able to be attached to the bone screw at any orientation or position. This allows the screw to be placed in the vertebra in an anatomically optimal position, without any additional constraint imposed by its method of attachment to the longitudinal element. This also allows the screws to be used as a means of intraoperative realignment (e.g., for fracture/dislocations or spondylolisthesis) and still to be attachable in their new position to the longitudinal element.

Three-Dimensional Positional Control

One major purpose of any fixation device is to increase the likelihood of achieving successful bone fusion. There are no data to suggest that motion in any particular direction is better or worse than in any other, in terms of achieving fusion. Thus, fully three-dimensional fixation becomes a logical objective. A second purpose of a fixation device is to limit intervertebral motion so as to prevent nerve-root or spinal cord pressure. This may potentially be produced by any one of various displacements (either rotations or translations), so again three-dimensional fixation becomes the objective.

Despite this, most current spinal posterior implants do not produce such three-dimensional fixation. This occurs for one or more of three reasons: (1) absence of a rigid attachment to the vertebra itself; (2) reliance on soft tissues to not stretch out or "creep"; or (3) absence of rigid attachment between components of the device.

The most commonly used spinal implant, the Harrington rod system, has all three of the above characteristics. The hooks simply push (or pull) against their attachment sites, and they rely on soft-tissue resistance[2,3,9] as well as external trunk support (bracing) to produce sufficient vertebral-motion limitation. As a result, lordosis flattening in the lumbar spine[67,117] or overdistraction at a fracture site[2,3,9] can occur. Once displacement occurs, the hooks may detach from the rod. Modified hooks[13,49,74] or segmental wiring[41,104,164] represent significant improvements, but flexion/extension can still occur by means of the lamina rotating within the hook or wire loop. This lack of three-dimensional fixation at the attachment sites of Harrington hooks (for Luque wires, for that matter), is a part of the reason that these implants must span five, six, or even seven vertebrae to develop adequate stability.

With posterior plates and screws, the screw does provide a rigid grip on the vertebra. However, the screw is not rigidly mechanically linked to the plate. Rather, sufficient compression between plate and underlying bone is needed to prevent "toggle" of the screw in its plate hole[153] or excessive shearing forces on the screw. The occurrence of this toggle is probably related to the fall-off in screw tension known to occur in vivo.[12] This issue is a concern even when these plates are mounted onto broad surfaces such as the femur or tibia.[26] The problem becomes even greater when the plates are attached to the spine, where the bone bed is quite irregular.[68,181] This results in relatively small bone-plate contact areas and thus high contact pressures, increasing the likelihood of bending or shear loads being applied to the screws. These plates, of course, overlay a significant portion of the surface normally used as a graft bed.[181] As with the rods, here also, five vertebrae must be instrumented for adequate control of significant instability.[143,145]

The Magerl external fixator[106,107,152,181] was the first device to provide a secure grip on the vertebrae to which it was attached, to not rely on soft tissues to provide three-dimensional adjustability, and to provide secure three-dimensional positional control. Thus, this device represents a major advance in spinal implants. It does have the characteristics of any external fixator in that pin-track infections may occur and the posterior prominence of the device is an inconvenience. The flexibility due to the unsupported span of the Schanz pins has been conjectured to provide a certain "shock-absorbing" quality. However, this same characteristic also has led its developers to recommend the use of supplemental internal fixation in more unstable cases, which limits the range of cases in which the pins may be applied percutaneously. In addition, this flexibility often requires the device to be used as either a distractor or a compressor, rather than as a fixator. Thus, it relies on soft tissues being sufficiently intact to prevent excessive creep.

Spinal-Canal Avoidance

Deliberate encroachment into the spinal canal is a routine part of most device implantation, either with hooks (e.g., Harrington, Weiss, Knodt) or wires (e.g., Luque) or both. Use of hooks alone has been quite safe, although problems do occur,[60,110] and there is the always-present risk of intraoperative errors when working within the spinal canal. The use of laminar wires has caused some major complica-

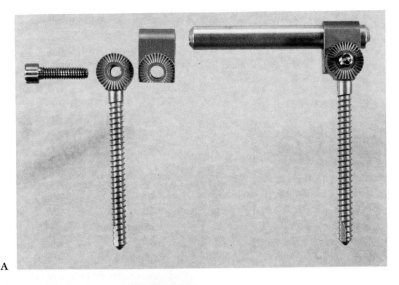

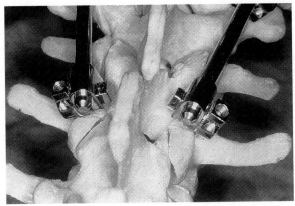

Fig. 87-1

A, VSF components consist of bone screw, articulating clamp, clamp bolt, and connecting rod. **B,** VSF assembled is compact and allows "up and in" screw placement to avoid facet-joint impingement, allow longer screw depth of penetration, and produce greater screw-bone interface strength.

tions either during their placement[75,142,175] or removal,[11,126] or when used in combination with Harrington hooks.[142,175]

All these complications are related to deliberate violation of the spinal canal during the process of implanting these devices. In contrast, bone-screw placement does not require entrance into the canal. Extensive experience with the safety of this method has been gathered, either with plates, external fixators, or facet-joint fusions.[16,82,130] The risks of screw placement too far medially or too far anteriorly do exist, but modern image intensifiers allow good intraoperative visualization to guard against both these risks. A further safeguard to keeping the screw within the pedicle is the fact that the medial and inferior pedicle borders may be easily and safely palpated intraoperatively.[108,109,143]

Use of Safest Surgical Approach

The choice between anterior- and posterior-approach devices depends on many factors, but certainly there are advantages to avoiding the abdominal or thoracic cavities. For cases in which the anterior approach is selected primarily in order to perform spinal-canal decompression, a variety of stabilizing devices are becoming available.* These involve only a limited segment of spine and do not require spinal-canal encroachment. At least one of them[42] provides full three-dimensional rigid fixation, although anterior prominence and proximity to the aorta is an issue about which some concern exists.

In order to achieve all five of the above design objectives simultaneously, the authors' approach has been to devise an "internal fixator" (Fig. 87-1) that (1) could be adjusted to span as short as a single motion segment; (2) provides truly three-dimensional positional adjustability; (3) provides secure three-dimensional fixation by attachment through the pedicle into the vertebral body; (4) does not violate the spinal canal; and (5) utilizes the posterior approach.

*References 14, 42, 59, 62, 78, 133, 137, 140, 143, 145, and 148.

Design Issues

To achieve the above five objectives, six major design issues were identified for further investigation as discussed below.

In Vivo Loads

Few data are available concerning the loads that the implant needs to support. Schläpfer and co-workers[152,181] have presented their results using an external spinal fixator as a load transducer, but the data are not fully three-dimensional and do not allow full separation of the various load components. This important work, however, does suggest that the implant is very largely "shielded" from bending loads by the trunk extensor muscles. Other in vivo measurements have been made using strain gauges on Harrington rods in humans[123,138,169] and in sheep,[124] or on Dwyer cables in dogs,[156] but these are difficult to convert into loads acting at the site of instability. "Free-body analysis" estimates of in vivo loads are only as good as the estimates on which they are based, and do not deal at all with load sharing between vertebrae and muscles.

Thus, for present purposes, the best answer to the question "How strong should the implant be?" comes from the empirical clinical experience that has been accumulated in five areas. First, Roy-Camille posterior plates are typically attached[143,145,146] using 3.5- to 4.5-mm cortical screws. Although ideally these screws are protected from all but pure tensile loads, in practice this seems to be quite unlikely, especially for the screws at the ends of the plates. As noted earlier, these screws are almost surely exposed to some shearing and cantilever bending loads. Although screw breakage has been reported in a substantial number of cases,[147] in the majority of cases breakage does not occur. Thus, even though the in vivo loads are unknown, 3.5- to 4.5-mm screws appeared to provide adequate strength in many of Roy-Camille's cases.

Secondly, in vivo bending of the plates themselves has not been reported to be a problem. Mechanical testing in vitro[99,100] has shown that plastic deformation of the Roy-Camille plates occurs at only 11.3-nm (8.3 ft-lb). For comparison, this is even weaker than the bending strength (14.7 Nm, or 10.85 ft-lb) of the 5-mm portion of the Schanz pins used in the external fixator (see below). Thus, in vivo bending loads taken by the plate must be less than 11.3 nm.

Thirdly, Cyron and co-workers[28] have shown in vitro that spondylolysis can be produced with a mean moment of 35 Nm for L5 vertebrae and 28 Nm for L1 vertebrae. These must represent upper limits to in vivo moments, since spondylolysis does not routinely develop after spinal injuries, even with complete paraplegia in which trunk muscle paralysis occurs.

Fourthly, significant experience has been reported for facet-joint fusions with a screw placed obliquely across the facet joint in conjunction with posterior bone graft for various nontraumatic conditions. Boucher[16] encountered only two broken screws out of a total of 482. Of 44 L5-S1 fusions, King[82] does not describe any breakages. In the 150 patients of Pennal et al.,[130] only one screw broke. In the first two studies, screw diameters were not specified, but were probably approximately $\frac{1}{8}$ in. In the last study, screw minor diameter was $\frac{1}{8}$ in.

Fifthly, the external spinal fixator[108,109,152,153] uses 6-mm Schanz pins thinned down to 5 mm along their anterior 6 cm. These pins, of course, are fully exposed to all the loads taken by the fixator. Breakage or bending of these pins has not been reported. This should probably not be surprising, since the bending strength (load needed to produce plastic deformation) of the 5-mm portion of pin is 14.7 Nm per pin or 29.4 Nm per pair. Thus, it can be seen empirically that 5 mm certainly seems to be strong enough. If an even larger size could be used, the margin of safety would only increase.

Vertebral Morphometry

The pedicle seems to be the strongest site accessible posteriorly through which to obtain a three-dimensionally rigid "grip" onto the vertebra. Certainly, no other site with this property seems to have been proposed. The limiting factor to the size of the screw that can be placed from posteriorly through the pedicle into the vertebral body is the mediolateral width of the pedicle. Saillant[149] has reported certain important cadaveric data, but these data have certain drawbacks. First, only average values were given and not the ranges or standard deviations. Second, bone-screw path length was reported only for a purely sagittal screw placement; other screw placement angles may be preferable[108,109] and would alter this length. Third, only the pedicle diameter perpendicular to the pedicle axis was reported: for screws placed at any other direction than along the pedicle axis, an effectively smaller pedicle diameter may be present. Thus, a morphometric study addressing these issues was undertaken. The major findings are presented below, and full details are reported elsewhere.[97]

Bone-Screw Design

Bone-screw interface strength is commonly the limiting factor in the overall strength of a stabilizing implant, at least over the first few days or weeks (fatigue of metal or resorption of bone may become a problem later on). Some testing of mechanical characteristics of bone screws has been performed. Lavaste[99,100] compared various commercially available screws in pull-out tests. Zindrick et al.[185] compared certain commercially available screws, and also the effects of various details of screw placement technique.

The optimizing of bone-screw strength requires a controlled study in which various screw design features are varied systematically to allow assessment of individual design variables. This has not previously been reported for bone screws. Furthermore, despite a fairly sizable literature characterizing the pull-out strength of various screw designs in limb bones, it does not appear that a systematic study has been done that independently varies the different screw design features such as tooth profile, pitch, and minor diameter. Bechtol[8] compared pull-out strength from dog limb bones of screws with one each of eight different tooth profiles, but the minor diameters were unspecified and various pitches were used in such a way as to not allow the effect of this variable to be isolated. Koranyi et al.[83] reported equal pull-out strengths for both V-toothed Sherman screws and buttress-toothed Synthes screws, using dog or cattle femora. However, neither major nor minor diameters were specified, although tooth heights were the same. Lyon et al.,[105] Nunamaker and Perren,[127] and Schatzker et al.[151] each studied various groups of different commercially available screws, but the individual effects of pitch, major diameter, and minor diameter could not be segregated, since these parameters were not systematically varied.

In order to design a screw with optimal bone-metal interface strength, the authors undertook a study,[92] using various combinations of pitch, minor diameter, and tooth profile, for each of various major diameters. Pull-out testing was utilized, since this load type would be most sensitive to thread-design variations. Of course, pure pull-out loads alone are not likely to occur in vivo, since additional kinds of loads (bending, shearing) would usually occur simultaneously.

Articulating Clamp

Some sort of mechanism is needed to link the four screws rigidly after they are placed into the vertebra above and the vertebra below the site of instability.

The four most important design objectives were thought to be three-dimensional adjustability, strength, compactness, and security of three-dimensional positional control. Adjustability in all three dimensions was sought, since this would simplify screw insertion: no special alignment between the screws would need to be maintained during their insertion to allow later connection of the screws to a longitudinal rod. Three-dimensional adjustability also allows the reduction (in the case of fractures or spondylolisthesis) to be "unconstrained" and can be performed in a controlled fashion with the fixator already in place (but before tightening the locking mechanism). The strength of this articulating clamp should exceed that of the screw, so as not to become the limiting factor to overall implant strength. Compactness is obviously important for comfort and for normal muscle function. Finally, "security" means that the likelihood for loosening during postoperative in-vivo repetitive loading should be extremely low.

To prevent loosening, the threads that the clamp bolt engage inside the rod clamp are of a special pattern known as Spiralock.* This state-of-the-art thread is primarily used in aircraft and other critical high-vibration applications. Other advantages of this thread besides security against loosening include (1) it may be repeatedly tightened, loosened, and retightened without degradation; (2) it has a much better distribution of loads along the engaged bolt threads compared to standard threads; and (3) a separate locking nut is not needed.

In order to achieve the four design objectives for the clamp, a series of clamping systems were designed and tested by mock-up cadaver implantation. The final articulating clamp type is that shown in Fig. 87-2 (see also Fig. 87-1). Note that fine, stepwise adjustability exists for rotation about the transverse axis in increments of 6 degrees, since there are 60 radially arranged teeth on the "face gear" on the head of the bone screw. Infinite adjustability exists for longitudinal axis rotation and longitudinal translation or lengthening. Mechanical testing (static and fatigue) was performed[10] and is summarized here.

Depth of Screw Penetration into Vertebra

How close to the anterior cortex should the tip of the pedicle screw be placed? The greater the depth of penetration (Fig. 87-3), the more secure the screw "grip" on bone, but the greater the risk of cortical breakthrough and damage to aorta or other structures.

*Kaynar: A MicroDot Company, Fullerton, CA.

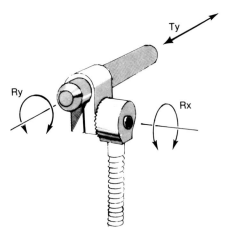

Fig. 87-2

Articulating clamp assembly showing adjustability between components: flexion/extension (x-axis rotation, *Rx*), axial rotation (y-axis rotation, *Ry*), intervertebral separation (y-axis translation, *Ty*).

FLEXION

TORSION

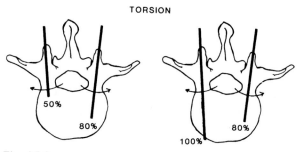

Fig. 87-3

Experimental design for study of depth versus strength. Opposite pedicles of each vertebra had screws implanted to different depths: 50% and 80% depth in half the specimens; 80% and 100% (to cortex) in the other half. One each of the two bending moments were then sequentially applied to opposite screws in each vertebra: "torsion," tending to move screw tip laterally; and "flexion," tending to move screw tip cephalad.

Magerl[109] recommends placement of the screw tip just into but not through the anterior cortex. Mechanical testing of various depths of placement, however, does not appear to have been done. Roy-Camille,[143,145,146] on the contrary, does not recommend a close approach to the anterior cortex. His

clinical reports do not describe in detail the depth of penetration actually used, but illustrative roentgenograms show penetration of approximately 50% to 60% depth. Screw loosening has not been reported as a significant problem. Mechanical testing in vitro by Lavaste[99,100] suggested that anterior cortex engagement did not add significantly to the pull-out strength of the screws.

Because of these conflicting recommendations concerning depth of screw penetration, specific investigation of this issue has been carried out[93] and is summarized here.

Screw Placement

What is the best method for screw placement below the L5-S1 disc? Although Magerl placed screws into the posterior ilia,[106-109] subsequent investigators have generally placed them into the sacrum as a way of avoiding potentially troublesome immobilization across the ungrafted sacroiliac joint. Some recommend that S1 screws be aimed anteromedially toward the sacral promontory[36-38]; others recommend an anterolateral obliquity into the sacral ala.[46,47] These and other recommendations are tabulated elsewhere.[89]

When Asher and Strippgen measured the path lengths of various screw placements in the sacrum, they found that the length anteromedially to the sacral promontory was 47 mm in women and 50 mm in men; the length anterolaterally into the S1 ala was 37 mm in women and 39 mm in men.[5] From these length data, the authors inferred that the stronger screw would be the one directed anteromedially into the promontory. They made no direct measurements of strength, however, to confirm this inference. Zindrick and associates did perform strength measurements, using 6.5-mm screws placed into various sites in the sacrum.[185] Unfortunately, although they noted a very high interspecimen variation, they did not do right-left comparisons of different screw sites within the same specimen. Thus, it is not clear whether the mean differences observed between screw sites were significant. Also, the load used was pull-out of the screw along its own axis, and this does not appear to be a major mode of clinical failure.

In summary, none of the above recommendations are based on direct testing with known statistical significance. To provide further understanding of this issue we undertook on anatomic, morphologic, and biomechanical study of different sacral screw locations. This has been reported previously[40] and is summarized here.

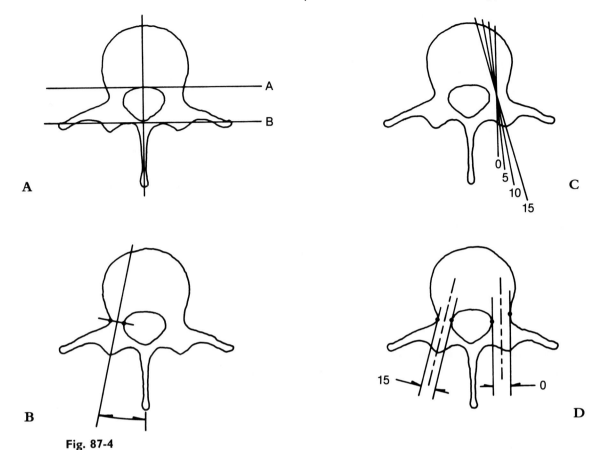

Fig. 87-4

Construction lines used to obtain measurements from vertebral CT scans. **A,** Vertebral body length from anterior cortex to line *A,* pedicle length from line *A* to posterior cortex or to line *B* ("facet corrected"). **B,** Pedicle axis angle measured from sagittal plane (anteromedial positive), pedicle diameter along a perpendicular to axis. **C,** Screw-path length (or chord length) from anterior to posterior cortex at 0 degrees, 5 degrees, 10 degrees, or 15 degrees posterolaterally from the sagittal plane. **D,** Pedicle diameter at 0 degrees and 15 degrees: note that bone contact points do not fall along common perpendicular to axis.

Methods

Vertebral Morphometry

A retrospective review was performed of CT scans of 92 vertebrae from T9 to L5, for evaluation of 41 patients for various spinal conditions (10 single-level fractures, 12 herniated or bulging discs, 3 unspecified cord lesions, 2 bony degenerative changes, and 14 negative studies). Individual vertebrae with positive findings were excluded. The age range was 18 to 75 years (mean of 36 and median of 28 years); there were 14 women and 27 men. The number of specimens at each level were as follows: 7 at T9, 9 at T10, 11 at T11, 12 at T12, 11 at L1, 7 at L2, 12 at L3, 12 at L4, and 10 at L5. A Siemens Somatom-2 third-generation scanner (Siemens, Inc., Erlangen, Germany) was used, with 4-mm cuts and a 5-second scan time.

The CT image was selected on which the width of both pedicles appeared the largest (thus passing through the midheight of both pedicles). Measurements of the parameters defined in Fig. 87-4 were obtained directly from the film and were corrected to lifesize by the appropriate scale factor of 1.25. Three parameters are of particular interest here. Firstly, pedicle axis angle was measured relative to the sagittal plane, with positive values for anteromedial angulation (Fig. 87-4, *B*). Secondly, pedicle diameter was measured both perpendicular to the pedicle axis (Fig. 87-4, *B*), and at the specified approach angles of 0 degrees and 15 degrees (Fig. 87-4, *D*). Thirdly, screw-path length (chord length) was measured between anterior and posterior cortices along a line passing through the middle of the pedicle and inclined at 0, 5, 10, and 15 degrees (Fig. 87-4, *C*). Other measured parameters and further methodologic details are reported elsewhere.[97]

To establish the validity of the CT scan measurements, eight cadaver vertebrae (1 T12, 3 L2, 3 L3, 1 L4) had their inferior end plates embedded in polymethylmethacrylate and were attached to a positioning jig and CT scanned in a manner identical to the patient CT scans. The vertebrae were then sectioned through the midpedicle transverse plane and other measurements of selected parameters were obtained, which were then correlated to the CT scan measurements.

Screw-path length cannot be directly measured from routing lateral roentgenograms. Occasionally it may be useful to predict screw-path length when CT scans are not available. For this reason, the ratios between path length and midsagittal anteroposterior diameter of vertebral body (which can be measured on lateral roentgenograms) were calculated for various approach angles.

Bone-Screw Design

The pedicle diameter dictates the maximum major diameter for the screw, but choice remains concerning minor diameter (root diameter), pitch, and tooth profile. Two values for each of these three parameters were selected for study for the 6-mm major-diameter screws, giving a total of eight possible screw designs. The values were: thread profile either V or buttress, minor diameter of 3.8 or 5 mm, and pitch of 2 or 3 mm. For the 7-mm major-diameter screws, the values were: thread profile buttress only, minor diameter of 5 or 6 mm, and pitch of 2 or 3 mm. Two screw types that differed by only one screw design variable at a time were directly compared by placement into the right and left pedicles of individual cadaveric vertebrae, which had been embedded in base blocks of polymethylmethacrylate. Predrill diameter was 85% of the minor diameter of the screw. Predrilling was done along the pedicle axis and to the same depth as subsequent screw penetration, which was 80% of path length. No pretapping was performed. Thread-cutting flutes were present on the tips of all screws. The polymethylmethacrylate blocks were then attached to an MTS machine for pull-out testing of each screw, one at a time, with the pull-out direction along the long axis of the screw.

A randomized balanced incomplete block experimental design was used (Tables 87-1 and 87-2). This was chosen because (1) there were three variables of interest but only two pedicles per vertebra, and (2) significant variation between vertebral specimens was noted on preliminary experiments. Three blocks were defined, each one consisting of a subgroup of four screw types (see Table 87-1). For each

Table 87-1

Test design for pull-out of 6-mm screws*

Screw Type	Tooth Profile	Minor Diameter (mm)	Thread Pitch (mm)	Block 1	2	3
1	V	3.8	2	X		X
2	V	3.8	3	X		X
3	V	5.0	2	X		
4	V	5.0	3	X		
5	B	3.8	2		X	X
6	B	3.8	3		X	X
7	B	5.0	2		X	
8	B	5.0	3		X	

*Eight experimental screw types resulted from using two values for each of three design variables (tooth, minor diameter, and pitch). In each block, one variable was held constant. In Block 1, only screws with V threads were used, allowing the effect of minor diameter and pitch to be studied. Block 2 was similar, but for buttress (B) screws alone. In Block 3, only screws with a minor diameter of 3.8 mm were used, allowing the effect of tooth profile and pitch to be studied.

subgroup, there were six possible combinations of screw types taken two at a time (see Table 87-2). Each combination was studied by placement into the two pedicles of a vertebra, two vertebra per combination were used to provide duplicate measurements, for a total of 24 pull-outs per block. A direct

Table 87-2

Test design for right-left pedicle pairings of experimental screws for pull-out*

Vertebral Group	Block 1 Right	Left	Block 2 Right	Left	Block 3 Right	Left
A	1	2	5	6	1	2
B	1	3	5	7	1	5
C	1	4	5	8	1	6
D	2	3	6	7	2	5
E	2	4	6	8	2	6
F	3	4	7	8	5	6

*In Block 1, each of the six possible pairings (A-F) of screw types no. 1, 2, 3, and 4 were placed respectively into the right and left pedicles of individual vertebral specimens. In Block 2, a similar arrangement was used, for screw types no. 5, 6, 7, and 8. In Block 3, screw types no. 1, 2, 5, and 6 were studied. Each vertebral group consisted of two vertebral specimens, giving a total of 36 vertebrae (72 pedicles) tested.

comparison of 6-mm versus 7-mm major-diameter screws was not performed, since the strengthening effect of major diameter has already been established.[105,127] Further details of the test procedure and data analysis are presented elsewhere.[92]

Articulating Clamp

Static testing involved three different load types, as shown in Fig. 87-2, which also shows the coordinate system used in the testing. Moments about the transverse axis (flexion/extension [Mx]) are probably the largest loads to which the device will be exposed. Axial torsional moments (twisting [My]) may also be significant. Finally, although axial compression forces (Fy) probably will be located anterior to the rod, tending to produce a "jamming" effect of the clamp on the rod, nonetheless they may be quite large in magnitude. As has been pointed out,[94] the in vivo loads to which this device will be exposed are really not known. This is emphasized by the large disparity between the in vivo strain-gauge measurements from the external spinal fixator and typical predictions from free-body analysis. The former showed peak bending moments of only 8 nm,[180] while the latter predicts bending moments of 91 nm at 40 degrees flexed posture.[119,173]

Depth of Screw Penetration into Vertebra

Vertebral specimens were prepared in a manner identical to that used in the screw design study. In all cases, the screws were 6 mm in major diameter, 5 mm in minor diameter, 2 mm in pitch, and buttress toothed. One screw was implanted into each of the right and left pedicles, but using a different depth of penetration on each side (see Fig. 87-3). Some specimens were used to compare 50% versus 80% penetration, others were used to compare 80% versus 100% penetration. Loading to failure was then performed using a pure moment about either (1) the transverse or x-axis ("flexion" loading, tending to force the screw tip up through the superior endplate), or (2) the longitudinal or y-axis ("torsion" loading, tending to force the screw tip out through the lateral cortex of the vertebral body). The moments were applied about a point near the center of the pedicle, in such a way as not to constrain subsequent screw motion. Four specimens were used for each load type. These load types were chosen because we believed they would be the most sensitive to different depths of penetration and would be at least as realistic as pull-out loading.

Sacral Screw Placement

A three-dimensional electromechanical digitizer was used to measure in 38 human pelves the locations of major neurovascular structures relevant to sacral bone-screw placement, as well as the screw path lengths for three specific sacral screw locations: S1 pedicle to promontory, S1 pedicle to ala, and S2 pedicle to ala.

In nine human pelves, right-left (randomized) comparisons were made of screw-bone interface stiffness of 7-mm major-diameter VSF screws exposed to a flexion torque about an axial passing 1 mm anterior to the posterior cortex at the screw entry site. The screw on one side was aimed into the promontory and on the other side into the ala.

Results

Vertebral Morphometry

Pedicle axis angle data are shown in Fig. 87-5. The minimum angulation is at T12, with a value of −0.6 degrees (i.e., very slight anterolateral angulation). The maximum is at L5 with an angulation of +27.2 degrees. In rough terms, the axis angle is 0 to 10 degrees in the lower thoracic spine, and gradually increases caudally throughout the lumbar region.

Standard deviations for our study are fairly small (typically, 3 to 5 degrees). The data of Saillant[149] are shown for comparison: good agreement exists except for L1-L4, where the authors' data show substantially larger pedicle axis angles.

Pedicle diameter data are shown in Fig. 87-6 and Table 87-3. The former shows the results of all three different methods for measuring pedicle diameter. It may be seen that (1) pedicle diameter is almost constant from T9-L1, with a mean at each level of approximately 7 mm; (2) a gradual increase in diameter occurs from L1-L5; (3) very similar results are obtained from the three different measures of pedicle diameter; (4) the standard deviations at each vertebral level are quite small (most are less than 2 mm); and (5) quite good agreement exists with the data of Saillant,[149] although the authors' mean values tend to be somewhat smaller.

Table 87-3 shows for each vertebral level the distribution by size of pedicle diameters (measured perpendicular to the pedicle axis). Note that (1) pedicles smaller than 5 mm were never encountered below T10, with the exception of L1, and elsewhere they were infrequent, and (2) pedicles 8 mm or larger were encountered in significant numbers at all levels, from 35% at T9 up to 100% at L5.

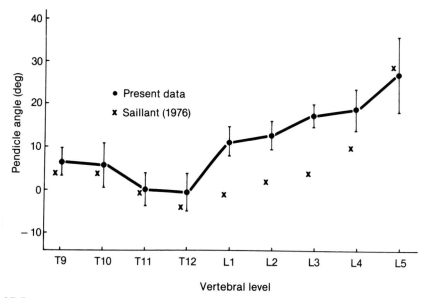

Fig. 87-5

Pedicle axis angle relative to sagittal plane for each vertebral level. Means ±1 SD are shown, compared to means (*x*) from Saillant.[149]

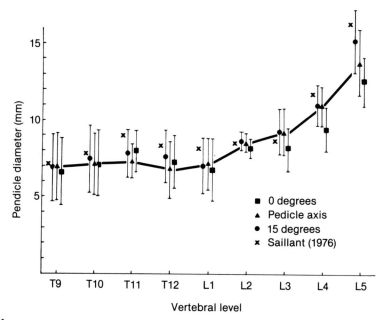

Fig. 87-6

Pedicle diameter means ±1 SD for each vertebral level, measured three different ways (see Figs. 87-1, *B* and 87-1, *D*) and compared to means (*x*) from Saillant.[149]

Screw-path length (chord length) data are shown in Fig. 87-7 for both the 0-degree and the 15-degree approach angles. Major features of these results include (1) a slightly longer path length always results from the more steeply inclined approach (15 degrees); (2) path length is almost constant over the vertebral levels studied, with a small decrease occur-ring caudally (45.1 mm at T9, 36.4 mm at L5); (3) standard deviations are relatively small; and (4) good agreement is present with the data of Saillant.[149]

The accuracy of the CT scan measurements is illustrated in Fig. 87-8. The various measurements obtained by CT scanning of cadaver vertebrae are plotted against the same measurement obtained by

Table 87-3
Pedicle diameter and distribution by size

Level	Mean	SD	No.	3-3.9 mm	4-4.9 mm	5-5.9 mm	6-6.9 mm	7-7.9 mm	8-19.4 mm
T9	6.88	2.23	14	14%	7%	14%	21%	7%	35%
T10	7.47	2.24	18	11		11	39		39
T11	7.83	1.56	22			14	18	14	55
T12	7.63	1.79	24			21	21	12	46
L1	7.01	1.84	22	9		18	18	14	41
L2	8.67	0.64	14					7	92
L3	9.30	1.51	24				8	12	79
L4	11.03	1.36	24						100
L5	15.15	1.97	20						100

Pedicle diameter and distribution by size. Diameter was measured perpendicular to pedicle axis (Fig. 34-1, *B*). Means (± 1 SD) are graphed in Fig. 87-6. Note large number of pedicles 8 mm or larger, especially at lower vertebral levels.

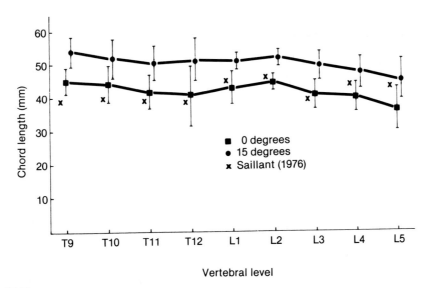

Fig. 87-7
Screw-path length (chord length) measured along a line at 0 and 15 degrees relative to the sagittal plane (see Fig. 87-1, *C*), and compared to means (*x*) from Saillant.[149]

calipers. All these data are seen to fall very close to the y = x line, with an apparently high correlation coefficient. This indicates similarity of CT to direct caliper measurement.

The ratio between screw path length and anteroposterior diameter of vertebral body was calculated for both the 0- and the 15-degree approach angle. The mean (± 1 SD) at 0 degrees was 1.32 ± 0.12, and at 15 degrees was 1.60 ± 0.9. In other words, the path length is approximately one third longer than the anteroposterior body diameter for a 0-degree approach angle, and two thirds longer for a 15-degree approach angle.

Bone-Screw Design

Table 87-4 shows the significance of each screw design variable. Minor diameter is significant for 6-mm screws, both for the **V** tooth and **B** tooth subgroups. In each case, the smaller minor diameter (3.8 vs. 5 mm) is somewhat stronger: 26% for the **V** tooth (1093 N vs. 1181 N adjusted mean strengths). However, for 7-mm screws with **B** threads, minor diameter was not significant.

Pitch was significant only for 6-mm **B** threads: 2-mm pitch screws were 21% stronger than 3-mm pitch (1416 N vs. 1174 N adjusted mean strengths). This

Table 87-4

Significance of screw design variables on pull-out strength of 6-mm and 7-mm screws

Variable	Major Diameter (mm)	Block 1 (V-Tooth Subgroup)	Block 2 (B-Tooth Subgroup)	Block 3 (3.8 Minor Subgroup)
Minor	6	$p = 0.05*$	$p = 0.01†$	—
	7	—	NS	—
Pitch	6	NS	$p = 0.01‡$	NS
	7	—	NS	—
Tooth	6	—	—	NS
	7	—	—	—
Minor and pitch	6	NS	NS	—
	7	—	NS	—
Pitch and tooth	6	—	—	NS
	7	—	—	—

NS = not significant; ($p = 0.05$); — = variables the significance of which were not tested.
*1093 N vs. 864 N adjusted mean pull-out of 3.8 mm and 5.0 mm minor diameter screws, respectively.
†1408 N vs. 1181 N adjusted mean pull-out of 3.8 mm and 5.0 mm minor diameter screws respectively.
‡1416 N vs. 1174 N adjusted mean pull-out of 2 mm and 3 mm pitch screws respectively.
The significance level is noted for each design variable and certain combinations of variables, for each of the Blocks (1, 2, and 3) and for each of the 6- and 7-mm diameter sizes.

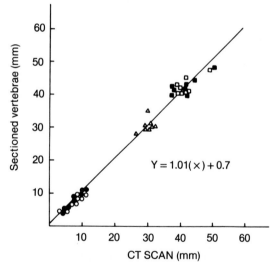

Fig. 87-8

Correlation between caliper measures and CT scan measurements on cadaver vertebrae.

effect was not seen for 6-mm V threads or 7-mm B threads.

Tooth pattern (V vs. B) was not significant for the one subgroup tested, which was the 6-mm major, 3.8-mm minor screws. Finally, the interaction between variables (minor and pitch, pitch and tooth)

can also be seen to be not significant (NS) in the areas tested.

Table 87-5 shows the mean pull-out strengths of the various crew types studied, with no adjustment for vertebral specimen bone density, size, or donor age, and with no consideration given to the right-left pedicle pairing used in the analysis to produce Table 87-4. Because of this, direct comparison between means must be made very cautiously. Nonetheless, it is valid to note that the screw type with lowest mean value is still substantial at 715N (161 lb), that many of the means are over 1000 N, and that the highest mean is 1978 N (440 lb).

Articulating Clamp

Static testing has been performed for each of three different load types (see Fig. 87-2). To produce rotation of the bone screw relative to the articulating clamp about the clamp bolt (x-axis rotation, or flexion/extension), moments must exceed 149 nm (110 ft-lb). For rotation of the connecting rod within the articulating clamp (y-axis rotation, or axial twisting), moments of 27.5 nm (20.3 ft-lb) may be sustained. Finally, sliding of the rod within the clamp (y-axis translation or axial collapse) requires loads of at least 4878 N (1095 lb) for 6-mm diameter rods, and at least 10690 N (2400 lb) for 8-mm diameter rods.

Table 87-5

Mean pull-out strengths of various experimental screw types*

Screw Type	Tooth Profile	Major Diameter (mm)	Minor Diameter (mm)	Thread Pitch (mm)	Mean	SD	Pull-out (N) Range	No.
1	V	6	3.8	2	1326	692	818-2942	13
2	V	6	3.8	3	1645	944	625-3592	13
3	V	6	5.0	2	976	330	630-1580	6
4	V	6	5.0	3	715	253	395-1101	6
5	B	6	3.8	2	1978	868	700-3494	12
6	B	6	3.8	3	1435	624	700-2747	12
7	B	6	5.0	2	1132	600	550-2063	6
8	B	6	5.0	3	1248	440	600-1840	6
1	B	7	5.0	2	1675	41	1120-2014	6
2	B	7	5.0	3	1410	464	825-2000	6
3	B	7	6.0	2	1288	456	743-1839	6
4	B	7	6.0	3	1387	213	1123-1645	6

*The mean pull-out strength of each experimental screw type is presented, as well as the standard deviation (SD), range, and number of screw pull-outs performed. No adjustment has been made for vertebral specimen age, size, or bone density. All screws were placed along the pedicle axis to a depth of penetration equal to 80% of the vertebral path length.

Table 87-6

Mean strength by load type and depth of penetration

Load Type	Depth (%)	Mean Strength (nm)	Relative Strength (nm)	p Value (Matched-pairs)
Flexion	50	6.5	77	
	80	8.4	100	< 0.05
	80	6.9	100	
	100	10.6	154	< 0.05
Torsion	50	6.6	75	
	80	8.8	100	< 0.05
	80	5.7	100	
	100	7.1	124	< 0.05

Fatigue testing showed that even up to 1 million cycles, no loosening of the clamp could be produced. The site of failure, when applied loads were high enough to produce failure at less than 1 million cycles, was always at the first thread, consistent with expected material behavior notch sensitivity.

Depth of Screw Penetration into Vertebrae

Analysis of the data was performed using matched pairs t-testing. Results are shown in Table 87-6 and Fig. 87-9. Table 87-6 shows that there was a signif-icant difference for 50% vs. 80% and also for 80% vs. 100% depths of penetration, both for flexion and for torsion loads. The amount of difference seems worth noting: the 100% depth screws are almost twice as strong as the 50% depth screws (77% vs. 154% for flexion loads, 75% vs. 124% for torsion loads) and the 80% depth screws are 25% to 30% stronger than the 50% depth screws.

Screw Placement

The morphometric portion of this study showed that a large interspecimen variation exists for screw path length, diameter, and angulation. The regions ("safe zones") along the arcuate line over which no major neurovascular structures cross are very small and variable. Anterior cortical screw penetration would probably put such structures at significant risk.

The biomechanical portion of this study showed no significant difference by side-to-side matched pairs t-testing of the stiffness of the two screw sites at deflections of 0.1 degree of rotation. However, at 1.0 degree of rotation, the promontory screws were significantly ($p < 0.01$) stiffer.

Current Design

Based substantially on the above studies, VSF components for human use were fabricated, and under

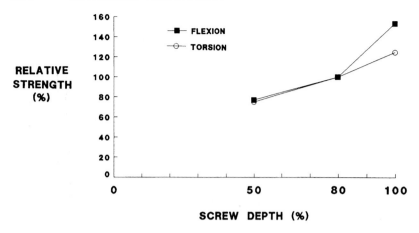

Fig. 87-9

Mean strength of the 100% and 50% depth screws relative to mean strength of 80% depth screws from their respective test blocks, plotted against % depth of penetration, both for flexion and for torsion loads.

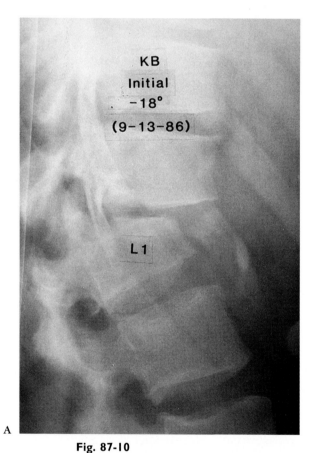

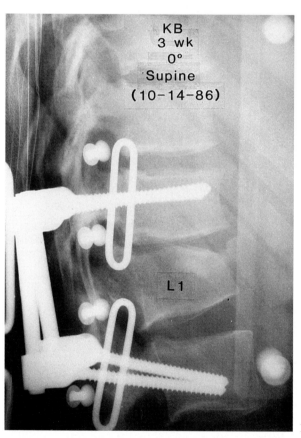

Fig. 87-10

Trauma reduction and fixation. Fracture-dislocation at T12-L1. **A,** Initial lateral x-ray film. **B,** Postoperative lateral x-ray film after realignment and VSF placement.

a research protocol approved by the University of Vermont Human Experimentation Committee, implantation was begun in 1986. Clinical results are reported elsewhere[90,91,139] and are discussed below. Representative radiographs are shown in Figs. 87-10 and 87-11.

Discussion

An important principle that relates to spinal instrumentation is that normal tissue disruption should be avoided when feasible: the implant should involve ideally only the abnormal motion segment(s) and no

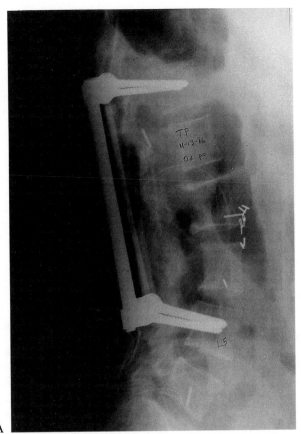
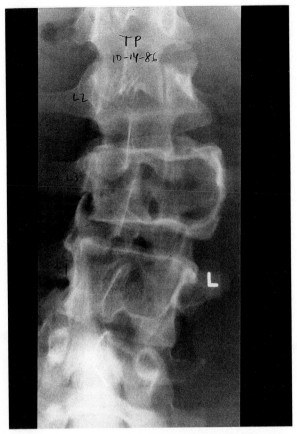

Fig. 87-11

Multiple motion-segment fusion. Ganglioneuroma that has replaced L2, L3, and L4 bodies. **A,** Preoperative anteroposterior x-ray film. **B,** Postoperative lateral x-ray film. Note absence of screws into L2, L3, and L4.

additional ones just for the sake of adequate mechanical performance by the implant. Secondly, a controlled and safe way to produce realignment between vertebrae (e.g. from trauma or spondylolisthesis should be available.) A third principle is that the implant should be a fixator rather than, for example, a distractor or a compressor, in order to provide secure positional control without dependence on soft-tissue intactness. Since motion can occur in any direction,[54,55,135] the fixation produced should be three-dimensional. Finally, the safety of the implantation process should be maximized.

Placement of screws through the pedicle is considered by some to be particularly dangerous. To the contrary, this procedure has certain aspects that render it particularly safe. First, this method completely avoids the need for violation of the spinal canal, such as passage of circumlaminar wires or placement of Harrington hooks with the potentially associated neurologic complications.[75,142,175] Second, device removal (either for intraoperative repositioning or as a separate procedure) is even safer than device placement, quite in contrast to the situation with cir-

cumlaminar wires.[11,126] An additional commentary on the safety of the pedicle route is that (1) there has been extensive clinical experience with screw fixation into the pedicle*; (2) biopsies of the vertebral body are commonly done through the pedicle[27] for the thoracolumbar and lumbar spine; and (3) the pedicle has been used as a surgical route either for placement of vertebral body bone grafts[29,30] or for "shelling out" of cancellous bone from the vertebral body for management of scoliosis.

A final observation concerning bone-screw placement safety is that even if the pedicle cortex is disrupted, neurologic damage does not necessarily follow. In a retrospective roentgenographic study of patients with Roy-Camille plates and pedicle screws, Saillant[149] noted that 10% of 375 screws in 56 patients were outside the pedicle cortex, and yet there were only two cerebrospinal fluid leaks (which spontaneously resolved), and there were no neurologic deficits produced. Adding further to this benign ex-

*References 46, 68, 103, 108, 109, 137, 143, 145, 158, and 166.

perience, it should be noted that correct screw placement is much easier with the VSF, since there is no plate with fixed-position screw holes to "force" the screws into anatomically undesirable positions. This feature, as well as use of a C-arm image intensifier to provide a coaxial view,[22,87,89,95] have resulted in a very low rate (1/216 = 0.5%) of VSF screws out of the pedicle.[91,139]

The issue of anterior versus posterior surgical approach is, of course, a complex one. Although significant advances have been made in the design of anterior spinal implants, the exact indications for the use of anterior implants remain to be established and will depend partially on the availability of alternative posterior implants.

Vertebral Morphometry

The new data presented here[97] extend significantly the previously available dimensional information[149] concerning spinal-fixation devices. CT scanning has been shown to be highly accurate (not surprisingly) compared to direct measurements, allowing us to depend on preoperative measurements. The pedicle axis (see Fig. 87-5) is almost always anteromedially directed, and gradually increases to substantial levels between L1 (11.5 degrees) and L5 (27.2 degrees), a finding differing somewhat from Saillant.[149] Subsequent work by others[118,184] has confirmed and extended these results. Our data support the recommendation of Magerl[108,109] that bone screws be angulated anteromedially, following the axis of the pedicle. This angulated placement results in the right and left bone screws being nonparallel, which produces a "toe-nailing" effect that should substantially increase pull-out strength of the fully assembled fixator and also should allow the vertebral body to function as a cross bridge, which provides resistance to lateral pushover.[87-89] Testing of both these effects is presently underway in our lab.

Previously available screws vary from 3.2 mm in minor diameter[130] up to 5.0 mm in major diameter.[108,109] Our data (see Fig. 87-6 and Table 87-3) show that substantially larger screws may be safely accommodated by the pedicles at many vertebral levels, which is the basis for VSF screws being made in 5-, 6-, and 7-mm major diameters. Whether it is mechanically beneficial to use a diameter larger than 5 mm remains to be established. Future experience with various-sized screws, or alternatively, measurement of the loads acting on the fixator in vivo, will be needed to resolve this issue.

Pedicle diameter is not much influenced by screw approach angle. This is helpful for intraoperative safety in screw placement, since it shows that an exact screw placement angle is not necessary.

The fairly constant screw path length (see Fig. 87-7) found from T9 to L5 reduces the range of screw lengths needed to achieve consistently screw tip placement fairly close to the anterior cortex (to take advantage of the increased strength shown here to be achievable with increased depth of penetration). Use of a C-arm image intensifier and a "near-approach view"[89,95] allows direct visualization of the true relationship between screw tip and anterior cortex. Intraoperative safety in screw placement is further aided by the observation that screw-path length is consistently longer for more anteromedial screw angulation; a strategy of "erring medially" should help in preventing anterior cortex penetration.

Bone-Screw Design

The screw design experiments reported here were undertaken because certain major questions remained unanswered by the fairly extensive literature on bone screws. Our data (see Tables 87-4 and 87-5) certainly do not provide the complete answers, but the test approach used here is a valuable one, since for the first time it allows the effect of various individual screw-design variables to be analyzed independently.

The issue of minor diameter is particularly important when the screw is subjected to bending and shear loads, as is almost surely the case for bone screws. A larger minor diameter increases the screw's resistance to bending, but its effect on pull-out strength has apparently not been tested previously, even though recommendations for a deep thread have been made[32,131] for cancellous screws. We predicted that changing the minor diameter should have no effect on pull-out for the following reason. Screw pull-out causes shear failure of a cylinder of bone, equal to or somewhat greater than the major diameter of the screw.[83] The force needed for pull-out is related to the surface area of this cylinder, which is determined only by the major diameter and depth of penetration of the screw. Note that the minor diameter (thus a deeper thread) does not change the area of that which must be sheared off, and thus does not affect pull-out strength. A smaller diameter does produce a larger volume of bone interposed between the metal threads, but it is not clear that this is an important parameter.

Although we predicted that minor diameter would be a nonsignificant variable, the results do not provide a clear-cut answer: minor diameter is significant for the 6-mm-major-diameter screws, but is not significant for the 7-mm screws. The explanation for this difference is not yet clear. One factor that may be important is the range of minor diameters used in the experiments. For the 7-mm major-diameter screws, the range was only 1 mm, while for the 6-mm-major-diameter screws the range was slightly larger, namely, 1.2 mm. Perhaps this was just enough to produce the insignificance of minor diameter seen in the 7-mm screws. A larger sample size may also help resolve this issue.

From these data, the obvious choice to maximize pull-out strength would be the 3.8-mm minor diameter for the 6-mm screws. However, this would produce a screw with a bending strength, compared to that of a 5-mm-minor-diameter screw, of only approximately 44% ($[3.8/5]^3 = 0.44$). The proper balancing between bending and pull-out strengths requires knowing the in vivo loads acting on the fixator. In the absence of such data, we selected for the VSF a minor diameter of 5 mm for the 6-mm-major-diameter screws, for two reasons. First, the actual pull-out strength of even the 5-mm-minor-diameter screw is quite strong (1132 to 1248 N, or 514 to 567 lb, for the buttress threads). Second, we believed that higher demands would be made on the implant in vivo from loads tending to produce screw bending than from those tending to produce screw pull-out.

We predicted that pitch would also be a variable that does not have a significant effect on pull-out strength. The surface area of the cylinder of bone that must be sheared off during screw pull-out (as discussed above) is not affected by the pitch: for the smaller pitch, each tooth of bone is smaller, but the larger number of them exactly counterbalances this. This argument is particularly true for metal screws in bone, since the relatively high stiffness of metal produces a fairly uniform load distribution along the entire length of the screw.

The data fairly strongly support this prediction. Pitch is insignificant in three of the four areas in which it was tested (6-mm V-tooth subgroup, 6-mm 3.8-minor-diameter subgroup, and 7-mm B-tooth subgroup). Pitch was significant only in the 6-mm B-tooth subgroup. Surprisingly, it was the smaller pitch that was stronger (21%). This is in contrast to the view that widely separated threads (i.e., a large pitch) provide greater resistance to pull-out,[131] a view that apparently has not been supported by biomechanical testing. Why pitch is a significant variable for the 6-mm-major and not the 7-mm-major B-tooth subgroup (Subexperiment II) is not clear. Furthermore, why it should occur for the 6-mm-major B-tooth subgroup but not the V-tooth subgroup

is also not clear. Further testing will be needed to resolve this issue.

For the VSF design, we selected a pitch of 2 mm for the 6-mm-major-diameter screws. The reasons are (1) we chose the B (buttress)-tooth pattern as discussed below, and it is for this subgroup that the lower pitch appears to be stronger, ad (2) only minimally increased effort is involved in fabrication or implantation of the lower pitched screw. For the 7-mm-major-diameter screws, we have also chosen 2-mm pitch, for similarity to the 6-mm screws.

Concerning tooth profile, it seems to have been widely accepted that buttress (B) threads are superior to more traditional V threads. The essential features of the buttress thread are (1) the leading edge is perpendicular (or very nearly so) to the long axis of the screw while the trailing edge is inclined, and (2) the space between adjacent teeth is significantly greater than the space occupied by the teeth themselves.

However, it is not at all clear that the buttress thread actually is mechanically superior. The only directly applicable experimental work that seems to have been reported is that by Koranyi et al.[83] Comparison was made of V and B threads of identical tooth height, but major diameters were not stated: probably the most logical assumption is that they were the same. No rationale for use of buttress threads is mentioned by Müller et al.[120] or Perren.[131] This latter work cites the extensive, pioneering experience of Danis[31,32]; however, neither of these monographs contains or cites experimental work related to this issue. Rather, the stated rationale for the asymmetric tooth profile is only that this thread pattern was used for the screws that attach the rails to the wooden ties in the European railways.[31] Danis modified this screw design somewhat, by steepening the slope of the trailing edge of each tooth enough that the interspace between teeth was six times larger than the space occupied by the teeth themselves. The rationale for this modification was that bone is only one sixth as strong as metal.[32] Apart from the apparent absence of experimental support for this design, even on theoretical grounds this latter reason is not clearly valid: increasing the space between teeth does not alter the surface area of the cylinder of bone that must be sheared off to produce pull-out (as discussed above regarding pitch), and thus should not affect pull-out strength.

Our data (see Table 87-4) fail to show any significant difference between V and B threads for any of the subgroups tested. This confirms our initial hypothesis. Since there is no difference between these thread profiles, for the VSF we chose to use a buttress thread, simply for the reasons that they may be slightly easier to implant, because a smaller volume of bone is crushed by the less-voluminous teeth, and many surgeons seem accustomed to using buttress threads.

We prepared the screw entry site by using a drill bit rather than a curved probe. The reason for this was our belief that a drill bit more dependably produces an appropriately shaped pilot hole than does a curved probe. We compared a straight 3-mm-diameter probe and a powered 4-mm-diameter drill bit; no difference in pullout strength resulted.[96]

Articulating Clamp

The three-dimensional positional adjustability of the articulating clamp (see Figs. 87-1 and 87-2) provides a number of benefits: (1) safer bone-screw placement and avoidance of facet-joint impingement, because anatomically defined placement is unconstrained by the VSF design; (2) easier bone-screw placement, because no special alignment between screws is required; (3) the screws can be used to produce realignment of fracture/dislocations or spondylolisthesis, and the rods can still be readily attached to the screws in their new positions after realignment; and (4) accommodation to unusual anatomic configurations or only partially reducible fractures. The three-dimensional positional control of the clamp prevents loss of intervertebral alignment and provides improved screw-bone interface strength, because of improved load distribution along the screw length.[22]

Based on clinical experience as well as subjective comparison with existing implants, the compactness of this device seems to be more than adequate. This is particularly true when one considers the substantially decreased length of this device, compared with many currently used implants.

Although the in vivo loads to which this device will be exposed are not known for sure, the articular clamp component of the VSF certainly appears not to be the "weak link" in the overall system. A screw placed at 80% depth of penetration can tolerate up to 8.72 nm (6.41 ft-lb) of "torsion" or y-axis moment. The connecting rod, however, requires moments of 27.5 nm (20.3 ft-lb) before slippage occurs. This is a safety factor of more than three. An even greater safety factor exists for "flexion" or transverse axis moments. The screw can tolerate 8.41 nm (6.12 ft-lb), while the articulating clamp attached to the head of the screw can tolerate 149 nm, a safety factor of 18.

Depth of Screw Penetration into Vertebrae

Mechanical testing of various bone-screw depths of penetration has been performed, which addresses the conflict between recommendations in the literature concerning this issue. Compared to those at 50% penetration, screws at 80% depth of penetration are 25% to 30% stronger and those at 100% depth are 100% stronger. Whether this is functionally significant will require clinical comparative testing or knowledge concerning in vivo implant loads. To improve safety, a "near approach view" has been described[95] for intraoperative radiographic monitoring of screw placement close to the vertebral body anterior cortex.

Screw Placement

Should sacral screws be placed through the anterior sacral cortex? The neurovascular structures seem, based on our work, to be very much at risk, yet anecdotal experience suggests that one can "get away with it." Biomechanical testing of "to" versus "through" cortex remains to be done.

Our data show that screws oriented anteromedially, into the promontory, are stiffer. Since this also is an orientation that probably can be more easily monitored radiographically, this is the method that has been used for all the VSF patients. Further clinical experience will be useful to address this issue more fully.

In Vivo Loads

How strong does a spinal implant really need to be? Although significant research has been done concerning loads on the normal spine, only limited and partial information is known* concerning loads acting at the site of injury or other types of instability. Major unresolved issues include: (1) To what extent does muscle activity alter the loads to which the implant is exposed? (2) To what extent can the unstable motion segment safely bear loads? and (3) What is the time course of healing and return to normal load-bearing capacity?

It is only after such in vivo loads are known that optimal design of a spinal fixator can be completed.[94] The morphometric data presented here define the upper limits for screw diameter and length, but the question remains of what the dimensions actually should be. To answer this question, loads need to

---

*References 123, 124, 138, 152, 153, 156, 169, and 181.

be known. We have shown the relative strengths of various screw designs, but a final selection among these designs requires knowledge of the loads. The static strength of the articulating clamp in the current prototype has been measured, but to what extent it may be "overdesigned" depends upon the in vivo loads. Finally, we have measured the strengthening effect of depth of screw penetration, but how much strength is actually needed? Again the knowledge of the in vivo loads is required.

Clinical Experience

The initial study group of 54 patients had diagnoses as follows: 20 trauma (15 burst fractures), 15 pseudarthroses, 8 spondylolysis/spondylolisthesis, 9 disc degeneration and/or stenosis, 1 tumor, and 1 infection. The major objectives for these implantations were to obtain: (1) a bone fusion spanning only the abnormal motion segments, using instrumentation that does not extend beyond the fusion; (2) a satisfactory or better alignment across the grafted vertebrae; and (3) an acceptably small incidence of device-related complications. The major indication for entry into the study was the presence of mechanical insufficiency suspected to be the cause of debilitating back pain or of significant risk to neural elements.

The treatment and follow-up program was as follows. A bivalved thoracolumbar orthosis (no thigh extension) was worn for 6 months (during recumbency for at least the first 6 weeks). Mobilization was done as rapidly as tolerated by symptoms (usually 2 to 3 days postoperatively), and activities gradually progressed to normal at 6 months. Follow-up clinically and radiographically was done at 1 week, 6 weeks, 3 months, 6 months, 9 months, and 12 months. The implant was then removed (in 29 of 54 cases), typically at 12 months, and follow-up continued until at least 6 weeks after removal. Cases in which removal did not occur were generally followed until at least 24 months postimplantation.

Radiographic assessment early in the series included lateral x-ray films obtained with the patient both supine and upright. Since no difference in kyphosis angle was seen between these films on any patients, this was discontinued. Lateral x-ray films in the upright posture were subsequently obtained at 1 week, 6 weeks, and 3 months. Flexion/extension laterals were obtained at 6 months, 9 months, 12 months, and after removal. CT scans were obtained

before implantation on all patients and after implantation on most of those whose VSF was removed.

Implantations have been as high up as T9 and as low down as the sacrum, the latter of which were all onto the promontory through the S1 pedicle. Note that most of the trauma implantations occurred in the thoracolumbar region, and most of the nontrauma implantations were in the lumbosacral region.

The number of vertebrae spanned by the VSF and bone graft were: 2 vertebrae in 10 cases, 3 in 39 cases, 4 in 3 cases, and 5 in 2 cases. The compact size of the VSF easily allows immobilization of only a single motion segment. Most implantations were for abnormalities involving two adjacent motion segments (e.g., burst fracture involving both end plates, or two-level pseudarthrosis), and thus the most common number of vertebrae spanned was three. Even in the cases involving four or five vertebrae, the strength of the screw-bone interface and of the implant itself obviates the need for screws into the intermediate spanned vertebrae.

The results in terms of fusion rate have been as follows. In the 34 cases in which device removal was undertaken, 29 had a solid fusion, and 5 were found to have a nonunion. Regrafting was done in all five patients with nonunion. Four of them had the VSF removed 1 year later, and graft inspection revealed a solid fusion in all four. One of the five (the patient on renal dialysis) has not yet had the VSF removed, although there is no radiographic or clinical evidence for nonunion. Of the 20 cases in which device removal was declined by the patient, there is also no radiographic or clinical evidence for nonunion (this includes flexion/extension lateral x-ray films). Thus, the known number of nonunions after the initial VSF implantation is $5/54 = 9.3\%$ for all patients. For the trauma subgroup it is $2/20 = 10\%$.

The complications have been as follows. In one patient, one of the L4 transverse processes split during screw placement ($1/216$ screws = 0.46%), as a result of which the screw was placed into the next vertebra (L3). One patient had one screw at L3 ($1/216$ screws = 0.46%) cause radicular dysesthesia that resolved after device removal. One patient had one screw placed through the medical cortex of the S1 pedicle ($1/216$ screws = 0.46%), which caused both dysesthesia and motor weakness that have only partially resolved after device removal. There has been one infection as a result of device placement ($1/54$ patients = 1.9%) and one infection as a result of device removal ($1/29$ patients = 3.4%).

Summary

Presented here is a summary of the biomechanical testing of and clinical experience with the Vermont Spinal Fixator, a posterior spinal implant for managing with various types of mechanical insufficiency (e.g., fractures, spondylolisthesis, degenerative "instability"). The major characteristics of this device are (1) three-dimensional adjustability, which allows anatomically and biomechanically optimal screw placement (without having to align screws to holes or slots in a plate) and also easy reduction of fracture/dislocations or spondylolisthesis; (2) three-dimensional fixation, which prevents loss of alignment, even without anterior intervertebral body load sharing; (3) compact, simple design with very few parts, to reduce "fiddle factor," allow only single motion-segment instrumentation, and reduce adjacent soft-tissue irritation; and (4) use of screws for attachment, which eliminates deliberate encroachment into the spinal canal (e.g., Luque wires or Harrington hooks) and allows much more secure fixation than do hooks, even to the sacrum or to laminectomized vertebrae.

New experimental data are reported concerning pertinent vertebral dimensions. These data show that the pedicle can safely accommodate a vertebral screw of ample diameter in almost all cases. Safety is further enhanced by the near constancy in screw-path length at different vertebral levels, the dependable orientation and diameter of the pedicles, and the knowledge that path length is longer with anteromedial angulation of the screw.

Mechanical testing was performed on a variety of experimental bone-screw designs, using various combinations of minor diameter, pitch, and tooth pattern. A special experimental design allowed the effect of each variable to be isolated. Minor diameter appears to be a significant variable for 6-mm but not 7-mm screws. Pitch is insignificant in three of four areas tested, and tooth pattern is insignificant in all areas tested.

The strength of the articulating clamp has been determined for static and dynamic loading. This device can readily accommodate loads that are high compared to bone-screw attachment strength, which in turn has been shown by extensive clinical experience to be adequately secure.

Clinical experience to date has been very encouraging. The fusion rate, maintenance of alignment, and complication rate have all been good.

Future research directions include biomechanical investigation of the cross-bridging role of the vertebral body resulting from oblique screw placement, investigation of various methods to further improve bone-screw interface strength, progress toward in vivo load measurements, and acquisition of further clinical experiences.

References

1. Akbarnia BA, Fogarty JP, Tayob AA: Contoured Harrington instrumentation in the treatment of unstable spinal fractures: the effect of supplementary sublaminar wires, *Clin Orthop Relat Res* 189:186, 1984.

2. Amis J, Herring JA: Iatrogenic kyphosis: a complication of Harrington instrumentation in Marfan's syndrome: a case report, *J Bone Joint Surg* 66A:460, 1984.

3. Anden U, Lake A, Nordwall A: The role of the anterior longitudinal ligament in Harrington rod fixation of unstable thoracolumbar spinal fractures, *Spine* 5:23, 1980.

4. Armstrong GWD: *Harrington instrumentation for spinal fractures.* Presented at the Scoliosis Research Society Annual meeting, Toronto, Ontario, Canada, September 4-6, 1976.

5. Asher MA, Stripgen WE: Anthropometric studies of the human sacrum relating to dorsal transsacral implant designs, *Clin Orthop* 203:58, 1986.

6. Attenborough CG, Reynolds MT: Lumbosacral fusion with spring fixation, *J Bone Joint Surg* 57B:283, 1975.

7. Barrack RL, Skinner HB, Stephen D, et al: *Retrieval and analysis of failed Harrington rods.* Presented at the Orthopedic Research Society meeting, Las Vegas, Nevada, January 30-February 1, 1983.

8. Bechtol CO: *Internal fixation with plates and screws.* In Bechtol CO, Ferguson AB Jr, Laing PB, editors: *Metals and engineering in bone and joint surgery,* Baltimore, 1959, Williams & Wilkins, p 152.

9. Benner B, Moiel R, Dickson J, Harrington P: Instrumentation of the spine for fracture dislocations in children, *Childs Brain* 3:249, 1977.

10. Beynnon BD, Krag MH, Pope MH, et al.: *Fatigue evaluation of a new spinal implant,* American Society of Mechanical Engineering winter annual meeting, Anaheim, CA, 1986.

11. Blackman R, Toton J: *The sublaminal pathway of wires removed in SSI.* Presented at the Scoliosis Research Society annual meeting, 1984.

12. Blumlein H, Cordey J, Schneider UA, et al.: Longterm measurements of axial tension in bone screws in vivo (in German), *Zeitschr Orthop* 115:603, 1977.

13. Bobechko WP: *The instant Harrington.* Presented at the Scoliosis Research Society annual meeting, Montreal, Quebec, Canada, September 16-18, 1981.

14. Bohler JL: Operative treatment of fractures of the dorsal and lumbar spine, *J Trauma* 10:1119, 1970.

15. Bohlman HH: Current concepts review: treatment of fractures and dislocations of the thoracic and lumbar spine, *J Bone Joint Surg* 67A:165, 1985.

16. Boucher HH: A method of spinal fusion, *J Bone Joint Surg* 41B:248, 1959.

17. Bridwell KH: *The treatment of flexion/distraction spinal fractures with SSI and Luque Rectangles.* Presented at the Scoliosis Research Society annual meeting, Orlando, Florida, September 19-22, 1984.

18. Brown CW, Donaldson DH, Odom JA: *A new approach to low lumbar fractures.* Presented at the Scoliosis Research Society annual meeting, Orlando, Florida, September 19-22, 1984.

19. Brunski JB, Hill DC: *Stresses in a Harrington distraction rod: their origin and relationship to fatigue fractures in vivo.* Presented at the Orthopedic Research Society meeting, Anaheim, CA, March 8-10, 1983.

20. Bryant CE, Sullivan JA: Management of thoracic and lumbar spine fractures with Harrington distraction rods supplemented with segmental wiring, *Spine* 8:532, 1983.

21. Cabot JR, Fairén M, Roca J, et al.: La panarthrodése lumbo-sacrée avec la plaque crabe, *Acta Orthop Belg* 47:657, 1981.

22. Carlson GD, Abitbol JJ, Anderson DR, et al.: Screw fixation in the human sacrum: an in vitro study of the biomechanics of fixation, *Spine* 17(suppl 6): 196, 1992.

23. Casey MP, Jacobs RR: *Internal fixation of the lumbosacral spine: a biomechanical evaluation.* Presented at the annual meeting of the International Society for Study of the Lumbar Spine, Montreal, Quebec, Canada, June 3-7, 1984.

24. Casey M, Jacobs RR, Asher M: *The rod-long fuse-short technique in the treatment of thoraco-lumbar and lumbar spine fractures.* Presented at the Scoliosis Research Society annual meeting, Orlando, Florida, September 19-22, 1984.

25. Convery FR, Minteer MA, Smith RW, Emerson SM: Fracture-dislocation of the dorsal-lumbar spine: acute operative stabilization by Harrington instrumentation, *Spine* 3:160, 1978.

26. Cordey J, Perren SM: *Limits of plate on bone friction in internal fixation of fractures.* Presented at the Orthopedic Research Society annual meeting, Las Vegas, Nevada, January 21-24, 1985.

27. Craig FS: Vertebral body biopsy, *J Bone Joint Surg* 38A:93, 1956.

28. Cyron BM, Hutton WC, Troup JDG: Spondylolytic fractures, *J Bone Joint Surg* 58B:462, 1976.

29. Daniaux H: Technik und Erste Ergebnisse der transpedikulären Spongiosaplastik bei Kompressionsbrüchen im Lendenwirbelsäulebereich, *Acta Chir Aust Suppl* 43:79, 1982.

30. Daniaux H: Technik und Ergebnisse der transpedikulären Spongiosaplastik bei Brüchen im thorakolumbalen Übergangs- und lendenwirbelsäulenbereich, *Hefte Unfallheilkd* 165:182, 1983.

31. Danis R: *Technique de l'osteosynthese: etude de Quelque Procedes,* Paris, 1932, Masson.

32. Danis R: *Theorie et pratique de l'osteosynthese,* Paris, 1949, Masson.

33. Denis F, Armstrong SWD, Searls K, Matta L: Acute thoracolumbar burst fractures in the absence of neurologic deficit: a comparison between operative and nonoperative treatment, *Clin Orthop* 189:142, 1984.

34. Denis F, Ruiz H, Searls K: Comparison between square-ended distraction rods and standard round-ended distraction rods in the treatment of thoracolumbar spinal injuries: a statistical analysis, *Clin Orthop Relat Res* 189:162, 1984.

35. Dewald RL: Burst fractures of the thoracic and lumbar spine, *Clin Orthop* 189:150, 1984.

36. Dick W: The "fixateur interne" as a versatile implant for spine surgery, *Spine* 12:882, 1987.

37. Dick W: *Innere Fixation von Brust und Lendenwirbelfrakturen,* Bern, Switzerland, 1984, Hans Huber Verlag.

38. Dick W, Kluger P, Magerl F, et al.: A new device for internal fixation of thoracolumbar and lumbar spine fractures: the "fixateur interne," *Paraplegia* 23:225, 1985.

39. Dickson JG, Harrington PR, Erwin WD: Results of reduction and stabilization of the severely fractured thoracic and lumbar spine, *J Bone Joint Surg* 60A:799, 1978.

40. Dohring EJ, Krag MH: *Sacral screw fixation: a morphologic, anatomic and mechanical study.* Presented at the American Academy of Orthopedic Surgery annual meeting, Anaheim, CA, March 8, 1991.

41. Drummond D, Adamson B, Sponseller P, Keene J: *Interspinous segmental spinal instrumentation for unstable fractures.* Presented at the Scoliosis Research Society annual meeting, Orlando, Florida, September 19-22, 1984.

42. Dunn HK: Anterior stabilization of thoracolumbar injuries, *Clin Orthop* 189:116, 1984.

43. Dunn HK, Bolstad KE: Fixation of Dwyer screws for the treatment of scoliosis, *J Bone Joint Surg* 59A:54, 1977.

44. Dunn HK, Daniels AU, Goble EM, Gardiner RJ: *A comparison of spinal bending stability with posterior and anterior fixation devices.* Presented at the Scoliosis Research Society annual meeting, Seattle, Washington, September 12-14, 1979.

45. Edwards CC: *The spinal rod sleeve. Its rationale and use in thoracic and lumbar injuries.* Presented at the Scoliosis Research Society annual meeting, Montreal, Quebec, Canada, September 16-18, 1981.

46. Edwards CC: *Sacral fixation device: design and preliminary results.* Presented at the Scoliosis Research Society annual meeting, Orlando, Florida, September 19-22, 1984.

47. Edwards CC: Spinal screw fixation of the lumbar and sacral spine: early results treating the first 50 cases, *Orthop Trans* 11:99, 1987.

48. Edwards CC, Griffith P, Levine AM, DeSilva JB: *Early clinical results using the spinal rod sleeve method for treating thoracic and lumbar injuries.* Presented at the American Academy of Orthopedic Surgeons annual meeting, Washington, DC, January 27-29, 1982.

49. Edwards CC, Levine AM, York JJ, Holt ES: *A new spinal hook: rationale and clinical trials.* Presented at the Scoliosis Research Society annual meeting, Orlando, Florida, September 19-22, 1984.

50. Edwards CC, York JJ, Levine AM: *Determinants of hook dislodgement: rigidity of fixation, rod clearance, and hook design.* Presented at the International Society for Study of Lumbar Spine meeting, Montreal, Quebec, Canada, June 3-7 1984.

51. Erwin WD, Dickson JH, Harrington PR: Clinical review of patients with broken Harrington rods, *J Bone Joint Surg* 62A:1302, 1980.

52. Flesch JR, Leider LL, Erickson DL, et al.: Harrington instrumentation and spine fusion for unstable fractures and fracture-dislocations on the thoracic and lumbar spine, *J Bone Joint Surg* 59A:143, 1977.

53. Floman Y, Yosipovitch Z, Shiloni E, Robin GC: *The simultaneous application of a compressive wire and Harrington distraction rods in the treatment of fracture dislocation of the thoracolumbar spine*. Presented at the Israel Orthopedic Society meeting, Haifa, Israel, October 20-22, 1980.

54. Frymoyer JW, Krag MH: *Spinal stability and instability: definitions, classification, and general principles of management*. In Dunsker SB, Schmidek HH, Frymoyer JW, Kahn A III, editors: *The unstable thoracic and lumbosacral spine*. New York, 1986, Grune & Stratton.

55. Frymoyer JW, Selby DK: Segmental instability: rationale for treatment, *Spine* 10:280, 1985.

56. Gaines RW, Breedlove RF, Munson G: Stabilization of thoracic and thoracolumbar fracture-dislocations with Harrington rods and sublaminar wires, *Clin Orthop Relat Res* 189:195, 1984.

57. Gaines RW, Humphreys WG: A plea for judgement in management of thoracolumbar fractures and fracture-dislocations: a reassessment of surgical indications, *Clin Orthop* 189:36, 1984.

58. Gaines RW, Munson G, Satterlee C, et al.: *Harrington distraction rods supplemented with sublaminar wires for thoracolumbar fracture dislocation. Experimental and clinical investigation*. Presented at the Scoliosis Research Society annual meeting, Denver, Colorado, September 22-25, 1982.

59. Gardner ADH: *Four years experience with an anterior spinal distraction device for the correction of kyphotic deformities, and its use as a permanent implant*. Presented at the Scoliosis Research Society annual meeting, Denver, Colorado, September 22-25, 1982.

60. Gertzbein SD, MacMichael D, Tile M: Harrington instrumentation as a method of fixation in fractures of the spine: a critical analysis of deficiencies, *J Bone Joint Surg* 64B:526, 1982.

61. Goel VK, Panjabi MM, Takeuchi R: *Biomechanics of the Harrington instrumentation for injuries in the thoraco-lumbar spine*. Presented at the International Society for Biomechanics, Waterloo, Ontario, Canada, June, 1983.

62. Hall JE: Dwyer instrumentation in anterior fusion of the spine: current concepts review, *J Bone Joint Surg* 63A:1188, 1981.

63. Hannon KM: Harrington instrumentation in fractures and dislocations of the thoracic and lumbar spine, *South Med J* 69:1269, 1976.

64. Hardy AG: Treatment of paraplegia due to fracture-dislocation of the dorsolumbar spine, *Paraplegia* 3:112, 1965.

65. Harrington PR: Instrumentation in spine instability other than scoliosis, *S Afr J Surg* 5:7, 1967.

66. Harrington PR: History and development of Harrington instrumentation, *Clin Orthop Relat Res* 93:110, 1973.

67. Hasday C, Passoff T, Perry J: *Gait abnormalities arising from iatrogenic loss of lumbar lordosis secondary to Harrington instrumentation in lumbar fractures*. Presented at the Scoliosis Research Society annual meeting, Denver, Colorado, September 22-25, 1982.

68. Herrmann HD: Transarticular (transpedicular) metal plate fixation for stabilization of the lumbar and thoracic spine, *Acta Neurochir* 48:101, 1979.

69. Jacobs RR, Asher MA, Snider RK: Thoracolumbar spinal injuries: a comparative study of recumbent and operative treatment in 100 patients, *Spine* 5:463, 1980.

70. Jacobs RR, Casey MP: Surgical management of thoracolumbar spinal injuries. General principles and controversial considerations, *Clin Orthop* 189:22, 1984.

71. Jacobs RR, Dahners LE, Gertzbein SD, et al.: A locking hook-spinal rod: current status of development, *Paraplegia* 21:197, 1983.

72. Jacobs RR, Gertzbein SD, Nordwall A: *A locking hook-spinal rod: a preliminary clinical report on its use in thirty thoracolumbar spinal injuries*. Presented at the International Society for Study of Lumbar Spine, Toronto, Ontario, Canada, June 6-10, 1982.

73. Jacobs RR, Nordwall A, Nachemson A: Reduction, stability and strength provided by internal fixation systems for thoracolumbar spinal injuries, *Clin Orthop Relat Res* 171:300, 1982.

74. Jacobs RR, Schlaepfer F, Mathys R Jr, et al.: A locking hook spinal rod system for stabilization of fracture-dislocations and correction of deformities of the dorsolumbar spine: a biomechanic evaluation, *Clin Orthop Relat Res* 189:168, 1984.

75. Johnston CE II, Norris R, Burke SW, et al.: *Delayed paraplegia following segmental spinal instrumentation*. Presented at the Scoliosis Research Society annual meeting, Orlando, Florida, September 19-22, 1984.

76. Kahanovitz N, Arnoczky SP, Levine DB, Otis JP: The effects of internal fixation on the articular cartilage of unfused canine facet joint cartilage, *Spine* 9:268, 1984.

77. Kahanovitz N, Bullough P, Jacobs RR: The effect of internal fixation without arthrodesis on human facet joint cartilage, *Clin Orthop Relat Res* 189:204, 1984.

78. Kaneda K, Abumi K, Fujiya M: Burst fractures with neurologic deficits of the thoracolumbar-lumbar spine: results of anterior decompression and stabilization with anterior instrumentation, *Spine* 9:788, 1984.

79. Kaneda K, Abumi K, Hashimoto T: *Biomechanical study of the anterior spinal fixation device in pig spine*. Presented at the Scoliosis Research Society annual meeting, Orlando, Florida, September 19-22, 1984.

80. Keene JS, Drummond DS, Narechania RG: *Mechanical performance of the Wisconsin compression system*. Presented at the Orthopedic Research Society annual meeting, Atlanta, Georgia, 1980.

81. Kempf I, Jaeger JH, Ben Abid M, et al.: Osteosynthesis of dorso-lumbar spinal fractures: biomechanical approach and comparative study: reversed Harrington pins and hooks: Roy-Camille bone plates, *Rev Chir Orthop* 65(11):43, 1979.

82. King D: Internal fixation for lumbosacral spine fusions, *J Bone Joint Surg* 30A:560, 1948.

83. Koranyi E, Bowman CE, Knecht CD, Janssen M: Holding power of orthopaedic screws in bone, *Clin Orthop Relat Res* 72:283, 1970.

84. Kostuik JP, D'Angelo G, Fernie G, et al.: *Comparison of spinal fracture fixation devices under dynamic cyclical loading of calf spines.* Presented at the Scoliosis Research Society annual meeting, Orlando, Florida, September 19-22, 1984.

85. Kostuik JP, Gleason TF, Errico TJ, et al.: *Posterior segmental spinal instrumentation in adults.* Presented at the Scoliosis Research Society annual meeting, Orlando, Florida, September 19-22, 1984.

86. Krag MH: *Internal fixation of lumbosacral spine, experience with the Vermont spinal fixator.* In Lin PM, Gill K, editors: *Lumbar interbody fusion* (principles & techniques of spine surgery), Rockville, MD, 1989, Aspen Publishers, p 251.

87. Krag MH: *Biomechanics of transpedicle spinal fixation.* In Weinstein JN, Wiesel S, editors: *The lumbar spine,* Philadelphia, 1990, W. B. Saunders, p 916.

88. Krag MH: *Spinal fusion: overview of options and posterior internal fixation devices.* In Frymoyer JW, editor: *The adult spine,* New York, 1991, Raven Press, p 1919.

89. Krag MH: Biomechanics of thoracolumbar spinal fixation (#8902.0), *Spine* 16(suppl 3):S84, 1991.

90. Krag MH: *The Vermont spinal fixator.* In An HS, Cotler JM, editors: *Spinal instrumentation,* Baltimore, 1992, Williams & Wilkins, p 237.

91. Krag MH: *The vermont spinal fixator.* In Lonstein J, Arnold D, editors: *Internal pedicular fixation of the lumbar spine,* Spine State Art Rev, 1992.

92. Krag MH, Beynnon BD, Pope MH, et al.: An internal fixator for posterior application to short segments of the thoracic, lumbar, or lumbosacral spine: design and testing, *Clin Orthop* 203:75, 1986.

93. Krag MH, Beynnon BD, Pope MH: Depth of insertion of transpedicular vertebral screws into human vertebrae: effect upon screw vertebra interface strength, *J Spinal Disord* 1:287, 1988.

94. Krag MH, Pope MH, Wilder DG: *Mechanisms of spine trauma and features of spinal fixation methods. Part I: Mechanisms of injury.* In Ghista D, editor: *Spinal cord medical engineering,* Springfield, IL, 1986, Charles C Thomas, p 133.

95. Krag MH, Van Hal ME, Beynnon BD: Placement of transpedicular vertebral screws close to anterior vertebral cortex: description of methods, *Spine* 14:879, 1989.

96. George DC, Krag MH, Johnson CC, et al.: Hole preparation techniques (drill versus probe) for transpedicular screws: effect upon pullout strength from human cadaveric vertebrae, *Spine* 16:181, 1991.

97. Krag MH, Weaver DL, Beynnon BD, Haugh LD: Morphometry of the thoracic and lumbar spine related to transpedicular screw placement for surgical spinal fixation, *Spine* 13:27, 1988.

98. Laborde JM, Bahniuk E, Bohlman HH, Samson B: Comparison of fixation of spinal fractures, *Clin Orthop Relat Res* 152:303, 1980.

99. Lavaste F: *Etude des implants rachidiens: mémoire de biomechanique.* Master's thesis, Paris, 1979, "Ingeneur" Ecole Natl Supér des Arts et Metiers à Paris.

100. Lavaste F: Biomechanique du rachis dorso-lombaire, *Deux J Orthop Pitie* 19, 1980.

101. Lewis J, McKibbin B: Treatment of unstable fracture-dislocations of the thoracolumbar spine accompanied by paraplegia, *J Bone Joint Surg* 56B:603, 1974.

102. Liu YK, Goel VK, Dejong A, et al.: Torsional fatigue of the lumbar intervertebral joint, *Spine* (in press).

103. Louis R: *Single-staged posterior lumbo-sacral fusion by internal fixation with screw-plates.* Presented at the International Society for Study of Lumbar Spine, Sidney, Australia, April 14-18, 1985.

104. Luque ER, Cassis N, Ramirez-Wiella G: Segmental spinal instrumentation in the treatment of fractures of the thoracolumbar spine, *Spine* 7:312, 1982.

105. Lyon WF, Cochran JR, Smith L: Actual holding power of various screws in bone, *Ann Surg* 114:376, 1941.

106. Magerl F: *External skeletal fixation of the lower thoracic and the lumbar spine.* In Uhthoff HK, Stahl E, editors: *Current concepts of external fixation of fractures,* New York, 1982, Springer-Verlag, p 253.

107. Magerl F: *Clinical application on the thoracolumbar junction and the lumbar spine.* In Mears DC, editor: *External skeletal fixation,* Baltimore, 1983, Williams & Wilkins.

108. Magerl FP: Stabilization of the lower thoracic and lumbar sine with external skeletal fixation, *Clin Orthop Relat Res* 189:125, 1984.

109. Magerl F: *External spinal skeletal fixation.* In Weber B, Magerl F, editors: *The external fixator,* New York, 1985, Springer-Verlag, p 290.

110. McAfee PC, Bohlman HH: *Complications of Harrington instrumentation in thoracolumbar fractures: ten year experience.* Presented at the Scoliosis Research Society annual meeting, Orlando, Florida, September 19-22, 1984.

111. McAfee PC, Bohlman HH, Werner FW, Glisson RR: *A biomechanical analysis of spinal instrumentation systems in thoracolumbar fractures: comparison of traditional Harrington distraction instrumentation with segmental spinal instrumentation.* Presented at the Scoliosis Research Society annual meeting, Orlando, Florida, September 19-22, 1984.

112. McAfee PC, Bohlman HH, Yuan HA: Anterior decompression of traumatic thoracolumbar fractures with incomplete neurological deficit using a retroperitoneal approach, *J Bone Joint Surg* 67A:89, 1985.

113. McAfee PC, Werner FW, Glisson RR: A biomechanical analysis of spinal instrumentation systems in thoracolumbar fractures: comparison of traditional Harrington distraction instrumentation with segmental spinal instrumentation, *Spine* 10:204, 1985.

114. McAfee PC, Yuan HA, Lasda NA: The unstable burst fracture, *Spine* 7:365, 1982.

115. Miller F, Reger SI, Wang GJ, Boychuck L: *Biomechanical analysis of segmental spine fixation in a fracture model.* Presented at the Orthopedic Research Society, Anaheim, CA, March 8-10, 1982.

116. Mino DE, Stauffer ES, Davis PK: *Torsional loading of Harrington distraction rod instrumentation compared to segmental sublaminar and spinous process supplementation.* Presented at the Scoliosis Research Society annual meeting, Orlando, Florida, September 19-22, 1984.

117. Moe JH, Denis F: The iatrogenic loss of lumbar lordosis, *Orthop Trans* 1:131, 1977.

118. Moran JM, Berg WS, Berry JL, et al.: Transpedicle screw fixation, *J Orthop Res* 7:107, 1989.

119. Morris JM, Lucas DB, Bresler MS: Role of the trunk in stability of the spine, *J Bone Joint Surg* 43A:327, 1961.

120. Müller ME, Allgöwer M, Schneider R, Willenegger H: *Techniques recommended by the AO group: manual of internal fixation*, ed 2 rev, Berlin, 1979, Springer-Verlag.

121. Munson G, Satterlee C, Hammond S, et al.: Experimental evaluation of Harrington rod fixation supplemented with sublaminar wires in stabilizing thoracolumbar fracture-dislocations, *Clin Orthop* 189:97, 1984.

122. Murphy MJ, Southwick WO, Ogden JA: *Treatment of the unstable thoracolumbar spine with combination Harrington distraction and compression rods.* Presented at the Scoliosis Research Society annual meeting, Montreal, Quebec, Canada, September 16-18, 1981.

123. Nachemson A, Elfstrom G: Intravital wireless telemetry of axial forces in Harrington distraction rods in patients with idiopathic scoliosis, *J Bone Joint Surg* 53A:445, 1971.

124. Nagel DA, Cordey J, Schneider E, et al.: *In vivo measurement of load on Harrington distraction rods in sheep spines with and without fusion.* Presented at the Orthopedic Research Society meeting, 1984.

125. Nagel DA, Koogle TA, Piziali ED, Perkash I: Stability of the upper lumbar spine following progressive disruptions and the application of individual internal and external fixation devices, *J Bone Joint Surg* 63A:62, 1981.

126. Nicastro JF, Traina J, Hartjen CA, Lancaster JM: *Intraspinal pathways of sublaminar wires during surgical removal.* Presented at the Scoliosis Research Society annual meeting, Orlando, Florida, September 19-22, 1984.

127. Nunamaker DM, Perren SM: Force measurements in screw fixation, *J Biomech* 9:669, 1976.

128. Ogilvie JW, Bradford DS: *Lumbar and lumbosacral fusion with segmental fixation.* Presented at the Scoliosis Research Society annual meeting, 1984.

129. Osebold WR, Weinstein SL, Sprague BL: Thoracolumbar spine fractures: results of treatment, *Spine* 6:13, 1981.

130. Pennal GF, McDonald GA, Dale GG: Method of spinal fusion using internal fixation, *Clin Orthop Relat Res* 35:86, 1964.

131. Perrren SM: Physical and biological aspects of fracture healing with special reference to internal fixation, *Clin Orthop* 138:175, 1979.

132. Pietruszka I: Early rehabilitation after fracture fixation using Daab's serrate plate and cancellous autotransplants, *Chir Narzadow Ruchu Ortop Pol* 45:507, 1980.

133. Pinto WC, Avanzi O, Winter RB: An anterior distractor for the intraoperative correction of angular kyphosis, *Spine* 3:309, 1978.

134. Pope MH, Krag MH, Wilder DG: *Mechanisms of spine trauma and features of spinal fixation methods. II: Fixation mehods.* In Ghista DN, editor: *Spinal cord injury medical engineering*, Springfield, IL, 1986, Charles C Thomas.

135. Pope MH, Panjabi M: Biomechanical definitions of spinal stability, *Spine* 10:255, 1985.

136. Purcell GA, Markolf KL, Dawson EA: Twelfth thoracic-first lumbar vertebral mechanical stability of fractures after Harrington rod instrumentation, *J Bone Joint Surg* 63A:71, 1981.

137. Puschel J, Zielke K: *Transpedicular vertebral instrumentation using VDS instruments in ankylosing spondylitis.* Presented at the Scoliosis Research Society annual meeting, Orlando, Florida, September 19-22, 1984.

138. Quintin J, Burny F, Bourgois R, et al.: Mesure de la deformation des implant in vivo, *Acta Orthop Belg* 48:688, 1982.

139. Reinsel T, Krag MH: The Vermont Spinal Fixator in the treatment of trauma and degenerative disorders—a 2 year follow-up (Manuscript in preparation).

140. Rezaian SM, Dombrowski ET, Ghista DN: Spinal fixator for the management of spinal injury (the mechanical rationale), *Eng Med* 12:95, 1983.

141. Roaf R: A study of the mechanics of spinal injuries, *J Bone Joint Surg* 42B:810, 1960.

142. Rossier AB, Cochran TP: The treatment of spinal fractures with Harrington compression rods and segmental sublaminar wiring: a dangerous combination, *Spine* 9:796, 1984.

143. Roy-Camille R, Saillant G, Berteaux D, Marie-Anne S: *Early management of spinal injuries.* In McKibbin B, editor: *Recent advances in orthopaedics*, New York, 1979, Churchill-Livingstone.

144. Roy-Camille R, Saillant G, Berteaux D, et al.: Vertebral osteosynthesis using metal plates: its different uses, *Chirurgie* 105:597, 1979.

145. Roy-Camille R, Saillant G, Berteaux D, Salgado V: Osteosynthesis of thoracolumbar spine fractures with metal plates screwed through the vertebral pedicles, *Reconstr Surg Traumatol* 15:2, 1976.

146. Roy-Camille R, Saillant G, Marie-Anne S, Mamoudy P: Behandlung von Wirbelfrakturen und -luxation am thorako-lumbalen Übergang, *Orthopaedie* 9:63, 1980.

147. Roy-Camille R, Saillant G, Mazel C: Internal fixation of the lumbar spine with pedicle screw plating, *Clin Orthop* 203:7, 1986.

148. Ryan MD, Taylor RKF, Sherwood AA: *New instrumentation for anterior lumbar and thoracolumbar interbody spinal fusion.* Presented at the Scoliosis Research Society annual meeting, 1981.

149. Saillant G: Anatomical study of vertebral pedicles: surgical application (in French). *Rev Chir Orthop* 62:151, 1976.

150. Savastano AA, Corvese LA, Davignon RP: Experiences with Harrington instrumentation for unstable fractures of the truncal spine, *R I Med J* 62:325, 1979.

151. Schatzker J, Sanderson R, Murnaghan PJ: The holding power of orthopaedic screws in vivo, *Clin Orthop Relat Res* 108:115, 1975.

152. Schläpfer F, Magerl F, Jacobs R, et al.: In vivo measurements of loads on an external fixation device for human lumbar spine fractures, *Inst Mech Eng* C131/80:59, 1980.

153. Schläpfer F, Wörsdörfer O, Magerl F, Perren SM: *Stabilization of the lower thoracic and lumbar spine: comparative in vitro investigation of an external skeletal and various internal fixation devices.* In Uhthoff HK, Stahl E, editors: *Current concepts of external fixation of fractures,* New York, 1982, Springer-Verlag.

154. Schlicke L, Schulak J: The simultaneous use of Harrington compression and distraction rods in a thoracolumbar fracture-dislocation, *J Trauma* 20:177, 1980.

155. Schmidek HH, Gomes FB, Seligson D, McSherry JW: Management of acute instable thoracolumbar (T11-L1) fractures with and without neurological deficit, *Neurosurgery* 7:30, 1980.

156. Shapiro FD, McDonald CW, Dwyer AP, et al.: Telemetric monitoring of cable tensions following Dwyer spinal instrumentaton in dogs, *Spine* 3:213, 1978.

157. Shen G, Gilbertson L, Hite J: *Biomechanical aspects of Harrington spinal instrumentation.* Presented at the Scoliosis Research Society annual meeting, Baltimore, Maryland, November 30-December 2, 1978.

158. Sijbrandij S: A new technique for the reduction and stabilisation of severe spondylolisthesis, *J Bone Joint Surg* 63B:266, 1981.

159. Slot GH: *A new distraction system for the correction of kyphosis using the anterior approach.* Presented at the Scoliosis Research Society annual meeting, Montreal, Quebec, Canada, September 16-18, 1981.

160. Stauffer ES: Current concepts review. Internal fixation of thoracolumbar spine fractures, *J Bone Joint Surg* 66A:1136, 1984.

161. Stauffer ES, Neil YL: Biomechanical analysis of structural stability of internal fixation in fractures of the thoracolumbar spine, *Clin Orthop* 112:159, 1975.

162. Sullivan JA: Sublaminar wiring of Harrington distraction rods for unstable thoracolumbar spine fractures, *Clin Orthop* 189:178, 1984.

163. Taylor TKF, Cummine J: Harrington instrumentation for fractures and dislocations of the thoracolumbar spine, *J Bone Joint Surg* 60B:289, 1978.

164. Tello CA: *Early results with a variation of spinal instrumentation.* Presented at the Scoliosis Research Society annual meeting, Orlando, Florida, September 19-22, 1984.

165. Trias A, Massoud M, Ghibely A: *Modified Harrington rod.* Presented at the Scoliosis Research Society annual meeting, Denver, CO, September 22-25, 1982.

166. Vercauteren M, DeGroote W, Van Nuffel J, et al.: Reduction of sondylolisthesis with severe slipping, *Acta Orthop Belg* 47:502, 1981.

167. Ward JJ, Nasca RJ, Lemons JE: *Biomechanical evaluation of the neural arch.* Presented at the Scoliosis Research Society annual meeting, Orlando, Florida, September 19-22, 1984.

168. Ward JJ, Nasca RJ, Lemons JE, Bidez MW: *Cyclic torsional testing of Harrington and luque sinal implants.* Presented at the Scoliosis Research Society annual meeting, Orlando, Florida, September 19-22, 1984.

169. Waugh TR: Intravital measurements during instrumental correction of idiopathic scoliosis. *Acta Orthop Scand Suppl* 93, 1966.

170. Weiss M: Dynamic spine alloplasty (spring-loading corrective devices) after fracture and spinal cord injury, *Clin Orthop Relat Res* 112:150, 1975.

171. Wenger DR, Carollo JJ, Wilkerson JA Jr, et al.: Laboratory testing of segmental spinal instrumentation versus traditional Harrington instrumentation for scoliosis treatment, *Spine* 7:265, 1982.

172. Wenger D, Miller S, Wilkerson J: *Evaluation of fixation sites for segmental instrumentation of the human vertebra.* Presented at the Scoliosis Research Society annual meeting, Montreal, Quebec, Canada, September 16-18, 1981.

173. White AH, Wynne G, Taylor LW: Knodt rod distraction lumbar fusion, *Spine* 8:434, 1983.

174. Whitesides TE Jr, Shaw SGA: On the management of unstable fractures of the thoracolumbar spine: rationale for use of anterior decompression and fusion and posterior stabilization, *Spine* 1:99, 1976.

175. Wilber RG, Thompson GH, Shaffer JW, et al.: Postoperative neural deficits in segmental instrumentation: a study using spinal cord monitoring, *J Bone Joint Surg* 66A:1178, 1984.

176. Wilder DG, Pope MH, Frymoyer JW: *Cyclic loading of the intervertebral motion segment.* Presented at the Northeast Bioengineering Conference, Hanover, NH, 1982.

177. Willen J, Lindahl S, Irstam L, et al.: Thoracolumbar crush fracture: an experiemental study on instant axial dynamic loading: the resulting fracture type and its stability, *Spine* 9:624, 1984.

178. Willen J, Lindahl S, Irstam L, Nordwall A: Unstable thoracolumbar fractures: a study by CT and conventional roentgenology of the reduction effect of Harrington instrumentation, *Spine* 9:214, 1984.

179. Williams EWM: *Traumatic paraplegia.* In Matthews DN, editor: *Recent advances in surgery of trauma,* New York, 1963, Churchill-Livingstone, p 171.

180. Wilson PD, Straub LR: Lumbosacral fusion with metallic-plate fixation, *Am Acad Orthop Surg Instruct Course Lect* 9:53, 1952.

181. Wörsdörfer O: *Operative Stabilisierung der thorakolumbalen und lumbalen Wirbelsäule: Vergleichende biomechanische Untersuchungen zur Stabilität und Steifigkeit verschiedener dorsaler Fixations-Systems.* Master's thesis, 1981, Medizinisch-Naturwissenschaftliche Hochschule der Universität Ulm.

182. Yamagata M: Biomechanical study of posterior spinal instrumentation for scoliosis, *J Jpn Orthop Assoc* 58:523, 1984.

183. Yosipovitch Z, Robin GC, Makin M: Open reduction of instable thoracolumbar spinal injuries and fixation with Harrington rods, *J Bone Joint Surg* 59A:1003, 1977.

184. Zindrick MR, Wiltse LL, Doornik A, et al.: Analysis of the morphometric characteristics of the thoracic and lumbar pedicles, *Spine* 12:160, 1987.

185. Zindrick MR, Wiltse LL, Widell EH, et al.: Biomechanical study of interpedicular screw fixation in the lumbosacral spine, *Clin Ortho Relat Res* 203:99, 1986.

Chapter 88

Posterior Lumbar Interbody Fusions by Implanted Threaded Titanium Cages

Charles D. Ray

**Advantages of Posterior Lumbar
  Interbody Fusion**

**Disadvantages of Posterior Lumbar
  Interbody Fusion**

The Ray TFC Device

  advantages
  patient selection
  implantation technique
  follow-up
  outcome

Advantages of Posterior Lumbar Interbody Fusion

Posterior lumbar interbody fusions (PLIFs) have certain, distinct mechanical and surgical advantages when compared with other methods (e.g., posterior, posterolateral, or intertransverse process fusions).[3-5,7,12-14,22] There are three primary reasons: (1) The interbody bone is placed in the center of segmental motion, where the movement is the most restricted; that is, the lever arm of vertebral motion is the shortest, giving the interbody method the greatest theoretical potential for inhibiting motion. (2) The smallest volume of bone is required to achieve fusion. (3) The graft bone is virtually surrounded by essentially consistent circulation from viable bone, that is, the cancellous portions of the opposing vertebral bodies, from which the graft bone will receive its nutrition. Noninterbody fusion methods have longer leverage arms, since the bone is placed some distance from the movement center, a relatively large graft volume is required (since much of the graft bone normally will be absorbed) and the somewhat uncertain nutritional source for circumvertebral placed graft bone is the undersurface of the surgically injured muscle. Inherently, therefore, PLIFs are potentially more stable and should enjoy faster fusion development.

Disadvantages of Posterior Lumbar Interbody Fusion

PLIFs do not always fulfill their potential; negative aspects are well known. Most notably, there is a documented significant risk for nerve-stretch injury arising from the retraction required to bypass the root, ganglion, and dura during cutting of the recipient hole and placement of the graft. Collapse, slippage, displacement, or frank extrusion of the carefully fitted graft bone is not rare, and each represents a potentially hazardous complication, reportedly occurring altogether in about 3% to 10% of cases.[4,10,13,14,16] Fracture or fibrotic infiltration of the graft is also not rare, and when it occurs, it commonly leads to fusion failure.[4,10,13] Sterile prepared bank bone, such as homologous, freeze-dried bone dowels or tricortical grafts, are often used because they are stronger than equivalent autologous bone and eliminate the need for intraoperative graft harvesting. However, they are rather brittle, often rather porous and expensive. Ethylene oxide sterilized bone shows a poor propensity for osteoinduction and fresh-

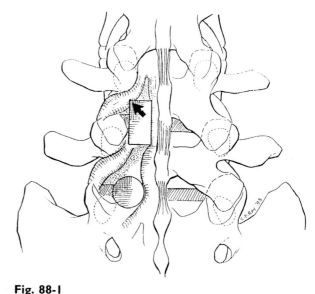

Fig. 88-1

Diagram showing rectangular and round inserts or grafts and neural element retraction required for their placement. Particularly hazardous upper-outer rectangular corner is shown (*arrow*) compressing ganglion, an unlikely situation when using round implants.

frozen homologous bone bears a small risk of virus infection to the recipient patient.[9,11] Henssge found that interbody grafts that fracture or fibrose may have an ingrowth of surrounding, remnant nuclear tissue invading and essentially attacking the graft and leading to the failure.[8]

Many studies have shown that fresh autologous cancellous bone is the material of choice for nearly all fusion grafting but has inadequate mechanical strength for interbody applications and may collapse or be extruded quite early. Such graft material therefore requires some means of structural support, such as a shell or vertical (axial) columns. Tricortical grafts fulfill the latter by their inherent struts of strong cortical bone margins. Thus, the cortical portions serve as supports, but they integrate into the fusion very slowly. Rectangular tricortical grafts require significant skill and special instruments for precise cutting of both the grafts and recipient holes. If improperly cut, the close fit between them, essential for a good, rapid development of the fusion will be jeopardized.[4,10,14,16] Further, rectangular grafts or inserts have sharp lateral-superior corners that during insertion may compromise or potentially induce injuries to the root, ganglion, or dura (Fig. 88-1).

To overcome the difficulties of cutting a precise rectangular graft and holes, a number of authors, following Wiltberger, developed and successfully used round bone dowels.[4,13,16-18,23] These dowels suf-

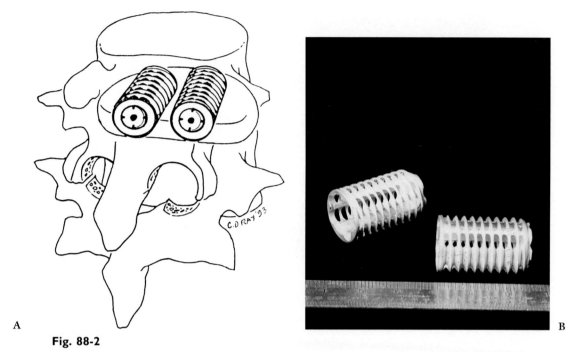

Fig. 88-2

A, Diagram showing Ray Threaded Fusion Cages (TFCs) in position at the L4-L5 level. Note semicircular laminotomies. **B,** Photograph of TFCs showing high degree of perforation of walls. Note internal axial ribs blocking perforations on lateral walls of cages.

fered the problems mentioned above, so Bagby developed stainless steel cylinders with multiple perforations drilled through their smooth walls.[1,5] He drove these devices into intervertebral holes drilled into the necks of horses who suffered from a chronic cervical spine subluxation disease called "wobbler syndrome." The unstable cervical segments would intermittently slip, producing cord compression and often paralysis. Bone chips from the intervertebral drilling process were returned to and packed (along with other bone chips) inside these smooth, perforated "baskets." Fusions developed from one vertebra through the device and into the opposite vertebra. The drilling and hammering required for insertion proved hazardous at times; several vertebrae were fractured, and about 7% of the baskets became displaced.[5]

The Ray TFC Device

The insertion by hammering into the hole and the relatively thick, smooth walls having discretely drilled holes were not, in my opinion, reasonable constructs for human use, therefore I developed the threaded fusion cage (TFC)[19,20] (Figs. 88-2, *A* and *B*). This new device was related to and an essential refinement of a combination of the Bagby basket and a more recent threaded cervical interbody bone dowel as re-

ported by Otero-Vich[17] and the author's personal experience with a method of transfacet fusion.[17] Further, for practical, safe clinical applications in the lumbar spine, a significant new system of surgical instrumentation had to be developed[19,20] (Fig. 88-3).

The Ray TFC devices, presented here, are threaded, abundantly perforated (70% of walls) cylinders whose perforations are not drilled through but are formed by the internal machining and subsequent external threading of solid rods of medical alloy titanium. It is important that these machined perforations are cut through the devices such that the apex of each thread in the recipient vertebral bone bed projects through the shell and will thus remain in contact with the valley of the same thread occupied by the internally impacted bone graft material. Thus, unlike any other interbody or epivertebral instrumentation, the mere internal packing of the soft, loose graft bone presses it against the internally projecting, threaded recipient bed of the vertebral spongiosa. Further, although the superior and inferior walls of each TFC has such perforations, the lateral walls do not. Thus, when screwed into proper position, the perforations face only the spongiosae and the lateral blockage prevents nuclear tissue ingrowth.[2,8,19] These lateral struts also strengthen the entire load-bearing construct, spanning the disc space. The TFCs, seated tightly inside the exactly

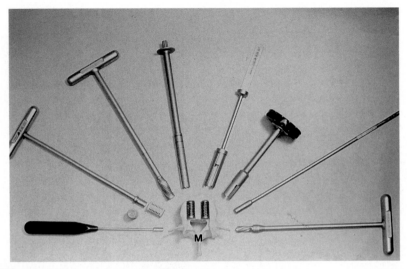

Fig. 88-3

Photograph of special instruments used during implantation of Ray TFCs. Plastic spinal model (*M*) with two cages in situ, lies in center of the display. Dark-handled instrument at left is graft-packing and plastic-cap-applying device. Counter clockwise from the right are the pilot rod, lamina cutter with ratchet placed on it, C-retractor with seating punch inside, vertebral body cutter, spiral-fluted tap, cage and insertion tool, and the cap applier.

matched, adjacent threaded vertebral bodies, are totally prohibited from dislodgment or expulsion. Animal pull-out testing showed that the cages cannot be avulsed, short of vertebral body disintegration.

Advantages

The advantages of the Ray TFCs are (1) The cylindrical shape of the device permits ease of cutting deeply through the adjacent end plates and into the vertebral spongiosa. (2) Tapping of the recipient beds prevents displacement and prepares the apices of threads for direct contact with the internally packed graft bone. (3) The large perforations (1.5 × 3.5 mm) are expected to prevent or reduce stress shielding of the fusion bone. (4) Soft, cancellous bone is used for the graft, well supported during fusion formation by the metal shell (about six times stronger than the recipient bed bone). (5) The round construct permits safer nerve retraction than a rectangular one. (6) The new instrumentation system guides and controls all drilling, tapping, and insertion of the TFC by utilizing a pilot drill and rod over which each subsequent instrument is placed during use. (7) Unique retractors hold and protect the ganglion, dura, and traversing nerve during the procedure. (8) Stabilization occurs instantly, requiring no additional interbody or posterolateral grafting or additional instrumentation. (9) The devices are not removed subsequently, obviating a second procedure as is often required for posterior or posterolateral in-

strumentation and bone screws. (10) The cylindrical TFC, acting as opposing arches inside the two vertebrae, is more supportive of body loading than a rectangular device of equal width could. (11) The implantation procedure is significantly faster and less expensive than anterior-posterior fusion procedures, especially if posterior instrumentation is used. (12) Titanium is the most tissue-compatible metal and is significantly more radiolucent than stainless steel in CT or MRI scans. Hydroxyapatite and synthetic bone substitutes packed inside TFCs have been investigated and will likely be used more extensively in the future, with or without bone-growth-inducing factors, hopefully eliminating the need for any graft bone.[15,24] This will further simplify and shorten the surgical time.

In general, the RAY TFC procedure may well be the fusion method of choice in appropriately selected patients. As a note of precaution, however, the most important technical detail that may limit a good outcome is that the disc space must be distracted, to stretch the anulus and each TFC *must* penetrate both respective vertebral end plates by 3 mm or more; otherwise, the cage may be loose and both the graft and recipient bed may not grow together properly. Larger TFCs for matched-pair anterior implantation, especially in very high disc spaces, will be in clinical application in the near future.

Ray TFCs are supplied in 12-mm, 14-mm, 16-mm, and 18-mm diameters and 21-mm and 26-mm lengths, the appropriate diameter and length being selected according to the measurements made from preoperative imaging studies.

Patient Selection

Published "appropriate" patient selection criteria for any form of spinal fusion are not fully acceptable by all surgeons or agencies. In general, the most agreeable criteria for lumbar fusions (outside of patients presenting with a major traumatic instability or displacement with signs of progressive neurologic loss) are patients with severe disabling low-back pain of discogenic (sometimes of facetogenic) origin from diseased discs, that is, having significant loss of both height and mobility of the segment in accompaniment with the disabling back pain. The cases in question should have had a vigorous, appropriate attempt at nonsurgical treatment methods. Equally important is to select patients who have few if any negative variables, such as a chronic pain syndrome, psychosocial disorders or economic/legal entanglements to their dysfunction. Thus, the history and physical examination are done in detail and carefully considered; a specific work-up then ensues. Screening studies should include x-ray studies and a structural imaging technique such as a CT scan or preferably an MRI. Additionally, functional (inhibitory or provocative painful injections, e.g., facet-joint injections, discography) studies are important, since the correlation between structural changes and symptoms may be low or misleading. Ancillary trials using a rigid brace, cast or external fixation may be of some benefit in selecting patients but they are not absolutely reliable, either.

The height of the target disc space should not exceed 6 mm for a 12-mm diameter cage, 8 mm for a 14-mm diameter cage to be implanted, 10 mm for a 16-mm diameter TFC, or 12 mm for an 18-mm diameter cage, otherwise the purchase into each adjacent vertebra may be inadequate. Higher disc spaces can be TFC implanted only via an anterior approach using larger cages. TFCs can be implanted by an anterior or posterior approach.

There have been 240 US TFC implant cases to date (Sept. 1994) and approximately 2500 have been implanted abroad. Patients have ranged in age from 18 through 79 (mean age, 41 years); follow-up periods have ranged from a few months to nearly 6 years; males were twice as likely as females to be selected for the fusions in the United States, which were performed at the L5-S1 level in 57%, L4-L5 in 40%, and L3-L4 in 3%. Females outnumbered males in the Far Eastern cases, and the most often operated level was L4-L5. In 96% of all cases the predisposing consideration was low-back pain with 74% showing degeneration of the anulus. Herniated discs were present in 57% of the patients, 21% had vertebral endplate osteophytes, and 43% had disc height loss of greater than 10%. Clinical outcomes are discussed below.

Implantation Technique

Technically, the new method is quite straightforward, primarily since the author has developed special instruments to protect the neural structures and to guide the lamina cutting, disc-space drilling and tapping, and TFC insertion and for packing the graft material inside the cages. Before beginning the procedure, the necessary measurements are taken from the x-ray films and scans—namely, disc height, anterior-posterior diameter, and width of the vertebral end plates. The angulation of the disc space from horizontal is noted.

Generous laminotomies out to and involving at least one-half of the medial aspect of the facet are first performed bilaterally at the target space. The ventral two thirds (and no more) of the interspinous ligament is removed along with the entire posterior ligamentum flavum from both sides, leaving a dorsal ligamentous band between the spinous processes and a Cloward laminar spreader is placed on one side stretching the anulus. Venous bleeding (the principal source of blood loss) is controlled. A round hole is then cut in the anulus with a number 11 blade bilaterally both sides midway between the spinous process and each pedicle. Exposing both sides simultaneously permits a careful bilaterally balanced approach for placing the pair of cages.

On one side at a time, a pilot drill of proper diameter, maintained at the proper angle, paralleling both the disc space (cephalocaudally) and the midline (mediolaterally), is used to bore through each of the anular holes and into the nucleus, to a depth of 25 mm. A slightly confluent angulation of the two drillings toward the midline is often used. The location and angle of the drill is quite important and must pass through the disc equidistant to its walls, as it will then orient the remaining steps. A matching pilot rod is inserted into the hole, a circular end-cutting lamina cutter is passed over the pilot rod and guides the semicircular scoring of the lamina. The remaining laminotomy is completed by a turbine drill or punches. Once the laminotomy is fully and exactly concentric with the pilot rod, the dura is retracted by passing a Penfield dissector number 2 or equivalent, under the interspinous ligament band across from the other side, and the dura is levered

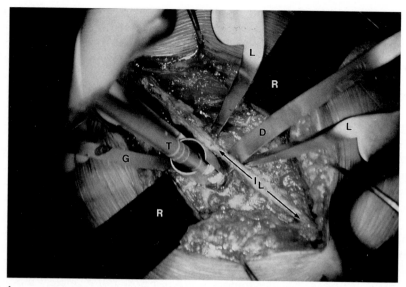

Fig. 88-4

Intraoperative photograph showing wide lateral retractors (*R*), narrow ganglion (*G*) and wider dural (*D*) retractor, the Cloward (*L*) lamina spreader, and the protective **C** retractor. Inside **C**-retractor can be seen spiral tap (*T*) entering intradiscal hole. Tap has its own T-handle and does not use a ratchet. Note markings, as engraved bands around shaft of tap, indicating intradiscal depth referable to top of **C**-retractor. Also note intact interspinous ligament (*IL*).

away from the pilot rod. A protective ganglionic retractor may also be placed if needed. When all the neural structures are clear, a tall, cylindrical **C**-retractor (shown in Fig. 88-4) is placed concentrically with the pilot rod and nailed equally into the posterior vertebral bodies, spanning the disc space. The cutting of the hole equally into the two vertebral bodies is controlled by an end-cutting vertebral body cutter, also passed along the axis of the pilot rod. Further, the pilot rod is stabilized by a removable handle held and controlled by the assistant surgeon, helping the surgeon to stay exactly on the desired track. All the manual cutting force is applied axially by the surgeon using a hand-operated circular ratchet forced against a collar attached to the external end of each cutting instrument. At a depth of 1 cm below the vertebral surface, the cutting instrument is removed and the purchase into each vertebra is checked by looking down through the **C**-retractor. If the purchase is not equal, it can be corrected somewhat as the cutting continues to the proper depth, usually 3 cm, but sometimes less (depending on vertebral body size and the TFC length to be used). The disc material should be cleared out as one progresses inwardly. At a depth of 2 cm, the pilot rod serves no further purpose and is removed. After reaching the 2.5- or 3-cm desired depth all loose tissue is removed and the spiral vertebral tap then threads the hole, being careful not to strip out

the bone threads or overbore the vertebra. A TFC having the correct diameter (14, 16, or 18 mm) and length (21 or 26 mm) is screwed into the threaded hole, seated at least 3 mm below the posterior surface of the vertebral body and all retractors are removed. The Cloward retractor is then no longer needed, as the first TFC placed maintains the intradiscal space. The opposite side is then operated on in the same way as the first.

When all cages are placed (at one or two levels), a cross-table lateral x-ray film is taken to permit adjusting the correct depth of the cages. Cancellous bone is obtained from one ilium by laterally stretching the midline wound over to the desired posterior superior iliac crest and outling a flap of its cortex to gain access inside. The volume of cancellous bone required to pack the TFCs is estimated (from a low of 2 ml for a 12-×-21-mm cage and 3 ml for a 14-×-21-mm cage to 8 ml for a 18-×-26-mm cage), and the bone is collected from within the iliac tables and placed inside a 20- or 30-ml disposable syringe. The volume is measured by moderate compression of the graft bone, pressing the syringe plunger within the syringe barrel. Each cage is reexposed in turn and tightly packed with the cancellous chips. A polyethylene plastic cap is applied, to retain the bone, and the procedure is finished.

The average blood loss (400 ml to 600 ml) has been greater than was initially expected and appar-

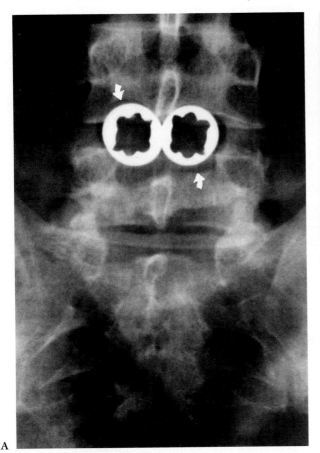

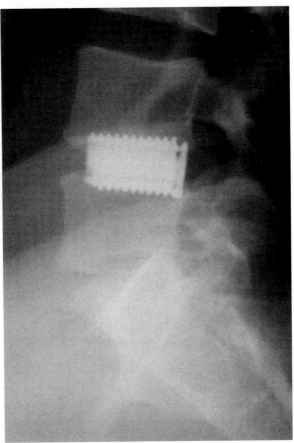

A   B

Fig. 88-5

A, Anteroposterior x-ray film of lumbar spine with cages in place at L4-L5 level, 6 months postoperatively. Note ease of viewing through implants (15-degree Ferguson view), a means to determine bone graft substance inside cages. Arrows point to semicircular laminotomies, not to be mistaken for possible dark halos around implants. **B,** Lateral film from patient in Panel A. Note absence of halo formation, sclerosis, or vertebral body changes.

ently arises from epidural venous bleeding (not ordinarily encountered with anterior or posterolateral fusion procedures) along with losses from both donor and recipient sites. The learning curve has been rather short, but with some experience surgeons should be able to complete a one-level TFC procedure in about 2 hours and a two-level case in about 3 hours, leading to a considerable cost savings as compared with standard fusion methods.

Follow-Up

Patients are seen at 6 weeks and then at 3, 6, 12, 18, and 24 months and yearly as indicated thereafter. Anteroposterior, lateral, and Ferguson (15-degree caudal angulation) views are taken at each visit and flexion/extension films at 6, 12, and 24 months (Fig. 88-5). The success of fusion is estimated by (1)

continued presence of visible bone within each cage, seen on the Ferguson view, (2) absence of a dark halo around or inside each cage, seen on anteroposterior and lateral views, (3) absence of more than 2 degrees of angular change at the fused segment on lateral flexion/extension views, (4) disc-space settling of less than 1.5 mm, seen on a lateral x-ray film, or (5) absence of significant end-plate or vertebral-body bony sclerosis around the TFC. Criterion 3, above, is the most difficult to determine with accuracy and has led to the introduction of a variety of measurement methods among those concerned with the TFC cases. Since the graft bone inside the cages remains fully visible after months or years, the bone bridging (fusion) is believed to develop a union rather rapidly across the disc space.

Another valuable benefit from these thin titanium cages is the remarkably reduced metallic artifact seen on CT scans or MRI; the bone inside the cages can be visualized using either technique or with antero-posterior plain x-ray films[21] (Fig. 88-6).

Outcome

All of my cases were evaluated postoperatively by myself, my physician's assistant, Matt Garner, PA-C and a radiologist, Kenneth Heithoff, Minneapolis; observations were independently recorded and then compared. Only minor discrepancies have been seen in our notes, except as regards criteria of flexion/extension movement, in a few cases. Indeed, motion on flexion/extension films was judged an unreliable criterion for segmental fusion, therefore the absence of a dark halo around the cage(s) (which would indicate the lack of proximate bone growth) and visible bone inside the cavity, on routine lumbar spine x-rays, have served as principal criteria. Four of the 55 patients upon whom I have operated, had halos and persistent back pain, related to the use of smaller cages with insufficient purchase into adjacent vertebral bone beds. These cases had subsequent pedicle screws and rods placed, bridging the cage fusion space, and the halos slowly disappeared. At time of that second surgery, cages in three were biopsied (6 to 9 months post-op), all showing viable bone inside. Many cases now over two years post-operative show bone growth across the anulus, anteriorly or posteriorly or both, obliterating any possible mobility, further confirming the assumptions of fusion from the above criteria.

Among the original 10 cases, operative complications were minimal. One had a marked foot drop requiring 6 months to clear by 95%. Another patient of this group returned to work as a truck driver after 6 weeks postoperative and remains at work after 5 years. Postoperatively, these patients wore a corset with stays but no brace. Subsequent cases have worn rigid braces. After 5 1/2 years to 4 3/4 years follow up period in this cohort of 10 cases, there has been no device displacement, no infection (discitis or osteomyelitis) and no persistent neurological injury.

Combining these 10 with an additional 45 cases upon whom I have operated over the last 2 1/2 years (a personal experience involving 157 cages inserted), none has required additional surgery except the 4 discussed above. All of the cages implanted for more than 6 months (the protocol decision point for fusion), save the above 4 plus one other, involving 50 of the 55 cases, apparently had early segmental fusion, whether or not they were smokers. All cases over 12 months, save one, have returned to some

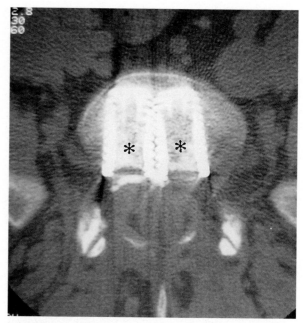

Fig. 88-6

CT scan (using bone algorithm in General Electric 9800 scanner) image through TFC, 3 months postoperatively. Note remarkably minimal artifact and clear presence of graft bone packed inside (*asterisks*). Graft bone shows some normal variation in density.

work, including workman's compensation cases. One patient in the more recent 45 patient cohort, showed a change in flexion/extension disc angulation greater than 2 degrees, and required a year before the fusion was declared solid. Simultaneously, there was an abatement of symptoms. Only one patient among the 45 had a foot weakness lasting more than a few days but less than a few months; no others had any neurological change, even briefly after surgery. As required in the new protocol, all patients were provided a rigid shell (TLSO or Boston overlap) brace to wear for 3 months.

During 1992, Gill also implanted Ray-TFCs in 28 patients whose age averaged 37 years. These cases were implanted primarily for degenerated herniated discs at L4 or L5.[6] Discography was seldom used in his patient selection. One-third of these cases had prior discectomies. Blood loss ranged from 150 to 450 ml and no complications occurred. At the L4-5 level the average operating time for one level was about 100 minutes.

Y-S Kim of Seoul, Korea (personal communication) implanted 310 patients in 1993. Other than there being a slightly greater proportion of female patients and those operated at the L4-5 level, rather than L5-S1, his cohort was quite closely matched as to selection and to reported outcome, when compared with the USA FDA-IDE study.

An FDA-Investigational Device Exemption (IDE) USA study of 240 cases with 13 investigators at 9 investigating centers has been done. Standardized reporting was utilized in all cases and all x-rays were read by Drs. Kenneth Heithoff, Minneapolis and Clyde Helms, San Francisco. The results as of Sept. 1994 are as follows:

Total Cases Implanted: 240

FOLLOW-UP PERIOD	6 months	12 months	24 months
NUMBER OF CASES (Data Received/Data Due)	182/226	130/160	19/27
FUSION RATE %	78/80%	91/90%	95/97%
PAIN RELIEF (Fair, Good, Excellent)	77%	83%	84%
& FUNCTION (Poor)	23%	17%	16%

COMPLICATIONS: 5 Superficial wound infections, 1 deep infection. All cleared.

PERSISTENT NEUROLOGICAL DEFICIT: None.

DEVICE DISPLACEMENT OR MIGRATION: None.

DEVICE BREAKAGE: One.

DEVICES REMOVED: None.

INTRAOPERATIVE SUPPLEMENTAL FUSION AND GRAFTING USED: None.

DEPTH OF GREATEST END-PLATE SETTLING: 1.5 mm.

It is estimated that over 2,500 Ray-TFC cases have been performed outside the USA, in the Far East, Middle East, Pacific Basin, Europe, Africa and South America, with reportedly similar case selection criteria and clinical outcomes. In conclusion, the method appears to take its place among other major techniques for lumbar fusion. C. V. Burton (personal communication) has also found the TFC method to be more cost-effective and safer than many other instrumented fusions, especially those using pedicle screws and plates or rods, particularly if anterior-posterior fusions are performed. Cervical applications of the TFC are planned.

Full Disclosure: The author developed and patented the cages and instruments reported here; all rights are now owned by Surgical Dynamics, Inc. The author has an indirect financial interest in (royalties from) these devices. The Ray-TFC (earlier designated as The Optifuse), Threaded Fusion Cages and surgical instrument system are Manufactured by Surgical Dynamics, Inc., 2575 Stanwell Dr., Concord, CA 94520.

References

1. Bagby GW: *Stainless steel implants for intervertebral body fusions.* Presented at the North American Spine Society annual meeting, June 27, 1987.
2. Brantigan JW, Steffe AD: *A carbon fiber implant to aid interbody lumbar fusion: 1-year clinical results in 26 patients.* Presented at the North American Spine Society annual meeting, July 9, 1992.
3. Cloward RB: The treatment of ruptured lumbar intervertebral discs by vertebral body fusion, *J Neurosurg* 10:154, 1953.
4. Collis JS: Total disc replacement: a modified posterior lumbar interbody fusion, *Clin Orthop* 193:64, 1985.
5. DeBowes RN, Grant BD, Bagby GW, et al.: Cervical vertebral interbody fusion in the horse: A comparative study of bovine xenografts and autologous supported by stainless steel baskets, *Am J Vet Res* 45:191, 1984.
6. Gill K, Ray CD: *Current experience with Optifuse, the threaded fusion cage.* Presented at the Japanese Orthopedic Society annual meeting, Osaka, Japan, April 8, 1993.
7. Goel VK, Kim YE, Lim T-H, Weinstein JN: An analytical investigation of the mechanics of spinal instrumentation, *Spine* 14:1003, 1989.
8. Henssge EJ: Fate of interbody bone in PLIF failures, *Dtsch Med Wochenschr* (personal communication), 1989.

9. Herron LD, Newman MH: The failure of ethylene oxide gas-sterilized freeze-dried bone graft for thoracic and lumbar spinal fusion, *Spine* 14:496, 1989.

10. Jaslow IA: Intercorporal bone graft in spinal fusion after disc removal, *Surg Gynecol Obstet* 82:215, 1946.

11. Leads from the MMWR: Transmission of HIV through bone transplantation: case report and public health recommendations, *JAMA* 260:2487, 1988.

12. Lee C: *Clinical biomechanics of lumbar spine surgery.* In White AH, Rothman RH, Ray CD, editors: *Lumbar spine surgery, techniques and complications*, St. Louis, 1987, Mosby, p 35.

13. Lin PM, et al.: Posterior lumbar interbody fusion, *Clin Orthop* 180:154, 1983.

14. Ma GW: Posterior lumbar interbody fusion with specialized instruments, *Clin Orthop* 193:57, 1985.

15. Mooney V, Derian C: Synthetic bone graft. In White AH, Rothman RH, Ray CD, editors: *Lumbar spine surgery, techniques and complications*, St. Louis, 1987, Mosby, p 471.

16. Mosdal C: Cervical osteochondrosis and disc herniation: eighteen years' use of interbody fusion by Cloward's technique in 755 cases, *Acta Neurochir* 70:207, 1985.

17. Oretero-Vich JMO: Anterior cervical interbody fusion with threaded cylindrical bone, *J Neurosurg* 63:750, 1985.

18. Ray CD: Transfacet decompression and dowel fixation: a new technique for lumbar lateral spinal stenosis, *Acta Neurochir Suppl* 43:48, 1988.

19. Ray CD: *Threaded fusion cage: new technique for lumbar interbody fusions.* Presented at the North American Spine Society annual meeting, Quebec City, June 29, 1989.

20. Ray CD: *Lumbar interbody threaded prostheses.* In Brock M, Mayer HM, Weigel K, editors: *The artificial disc*, Berlin, 1991, Springer Verlag, p 53.

21. Romner B, Olsson M, Ljunggren B, et al.: Magnetic resonance imaging and aneurysm clips: magnetic properties and image artifacts, *J Neurosurg* 70:426, 1989.

22. White AH, Rothman RH, Ray CD: *Lumbar spine surgery, techniques and complications*, St. Louis, 1987, Mosby.

23. Wiltberger BR: Intervertebral body fusion by the use of posterior bone dowel, *Clin Orthop* 35:69, 1964.

24. Wozney JM, Rosen V, Celeste AJ, et al.: Novel regulators of bone formation: molecular clones and activities, *Science* 242:1528, 1989.

Chapter 89
Anterior Lumbar Instrumentation and Fusion

John D. Schlegel

Rand L. Schleusener

Hansen A. Yuan

History

Indications

Technique

approach
decompression
bone grafting
internal fixation

Types of Devices

plate systems
cable systems
rod systems

Biomechanics of the Device

Management of Specific Conditions

posttraumatic kyphosis
iatrogenic lumbar kyphosis (flatback
  deformity)
lumbar scoliosis
failed posterior surgery
burst fractures/neoplastic conditions

Complications

Summary

Techniques and instrumentation systems associated with spinal fixation have escalated in number and popularity over the past few years. Though posterior fusion and instrumentation remains a mainstay procedure in spinal surgery, anterior approaches for certain conditions are extremely valuable. The authors feel that certain pathologic conditions, especially neoplastic and traumatic disorders, may be better handled by the use of anterior surgery.

Supplemental internal fixation is an accepted procedure in many orthopedic conditions. It has, until recently, maintained a less popular acceptance in spinal fusion. When vertebrectomy is performed, internal fixation anteriorly is an integral portion of the procedure. The chapter will discuss the indications, techniques, and biomechanical background associated with anterior spinal fusion and internal fixation.

History

Posterior spinal fusion dates back to the early 1900s. Hibbs and Albee described surgical techniques for fusion in 1911.[1,3] Posterior fixation devices including wire techniques were described by Hadra in 1891 and Lang in 1909.[3] Posterior surgery was the procedure of choice until the mid-1930s. During this time, anterior surgery became a viable alternative to address the problems of Pott disease, degenerative disorders, and spondylolisthesis.*

Internal fixation for anterior procedures has been much slower to gain acceptance. Humphries et al. developed a slotted contoured plate that was used for anterior fixation in 1961.[27] Their clinical results reported in 27 patients were moderately successful. Werlinich reported good results in 127 patients with anterior fusion and fixation with an associated staple.[56] Beginning in 1964, Dwyer used a cable system for anterior spinal instrumentation.[14–16,23,50] Subsequent to this, Zielke, Dunn, Yuan, Black, Kostuik, Kaneda, and other authors have developed fixation devices for anterior procedures.[4,8,11–13,30–37,45,48] These are used for patients with instability, for patients who have had a vertebrectomy, or in situations to correct significant deformity.

The available systems can be divided into three types: cable systems, rod systems, and plate systems.[49] Cable systems were initially developed by Dwyer. They are easy to use and have adequate stability. Unfortunately they have a tendency to place the thoracolumbar spine in kyphosis.[23] Multiple rods systems are in use. They show excellent stability on biomechanical testing and provide adequate fixation.

*References 5, 7, 18, 24 to 26, 29, 44, 51, and 52.

Unfortunately, many are bulky and have been associated with complications. Plate systems make up the final category of devices. Though deformity has to be corrected manually, they are low profile and technically are quite easy to use.[22] This chapter will describe the techniques and indications for anterior lumbar instrumentation and fusion.

Indications

The indications for anterior lumbar surgery are fairly well known. Degenerative disc disease has been treated with anterior discectomy for some time with varying results[6,20,54]; most authors do not think supplemental anterior fixation is necessary for these conditions.

The potential goals of supplemental anterior fixation for anterior fusion are (1) correction of deformity and reduction of risk of neurologic impairment, (2) maintenance of rigidity and anatomic alignment, (3) decreased pseudoarthrosis rate, and (4) enhanced postoperative patient mobilization and rehabilitation.

Indications for anterior fusion and internal fixation are (1) thoracolumbar burst fracture with or without neurologic deficit, (2) iatrogenic lumbar kyphosis (flat-back syndrome), (3) one- or two-level neoplastic disorder with or without neurologic deficit, (4) repair of failed posterior fusion, (5) instability, possibly secondary to wide laminectomy and posterior decompression, (6) high-grade spondylolisthesis or spondyloptosis, and (7) spinal osteotomy.[49]

Many authors favor a posterior approach to many traumatic neoplastic conditions.[53] Though decompression of the spinal canal can be accomplished indirectly via distraction[19] and directly via the posterolateral approach, we feel strongly that in conditions in which the pathology is largely anterior (i.e., burst fracture or metastatic neoplasm) anterior surgery is the safest and most effective way to decompress the canal completely. In traumatic situations in which posterior distraction is used the canal certainly is decompressed, but usually not to a maximum effect. This has been supported by the work of Gertzbein and others.[17,20,21,58] Especially in the patient with neurologic impairment, this is not optimal. Therefore, there exists a strong rationale for the anterior approach.[9,10,17,41]

When more than one vertebral body has to be removed, supplemental anterior internal fixation in addition to fusion is a very important adjunct to the procedure. The force placed on the thoracolumbar spine above the level of the waist can approach 2.5

to 3 times body weight. When simple bone grafting without fixation is performed, collapse and reproduction of deformity can occur. Bone graft material may require 6 months to 1 year to incorporate fully. The use of supplemental fixation maintains anatomic alignment during this healing process and can be done safely with very low risk.

Technique

Approach

The anterior approach to the spinal column is not difficult.[55] For illustrative purposes, the described approach will be for an injury of the L1 vertebral body. Various surgeons use either right or left approach. We prefer a left approach, since mobilization of the liver on the right side makes that approach somewhat more technically demanding. The patient should be placed in a right lateral decubitus position. Spinal cord monitoring is used. All bony prominences are protected. The table is broken at the level of the lower rib-cage and angulated about 20 degrees. The appropriate ribs are palpated and the tenth rib is selected as the entrance point for the surgical dissection. A skin incision is made over the tenth rib from the posterior margin of the erector spinae muscles to the costochondral junction. The incision is then extended distally in line with and parallel to the lateral border of the rectus abdominal muscle. The external thoracic muscles are divided with electrocautery over the tenth rib to expose the periosteum of the rib. The rib is dissected free of periostium and removed. The rib is excised at the costocartilage junction, which is the key to exposing the diaphragm.

The costal cartilage is then split longitudinally with a knife. Stay sutures are placed to aid in retraction and subsequent closure. The chest cavity is then entered and rib spreaders are placed. Using the gateway created by splitting the cartilage tip of T10, blunt finger dissection is used to dissect the abdominal contents away from the diaphragm in the retroperitoneal space. It is difficult to complete the entire dissection without dividing the anterior portion of the diaphragm. The diaphragm is visualized both inferiorly and superiorly prior to division 1 to 1.5 cm from the costal insertion. Innervation is from the phrenic nerve centrally, allowing for little denervation and loss of function. Sutures are placed on both sides of the divided diaphragm to aid in accurate reapproximation of the diaphragm during closure. Only the portion of the crus necessary for exposure is removed from the spine.

Once the chest activity is entered, the level is confirmed by palpating the ribs on the interior of the chest cavity, which is much more reliable than external palpation. The vertebral bodies and discs are easily palpable under the pleura. The vertebral bodies are recognizable by their concavity (valleys), and the discs by their convexity (hills). An 18-gauge spinal needle bent at double right angles is then inserted in the desired disc and anteroposterior x-ray scanning is done to confirm the correct level.

Once the level has been confirmed by x-ray scanning, rib spreader retractors are placed over the moist lap sponges on the skin to avoid damage to the segmental vessels. The lung is packed off with a moist lap and may be held in place with a malleable retractor clamped to the rib spreader. The malleable retractor must not be allowed to lie on the pulsating aorta, as this is a potential source of vascular erosion.

The pleura is incised longitudinally over the lateral aspect of the vertebral column. Sharp dissection is used to open the pleura directly over a disc. The dissection is extended as far as needed, taking care to avoid damage to the segmental vessels, which are located directly over the midportion of the vertebral body. The segmental vessels are then ligated and transsected with 2-O silk and at the midportion of the body. The segmental vessels must not be ligated too close to the aorta, which would risk avulsion of the artery, or too close to the spinal column, which would risk damage to the collateral circulation of the spinal cord. Once the segmental vessels are ligated, the pleura and soft tissue can be dissected off the spine with a Cobb elevator. The pleura can then be retracted using a stay suture to expose the spine.

Decompression

Vertebrectomy is then performed. Anatomic landmarks are identified. The pedicle of L1 is an excellent anatomic landmark and can be removed with a Kerrison rongeur, exposing the posterior aspect of the body more visibly. A number 15 blade is used to resect the disc between T12-L1 and L1-L2. This is done, and pituitary rongeurs are used to evacuate the disc totally. A burr or osteotomes are then used to remove the middle portion of the vertebral body of L1. We prefer to try to preserve the very anterior aspect of the body as well as the anterior longitudinal ligament to help provide stability. Certain points need to be emphasized at this juncture: If the patient has an old fracture, if there is significant canal stenosis, or if there is kyphosis of greater than 20 degrees, it is very important to remove a significant aspect of the mid and anterior vertebral bodies prior to canal debridement. We prefer to take an anterior and middle trough resected down to the opposing cortex of the body. If the dural sheath is exposed on the side of surgical entry, or if a wide trough is not cut, then the dura can buttonhole through this entry point, migrate anteriorly, and make surgical decompression of the remainder of the canal essentially impossible. This point cannot be overemphasized. We prefer to cut a deep trough while doing a vertebrectomy and to approach the dural tube, either at its mid or opposite aspect. After that, we burr back to the posterior cortical margin and use a curette or small Kerrison rongeur to try to remove the posterior wafer of the vertebral cortex. Again, if the dura is exposed on the side of surgical entry (in this case left), it will buttonhole, making decompressions of the far side of the canal difficult.

Bone Grafting

After the spinal decompression is complete, fixation of the spine may be necessary. Anterior strut fusion has a basic biomechanical advantage over posterior fusion as the bone graft is under compression. Posterior fusions, especially in kyphotic situations, are more likely to absorb or progress to pseudoarthrosis, as the graft is under tension. Even with the biomechanical advantage of compression, strut grafting alone in certain pathologic conditions is insufficient without supplemental internal fixation. At the thoracolumbar junction, stresses on the vertebral body can approach three times body weight. Bone graft material is a nonphysiologic entity, which has to revascularize and heal. This is excessive force to be placed on graft material, and augmentation with instrumentation is necessary. Laboratory data support this philosophy.[40,42]

The technique for bone grafting is simple, yet important. A slot is fashioned in the vertebral bodies above and below. A trough is fashioned on the undersurface of the T12 vertebral body, as well as the superior surface of the L2 vertebral body. This slot should be cut directly left to right with no migration, either toward the spinal canal or anterior toward the vascular structures. We actually prefer to start the slot slightly posterior to the midportion of the body of the associated vertebrae and carry it slightly anteriorly as we go across the body. This helps prevent graft migration or dislodgement. A slot cut beginning at the area of danger and working away from it is the safest and best. After impact has been made on the graft, the table is leveled and the graft is checked for stability. If the graft can be mobilized with a clamp, we redo the entire procedure.

The graft should be stable, it should not be allowed to move, and it should be in anatomic position. Anterioposterior and lateral radiography are performed at this time.

Internal Fixation

Anterior instrumentation has been controversial over the years. It was used in the 1930s and 1940s to augment a fusion for spondylolisthesis.[5,7] It was gaining favor until certain rare and untoward consequences occurred approximately 10 years ago.[28,43] It is our opinion that technical factors, rather than the hardware itself, are responsible for many of these failures. Realize that there is an important specified margin of safety that allows for placement of this hardware.

From a technical standpoint, instrumentation associated with bony fusion is not a new concept. It is routinely used almost without exception in injuries to upper and lower extremities. We have had a much slower acceptance of that in reference to spinal problems. Obviously, potential complications play a role in that. But acceptance of intervertebral fixation for cervical procedures as well as more recently, again, for thoracolumbar procedures appears to be gaining popularity.

Various instrumentation systems exist for anterior thoracolumbar surgery.[15] They fall into two categories: plating systems (I plate, DCP plate, ALPS plate, Armstrong plate) and rod systems (Dunn Device, Kaneda Device, TSRH system, CD system, Zielke system). Whichever system is chosen, it is important to recognize that placement of the device is crucial (Fig. 89-1). The exact margin of safety is shown, illustrating the risk points in reference to neural structures as well as vascular structures. If bulkier devices are used (i.e., Dunn Device, Kaneda device, TSRH system), then the right-sided approach is safer, as it lessens the chance of vascular complications.

The technique for anterior instrumentation is quite simple. A subperiosteal exposure of the entire vertebral body above and below is necessary. Most anterior systems require some type of screw placement into the vertebral body above and below the injured levels. Some require fixation of the opposing cortex, though this needs to be done carefully. It is important for wide exposure to be obtained, and this necessitates the entire body of T12 and L2 to be exposed in this particular situation. It is important to try to reduce the kyphosis and restore the spinal column to as normal an anatomic alignment as possible. After this is done, the device is secured

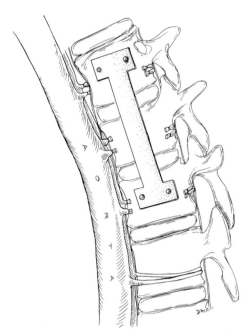

Fig. 89-1

Direct lateral placement of the Syracuse I plate. *(From Schlegel J, Yuan H, Fredrickson B: Anterior interbody fixation devices. In Frymoyer J, editor: The adult spine, New York, 1991, Raven Press.)*

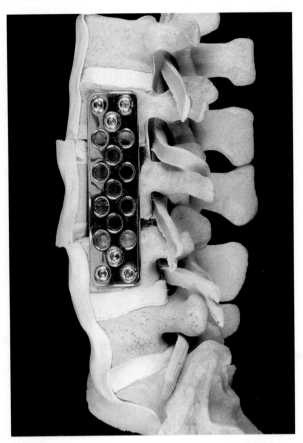

Fig. 89-2

Contoured anterior spinal fixation system. *(From Schlegel J, Yuan H, Fredrickson B: Anterior interbody fixation devices. In Frymoyer J, editor: The adult spine, New York, 1991, Raven Press.)*

to the T12 and L2 bodies and anatomic reduction is restored.

X-ray films are obtained at the time closure has begun. The posterior parietal pleura is closed over the fixation device with absorbable suture. The hemidiaphragm is repaired, utilizing O-silk in an interrupted figure-eight fashion, and oversewn with a running stitch. A chest tube is placed, and the parietal pleura is closed anteriorly. Muscular layers are closed utilizing O-Vicryl or a similar absorbable stitch. The skin is closed using skin staples. The patient is usually able to be extubated and returned to the intensive care unit where he/she will be monitored overnight, and then will be moved to a regular hospital ward. Careful observation of the patient's neurologic status is carried out. A CT scan is usually obtained 1 day postoperatively to assess the decompression and efficiency of the surgical procedure.

Types of Devices

Plate Systems

With adequate technique and exposure, plates can be easily and safely applied to the lumbar spine. Conventional DCP plates can be used as advocated by proponents of the AO system. In 1986, Ryan et al.[48] reported their techniques and results using a bolt-plate fixation device for anterior fusion. This device consists of two transvertebral bolts placed in the coronal plane and connected by one lateral slotted plate. The system is made of pure titanium. It can be used for stabilization after discectomy or one-level vertebrectomy. A postoperative orthosis is required.

In 1988, Black et al.[4] described a low-profile longitudinal rectangular plate that could span two or three adjacent vertebrae (Fig. 89-2). The plate is made of 316 LVM and contours easily to the vertebral bodies. Early results with its use in seven patients were encouraging.

The early experience with Syracuse I plate has equally been positive.[2,59] The device is a 3.5-mm stainless steel plate in the shape of an I that is attached to the vertebral body with four 6.5-mm cancellous screws. Clinical experience with its use has been reported in 16 cases with no major complications. An illustrative case is presented in Fig. 89-3.

Other plating systems are available. The Z plate is a titanium-based plate with multiple advantages. It allows for postoperative magnetic imaging. Can-

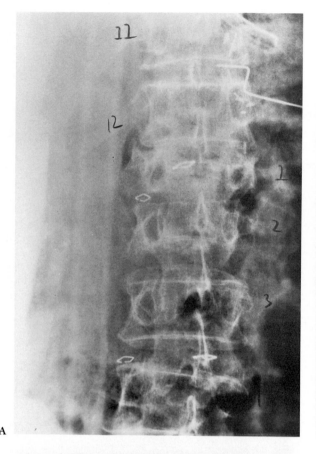

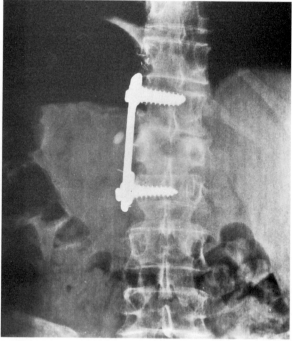

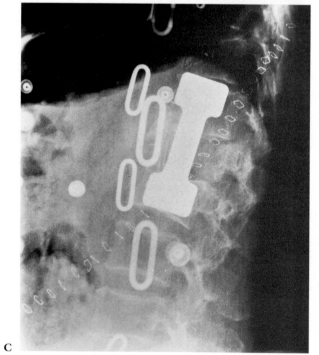

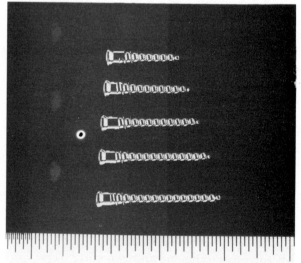

Fig. 89-3

29-Year-old male with L1 burst fracture. Anterior vertebrectomy, instrumentation, and fusion were carried out using Syracuse I plate. Various sizes and screw configurations for I plate are demonstrated. **A,** Anteroposterior radiograph showing burst fracture at L1. **B,** Postoperative anteroposterior radiograph showing anterior instrumentation and fusion utilizing I plate. **C,** Lateral radiograph showing lateral placement of I plate. **D,** Cancellous fixation screws for I plate.

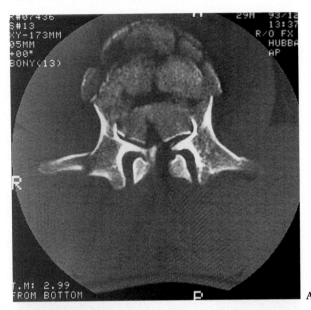

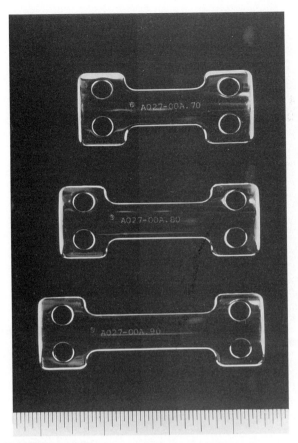

Fig. 89-3, cont'd

E, Various sizes of Syracuse I plate.

cellous screws (6.5 mm) are inserted prior to plate placement. A distraction device can be placed over the screw extenders, allowing for reduction of deformity. The slotted plate can be then introduced and secured. The screws are convergent, producing a more stable construct (Fig. 89-4).

The anterior locking plate system (ALPS) is made of 316 LVM stainless steel. It consists of a combination of straight and contoured rectangular vertebral plates, vertebral double-locking screws and self-locking screws. The plates are 3 mm thick and 25 mm wide. There are two columns of holes in each plate; one column is elliptical and the other round. The elliptical holes are designed to receive the double-locking screws, and the four round holes are designed for the self-locking screws. A center hole is present in all plates and is used for the plate holder; the straight vertebral locking plates are available in seven lengths, ranging from 50 to 110 mm. The contoured plates are used in situations in which the vertebral bodies are misaligned up to 5 degrees; they are available in six lengths, ranging from 60 to 110 mm.

Plate systems have an important use in anterior

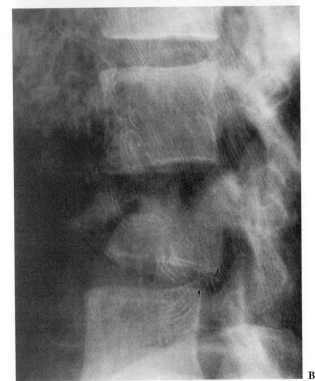

Fig. 89-4

29-Year-old male who suffered burst fracture of L3 vertebral body with significant neurologic compromise. Anterior decompression, vertebrectomy, instrumentation, and fusion were carried out using Z plate. Patient had excellent restoration of his spinal canal and obtained neurologic recovery. Note lateral placement of device and screw incorporation into opposing vertebral cortex. **A,** Severe 100% canal compromise. **B,** Lateral x-ray film of L3 fracture.

spinal fixation when they span two or three vertebral segments. However, reduction of deformity

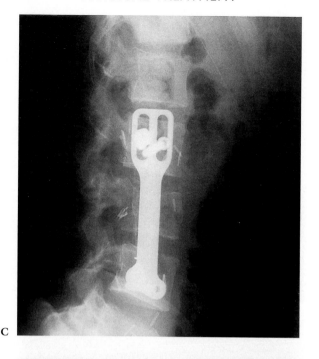

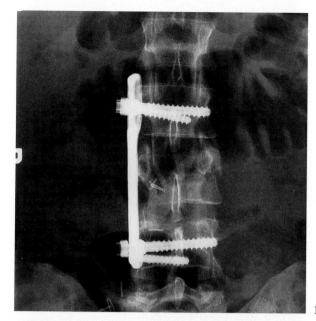

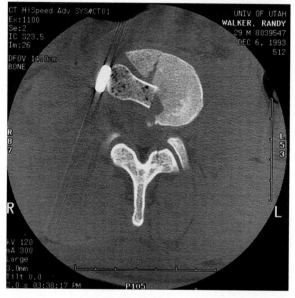

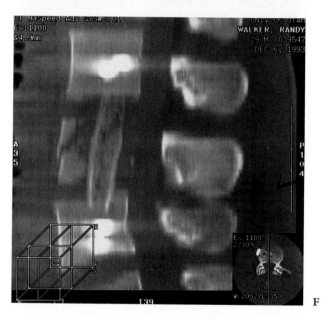

Fig. 89-4, cont'd

C, Postoperative x-ray film showing restoration of sagittal alignment with Z-plate fixation. D, Antero-posterior postoperative film. E, Postoperative CT scan decompression of canal. F, Sagittal reconstruction showing bone graft and canal decompression.

must be carried out manually. They have application in posttraumatic kyphosis, iatrogenic flatback deformity, and failed posterior surgery or pseudarthrosis. They have no place in scoliotic or rotational deformities.

The major difficulty with plates is screw backout even after solid arthrodesis has been achieved. With the I plate the proximal part of the screw (distal to the head) completely fills the plate screw hole, producing a "press-cold weld" fit and decreases the incidence of screw backout noted with other 6.5-mm cancellous screws. Other devices employ a crossing technique to lock the screws or recommend engaging the opposing vertebral cortex.

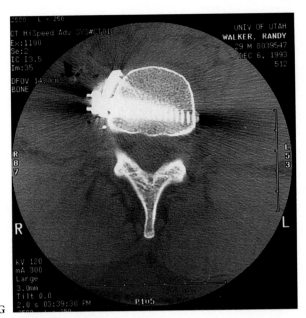

Fig. 89-4, cont'd

G, CT scan documenting screw placement.

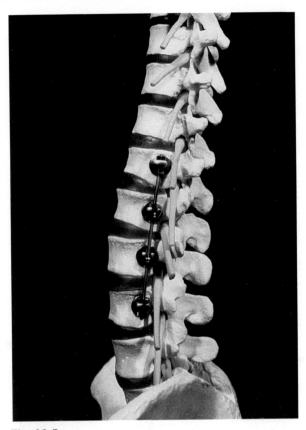

Fig. 89-5

Zielke device. (From Schlegel J, Yuan H, Fredrickson B: Anterior interbody fixation devices. In Frymoyer J, editor: The adult spine, New York, 1991, Raven Press.)

Cable Systems

In 1964, Dwyer first used a cable system for anterior spinal instrumentation.[23] Developed largely for scoliosis, the system gained widespread popularity. A special screw-staple assembly was drilled into each vertebral body on the convex side of the curvature. A braided titanium cable was passed through the screw heads and tension was applied. This device was a major conceptual breakthrough in anterior spine surgery and has been used extensively. Excellent results have been reported with its use.[14,16] Dwyer reported only two cases of pseudoarthrosis in 51 patients. Simmons et al. reported on over 80 patients with Dwyer instrumentation.[50] Unfortunately, problems and complications have presented. Dwyer et al. reported a 43% complication rate in 77 patients,[16] including progressive kyphosis (18 patients), loss of correction (22 patients), nonunion (15 patients), implant failure (5 patients), and deep paravertebral infection (3 patients). The pull-out strength of the screw system, especially in osteoporotic bone, has also been questioned. Finally, serious vascular and urologic complications have been documented.[43]

Rod Systems

Zielke Device

In 1975 Zielke modified the Dwyer system.[8] This system was made of stainless steel rather than tita-

nium and appeared to have better pull-out characteristics (Fig. 89-5). The screws have slotted heads and are either top-opening (in between vertebra) or side-opening (top and bottom vertebra). A threaded, 3.2-mm-diameter flexible rod is attached to the screws. An outrigger device can be applied to produce lordosis (or reduce iatrogenic kyphosis) during curve correction, which is a distinctive benefit not available with plate systems.

During curve correction, compression is initiated at the apex of the curve. The nuts on the compression side of the device are then tightened and the surgeon works sequentially away from the apex of the curve. The screws must be inserted slightly posteriorly in the body because anterior placement will accentuate kyphosis. A 10% to 15% correction per disc level of scoliosis can be obtained in most cases.

We believe this is probably the implant of choice for correction of lumbar degenerative scoliosis. Moe et al.[45] reported its use in 66 patients. Kaneda et al. reported its use in 31 patients (only 8 adults).[31] A 59% correction of curve was obtained in the adult population. Kyphosis was also corrected (21 degrees to 8 degrees). Pseudarthrosis later developed in two of the adult patients. No major complications were encountered.

Kostuik et al. think the Zielke instrumentation is useful for symptomatic pseudoarthrosis after attempted posterolateral fusion.[35] They recommend the placement of two parallel Zielke rods under compression.

The Zielke system is best used when the system is under tension and the bone is under compression, as in scoliosis surgery. Used as a stabilizing device only, Kostuik et al. noted an 18% incidence of pseudarthrosis with single rods, and a 9% incidence with double rods when interbody grafts were used in cases of salvage low-back surgery.

Kostuik-Harrington Device

Kostuik has developed and extensively used an anterior modification of the classic posterior Harrington instrumentation.[32–37] In this procedure, Kostuik spinal screws are inserted into the appropriate vertebral bodies, and a Harrington distraction rod placed through the screw holes and distracted in the usual fashion (Fig. 89-6). When optimal distraction is maintained, **C** washers lock the rod into place. A second, heavier Harrington compression rod is then placed posteriorly to the first rod. This was his classic description in the treatment of burst fractures. The system is adaptable and can be used for distraction, compression, or stabilization alone.

Its use has been reported extensively and is an excellent method for treating kyphotic and flatback deformities. Kostuik has reported 279 cases using this technique.[34] Complications have included 35 screw breakages (12.5%; 24 of these were with the older, thin-shanked screw), 2 fractured distraction rods (0.7%), and 8 vertebral body fractures (2.8%), without untoward effects. No vascular or neurologic injuries were reported. This device is a very acceptable system for the treatment of posttraumatic kyphosis, pseudarthrosis, iatrogenic flatback, and burst fractures.

Kaneda Device

In 1984, Kaneda et al. reported a series of unstable lumbar fractures treated with a new device.[30] This device consists of two vertebral plates of a trapezoidal configuration each having four spikes (Fig. 89-7). Two screws pass through each plate, securing it to the appropriate vertebra (one above and one below). A vertebral body spreader can be placed between the

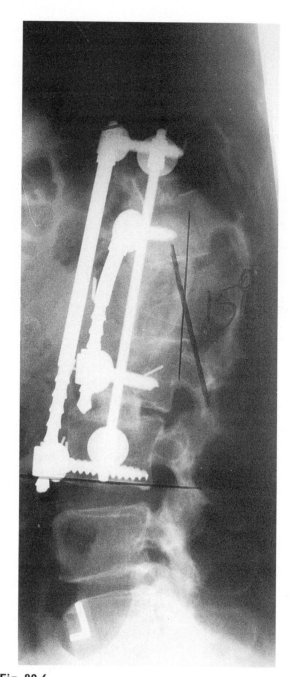

Fig. 89-6

Instrumentation and fusion with the Kostuik-Harrington device. *(From Schlegel J, Yuan H, Fredrickson B: Anterior interbody fixation devices. In Frymoyer J, editor:* The adult spine, *New York, 1991, Raven Press.)*

screw heads to assist with reduction. Two rigid threaded rods with eight nuts (four nuts to each rod) are then used to connect the rods to the screws. The nuts can also be adjusted to allow for curve correction or compression. This device holds up well under biomechanical testing and would appear to be a good option for degenerative one- or two-level de-

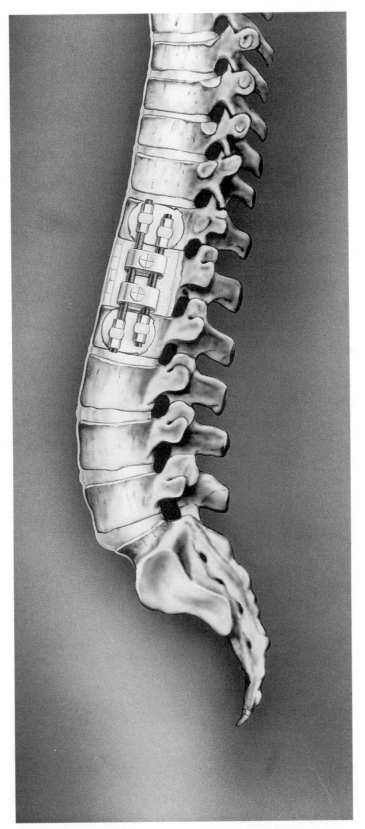

Fig. 89-7

Kaneda device. *(From Schlegel J, Yuan H, Fredrickson B: Anterior interbody fixation devices. In Frymoyer J, editor: The adult spine, New York, 1991, Raven Press.)*

formity (kyphosis, pseudoarthrosis, and burst fracture).

Other Systems

Multiple other anterior systems now exist. Most of the posterior pedicular instrumentation systems can be easily adapted for anterior usage. A sampling of these systems include TSR, Modulack, and CD.

Biomechanics of the Device

The underlying biomechanical concept of anterior fusion surgery is that compression is placed directly on the graft material. Posterior fusion, especially in kyphotic situations, is under tension, and this is subject to plastic deformation, fracture, or pseudarthrosis. Although the benefit of anterior bone grafting and fusion is through compressive forces, the loads in the lumbar spine can sometimes approach three times the body's weight. In certain pathologic conditions, we think this is an excessive load to be placed on the graft material and that internal fixation is necessary to enhance stability. However, limited comparative biomechanical data exist to prove our assertion. Mann et al.[40] performed a laboratory evaluation of anterior fixation devices. Anterior vertebrectomy (with preservation of the anterior longitudinal ligament) was performed in nine fresh cadaver specimens. The grafted specimen alone, along with specimens internally fixed with the Kostuik Device, Kaneda device, and I-plate systems were compared with the intact spine in flexion, extension, and right and left lateral bending. The relative stability of each device is shown in Table 89-1. We believe these results indicate that the use of bone graft without additional instrumentation does not provide adequate support to the spine with the gross instability produced by vertebrectomy. All the devices tested returned stability to at least that of the intact spine. The Kaneda device and I plate provided the greatest increase in stiffness. Supplemental work by McGowan et al.[42] shows that if significant posterior element disruption is present, then anterior instrumentation alone does not provide appropriate support, and additional posterior fixation will be required. This is also supported by the clinical work of Kostuik.

Kostuik has also shown that the holding power of screws in vertebral bodies is doubled if the contralateral cortex of the vertebral body is perforated. A 6.5-mm cancellous thread is preferable. In osteoporotic bone, the addition of bone cement will greatly enhance the fixation of the screws.

Table 89-1
Bending moments of the average percent increase in stiffness of each device over the normal spine in each of the tested modes*

	Flexion (14 N-m)	Extension (12 N-m)	RL Bend (10 N-m)	LL Bend (10 N-m)
Graft	−6.8% (NS)	−10.0% (NS)	−48.6% ($p < 0.0025$)	−12.2% ($p < 0.1$)
Kostuik	−24.2% ($p < 0.1$)	5.3% (NS)	7.5% (NS)	20.1% ($p < 0.05$)
Kaneda	9.6% (NS)	3.3% (NS)	16.1% ($p < 0.02$)	37.2% ($p < 0.01$)
I plate	12.4% ($p < 0.15$)	8.6% (NS)	6.8% (NS)	25.5% ($p < 0.01$)
Revised I plate	16.3% ($p < 0.1$)	8.7% (NS)	16.9% ($p < 0.01$)	29.0% ($p < 0.01$)

*Results for the grafted spine alone without instrumentation are included. Negative numbers indicate a percent decrease in stiffness when compared to the intact spine. Statistical significance levels when compared to the normal spine are listed in parentheses.
RL = right lateral; LL = left lateral; NS = not significant.

Management of Specific Conditions

Posttraumatic Kyphosis

Last posttraumatic problems following fracture or injury to the thoracolumbar spine are not uncommon. McAfee et al.[41] reported excellent results with anterior decompression in patients with incomplete neurologic lesions, both acute and chronic. Although some authorities still advocate conservative acute management of spinal fractures,[38] other reports document problems with late posttraumatic pain and neurologic compromise.*

Malcolm et al.[39] reported their results in 48 patients surgically treated for posttraumatic kyphosis. Their indications for surgery were a painful deformity (greater than 50 degrees kyphosis), instability, and/or neurologic compromise. Twenty-four of the patients had a previous laminectomy (50%). Anterior fusion alone was performed on 12 patients, with 6 failures occurring (50%). No internal fixation was employed, and the patients were ambulated early (1 week). Roberson and Whitesides[47] reviewed the cases of 34 patients with late posttraumatic kyphosis. Both anterior and posterior approaches were used. They thought that posterior fusion alone was

*References 34, 37, 39, 46, 47, and 57.

usually not sufficient treatment and that it did not fully address the problem. Eighteen of these patients had anterior fusion alone, with 17 of them obtaining solid fusion with no evidence of a further progression of the kyphosis. Roberson and Whitesides recommended 2 to 3 months of postoperative rehabilitation. Kostuik has done extensive work with posttraumatic kyphosis. He has reported on 45 patients with posttraumatic kyphosis treated with anterior surgery and instrumentation with the Kostuik-Harrington system. Pain relief was good or excellent in 37 of 45 patients (82%). Screw breakage occurred in 3 of 45 patients (6.7%). Four of 10 residual paraparetics improved by more than one Frankel grade after surgery.

The present indications for surgery in cases of posttraumatic kyphosis are significant back pain, deformity, instability, progression of deformity, or current or progressing neurologic compromise. Supplemental posterior surgery does not need to be considered unless significant posterior instability is present. Rod systems (Kostuik, Kaneda, Zielke) are the preferable devices because they provide distraction forces for reduction of the kyphosis. Plates are also very applicable, through the reduction must be done manually, and no more than 2 to 3 segments can be bridged.

A representative case is shown in Fig. 89-8. This is a 28-year-old man with a previous L1 fracture treated at an outside facility. He had persistent kyphosis with back and significant lower-extremity pain on activity. He underwent simultaneous anterior/posterior corrective osteotomy with instrumentation (TSRH). Preoperative and postoperative radiograms are shown in Fig. 89-8.

Iatrogenic Lumbar Kyphosis (Flatback Deformity)

Iatrogenic loss of lumbar lordosis following posterior distraction instrumentation and fusion for scoliosis has been well documented[34,36] and presents a major functional problem in patients with posterior fusion that extends to the lower lumbar spine or sacrum. Extension osteotomy is the accepted procedure of choice when these patients become symptomatic. Classically, these patients report back pain and an inability to stand erect without flexing the knees and hips. With fusion to the sacrum, Kostuik[36] reported a 49% loss of lordosis following Harrington instrumentation. He also noted that treatment by posterior osteotomy alone showed excellent early correction but that 50% of patients later showed loss of correction.

Because of these problems, the symptomatic patient with flatback deformity is better treated by single-stage anterior-opening wedge osteotomy with internal fixation followed by posterior-closing wedge osteotomy. Kostuik reported significant pain relief in 90% of patients treated by this approach. The acceptable devices are the distraction rod systems (Kostuik, Kaneda, Zielke). Plating systems can also be used but, as mentioned previously, have the disadvantages that the reduction and positioning must be done manually.

Lumbar Scoliosis

Degenerative scoliosis of the adult lumbar spine can be disabling and painful condition (see Chapter 65). Posterior surgery alone is often insufficient to correct the curve and has a high rate of pseudarthrosis. Posterior distraction instrumentation and fusion to L4 or below are contraindicated especially in patients with thoracic hypokyphosis. Because pain is the major disabling problem of these patients, careful preoperative evaluation is very important. Facet blocks and discography are useful to identify the possible sources of pain and to plan the levels of fusion accurately. Kostuik et al.[34,35] and Kaneda et al.[31] have reported and recommended anterior instrumentation and fusion for painful lumbar scoliosis.

Painful adult scoliosis greater than 40 to 50 degrees or painful progressive scoliosis of the lumbar spine should be managed with anterior instrumentation and fusion after careful preoperative evaluation and counseling. For curves greater than 80 degrees, a combination of anterior and posterior procedures may be needed. The preferred implant system anteriorly is the Zielke implant. Ten to fifteen degrees of curve correction per disc level can usually be obtained, although this varies as a function of age, spinal stiffness, and neurologic systems.

Failed Posterior Surgery

Much attention is focused on unfortunate patients with failed posterior surgery (Chapter 98). Failed posterior surgery is a major cause of disability in this country. With the popularity of bone-screw fixation and the 360-degree technique of fusion, anterior internal fixation is now rarely required. Nevertheless, in cases of significant posterior adhesion formation, extensive laminectomy, and loss of bone stock or posterior pseudarthrosis, anterior internal fixation and fusion remains a viable option.[34,35] Anterior fusion and instrumentation have particular utility in cases with associated kyphosis or deformity that

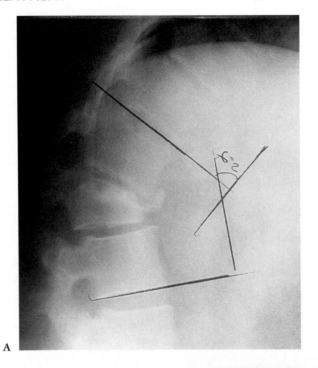

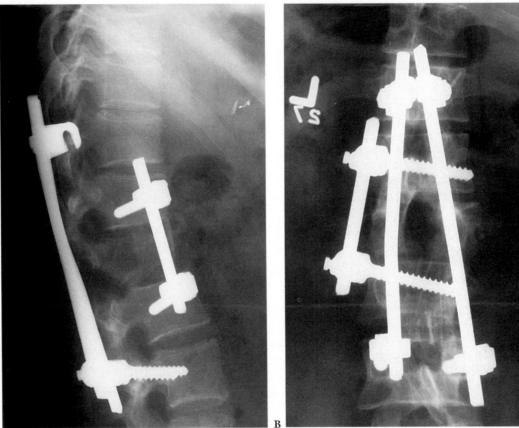

Fig. 89-8

28-Year-old man with previous L1 burst fracture. Patient had posttraumatic kyphosis. Because of persistent pain and problems, patient underwent simultaneous anterior/posterior osteotomy and correction of sagittal alignment. **A,** Kyphotic deformity of 62 degrees. **B,** Lateral (*left*) and anteroposterior radiograph (*right*) of postoperative reconstruction.

needs correction. Both rod systems or plate systems can be used depending on the extent and type of deformity. Long-term clinical trials in this population, however, are lacking at present.

A 63-year-old woman presented with severe low-back and lower-extremity pain. She had multiple previous posterior decompressions and attempted fusions. Obvious lateral listhesis was present at L4-L5. She underwent anterior discectomy, instrumentation and fusion from L3 to L5. Her pain relief at 1 year postoperatively is good, and her function has increased (Fig. 89-9).

Burst Fractures/Neoplastic Conditions

Anterior- and middle-column pathology with neurologic deficit is best treated by anterior surgery. Though posterior distraction can produce canal debridement, this is sometimes unpredictable. Patients with burst fractures and neoplastic disorder require anterior vertebrectomy and fusion. Supplemental instrumentation is crucial in providing stability and maintenance of alignment.

Figure 89-3 shows a 29-year-old man with an L3 burst fracture. He has weakness of all musculature

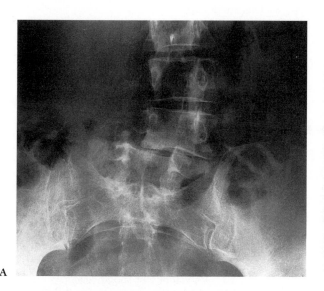

A

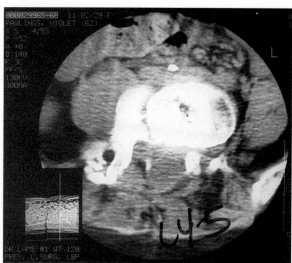

B

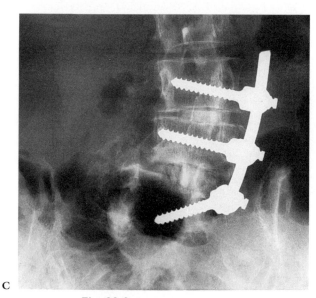

C

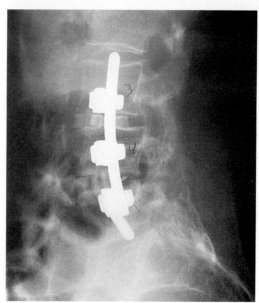

Fig. 89-9

63-Year-old woman with multiple previous posterior decompressions. She had severe lateral listhesis at L4-L5. She underwent anterior discectomy, instrumentation, and fusion from L3 to L5. **A,** Lateral listhesis at L4-L5. **B,** CT scan showing listhesis and lack of posterior elements. **C,** Postoperative anteroposterior radiogram (*left*) and lateral radiogram (*right*) showing lumbar fusion.

distal to the quadriceps. He underwent a right anterior retroperitoneal approach and L3 vertebrectomy. Instrumentation and fusion was performed and the patient had complete neurological return and full function.

Complications

Throughout this chapter, we have stressed the potential complications associated with the various fixation devices (see box opposite) and paid particular attention to operative technique and device placement. The most devastating complications are vascular and neurologic. Kostuik reported 2 iliac vein lacerations in 79 patients treated with anterior decompression (2.5%).[32] In a larger series of patients (279) treated for a variety of kyphotic deformities, he reported 3 cases of vascular insult (1.1%) and 2 cases of neurologic deterioration (0.7%).[34] The vascular injuries occurred during surgery and were not due to the fixation devices. However, significant vascular injuries led to the removal of the Dunn device from widespread commercial use.[26] Whether technical or implant design features (or both) were responsible for these is not known. Urologic complications have been documented after Dwyer instrumentation,[43] although the one case presented involved obstruction of the left ureter by scar tissue, and not by the device itself.

Prevention of complications is essential. Meticulous placement of the device with mobilization of the great vessels and adequate neurologic decompression are mandatory. Spinal cord monitoring or the wake-up test should be routinely used. Careful preoperative planning and patient selection cannot be overemphasized.

Summary

Internal fixation in general is widely accepted by orthopedic surgeons to provide rigidity, improve fusion rates, reduce postoperative morbidity, and correct deformity. Anterior lumbar surgery for a variety of indications has gained popularity in most centers throughout the world. The indications for anterior lumbar surgery augmented with internal fixation currently are few; but when the procedure is indicated, it is invaluable in dealing with very difficult surgical problems. Detailed knowledge of the approach, indications, and implant characteristics are most important. Even more important is careful patient evaluation, selection, and documentation. Further scientific investigation with implant and technical modification will help make anterior internal fixation a more acceptable, safer procedure in the future.

Complications

- Retroperitoneal fibrosis
- Urologic dysfunction
- Major vascular injury/aneurysm
- Neurologic impairment
- Implant failure
- Sympathetic nerve injury
- Infection
- Graft migration
- Pseudarthrosis
- Deep venous thrombosis/embolism

References

1. Albee FH: Transplantation of a portion of the tibia into the spine for Pott's disease, *JAMA* 57:885, 1911.
2. Bayley JC, Yuan H, Fredrickson B: The Syracuse I plate, *Spine* 16:120, 1991.
3. Bick EM: An essay on the history of spine fusion operations, *Clin Orthop* 35:9, 1964.
4. Black RC, Gardner VO, Armstrong GWD, et al.: A contoured anterior spinal fixation plate, *Clin Orthop* 227:135, 1988.
5. Burns BH: Operations of spondylolisthesis, *Lancet* 1:1233, 1933.
6. Calandruccio RA, Benton BF: Anterior lumbar fusion, *Clin Orthop* 35:63, 1964.
7. Capener N: Spondylolisthesis, *Br J Surg* 19:374, 1932.
8. Chan DP: *Zielke instrumentation*, AAOS Instruct Course Lect 32:208, 1983.
9. Clohisy JC, et al.: Neurologic recovery associated with anterior decompression of spinal fractures at the thoracolumbar junction (T_{12}-L_1), *Spine* 17:325, 1992.
10. Denis F: The three column space and its significance in the classification of acute thoracolumbar spinal injuries, *Spine* 8:817, 1983.
11. Dunn HK: Spinal instrumentation. I. Principles of anterior and posterior instrumentation, *AAOS Instruct Course Lect* 32:192, 1983.
12. Dunn HK: Anterior stabilization of thoracolumbar injuries, *Clin Orthop* 189:116, 1984.
13. Dunn HK: Anterior spine stabilization and decompression for thoracolumbar injuries, *Orthop Clin North Am* 17:113, 1986.
14. Dwyer AF, Newton NC, Sherwood AA: An anterior approach to scoliosis, *Clin Orthop* 62:192, 1969.
15. Dwyer AF: Anterior instrumentation in scoliosis, *J Bone Joint Surg* 52B:782, 1970.
16. Dwyer AP, O'Brien JP, Seal PP, et al.: The late complications after the Dwyer anterior spinal instrumentation for scoliosis, *J Bone Joint Surg* 59B:117, 1977.

17. Essess SI, Botsford DJ, Kostuik JP: Evaluation of surgical treatment for burst fractures, *Spine* 15(7):667, 1990.

18. Fang HS, Ong GB, Hodgson AR: Anterior spinal fusion: the operative approaches, *Clin Orthop* 35:16, 1964.

19. Fredrickson BE, et al.: Vertebral burst fractures: an experimental, morphologic, and radiographic study, *Spine* 17:1012, 1992.

20. Freebody D, Bendall R, Taylor RD: Anterior transperitoneal lumbar fusion, *J Bone Joint Surg,* 53B:617, 1971.

21. Gertzbein SD, Crowe PJ, Fazi M, et al.: Canal clearance in burst fractures using the AO internal fixation, *Spine* 17:558, 1992.

22. Haas N, Blauth M, Tscherne H: Anterior plating in thoracolumbar spine injuries, *Spine* 16:100, 1991.

23. Hall JE: Dwyer instrumentation in anterior fusion of the spine, *J Bone Joint Surg* 63A:1188, 1981.

24. Harmon PH: Anterior excision and vertebral body fusion operation for intervertebral disk syndromes of the lower lumbar spine, *Clin Orthop* 26:107, 1963.

25. Hodgson AR: Results of anterior fusion, *J Bone Joint Surg* 48B:595, 1966.

26. Hodgson AR, Stock FE: Anterior spinal fusion: a preliminary communication on radical treatment of Pott's disease and Pott's paraplegia, *Br J Surg* 44:266, 1956.

27. Humphries AW, Hawk WA, Berndt AL: Anterior interbody fusion of lumbar vertebrae: a surgical technique, *Surg Clin North Am* 41:1685, 1961.

28. Jendrisak MD: Spontaneous abdominal aortic rupture from erosion of a lumbar spine fixation device: a case report, *Surgery* 99:631, 1986.

29. Jenkins JA: Spondylolisthesis, *Br J Surg* 24:80, 1936.

30. Kaneda K, Abumi K, Fujiya M: Burst fractures with neurologic deficits of the thoracolumbar-lumbar spine, *Spine* 8:788, 1984.

31. Kaneda K, Fujiya N, Satoh S: Results with Zielke instrumentation for idiopathic thoracolumbar and lumbar scoliosis, *Clin Orthop* 205:195, 1986.

32. Kostuik JP: Anterior spinal cord decompression for lesions of the thoracic and lumber spine, techniques, new methods of internal fixation results, *Spine* 8:512, 1983.

33. Kostuik JP: Anterior fixation for fractures of the thoracic and lumbar spine with or without neurologic involvement, *Spine* 13:286, 1984.

34. Kostuik JP: Anterior Kostuik-Harrington distraction systems for the treatment of kyphotic deformities, *Iowa Orthop J* 8:68, 1989.

35. Kostuik JP, Errico TJ, Gleason TF: Techniques of internal fixation for degenerative conditions of the lumbar spine, *Clin Orthop* 203:219, 1986.

36. Kostuik JP, Maurais GR, Richardson WJ, Okajima Y: Combined single stage anterior and posterior osteotomy for correction of iatrogenic lumbar kyphosis, *Spine* 13:257, 1988.

37. Kostuik JP, Matsusaki H: Anterior stabilization, instrumentation, and decompression for posttraumatic kyphosis, *Spine* 14:379, 1989.

38. Krompinger WJ, Fredrickson BE, Mino DE, Yuan HE: Conservative treatment of fractures of the thoracic and lumbar spine, *Orthop Clin North Am* 17:161, 1986.

39. Malcolm BW, Bradford DS, Winter RB, Chou SN: Post-traumatic kyphosis, *J Bone Joint Surg* 53A:628, 1981.

40. Mann KA, Found EM, Yuan HA, et al.: *Biomechanical evaluation of the effectiveness of anterior spinal fixation systems.* Presented at the Orthopaedic Research Society 33rd annual meeting, San Francisco, 1987.

41. McAfee PC, Bohlman HH, Yuan HA: Anterior decompression of traumatic thoracolumbar fractures with incomplete neurological deficit using a retroperitoneal approach, *J Bone Joint Surg* 67A:89, 1985.

42. McGowan DP, Mann KA, Yuan HA, et al.: *A biomechanical study of anterior spinal fixation for thoracolumbar burst fractures with varying degrees of posterior disruption.* Presented at the International Society for the Study of the Lumbar Spine meeting, 1987.

43. McMaster WC, Silbert I: An urological complication of Dwyer instrumentation, *J Bone Joint Surg* 57A:710, 1975.

44. Mercer W: Spondylolisthesis, *Edinb Med J* 43:545, 1936.

45. Moe JH, Purcell GA, Bradford DS: Zielke instrumentation (VDS) for the correction of spinal curvature: analysis of results in 66 patients, *Clin Orthop* 93:207, 1973.

46. Myllynen P, Bostman O, Riska E: Recurrence of deformity after removal of Harrington's fixation of spine fracture, *Acta Orthop Scand* 59:497, 1988.

47. Roberson JR, Whitesides TE: Surgical reconstruction of late posttraumatic thoracolumbar kyphosis, *Spine* 10:307, 1985.

48. Ryan MD, Taylor TKF, Sherwood AA: Bolt-plate fixation for anterior spinal fusion, *Clin Orthop* 203:196, 1986.

49. Schlegel J, Yuan H, Fredrickson B: *Anterior interbody fixation devices,* In Frymoyer J, editor: *The adult spine,* New York, 1991, Raven Press, 1947.

50. Simmons EH, Sue-A-Quan EA, O'Leary PF, Garside HJ: An analysis of Dwyer instrumentation of the spine with assessment of its place in spinal surgery, *J Bone Joint Surg* 59B:117, 1977.

51. Southwick WO, Robinson RA: Surgical approaches to the vertebral bodies in the cervical and lumbar regions, *J Bone Joint Surg* 39A:631, 1957.

52. Speed K: Spondylolisthesis, *Arch Surg* 37:175, 1938.

53. Starr JK, Hanley EN: Junctional burst fractures, *Spine* 17:551, 1992.

54. Stauffer RN, Coventry MB: Anterior interbody lumbar spine fusion, *J Bone Joint Surg* 54A:756, 1972.

55. Watkins RG: *Surgical approaches to the spine,* New York, 1983, Springer-Verlag.

56. Werlinich M: Anterior interbody fusion and stabilization with metal fixation, *Int Surg* 59:269, 1974.

57. Whitesides TE Jr: Traumatic kyphosis of the thoracolumbar spine, *Clin Orthop* 128:78, 1977.

58. Willen J, Lindahl S, Irstam L, Nordwell A: Unstable thoracolumbar fractures, *Spine* 9:214, 1984.

59. Yuan HA, Mann KA, Found EM, et al.: Early clinical experience with the Syracuse I-plate: an anterior spinal fixation device, *Spine* 13:278, 1988.

Chapter 90
Lumbar Pathoanatomy: Soft- and Hard-Tissue Decompression
Charles D. Ray

Concepts and Indications

guiding principles in tissue resections
the inaccessible zone
planning the approach, making the incision
dissection and decompression
the poor man's laser
bone cutters
impaction

Working Inside the Inaccessible Zone

Paralateral Approach

Arthroscopic/Laparoscopic Techniques and Stereotaxia

Concepts and Indications

Guiding Principles in Tissue Resections

The decompression of soft tissue in the lumbar spine clearly involves the removal of hard tissues as well. Because of the protective nature of bone overlying nerve, dura, and other soft structures, one must open a door or a window before going through to the target. The key element here is an appropriate approach guided by anatomic structures (especially bony ones), in order to identify target lesions in their locations relative to that bone. Although the major goal in all such dissections is to relieve the offending lesion, the other equally important goals are the prevention of injury in the process of the dissection or resection and the prevention of future problems that might be caused by excessive destruction of the bone, ligaments, and other supporting elements.*

Lumbar decompressions involving a significant removal of bone, especially in patients with large herniations or those requiring a detailed exploration for any soft-tissue lesion, a central or lateral stenosis generally run risks that might well result in destabilization of the segment. Destabilization may occur in the process of the exposure itself but is more likely to occur during the exploration. Extensive decompressions performed from the posterior midline approach are sometimes deceptively easy to perform; one may get carried away with the clarity of exposed anatomy, but a significant number of these patients may have immediate or delayed postoperative instability. Although inadvertent loss of stability is unusual in most spine surgery, it can have significant and debilitating results. Instability is highly unlikely in patients who have advanced autostabilization from collapsed or highly degenerated disc spaces, so one must be more careful when the exposure is large and the bone is soft in patients who also have open, flexible disc spaces.

For the purposes of this chapter, instability may be defined as a painful, disabling, motion-related (usually micro motion) disorder of one or more vertebral segments resulting from a loss of the mechanical integrity of stabilizing structural components of that segment. Very often there is a combined loss of several stabilizing components producing the instability; these may include a mixture of facet joints, dorsal spinous processes or interspinous ligaments, a pedicle, a pars interarticularis, or the disc anulus. Painless, nondisabling, or otherwise asymptomatic loss of mechanical integrity is excluded from this consideration.

It has been pointed out by David Selby, at Dallas Spine Institute, (personal communication) that all surgical procedures should have the following characteristics:

1. Good anatomic dissection, good hemostasis, adequate exposure.
2. Gentle handling of the tissues.
3. Good instrumentation to shorten the procedure and achieve good results.
4. Versatility in surgical approaches as required by the pathology, including the consideration for possible instability.
5. Meticulous postoperative care with early, well-planned rehabilitation.

Further, good imaging studies are necessary to determine the anatomic condition and in planning the approach.[6,7,10] Films from these imaging studies should be present in the operating room and frequently referred to during the course of the procedure. Variations on an approach should be made if they permit a better exposure of the target lesion with less destruction of the supporting tissues. The operating physician should have a good understanding of anatomy, biomechanics and clinical results and how they interact.

Inherently, bone is a very fibrous, hard tissue, having a distinct "grain structure." The surgeon should be acquainted with the planes of the grain structures native to each bony part and base his or her dissection on them with preservation of structures. In a real sense, bone behaves as wood and a good carpenter or cabinetmaker would probably make a very good bone-removal surgeon. Destruction of more than one third of the facet joint (usually most of the medial aspect of a facet), for example, may often predispose the joint to ultimate fracture with instability, or rarely, a facet joint that "locks" in hyperflexion or rotation. Ordinarily, the soft-tissue components of a facet capsule regenerate rather quickly if lacerated, showing rapid restitution of the synovial lubricant function and no instability.

The Inaccessible Zone

The majority of nerve entrapments occur in the vicinity of the pedicle, ventral to the facet and lamina. Because of the bony protective covering of the nerve root and ganglion they are indeed inaccessible.[18] The preganglionic root sleeve begins to form at the medial aspect of the pedicle, almost encircling it to pass caudally or inferiorly to the pedicle like a

*References 6, 7, 9, 13, 15, 16, and 18.

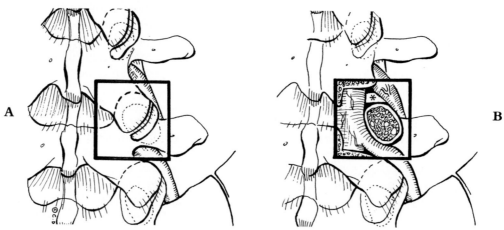

Fig. 90-1

The "inaccessible zone." **A,** Inside boxed area, right lumbar 4 level, lies zone, centered around pedicle. Most lesions of lumbar spine are found beneath (ventral to) laminas here. **B,** Facet joint and laminas have been removed in boxed area of **A.** Beneath are shown L4 and L5 roots and relationship of each to base of pedicle. Disc at L4-L5 is indicated at asterisk. Illustration is only for clarification of anatomy; surgical decompression to this extent would likely produce some degree of instability, probably torsional.

rope passing around a pulley (Fig. 90-1). The four sides of the upper part or true neural foramen consist of the pedicle of that segment, cephalad; the pedicle of the segment below, caudad; the facet joint, dorsally; and the vertebral body, ventrally (Fig. 90-2). After emergence from the foramen, the nerve once again may be vulnerable to compression or entrapment, but at very few locations. If a lesion is lateral or distal to the ganglion (such as with the far lateral herniation disc or a lateral stenosis), plain films or myelograms are usually of no value. Depending on whether the offending lesion is principally bony or soft tissue in type, the CT or MRI scan will usually reveal and define the lesion and its relationship to the bony anatomy. Inside the boxed area shown in Fig. 90-1, is the "inaccessible zone." Most lesions of the lumbar spine are found within this region, ventral to the facet joint and medial, or caudad (rarely, cephalad) to the pedicle. Relatively easy access to the lesion is obtained by taking off the bone within this boxed area, but this is the very area where such destruction may well lead to segmental instability, especially if the disc space of that segment is open and movable.

Planning the Approach, Making the Incision

In many decompressions, particularly the more limited ones such as a microdiscectomy, the skin overlying the target may be marked with a tissue dye injected under fluoroscopic control, prior to the patient's arriving at the operating room. Such a

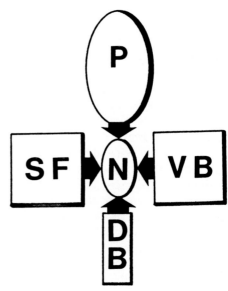

Fig. 90-2

Components of normal lateral neural foramen. Walls are composed of pedicle *(P),* superior facet *(SF),* vertebral body *(VB),* and in case of most common foraminal stenosis, disc bar (or uncinate spur) *(DB).* Nerve *(N)* may be held hostage by diametrically opposing members of this diagram.

marking injection may consist of Lymphazurin 1% (isosulfan blue for lymphography, 0.3 ml) injected into both the deeper structures (such as down to the dorsal tip of the target spinous process and the adjacent interspinous ligament) and the overlying dermis. This gives a double reference (superficial and deep) before and during the initial incision and dissection. (Note that in obese patients, this skin marking usually is pulled down almost one segment by the patient being operated on in a kneeling position.) The radiologist who performs the marking injection should be keenly aware of the number of movable segments, the presence of congenital anomalies, and whatever else might be misunderstood between the apparent radiologic anatomy and the location of the actual lesion underneath. An order or a diagram from the surgeon directing the radiologist to the level and location of the injection should be written in the patient's chart. The length of the skin incision is determined largely by the number of spinal segments to be operated on plus some additional length dictated by the depth to the target, the flexibility of overlying tissues, the difficulty of the procedure, and the anticipated extent of the lateral dissection.[9]

One should remember that the cosmetic appearance of the final wound is quite dependent on the initial incision and the method used for closing the skin, with some dependency on the method of retraction and the technique of dealing with superficial bleeding. Once the extent of the incision is marked on the skin, or on the overlying protective plastic drape (if used), a long straight-edged device such as an osteotome is laid on the skin, spanning the limit marks of the incision, and a large scalpel blade is used to cut along the straight edge. This makes a neat, singular incision with a cut perpendicular to the skin. Such an incision is not only easier to close but is less likely to be overlapped during suturing, and definitely has a better cosmetic appearance than most free-hand incisions. One may coagulate just below the epidermis with an electrosurgical tip (or a bipolar coagulator tip), being careful not to burn the dermis itself. Just below the surface of the skin, one may also obtain an acceptable, small, fat or fat and paratenon graft for use in covering exposed dura of nerve (see Chapter 65 on grafts used in covering neural tissues to prevent fibrosis).

If a patient has recently taken aspirin (which has a long-term effect, e.g., over the lifetime of platelets, in altering their "stickiness" to internal vascular walls) or a nonsteroidal antiinflammatory medication (having a shorter-lived effect on anticoagulation), the tissues may continue to ooze. Generally, however, the application of stable retraction will stop this. By sweeping away the dorsal fascial fibers near the midline, one can see the unique crisscrossing of these fibers just dorsal to the interspinous ligaments and processes. This crossing occurs at the exact midline. The dorsal fascia is cut close on one or both sides of each spinous process, as needed, at the target levels. This cutting is best performed with the use of a

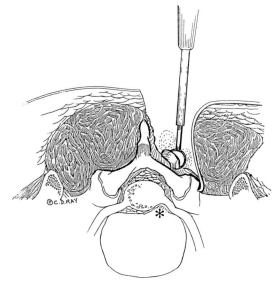

Fig. 90-3

Diagram of cross section at L5-S1 level during process of reoperation, long after wound healing and scar formation. Hot wire RF cutting loop (attached to standard ES coagulation-cutting knife handle) is shown dissecting flap or slab of scar tissue away from dorsal surface of lamina and facet capsule. Smoke that evolves is suctioned away. Bleeding vessels can also be coagulated with the same loop. An ES knife handle with built-in, finger-operated switches is preferred. Loop is attached to long extension. Herniated disc is shown at asterisk; it displaces and entraps emerging root. Unilateral exposure is held open using two-toothed Raylor (malleable, Taylor-like) retractor passed lateral to facet joint and pedicle.

hot cautery tip or a circular wire loop that cuts the tissue is a fashion similar, large to a laser, that is, with little or no eschar formation (Fig. 90-3).

Stripping of the muscle away from the midline (which gives the procedure the name of "subperiosteal dissection") is best performed using a broad-bladed Cobb or similar dissector. The muscle stripping is both from the spinous processes and the laminas, out to the facets. In the case of the patients who have had prior surgery, this stripping may be more difficult because of fibrous adhesions. This retrolaminar scar tissue is also very well dissected or removed with the hot wire loop technique shown in Fig. 90-3.

Dissection and Decompression

In general the important elements to consider in performing a spinal decompression are (1) removal of pressure from the neural element, (2) maintenance of the stability of the spinal segment, (3) avoidance of injury, and (4) prevention of future problems.

The attachment of soft tissues to bone can present difficulties in dissection, or the "freeing up" of

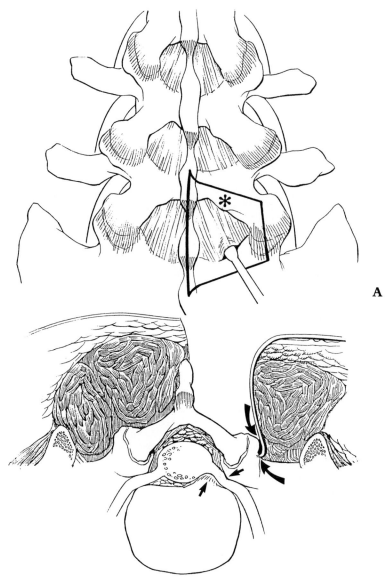

Fig. 90-4

A, Diagrams of a limited exposure laminotomy (essentially a microdiscectomy) at L5 to S1 space. A 2-cm wide Taylor-like retractor has been placed lateral to facet joint *(curved arrows)*. Lateral herniation and facet joint *(small arrows)* mutually compromise emerging ganglion. Small but adequate window of access *(asterisk)* is indicated by outlined area.

structures. The detachment of ligamentum flavum, scar tissue, or anulus from bony insertions or attachments can be trying, even resulting in possible injury or tears in root sleeves or the dura. These complications can occur regardless of the technique employed, i.e., dull or sharp dissection. Instruments with sharp edges may inadvertently cut nerve sheath or dura. Generally, the best instruments for dissection of tissue (especially fibrosis or scar) from bone are small curettes. Next in line are blunt dissectors (which actually bluntly strip tissue from bone); blunt

dissection, however, does not always work, particularly when the adhesions are dense (Fig. 90-4). Unusual, but very practical instruments for such dissection are up-or down-cutting osteophyte elevators (Surgical Dynamics, Inc., Concord, CA). These tools resemble right-angled, elongated blunt dissectors but are half-round in cross-section, that is, on the down-cutting type where the flat surface is faced ventrally, away from the handle; the device resembles a human leg and narrow foot wearing a flat-soled shoe. The rounded upper surface faces the dura while the

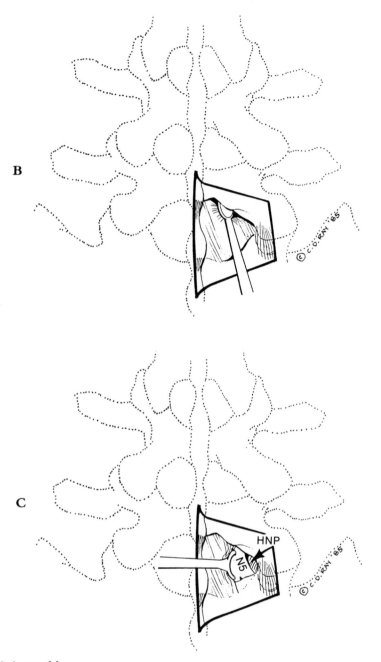

Fig. 90-4, cont'd

B, Through small access superior attachment of ligamentum is dissected free from ventral surface of L5 lamina using curette, cutting edge facing dorsally. **C,** Laterally freed ligamentum is retracted medially revealing displaced, tightened L5 nerve root *(N5)*. Herniated disc *(HNP)* is now becoming visible. Small medial facetectomy is made to give exposure further lateral to root.   *Continued.*

sharp flat surface faces the dorsum of the vertebral body or anulus. This dissector can be pressed against an old adherent disc bar, for example, and by a sweeping, rotary dissection it will cut the adherent disc scar away from the dorsally overlying dura. The up-cutting type has its flat surface facing dorsally toward the handle, on top of the foot; thus it should, for example, be placed between the lamina and the attached, underlying ligamentum flavum. With the flat cutting surface facing upward against the underside of the overlying laminar bone and rotating this edge in a circular sweep, the up-cutting elevator can be used to dissect the ligamentum safely away from the lamina.

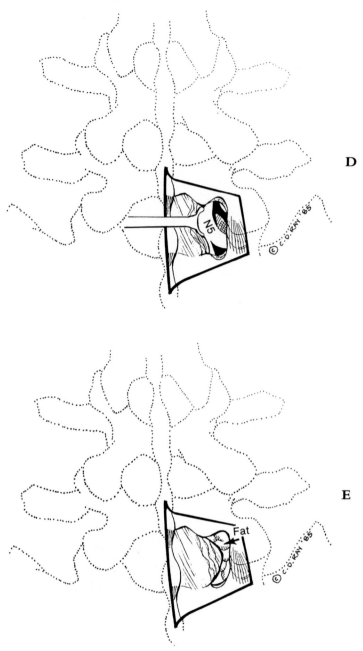

Fig. 90-4, cont'd

D, Small laminotomies, inferior L5 and superior S1, together with medial facetectomy, usually provide excellent visualization and root mobility. Ligamentum remains largely attached. Herniation is now removed. **E,** Ligamentum is again laid over exposed dura; it has retracted since its elastic fibers (comprising about 80% of its bulk) shorten when detached from bone. A small fat or fat/fascia graft (about 5 ml) is placed near or around exposed nerve sleeve; a larger additional free graft (10 to 20 ml) will be placed over laminotomy site and wound closed.

The Poor Man's Laser

Soft-tissue dissection and resection using an electrosurgical-radiofrequency (RF) current applied to the tip of a switch-controlled cutting blade attached to insulated handles is an excellent means for quick dissection through most soft tissues.[1,15] This method is especially valuable for debulking scars and for clean removal of tissue attached to bone as shown in Fig. 90-3. For such a purpose, the electroknife hot loop is more useful than is a narrow vaporizing beam from a laser unit. This electrosurgical dissection uses an 8-mm or smaller loop of stiff, high-temperature wire (as is often applied in neurosurgery for the resection of meningiomas). The thin wire loop operates at very high RF current (75% of maximum or more) from a standard electrosurgical generator, and thus has a very high current density along its surface. The temperature at that junction rises very high and very rapidly, although with a low heat mass. The frequency of the current (about 1 MHz) produces relatively little stimulation of muscle or nerve. As the current flows at the tissue-wire interface, there is rapid boiling and desiccation; the tissue simply evaporates apart, also giving the surface a self-cleaning effect. Thus, tissue is cut but not particularly burned, similarly to cutting with a laser beam. However, if allowed to remain stationary for any length of time, the cutting tip will char the tissue and stick to it.

With experience and caution, the electrosurgical hot loop can uniquely and easily clean connective tissue and much of the attachment of ligaments from spinous processes, the dorsal surface of laminas, and elsewhere adjacent to bone. For example, using extreme caution not to injure nerve or cut the dura nearby, the ragged anulus within the disc space can be cut free from its attachment to the end plates. In doing this, there may be some stimulation of posterior primary nerves causing the back to jump slightly, but even in the locally anesthetized patient, this has no undesirable or persistent effect. The technique compares well histologically with laser cutting of soft tissues, that is, the depth of the eschar and the changes in the cut tissue appear almost identical with these two methods.[2,3] I therefore refer to the hot loop as "a poor man's laser." With variously shaped hot-cutting loops, many of the popular laser cutting techniques in use today may be replaced by the RF method and are now being studied. Most spine surgeons will be pleased with the success in tissue incision or removal coming from this method. Cutting through fat (a poorly conductive tissue due to its low water and salt content) is not as successful with a hot loop, however.

One interesting potential complication arising from the use of the hot loop may come from the smoke generated by the cutting action. Similar to the effect of laser cutting, the smoke and accompanying water and tissue vapors (smoke plume) billowing from the cut tissue may contain live viruses. This potential has been documented in surgeons using laser cutting who contracted human papillomavirus by way of their nasopharynx by inhaling the laser plume. Therefore, when using hot-loop or laser-beam cutting, the surgeon and assistants should continuously suction out the plume and wear a laser particle surgical face mask as a precaution.

Bone Cutters

The cutting of bone remains the domain of rongeurs, punches, shears, sharp osteotomes, curettes, reciprocating saws, rasps, files, or high-speed rotary, electric drills or gas turbines (with a precaution regarding noise in the surgeon's or patient's ears).[17] The cutting and removal of bone are essential elements during soft-tissue dissection or decompressions, since the bone acts as a supporting and organizing structure to house and protect vascular and neurologic elements and often to provide a support for their circulatory supply. At present, the major mechanical methods indicated above remain the techniques of choice for bone removal. I personally prefer small osteotomes and chisels (as narrow as 2 mm wide, with or without curved tips) as the most useful instruments for cutting small areas of bone such as osteophytes or portions of facets, spurs or pedicles. Indeed, a sharp osteotome approximately 4 mm wide can well be used during virtually all of a standard laminotomy or laminectomy procedure. Again, one must be familiar with the "grain" of the bone when making cuts, to prevent inadvertent fracturing or undesirable splitting of the bone. Time would be well spent by the spine surgeon in experimenting with the cutting of highly grained wood using surgical instruments, for example, osteotomes or high-speed turbines, to gain an appreciation for the laminar grain structure of living bone.

Unfortunately, the laser is not appropriate for cutting bone since a so-called rapid super pulse technique is required.[4] In such cases, the energy is so high that there is a great danger of overpenetration of both bone and underlying soft tissue; that is, laser energy cannot be easily contained once it passes through bone. The development of a superpressure (approximately 3700 atmospheres), very-fine-water-stream cutter has been reported to cut bone well, but has yet to be practically applied.[8] A sonic curette, axially vibrated by a magnetostrictive or piezoelectric generator, operating at about 25 kHZ to reduce the frictional interface of the cutting tip, has been reported, but one finds that a dull sonic curette cuts bone no better than an ordinary dull bone curette; thus, the continued sharpness of the cutting edges is still the critical element.

Optical magnification (by eyeglass-mounted telescopes, by "loupes" or via a surgical microscope), provides a distinct advantage for the deep dissection

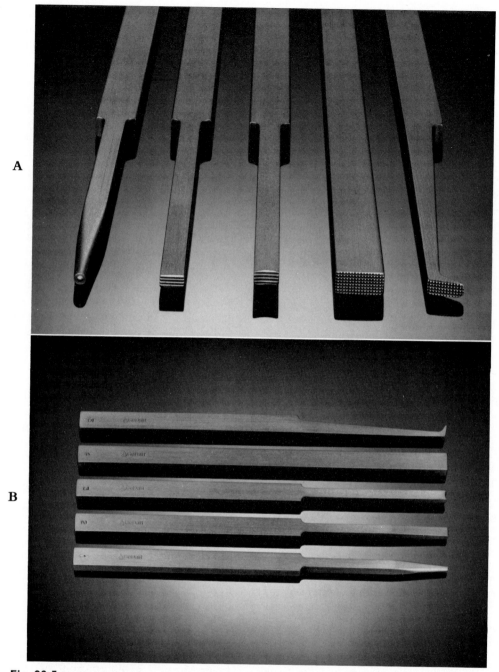

Fig. 90-5

Bone impactor instruments for decompression of offending bony excrescences, disc bars, or osteophytes. **A,** Full-length view of impactors; overall length is 25 cm. **B,** Close-up view of tips of impactors showing small rounded, small rectangular, and curved tip (to fit contour of pedicle), large rectangular, and footed types. Note that all have nonslip knurling on the bone-striking surfaces to prevent slippage when impacting bone. Large rectangular impactor is also used to drive bone fusion dowels and bone chip tamper for fusions. Toe of footed impactor is passed beneath (ventral to) dura or entrapped ganglion to decompress by impaction of osteophyte. (See also Fig. 90-6, *B.*)

and tissue removal often demanded in spine surgery. Coaxial fiber optic illumination, used in conjunction with the eyeglass-fitted optical magnifying telescope also provides an important improvement in the deep visualization of these tissues.

Impaction

On occasion, cortical bone or hyperostotic spurs may be resected away from their tight grip on neural structures by the method of impaction. Thus, spurs,

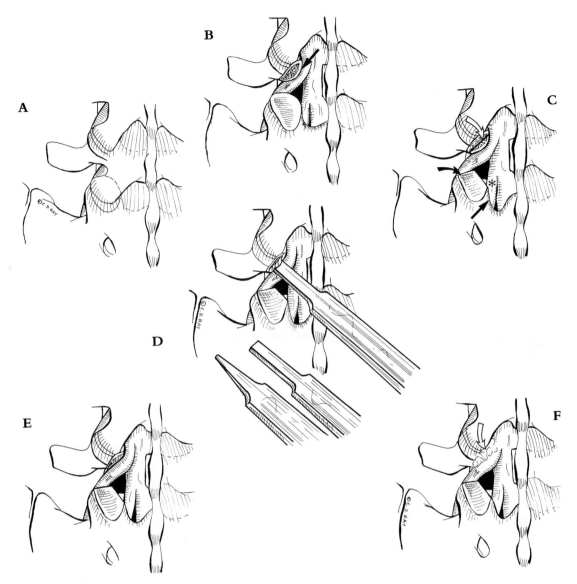

Fig. 90-6

Impaction for decompression of inferior pedicle. **A,** Exposure of left-sided L4-L5 and L5-S1 is diagrammed. **B,** Full left hemilaminectomy has been performed, showing tight situation of L5 nerve as it passes around its pedicle *(arrow),* somewhat as rope would pass around a pulley. Exposures are ordinarily not this extensive. Disc space should have been found to be quite stable so that total facetectomy will not destabilize segment. **C,** Tip of superior facet *(curved black arrow)* at S1 has been cut. Inferior pedicle *(open white arrow)* has been cut across (slotted) with osteotome. S1 root passing over L5-S1 disc margin is indicated by asterisk. (If subarticular stenosis of L5-S1 were present, location of appropriate decompression would be indicated by straight black arrow.) **D,** Impactor, shaped to fit inferior curve of pedicle, is tapped with nylon mallet, aiming upward and laterally, driving cortical portion of pedicle away from root, allowing it to relax. Root is carefully protected from possible pinching by impactor as it is struck. Two other types of impactors (see Fig. 90-4) are also shown. (Also see chapter 16.) **E,** Root is now relaxed as it passes around impacted pedicle. If need be, more of pedicle can be resected and impacted. Exposure is often sufficient to permit exploration and impaction of possible disc spur or bar at L5-S1 level. **F,** Small fat graft has been placed between impacted pedicle and L5 root/ganglion.

ridges, or bars of soft or medium hardness bone may be reduced in prominence by driving them into the underlying bone.[11] Impaction devices of several shapes may be used depending on need within the central canal, along the neural path through a foramen or laterally (Figs. 90-5 and 90-6). Particularly valuable is the footed impactor, which can be placed ventrally to extend underneath a root or ganglion and used to crush a small bony prominence out of harm's way. When the bony element is hard

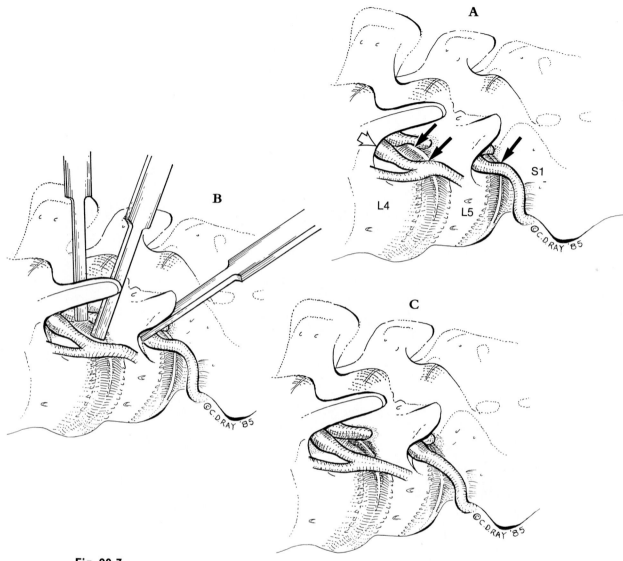

Fig. 90-7

Lateral approach to impaction of pedicles and disc bars or spurs. Shown are left side of vertebral bodies at the L4, L5, and S1 levels. **A,** Tight pedicle situation, as shown in Fig. 90-5, is indicated by open arrow at L4. Similar compression is located at L5 but not indicated with an arrow. Disc bars and spurs are indicated by solid arrows, covered with annular fibers so that they appear as smooth mounds elevating spinal nerves, L4 and L5. **B,** Impactors being used to decompress nerves by driving spur or bar into vertebral body. Impaction of inferior aspect of pedicle of L5 is shown; this has already been done at L4 in this diagram. A footed impactor (Fig. 90-4) is particularly useful for impacting spurs beneath the dura, ventral to a ganglion or a spur inside a foramen. **C,** Postimpaction situation showing relaxed position of L4 and L5 nerves as they now pass over impacted bony ridges, caudad to impacted pedicles.

or brittle, fragmentation may occur during impaction; the loose fragments should all be removed. In some cases of lateral stenosis, parts of the inferior surface of a pedicle may have to be similarly resected. This can be performed by cutting into the body of the pedicle with a narrow osteotome and forcing or impacting the cortical portion inward, into the central cancellous portion of the pedicle (see Fig. 90-6).

Via a lateral laminotomy, impaction of a lateral uncinate spur or discal bar may be performed (Fig. 90-7).

Working Inside the Inaccessible Zone

It can indeed be a technical challenge to reach and work effectively within the inaccessible zone with-

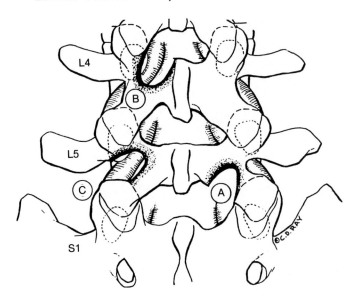

Fig. 90-8

Typical laminotomies and their primary applications. **A,** Inferior laminotomy (most common, for removal of HNP). **B,** Superior laminotomy (used in decompressions for subarticular stenosis but useful in certain cases of lateral stenosis to achieve good access to inferior medial aspect of pedicle). **C,** Lateral laminotomy (used for lateral stenoses and offending lateral osteophytes). I refer to this as a midline paramedial approach. After exposure is made to osteophyte, a bone impactor is usually used in decompression.

out excessive bone removal. A laminotomy (possibly a laminectomy) may need to be enlarged as needed to gain adequate access to the underlying soft tissues without having to apply undue traction on the nerve or dura. The major types of laminotomies useful for "windowing" the bone to approach underlying lesions are shown in Fig. 90-8. Inferior laminotomy, the most commonly used procedure for removal of a herniated disc, allows limited lateral access to stenotic spurs unless significant undercutting of the facet is performed. By the superior laminotomy approach, decompressions for subarticular or central recess stenosis are best achieved. However, for decompression of lateral stenosis, lateral herniations and for resection of certain lateral spurs, the lateral laminotomy is often the best approach. This is particularly true at the L3-4 level and above. One must be careful not to remove too much of the lamina by any of these three approaches, otherwise a laminar or pars fracture may occur during the procedure or later. Instruments for the impaction or disruption of bone spurs may be used in conjunction with any of these approaches in order to decompress bony prominence that may compress the nerve or dura from their ventral aspect.

Although there is some controversy, it appears important to preserve the interspinous ligament to maintain a greater degree of flexion-stability of the posterior segmental structures. As a potential ad-junct, the ligamentum flavum may be detached from its origin beneath the upper lamina and its insertion dorsal on the lamina caudally and detached laterally at the facet, thus being preserved almost in toto. This flap of ligamentum is retracted medically during the procedure and is restored to its initial position, later. When the ligamentum is allowed to fall back into position, after the decompression, it acts as an excellent, even though partial, cover for the exposed dura, and will generally reattach to its original bony insertions. The potential use of autologous fat or other dural covering agents is discussed in the chapter on grafts and other barriers to fibrous ingrowth.

Paralateral Approach

If one carefully examines a full-body CT scan section at a level above the crest of the ilium, one can draw a line of approach to the target lesion from the skin surface, along the line of best intermuscular tissue dissection down to the lateral aspect of the targeted foramen. This line begins about 12 to 15 cm lateral to the midline and passes through the septum between the two paraspinal erector muscles (iliocostalis and longissimus) to define the paralateral approach.[12,14] This differs from the paraspinal approach described by Leon Wiltse and his colleagues; they use a midline skin incision, but deep in the sub-

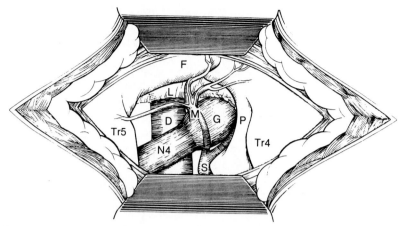

Fig. 90-9

Diagram of paralateral approach, right L4-L5 level. L4 to L5 disc margin (*D*); superior facet of L5 (*F*); ganglion of L4 (*G*); ligamentum flavum (*L*); neurovascular medusa of L4 posterior primary nerve branch (*M*); L4 nerve (*N4*); pedicle of L4 (*P*); segmental artery (*S*); and the transverse processes of L4 (*Tr4*) and L5 (*Tr5.*)

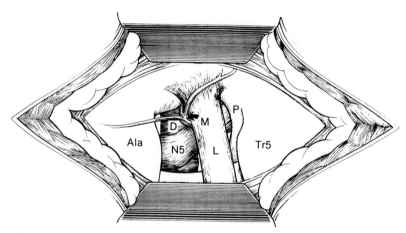

Fig. 90-10

Diagram of approach to the right L5-S1 space. L5 nerve (*N5*) and ganglion are trapped between lateral disc bar (*D*) or spur and an iliolumbar ligament (*L*.) Posterior primary neurovascular bundle, or medusa (*M*), is displaced caudad around ligament. Also indicated are pedicle (*P*) and transverse process of L5 (*Tr5*) and sacral ala.

cutaneous region the dissection is carried laterally between the longissimus and multifidus muscles.[19] Thus, their approach path is parallel to the midline in a plane roughly over the lateral edge of the facet joint. The paralateral approach is considerably further lateral. In Figs. 90-9 and 90-10 a paralateral approach at the L5-S1 disc level is shown. (Also see Chapter 80 on lateral stenosis.) This procedure works much better for lesions found lateral to the disc margin at L3-L4 or L4-L5. Localization of the target is facilitated by an injection of marking dye into the skin overlying the tip of the transverse process of the target vertebra, thus indicating the lower aspect of the approach. That is, L5 for an L4-L5 approach, and L4 for an L3-L4 approach.

A small, slightly J-shaped incision of perhaps 5 or 6 cm length is positioned near the palpable deep muscle margin, between 10 and 16 cm from the midline (Fig. 90-11). On reaching the lateral fascia, it is divided with an electrosurgical knife; one then inserts an exploring finger to identify the tip of the transverse process. The two transverse processes defining the segment should be palpated and the anteroposterior lumbar preoperative plane film consulted to check on the agreement between the x-ray anatomy and the palpable structures. Other

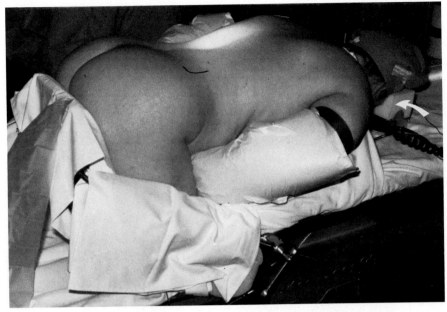

Fig. 90-11

Prone-sitting frame of author's design used for paralateral and other lumbar spinal surgical cases. Patient is face down on special forehead/chin rest *(white arrow)*, adjustable to permit normal lordosis of the neck. Paralateral incision is indicated.

anatomic details may be compared with the scans as well. Should there remain some uncertainty, a marking needle is inserted through the dorsum of the skin and directed perpendicularly down to either of these transverse process. A cross-table lateral x-ray film is then made.

Retraction for deep visualization may be difficult but is most important. Small Hibbs-like retractors using an upward pull are particularly helpful in this lateral exposure. The dissection at the target space then begins at the superior edge of the inferior transverse process near the location of the disc, close to where the postganglionic nerve emerges from the foramen (through the lateral curtain of the ligamentum flavum). A small portion of the ventral aspect of the facet may be removed with a punch. The ganglion is dissected free, to clarify the lateral anatomy. The intended dissection and decompression are then performed.

With good retraction, the paralateral approach permits a good view of foraminal and postforaminal anatomy. A very far lateral herniated disc can be well decompressed via this approach (Fig. 90-12). Far lateral stenoses or herniations may also be approached by this method, provided that the lesion does not extend medial to the pedicle.[5] Nevertheless, paralateral procedures especially for stenotic decompressions may be particularly challenging initially because of the relative strangeness of this deep

anatomy, the limited exposure, and the fact that few, if any, bony landmarks are visualized. Closed drainage is generally used for 2 days because the lateral tissue spaces are filled only with muscle and fat, with an absence of tough ligaments or muscular compartments as are found in midline approaches to the lumbar spine.

Arthroscopic/Laparoscopic Techniques and Stereotaxia

The use of guiding tubes to provide a protected access to a surgical target, as in knee or abdominal laparoscopy, is already well established in spinal surgery, primarily for discectomies. Such discectomies have employed remotely operated disc tissue cutters, aspirators, grabbing tools (similar to bronchial or lung biopsy instruments), and laser desiccation beams. In some cases, the cutting or dissecting or desiccating instruments are inserted in one side and the visualizing optical fiber bundle in the other side of the disc space (biportal approach). Since there is no clear correlation between the mass of disc tissue removed and clinical result, further analysis of large groups of patients will need to be performed via each technique in order to determine relative efficacy and safety. Many cases of arthroscopic intradiscal "fusions" have been reported but are not

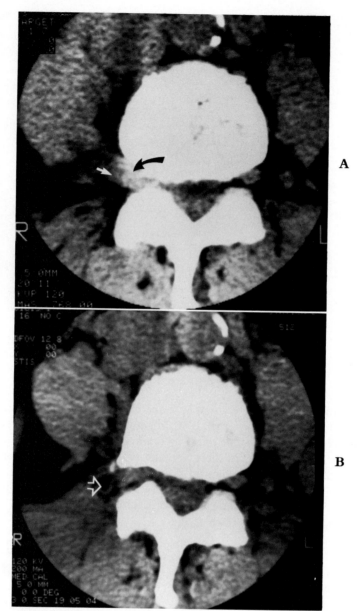

Fig. 90-12

A, Preoperative and **B,** postoperative CT scans of far lateral extruded disc *(long arrow)* at right L4-L5 space elevating and compressing nerve *(short arrow)*. Small fat graft is indicated *(open arrow)*.

as yet validated. If the graft bone is packed inside a tubular device, such as a threaded person cage, laparoscopic implantation and fusion will become a reality. (See chapter on the threaded fusion cage.)

It is anticipated that true spinal stereotaxia will develop in the near future so that through very small apertures (similar to the laparoscopic techniques) a variety of procedures may be performed, probably under fluoroscopic or ultrasonic imaging guidance. Robotics will ultimately be coupled with such procedures, performing them with greater control and finesse than

can be done by human operators alone. Lateral lesions in particular may thus be approached with very minimal dissection, a very short hospitalization (outpatient day surgery), and a quick return to work. Micro methods of tissue dissection, resection, stabilization, and insertion of ancillary devices (such as an artificial disc, prosthetic nucleus, or restorative medications) are currently being developed to address lesions involving both hard and soft tissues. Intraspinal laparoscopic visualization and certain limited procedures, primarily neurosurgical, are now being reported.

References

1. Arnaud JP, Adloff M: Electrosurgery and wound healing: an experimental study in rats, *Eur Surg Res* 12:439, 1980.

2. Bellina JH, et al.: Carbon dioxide laser and electrosurgical wound study with an animal model: a comparison of tissue damage and healing patterns in peritoneal tissue, *Am J Obstet Gynecol* 148:327, 1984.

3. Castro DJ, et al.: Wound healing: biological effects of Nd:YAG laser on collagen metabolism in pig skin in comparison to thermal burn, *Ann Plast Surg* 11:131, 1983.

4. Clayman L, et al.: Healing of continuous wave and rapid super pulsed carbon dioxide laser-induced bone defects, *J Oral Surg* 36:932, 1978.

5. Godersky JC, et al.: Extreme lateral disc herniation: diagnosis by computed tomographic scanning, *Neurosurgery* 14:549, 1984.

6. Heithoff KB, Ray CD: Principles of the computed tomographic assessment of lateral spinal stenosis. In Genant HK, et al., editors: *Spine update* 1987, San Francisco, 1987, Radiology Research and Education Foundation, p 191.

7. Heithoff KB, Ray CD, Schellhas KP, Fritts HM: CT and MRI of lateral entrapment syndromes. In Genant HK, et al., editors: *Spine update* 1987, San Francisco, 1987, Radiology Research and Education Foundation, p 203.

8. Helwig D: 55,000-psi water jet cuts better than steel, *Pop Sci* 226:76, 1985.

9. Morris JM: Surgical management of lumbar disc disease. In Genant HK, et al., editors: *Spine update* 1987, San Francisco, 1987, Radiology Research and Education Foundation.

10. Ray CD, Heithoff KB: Techniques for decompression of lumbar spinal stenosis "guided" by high-resolution CT scans, *Mod Neurosurg* 1:31, 1982.

11. Ray CD: Bone impactors: new instruments for spinal decompression, *Spine* 11:1051, 1986.

12. Ray CD: *The paralateral approach to decompression for lateral stenosis and far lateral lesions of the lumbar spine.* In Watkins RG, Collis JS Jr, editors: *Lumbar discectomy and laminectomy,* Rockville, MD, 1987, Aspen Publishers, Inc., p 418.

13. Ray CD: *Extensive lumbar decompression: patient selection and results.* In White AH, Rothman RH, Ray CD, editors: *Lumbar spine surgery: techniques and complications,* St. Louis, 1987, Mosby, p 164.

14. Ray CD: *Far lateral decompressions for stenosis: the paralateral approach to the lumbar spine.* In White AH, Rothman RH, Ray CD, editors: *Lumbar spine surgery: techniques and complications.* St. Louis, 1987, Mosby, p 175.

15. Ray CD: *Methods of tissue dissection and resection in lumbar surgery.* In White AH, Rothman RH, Ray CD, editors: *Lumbar spine surgery: techniques and complications,* St. Louis, 1987, Mosby, p 208.

16. Ray CD: *Decompression of lumbar osteophytes, spurs and bony encroachment.* In White AH, Rothman RH, Ray CD, editors: *Lumbar spine surgery: techniques and complications,* St. Louis, 1987, Mosby, p 230.

17. Ray CD, Levinson R: Noise pollution in the operating room: a hazard to surgeons, personnel and patients, *J Spinal Disord* 5:485, 1992.

18. Ray CD: *Decompressions and the "inaccessible zone."* In Hardy RW Jr, editor: *Lumbar disc disease,* ed 2, New York, 1992, Raven Press, pp 123–137.

19. Wiltse LL, et al.: The paraspinal sacrospinalis-splitting approach to the lumbar spine, *J Bone Joint Surg* 50A:919, 1968.

Chapter 91
Degenerative Spondylolisthesis
Paul J. Slosar
James B. Reynolds

Prevalence and Etiology

Signs and Symptoms

Pathologic Process

Conservative Care

Radiology

Indications for Surgery

Operative Treatment

      selection of fusion levels
      instrumentation
      surgical techniques
      bone graft

**Degenerative Spondylolisthesis and
   Degenerative Scoliosis**

Summary

Degenerative spondylolisthesis is a forward slippage of one vertebra over the next as a result of degenerative changes in the intervertebral disc and/or articular facet joints. Junghanns[21] identified several cases of "pseudospondylolisthesis" among Schmorl's collection of cadaveric spines. He noted that facet arthrosis usually occurred at the fourth lumbar level and commented on an abnormal pedicle facet angle. Macnab[27] described the clinical entity as "spondylolisthesis with an intact neural arch." His recommendations for treatment are relevant today. Newman and Stone[29] objected to the name proposed by Macnab, since it is not the only form of spondylolisthesis with an intact arch. They proposed the currently accepted descriptive term, *degenerative spondylolisthesis.*

Prevalence and Etiology

Degenerative spondylolisthesis predominantly occurs in females (3:2) greater than 50 years of age, with the most frequent site of anterolisthesis at L4 over L5 (90%).[28,31]

Degenerative spondylolisthesis seldom exceeds a Grade 1, or 25% slip.[29,32] The forward slipping of the fourth lumbar vertebra ceases when the intact lamina and inferior articular facets of L4 come to rest against the body of L5. It has been observed that in degenerative spondylolisthesis an abnormal relationship exists between the L4-L5 disc space and the top of the pelvis.[10] Normally, the caudal quarter of the L4 vertebral body crosses the intercrestal line or horizontal plane formed by the superior aspect of the pelvic crests. In degenerative spondylolisthesis, the L4-L5 disc space is generally above this intercrestal line and assumes a horizontal position. With the disc being relatively out of the pelvis and oriented horizontally, added mechanical stress is placed on the L4-L5 level. A fourfold increased incidence of sacralization is observed in these patients, which further increases the stress to this vulnerable L4-L5 disc level.[31]

Facet joint orientation may predispose an individual to develop degenerative anterolisthesis.[1,29,33] Coronal orientation of the lumbosacral (L5-S1) articular processes confers a ventral-dorsal stability, while the more oblique or sagittally oriented facet joints of the L4-L5 articulation allow more relative anterior displacement. Sato and colleagues[33] reported that patients with degenerative spondylolisthesis were often found to have a relatively narrow inferior articular process. This narrow articulation may be a less effective check-reign mechanism for preventing the L4 vertebra from slipping forward on the L5 vertebra below.

Signs and Symptoms

The patient with degenerative spondylolisthesis often has a protracted history of low-grade back pain that is intermittently intense, but rarely causes severe disability. As the pathology progresses, the patient's symptoms evolve into neurogenic claudication and, more commonly, sciatica. This reflects the canal stenosis and nerve root compromise found surgically and radiographically.[9]

On physical examination these patients are quite flexible, usually able to touch the floor on forward bending with their knees locked. Most frequently, they do not have a neurologic abnormality, and straight-leg raising is usually negative.

Pathologic Process

Primary disc degeneration and an intact pars interarticularis differentiate degenerative from isthmic spondylolisthesis, in which a structural defect in the pars allows anterolisthesis of the anterior elements or body.

Degenerative spondylolisthesis is the result of a cascade of events that begins with degeneration of the intervertebral disc.[7] As discussed previously, the pars interarticularis remains intact as the superior vertebra migrates anteriorly.

As disc degeneration progresses, a predictable pattern of events is observed. Alteration in the facet articulation occurs as disc height is lost. Advanced degeneration of the malaligned facet joints with osteophyte formation and synovial hypertrophy predictably follows. Gradually, the L4-L5 facet joint remodels and hypertrophies as the vertebral body continues to slip forward. The inferior facet of the cephalic vertebra erodes through the superior articular process of the caudal vertebra as the slip progresses. Facet joint hypertrophy is the main cause of stenosis both in the central canal and neural foramina. Stenosis is also due to thickening of the facet capsule, ligamentum flavum, and posterior longitudinal ligament. As the disc collapses, the thickened ligamentum flavum becomes redundant, encroaching further on the stenotic canal. Closely related to this disc collapse is the development of foraminal stenosis. Narrowing of the superior-inferior dimensions of the foramina occurs with loss of disc-space height, as does foraminal narrowing in the anterior-posterior width as the anterolisthesis advances and

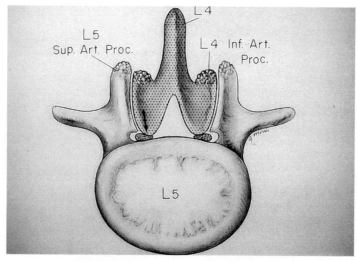

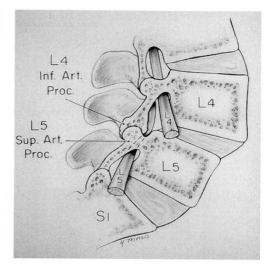

Fig. 91-1

Axial and sagittal views at the level of anterolisthesis. **A,** Note the sagitally oriented facet joints. **B,** The compression of the traversing L5 nerves by the subluxing L4 inferior articular processes. (From Wiltse LL, Kirkaldy-Willis WH, McIron GW: The treatment of spinal stenosis, *Clin Orthop* 115:83, 1976.)

the facet enlarges. A bulging anulus fibrosis can also be found buckling into the inferior portion of the foramina. The midline of the canal narrows as the lamina of L4 and hypertrophic ligamentum flavum slide toward the body of L5.[6,8,9] Compression of the cauda equina against the body of L5 may occur as the lamina and inferior articular process of L4 slide forward. The inferior articular process of L4 will frequently entrap the L5 nerve root in the lateral recess (Fig. 91-1, *A, B*).

An intraspinal synovial cyst originating from the facet joint can be a source of stenosis. These synovial cysts can occur in association with the hypertrophic degenerative changes at the facet joints, found in degenerative spondylolisthesis (Fig. 91-2, *A, B*). Treatment for isolated cysts includes aspiration, injection of corticosteroids, or rupturing the cyst with hydrostatic pressure via injection. If surgical intervention is indicated for the degenerative spondylolisthesis, then the synovial cyst may be excised at that time.

Conservative Care

As degenerative spondylolisthesis occurs in stages, each with its characteristic symptomatology and radiographic appearance, the treatment should be specific for the appropriate stage. Patients with minimal impairment and early stages of disc degeneration respond best to a physical therapy stabilization program. Rarely, lumbosacral corsets may help.

The intermediate stages with facet degeneration respond to nonsteroidal antiinflammatory medications, and in some cases, facet injections of corticosteroids or rarely facet rhizotomy.[4]

The advanced stages of degenerative spondylolisthesis with central canal, lateral recess, and foraminal stenosis may respond to epidural or selective nerve root injections. When the stenosis becomes severe, the effectiveness of epidurals may be reduced because of the difficulty in diffusion of the medication uniformly about the dura. If this occurs, patients may respond to selective nerve root injections.

Radiology

Routine standing anteroposterior, lateral, and oblique roentgenograms will establish certain criteria for the diagnosis of degenerative spondylolisthesis. It is imperative that these radiographs be taken in the standing position to axially load the spine and stress the slip (Fig. 91-3, *A, B, C*).[26] Associated, but not diagnostic, changes that may be seen on plain radiographs include hypertrophic changes in the zygoapophyseal joints, foraminal and disc-space narrowing, and characteristic impingement of the inferior articular process of L4 into the superior articular process of L5.

There are many ways to assess stability in degenerative spondylolisthesis. Comparison of the supine lateral radiographs or a lateral scout film of the patient's CT scan or MRI against the standing lateral

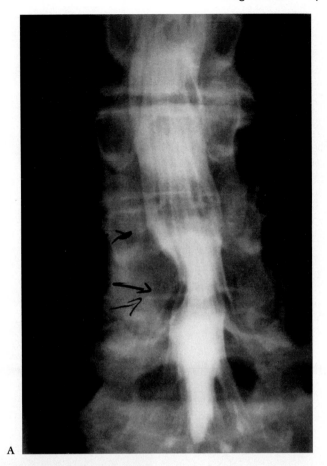

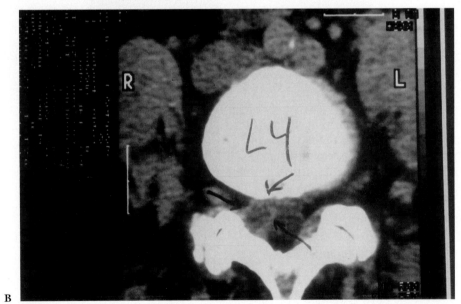

Fig. 91-2

Intraspinal synovial cyst demonstrated by myelogram and CT scan. **A,** Note the significant thecal sac impingment on myelogram. **B,** CT scan demonstrates a ballooning of the facet capsule with cystic degeneration of the facet joint.

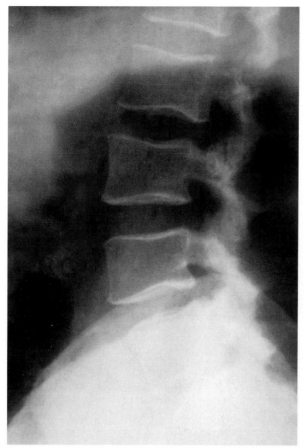

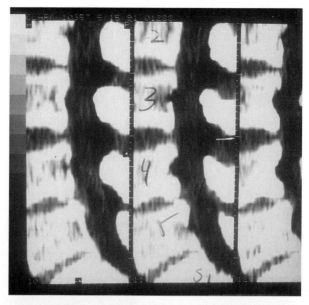

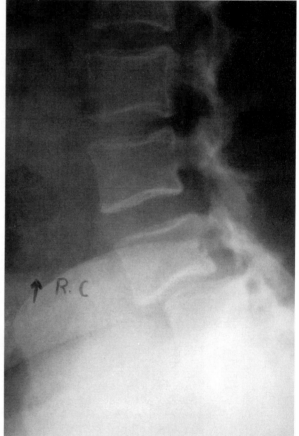

Fig. 91-3

Sagittal views of a patient supine compared with standing. **A,** Standard lateral lumbar radiograph demonstrates the reduced anterolisthesis in the supine position. **B,** CT scan of the same. **C,** A weight-bearing (standing) lateral radiograph of the same patient. This unstable degenerative spondylolisthesis was not appreciated until the standing radiograph was taken.

radiograph of the lumbar spine is helpful. Patients with a proportionally greater slip on the radiograph compared with the lateral scout film would be considered to have instability. A similar comparison can be made between supine and standing lateral radiographs.

Occasionally, a vacuum sign can be seen in the disc space of the lumbar spine, on plain radiographs, and particularly on CT scans. This finding is strongly suggestive of instability.

Vertebral body translation on comparison of standing lateral flexion and extensive views of the lumbar spine is an indication of instability. The severity of symptoms does not appear to correlate with the amount of slip.[5,16]

Traditionally, patients with degenerative spondylolisthesis and symptoms of spinal stenosis have been evaluated with myelogram and postmyelogram CT

scan.[17] The extent of stenosis and nerve-root entrapment can be evaluated with this study. Non–contrast-enhanced CT scan gives the most accurate demonstration of the bony pathology, making it the imaging procedure of choice. Sagittal and coronal

CT reconstructions clearly outline the bony impingement of the nerve root, usually L4, in the L4-L5 foramina, or the L5 root in the lateral recess. Note that the true extent of pathology may not be revealed by the CT or MRI scans. The patient is in the supine position during imaging, and thus the spondylolisthesis may be reduced.

In our experience, CT scans with high-quality sagittal and coronal reconstructions best demonstrate central canal and forminal stenosis. MRI scans do not demonstrate the bone detail as well as CT scans and are therefore less useful in the evaluation of spinal stenosis.

Historically, myelograms were the imaging procedure of choice, but they do not give an accurate visualization of the pathology. Anteroposterior views usually show two large bulbous masses protruding into the midline (Fig. 91-4, *A*). These masses are hypertrophied facets. They entrap the nerve in the lateral recess. The lateral view (Fig. 91-4, *B*) shows an anterior indentation from the bulging disc and superior aspect of the inferior vertebra at the level of the slip. A posterior indentation is from the lamina of the superior vertebra and the thickened ligamentum flavum.

Myelograms, when done in the standing position, may show dramatic abnormalities, particularly in patients with a large degree of anterior translation. Currently, myelogram or contrast-enhanced CT scan is used only rarely, typically in patients with previous lumbar spine surgery.

Indications for Surgery

The major indication for surgery is persistent pain after a trial of conservative care. Incapacitating neurogenic claudication or radiculopathy are common indications for surgery. Two thirds of the patients who require surgery do so because of constant leg pain.[30] The other one third have surgery because of neurogenic claudication that significantly interferes with their lifestyle.

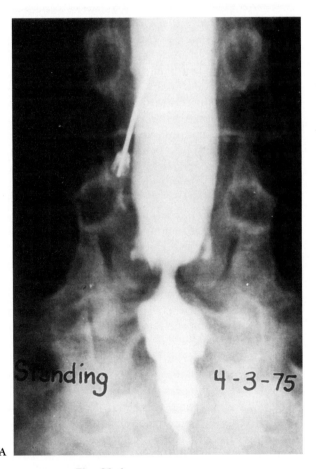

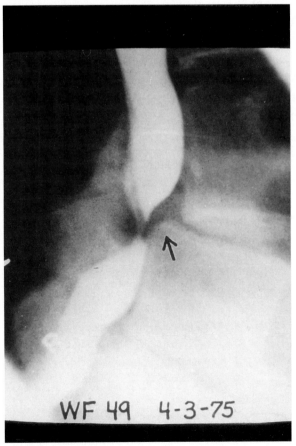

A   B

Fig. 91-4
Myelograms, when done in the standing position, may show dramatic abnormalities, particularly in patients with a large degree of anterior translation. **A,** Anteroposterior view. **B,** Sagittal view.

Less frequently, objective neurologic loss in the form of motor weakness is documented, and this is a strong indication for surgical intervention. Mild sensory deficits or mild nonprogressive motor weakness can be followed clinically if symptoms are tolerable to the patient.

Any history of urinary incontinence or sensory loss in the perineum may require medical evaluation with urodynamic studies. Patients with this clinical presentation may quickly develop cauda equina syndrome and should be considered strongly for surgical intervention. Patients may develop transient numbness in the perineum while walking. This neurogenic claudication occurs only in patients with severe stenosis. These patients should undergo timely surgical decompression, or be monitored closely.

A number of factors influence surgical decision-making in degenerative spondylolisthesis (Table 91-1). Overall patient health must be evaluated in conjunction with the presenting symptoms and objective physical findings. Patients with concomitant diseases, including diabetes with peripheral neuropathy and peripheral arterial occlusive disease,

Table 91-1

Factors relevant to surgical intervention in degenerative spondylolisthesis

Factors	Pro	Con
Pain	Constant leg pain	No pain with sitting or lying
	Pain at rest	Intermittent leg pain
Neurologic	Cauda equina compression	Stable sensory deficit
	Progressive motor loss	
	Motor weakness	
Health	Age (physiologic) ≤ 75 years	Age (physiologic) > 75 years
	Peripheral neuropathy*	Peripheral vascular disease
Radiographic	Progression of anterolisthesis	

*Patients with peripheral neuropathy have a reduced ability to recover neurologically, and may benefit from earlier surgical decompression. Obviously, the peripheral neuropathic component of their pain may not improve postoperatively, and this must be discussed with the patient.

must be identified preoperatively. The presence of peripheral neuropathy decreases a patient's ability to recover from a more central/proximal insult, possibly supporting an earlier surgical intervention. On the other hand, patients with arterial occlusive disease are typically a high-risk surgical group and usually have less active lifestyles. These factors may urge the caregiver to follow a more conservative course in this population.

Patients with pain while ambulating, but not at rest, must decide whether their quality of life is compromised to the point where surgical treatment is warranted. Patients who have no pain at rest, and can sit painlessly, can be treated conservatively much longer than those who experience difficulties while sitting. Postoperatively, back pain while sitting can occur as a direct result of the surgery, and this should be discussed with the patient. Substituting sitting pain for walking pain can confound the outcome of a technically successful surgery.

Operative Treatment

Surgical treatment usually consists of adequate posterior decompression at the level of spondylolisthesis and possibly arthrodesis.

Laminotomy has been used successfully for decompression of degenerative spondylolisthesis. It has the advantage of leaving the midline structures intact. Preservation of the spinous process and intraspinous and supraspinous ligaments confers some degree of stability, and patients seem to rehabilitate more easily postoperatively. The disadvantage of performing only a laminotomy is the difficulty in attempting to remove the thickened ligamentum flavum. In addition, adequate decompression of the lateral recesses and foramina may be technically impossible. We have observed a higher incidence of residual stenosis and persistent symptoms of nerve-root compression when a laminotomy is used.

The benefits of decompression are accepted by all authors, but controversy still surrounds the role of fusion. A review of the literature illustrates the evolution to the present-day techniques of decompression. Midline posterior decompression, which consists of removal of the lamina of L4 and L5 with preservation of the pars interarticularis and facets, is generally well accepted (Fig. 91-5).[5,15,30,38] Several authors reported satisfactory results with localized decompressive procedures, which included partial excision of lamina and spinous processes with medial facetectomies.[12,28,32] Rosenberg[31] initially decompressed only the nerve roots on the symptomatic side, but found improved results with bilateral de-

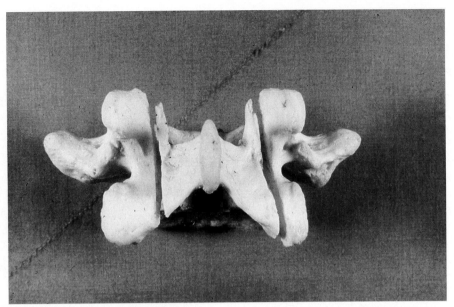

Fig. 91-5
Midline posterior decompression with preservation of the pars interarticularis and facet joints.

compression. Kaneda and associates[22] make the point that the muscle weakness, sensory loss, and decreased reflexes seen in postoperative failures originate in the nerve roots, not the cauda equina. He stresses the importance of removal of the medial part of the degenerated hypertrophied facet joints that encroach on the nerve roots and canal.

It has been well demonstrated that patients with degenerative spondylolisthesis will have some progression in the amount of anterolisthesis after decompression.* There is a wide variation in both the incidence of slip increase as well as the degree of slip progression. It must be noted that not all increasing slips are symptomatic.[20] Of the studies reporting increased slips postoperatively, the authors have been unable to correlate statistically the slip with a poor outcome.† White and Wiltse documented a 65% incidence of postoperative instability after decompression in patients with degenerative spondylolisthesis, but only a 2% incidence in patients without degenerative spondylolisthesis.[36]

Comorbid conditions including rheumatoid arthritis, primary neural disorder, and recurrent

trauma after decompression were also associated with a poor outcome and postoperative instability.[36] Katz and associates[23] found a relatively constant increase in probability that with the passage of time, patients with degenerative spondylolisthesis (treated with decompression only) would need a repeat operation. None of the patients who were fused primarily came to a second surgery. Verbiest[35] concluded that as the number of levels needing decompression increased, the satisfactory results decreased.

As it has been difficult to correlate an increase in postoperative slip with a poor outcome, the advocates of fusion have been able to demonstrate improved outcomes with the addition of posterolateral fusion* Among the advocates of fusion, disagreement still exists. Strong advocates of fusion recommend the procedure in all patients with degenerative spondylolisthesis who undergo decompression.† Others have less rigid indications for fusion, but tend to perform them in patients requiring extensive decompression, these less than 65 years old, and those with large preoperative anterolisthesis (greater than 10 mm).[12,23,30] Spengler[34] has not performed any

*References 3, 5, 20, 22, 23, 28, 30, 31, 36, and 38.
†References 3, 11, 12, 18, 20, 30, and 31.

*References 11, 17, 23, 25, 28, 36, and 37.
†References 3, 11, 22, 25, 27, 32, and 36 to 38.

Table 91-2

Fusion criteria in degenerative spondylolisthesis

Factors	Pro	Con
Age	Young (< 65 years)	Older (> 65 years)
X-Ray		
Disc height	Normal, slight narrowing	Marked narrowing
Supine vs. standing	Anterior translation	No anterior translation
Flexion/ extension	Translation > 2 mm	No motion
Vacuum sign	Present	Absent
CT Scan		
Facet orientation	Sagittal	Coronal
Foraminal stenosis[*]	Present— moderate to severe	Absent/minimal
Vacuum sign	Present	Absent

[*]Moderate to severe foraminal stenosis usually requires facet removal for decompression, which increases segmental instability.

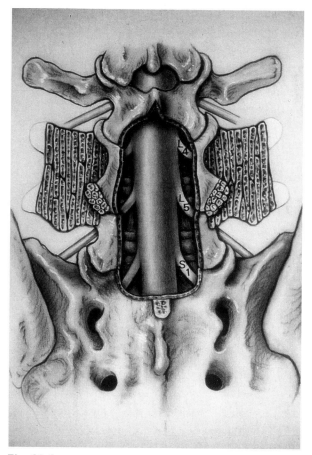

Fig. 91-6

Drawing of an L4-L5/L5-S1 decompression with an in situ posterolateral fusion of L5-L5. (From Wiltse LL, Kirkaldy-Willis WH, McIron GW: The treatment of spinal stenosis, *Clin Orthop* 115:83, 1976.)

posterior stabilization procedures after decompression in this patient population.

We have found the criteria listed in Table 91-2 to be useful in determining which patients would benefit from a fusion at the time of arthrodesis. Sagittal facet orientation predisposes the vertebral body to progressive anterolisthesis; this should be noted on a preoperative CT scan. Lateral flexion-extension radiographs that demonstrate any translatory motion indicate segmental instability. More than 2 mm or 3 mm of motion indicates significant instability. A more subtle but useful factor is a change in position of the anterolisthesis, which may be noted by comparing supine and standing radiographs. In our experience, a vacuum sign present on CT or x-ray study is also indicative of segmental instability.

Preservation of disc-space height implies that more motion potential remains in the segment as compared with a relatively collapsed or narrowed disc space. These patients are more likely to show a pro-

gressive postoperative anterolisthesis. Fusion should be considered more strongly in younger, healthier patients, particularly if they have a wide disc space. A schematic drawing of a decompression and in situ fusion is shown in Fig. 91-6.

A fusion without decompression is almost never indicated in the patient with degenerative spondylolisthesis, as the symptoms are primarily due to stenosis. The rarely encountered young patient with single level instability due to facet arthrosis may develop degenerative spondylolisthesis. In the absence of neurologic involvement, a single level arthrodesis may be indicated.

Selection of Fusion Levels

For degenerative spondylolisthesis, it is usually necessary to fuse only the involved level. Multiple levels may be fused if the patient demonstrates multiple levels of symptomatic disc degeneration or multiple level wide decompressions are performed. If fusions at L3-L4 and L4-L5 are indicated, it is probably best to include L5-S1 in the fusion. It has been our experience that arthrodesis two levels above the lumbosacral joint will cause symptomatic disc degeneration to occur at this level. In a select population of patients with an abnormal disc at L5-S1, degenerative spondylolisthesis at L4-L5, and normal discs above, we have found that the best results occur when both abnormal levels are fused.

Instrumentation

Among the advocates for fusion after decompression, disagreement exists regarding the need for spinal instrumentation. Spinal instrumentation is used to maintain vertebral alignment, augmenting stability until a solid fusion occurs. We do not advise an attempt to correct the anterolisthesis. Attempting to correct the slip puts a great deal of force on the screw–bone interface. The bone in these patients is usually soft and will not tolerate such force. Pedicle fracture or implant loosening may occur with reduction maneuvers.

Hanley[16] and Frymoyer and Selby[13] described a rotational component in addition to the translation deformity observed in degenerative spondylolisthesis. The rotation places traction on the neural elements, in addition to the stenotic compression from the bone and ligamentous hypertrophy. In situ fusion alone would not correct this rotational deformity. Hanley advocated Harrington distraction for correction, but cautioned against excessive distraction. He also noted an increase in the slip postoperatively, but this was not associated with a poor outcome. Kaneda[22] and Fujiya[14] and their associates advocate a posterolateral fusion with a combined distraction and compression rod technique, which gave a 97% fusion rate and prevented significant advancement of the slip postoperatively. Apparently, the immediate surgical correction of the anterolisthesis was lost at follow-up, as the segments returned to their preoperative position. Instrumentation, in this condition, may not be able to maintain a significant deformity correction, but appears to minimize the postoperative instability while providing an adjunct to fusion.

Bone screw fixation has the ability to correct and maintain rotational and translatory deformity, but prospective studies defining their role in this condition are still awaited.

A recent study by Kim and associates[24] found significant improvement in fusion rates with combined anterior and posterior fusion. Inoue and associates[19] report that anterior interbody fusions in patients younger than 60 years of age are a reliable surgical option. Anterior interbody fusion is able to correct malalignment, restore disc height, and reduce nerve-root compression by enlarging the stenotic canal. This procedure does not directly address the hypertrophic ligatum flavum or facet joints. The anterior approach carries with it increased risk of complications in this patient population. Calcified vascular structures that must be mobilized during the anterior approach are at greatest risk for thrombosis postoperatively.

Surgical Techniques

After incising the skin with a scalpel, electrocautery is used to minimize bleeding; use a fairly high setting with equal coagulation and cautery and a Blend 2 setting. The fascia is incised on either side of the midline. A Cobb elevator is used to maintain tension on the muscle, while the cautery is used to dissect the tissue away from the spinous processes and lamina. The pars interarticularis should be completely exposed. If a fusion is to be performed, exposure of the transverse processes should be completed at this time. A Meyerding retractor is used by the surgeon on the opposite side of the table to keep tension on the muscle and facilitate exposure of the tips of the transverse processes. Electrocautery may continue to be used for this exposure, but do not dissect deep to the transverse process or pars, for the nerve roots are most vulnerable to injury in these areas. Bipolar cautery is used in the area of the pars interarticularis to prevent bleeding of the small deep radicular vessels. Only bipolar cautery should be used in this area to minimize potential thermal injury to the nerve root directly below this landmark.

If there is any question regarding the level at which the surgery is to be done, a localizing radiograph should be taken to confirm the level before any bone is resected. Decortication is performed with a high-speed burr or curette on the transverse processes. Chisels are used for decortication of the pars interarticularis and lateral faces of the articular processes. Thorough decortication of the lateral face of the facets, pars interarticularis, and transverse processes is essential for a successful lateral fusion. The high-speed burr is less likely to fracture the transverse process than a curette.

Intermittent irrigation should be used to keep the burr tip and tissues cool during decortication.

Decortication is performed at this point in the operation because the lamina are still intact. This minimizes the chance of injury to the cauda equina with the burr. The area can then be packed with a sponge to tamponade bleeding.

The lamina and ligamentum flavum are thinned with a rongeur and removed with a Kerrison rongeur. If the canal is very stenotic, a Cloward chisel can be used to separate small pieces of lamina. These fragments can then be removed with a large pituitary rongeur. This can be continued until there is room for a Kerrison rongeur, or until an adequate amount of lamina has been resected. Care must be taken to preserve 5 mm of the pars to prevent fractures in the future.

Attention is now turned to the facet joints. The medial one third of the facet is often very difficult to remove using Kerrison rongeurs. The Cloward chisel can be used to safely resect the medial one third of the facet. The ligamentum flavum is between the chisel and the dura once the bone has been broken through. The chisel is beveled so that it will break off the bone before it cuts completely through. An osteotome is smooth and tapered. It will not separate the bone before plunging completely through. The Cloward chisel also has a very long round handle that makes it easy to control.

The caudal half of the foramina at the slip level is often very stenotic because the superior facet at the slip level hypertrophies. It is important to resect that portion of the facet over the disc space back to the level of the pedicle. This can be done easily and quickly with a Cloward chisel. Place the chisel on the anterior one third of the facet joint over the disc space and aim toward the pedicle. This will usually remove the entire portion of the hypertrophied superior facet. The disc is bulging into the inferior half of the foramina. If soft, it may be removed by a knife and pituitary ronguer. If the disc is hard or calcified, use a chisel. It should be quite safe since the nerve root is in the upper half of the foramina. Of course, one should visualize and protect the nerve root before embarking on this type of decompression. At times, the body of the caudal vertebra has osteophytes, projecting laterally from its superior portion. This impinges the nerve root at the exit zone or just beyond the exit zone. This can only be removed if the facet is first removed.

If an instrumented fusion is performed, a final way of decompressing a foramina is by spreading or distracting the bone screws as they are being tightened to the plate or rod. This should only be done a small amount, or there is too great a pressure on the screws.

The starting hole for the screw is made with a 4 mm high-speed burr. A blunt probe is placed into the pedicle. Bone screw landmarks are identified by palpating and visualizing the inner wall of the pedicle and the superior and inferior walls with an angled probe through the laminectomy site. Different markers are placed in the left and right pedicles so that with one radiograph, the surgeon can determine whether the probes, and thus the pilot holes in the pedicles, are in the proper position and direction. Before the pedicles are tapped the probes are placed in the pilot holes and a lateral radiograph is taken. The bone graft is taken while waiting for the x-ray film to be developed.

Bone Graft

Bone graft should be taken through the midline incision and not through a separate incision over the iliac crest. It will give a better cosmetic result and be less painful. The midline incision will need to be extended distally. The graft is taken from the posterior superior iliac crest and four finger-breadths anteriorly. This will avoid injuring the cluneal nerves.

The skin and the subcutaneous tissue are elevated off the fascia over to the iliac crest. The midline incision must be distal enough to allow complete exposure of the posterior superior iliac crest. The fascia is incised with cautery midway between the inner and outer table. The periosteum is elevated off the ilium and outer table and thus the gluteal muscle is also elevated about four finger-breadths anteriorly along the crest of the ilium. By taking the periosteum, good strong tissue is present to permit a good repair of the gluteal muscle. A Taylor retractor placed to the depth of the reflected gluteus will allow good exposure.

A 1-in. straight osteotome is used to osteotomize the crest from the posterior superior iliac crest and four finger-breadths anteriorly. Going further anterior four finger-breadths markedly increases the risk of injury to the cluneal nerves, which may produce a painful graft site. Beyond this boundary, the inner and outer tables are quite close together, and thus little bone graft can be obtained here.

A 1-in. wide osteotome is used to take the outer half of the crest. The deep part of that cut is made by a curved osteotome, so that the deep part of the cortex separates cleanly. Small straight gouges cut small thick strips of cancellous bone. Curettes are used to take the remaining cancellous bone, and are not as likely to penetrate through the inner table as the osteotomes or gouges. Curettes can also obtain bone between the inner and outer table at the edges

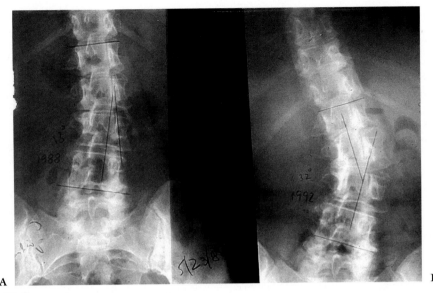

Fig. 91-7

Patient with degenerative scoliosis and spondylolisthesis. **A,** Extent of curvature in 1988. **B,** Progression as seen in 1992.

of the donor site and under the crest of the ileum. A block of Gelfoam placed in the ilium donor site will reduce bleeding.

Bone graft is placed between the transverse process. If bone screws are used, the bone graft is placed after the screws are in place, but before the saddles, rods, or plates are installed. If all the iliac bone graft is in place, and the instrumentation has been installed, additional bone graft obtained from the laminectomy can be added to the fusion site. This bone must be absolutely free of any soft tissue or cartilage.

The iliac donor site is closed over suction drainage with three or four interrupted sutures. A #1 absorbable suture is placed through the periosteum and fascia of the gluteal. The two outer sutures are pulled tight by an assistant, and the surgeon ties the middle suture or sutures. A suction drain is also placed deep to the midline fascia. Closure of the midline fascia is then completed with a large running absorbable suture. Meticulous subcutaneous and subcuticular closure is accomplished with running absorbable sutures respectively. The skin is covered with steri-strips and a large compressive dressing.

Degenerative Spondylolisthesis and Degenerative Scoliosis

Degenerative scoliosis is often seen in patients with degenerative spondylolisthesis. The treatment of a patient with both degenerative spondylolisthesis and degenerative scoliosis is much more complex than when either condition exists alone. The combination of spondylolisthesis and scoliosis creates a multidirectional instability with anterolisthesis, lateral translation, and rotational instability. In older patients these are unstable situations in which there is likely to be significant progression of the deformity.

These patients may develop radicular symptoms, with the most frequently compromised nerve being L5. Compression of the L5 nerve root may be caused by a degenerative spondylolisthesis at L4-L5 or a degenerative scoliosis producing foraminal and far-out stenosis of the L5 foramina. The symptomatic nerve compression is usually found on the convex side of the major lumbar curve. The far-out stenosis occurs as the result of a short compensatory curve at L5-S1. The concavity of the compensatory curve at L5-S1 is on the same side as the convexity of the major curve. In Fig. 91-7, the degenerative scoliosis has a left convex curve from L1 to L4. The short compensatory curve at L5-S1 is concave on the left side. This creates a far-out stenosis as the transverse process of L5 angles toward the sacral ala, compressing the exiting L5 nerve.

Patients less than 70 years of age are ideally treated with an extraforaminal decompression. When there is no central stenosis and only one nerve root is compressed in a foramen or extraforaminally, isolated decompression of the nerve is indicated. If significant central stenosis and foraminal stenosis are present, a decompression-fusion is indicated. A word of caution: when doing a central lumbar decompression in patients with both degenerative spondylolisthesis and scoliosis, a fusion is usually indicated because of the instability created by the decompression. Dramatic progression of these curves is the rule rather than the exception in these cases. In many cases, recurrent stenosis has been observed. The extraforaminal decompression does not cause this instability and hence fusion is not needed.

Patients 70 years and over will typically fail with traditional surgical treatment. A central decompression causes progression of the curve and the instrumentation used for fusions may fail because the bone is too soft. Nonunion and loss of fixation are common in this situation. Our recommendation for this group of patients is facet blocks with rhizotomies for back pain and spinal cord stimulators for leg pain.

Summary

Degenerative spondylolisthesis is common in females 50 years of age and older and usually occurs at the L4-L5 level. The typical patient has a long history of back pain that responds well to conservative therapy.

When surgical treatment is indicated it is usually for sciatica or pseudoclaudication. A wide bilateral decompression is the best treatment. The outcome is improved in many cases with an intertransverse fusion. In cases with significant instability, bone screw instrumentation is indicated. Patients with a combination of degenerative spondylolisthesis and degenerative scoliosis should be treated with conservative care as long as possible because of the tendency to have a less predictable outcome from surgical intervention.

References

1. Albrook D: Movements of the lumbar spinal column, *J Bone Joint Surg [Br]* 39:339, 1957.
2. Bolender N, Schonstrom N, Spengler D: The role of computed tomography and myelography in the diagnosis of central spinal stenosis, *J Bone Joint Surg* 67A:240, 1985.
3. Bolesta MJ, Bohlman HH: Degenerative spondylolisthesis: the role of arthrodesis, *Orthop Trans* 13:564, 1989.
4. Brown MD, Lockwood JM: Degenerative spondylolisthesis, *Intr Course Lect Am Acad Orthop Surg,* St. Louis, Mosby, 32:162, 1983.
5. Cauchoix J, Benoist M, Chassaing V: Degenerative spondylolisthesis, *Clin Orthop* 115:122, 1976.
6. Ehni G: Effects of certain degenerative diseases of the spine, especially spondylolysis and disc protrusion on the neural contents particularly in the lumbar region: historical account, *Mayo Clin Proc* 50:327, 1976.
7. Epstein JA, Epstein BS, Lavine L: Nerve root compression associated with narrowing of the lumbar spinal canal, *J Neurol Neurosurg Psychiat* 25:165, 1962.
8. Epstein JA et al.: Lumbar nerve root compression at the intervertebral foramina caused by arthritis of the posterior facets, *J Neurosurg* 39:362, 1973.
9. Epstein NE et al.: Degenerative spondylolisthesis with an intact neural arch: a review of 60 cases with an analysis of clinical findings and the development of surgical management, *Neurosurgery* 13:555, 1983.
10. Farfan HF, Kirkaldy-Willis WH: The present status of spinal fusion in the treatment of lumbar intervertebral joint disorders, *Clin Orthop* 158:198, 1981.
11. Feffer HL et al.: Degenerative spondylolisthesis: to fuse or not to fuse, *Spine* 10:287, 1985.
12. Fitzgerald JA, Newman PH: Degenerative spondylolisthesis, *J Bone Joint Surg [Br]* 58:184, 1976.
13. Frymoyer JW, Selby DK: Segmental instability: rationale for treatment, *Spine* 10:280, 1985.
14. Fujiya M et al.: Clinical study on stability of combined distraction and compression rod instrumentation with posterolateral fusion for unstable degenerative spondylolisthesis, *Spine* 15(11):12, 1990.
15. Gertzbein SD: *Degenerative spondylolisthesis.* 52nd AAOS Instructional Course Lectures, Las Vegas, NV, January, 1995.
16. Hanley EN: Decompression and distraction-derotation arthrodesis for degenerative spondylolisthesis, *Spine* 11:269, 1986.
17. Herkowitz HN, Kurz LT: Degenerative lumbar spondylolisthesis with spinal stenosis, *J Bone Joint Surg* 73A:802, 1991.
18. Herron LD, Trippi AC: L4-5 degenerative spondylolisthesis: the results of treatment by decompressive laminectomy without fusion, *Spine* 14:534, 1989.
19. Inoue S and others: Degenerative spondylolisthesis: pathophysiology and results of anterior interbody fusion, *Clin Orthop* 227:90, 1988.
20. Johnsson KE, Wilner S. Johnsson K: Post-operative instability after decompression for lumbar spinal stenosis, *Spine* 11:107, 1986.
21. Junghanns H: Spondylolisthesen ohne spalt in zwischengelenkstueck, *Arch fuer Orthopaedische Unfallchir* 29:118, 1930.
22. Kaneda K et al.: Follow-up study of medial facetectomies and posterolateral fusion in isthmic spondylolisthesis: 53 cases followed for 18–89 months, *Clin Orthop* 203:159, 1986.
23. Katz JN et al.: The outcome of decompressive laminectomy for degenerative lumbar stenosis, *J Bone Joint Surg* 73A:809, 1991.
24. Kim SS et al.: Factors affecting fusion rate in adult spondylolisthesis, *Spine* 15(9):979, 1990.
25. Lombardi JS et al.: Treatment of degenerative spondylolisthesis, *Spine* 10:821, 1985.

26. Lowe RW et al.: Standing roentgenograms in spondylolisthesis, *Clin Orthop* 117:80, 1976.

27. Macnab I: Spondylolisthesis with an intact neural arch: the so-called pseudo-spondylolisthesis, *J Bone Joint Surg* 32:325, 1950.

28. Newman PH: Surgical treatment for spondylolisthesis in the adult, *Clin Orthop* 117:106, 1976.

29. Newman PH, Stone KH: The etiology of spondylolisthesis with a special investigation, *J Bone Joint Surg [Br]* 45:39, 1963.

30. Reynolds JB, Wiltse LL: Surgical treatment of degenerative spondylolisthesis, *Spine* 4:148, 1979 (abstract).

31. Rosenberg NJ: Degenerative spondylolisthesis: predisposing factors, *J Bone Joint Surg [Am]* 57:467, 1975.

32. Rosenberg NJ: Degenerative spondylolisthesis: surgical treatment, *Clin Orthop* 117:112, 1976.

33. Sato K et al.: The configuration of the laminas and facet joints in degenerative spondylolisthesis: a clinicoradiologic study, *Spine* 14:1265, 1989.

34. Spengler DM: Current concepts review: degenerative stenosis of the lumbar spine, *J Bone Joint Surg* 69A:305, 1987.

35. Verbiest H: A radicular syndrome from developmental narrowing of the lumbar vertebral canal, *J Bone Joint Surg* 36B:230, 1954.

36. White AH, Wiltse LL: Spondylolisthesis after extensive lumbar laminectomy, *J Bone Joint Surg [Am]* 58:727, 1975.

37. Wiltse LL: *Degenerative spondylolisthesis.* 51st AAOS Instructional Course Lectures, Atlanta, GA, February, 1984.

38. Wiltse LL, Kirkaldy-Willis WH, McIron GW: The treatment of spinal stenosis, *Clin Orthop* 115:83, 1976.

Chapter 92

Spondylolisthesis: Isthmic, Congenital, Traumatic, and Post-Surgical

James B. Reynolds
Paul J. Slosar, Jr.

Classification

  classification system

Isthmic Spondylolisthesis

  incidence and pathogenesis
  natural history
  physical findings
  radiographic analysis
  radiographic measurements
  nonoperative treatment
  surgical treatment
  distribution of pain/foraminal stenosis
  herniation at the level of a spondylolisthesis
  stability/disc space height

High-Grade Spondylolisthesis

  surgical techniques

Congenital Spondylolisthesis (Type I)
Traumatic Spondylolisthesis (Type IV)
Postoperative Spondylolisthesis (Type VI)
Summary

Spondylolisthesis was first recognized by obstetricians in the 1700s and 1800s. They noted the occurrence of severe spondylolisthesis because of the obstruction to the birth canal that occurred during labor. During this period, spondylolisthesis was thought to occur only in females.[10,11] It was not until 1920 that radiographic equipment was of sufficient quality to image a lateral view of the lumbar spine. Between 1920 and 1930 the Mayo Clinic had accumulated a large number of x-ray films of the lumbar spine and began identifying patients with spondylolisthesis. After analyzing these x-ray films, Meyerding, an orthopedic surgeon at the Mayo Clinic, wrote a classic paper categorizing the degrees of slip.[13] He noted that spondylolisthesis, although present in both women and men, is more common in men. Meyerding also discussed fusion as a surgical treatment.

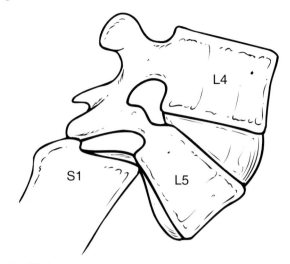

Fig. 92-1
Congenital spondylolisthesis (type IA).

Classification

Wiltse, Newman, and MacNab[23] described and classified spondylolisthesis. In 1976 they collaborated to produce the classification system currently in use. Wiltse and Rothman[24] have made minor modifications, some of which are based on additional information provided by CT scans.

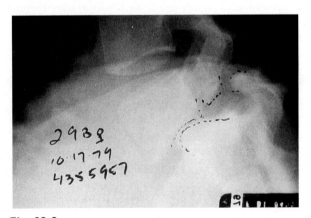

Fig. 92-2
Isthmic spondylolisthesis (type IIA, lytic).

Classification System

Type I. Congenital or dysplastic—Due to dysplastic articular elements at the lumbosacral junction.

A. Dysplastic, axially (horizontal) oriented facets at the level of the slip (Fig. 92-1). This subtype is frequently associated with spina bifida and frequently becomes symptomatic at age 10 years.

B. This subtype has sagittal orientation of the facets that allow spondylolisthesis to occur at the involved level. This subtype is most frequently symptomatic about age 30 years.

Type II. Isthmic

A. Lytic—This is a classic pars interarticularis defect due to a nonunited stress fracture (Fig. 92-2).

B. Elongated—Repeated episodes of fracture, slip, and healing produce an elongated pars interarticularis (Fig. 92-3). (This lesion has been described as similar to a taffy pull.)

C. Acute traumatic pars fracture.

Type III. Degenerative—This type occurs as a result of segmental instability and is marked by degenera-

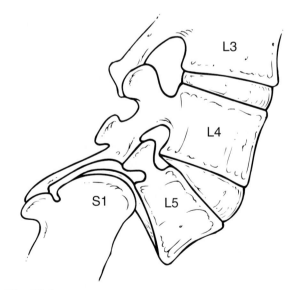

Fig. 92-3
Isthmic spondylolisthesis (type IIB, elongated).

tive facet joints. The pars interarticularis remains intact (see Chapter 91).

Type IV. Traumatic—This is due to a fracture in the posterior restraint system (pedicle or facet) other than the pars.

Type V. Pathologic—Due to a localized or generalized bone disease.

Type VI. Postsurgical—Due to loss of stability either from the disc or facets; or a postoperative stress fracture of the inferior articular process.

There are additional complexities to the standard classification as presented above. Isthmic spondylolisthesis is much more common than any other form of spondylolisthesis. The evaluation and treatment of isthmic spondylolisthesis does vary with the severity of the spondylolisthesis. This is best divided into high-grade slips and low-grade slips. As indicated by radiographic measurements, grades I and II are considered low-grade slips and grades IV and V are considered high-grade slips. Grade III is intermediate. High-grade slips have some symptoms and physical findings different from low-grade slips, and the treatment becomes more difficult as the slip becomes greater. Otherwise, the general description of symptoms and treatment apply to all isthmic spondylolisthesis unless otherwise stated.

Isthmic Spondylolisthesis

Incidence and Pathogenesis

The incidence of isthmic spondylolisthesis is as high as 6% in North American males of European descent. Other ethnic groups have a lower incidence, with the lowest found in Oriental females. While the ratio of involvement is 2:1 (male:female), it appears that adolescent females have a strong disposition toward developing high-grade slips.[17] Isthmic and congenital spondylolisthesis are transmitted genetically. Both types are found in members of the same family, and frequently multiple generations will be affected, supporting the genetic link.[28]

Isthmic spondylolisthesis is not truly congenital, but is more developmental in nature. The incidence in newborns, as well as patients who have never walked, has been reported to be near zero. Patients with isthmic spondylolisthesis appear to be predisposed to the lesion developing. The defect in the pars interarticularis is due to a stress fracture that usually occurs around age 6. The slip occurs typically during the adolescent growth spurt, which is earlier for girls (11 to 13 years) than boys (13 to 15

years).[6] The most common level for spondylolisthesis, in both congenital and isthmic types, is L5-S1. It can occasionally be seen at L4-L5, but rarely above that. This is in distinction from degenerative spondylolisthesis, which is typically seen at the L4-L5 interspace.

Natural History

It is the rare child who presents to a physician with complaints of pain, deformity, or disability directly related to isthmic spondylolisthesis. The vast majority of children in whom lytic defects of the pars interarticularis develop are usually asymptomatic. Most studies in the literature are directed toward the symptomatic child or adolescent with spondylolisthesis. While these patients are by far the minority, they do represent those who more frequently require treatment. It is also important to understand the natural history of the asymptomatic patients as well.

Baker and Frederickson and their colleagues performed a prospective study evaluating 500 children on a routine 5-year basis through adolescence and into adulthood.[1,6] They noted that the defect typically occurred around the age of 5 or 6 in most individuals, but isolated cases occurred during adolescence. They found a general incidence similar to the other reports of the literature approximating 5% or 6%. It must be noted that this was a study of a normal, asymptomatic population. Pain was not found to be reported by any of the patients enrolled in this study through childhood or adolescence. Anterolisthesis was observed in the majority of patients with a bilateral pars defect but not in any of those with a unilateral defect. The majority of their patients had stable slips, meaning that the initial degree of slip tended not to progress. Overall, the percentage of anterololisthesis ranged from 0 to 30% in this study.

Children who present for medical evaluation will often have a precipitating minor trauma prior to their presentation. They will come in because of pain or deformity due to the isthmic spondylolisthesis. Physical findings in these children or adolescents are distinctly different from their adult counterparts. They may present with or without back pain. Often the patient's parent or school physician will identify a postural deformity or abnormal gate. Tightness of the hamstrings may be marked, which accentuates both the postural or cosmetic deformity as well as the typical (waddling gait) that these patients demonstrate. Signs and symptoms may be aggravated by repetitive activity or sports participation. Radicular symptoms are not typically seen.

Physical Findings

On physical examination, tenderness in the low lumbar region is variable. Scoliosis may be seen in a small number of these patients with symptomatic spondylolisthesis. It must be noted that this scoliosis is generally not structural, but is usually due to lumbar spasm. Symptom resolution should improve the scoliosis in these cases. Patients with high-grade slips may have a palpable step-off noted on examination of the lumbar spine (see Fig. 92-9B and C). These patients may demonstrate the classic heart-shaped buttocks, an abdominal crease, and hamstring tightness. These are patients with severe slips and thus marked deformity at the lumbosacral junction. Objective neurologic deficits are extremely rare in the vast majority of patients with isthmic spondylolisthesis.

Adults also may present after an acute traumatic event, usually twisting or lifting. They often have more severe low-back pain with or without sciatica. If radicular symptoms are present, the L5 root is most commonly involved in those with isthmic defects at L5, while those with defects at L4 will have dermatomal changes in the L4 distribution. The presence of these sometimes severe radicular symptoms is in contrast to the children presenting with painful isthmic spondylolisthesis. Adults may also have more persistent and more frequently recurring pain even after the elimination of repetitive trauma. The vast majority of adults will respond to rest and antiinflammatory medication.

Radiographic Analysis

Anteroposterior and lateral x-ray films of the lumbar spine in patients with spondylolisthesis should always be taken in the standing position. Approximately one-quarter of these patients show a significant increase in slip, or slip angle, on a standing lateral x-ray film as compared with the same film taken in a supine position (Fig. 92-4, A and B).[12] Most lateral films are taken with the patients lying on their sides. A better technique is to take the lateral film of the lumbar spine in the supine position. The weight of the pelvis may reduce the spondylolisthesis. It is technically difficult to take a lumbar film in the supine position. The scout film of the CT or MRI scan is a lateral view taken in the supine position. Although on different scales, the percentage of slip and angular rotation can be compared to the standing lateral of the lumbosacral spine.

Lateral flexion-extension bending films rarely show a significant change in the slip unless it is quite

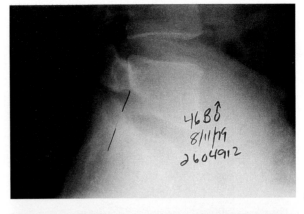

A

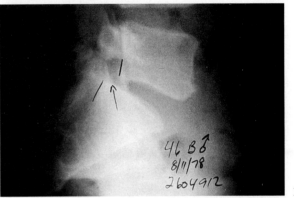

B

Fig. 92-4

A, Supine radiogram of patient with isthmic spondylolisthesis and no apparent slip. **B,** Standing radiogram of same patient with obvious anterololisthesis.

unstable.[12] A standing spot lateral film of L5-S1 can be helpful when measuring the percentage of slip or the angulation. Oblique x-ray films usually demonstrate the pars interarticularis defect, but reformatted CT scans will more clearly demonstrate the pars defect, making oblique films unnecessary (Figs. 92-5, A, B, and C). The CT scan should be reformatted to produce high-quality sagittal and coronal images as well as the standard axial image. MRI will demonstrate a pars defect but the quality of bone resolution is inferior to CT scanning, making a high-quality CT scan the preferred study for patients with spondylolisthesis.

Technetium bone scanning is valuable when looking for the occult pars fracture that can occur in the young patient. This is of particular value in a young patient with unexplained back pain.[26] Increased uptake of the radionucleide technetium in the area of the pars may indicate that a fracture is acute. MRI scans have recently been reported to demonstrate the occult pars fractures in young patients with spondylolysis.

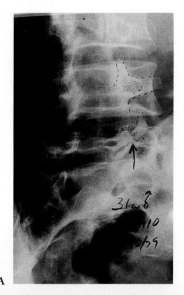

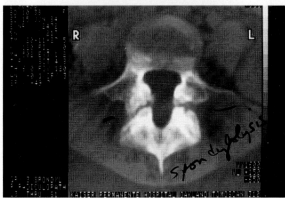

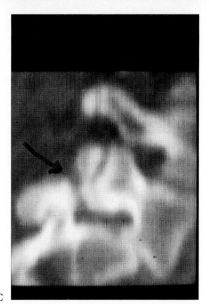

Fig. 92-5

A, Oblique radiogram demonstrating classic "collar" around "scotty dog's" neck seen in lytic spondylolisthesis. **B,** Axial and **C,** sagittal CT scan reconstructions demonstrating similar lytic defect in pars interarticularis.

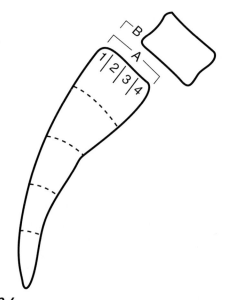

Fig. 92-6

Illustration of "grade of slip" and "percentage slip": grade I = 0 to 25%; grade II = 25% to 50%; grade III = 50% to 75%; grade IV = 75% to 100%.

Radiographic Measurements

The measurement of spondylolisthesis was first discussed by Meyerding.[13] He divided the top of the sacrum into four equal parts. The grade of slippage is determined by the relative position of the posterior L5 vertebral body over the sacrum (Fig. 92-6). Increasing grades (I to IV) indicate a more severe anterololisthesis. A grade V slip is a spondyloptosis, where the L5 vertebrae has slipped entirely off the sacrum.

Other methods measure this anterololisthesis by the percentage of slip. The percentage is derived by making the maximum width of the sacrum on the lateral view the denominator and the distance between the posterior cortex of S1 and the posterior cortex of L5 (in an L5-S1 spondylolisthesis) the numerator.[27] Percentage slip is derived by multiplying this result by 100. The point on the top of the sacrum where the back of the L5 vertebra is marked is determined by following a perpendicular line from the sacrum to the posterior inferior corner of L5 (see Fig. 92-6).

The sagittal rotation, or slip angle, measures the rotation of the superior vertebrae relative to the inferior vertebrae. L5-S1 is the only level at which this measurement is significant. The slip angle, formed by a perpendicular line drawn from a line along the back of the sacrum, starts at the posterior corner of S1 as viewed on the lateral x-ray film. The second line is drawn on the superior end plate of L5. The inferior end plate of L5 should not be used because it is often deformed. The angle formed by these two intersecting lines is the sagittal rotation angle. An increased slip angle predicts slips that are more likely to progress.[2,17] All measurements should be made from standing films (Fig. 92-7). Wiltse and Winter recommend measuring this angle from the anterior border of L5, as seen in Fig. 92-8.[27]

Nonoperative Treatment

Once the diagnosis has been established, the goal of treatment is symptom resolution or control. The nonoperative treatment of isthmic spondylolisthesis should include exercise and/or bracing. Some patients may need a short period of decreased activity and possibly complete avoidance of strenuous activity until symptoms have resolved. A short course of nonsteroidal antiinflammatory medications is sometimes helpful. Once symptoms have resolved, the child may resume normal activities.

Young patients with grade I spondylolisthesis have had a 78% success rate in terms of symptom resolution when treated with a modified Boston brace (worn full time for 6 months and then weaned over the subsequent 6 months). A small percentage of the patients had their pars defects heal radiographically.[21] Adults may receive symptomatic relief from the standard canvas lumbosacral corset. Exercise can improve or relieve a patient's symptoms. Stabilization exercises with a flexion bias should be emphasized, as they have been shown to achieve better results in patients with spondylolisthesis.[19]

In conjunction with stabilization training exercises, epidural or selective nerve root injections should be used for adults who have leg pain. The selective nerve root block is usually more effective than a traditional epidural injection in patients with spondylolisthesis. The epidural injection will take the path of least resistance and therefore may not travel into a stenotic foramen.

When treating children with isthmic spondylolisthesis, activity limitation should be short term. If symptoms continue after several months of appropriate activity modification and bracing, these children must be considered for surgical intervention. If symptoms effectively resolve with nonoperative treatment, but then quickly resume as the child resumes full-level activity, an individual decision between the patient, the family, and the treating physician must be made as to the risk versus the benefits of surgical intervention. Interval lateral radiography at L5-S1 should be performed at 6-month intervals until it is clear that severe slip progression will not develop. These are especially appropriate during the growing years, when the risk for progression is great-

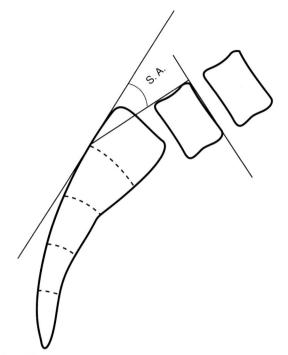

Fig. 92-7
Slip angle calculated by determining angle between line along posterior upper sacrum and line perpendicular to cephalad end plate of L5.

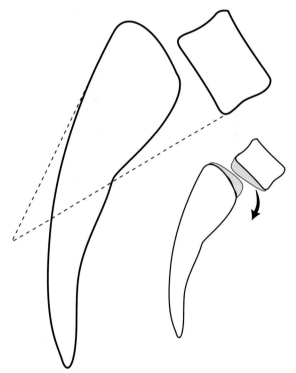

Fig. 92-8
Sagittal rotation (slip angle) may also be determined by extending line along anterior body of L5 until it intersects line drawn along posterior body of S1.

est. More frequent follow-up, with close monitoring, is indicated for patients who have demonstrated a clear slip with or without progression. As slips on the order of grade II develop in children, they began to have significant structural abnormalities as well as sagittal plane asymmetry. Most spine surgeons adopt a reasonably aggressive approach in these patients because the results of an in situ fusion are relatively predictable for these low-grade slips. Attempted fusions and/or surgical reductions of the higher-grade slips is much more complicated and far less predictable. Ideally, the goal of conservative care, as well as operative care, is to prevent childhood slips from progressing beyond a grade II.[9]

Surgical Treatment

General Principles

There are several factors that must be considered when contemplating surgical intervention. Patient age, pain distribution, the amount of slip, as well as disc height and stability at the level of spondylolisthesis are all relevant variables.

Under 30 Years of Age

The vast majority of patients below 30 years of age can be treated with a noninstrumented in situ fusion, regardless of symptom location (back pain, leg pain, or both).[16,17] Attention to the surgical technique is quite important. The paraspinal approach should be used for in situ fusion because it retains

the midline structures and therefore retains stability. This technique minimizes slip progression while waiting for fusion to occur. Neurologic deficits in young patients with spondylolisthesis are usually minor and will resolve once the fusion is solid. Hamstring tightness, a common finding in these patients, will usually resolve within the first postoperative year (see Fig. 92-9, C and E). Radicular pain also will resolve when the fusion is solid.

Instrumented fusion should be done in patients between ages 20 and 30 who have greater than 3 mm of translation noted on comparison of supine and standing radiograms. Those rare patients with isthmic spondylolisthesis above L5-S1 can be treated similarly. In these cases, bone screw instrumentation should be used through a paraspinal approach.[25]

Over 30 Years of Age

In patients over the age of 30, we have found it useful to determine the appropriate surgical procedure based on the specific symptoms and pathology noted in Table 92-1. A wide variety of symptom constellations exists in these patients and categorizing them by location and diagnostic pathology is appropriate. Evaluation of foraminal stenosis or lateral recess stenosis is paramount in this patient population. High quality, reformatted sagittal and axial CT scans are invaluable for this evaluation. Of note, almost everyone in this age category is treated with a fusion. Attention to appropriate stenosis decompression must be individualized.

Table 92-1

Surgical options in patients over 30 years of age who have isthmic low-grade spondylolisthesis

Symptoms	Radiographic Findings	Treatment
Back pain	No stenosis; no translation	In situ fusion/paraspinal
Back pain	No stenosis; ≥3 mm translation	In situ fusion with instrumentation/paraspinal
Back and unilateral leg pain/numbness	Unilateral foraminal/lateral recess stenosis; no translation	Posterior midline and unilateral foraminal decompression; unilateral or bilateral in situ fusion
Bilateral leg pain/numbness	Bilateral foraminal/lateral recess stenosis	Posterior midline and bilateral foraminal decompression; fusion with instrumentation; possible Anterior Interbody Fusion
Elderly (>60 years)/ back pain	Narrow disc space; osteophytes; no translation; mild to moderate foraminal stenosis	Posterior midline and facet preserving foraminal decompressions ± fusion

Surgical Summary

Isthmic spondylolisthesis is successfully treated in the majority of patients with conservative measures. In the young, a Boston brace is effective. In the adult population, stabilization exercises are used. The surgical treatment for patients up to 30 years of age is fusion through the paraspinal approach. In patients over 30, most have a combination of leg and back pain. These patients will need decompression and fusion with instrumentation. Combined anterior-posterior fusion may be necessary in selected patients.

Distribution of Pain/Foraminal Stenosis

Consideration of the patient's pain distribution is especially relevant in patients over the age of 30. Patients with significant leg pain will usually have a component of foraminal stenosis that needs to be decompressed. In patients with a narrowed disc space, the anulus may heap up and occupy the inferior portion of the foramina. Further laterally, the anulus can also bulge out against the L5 root. Osteophytes off the vertebral body of S1 may project laterally, impinging the L5 nerve. A traction spur off the body of L5 can project under the root. It is therefore essential in these patients to inspect the foramina anterior to the L5 root.

The most lateral structure to impinge on the L5 root in an L5-S1 spondylolisthesis is the transverse process. This "far-out stenosis" as described by Wiltse is often found in patients with grade II or greater spondylolisthesis. This far-out stenosis can trap the L5 root between the transverse process and sacral ala.[22]

Patients with a preponderance of back pain may not have a significant amount of foraminal stenosis, but this must be verified by CT scan. If the foramen and lateral recesses are clear then decompression is not necessary. These patients with predominantly back pain usually have low-grade (grade I) slips and tend to do well with posterolateral fusing through a paraspinal approach.

Herniation at the Level of a Spondylolisthesis

Treatment of a herniation at the level of a spondylolisthesis should include a laminectomy, a discectomy, and a fusion. The Gill fragment should be excised and the level fused with instrumentation. After a thorough discectomy, bone is placed in the disc space (interbody fusion) through an anterior or posterior approach.

Stability/Disc Space Height

Isthmic spondylolisthesis should be considered an unstable condition. A vacuum sign in the disc space, present on a plain x-ray film or on a CT scan, is a strong indicator of instability. All spondylolistheses in patients younger than 18 years are unstable.[12] The older patient, over 60 years of age, with a very narrow disc space and large osteophytes on the anterior vertebral body may have a stable spondylolisthesis. If comparative films of standing and lying show no increase in slip, and there is no vacuum sign on CT or plain x-ray films, it is usually a stable spondylolisthesis.

Surgical intervention in the way of posterior midline decompression (Gill procedure) will sacrifice stability. This type of decompression without fusion is to be avoided in patients with spondylolisthesis. Rapidly progressive, high-grade slips are seen postoperatively in these patients. When decompression is required, segmental stability must be restored either by instrumentation and posterior fusion or by combined anterior and posterior fusions. Posterior interbody fusion can be considered for a one-level fusion at L5 S, only after decompression of the disc if the slip is less than 5 mm.

High-Grade Spondylolisthesis

We have outlined the treatment principles for patients with low-grade (I to II) slips. For more severe slips at L5-S1 (grades III to IV) incorporation of the L4-L5 inner space is essential. As the L5 transverse processes have slipped forward and rotated sagittally, they become less accessible for gaining a successful posterior lateral fusion to the sacrum. Evaluation of the sacral angle is also helpful in these cases. As the angle approaches 50 degrees, the likelihood of obtaining a solid arthrodesis between L5 and the sacrum decreases dramatically. It is in these cases of high-grade spondylolisthesis that extension of the fusion to incorporate the next proximal motion segment is indicated. There are various technical difficulties unique to these high-grade slips that will be discussed further in the section on surgical techniques. The treatment of a grade V spondyloptosis usually involves an anterior vertebrectomy of the dislocated L5 vertebrae. L4 is then fused to the sacrum anteriorly and posteriorly.

It must be emphasized that the surgical treatment of patients with high-grade spondylolisthesis and/or spondyloptosis is exceptionally difficult and should not be undertaken lightly. These patients have distorted anatomy and often malformed pedicles, which makes instrumentation of these segments difficult. The clinical results and fusion rates of the higher-grade slips is often unpredictable. The best results are found in centers that frequently encounter these types of patients.

Surgical Techniques

General Principles

Schoenecker et al.[18] have reported on cauda equina syndromes after in situ fusions for high-grade slips. Possible slip progression intraoperatively with the children under anesthesia was given as an etiology for these deficits. It is therefore recommended that instead of using the spinal frame, the patients be positioned on chest rolls. Lateral chest and abdominal rolls will give better support, minimizing the chances for an intraoperative slip progression. The midline approach was also believed to contribute to instability in these patients. The paraspinal approach should be used to avoid destabilizing these patients. If a midline approach is necessary, instrumentation should be used (see Chapter 86).

Postoperative immobilization is still controversial. Immobilization may consist of a simple lumbosacral corset, a thoracolumbarsacral orthosis (TLSO) with thigh extension, or a mini-hip spica cast. It makes sense to immobilize young patients with in situ fusions to assist them in complying with activity modification for the first 3 months. As the data are still controversial regarding the ability of these orthoses actually to immobilize the lumbosacral junction, we can only comment on the observations that some type of immobilization does slow these children down during the immediate postoperative period. After the first 3 months, the patients may be allowed unprotected ambulation and low activity. They should continue to be prohibited from participation in sports and physical education until a mature fusion mass is noted radiographically.

Foraminal Decompression

Removal of the Gill fragment, which is the lamina, spinous process, and inferior articular process, is only the beginning of a posterior decompression. As noted above, there are multiple structures (annulus, osteophytes, traction spurs, and transverse process of

L5), which can compress the exiting spinal nerve. These nerves are tethered to the vertebral body by ligaments in the midzone to the exit zone of the foramina. These ligaments prevent the nerve from being easily mobilized. Care must be taken to work from proximal in the entrance zone to distal beyond the exit zone. A Cloward chisel can be used to remove heaped-up anulus and osteophytes anterior to the nerve root. Dorsal to the exiting roots, at the level of the spondylolysis, heaped-up inflammatory cartilaginous tissue should also be carefully mobilized off the nerve root. Any remaining part of the pars interarticularis should be removed up to the level of the pedicle.

Reduction

The reduction of a high-grade spondylolisthesis has great biomechanical and esthetic appeal. Reduction with circumferential fusion[15] and reduction with posterior interbody fusion[5,20] have given reasonable rates of fusion, but carry a significant added risk of neurologic injury. L5 vertebrectomy has been used in cases of spondyloptosis.[7] The rationale for reduction is the improved cosmetic appearance and reduction of the deforming forces that may cause progression in the face of a solid fusion.

Reynolds, Banta, and Wiltse[17] reported on 27 patients between the ages of 10 and 24, with high-grade (III to V) spondylolisthesis or spondyloptosis. All patients were treated with an in situ fusion through a paraspinal approach. No attempt was made to reduce the anterolisthesis. There was no significant progression of the slip or slip angles postoperatively. Patients were restricted to bed rest until pain subsided and then restricted to home ambulation for 4 to 6 weeks. After the first month their activity was increased gradually. None of the patients was treated with a corset, orthosis, or cast. These patients had a good cosmetic result with complete resolution of neurologic dysfunction. The cosmetic improvement is thought to occur because the hamstring tightness resolves when the fusion occurs (Fig. 92-9, A to E).

Pars Interarticularis Repair

Direct repair of a pars defect is indicated in selected cases. At the L5-S1 interspace, there is no advantage to isolated repair of the defect compared to a fusion (from the sacral ala to the transverse process of L5). At levels proximal to L5-S1, with a low-grade slip

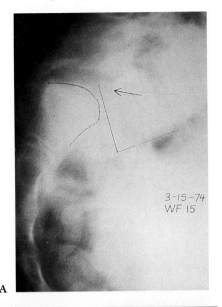

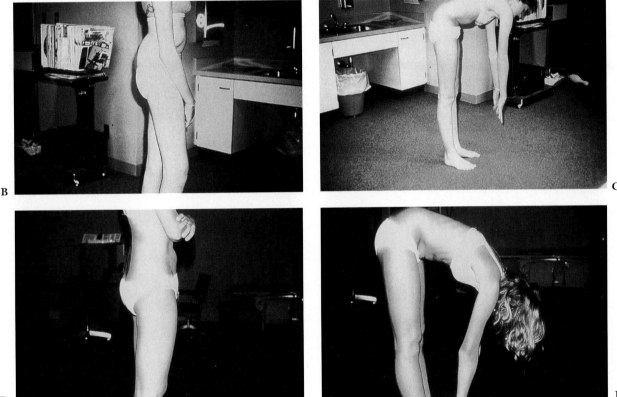

Fig. 92-9

A, Preoperative radiogram of adolescent with high-grade (73%) isthmic spondylolisthesis. **B** and **C,** Clinical examination of same patient, illustrating preoperative cosmetic deformity (flat buttocks and abdominal crease) and hamstring tightness. **D** and **E,** Post-operative clinical examination at 1 year after in situ fusion through paraspinal approach. Note improvement in cosmetic appearance as well as resolution of hamstring tightness.

and normal disc height, repair may be attempted. In patients older than 18 years, a discogram is indicated and should be normal. Various techniques have been used for the repair of the defect, including a 4.5 malleolar screw and hook plate system.[14] The direct repairs have excellent results.[4,8] One of the safest and easiest techniques uses a stainless steel wire. The wire is passed inferior to the spinous process of the vertebra with the spondylosis and up around the transverse processes of the same vertebrae.

A

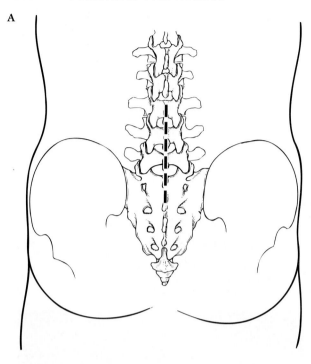

Fig. 92-10

A, Paraspinal muscle splitting approach. Midline incision is made and dorsal lumbar fascia is incised two fingerbreadths (approximately 2 cm) laterally to midline. Blunt finger dissection is carried out, splitting muscle down to level of facet joints.

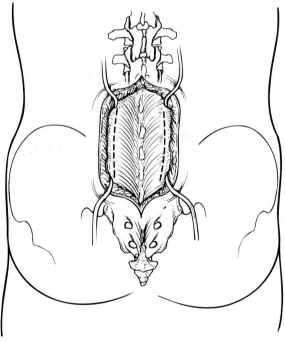

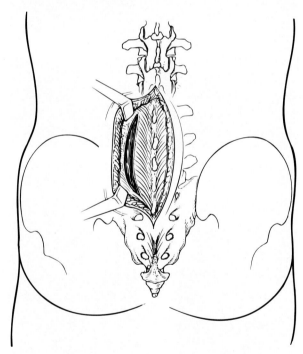

Midline Approach

This dissection has been described in detail in Chapter 91 on Degenerative Spondylolisthesis.

Paraspinal Approach

The paraspinal approach has been well described by Wiltse and Spencer[25] (Fig. 92-10, *A, B,* and *C*). The

sacral ala is the lighthouse to this approach. A slightly longer than usual midline skin incision is made. The skin is undermined laterally and the fascia is incised two fingerbreadths from the midline. There is a natural cleavage plane between the multifidus and longissimus that can be found easily with blunt finger dissection. A finger can reach down and separate the muscles. Near the sacrum some muscle must be cut. The ala of the sacrum and transverse process

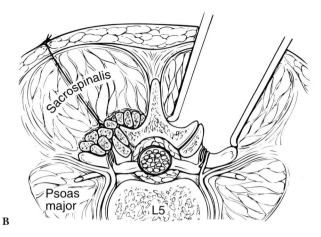

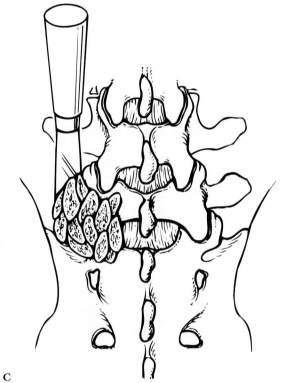

Fig. 92-10, cont'd

B, Two deep Gelpi retractors provide best visualization for this approach. **C,** In situ fusion between sacral ala and transverse process of L5. *(Redrawn from Wiltse LL, Spencer CW: Spine 13:696, 1988.)*

of L5 are palpated. Deep Gelpi retractors are placed for visualization. A generous amount of muscle must also be resected from the areas over the ala, facets, and pars. This allows adequate exposure and creates room for the bone graft. Muscle is then reflected off the transverse process, facets, and pars intraarticularis. Decortication of these structures is then carried out. A flap of bone is cut from the ala and turned up to the transverse process of L5 as described by

Wiltse. Bone graft is added to the areas of decortication and lightly tamped into place. If instrumentation is to be used, the pedicles of L5 and S1 are easily accessible through this approach.

Anterior Interbody Fusions

Indications In cases in which a Gill procedure has been done, a large gap exists between the transverse process of L5 and the sacral ala. An anterior interbody fusion provides additional stability and additional area of bone-to-bone contact for fusion to occur (see Chapter 83). Patients with nonunions or delayed unions posteriorly will benefit from the addition of an anterior interbody fusion. Indications for a primary combined anterior interbody fusion/posterior lateral fusion are seen in the box below. Some patients will demonstrate a significant psychological, social, or economic hardship if resolution of their pre-op symptoms persists after surgery. This is often seen in patients when only a posterior fusion was attempted. Patients referred to us with persistence of symptoms after a posterior-only procedure, will usually come to an anterior interbody fusion as a salvage procedure. A conscious effort can be made to incorporate certain subjective aspects of a patient's life into the decision to recommend a combined anterior and posterior fusion as a primary procedure. In many of our patients, this combined procedure brings about a more reliable and timely resolution of their symptoms.

Indications for Primary Combined Anterior Interbody Fusion/Posterior Lateral Fusion in Patients with Isthmic Spondylolisthesis

1. Very active patients.
2. Obese patients.
3. Patients needing an extensive posterior decompression.
4. Patients in whom an extended delay in resolution of symptoms outweigh the risk of an anterior surgical procedure.
5. Patients with prior failed posterior procedures.
6. Grades II through IV spondylolisthesis.

General Principles The combined anterior and posterior procedure should be performed only by surgeons who have had a great deal of experience with the procedure, at a hospital that has dedicated personnel to expedite the transition from anterior to posterior procedures. Turnover time from skin closure on the first procedure to skin incision on the second procedure is ideally 30 minutes and absolutely no more than 60 minutes. The total time for the combined procedures should be no more than 10 hours.

The anterior procedure is best completed first. By doing the anterior procedure first, the disc space can be opened by raising the kidney rest, allowing better evacuation of the nucleus and optimal placement of the bone graft. By doing the posterior procedure second, the bone screw fixation may be distracted to place compression on the anterior graft.

In patients over 45 years of age, the anterior-posterior procedures should be staged to reduce complications. The time between procedures should be 6 to 12 weeks. In patients below the age of 45, staged procedures are indicated if the patient's physical condition is less than optimal.

In a combined anterior-posterior procedure for high-grade spondylolisthesis, it is best to do the posterior procedure first. The anterior procedure for these cases will frequently use a fibular dowel graft or a bone block from L5 to S1. Attempts to enlarge the foramina by bone screw distraction posteriorly would disrupt or possibly fracture these anterior grafts.

The anterior interbody fusion can be performed by several methods, which differ mainly in the types of interbody grafts used. The type of anterior fusion is determined by the degree of slip, disc space height, and angulation. In low-grade slips (grade I) with parallel end plates at L5 and S1, the disc space can be filled with allograft or autogenous graft. Allografts may be in the form of femoral rings, Crock dowels, or tricortical iliac crest grafts. Autogenous graft can be fashioned from tricortical block grafts or Crock dowels. Crock dowels are especially easy to use when the disc space is narrow. Tricortical iliac crest grafts or femoral rings are easiest to use when the disc space is wide. Femoral dowel allografts should not be used because they tend to resorb.

Traditional anterior interbody fusions are technically difficult or impossible in patients with high-grade slips. As the body of L5 slips forward, it also tends to roll sagittally into a segmental kyphosis, making the disc space inaccessible. There are two techniques to be used in these higher-grade slips. The autogenous fibula can be used as a dowel between L5 and S1. The other method uses an iliac crest graft slotted from L5 to the sacrum. Both methods can be

used simultaneously. Autogenous bone graft seems to be preferable for anterior procedures in patients with high-grade spondylolisthesis.

Techniques

Crock Dowels for Grade I Spondylolisthesis
Preoperative evaluation of disc space size is important. An anterior fusion in a narrow disc space is most easily performed in the manner described by Harry Crock.[3] The round cutting chisels create a space 2 mm smaller than the graft, allowing for a snug fit. Autogenous graft may be taken or commercially prepared allografts can be used. In a larger disc space, a femoral ring can be used. Once the disc is excised initial cuts in the disc space can be made by Crock chisels. Two parallel cuts are made with these chisels and then a high-speed burr or curette is used to fashion a slot for the femoral ring graft. The slot is typically 30 mm wide and 25 to 30 mm deep. Positioning the patient on top of an operating room table kidney rest allows for interoperative disc space opening. A rolled-up towel between the patient's lumbar spine and kidney rest is essential. If a kidney rest is elevated three-quarters of the way before the initial cuts are made, the graft can be made to fit much tighter.

Anterior Interbody Fusion with a Fibula Graft
In higher-grade ($\geq$ II) spondylolisthesis the fibula is used as a stabilizing graft (Fig. 92-11). Technically

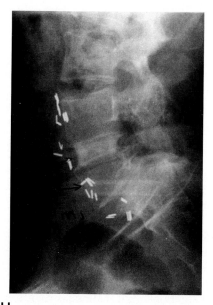

Fig. 92-11

Anterior fibular graft for high-grade spondylolisthesis at L5-S1. There is also anterior interbody fusion at L4-L5 with femoral ring allograft.

it is a straightforward procedure. As L5 is sitting anterior to S1, a Steinmann pin is drilled through the body of L5 across the disc space and into S1. This should be done under fluoroscopy. Care must be taken not to drill too far through the sacrum into the spinal canal. When a patient with a high-grade slip is supine on the operating room table, the direction of drilling is perpendicular to the floor. Starting in the middle of the body of L5, the Steinmann pin is directed through L5 across the disc space and into the sacrum. This is easily confirmed with lateral intraoperative fluoroscopy. Cannulated drills from an anterior cruciate ligament (ACL) reconstruction set are ideal for this procedure. The cannulated drill is placed over the guide pin to drill through L5 and into S1. The size of the cannulated drill is based on the size of the harvested fibula. The sizing rings in the ACL reconstruction set are placed over the fibula once its edges have been rounded. The smallest sizing ring that is easily fit over the fibula is chosen. The drill bit is 1 mm smaller than the sizing ring (usually a 10- or 11-mm drill bit). When drilling over the Steinmann pin a lateral fluoroscopic image should be obtained to be certain that the drill is not advancing the pin through to the sacrum and into the spinal canal. A depth gauge is used to measure the length of the hole, and the fibula is cut to size. The fibula is then placed into the hole and tamped into place. If a small corner of the fibula protrudes, it should be trimmed off so that the end of the fibula is flush with the anterior portion of the body of L5. An autogenous fibula is preferable to an allograft fibula because autogenous graft is less brittle. As the fibula is cortical bone, the autogenous graft appears to incorporate in a more timely and reliable manner than allograft.

The graft is harvested by resecting 6 cm from the middle portion of the fibula. This is a relatively benign procedure, with few sequelae. The fibular ends are rounded with a high-speed burr. The fibula is then sized for width as noted above with the ACL reconstruction sizing rings.

Iliac Crest Graft For high-grade (II through V) spondylolisthesis, an iliac crest graft can be used between L5 and S1. The L5-S1 disc is removed anteriorly. The cartilaginous end plate of L5 is removed. A slot is made in the anterior portion of the sacrum and the inferior body of L5. A tricortical piece of iliac crest is harvested. The iliac crest graft is fashioned to fit into the spot between these two vertebral bodies. A screw can be placed through the graft into the body of L5 or into the body of S1 to hold the graft in position.

Congenital Spondylolisthesis (Type I)

Patients with congenital spondylolisthesis (type IA) (see Fig. 92-1) usually become symptomatic at about 10 years of age. These patients usually have the spondylolisthesis at L5-S1. The facets are hypoplastic and axially oriented. Frequently, more leg pain develops than back pain. They tend to become symptomatic at a smaller percentage of slip as compared with patients with (type II) isthmic spondylolisthesis. As the lamina is intact, the slip causes not only foraminal stenosis but central stenosis. This group of patients has predominantly leg pain, hamstring tightness, or altered gait. If they do have back pain, it is less severe than the leg pain. Surgery should be considered for all these patients because the spondylolisthesis almost never resolves with conservative care. The surgical treatment is an in situ fusion through a paraspinal approach. Expect gradual resolution of hamstring tightness, gait abnormalities, and leg pain.

Patients with congenital spondylolisthesis, type IB, usually become symptomatic around age 30. In this subtype, the facets are hypoplastic and sagittally oriented. This group of patients will also experience more leg pain than back pain. If conservative treatment fails, posterior decompression and fusion are indicated.

Traumatic Spondylolisthesis (Type IV)

Traumatic spondylolisthesis consists of acute traumatic fracture of the pars interarticularis and acute traumatic fracture of the pedicles or facets. This type of spondylolisthesis is quite prone to progress rapidly once a patient is ambulated. If the spondylolisthesis reduces, conservative care, including a one-leg spica cast and bed rest, may produce a good result. The patient would need a cast and bed rest for as long as 3 months, and then be allowed up in the cast for another 3 months. The more accepted manner of treatment is surgical, with a posterior fusion at the involved motion segment.

Postoperative Spondylolisthesis (Type VI)

Extensive, facet-sacrificing midline decompression is the usual cause of this spondylolisthesis. Attention to preserving the facets may decrease this occurrence. All these patients need to undergo fusion. A few patients with this type of spondylolisthesis have a marked increase (up to 50%) of the slip when standing. A great amount of translation may be seen when comparing supine to standing lateral x-ray films. The anterolisthesis may reduce almost anatomically when supine. In these cases, an anterior interbody fusion with anterior plate fixation will hold the spondylolisthesis reduced and graft in place. Depending on the patient's symptoms and the rigidity of the fixation, a posterior fusion with instrumentation may be indicated.

Summary

There are other chapters in this book to which the reader can refer for extensive discussions with regard to specific types of spondylolisthesis and the surgical techniques used to treat them. Chapter 83 on Anterior Lumbar Interbody Fusion and Combined Anteroposterior fusion discusses a common surgical technique for all types of spondylolisthesis, especially high-grade slips. Chapter 85 on Anatomic Strategies of Internal Fixation is applicable because most spondylolisthesis surgery requires internal fixation. Similarly, Chapter 86 deals with Instrumented Posterior Lumbar Surgery. Chapter 91 on Degenerative Spondylolisthesis discusses a subtype of spondylolisthesis referred to in this chapter in the section on Classification. Chapter 110 on Adult Scoliosis also deals to some extent with various forms of spondylolisthesis with its attendant surgical treatment.

References

1. Baker DR, McHolick W: Spondylolysis and spondylolisthesis in children, *J Bone Joint Surg* 38A:933, 1956.
2. Boxall D, Bradford DS, Winter RB, Moe JH: Management of severe spondylolisthesis in childen and adolescents, *J Bone Joint Surg* 61A:479, 1979.
3. Crock HV: Practice of spinal surgery, Wien, 1983, Springer-Verlag.
4. Bradford DS, Iza J: Repair of the defect in spondylolysis or minimal degrees of spondylolisthesis by segmental wire fixation and bone grafting, *Spine* 10:673, 1985.
5. Edwards C: Prospective evaluation of a new method for complete reduction of L5-S1 spondylolisthesis using corrective forces alone, *Orthop Trans* 14:549, 1990.
6. Frederickson BE, Baker D, McHolick WJ, et al.: The natural history of spondylolysis and spondylolisthesis, *J Bone Joint Surg* 66A:699, 1984.

7. Lehmer, Sm, Steffee, Gaines RW: Treatment of L5 S, spondyloptosis with L5 vertebrectomy and reduction of L4 onto the sacrum, *Spine* 19:1916-1925.
8. Hambley M, Lee CK, Gutteling E, Zimmerman MC, et al.: Tension band wiring—bone grafting for spondylolysis and spondylolisthesis: a clinical and biomechanical study, *Spine* 14:455, 1989.
9. Harris IE, Weinstein SL: Long-term follow-up of patients with grade-II and IV spondylolisthesis: treatment with and without posterior fusion, *J Bone Joint Surg* 69A:960, 1987.
10. Herbinaux G: *Traite sur diverse accouchemens laborieux et sur les polypes de la matrice*. Bruxelles, 1782, De Boubers.
11. Kilian JF: *Schilderungen neuer Backenformen und Ihrer Verhalten im Leben*, Mannheim, 1854, Bassermann und Mathy.
12. Lowe RW, Hayes TD, Kaye J, et al.: Standing roentgenograms in spondylolisthesis, *Clin Orthop* 117:80, 1976.
13. Meyerding HW: Spondylolisthesis, *Surg Gynecol Obstet* 54:371, 1932.
14. Morscher E, Gerber B, Fasel J: Surgical treatment of spondylolisthesis by bone grafting and direct stabilization of spondylolysis by means of a hook screw, *Arch Orthop Trauma Surg* 103:175, 1984.
15. O'Brien JP, Mehdian H, Jaffray D: *Reduction of severe lumbosacral spondylolisthesis: a report of 22 cases with follow-up from 4-12 years*. Presented at the International Society for the Study of the Lumbar Spine 15th meeting, June, 1988.
16. Peek RD, Wiltse LL, Reynolds JB, et al.: In situ arthrodesis without decompression for grade III or IV isthmic spondylolisthesis in adults who have severe sciatica, *J Bone Joint Surg* 71A:62, 1989.
17. Reynolds JB, Banta C, Wiltse LL: *High grade spondylolisthesis in the young: a long-term follow-up of in situ fusion*, Presented at the 59th annual meeting of the American Association of Orthopedic Surgeons, Washington, DC, Feb 20-25, 1992.
18. Schoenecker PL, Cole HO, Herring JA: Cauda equina syndrome after in situ arthrodesis for severe spondylolisthesis at the lumbosacral junction, *J Bone Joint Surg* 72A:369, 1990.
19. Sinaki M, Luttness MP, Ilstrup DM, et al.: Lumbar spondylolisthesis: retrospective comparison and three-year follow-up of two conservative treatment programs, *Arch Phys Med Rehab* 70:594, 1989.
20. Steffee AD, Sitkowski DJ: Reduction and stabilization of grade IV spondylolisthesis, *Clin Orthop* 227:82, 1988.
21. Steiner ME, Micheli LJ: Treatment of symptomatic spondylolysis and spondylolisthesis with the modified Boston brace, *Spine* 10:937, 1985.
22. Wiltse LL, Guyer RD, Spencer CW, et al.: Alar transverse process impingement of the L5 spinal nerve: the far-out syndrome, *Spine* 9:31, 1984.
23. Wiltse LL, Newman PH, Macnab I: Classification of spondylolysis and spondylolisthesis, *Clin Orthop* 117:23, 1976.
24. Wiltse LL, Rothman LG: Spondylolisthesis: classification, diagnosis, and natural history, *Semin Spine Surg* 1:78, 1989.

25. Wiltse LL, Spencer CW: New uses and refinements of the paraspinal approach to the lumbar spine, *Spine* 13:696, 1988.

26. Wiltse LL, Widell EH Jr, Jackson DW: Fatigue fracture: the basic lesion in isthmic spondylolisthesis, *J Bone Joint Surg* 57A:17, 1975.

27. Wiltse LL, Winter RB: Terminology and measurement of spondylolisthesis, *J Bone Joint Surg* 65A:768, 1983.

28. Wynne-Davies R, Scott JHS: Inheritance and spondylolisthesis: a radiographic family survey, *J Bone Joint Surg* 61B:301, 1979.

Chapter 93
The Use of Electrical Stimulation for Spinal Fusion
Kevin S. Finnesey

Mechanism of Action

Direct Current Stimulation

    clinical efficacy

    indications

    surgical procedure for implantation in
       bilateral lateral lumbar fusion

Pulsing Electromagnetic Fields

    clinical efficacy

    indications

    applying the device

    advantages and disadvantages

    cost and procedural codes

    safety

Summary

The first documented use of electrical stimulation in orthopedics dates back to the mid-1800s.[15] However, the systematic study of electrical stimulation of osteogenesis began with the work of Yasuda in 1953[36] and Bassett et al. in 1964.[3] The observation by Yasuda of endogenous electrical fields generated in bone under stress led him to hypothesize that the change of internal architecture of bone in response to stress (Wolff's law) is mediated through the action of these fields on the bone remodeling processes. That is, stresses exerted on bones are transformed into electrical energy, which in turn plays a role in the formation of callus. The origin of these stress-generated potentials (SGPs) was originally thought to be due to the piezoelectric properties of bone,[14] but several other mechanisms have also been proposed. It is now believed that the major component of the SGPs is due to streaming potentials, electric fields produced by the movement of fluid through the bone that displaces mobile charges loosely bound to the bones' surfaces.

The early work on the application of electric currents to bone growth involved long-bone nounions and congenital pseudarthrosis of the tibia. Dr. Allen Dwyer[11] of Australia was one of the early investigators in the application of direct current to spinal fusions, showing fusion in 40 of 47 patients, 27 of which were considered "difficult" patients who had multiple-level fusions or in whom fusion had been attempted previously.

Yasuda[36] also demonstrated that electrical signals of a magnitude comparable to those of SGPs applied externally, without the application of stress, could result in cellular responses mimicking those that occur during fracture healing and remodeling. New bone formation was stimulated at the electronegative cathode with bone resorption occurring at the positive anode. Subsequently, hundreds of cellular and animal studies demonstrated the ability of exogenous electric fields to modify the cellular processes involved in bone growth and fracture repair. These studies have led to the development of several devices now used clinically as an accepted therapeutic adjunct for the treatment of pseudarthrosis of long bones and to enhance the success rate of spinal fusions. Two such devices that will be highlighted in this chapter include the SpF Spinal Fusion Stimulator (EBI Medical Systems, Inc., Parsippany, NJ), and the Spinal-Stim PEMF Spinal Fusion System Model 8500 (American Medical Electronics, Inc., Richardson, TX), an externally worn device.

Three different techniques have been employed to generate electric fields in tissue: (1) direct current stimulation via implanted electrodes, (2) Inductively coupled electric fields induced from time-varying magnetic fields, and (3) Capacitatively coupled fields from external electrodes.[4] All three techniques produce electric fields at the fracture or fusion site on the order of 10 mV/cm, comparable to endogenous electric fields. At present, only inductively coupled and direct current stimulation devices are FDA approved and commercially available for use in lumbar spinal fusions.

Mechanism of Action

Despite intense research over the past 30 years a complete understanding of the mechanism by which cells detect and respond to electromagnetic fields is lacking. It has been demonstrated that when bone is stressed it develops an electric potential proportional to the applied stress; the bone generates an electric current when it is mechanically deformed. This electrical field in turn has an effect on cellular processes. Several theories have been proposed to account for the field-cell coupling but none of these have gained widespread acceptance by the scientific community.[1,23-25,29,30]

In the case of direct current stimulation, on the other hand, a large body of evidence suggests that the osteogenic response is, at least in part, a consequence of the Faradic reactions that occur at the cathode and may have little to do with the electrical field at all.

Direct Current Stimulation

During direct current stimulation, transfer of charge from the electrode into extracellular fluid occurs via a Faradic reaction in which chemical reactants are reduced at the cathode and oxidized at the anode. The nature of the reactants consumed and products generated depends on the electrode potentials and the chemical composition of the fluid in the vicinity of the electrodes. The concentration of the reactants consumed is decreased in the vicinity of the electrode, while the concentration of products is increased. The current being passed determines the rates of these reactions and consequently the degree to which the chemical environment around the electrodes is altered.

The primary reaction that occurs at the cathode under conditions that stimulate bone formation is one in which O_2 is consumed and OH^- is generated as described by the following reaction:

$$O_2 + 2H_2O + 4e^- \text{ yields } 4OH^-$$

Changes in O_2 and OH^- as predicted from this reaction have been measured in vitro[6] and in an in vivo rabbit medullary canal model.[2] Brighton and Friedenberg[7] proposed that the significant reduction of O_2 and increase in pH near the cathode as a result of this reaction are the osteogenic stimuli. This hypothesis is supported by several studies demonstrating that bone growth is optimal at low O_2 and elevated pH,[8] osteoblast metabolism is primarily anaerobic,[5] osteoclast activity is drastically reduced at elevated pH,[32] and the stimulation of new bone formation by direct current is more closely related to the decrease in oxygen tension than to the magnitude of the electric field.[2]

Clinical Efficacy

Animal Studies

In 1984 a double-blind study was performed by Nerubay et al.[28] on 30 1-month-old pigs that had spinal fusion performed at L5-L6. A direct current stimulator was implanted in all 30 pigs, with half the stimulators active and the other half inactive and used as controls. The pigs were further divided into one group that was killed at 1 month and another at 2 months. The results were evaluated by radiographic and histologic examination. A scoring system was devised based on the amount of graft consolidation present. The analysis consisted of active versus nonactive bone growth stimulators in the 1-month and 2-month groups and for all the pigs in the study. The 1-month group results did not allow statistical evaluation due to the sample size (n = 10). The 2-month group (n = 20) revealed a statistically significant increase in fusion score in the active bone growth stimulator group. A comparison of all the study groups showed a statistically significant increase in the 2-month group. The authors concluded that there was an increase of osteoblastic activity with bone formation in the group of animals that underwent a spinal fusion with concomitant electrical stimulation.

Kahanovitz and Arnoczky[16-18] reported their study of direct current stimulation in canine lumbar spinal fusions. Twelve mongrel dogs had posterior fusions bilaterally at L1-L2 and L4-L5. A 2-cm titanium electrode was placed through each facet. Half the electrodes were functional, while the others were identical but nonfunctional and served as controls. Two animals were killed at 2 and 4 weeks, and four animals were killed at 6 and 12 weeks postoperatively. Fusion success was determined by high-resolution x-ray studies and routine histology. Although there was little difference in the 2-, 4-, and 6-week

specimens, by 12 weeks all of the stimulated facet joints showed radiographic and histologic evidence of bone fusion, while none of the controls demonstrated evidence of osseous bridging at the fusion site. The authors concluded that direct current electrical stimulation appears to enhance the fusion success rate in the canine lumbar spine.

Clinical Studies

The first use of a direct current stimulator in a human spine was reported by Dwyer and Wickham in 1974.[11] Fusion was achieved in 40 of 47 patients (85%). Twenty-seven of these patients were difficult, requiring multiple-level fusions and having had a high incidence of prevous surgical procedures.

In 1982 a nonrandom multicenter study by Kane et al.[21] examining the results of direct current stimulation in 84 patients revealed a 91% fusion success rate. Over half the patients had a preoperative diagnosis of pseudarthrosis. A control group of age- and sex-matched patients had a fusion success rate of 81%. This control group had a much lower incidence of previous fusion surgery (19.5% vs. 56.1%), so the increase in the rate of fusion in the stimulated group was greater than one would expect. To gather further evidence and address the issues of investigator differences, a randomized prospective controlled trial was designed.[20] The objective of this clinical trial was to test whether the incidence of successful spinal fusion was higher when the direct current implantable stimulator was used as opposed to surgery alone. All patients admitted to this trial by the clinical investigator were in one or more of the following "difficult to fuse" categories:

1. One or more previous failed fusion attempts,
2. Grade II or worse spondylolisthesis,
3. Extensive bone grafting necessary for a multiple-level fusion, or
4. Other high-risk factors for failure of fusion, including gross obesity.

Each patient was randomized to undergo spine fusion surgery either with or without bone growth stimulator. The measurement of success was based on radiographic fusion. Flexion and extension lateral films were used to evaluate fusion; however, in certain circumstances a pseudarthrosis was confirmed operatively (in a refusion procedure). When it was of value or advantageous to verify fusion, other techniques, such as oblique stress films or additional anteroposterior views, were used. The radiographic assessment was confirmed by an independent radiologist to ensure a lack of investigator bias. Ninety-nine patients were entered into the trial, of which 63 were from investigators meeting the criterion of at least four patients (2 treated and 2 control). Of the 63 patients, 59 were available for follow-up, from seven investigators. There were 28 control patients and 31 stimulated patients. At 18 months after surgery, successful fusion was achieved in 25 of 31 treatment patients (81%) as compared with 15 of 28 control patients (54%). This result was statistically significant. Of the 36 patients from investigators not meeting the randomization criteria, 16 treated patients were available for analysis. Thirteen of the 16 (81%) had successful fusions, supporting a success rate seen in the adequately randomized group. In addition to the random study, a separate group of investigators participated in a nonrandom study to collect a broader base of safety and effectiveness data. The protocol for this open study was otherwise identical to the randomized study. Successful fusion was achieved in 108 of the 116 patients (93%). The poorest result was seen in the group recognized as having the highest risk, the previous failed fusion group, with success in 26 of 30 patients (87%).

Based on these results from the randomized and nonrandomized studies, the Food and Drug Administration approved the implantable direct current bone growth stimulator as "a spinal fusion adjunct to increase the probability of fusion success."[13]

In 1988, a technique for using the implantable direct current stimulator in anterior and posterior lumbar interbody fusion procedures was developed by Meril.[26] The modified Crock technique was used with tricortical iliac or patellar allograft material. One hundred fifty-six patients were followed prospectively. Fusion success was measured by multiplanar CT scan. The fusion success rate at an average of 21 months follow-up was 91% in the 98 patients without concomitant internal fixation.

Indications

The indications for use of the device vary among surgeons but primarily include patients with previous failed spine fusion or with established pseudarthrosis of a previous fusion; patients with high-degree spondylolisthesis; patients with metabolic bone disease that would make fusion difficult, including osteoporosis; patients who are heavy smokers; patients who are obese; and patients who require extensive removal of posterior elements to obtain an adequate decompression.

Surgical Procedure for Implantation in Bilateral Lateral Lumbar Fusion

The implantation of the SpF 2T device (EBI Medical Systems, Inc., Parsippany, NJ) is described.[35] This device may be used for fusions with and without lumbar instrumentation. It is critical that the surgical procedure be followed impeccably for the device to work properly.

Technique

The patient is placed prone on the operating table with chest rolls or knee chest frame as chosen by the operating surgeon. A standard midline longitudinal incision is made. The spinous processes, laminae, facets, and transverse processes are exposed in the routine fashion. Alternatively, a lateral Wiltse-type approach may be used, directly exposing the transverse processes. The facet joints, pars, and transverse processes are decorticated in the standard fashion. Bone graft is obtained from the posterior iliac crest through a separate fascial incision in the routine manner. Cortical cancellous strips of bone are obtained.

Prior to placement of the implant it is important to check the battery with the implant tester. To activate the stimulator before implantation, touch one of the two cathodes to the platinized circular anode on one side of the generator. Place the tester in a sterile bag and hold it within $1\frac{1}{2}$ in. of the SpF-2T generator. The reading should display: "Pre-implant OK." This can be checked on follow-up visits to be sure the device is still functioning.

The next step is implantation of the device. It is very important if internal fixation is used that the wires do not touch any of the internal fixation implants. After implantation of the device, electrocautery should not be used, so great care must be made to obtain adequate hemostasis prior to implantation of the device. The bone stimulator wires should be bent into a zig-zag pattern and must touch each transverse process as well as the ala of the sacrum. Spare titanium of the cathode should be flat against the transverse processes and not be allowed to bend. The plastic-covered lead must reach the edge of the fusion site, and the cathode must be completely within the fusion mass (Fig. 93-1). Place the connector at the proximal end of the fusion mass. The bone graft material is then tightly packed over the wire, which is in turn touching the transverse processes.

After placement of the leads the generator is placed subcutaneously in a pouch between the fas-

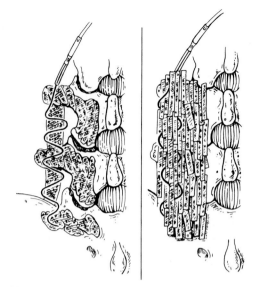

Fig. 93-1

Placement of direct current stimulator in fusion area. (*Courtesy EBI Medical Systems, Inc., Parsippany, NJ.*)

cia and the skin. The wound is then closed over drains. It is important that the generator battery is in soft tissue and not against bone. The anode area of the case should be 8 to 10 cm from the cathode.

The battery life is approximately 6 months. It can be checked with the implant tester on follow-up visits to check the function of the stimulator. When the battery is no longer working the battery can be removed on an outpatient basis under local anesthesia. The battery itself is removed, but it is unnecessary to remove the cathode wires.

Costs and Procedural Codes

Although there is some considerable cost to the use of these implants, the overall benefits can be considerable if one considers the cost of the necessity of a repeat lumbar fusion, hospitalization, etc. The cost of the SpF-2T device is $2,950. This is the exact same cost for all of the other implants, including the four-lead devices and others. The cost of implantation of the device is $1,000 (CPT-4 code is 20975); the cost of deep explantation of the device is $600 (CPT-4 code, 20680).

Pulsing Electromagnetic Fields

The second method used to deliver electric current to the fusion area involves the application of pulsing electromagnetic fields (PEMF) to the fusion site from a device containing electromagnetic coils placed externally.

Clinical Efficacy

Animal Studies

In 1964 Bassett et al.[3] demonstrated the effectiveness of PEMFs for treating nonunions of the tibia and femur in dogs. The effects of PEMFs on canine lumbar spine fusion were examined by Kahanovitz et al. in 1984.[17] The fusions were performed posteriorly and augmented with Harrington-type internal fixation. The histologic and radiologic studies showed an accelerated osteogenic response in the stimulated animals at 6 and 9 weeks. At 12 weeks, however, both the stimulated and nonstimulated groups had solid fusion and were indistinguishable.

In a more recent study, Kahanovitz et al.[19] evaluated the efficacy of PEMF on posterior facet fusions in 24 dogs. Eight dogs received PEMF for 30 minutes a day, another eight animals received 60 min/day. The last eight received no stimulation. When the animals were killed at 6 and 12 weeks, no statistical difference was found between the stimulated animals and controls. Although this appears significant, the stimulator periods are short in this study. The recommended stimulation time for the PEMF stimulator (Spinal-Stim, American Medical Electronics, Richardson, TX) is 4 hours.

Extensive studies have been done investigating the mechanism of action of how this electrical energy functions at the cellular level. Processes that may be altered by PEMFs include vascularization, synthesis of cartilage matrix, calcification in bone, and protein synthesis.

Clinical Studies

In 1985 Simmons[33] reported 13 patients with failed posterior lumbar interbody fusions treated with PEMFs. The average time since the last surgical fusion attempt was 40 months. These patients were treated with the external device only, a completely noninvasive treatment obviating the need for any hospitalization or surgical procedures and involving no morbidity. The device was worn by the patients for 8 to 10 hours per day. The total treatment period was 12 months. Simmons found that there was a "significant increase in bone formation in 85% (11 of 13) of the patients monitored." There was solid body-to-body fusion in 77% (10 of 13). Brodsky and Kahlil[9] reported a 36% fusion success rate in 30 patients with established lumbar spinal pseudarthrosis treated with PEMFs.

In 1990, Mooney[27] conducted a randomized double-blind prospective study of PEMFs for interbody fusions on 195 patients. There were 98 patients in the active group and 97 patients in the placebo group. Interbody fusions were done from either the anterior or the posterior approach. Patients with severe osteoporosis, inflammatory conditions of the spine, trauma, diabetes, renal dysfunction, or cancer were excluded from the study. The patients wore the Spinal-Stim device (American Medical Electronics, Richardson, TX) for at least 8 hours per day. The patients were not aware of whether the device was functional. When the grafts were reviewed by blinded radiographic evaluation, 92.2% of the patients receiving the active devices had a solid fusion. The placebo group had a fusion rate of 67.9%. This is a statistically significant difference. Factors including sex, age, level of the fusion, number of grafts, graft type, and internal fixation made no difference. Smoking was not an important factor. This study did not address a high number of patients with failed fusions. There was only one such patient in each group, and the patient in the active group with the failed fusion did not have fusion.

The use of PEMF in pseudarthrosis was examined by Lee[22] in 1989 in a group of 126 patients in a multicenter study. Sixty-seven percent of consistent users of the device had a successful fusion, whereas inconsistent users only had a 19.2% success rate.

It has been shown that smoking is a cause of symptomatic pseudarthrosis in spine fusion. Brown et al.[10] conducted a retrospective study looking at 50 smokers and 50 nonsmokers undergoing two-level lumbar fusions. He found a 40% pseudarthrosis rate in smokers versus an 8% pseudarthrosis rate in nonsmokers. He contributed the cause of the pseudarthrosis to lower pO^2 level and O^2 saturation in the arterial blood gasses of smokers. This in turn leads to inadequate oxygen levels in the blood flow to the graft. In Lee's study[22] nonstimulated smokers had a union rate of 60%, but PEMF-stimulated smokers had an 88.9% fusion rate. It was thought that PEMF may play a role in counteracting the effects of cigarette smoke on blood flow and oxygenation in the fusion area.

In 1989 Simmons et al.[34] participated in the same multicenter open trial in order to determine:

1. The fusion rates in patients receiving PEMF in conjunction with lumbar fusion surgery.

2. The effectiveness of this device with established nonunions.

The Spinal-Stim device again was used. Patients with cardiac pacemakers (a contraindication to use of the Spinal-Stim device), spinal trauma, spondylitis, Paget's disease, severe osteoporosis, metastatic cancer, diabetes mellitus, and renal dysfunction were excluded from the study. There were 190 patients in the study. Prognostic variables investigated were device use, sex, age, smoking, prior attempts at fusion, number of levels fused, surgical technique, graft material, internal fixation, and time since surgery. Fusion occurred in 76.7% of the patients who used the device consistently. Patients with inconsistent use (use for less than 3 months and less than 2 hours per day) had a fusion rate of 44.4%. Of interest in this part of the study is that smokers actually had a higher fusion rate than nonsmokers using PEMFs. The number of levels to be fused did not significantly affect the fusion rate. The conclusion from this study was that as a surgical adjunct and in nonoperative salvage, use of the Spinal-Stim consistently increased fusion rates. Age, sex, smoking, number of levels fused, and prior fusion attempts had no significant impact on fusion rates. Of interest is that internal fixation appeared to lower the success rate in multiple-level fusions.

Indications

The indications for applying the PEMF device are similar to those for the direct current stimulation device.*

Applying the Device

The Spinal-Stim device (Fig. 93-2) is a portable, lightweight device. It is applied just above waist level and has a strap for ease of use. Patients are able to work and participate in various recreational activities while wearing the device.

Advantages and Disadvantages

The obvious benefit for the Spinal-Stim device is that the treatment is not invasive and obviates the need for hospitalization and has no morbidity rate. An obvious disadvantage is that some patients may find it somewhat bulky and cumbersome. Compliance is also an issue and has been a problem for some patients as well, although compliance is not an issue

*Other uses for PEMF that have been investigated include use in osteonecrosis of the hip, infection, rotator cuff tendinitis of the shoulder, and spondylolysis.

with implanted direct current devices. The implantable devices, however, do require surgical procedures for implantation and removal. The Spinal-Stim device has a built-in patient compliance monitor that can be checked regularly with a printout. The system is recommended to be used for a minimum of 4 hours per day with a 12-week minimum treatment time. Two-hour-per-day use is recommended in some instances.

Cost and Procedural Codes

The device is rented by the company with a one-time flat fee, which is $4,850 at the time of this writing. This is apparently reimbursed by most insurance carriers. The CPT-4 code for application and monitoring of this device is 20974 with a physician fee of $500 to $700 for monitoring.

Safety

Issues have been raised regarding the safety of electromagnetic fields (EMFs).[31] There have been con-

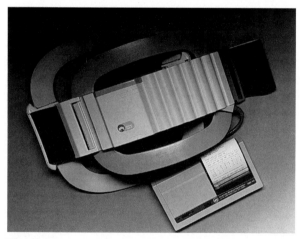

Fig. 93-2

Spinal-Stim™ device. (*Courtesy American Medical Electronics, Richardson, TX.*)

cerns by the public regarding whether harmful effects can result from EMFs, including cancer and other medical disorders. There is a spectrum of EMFs (Fig. 93-3) starting at the low end with computer displays and power levels on the order of 60 Hertz, to radiowaves (10/10 Hertz) to x-rays (10/20 Hertz). It is important to stress that there is a difference between EMFs and PEMFs. PEMFs are nonionizing, low-energy, time-varying magnetic fields found at the lower end of the electromagnetic spectrum. They are within the normal range found in living systems. PEMFs have been in clinical use for 20 years and to date no adverse long-term effects have been observed.[31]

Summary

Electrical stimulation of spinal fusions as presented in this chapter are in common use by many spine specialists today. There are several encouraging clinical studies. The recommended methods of using these technologies are changing, as are the surgical methods of performing spinal fusions.

The current failure rate in lumbar fusions for all patients is in the range of 20%.[12] Patients at a higher risk of failure include smokers,[10] obese patients, patients who have undergone multiple surgeries, patients with metabolic bone disease, patients with multiple level spondylolisthesis, and others. It is reasonable to add electrical stimulation to these high-risk patients. If another surgical procedure is contemplated in these patients, and electrical stimulation is to be used, a choice between implantable and externally worn devices needs to be made. Each has its own distinct advantages and disadvantages. Implantable stimulators have the advantage of automatic compliance and direct application of current to the fusion area. However, there is a disadvantage of a second surgical procedure for removal of the implant, although this is a simple procedure. Clearly,

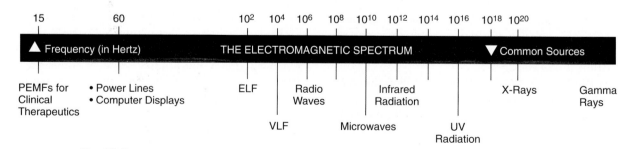

Fig. 93-3

PEMFs are at lower end of electromagnetic spectrum (*From* AME Today, *November 1992. American Medical Electronics, Richardson, TX.*)

more attention has been given to direct current stimulation in the literature.[19]

The externally worn PEMF devices have the advantage of being noninvasive, obviating the cost and morbidity of a surgical procedure and perhaps even avoiding the need for a repeat attempt at fusion in pseudarthrosis. The disadvantage with these devices is the issue of noncompliance. The usefulness of PEMF in interbody fusions is well documented in the literature.[27,33,34] The efficacy in bilateral lateral posterior fusions is less clear. PEMF also may play a role in counteracting the deleterious effect of smoking in lumbar fusion. Dr. Lee points out that in patients who have a pseudarthrosis who have undergone one or more previous surgeries and have multiple psychosocial behavioral problems, external electrical stimulation can be a much more attractive option than another extensive surgical procedure.

There is much to be gained and little to be lost from application of this technology to established pseudarthroses or in patients with risk factors for failure who are undergoing spinal fusions.

Lastly, as Kane et al.[21] have pointed out, these devices are designed as an adjunct to spinal fusion, not as a substitute for it. When performing a fusion, the surgeon must use meticulous technique in decortication, grafting, and placement of internal fixation when indicated.

References

1. Adair RK: Constraints on biologic effects of weak extremely-low-frequency electromagnetic fields, *Physiol Rev* 43:1039, 1980.
2. Baranowski TJ, Black J, Brighton CT: Microenvironmental changes and electrodic potentials associated with electrical stimulation of osteogenesis by direct current, *Trans Orthop Res Soc* 8:258, 1983.
3. Bassett CAL, Pawluk RJ, Becker RO: Effects of electric current on bone in vivo, *Nature* 204:652, 1964.
4. Black J: *Electrical stimulation: its role in growth, repair and remodeling of the musculoskeletal system,* New York, 1987, Praeger.
5. Borle AB, Nichols N, Nichols G: Metabolic studies of bone in vitro, *J Biol Chem* 235:1206, 1960.
6. Brighton CT, Adler S, Black J, et al.: Catholic oxygen consumption and electrically induced osteogenesis, *Clin Orthop Relat Res* 107:277, 1980.
7. Brighton CT, Friedenberg ZB: Electrical stimulation and oxygen tension, *Ann N Y Acad Sci* 238:314, 1974.
8. Brighton CT, Ray RD, Soble L, Keuttner KE: In vitro epiphyseal plate growth in various oxygen tensions, *J Bone Joint Surg* 51A:1383, 1969.
9. Brodsky AE, Kahlil MA: *Preliminary report on the use of the EBI pulsing electromagnetic field therapy for the treatment of pseudarthrosis of lumbar spine fusion,* Presented at the North American Spine Society meeting, Beoff, Canada, June 28, 1987.
10. Brown CW, Orme TJ, Richardson HD: The rate of pseudarthrosis (surgical non-union) in patients who are smokers and patients who are nonsmokers: a comparison study, *Spine* 2:942, 1986.
11. Dwyer AF, Wickham GG: Direct current stimulation in spinal fusion, *Med J Aust* 1:73, 1974.
12. Evans JH, Gilmore KC, O'Brien JP: How does fusion relieve low back pain? *Orthop Trans* 6:32, 1982.
13. Food and Drug Administration: *Summary of safety and effectiveness: Osteostim HS11 implantable bone growth stimulator.* Silver Spring, MD, 1987, Office of Device Evaluation.
14. Fukada E, Yasuda I: On the piezoelectric effect of bone, *J Psysiol Soc Jpn* 12:1158, 1957.
15. Hartshorne EM: On the causes and treatment of pseudarthrosis and especially of that form of it sometimes called supranumery joint, *Am J Med Sci* 1:121, 1841.
16. Kahanovitz N: In Rothman RH, Simeone FA, editors: *The spine,* ed 3, Philadelphia, 1992, W.B. Saunders Co.
17. Kahanovitz N, Arnoczky S, Hulse D, Shires P: The effect of postoperative electromagnetic pulsing on canine posterior spinal fusions, *Spine* 9:273, 1984.
18. Kahanovitz N, Arnoczky SP: The efficacy of direct current electrical stimulation to enhance canine spinal fusions, *Clin Orthop* 251:295-299, Feb. 1, 1990.
19. Kahanovitz N, Arnoczky S, Nemzek J, Shores A: The effect of electromagnetic pulsing on posterior lumbar spinal fusions in dogs, *Spine* 19:705, 1994.
20. Kane WJ: Direct current electrical bone growth stimulation for spinal fusions, *Spine* 13:363, 1988.
21. Kane WJ, Lunceford EM, Dyer AR: An analysis of the utility of implantable bone growth simulators in lumbar fusions, *Orthop Trans* 6:464, 1982.
22. Lee K: *Clinical investigation of the spinal stim system,* Presented at the annual meeting of the American Association of Orthopedic Surgeons, Las Vegas, NV, 1989.
23. Liboff AR, Mcleod BR: Kinetics of channelized membrane ions in magnetic fields, *Bioelectromagnetics* 9:39, 1988.
24. McLauchlan KA, Steiner UE: The spin-correlated radical pair as a reaction intermediate, *Mol Phys* 73:241, 1991.
25. Mcleod K, Rubin C: The role of polarization forces in mediating the interaction of low frequency electric fields with living tissues. In Blank M, editor: *Electricity and magnetism in biology and medicine,* San Francisco, 1992, San Francisco Press.
26. Meril AJ: *Tri-cortical and patellar allograft with a modified Crock technique in anterior and posterior direct current stimulation,* Presented at North American Spine Society meeting, San Diego, CA, 10-1–10-3, 1993.
27. Mooney V: A randomized double-blind prospective study of the efficacy of pulsed electromagnetic fields for interbody lumbar fusions, *Spine* 15:708, 1990.
28. Nerubay J, Marganit B, Bubin JJ, et al.: Stimulation of bone formation by electrical current on spinal fusion, *Spine* 11:167, 1986.
29. Pilla AA, Nasser PR, Kaufman JJ: The sensitivity of cells and tissues to weak electromagnetic fields. In Allen MJ, et al., editors: *Charge and field effects in biosystems III,* Boston, 1991, Birkhauser.

30. Polk C: Dosimetry of extremely-low-frequency magnetic fields, *Bioelectromagnetics* Suppl:209, 1993.

31. Reddy J: *Electromagnetic fields: are they harmful?* American Medical Electronics AME Today (in-house publication), 1993.

32. Shibutani T, Heersche J: Effect of medium pH on osteoclast activity and osteoclast formation in cultures and dispersed rabbit osteoclasts, *J Bone Miner Res* 8:331, 1993.

33. Simmons JW: Treatment of failed posterior lumbar interbody fusions (PLIF) of the spine with pulsing electromagnetic fields, *Clin Orthop* 183:127, 1985.

34. Simmons JW, Hayes MA, Cristensen KD, et al.: *The effect of postoperative pulsing on lumbar fusion: an open trial phase study,* Presented at North American Spine Society meeting, Quebec, Canada, June 29, 1989.

35. Wood GW: *Implantable monitorable spinal fusion stimulator, 2 lead telemetry model: Procedure for use of growth stimulator in bilateral lateral lumbar fusion,* Memphis, TN, 1990, Campbell Clinic Inc.

36. Yasuda I: Fundamental aspects of fracture treatment, *J Kyoto Med Soc* 4:395, 1953.

Section 4
Open Surgery of the Cervical Spine

94 Clinical Anatomy of the
    Cervical Spine

    Carson D. Schneck

95 Surgical Approaches to the
    Cervical Spine

    William Richardson
    Robert J. Spinner

96 Degenerative Disc Disease of the
    Cervical Spine: Degenerative
    Cascade and the Anterior Approach

    Steven C. Poletti
    John A. Handal

97 Degenerative Disc Disease of the
    Cervical Spine: Posterior Approach

    F. Todd Wetzel

98 Cervical Spondylotic Radiculopathy
    and Myelopathy: Anterior Approach
    and Pathology

    Sanford E. Emery

99 Cervical Spondylotic Radiculopathy
    and Myelopathy: Posterior Approach

    Richard S. Brower
    Harry N. Herkowitz

100 Cervical Fusions: Arthrodesis and
    Osteosynthesis of the Cervical Spine

    Henrik Mike-Mayer
    Howard B. Cotler
    Stanley D. Gertzbein

101 Anterior Instrumentation of the
    Cervical Spine

    Patrick J. Connolly
    Hansen A. Yuan

102 Sports Injuries of the Head and
    Cervical Spine

    F. Todd Wetzel
    Gregory A. Hanks
    P. Dean Cummings

Chapter 94
Clinical Anatomy of the Cervical Spine
Carson D. Schneck

Developmental Anatomy of the Cervical Spine

early development
prenatal development of the lower five cervical vertebrae
prenatal development of the occiput, atlas, and axis
postnatal development
congenital abnormalities

The Occiput-Atlas-Axis Complex

atlas
axis
atlantooccipital joints
atlantoaxial joints

Lower Cervical Spine

osteology
lower cervical spine intervertebral joints

Neural Relationships

Musculature of the Cervical Spine

anterior musculature
posterior musculature

Anterior Relationships of the Cervical Spine

A thorough three-dimensional appreciation of the bony, ligamentous, muscular, neural, and vascular relationships of the cervical spine complex provides insights into normal cervical spine function, the pathomechanics of cervical disorders, and the diagnosis and treatment of neck pain.

Developmental Anatomy of the Cervical Spine

Early Development

During the third week of development the mesoderm on either side of the neural tube and notochord becomes aggregated into a series of mesodermal blocks called "somites" (Fig. 94-1, *A*).[16,22] Shortly after its formation each somite becomes differentiated into a ventromedial part, the sclerotome, and a dorsolateral part, the dermatomyotome (Fig. 94-1, *B*). During the fourth week of development the sclerotomal cells shift their position to surround the neural tube and notochord, where they will form the vertebrae, ribs, and spinal ligaments (Fig. 94-1, *C*). The myotomal portion of the dermatomyotome will form the segmental musculature of the back and anterolateral body wall. The dermatomal portion of the dermatomyotome contributes to the dermis of posterior scalp, neck, and trunk.

Initially, each sclerotome consists of loosely aggregated cells cranially and densely packed cells caudally (Fig. 94-2, *A*). The sclerotomes are separated by very loosely organized intersclerotomal mesenchymal tissue into which the segmental arteries and veins grow. As each pair of sclerotomes surrounds the notochord and neural canal to form, respectively, the vertebral body and vertebral arch, a resegmentation occurs (Fig. 94-2, *B*). The condensed caudal half of each sclerotome fuses with the looser cranial half of the adjacent somite to form the definitive precartilaginous mesenchymal vertebra with the intersegmental mesenchyme becoming incorporated into the precartilaginous vertebral body. Hence, the definitive vertebral body becomes intersegmental in position (Fig. 94-2, *C*). The mesenchymal tissue that occupies the interval between two precartilaginous vertebral bodies forms the annulus fibrosus of the intervertebral disc. Where the notochord is surrounded by the developing vertebral bodies it degenerates and disappears. The portion of the notochord between the vertebral bodies becomes the embryonal nucleus pulposus.

The resegmentation of the sclerotomes into the definitive precartilaginous vertebrae causes the myotomes to bridge over the intervertebral discs, giv-

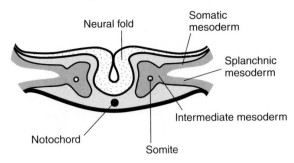

A

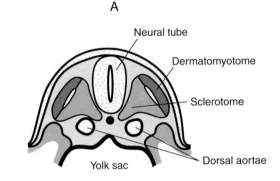

B

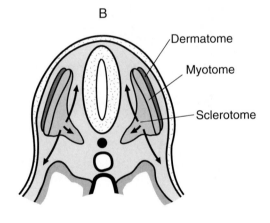

C

Fig. 94-1

Transverse sections of the embryo demonstrating the early differentiation of somites. **A,** Early-3-week embryo displaying somites forming on either side of developing neural tube and notochord. **B,** Late-3-week embryo showing division of somite into sclerotome and dermatomyotome portions. **C,** 4-week embryo demonstrating the migration of the sclerotomal cells about neural tube and notochord. *(Modified from Moore KL: The developing human, Philadelphia, 1982, WB Saunders, p 344.)*

ing the myotomes the ability to move the spine (Fig. 94-2, *C*). The developing segmental spinal nerves emerge behind the intervertebral discs to enter the

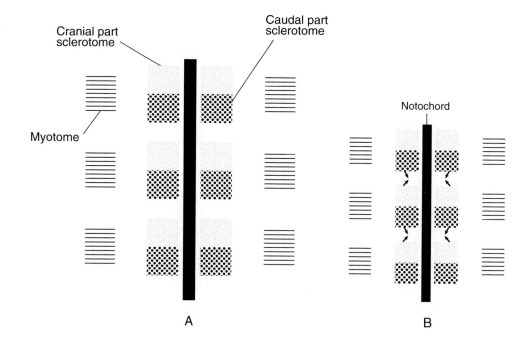

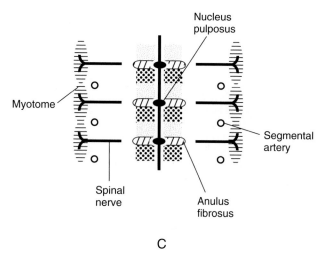

Fig. 94-2

Schematic representation of resegmentation of sclerotomes to form definitive vertebral bodies and their relationship to myotomes, spinal nerves, segmental arteries, and development of intervertebral disc. **A,** Loose cranial and dense caudal parts of sclerotome aligned opposite myotome. **B,** Caudal migration of dense caudal half of each sclerotome and cranial migration of loose cranial half of each sclerotome. **C,** Fused caudal and cranial halves of each sclerotome that form resegmented definitive vertebral body now located between mytomic segments. It also demonstrates formation of intervertebral disc from both interbody mesenchyme and notochord. Spinal nerves emerge behind discs, while intersegmental arteries are situated between fusing myotomes opposite middle of vertebral bodies. *(Modified from Sherk HH, Parke WE: Developing Anatomy. In The Cervical Spine Society Editorial sub-committee: The cervical spine. Philadelphia, 1983, JB Lippincott Co., p 2.)*

bridging myotomes. The intersegmental vessels come to be situated on either side of the vertebral bodies and the basivertebral veins will emerge from the middle of the posterior aspect of vertebral bodies.

The splittings and subsequent fusions of the sclerotomes explain two difficult questions: (1) How did the original eight cervical somites develop into seven cervical vertebrae? and (2) How are the eight cervical spinal nerves related to these seven cervical vertebrae?[14] The cranial half of the first cervical sclerotome fuses with the caudal portion of the fourth occipital somite to help form the basilar portion of the occipital bone (Fig. 94-3). Then the caudal half of the first cervical sclerotome fuses with the cranial half of the second cervical sclerotome to form the

first cervical vertebra. The same fusions are repeated down the length of the cervical spine, with the eighth cervical sclerotome contributing its cranial half to the seventh cervical vertebra and its caudal half to the first thoracic vertebra. Hence, half a sclerotome is lost from the top and bottom of the cervical spine, thereby reducing the eight cervical sclerotomes to seven cervical vertebrae. The sclerotomal segmentation leaves eight cervical spinal nerves exiting between the remaining seven cervical vertebrae to enter the eight cervical myotomes. Hence, the first cervical spinal nerve emerges between the occipital bone and the first cervical vertebra. The upper seven cervical spinal nerves will therefore emerge above the vertebrae of the same number. The eighth cervical

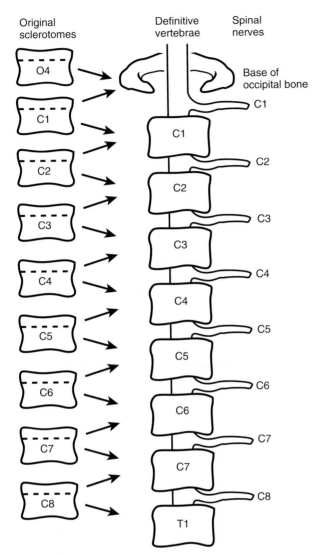

Fig. 94-3

Developmental process that results in eight cervical spinal nerves but only seven cervical vertebrae involves loss of two halves of original cervical sclerotomes. Cranial portion of first cervical sclerotome fuses with caudal portion of fourth occipital somite to form basilar part of occipital bone, while caudal portion of eighth cervical sclerotome fuses with cranial part of first thoracic sclerotome to form first thoracic vertebra. *(Modified from Larren WJ: Human embryology, New York, 1993, Churchill Livingstone, p 65.)*

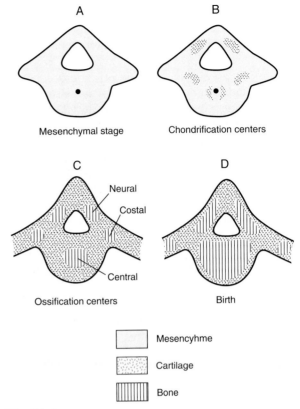

Fig. 94-4

Prenatal development of chondrification and ossification centers of lower five cervical vertebrae. **A**, Mesenchymal vertebra. **B**, Three paired chondrification centers that develop within mesenchymal vertebra. **C**, Ossification centers that develop within fully chondrified vertebra. **D**, State of expansion of ossification centers at birth. *(Modified from Sherk HH, Parke WE: Developing Anatomy. In The Cervical Spine Society Editorial Subcommittee: The cervical spine. Philadelphia, 1983, JB Lippincott Co., p 3.)*

nerve emerges between the seventh cervical vertebra and the first thoracic vertebra. As a result, below this level the thoracolumbosacral spinal nerves will be named for the vertebra above them.

Prenatal Development of the Lower Five Cervical Vertebrae

During the sixth fetal week chondrification begins at the cervicothoracic junction and progresses cra-

nially and caudally. In the lower five cervical vertebrae, two chondrification centers appear in the mesenchymal vertebral body on each side of the midline (Fig. 94-4, *A* and *B*).[16,24] Paired chondrification centers also develop in each side of the neural arch. These expand and by the end of the eighth week they fuse with each other posteriorly in the midline and anteriorly with the vertebral body (Fig. 94-4, *C*). Other chondrification centers develop in the mesenchymal costal processes, which protrude laterally from the posterior aspect of the vertebral body. The cartilaginous spinous and transverse processes develop as extensions of the chondrification centers in the vertebral arch. At about this time dorsal and ventral ossification centers develop within the cartilaginous vertebral body, and another pair of ossification centers forms in each half of the cartilaginous neural (vertebral) arch near the transverse process. The two centers in the body quickly fuse into a single center, so that each vertebra consists of three ossification centers connected together by hyaline cartilage. Each of these ossification centers expands during the last two prenatal trimesters. The vertebral arch ossification centers expand posteriorly into the laminae and anteriorly into the pedicles and even into the lateral portion of the definitive vertebral bodies, where they will form the uncinate process regions of the lateral vertebral body. At birth the neural arch ossification centers are joined together posteriorly by hyaline cartilage (Fig. 94-4, D). They are joined anteriorly via hyaline cartilage with the vertebral body ossification center, where they form a synchondrosis called the "neurocentral joint." The cartilage separating the ossification centers serves as epiphyseal plates so that growth of the neural arch will be able to accommodate the enlarging spinal cord.

Prenatal Development of the Occiput, Atlas, and Axis

The development of the occiput, atlas, and axis varies substantially from that of the lower five cervical vertebrae. Since the cranial part of the first cervical sclerotome fuses with the basiocciput, the first intervertebral disc is represented by the alar and apical ligaments of the dens. In the fusion of the caudal part of the first cervical sclerotome with the cranial part of the second cervical sclerotome, the portion homologous with the vertebral body of the atlas fuses with the body of the axis to form the odontoid process (dens). The lateral masses and posterior arch of the atlas are formed from the vertebral arch region of the mesenchymal atlas. A condensation of dense mesenchyme forms anterior to the developing vertebrae along the entire length of the spine. At atlas levels, this develops into the anterior arch of the atlas, the anterior atlantooccipital membrane and the anterior atlantoaxial ligament. At lower levels, this dense mesenchyme forms much of the anterior longitudinal ligament of the spine. Prior to birth, the atlas develops two primary ossification centers, one in each lateral mass (Fig. 94-5, A). These correspond to the paired vertebral arch centers of the lower cervical vertebrae. They expand into the posterior arch but remain as separate centers until after birth. The

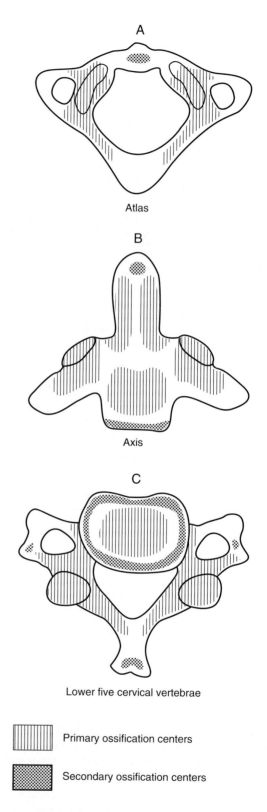

Atlas

Axis

Lower five cervical vertebrae

Primary ossification centers

Secondary ossification centers

Fig. 94-5

A and B, Prenatal development of primary ossification centers of atlas and axis and postnatal development of secondary ossification centers of anterior arch of atlas, dens apex, and ring epiphysis of inferior aspect of axis body. C, Postnatal development of primary and secondary ossification centers of lower five cervical vertebrae. Two constant secondary ring epiphyses develop within cartilaginous end plates on superior and inferior aspects of vertebral bodies. Inconstant secondary ossification centers may develop within tips of spinous and transverse processes. *(Modified from Sherk HH, Parke WE: Developing Anatomy. In The Cervical Spine Research Society Editorial Subcommittee: The cervical spine, Philadelphia, 1983, JB Lippincott, p 5.)*

axis develops from five primary ossification centers (Fig. 94-5, *B*). The odontoid ossifies from paired centers that fuse to form a single center by birth. The ossification centers for the body and vertebral arch of the axis develop as in the lower five cervical vertebrae.

Postnatal Development

The ossification centers in the lateral masses of the atlas that expand into the posterior arch join by about 3 years of age. A secondary ossification center develops in the anterior arch of the atlas by 1 year of age. It fuses with the lateral masses by 6 to 9 years. The odontoid process develops a secondary ossification center at its apex at 2 years of age, and this fuses with the primary ossification center of the odontoid by about 12 years. The primary ossification center of the odontoid begins to fuse with the primary ossification center in the axis body by 4 years of age, and the fusion is usually complete by the age of 7 years. However, about one third of normal adults have a persisting cartilaginous remnant between the odontoid and the body of the axis. A secondary ring epiphysis develops on the inferior aspect of the axis body in the same manner as those of the lower five cervical vertebrae, described below.

In the postnatal development of the lower five cervical vertebrae the primary ossification centers in each half of the vertebral arch typically fuse posteriorly during the first 3 to 5 years (Fig. 94-5, *C*). The neurocentral joints close during the third to sixth years. From late childhood up to shortly after puberty as many as five secondary ossification centers may appear: an inconstant one at the tip of the spinous process, an inconstant one at the tip of each transverse process and two constant ring (anular) epiphyses that develop as washer-like ossification centers within the cartilaginous end plates that cover the superior and inferior surfaces of the vertebral bodies. The secondary ossification center at the tip of the spinous process is frequently present in the sixth and seventh cervical vertebrae, but appears only sporadically in the third to fifth cervical vertebrae. Secondary ossification centers appear only rarely within the transverse processes of cervical vertebrae. The growth in height of the vertebral bodies occurs on the vertebral body side of the cartilaginous end plates. The secondary ossification centers typically fuse with the primary centers between 17 and 25 years. The fused ring epiphyses form a compact bony rim around the margins of the vertebral body ends. The central portion of the cartilaginous end plates that cover the rest of the superior and inferior as-

pects of the vertebral bodies remain throughout life as a component of the intervertebral disc. At cervical levels the costal process forms the anterior or costal element of the transverse process.

Congenital Abnormalities

Inducing substances produced by the notochord induce the sclerotomal mass around it to form the vertebral body, while inducing substances produced by the neural tube induce the formation of the vertebral arch. Defective induction of vertebral bodies on one side may produce hemivertebrae, which in turn can cause a type of congenital scoliosis.[12]

The cervical spine can also develop various defects in segmentation.[17] Occipitalization of the atlas is characterized by partial or complete fusion of the atlas with the circumference of the foramen magnum region of the occipital bone. The loss of atlantooccipital motion can increase the strain on the atlantoaxial ligamentous apparatus and produce atlantoaxial instability. This is particularly likely if there is an associated fusion of C2-C3 vertebrae. Atlantooccipital fusion can also bring the tip of the odontoid up into the foramen magnum, where it may encroach on the medulla-spinal cord junction.

Fusion of two or more cervical vertebrae can also cause Klippel-Feil syndrome. It can involve any or all of the cervical vertebrae. The intervertebral joints above and below the area of synostosis are subject to increased strain and hence may become hypermobile with significant instability or degenerative arthritis. These in turn can cause spinal cord or nerve root compression.

The odontoid process is subject to a number of congenital abnormalities. Agenesis or hypoplasia may occur if the fusion of the caudal part of the first cervical sclerotome goes awry. In odontoideum the odontoid is separated from the body of the axis by a wide gap and behaves as a free ossicle. This could be caused by an early embryonic failure of fusion of the odontoid sclerotomic mass with the body of the axis, or it could be produced by a postnatal failure of the synchondrosis that persists between the odontoid and the axis body until 4 to 7 years of age. Any of these odontoid abnormalities can cause atlantoaxial instability with spinal cord encroachment.

Faulty induction of the vertebral arch by inductive substances released from the neural tube can cause minor vertebral arch defects such as spina bifida occulta, in which there is a failure of only one vertebral arch to fuse, with no underlying involvement of meningeal or neural structures. This is less common at cervical than lumbosacral levels, and at cervical levels it most frequently involves the posterior arch of the atlas. If meninges bulge into a more extensive vertebral arch defect it is called "spina bifida with meningocele." If the spinal cord or spinal nerve roots are included in the meningeal sac, it is called "spina bifida with myelomeningocele." The most severe type of spina bifida is that accompanied by myeloschisis. In these cases, the vertebral arch defect is caused by a neural tube that fails to close, leaving the neural plate open on the skin surface.

In the development of a cervical rib, the costal element of the transverse process of the seventh cervical vertebra elongates to form a riblike structure. At times it may be long enough to reach the sternum. When present it can encroach on the scalene interval and produce a neurovascular compression syndrome involving the subclavian artery and brachial plexus.

The Occiput-Atlas-Axis Complex

A close examination of the three-dimensional morphology of the uniquely designed atlas and axis and their related atlantooccipital and atlantoaxial joints provides some interesting insights into their functional attributes as well as the pathomechanics of injuries to these structures.

Atlas

The atlas is a unique ringlike vertebra composed of paired lateral masses joined together by a short, relatively straight anterior arch and a long more highly curved posterior arch (Fig. 94-6, A and B.[3,8,25] The anterior arch occupies approximately the anterior one sixth of the ring, each lateral mass forms the anterolateral one sixth of the ring, and the posterior arch comprises about the posterior half of the ring.

The lateral masses form the thickest portion of the ring since they serve as the load-transmitting pathway from the occipital condyles to the superior articular facet of the axis. The lateral masses bear large ovoid or kidney-shaped superior articular facets that are concave from anterior to posterior and from medial to lateral (Fig. 94-6, A). They articulate with the reciprocally convex occipital condyles. The superior articular facets are obliquely situated, with their long axes converging anteriorly. They face superiorly, medially, and slightly posteriorly, just the opposite of the inferiorly, laterally, and anteriorly facing direction of the occipital condyles. Therefore, the loads transmitted from the occipital condyles to the superior articular facets will tend to be directed inferiorly, laterally, and slightly anteriorly. At times

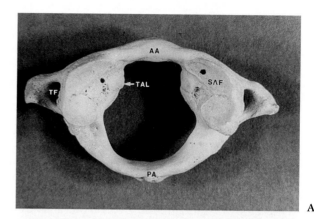

A

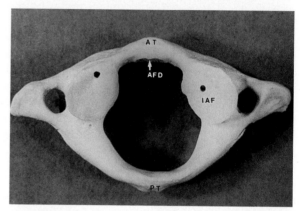

B

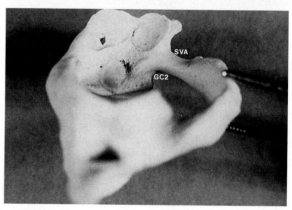

C

Fig. 94-6

Atlas. **A,** Superior view displaying the anterior arch (*AA*), posterior arch (*PA*), kidney-shaped superior articular facets (*SAF*) on superior aspect of lateral masses, tubercles for attachment of transverse atlantal ligament (*TAL*), and transverse foramina (*TF*) for transmission of vertebral vessels. **B,** Inferior view showing inferior articular facets (*IAF*), anterior tubercle (*AT*), articular facet for dens (*AFD*), and posterior tubercle (*PT*). **C,** Oblique superior and lateral view demonstrating thinning of posterior arch caused by superiorly situated sulcus of vertebral artery (*SVA*) and first cervical nerve and inferiorly located groove for second cervical nerve (*GC2*).

the superior articular facets are indented medially, where the transverse atlantal ligament attaches to a small tubercle on the medial aspect of the lateral mass

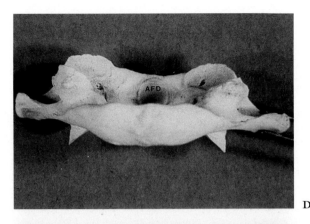

D

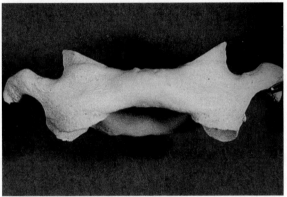

E

Fig. 94-6, cont'd

D, Posterior view visualizing ovoid articular facet for dens (*AFD*) and wedge shape of lateral masses. E, Anterior view also displaying wedge shape of lateral mass.

(Fig. 94-6, *C*). Less frequently they may be severely waisted at this point and almost divided into two articular surfaces.

In contrast, the inferior articular facets are round and face inferiorly and medially (Fig. 94-6, *B*), just the opposite of the superiorly and laterally facing superior articular facets of the axis. Therefore, loads transmitted from the atlas to the axis will be directed inferiorly and medially. In accord with Newton's third law, the equal and opposite loads transmitted from the axis to the atlas will be directed superiorly and laterally.

The anterior arch of the atlas is relatively transversely oriented with a prominent midline anterior tubercle that serves as a point of attachment for both the upward continuation of the anterior longitudinal ligament and the longus colli muscles. The posterior aspect of the anterior arch contains an oval or round articular facet for the dens or odontoid process of the axis (Fig. 94-6, *D*). This facet is concave from side to side, thereby allowing rotary motion to occur between the atlas and the dens. In a superior or inferior view the anterior arch tends to be thinnest where it joins the anterior aspect of the lateral mass. When cut in cross section this portion of the anterior arch is elliptical, with the major axis of the ellipse oriented in the vertical direction and the minor axis in the horizontal direction.[20] This implies it would be better able to withstand bending moments applied in a vertical plane than it would bending moments applied in the horizontal plane.

The posterior arch of the atlas forms about half of a circle. It has a midline posterior tubercle that is essentially a rudimentary spinous process and serves as the origin of the two rectus capitis posterior minor muscles. Its small size prevents it from interfering with extension at the atlantooccipital joints. At the point that the posterior arch joins the posterior aspect of the lateral mass it is deeply grooved on its superior aspect where the vertebral artery makes a hairpin turn medially and anteriorly around the posterior aspect of the lateral mass after coursing posteriorly from the transverse foramen of the atlas. This sulcus for the vertebral artery is the thinnest part of the posterior arch. The sulcus for the vertebral artery is best visualized in an oblique view of the atlas (Fig. 94-6, *C*). When cut in cross section this part of the posterior arch presents an elliptical profile, with the major axis of the ellipse in the horizontal direction and the minor axis in the vertical direction.[20] Hence, this portion of the posterior arch will be able to better withstand bending moments applied in the horizontal plane than it would bending moments applied in the vertical plane. At times the sulcus for the vertebral artery is converted into a foramen by a thin bony bar that extends from the posterior end of the superior articular process to the posterior arch.[18] The first cervical (suboccipital) spinal nerves exit from the spinal canal in this sulcus in close relationship to the vertebral artery. There is also a small groove along the inferior margin of the posterior arch just posterior to the inferior articular process. The second cervical spinal nerve emerges from the spinal canal in this groove. This further thins the posterior arch where it joins the lateral mass. Note that the first two cervical nerves emerge from the spinal canal posterior to the atlantooccipital and atlantoaxial joints, while all lower spinal nerves emerge from their intervertebral foramina anterior to the facet joints. This occurs because of the relatively anterolateral position of the atlantooccipital and atlantoaxial joints in contrast to the more posterolateral position of the facet joints.

The lateral masses of the atlas serve as load transmission struts for conveying loads between the occipital condyle and the superior articular facet of the axis. This type of dual-load transmission is unique.

The rest of the spine uses a tripod-load transmission system, with the anteriorly situated vertebral bodies and intervertebral discs transmitting the bulk of the loads, while the posterolaterally situated facet joints play a lesser load-transmitting role, but by their facing direction they help to determine the type and amount of motion possible at each level. It is interesting to observe that the dual-load-transmitting atlantooccipital joint-lateral mass-atlantoaxial joint complex is situated in the anterolateral wall of the spinal canal, where it is intermediate in position between the anteriorly situated vertebral bodies and the posterolaterally situated facet joints.

If the lateral masses are viewed from in front or behind they have a wedge-shaped configuration, with the apex of the wedge pointing medially (Fig. 94-6, *D* and *E*). Because of the obliquity of the superior and inferior facets, which tend to converge medially, the superior-inferior dimension of the medial aspect of the lateral mass is only about one fourth of the superior-inferior dimension of the lateral aspect of the lateral mass.

An appreciation of the three-dimensional morphology of the lateral masses and arches of the atlas provides good insight into the pathomechanics of Jefferson fractures. When compressive loads are transmitted from the occipital condyles to the superior articular facet of the atlas they are directed obliquely inferiorly, laterally, and slightly anteriorly (Fig. 94-7). As these loads are transmitted through the lateral mass of the atlas to its inferior articular facet they are directed onto the superior articular facet of the axis in an inferior and medial direction. In accordance with Newton's third law the superior articular facet of the axis imposes an equal and opposite force against the inferior facet of the atlas and this force is directed superiorly and laterally (Fig. 94-7). The result of these forces acting on the lateral masses of the atlas is a force directed laterally, which will tend to separate the lateral masses. This laterally directed resultant force is resisted in part by the anterior and posterior arches of the atlas, which act as tie rods that will resist any lateral displacement of the lateral masses. The transverse atlantal ligament also resists lateral displacement of the lateral masses, since it is stretched between tubercles on the medial aspect of the lateral masses. This ligament's attachments to the lateral masses are strategically placed in the center of the apex of the wedge of the lateral masses. Hence, the interaction of the injuring forces with the morphology of the atlas produces the clinical findings of a Jefferson fracture, which include separation of the lateral masses, two or more fractures involving the atlas ring, and a frequent avulsion or midsubstance tear of the transverse atlantal ligament. While the bony ring can fail at any point around its circumference, the thinnest parts of the ring are most prone to failure. Hence, fractures often occur where the arches approach the lateral masses.

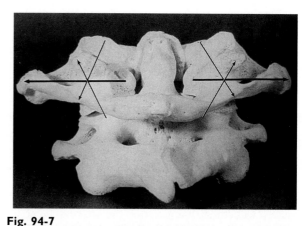

Fig. 94-7

Posterior view of atlas and axis illustrates vector forces imposed on lateral masses of atlas under compressive loading conditions. *Narrow arrows* depict downward and laterally directed forces produced by occipal condyles and upward and laterally directed forces applied by the superior articular facet of axis. *Thick arrows* demonstrate the laterally directed resultants of these forces that can produce Jefferson fractures.

The transverse processes of the atlas contain a transverse foramen for the transmission of the vertebral artery and its surrounding veins and sympathetic nerve plexus. This foramen divides the transverse process of the atlas into an anterior or costal element or process homologous to a rib and a posterior or transverse element homologous to the transverse process of the typical thoracic vertebra. Medially, the costal element attaches to the anterior part of the lateral mass, which is in a position homologous to the lateral part of the typical vertebral body. The transverse element attaches to the posterior part of the lateral mass at its junction with the posterior arch, which is homologous with the position of the pedicle-lamina junction of a typical thoracic vertebra. Laterally, the costal and transverse elements converge to end in a tubercle, which serves as a point of attachment of the obliquus capitis superior and inferior muscles and the rectus capitis lateralis muscle. The transverse process of the atlas is substantially longer than the transverse processes of the lower cervical vertebrae. It protrudes so far laterally that it can be palpated deeply just below the tip of the mastoid process in the interval between the mastoid process and the ramus of the mandible. The length of the transverse process increases the rotary torque capabilities of the muscles attaching to it by lengthening their moment arms. However, it also means that as the vertebral artery ascends from the transverse process of the axis to the transverse process of the atlas it must course laterally to reach the transverse foramen of the atlas, where it makes a laterally directed elbowlike bend. Then after the vertebral artery emerges from the transverse process of the atlas it courses posteriorly along the lateral margin of the superior articular process and then medially around its posterior margin. As it enters the spinal canal it angles forward. So after making a lateral bend through the atlas' transverse process it makes a posterior loop about the superior articular process. Because of the elbowlike lateral bend that the vertebral artery makes through the transverse foramen, during head rotation the rotation of the atlas on the more fixed axis can place tractional stresses on the vertebral artery. In patients with atherosclerotic changes in the vertebral circulation this can produce symptoms of vertebral-basilar insufficiency. Likewise, when the head is extended at the atlantooccipital joint the occipital bone closely approaches the posterior arch of the atlas, and this can compress the vertebral artery as it loops behind the superior articular process of the atlas. Injury to the vertebral artery in the vicinity of the atlantooccipital joint by trauma or manipulative therapy has been reported to produce ischemic stroke by causing intimal injury with a subsequent dissection that can result in thrombosis or embolism.[10]

Axis

The axis also has a number of unique features. It receives its name from the prominent dens that protrudes superiorly from its body and serves as an axis on which the atlas rotates. The axis is the thickest and strongest of the cervical vertebrae. It has the largest body and the thickest vertebral arch (Fig. 94-8, A and B). The anterior aspect of the body has a vertically running median ridge for the attachment of the anterior longitudinal ligament and the longus colli muscles. In an anterior or posterior view the body appears to have broad shoulders that support the medial part of the superior articular facets (Fig. 94-8, C and D). The lateral part of the superior articular facets is supported by the stout pedicles of the axis. The superior articular facets are round or oval and relatively flat. They face superiorly and laterally. The dual loads transmitted onto them from the inferior articular facets of the atlas must be split into the tripod-load-transmitting system that begins on the inferior aspect of the axis and continues to the lumbosacral junction.

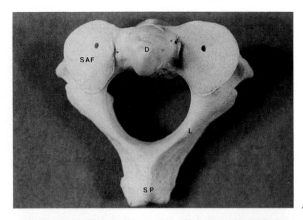

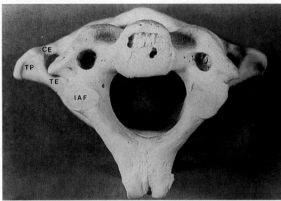

Fig. 94-8

Axis. **A,** Superior view. **B,** Inferior view. Labeled on these views are dens (*D*), superior articular facet (*SAF*), inferior articular facet (*IAF*), ridge (*R*) for attachment of anterior longitudinal ligament and longus colli muscles, pars interarticularis (*PI*), lamina (*L*), and spinous process (*SP*). Dens has facet on posterior aspect of its neck for articulation with transverse atlantal ligament (*FTAL*) and higher-level facet on anterior aspect of its bulbous portion for articulation with anterior arch of atlas (*FA*). Dens attachment sites of apical (*Ap*) and alar (*Al*) ligaments are indicated. Note obliquity of transverse processes (*TP*) and their transverse foramina (*TF*), which directs the vertebral vessels toward more laterally situated transverse foramina of atlas. Each transverse process has costal (*CE*) and transverse element (*TE*).

Therefore, the axis is a load-splitting vertebra. The oblique loads transmitted across the lateral atlantoaxial joints are largely directed inferiorly and medially onto the inferior aspect of the body of the axis. In a lateral view of the axis it is obvious that the inferior articular facets of the axis are more posteriorly situated than the superior facets (Fig. 94-8, E). Hence the smaller loads transmitted from the superior to the inferior facets must be directed posteriorly along the portion of the vertebral arch between these two facets. This part of the vertebral arch of the atlas is sometimes called its "pedicle" and at other times it is called the "pars interarticularis," because it bridges the two articular facets. The pars interarticularis of the axis differs from the better

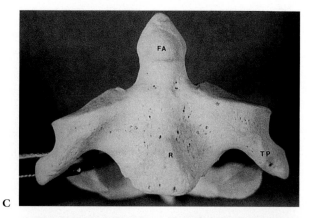

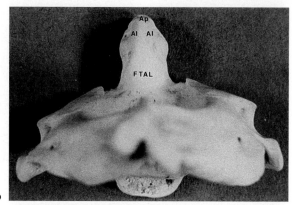

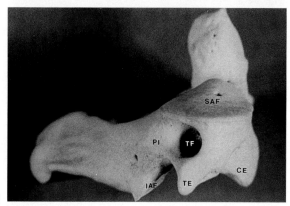

Fig. 94-8, cont'd

C, Anterior view. D, Posterior view. E, Lateral view.

known pars interarticularis of lumbar levels in that the axis pars interarticularis corresponds to its pedicle, while the lumbar pars interarticularis is the lateral portion of its lamina. Because the relatively vertically directed forces passing across the lateral atlantoaxial joints must be transmitted obliquely posteriorly to the C2-C3 facet joints before again assuming a vertical course through the articular pillars and facet joints of the lower cervical vertebrae, the pars interarticularis is subject to high shearing forces, not unlike those acting on the femoral neck. Hence

hyperextension, distraction, or even compression injuries can cause fractures of the pars interarticularis of the axis, which are called "hangman's fractures." The unusual thickness of the pedicles of the axis is likely a structural adaptation to the unique loads these pedicles convey.

The inferior articular facets of the axis are situated on the inferior aspect of the junction of the pedicle and lamina (Fig. 94-8, *B*). They are round or oval and relatively flat. They face inferiorly and anteriorly. The laminae of the axis are thick and strong. The thickness of the laminae is likely a structural adaptation to the significant muscular forces that must be conveyed from the spinous process to the body. Where the laminae join posteriorly they become continuous with a short thick spinous process that is deeply grooved on its inferior surface. The thickness of the spinous process is to accommodate all the muscles that attach to it, which include the rectus capitis posterior major, obliquus capitis inferior, interspinales, rotators, multifidus, and semispinalis cervicis muscles. The transverse processes of the axis are short, with costal and transverse elements that meet laterally to form a single tubercle to which the middle scalene, splenius cervicis, longissimus cervicis, semispinalis capitis, and intertransverse muscles attach. The transverse foramen is directed obliquely superiorly and laterally in anticipation of the vertebral artery's lateral inclination to reach the transverse foramen of the atlas.

The dens is a toothlike superior protrusion from the axis body that measures 12 to 15 mm in length.[3] It displays a slight constriction or neck where it joins the body. There is a small concave hyaline cartilage-covered facet on the posterior aspect of the neck of the dens for articulation with the transverse ligament of the atlas (Fig. 94-8, *D* and *E*). At a slightly higher level there is a larger oval or circular articular facet occupying much of the anterior aspect of the bulbous portion of the dens (Fig. 94-8, *C*). This articulates with the facet on the posterior surface of the anterior arch of the atlas. The fact that the facets on the anterior and posterior aspects of the dens are slightly offset implies that the intervening part of the dens could be subject to shearing stress in hyperflexion or hyperextension injuries. The apex of the dens is pointed for attachment of the apical ligament of the dens. The rough areas on the lateral aspect of the dens are for the attachment of the alar ligaments.

Atlantooccipital Joints

The ligamentous apparatus of this and all intervertebral joints must provide the necessary flexibility re-

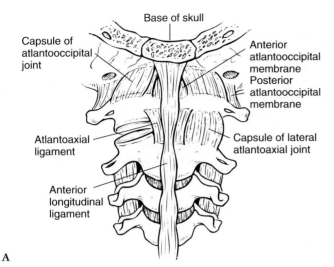

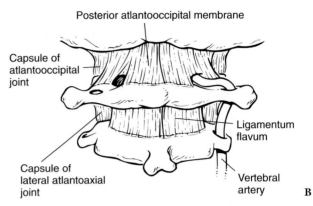

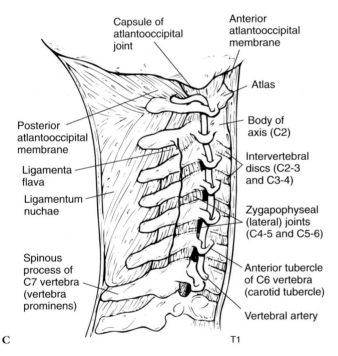

Fig. 94-9

Externally visualized craniovertebral ligaments. **A**, Anterior view; **B**, posterior view; and **C**, Lateral view of external aspect of ligaments uniting occipital bone with atlas and axis.

quired of that joint while maintaining a safe degree of stability. The surrounding musculature contributes to both the mobility and stability of these joints.

The atlantooccipital joints are paired synovial joints between the biconvex occipital condyles and the biconcave superior articular facets of the atlas. The major supporting ligaments are the articular capsules and the anterior and posterior atlantooccipital membranes. However, additional stability is provided by the ligaments that connect the axis to the occiput.[28]

The sleevelike articular capsule descends from the circumference of the occipital condyle to the circumference of the superior articular facet of the at-

las (Fig. 94-9). The articular capsules appear loosely fit in the neutral position, and the medial capsule is thin. The lateral capsule is reinforced by some obliquely running fibers that are sometimes referred to as the "lateral atlantooccipital ligament." They limit lateral bending to the opposite side.

The anterior atlantooccipital membrane is about 2 cm wide. It is composed of densely woven fibers that extend from the anterior margin of the foramen magnum to the superior border of the anterior arch of the atlas (Fig. 94-9, *A*). It is continuous laterally with the anterior capsule of the atlantooccipital joints. Anteriorly it is reinforced in the midline by a strong cordlike upward extension of the anterior longitudinal ligament that extends from the anterior tubercle of the atlas to the midline of the basilar part of the occipital bone.

The posterior atlantooccipital membrane is wider but thinner than the anterior atlantooccipital membrane.[23] It extends from the posterior margin of the foramen magnum to the superior margin of the longer posterior arch of the atlas. There is an opening in this membrane over the sulcus for the vertebral artery that permits the vertebral artery to enter and the first cervical nerve to exit the spinal canal. At times the upper border of this opening is ossified to create a bony foramen.

The tectorial membrane and the apical and alar ligaments of the dens, which extend from the atlas to the occipital bone, are two joint ligaments that could potentially constrain both atlantoaxial and atlantooccipital motion. They are described below with the atlantoaxial joint.

The synovium of the atlantooccipital joints has been described as frequently communicating medially with the joint between the dens and the transverse atlantal ligament.[3] The first cervical spinal nerve passes just posterior to the capsule of the atlantooccipital joint and provides its sensory innervation.

Flexion and extension is the most free motion of the atlantooccipital joints. Hence, these joints are sometimes referred to as the "yes" joints. Flexion and extension averages 13 degrees.[27] It occurs around a transversely oriented instantaneous axis of rotation. In the midline this axis passes just above the tip of the dens and then through the occipital condyles and the center of the mastoid processes laterally. Since the anterior atlantooccipital membrane is clearly anterior to this axis it should limit extension, while the posterior atlantooccipital membrane that is well posterior to this axis should limit flexion. The ligaments connecting the axis to the occipital bone are all close to the axis of rotation, but the tectorial membrane has been described as becoming taut in the extremes of both flexion and extension.[27]

Lateral bending at the atlantooccipital joints averages 8 degrees.[27] Its instantaneous axis of rotation is anteroposteriorly oriented in the midsagittal plane and situated about 2 to 3 cm above the tip of the dens. Lateral bending is largely constrained by the opposite lateral atlantooccipital ligament. Axial rotation at the atlantooccipital joints is negligible, as are translational movements.[27]

Atlantoaxial Joints

The atlas and axis articulate by three joints, a median and two lateral atlantoaxial joints. Some of the ligaments that restrain motion at these joints extend between the atlas and axis while others connect the axis to the occipital bone. The lateral atlantoaxial joints are formed between the inferior articular facets of the atlas and the superior articular facets of the axis. While the bony facets are relatively flat, the hyaline cartilage of both facets is convex. The articular capsule of the lateral atlantoaxial joints is thin and loose to permit relatively free motion. The capsule is reinforced posteromedially by an accessory ligament that extends from the back of the body of the axis just lateral to the attachment of the dens up to the medial aspect of the lateral mass immediately adjacent to the attachment of the transverse atlantal ligament (Fig. 94-10). The anterior atlantoaxial ligament is a strong membrane extending from inferior margin of the anterior arch of the atlas to the anterior aspect of the body of the axis (see Fig. 94-9). It is reinforced in the midline by a strong cord-like upward extension of the anterior longitudinal ligament that extends from the anterior surface of the body of the axis to the anterior tubercle of the atlas. It blends laterally with the anterior capsule of the atlantoaxial joints. The posterior atlantoaxial membrane is a wider and thinner membrane that extends from the inferior border of the posterior arch of the atlas to the upper border of the lamina of the axis. It is in a position comparable to the ligamenta flava of lower levels and is sometimes called a "ligamentum flavum."

The median atlantoaxial joint is a pivot joint between the dens of the axis and the anterior arch and transverse ligament of the atlas. It contains two synovial joints, each with an articular capsule and a separate synovial cavity. One joint is formed between the hyaline cartilage-covered concave facet on the posterior aspect of the anterior arch of the atlas and the hyaline cartilage-covered convex facet on the anterior aspect of the bulbous portion of the dens (Fig. 94-10, D). The other joint is between the smaller hyaline-cartilage covered facet on the posterior aspect of the neck of the dens and the transverse atlantal ligament.

The transverse atlantal ligament is a strong transversely oriented ligament attached on either side to tubercles on the medial aspect of the lateral masses (Fig. 94-10, B). It is widest at its middle, where two relatively narrow vertically running fasciculi are attached to it. The superior longitudinal fasciculus extends from the upper border of the transverse atlantal ligament to the anterior margin of the foramen magnum. An inferior longitudinal fasciculus extends from the inferior margin of the transverse atlantal ligament to the posterior aspect of the axis body.

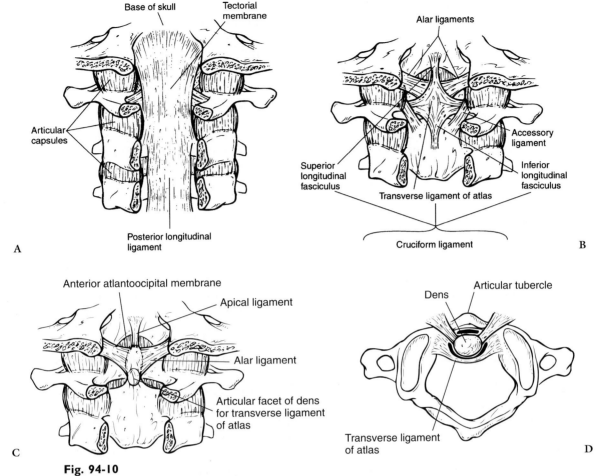

Fig. 94-10

Internal craniovertebral ligaments. **A,** Posterior view of anterior wall of upper cervical spinal canal. **B,** Posterior view with tectorial membrane removed to expose accessory, cruciform, and alar ligaments. **C,** Posterior view with cruciform and accessory ligaments removed to display fully apical and alar ligaments. **D,** Superior view displaying synovial and ligamentous features of median atlantooccipital joint.

The transverse atlantal ligament and the two longitudinal fasciculi together form a crosslike structure called the "cruciform ligament."

A very narrow cordlike apical ligament of the dens lies just external or anterior to the superior longitudinal fasciculus of the cruciform ligament (Fig. 94-10, C). It courses from the apex of the dens to the anterior margin of the foramen magnum. The majority of fibers in the alar ligaments extend from the lateral aspect of the dens to the medial aspect of the occipital condyles. They are situated anterior to the cruciform ligament. Each alar ligament is about 10 to 13 mm long. It is elliptical in cross section, measuring about 6 mm in superior-inferior dimension and 3 mm in anteroposterior dimension.[8] The direction of its fibers is variable and is dependent on the height of the dens relative to the occipital condyles. Contrary to standard textbook descriptions and illustrations, Dvorak and Panjabi reported that

as the ligaments coursed from the dens to the occipital condyles they were oriented craniocaudally in 9 of 19 specimens, horizontally in 6 specimens, and caudocranially in 4 specimens.[8] They also found that a majority of the alar ligaments (12 of 19) demonstrated a smaller ligamentous connection between the dens and the lateral mass of the atlas, which ran craniocaudally. They even found a small ligamentous connection between the dens and the anterior arch of the atlas in two specimens. They determined that each alar ligament functioned to limit rotation of the head to the opposite side. Each alar ligament was also tensed by lateral bending to the opposite side and by flexion. They concluded that simultaneous head flexion and rotation would cause maximal stretching of the contralateral alar ligament and hypothesized that these motions, which are common in whiplash, could cause rupture of the alar ligament.

The tectorial membrane lines the inner aspect of the anterior wall of the upper part of the spinal canal (Fig. 94-10, *A*). It is a broadened and strengthened upward continuation of the posterior longitudinal ligament, which tends to be hourglass-shaped at lower spinal levels. The tectorial membrane is fixed to the posterior surface of the body of the axis. From here it extends upward posterior to the cruciform ligament and dens to gain a broad superior attachment to the anterior and lateral margins of the foramen magnum, where the spinal dura fuses with it. It is a two-joint ligament that helps stabilize both the atlantooccipital and atlantoaxial joints.

In addition to these ligaments, the ligamentum nuchae can also help stabilize the atlantooccipital and atlantoaxial joints. It is a thin midline septum extending from the posterior tubercle of the atlas and spinous processes of the lower cervical vertebrae to the external occipital protuberance and median nuchal line.

Axial rotation is the most free motion at the atlantoaxial joints. It averages 47 degrees, and rotation at this joint makes up 50% of the total rotation that occurs in the cervical spine.[27] Most of the first 45 degrees of total neck rotation occurs at the atlantoaxial joints. Atlantoaxial rotation can be evaluated in relative isolation by testing rotation with the neck fully flexed, since the lower cervical vertebrae tend to be locked by neck flexion. Unlike most other cervical spine motions, atlantoaxial rotation does not decrease with age.[7] The instantaneous axis of atlantoaxial rotation is a vertical axis passing down the center of the dens. Atlantoaxial rotation is primarily limited by the alar ligaments with rotation to the right restrained by the left alar ligament and vice versa. The accessory ligament has also been described as resisting atlantoaxial rotation. Because of the biconvex nature of the cartilage-covered lateral atlantoaxial joints rotation is coupled with vertical translation.[27] In the neutral position, the maxima of both convexities are in approximation. When the head is rotated in either direction the inferior articular facets of the atlas move down the anterior or posterior slopes of the convexity of the superior articular facet of the axis. This causes a small downward vertical translation of the atlas.

A moderate amount of flexion and extension can occur at the atlantoaxial joints, amounting to an average 10 degrees of range of motion.[27] The instantaneous axis of rotation for flexion and extension is a transverse axis passing through the middle third of the dens. Flexion is primarily limited by the transverse atlantal ligament with potential contributions from the ligamentum nuchae, tectorial membrane,

and alar ligaments.[8] Extension is restrained by the anterior atlantoaxial ligament, alar ligaments, and tectorial membrane.[15,27] The amount of lateral bending that occurs at the atlantoaxial joints is negligible.[27]

Atlantoaxial instability can be a significant cause of myelopathy. It is best demonstrated on lateral cervical spine films taken in flexion, where it appears as a posterior displacement of the dens away from the anterior arch of the atlas. This carries the dens into the spinal canal, where it can encroach on the cervical spinal cord. In adults, the radiolucent interval between the posterior aspect of the anterior arch of the atlas and the posterior aspect of the dens should not exceed 3 mm, and it should not increase during flexion.[6,9] This radiolucent interval is called the "atlas-dens interval," and it is produced by the apposing hyaline cartilages of both articular surfaces. Because of the incomplete ossification in children under 8 years of age, the upper limit of normal for the atlas-dens interval is usually taken as 5 mm. The most common cause of atlantoaxial instability is disruption of the transverse atlantal ligament. Trauma can cause either avulsion or midsubstance tears, and inflammatory processes such as rheumatoid arthritis can cause ligament laxity. The other ligaments that resist flexion seem to offer little support when the transverse atlantal ligament is disrupted.

Lower Cervical Spine

The osteology, intervertebral joints, and mechanics of the lower cervical spine from the third to the seventh cervical vertebrae have many features in common, with only some quantitative differences from level to level.

Osteology

The lower five cervical vertebrae have many common bony features. Their bodies are smaller in all dimensions than thoracic and lumbar vertebrae. They generally increase in size from C3 to C7 levels to accommodate the increasing superincumbent loads (Fig. 94-11). The bodies are oval-shaped short cylinders. Their mediolateral dimensions are greater than their anteroposterior dimensions (Fig. 94-12, *A* and *B*). The anterior and posterior surfaces of the bodies are flat and of equal superior-inferior dimension. Hence, the normal cervical lordosis is produced by wedge-shaped intervertebral discs and not by wedge-shaped vertebral bodies. In anterior view the lateral margins of the superior surface of the vertebral bodies display prominent cranially projecting

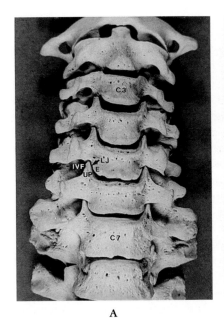
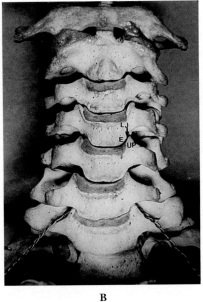
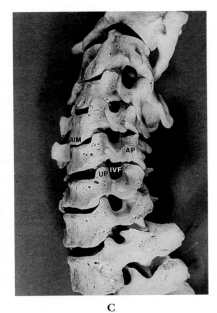

A   B   C

Fig. 94-11

Lower five cervical vertebra. **A,** Anterior view of articulated cervical spine without intervertebral discs. **B,** Anterior view of articulated cervical spine with felt pads occupying intervertebral disc spaces. **C,** Oblique left anterolateral view of articulated cervical spine to provide optional visualization of intervertebral foramina and their related boundaries. These views show progressively increasing size of vertebral bodies from C3 to C7, prominent uncinate processes (*UP*) that help form anterior boundary of intervertebral foramina (*IVF*), enchancrure (*E*), position of Luschka's joints (*LJ*), and articular pillars (*AP*). Inferiorly projecting anteroinferior margin of the vertebral bodies (*AIM*) is visualized on oblique view.

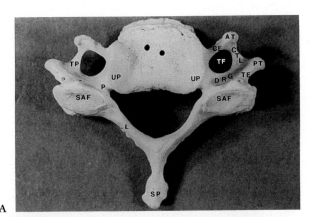
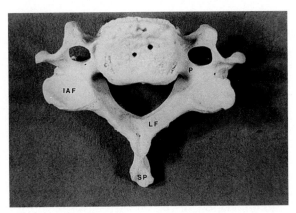

A   B

Fig. 94-12

Fifth cervical vertebra. **A,** Superior view. **B,** Inferior view. **C,** Left anterolateral view. Shown are uncinate processes (*UP*), superior articular facets (*SAF*), inferior articular facets (*IAF*), articular pillar (*AP*), pedicles (*P*), laminae (*L*), and spinous process (*SP*). **A** displays trough-shaped anterolaterally directed transverse processes (*TP*) formed by anterior costal element (*CE*) that ends in anterior tubercle (*AT*) and posterior transverse element (*TE*) that ends in posterior tubercle (*PT*). These are joined together distally by costotransverse lamella (*CTL*) to complete enclosure of transverse foramen (*TF*). Between transverse foramen anteriorly and superior articular facet and transverse element posteriorly there is curved groove that accommodates C5 dorsal root ganglion (*DRG*) and its spinal nerve roots as they fuse to form the spinal nerve. Note intimate relationship of these neural structures to uncinate process of Luschka's joint and vertebral vessels anteriorly and facet joint posteriorly. **B** shows roughened area on anterior aspect of inferior portion of lamina to which ligamenta flava (*LF*) attach. **C** demonstrates relatively equal superior and inferior notching of pedicle.

C

uncinate processes (Fig. 94-11, *A* and *B*). These cause the superior surface to demonstrate a mediolateral concavity that is most marked along the medial border of the uncinate processes. There is a reciprocal convexity on the lateral margin of the inferior surface of the next higher vertebral body. This convexity is sometimes called the enchancrure or anvil. It is in this position that the uncovertebral or Luschka's joints develop within the lateral part of the intervertebral discs, as will be described below. Where the anterior surface of the body joins the inferior surface there is a prominent inferior projection of the anteroinferior margin of the vertebra (Fig. 94-11, *C*). Hence, the inferior surfaces of the vertebral bodies tend to be concave in the anteroposterior direction. When the discs are not present it is obvious that the inferior surface of one vertebral body fits onto the superior surface of the next vertebral body in an interlocking fashion that tends to resist translational movements in any direction.

The pedicles of cervical vertebrae differ from those of thoracic and lumbar vertebrae in several respects. First, they tend to arise from the vertebral body closer to the midpoint between its superior and inferior surfaces. Therefore, the pedicles are equally grooved on their superior and inferior borders to form symmetrical superior and inferior vertebral notches that will create intervertebral foramina with substantial symmetry (Fig. 94-11, *C*, and 94-12, *C*). Second, the cervical pedicles originate from the posterolateral aspect of the body instead of from the posterior aspect as most thoracolumbar pedicles do. Third, the pedicles of cervical vertebrae are directed posterolaterally away from the midsagittal plane at an angle varying from 40 degrees at C3 to 29 degrees at C7.[19] This causes the intervertebral foramina to face obliquely anterolaterally. Both the posterolateral origin and the posterolateral inclination of the pedicles tends to increase the mediolateral dimensions of the cervical spinal canal to permit better accommodation of the elliptical cervical spinal cord, which has its major dimension in the mediolateral direction.

Because of the relatively equal superior and inferior notching of the cervical pedicles, the anterior wall of a cervical intervertebral (neural) foramen differs from those at thoracic and lumbar levels by being symmetrical. The upper third of the anterior wall is formed by the back of the body of the next higher vertebra. The intervertebral disc and Luschka's joint occupy the middle third of the anterior wall. The posterior aspect of the next lower vertebral body forms the lower third of the anterior wall. The other walls of the cervical intervertebral foramina are similar to

thoracolumbar intervertebral foramina, since both foramina are bounded above by the pedicle of the next higher vertebra, below by the pedicle of the next lower vertebra, and posteriorly by the facet joint.

The lower cervical laminae intersect the pedicles at nearly a right angle (Fig. 94-12, *A* and *B*). From the pedicles they are directed posteromedially to their point of junction. The lamina of one side is nearly parallel to the contralateral pedicle. The anterior aspect of the lower half of each lamina is roughened for the attachment of the ligamenta flava. Therefore, the lower part of each lamina overlaps the posterior aspect of the upper part of the next ligamentum flavum in a shingling type of pattern. As a result when the lower portion of a lamina is surgically removed one still cannot visualize the spinal canal until the ligamentum flavum is removed.

Lower cervical spinous processes are short but wide and bifid. Their shortness is an advantage in that they are not likely to interfere with extension. Their thickness and their bifid tips provide a large surface area to accommodate the many muscles that attach to them, including the semispinalis cervicis, multifidus, rotators, and interspinal muscles. The spinous process of the seventh cervical vertebra is larger and more prominent than any of the other cervical vertebrae. Therefore, it is more visible and palpable at the base of the neck. This has given the seventh cervical vertebra the name *vertebra prominens.*

The superior and inferior articular processes are stacked on top of each other and connected by a short, stout cylindrical articular pillar that is situated at the pedicle-lamina junction (Fig. 94-11, *B* and *C*, 94-12, *C*). All of the articular pillars are also stacked directly on top of each other, making them collectively look like one long pillar. Each superior articular facet faces obliquely superiorly and posteriorly and articulates with the next higher inferior articular facet that faces reciprocally inferiorly and anteriorly to form the zygapophyseal or facet joint. While the plane of the facet joint is only intermediate between the coronal and the horizontal plane, the cervical facet joints have the most horizontal orientation of any of the regional facet joints. Hence, these joints can be dislocated unilaterally or bilaterally without fracture. The relatively horizontal position of cervical facet joints and the thickness of the articular pillars connecting them together implies that they may be bearing greater loads than most thoracic and lumbar facet joints, which have a more vertical orientation in the coronal and sagittal planes, respectively.

The cervical transverse processes are directed anterolaterally and inferiorly. They are comprised of two distinct elements or processes separated by the transverse foramen. The transverse foramina of the third to sixth cervical vertebrae transmit the vertebral arteries, veins, and sympathetic plexus. The transverse foramen of the seventh cervical vertebra most commonly transmits only the vertebral veins. The barlike anterior element of the transverse process is called the "costal element" or "costal process." It arises from the lateral aspect of the vertebral body, just like the embryonic rib precursor from which it was derived. It ends distally in an anterior tubercle that serves as an attachment site for the longus and anterior scalene muscles. The posterior element of the transverse process is sometimes called the "transverse element" because it is homologous to the typical thoracic transverse process. Proximally, it attaches to the pedicle-lamina junction and distally it ends as a posterior tubercle that serves for the attachment of the splenius cervicis, iliocostalis cervicis, and longissimus cervicis muscles. Distally, the costal and transverse elements are connected by a costotransverse lamella. In a superior or oblique anterolateral view, the transverse processes are seen to be deeply grooved on their superior aspect (Figs. 94-11, D, and 94-12, A). The costal element forms the anterior lip of the groove and the transverse element forms the posterior lip of the groove. Since the vertebral vessels and nerves occupy much of the space in this groove or sulcus, the nerve roots, dorsal root ganglion, and ventral rami are crowded into the posterior part of the sulcus in a relatively narrow interval between the vertebral vessels anteromedially and the facet joint and transverse element of the transverse process posterolaterally (Fig. 94-12, A).

Lower Cervical Spine Intervertebral Joints

The intervertebral joints between the second and seventh cervical vertebrae include the major weight-bearing cartilaginous joints between the vertebral bodies and the paired synovial zygapophyseal or facet joints uniting the vertebral arches. The facet joints bear lesser loads, but by their facing direction they largely determine the permissible motions.

The interbody joints are comprised of the fibro-cartilaginous intervertebral disc, which is called a "symphysis type" of union. The disc is reinforced peripherally by anterior and posterior longitudinal ligaments.

Below the axis the anterior longitudinal ligament broadens to cover the anterior and part of the lateral aspect of the cervical vertebral bodies (see Figs. 94-9, A and B). It tends to be firmly attached to the intervertebral disc margins, where it blends with the outer layers of the anulus fibrosus. It is also firmly attached to the vertebral body margins immediately adjacent to the disc. It is less firmly adherent to the midportion of the vertebral bodies. Its most superficial fibers extend across four of five vertebrae, while the deeper ones pass only from one vertebra to the next. At cervical levels it has been described as being much thinner than it is at lower levels.[13] The anterior longitudinal ligament functions to resist spine extension and also serves to reinforce the anterolateral margin of the intervertebral disc.

The posterior longitudinal ligament extends along the posterior aspect of the vertebral bodies and therefore contributes to the anterior wall of the spinal canal (see Fig. 94-10, A). At cervical levels it is much wider mediolaterally than at lower spinal levels. It is firmly attached to the posterior aspect of the intervertebral discs and the adjacent posterior margins of the vertebral bodies. It has no significant attachment over the concavities of the bodies to permit the basivertebral veins to emerge from the posterior aspect of the vertebral bodies. At cervical levels the posterior longitudinal ligament is 2 to 3 mm thick. It is thicker than it is at thoracolumbar levels and even thicker than the cervical anterior longitudinal ligament.[1,13] The posterior longitudinal ligament functions to resist spine flexion and to reinforce the posterior aspect of the intervertebral disc.

In the young healthy spine the intervertebral discs contribute about 22% of the length of the cervical spine and are made up of a clearly delineated inner nucleus pulposus and an outer anulus fibrosus with hyaline cartilage end plates on its superior and inferior surfaces (Fig. 94-13).[4] However, with increasing age the anatomical and biochemical structure and the function of the intervertebral disc change substantially. The young nucleus pulposus occupies just under 50% of the cross-sectional area of the disc. It is a gelatinous material largely composed of glycosaminoglycans that bind large amounts of the water that makes up 90% of the young nucleus. The nucleus is surrounded peripherally by many concentric layers of the fibrocartilaginous anulus fibrosus. The collagen fibers in each lamina run obliquely vertically in a spiral fashion and insert into either the superior and inferior cartilaginous end plates or into the bony ring epiphysis. The fibers in each layer run in opposite directions, for example, upward and clockwise in one layer and upward and counter-clockwise in the next. They run on an angle of 30 degrees to the plane of the disc; hence, the fibers in each layer form a horizontal angle of 120 degrees and a vertical angle of 60 degrees with the fibers in the next layer (Fig. 94-13, D and E).[27] The vertical component of these helically running collagen fibers permits them to serve as tension resistors during flexion-extension and lateral bending motions, while their horizontal component resists the tensile stresses of rotary motions of the spine. Also, when the spine is under vertical load, the fibers of the anulus will resist the tensile stresses acting on the anulus that tend to cause it to bulge around its periphery.

Because the nucleus pulposus is enclosed about its circumference by the anulus fibrosus and bounded above and below by the hyaline cartilage end plates covering the vertebral body ends, the young nucleus will tend to behave as a fluid mass within a closed but somewhat distortable container (Fig. 94-13, *A* and *B*). As such it will obey Pascal's law, which says that given fluid in a completely closed container (e.g., water inside a balloon), if pressure is increased at one local point on the side walls of the container (e.g., press on the balloon with one finger), that local increase in pressure will be transmitted undiminished over the entire side walls of the container. Hence, whenever the cervical spine is bent in a given direction (e.g., flexion), there will be increased compressive load and stresses acting on that side of both the anulus and nucleus. Tensile stresses will be generated on the opposite side of the anulus and nucleus (Fig. 94-13, *C*). The young semifluid nucleus will be able to distribute the loads more evenly over the entire surface of the vertebral body to prevent undue load from being concentrated on the edge toward which the spine is being bent. If the interbody joint were a synovial joint the very high pressures that would be generated on the vertebral body edges toward which the spine is bent would tend to produce early hypertrophic degenerative changes. Therefore, the young intervertebral disc provides a hydraulic mechanism that functions as a self-contained fluid-elastic system, which will permit motion, absorb shock, and reduce pressures by distributing loads over a larger surface area.

As the disc ages, structural and chemical changes occur that makes the disc less able to perform its normal functions. All elements of the young healthy disc are present at birth, and at this time there is no evidence of Luschka's joints (Fig. 94-14, *A*). However, by adolescence bilateral degenerative clefts have developed in the posterolateral part of the anulus medial to the uncinate processes, thereby forming Luschka's joints (Fig. 94-14, *B*).[1,11] By 20 to 35 years of age these clefts gradually enlarge and spread toward the midline and the nucleus gradually suffers a reduction of glycosaminoglycans and desiccates (Fig. 94-14, *C*). By the age of 40 to 60 years, many of these clefts meet

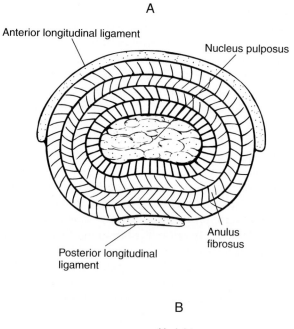

A

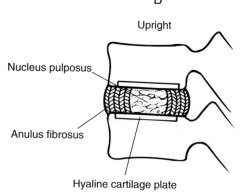

B

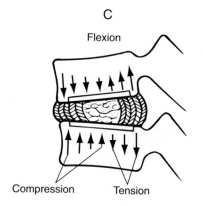

C

Fig. 94-13

Intervertebral disc. **A,** Transverse section of intervertebral disc and its reinforcing ligaments. **B** and **C,** Sagittal sections of intervertebral disc in upright and flexed positions, respectively.

in the midline and the nucleus has been largely replaced by ligamentous and fibrocartilage-like tissues and suffered a significant volume loss (Fig. 94-14, *D*).

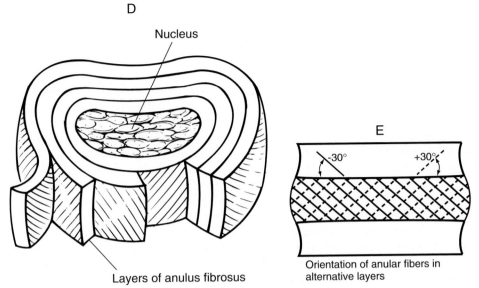

Fig. 94-13, cont'd

D, Anterosuperior peeled-away view of orientation of collagen fibers in alternate layers of anulus fibrosus. **E,** Schematic see-through anterior view of oblique angulation of collagen fibers in two adjacent layers of the anulus fibrosus. (Panels **D** and **E** modified from White AA, Panjabi MM: *Physical properties and functional biomechanics of the spine.* In White AA, Panjabi MM: *Clinical biomechanics of the spine,* Philadelphia, 1978, JB Lippincott Co., p 1.)

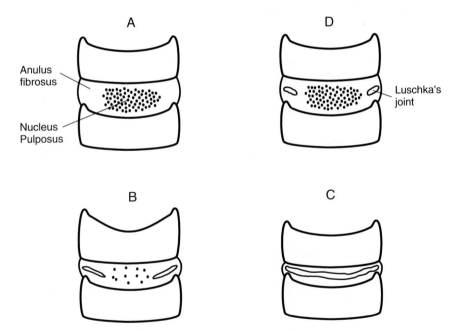

Fig. 94-14

Aging of the cervical intervertebral disc. **A,** In newborn, there is no evidence of degenerative clefts. **B,** By adolescence, degenerative clefts of Luschka's joints have usually developed in posterolateral anulus just medial to uncinate processes. **C,** By 20 to 35 years of age, degenerative clefts have enlarged and spread medially toward dehydrating nucleus pulposus. **D,** By 40 to 60 years of age, clefts have met in midline and intervertebral disc is commonly severely desiccated and disorganized with significant volume loss.

One interesting question is Why does the degeneration of the cervical disc begin laterally just medial to the uncinate process? A plausible explanation is that this is where the disc is thinnest and will therefore be subject to the greatest strain. Strain, in a physics sense, is by definition the change in length of an object (deformation) under load divided by the original length. Therefore, for the same displacement of the cervical spine in various directions (e.g., flexion, extension, lateral bending), the part of the disc that is narrowest or shortest to start with will show the greatest percentage change in length. As a result, it will be subject to the greatest strain and be the most likely to fail. Hence, while there may be other mechanical or chemical factors involved, it is not surprising that cervical disc degeneration starts in the area of Luschka's joints.

As the disc degenerates and loses its ability to distribute loads, loads will become more concentrated on the vertebral body edges toward which the spine is bent. With increasing pressures about the margins of the vertebral body hypertrophic degenerative processes can produce marginal osteophytes anywhere around the periphery of the vertebral body margins. When osteophytic bars develop posteriorly they may produce a myelopathy. When osteophytes extend posterolaterally they can produce foraminal stenosis. If they extend anteriorly they can encroach on the pharynx or esophagus to cause swallowing difficulties. Further, loss of disc height can cause a number of secondary complications that may produce neural encroachment. It can cause pedicle approximation that will narrow the superior-inferior dimension of the intervertebral foramen. It can also cause laminar approximation, which will produce bulging of the ligamenta flava into the spinal canal to further complicate any myelopathy. In addition, it can cause increased loading of the facet joints with resultant hypertrophic degenerative changes that may contribute to foraminal stenosis. Finally, as the inferior articular facet of the higher vertebra settles on the superior articular facet of the next lower vertebra, the obliquity of the cervical facet joints will cause the inferior facet to be displaced posteriorly. This may produce a retrolisthesis of the higher vertebra that will further narrow the spinal canal and intervertebral foramen.

Soft intervertebral disc herniation is less common at cervical levels than lumbar levels for a number of probable reasons. First, the superincumbent loads and hence the strains are less severe at cervical levels. Second, the uncinate processes tend to protect against posterolateral and lateral herniations. Third, the cervical posterior longitudinal ligament offers much more posterior reinforcement because of its greater width and thickness. Fourth, because degenerative changes appear earlier in cervical intervertebral discs, the earlier desiccation of their nucleus reduces the probability of soft-disc herniation.

The synovial facet joints between the vertebral arches are supported by their articular capsule and a number of extrinsic ligaments, including the ligamenta flava, interspinal, supraspinal, nuchal, and intertransverse ligaments.

The articular capsules are thin and loose and attach to the articular processes of adjacent vertebrae in a fashion that will permit relatively free motion (see Fig. 94-9, A and C). The ligamenta flava run from the anterior surface of the inferior half of the lamina of the higher vertebra to the superior margin and a little of the posterior surface of the lamina of the lower vertebra (Fig. 94-9, C). Hence, the ligamenta flava and lamina have an alternate shingling arrangement. The ligamenta flava form the greater share of the posterior wall of the spinal canal. Laterally, they blend insensibly with the anterior capsule of the facet joint. They have a high proportion of elastic fibers, which gives them their yellow color and physical properties. They resist spine flexion, but in hyperextension injury they can buckle into the spinal canal to traumatize the spinal cord.

Cervical interspinal ligaments are poorly developed thin membranous structures interconnecting adjacent spinous processes (see Fig. 94-9, A). In the cervical region the supraspinal ligaments that extend between the tips of the spinous processes are expanded into the ligamentum nuchae, which forms a thin midline fibrous sheet extending from the external occipital protuberance and median nuchal line to the spinous process of the seventh cervical vertebra (see Fig. 94-9, A). All these ligaments resist flexion. Poorly defined intertransverse ligaments connect adjacent cervical transverse processes. They presumably help resist rotary and lateral bending motions.[13]

Each of the intervertebral joints between the third and seventh cervical vertebrae permits some degree of flexion-extension, lateral bending, and rotation. Flexion and extension tend to be greatest at the C5-C6 and C6-C7 interspaces, where they total to 17 degrees and 16 degrees, respectively.[27] The large amount of flexion and extension permissible at the C5-C6 interval has been described as a potential cause for the high incidence of degenerative changes occurring at this level. Lateral bending and rotation are most free at C3-C4 and C4-C5 levels, where they total 11 to 12 degrees. Because of the obliquity of the facet joints, lateral bending and rotation tend to be coupled. For example, in lateral bending to the right, the right superior facet slides downward and backward and the left superior facet slides upward and forward. This causes the face to rotate toward the right. The uncinate processes play several possible roles in cervical spine motions. They appear to limit lateral translation. Uncinate processes are unnecessary at thoracic and lumbar levels, where lateral translation is limited, respectively, by the rib cage and the sagittal orientation of the lumbar facet joints. The uncinate processes also appear to limit lateral bending and serve as a guiding mechanism for flexion and extension and for anteroposterior translation.[15,27]

Neural Relationships

At the level of the atlas, the spinal cord occupies only approximately one third of the anteroposterior dimension of the inner circumference of the atlas ring. Another one third is occupied by the dens and transverse atlantal ligament, leaving the final one third for the meninges, cerebrospinal fluid, and epidural fat and veins. This latter one third has been called the "safe zone of Steele,"[26] implying that until encroachments at this level (e.g., atlantoaxial instability) intrude into the spinal canal by one third of that distance the spinal cord is likely to be spared. Even at lower levels of the normal cervical spine, the spinal cord comes nowhere near filling the spinal canal, not even at the level of the cervical enlargement (Fig. 94-15). In addition to this "free space" within the spinal canal, the cord is also protected by the water cushion effect of the cerebrospinal fluid, which slows accelerations and decelerations of the cord relative to the walls of the spinal canal. Further, the cord is somewhat stabilized by the denticulate ligaments, which are flange-like pial duplications extending from the lateral aspect of the cord. Its dentations penetrate the arachnoid to attach to the dura in the intervals between each set of emerging spinal nerve rootlets (Fig. 94-15, B).

The upper cervical cord segments are located at approximately the same level as their corresponding vertebrae (Fig. 94-15, A). Hence, their nerve roots pass transversely to exit from their intervertebral foramina. At lower cervical levels the spinal cord segments are one segment higher than the vertebral segment of the same number; that is, the C7 spinal nerve arises at the C6 vertebral level. As a result, the nerve roots descend obliquely to reach their intervertebral foramen (Figs. 94-15, A and B). Since the cervical intervertebral foramina are in the anterolateral wall of the spinal canal, the nerve roots course anterolaterally as they descend within the dural sac

(Fig. 94-15, C). They continue their descending anterolateral course as they enter their dural sleeve and the intervertebral foramen. The dorsal root ganglion and the ventral rami continue this descending anterolateral course as they exit the intervertebral foramen and enter the sulcus of the transverse process (Figs. 94-15, C and D). As the dorsal and ventral cervical nerve roots enter the intervertebral (neural) foramen they tend to occupy the lower part of the foramen at and below the level of the disc (Figs. 94-15, B and C).[5,21] The dorsal roots are located at the level of the disc and lie immediately adjacent to the superior articular facet, which forms the posterior wall of the foramen. They are situated cranial, dorsal, and lateral to the ventral roots. The ventral roots are located below the level of the disc, where they are caudal, ventral, and medial to the dorsal roots. This position brings the ventral roots into close contact with the uncinate process anteriorly and the pedicle of the next lower vertebra inferiorly. The upper portion of the intervertebral foramen is filled with fat and veins.

In the distal part of the intervertebral foramen the dorsal and ventral roots join to form the spinal nerve at the point where the swelling of the dorsal root ganglion begins. Grossly, the dorsal root ganglion appears to be situated on the spinal nerve and not on the dorsal root. At this point the dorsal root ganglion has the uncinate process anterior to it and the facet joint posterior to it. Since the length of cervical dorsal root ganglia typically exceeds 1 cm, they extend from the distal ends of the intervertebral foramen out into the sulcus of the transverse process, where they are situated posterior and lateral to the vertebral artery. At the distal end of the swelling of the dorsal root ganglion the spinal nerve terminates by splitting into dorsal and ventral rami. The ventral rami occupy the distal end of the sulcus of the transverse process, where they are situated mostly lateral to the vertebral artery (Fig. 94-15, D).

In a series of sagittal sections through a cervical spine with substantial degenerative changes these neural relationships and the potential effects of degenerative changes on the neural elements are well illustrated (Fig. 94-16). In the midsagittal section the C4-C5, C5-C6, and C6-C7 discs show substantial degenerative changes (Fig. 94-16, A). In the parasagittal section through the lateral part of the spinal cord there is a prominent osteophytic bar at the C5-C6 interval that intrudes into the anterior part of the spinal canal (Fig. 94-16, B). At the same C5-C6 interval there is a forward buckling of the ligamentum flavum into the posterior part of the spinal canal. The ligamenta flava of the C3-C4, C4-

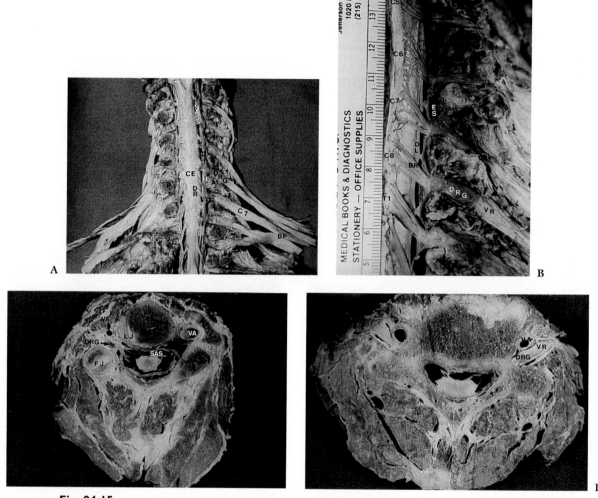

Fig. 94-15

Contents of spinal canal. **A,** Posterior view of cervical and upper thoracic portions of spinal canal with neural arches removed at level of pedicles (*P*). It shows cervical enlargement (*CE*) of spinal cord, subarachnoid space (*SAS*), dorsal roots (*DR*), dura (*D*), epidural space (*ES*), C2-T1 spinal nerves and dorsal root ganglia (*DRG*), and ventral rami forming brachial plexus (*BP*). **B,** Magnified posterior view of C5-T1 spinal cord levels, dorsal roots, dorsal root ganglia, and ventral rami (*VR*). Also visualized are dentations of denticulate ligament (*DL*) and subarachnoid and epidural spaces. Note that swellings of dorsal root ganglia are partly located outside intervertebral foramina within troughs of transverse processes. **C,** Cross section of C5-C6 vertebrae at level of their intervertebral foramen, demonstrating relatively generous subarachnoid space at this level. Dorsal root ganglion is visualized within one intervertebral foramen. Note that it is bounded anteriorly by vertebral artery (*VA*) and Luschka's joint (*LJ*) and posteriorly by facet joint (*FJ*). Also note common asymmetry in size of vertebral arteries of two sides. **D,** Cross section of another C5 vertebra at level of its pedicles. Note elliptical outline of cervical spinal cord and intimate relationship of dorsal root ganglia and ventral rami to vertebral arteries.

C5, C6-C7, and C7-T1 levels also show anterior buckling. In a sagittal section through the lateral part of the dural sac where the nerve roots enter their dural sleeves, the roots display an anterior relationship to the discs (Fig. 94-16, *C*). In a sagittal section at the point where the dorsal root ganglia emerge from the intervertebral foramen, the ganglia demonstrate an anterior relationship to the vertebral arteries and a posterior relationship to the facet joints

and articular pillars (Fig. 94-16, *D*). A sagittal section through the sulci of the transverse processes shows at higher levels (C3-C6) the ventral rami and at lower levels (C7-C8) the dorsal root ganglia lying in the sulci with the costal element of the transverse process anteriorly and the transverse element of the transverse process posteriorly (Fig. 94-16, *E*).

A coronal section through the vertebral bodies of another severely degenerated cervical spine shows

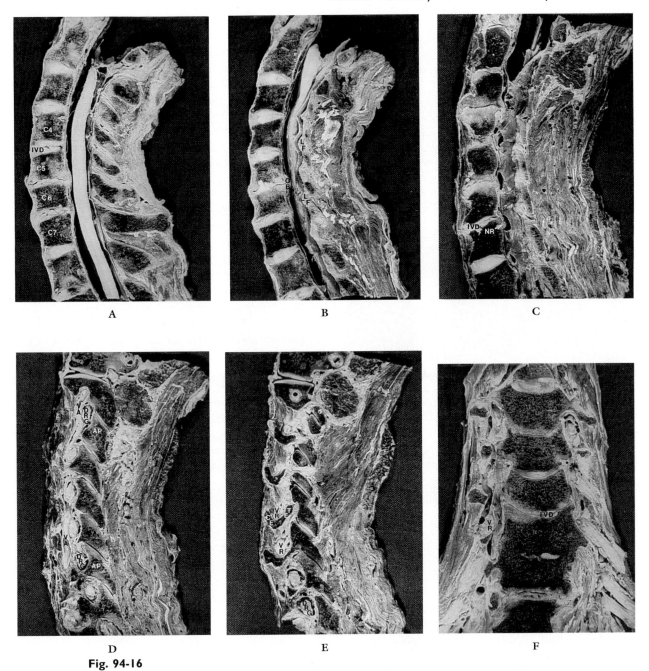

Fig. 94-16

Sagittal sections through cervical spine with substantial degenerative changes. **A,** Midsagittal section demonstrating major degenerative changes involving C4-C5, C5-C6, and C6-C7 intervertebral discs (*IVD*). **B,** Parasagittal section through lateral part of spinal cord. It shows prominent C5-C6 osteophytic bar (*OB*) that intrudes into anterior part of spinal canal. Degeneration of disc has caused forward buckling of a number of ligamenta flava (*LF*) into posterior part of spinal canal. **C,** Parasagittal section through lateral part of dural sac, where nerve roots (*NR*) enter their dural sleeve just posterior to posterolateral part of intervertebral discs. **D,** Sagittal section through point where the dorsal root ganglia (*DRG*) and spinal nerves are just exiting their intervertebral foramina. Note that these neural structures are bounded anteriorly by vertebral artery (*VA*) and posteriorly by articular pillars (*AP*). **E,** Sagittal section through sulci of the transverse processes showing ventral rami (*VR*) and dorsal root ganglia lying in sulci. They are bounded anteriorly by costal element (*CE*) and posteriorly by transverse element (*TE*) of transverse process. **F,** Anterior view of coronal section through cervical spine with severely degenerated intervertebral discs (*IVD*). Ventral rami are visualized lateral to vertebral artery.

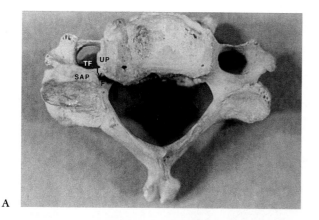

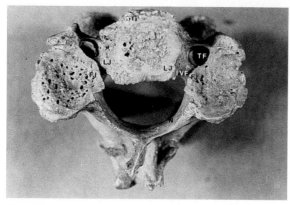

Fig. 94-17

Degenerated cervical vertebrae. **A**, Hypertrophic degenerative changes involving left uncinate process (*UP*) and left superior articular process (*SAP*), which encroach into both intervertebral foramen (*IVF*) and transverse foramen (*TF*). **B**, Even more severely degenerated cervical vertebra, showing bilateral hypertrophic degenerative changes of both Luschka's joint (*LJ*) and facet joints (*FJ*), causing bilateral encroachments into intervertebral and transverse foramina.

the right vertebral artery and veins with the ventral rami lateral to the artery (Fig. 94-16, *F*).

Specimens of degenerated cervical vertebrae demonstrate how hypertrophic degenerative changes involving the facet joints and Luschka's joint can not only encroach on the nerve roots and dorsal root ganglion within the intervertebral foramen, but they also have the potential to encroach on the dorsal-root ganglion, ventral rami, and vertebral vessels within the sulci of the transverse processes (Fig. 94-17). Encroachments on the vertebral artery can be significant since they supply the nerve roots, spinal cord, and brain stem.

Beyond the transverse processes the ventral rami of the upper four cervical nerves will continue anterolaterally to form the cervical plexus, while the ventral rami of the lower four cervical nerves will contribute to the brachial plexus.

The recurrent meningeal or sinovertebral nerve of Luschka provides the primary sensory innervation to the pain-sensitive walls and contents of the spinal canal. The sinovertebral nerve most commonly arises just outside the intervertebral foramen from the rami communicans that connect the spinal nerve or its ventral ramus to the sympathetic trunk. It then recurs through the intervertebral foramen to supply sensory innervation to the posterior longitudinal ligament, posterior portion of the anulus fibrosus, dura, epidural fat and vessels, ligamenta flava, and the periosteal lining of the vertebral canal.

Because of the position of the atlantooccipital and atlantoaxial joints anterior to the emerging C1 and C2 spinal nerves, their joint capsules are innervated by branches of the ventral rami of the C1 and C2 spinal nerves.[2, 28] The more posteriorly placed facet joints of the rest of the cervical vertebrae receive their sensory innervation from branches of the dorsal rami. The dorsal rami supply branches to both the facet joint capsule in the posterior wall of their intervertebral foramen and the next lower facet-joint capsule. The dorsal rami of most cervical spinal nerves divide into medial and lateral branches. The medial branches provide sensory innervation to the interspinal, supraspinal, and nuchal ligaments and end as cutaneous nerves to the posterior scalp and neck. They also provide sensory and motor innervation to the interspinal and multifidus muscles. The lateral branches supply sensory and motor innervation to the splenius capitis and cervicis, longissimus capitis, and semispinalis capitis muscles.

The sensory innervation of the anterolateral annulus of the intervertebral disc and the anterior longitudinal ligament is largely supplied by branches from the rami communicans to the sympathetic trunk.

Musculature of the Cervical Spine

The musculature capable of stabilizing and moving the cervical spine can be divided into anterior and posterior muscle groups. Obviously, anterior musculature will tend to be spine flexors and posterior musculature will be extensors. Since all muscles are situated on one side of the midsagittal plane they will laterally bend the spine to the ipsilateral side. Also, since almost all muscles have some obliquity to their pull they will rotate the spine to turn the face to either the ipsilateral or contralateral side. An appreciation of cervical musculature is important in understanding cervical spine function and the muscles encountered during surgery. Also, these muscles can be injured by cervical spine trauma.

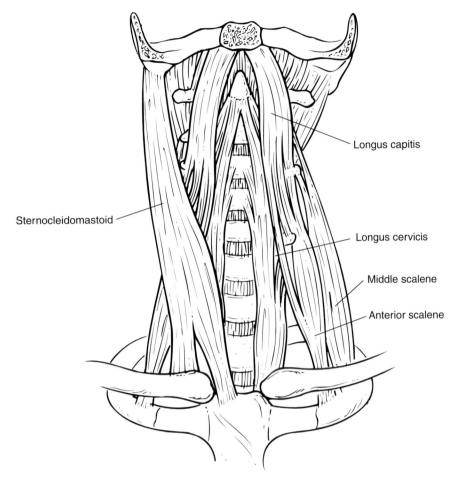

Fig. 94-18

Anterior musculature of cervical spine.

Anterior Musculature (Fig. 94-18)

The longus colli arise from the bodies of upper thoracic vertebrae and from the bodies and transverse processes of lower cervical vertebrae. They insert into the bodies and transverse processes of higher cervical vertebrae. The longus capitis arises from the anterior tubercles of the transverse processes of C3 to C6 and inserts into the basilar portion of the occipital bone. The longus muscles flex, laterally bend, and can rotate the spine in either direction. They are innervated by branches of the C1 to C6 ventral rami.

The rectus capitis anterior is a short muscle extending from the front of the lateral mass of the atlas to the basilar part of the occipital bone. The rectus capitis lateralis is a short muscle coursing from the transverse process of the atlas to the jugular process of the occipital bone. These muscles stabilize and, respectively, flex and laterally bend the atlantooccipital joints. They are innervated by C1 and possibly C2 ventral rami.

The anterior scalene muscle extends from the first rib to the anterior tubercles of the transverse processes of C3 to C6. The middle scalene courses from the first rib to the posterior tubercles of the transverse processes of C2 to C7. The posterior scalene stretches from the second rib to the posterior tubercles of the transverse processes of C4 to C6. The scalenes are clearly lateral benders of the spine. The anterior scalene may also flex and rotate the face contralaterally while the posterior scalene may extend and rotate the face to the same side. They are innervated by branches of the C3 to C8 ventral rami.

The sternocleidomastoid muscle arises from the medial clavicle and manubrium and runs posteriorly and laterally to insert on the mastoid process. Its major function is to rotate the face to the opposite side. It also laterally bends and flexes. It is innervated by the spinal portion of the accessory cranial nerve with most of its segmental input from the C2-C3 spinal cord level.

The infrahyoid or strap muscles that are situated on the front of the larynx and thyroid glands can also serve as accessory spine flexors. They extend from the upper ribs and manubrium to the thyroid cartilage and hyoid bone. While these muscles usually act on the larynx and hyoid in swallowing, when the hyoid is fixed they can participate in forced spine flexion. They are innervated by the ansa cervicalis that is derived from the C1 to C3 ventral rami.

Posterior Musculature (Fig. 94-19)

There are several oppositely coursing layers of posterior muscles that can move the spine. From approximately superficial to deep they include: (1) the upwardly and medially running trapezius, rhomboids, and levator scapulae muscles; (2) the upwardly and laterally coursing splenius cervicis and capitis, iliocostalis cervicis, and longissimus cervicis and capitis muscles; (3) the upwardly and mostly medially running semispinalis cervicis and capitis, multifidus, and rotator muscles; (4) the vertically coursing interspinal and intertransverse muscles; and (5) the variously running suboccipital muscles.

The upper trapezius extends from the clavicle and acromion upward and medially to the C7 spinous process, ligamentum nuchae, and superior nuchal line of the occipital bone (Fig. 94-19, A). It is innervated by the spinal portion of the accessory nerve with major segmental input from C3-C4 spinal cord segments. The rhomboids course from the lower medial scapular border to the upper thoracic and lower cervical spinous processes. The levator scapulae runs from the upper part of the medial border of the scapula to the C1 to C4 transverse processes. Both rhomboids and levator scapulae receive innervation mostly from the dorsal scapular nerve (C5), but levator scapulae also receives a branch from the C4 ventral ramus. With the scapula fixed, all these normally shoulder-moving muscles are potential spine extensors and lateral benders. Because the trapezius and rhomboids attach to the skull or spinous processes they rotate the face to the opposite side while the levator scapulae's transverse process attachment produces face rotation to the same side.

Splenius cervicis courses from upper thoracic spinous processes to the posterior tubercles of the transverse processes of C1 to C3 (Fig. 94-19, B). Splenius capitis extends from the lower ligamentum nuchae and lower cervical and upper thoracic spinous processes to the occipital bone and mastoid process. Both muscles extend, laterally bend, and rotate the face to the same side. They are innervated by lateral branches of middle and lower cervical dorsal rami.

Iliocostalis cervicis extends from the angles of the upper ribs to the posterior tubercles of the transverse processes of C4 to C6 (Fig. 94-19, B). Longissimus cervicis stretches from upper thoracic transverse processes to the posterior tubercles of the transverse processes of C2 to C6. Longissimus capitis runs from the upper thoracic transverse processes and lower cervical articular processes to the posterior margin of the mastoid process. These muscles are all parts of the erector spinae. They extend, laterally bend, and rotate the face to the same side. They are innervated by lateral branches of the cervical and upper thoracic dorsal rami.

The semispinalis cervicis arises from upper thoracic transverse processes and runs upward and medially to the C2 to C5 spinous processes (Fig. 94-19, C). The semispinalis capitis is the largest posterior neck muscle. It runs almost vertically upward from upper thoracic transverse processes to attach the occipital bone between its superior and inferior nuchal lines. The deeper multifidus muscles arise from upper thoracic transverse processes and lower cervical articular processes and course medially and upward across two to four vertebrae to insert on higher cervical spinous processes. Still deeper rotator muscles run from lower cervical articular processes to the next or second higher spinous processes. The semispinalis, multifidus, and rotator muscles are extensors and lateral benders and largely rotate the face to the opposite side. While the semispinalis gets innervated by both medial and lateral branches of cervical dorsal rami, the multifidus and rotators are innervated by medial branches.

Small paired interspinal muscles bridge between each of the C3 to T1 spinous processes (Fig. 94-19, D). They are minor spine extensors and receive innervation from the medial branches of cervical dorsal rami. There are paired anterior and posterior intertransverse muscles interconnecting, respectively, the anterior and posterior tubercles of the cervical transverse processes. The anterior muscles receive ventral rami innervation and the posterior muscles receive both dorsal and ventral rami innervation.

Four deep small suboccipital muscles interconnect the posterior aspect of the axis, atlas and occipital bone. All of these muscles are innervated by the C1 dorsal ramus (the suboccipital nerve), which emerges between them. The rectus capitis posterior major extends from the spinous process of the axis to the lateral part of the inferior nuchal line of the occipital bone. It extends and rotates the face to the same side. The rectus capitis posterior minor courses from the posterior tubercle of the atlas to the medial part of the inferior nuchal line. It is an extensor. The obliquus capitis inferior arises from the spinous process of the axis and

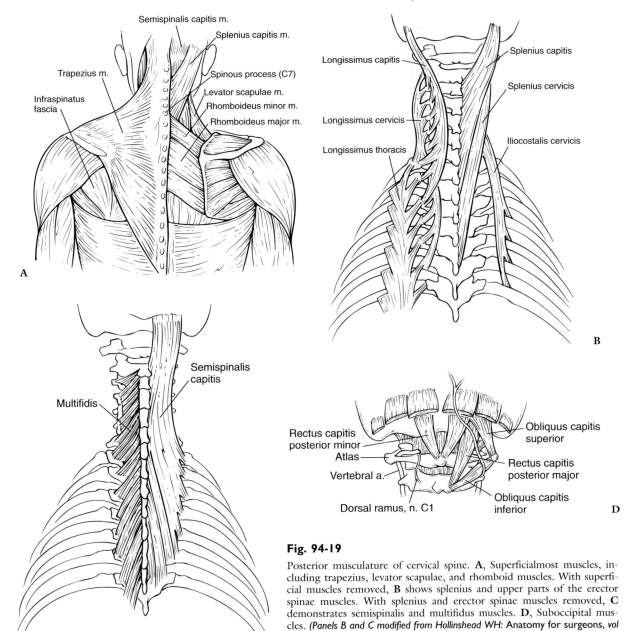

Fig. 94-19

Posterior musculature of cervical spine. **A,** Superficialmost muscles, including trapezius, levator scapulae, and rhomboid muscles. With superficial muscles removed, **B** shows splenius and upper parts of the erector spinae muscles. With splenius and erector spinae muscles removed, **C** demonstrates semispinalis and multifidus muscles. **D,** Suboccipital muscles. *(Panels B and C modified from Hollinshead WH:* Anatomy for surgeons, *vol 3,* Back and limbs, *New York, 1969, Harper & Row.)*

runs laterally to the transverse process of the atlas. It rotates the atlas to turn the face to the same side. The obliquus capitis superior runs from the transverse process of the atlas upward and slightly medially to attach to the occipital bone just above its inferior nuchal line. It extends and laterally bends the head.

Anterior Relationships of the Cervical Spine

Structures that are closely related to the anterior aspect of the cervical spine are of interest because they

are at times injured by hyperextension trauma to the cervical spine and because they are in the operative field in anterior approaches to the cervical spine (Fig. 94-20).

The sympathetic trunk runs longitudinally along the anterior aspect of the anterior tubercles of the transverse processes. Injuries to the sympathetic trunk will produce ipsilateral Horner's syndrome. The pharynx and esophagus are separated from the anterior aspect of the vertebral bodies only by the layers of the prevertebral fascia between which the retropharyngeal space is situated. The larynx is only additionally separated from the vertebral bodies by

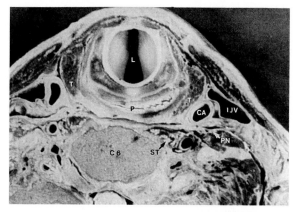

Fig. 94-20

Anterior relationships of cervical spine. Cross section of neck at the C6 level shows anteriorly related sympathetic trunk (*ST*), pharynx (*P*), larynx (*L*), lateral lobes of the thyroid gland (*T*), common carotid artery (*CA*), internal jugular vein (*IJV*), and phrenic nerve (*PN*).

the pharynx. At lower cervical levels the lateral lobes of the thyroid gland extend lateral to the lower pharynx and upper esophagus. Therefore, they are not far removed from the lateral part of the vertebral bodies and transverse processes. The carotid sheath structures are situated anterolateral to the transverse processes. The carotid sheath contains the internal jugular vein, vagus nerve, and the common carotid artery at lower levels and the internal carotid artery at higher levels. The phrenic nerve descends on the anterior surface of the anterior scalene muscle, which is located just anterior to the transverse processes.

References

1. Bland JH, Boushey DR: Anatomy and physiology of the cervical spine, *Semin Arthritis Rheum* 20:1, 1990.
2. Bogduk N: The clinical anatomy of the cervical dorsal rami, *Spine* 7:319, 1982.
3. Clemente CD: *Anatomy of the human body*, Philadelphia, 1985, Lea & Febiger, p 130.
4. Connell MD, Weisel SW: Natural history and pathogenesis of cervical disc disease, *Orthop Clin North Am* 23:369, 1992.
5. Daniels DL, Hyde JS, Kneeland JB, et al.: The cervical nerves and foramina: local coil MR imaging, AJNR *Am J Neuroradiol* 7:129, 1986.
6. Dickman CA, Mamourian A, Sonntag VKH, Drayer BP: Magnetic resonance imaging of the transverse atlantal ligament for the evaluation of atlantoaxial instability, *J Neurosurg* 75:221, 1991.
7. Dvorak J, Antinnes JA, Panjabi M, et al.: Age and gender related motion of the cervical spine, *Spine* 17:S393, 1992.
8. Dvorak J, Panjabi M: Functional anatomy of the alar ligaments, *Spine* 12:183, 1987.
9. Fesmire FM, Luten RC: The pediatric cervical spine: developmental anatomy and clinical aspects, *J Emerg Med* 7:133, 1989.
10. Frisoni GB, Anzola GP: Vertebrobasilar insufficiency after neck motion, *Stroke* 22:1452, 1991.
11. Hayashi K, Yabuki T: Origin of the uncus and of Luschka's joint in the cervical spine. *J Bone Joint Surg* 67A:788, 1985.
12. Hollinshead WH: *Anatomy for surgeons*, vol. 3, *The back and limbs*. New York, 1971, Harper & Row, p 127.
13. Johnson RM, Crelin ES, White AA, et al.: Some newer observations on the functional anatomy of the lower cervical spine, *Clin Orthop* 111:192, 1975.
14. Larsen WJ: *Human embryology*, New York, 1993, Churchill Livingstone, p 65.
15. Milne N: The role of zygapophyseal joint orientation and uncinate processes in controlling motion in the cervical spine, *J Anat* 178:189, 1991.
16. Moore KL: *The developing human*, Philadelphia, 1982, WB Saunders, p 344.
17. Netter FH: *Musculoskeletal system: congenital and developmental disorders.* In Ciba collection of medical illustrations, vol. 8, part 1, Summit, NJ, 1990, Ciba, p 26.
18. Netter FH. *Musculoskeletal system: normal anatomy.* In Ciba collection of medical illustrations, vol. 8, part 1, Summit NJ, 1990, Ciba, p 1.
19. Panjabi MM, Duranceau J, Goel V, et al. Cervical human vertebrae: quantitative three-dimensional anatomy of the middle and lower regions, *Spine* 16:861, 1991.
20. Panjabi MM, Oda T, Crisco JJ, et al.: Experimental study of atlas injuries. I. Biomechanical analysis of their mechanisms and fracture patterns, *Spine* 16:S460, 1991.
21. Pech P, Daniels DL, Williams WL, Haughton VM: The cervical neural foramina: correlation of microtomy and CT anatomy, *Radiology*, 155:143, 1985.
22. Sadler TW: *Langman's medical embryology*, Baltimore, 1985, Williams & Wilkins, p 133.
23. Schweitzer ME, Hodler J, Crevilla V, Resnick D: Craniovertebral junction: normal anatomy with MR correlation, *AJR Am J Roentgenol* 158:1087, 1992.
24. Sherk HH, Parke WE: Developmental anatomy. In Cervical Spine Research Society Editorial Subcommittee: *The cervical spine*, Philadelphia, 1983, JB Lippincott Co., p 1.
25. Sherk HH, Parke WH: Normal adult anatomy, In Cervical Spine Society Editorial Subcommittee: *The cervical spine*, Philadelphia, 1983, JB Lippincott Co., p 8.
26. Steel HH: Anatomical and mechanical considerations of the atlanto-axial articulations, *J Bone Joint Surg* 50A:1481, 1968.
27. White AA, Panjabi MM: *Clinical biomechanics of the cervical spine*, Philadelphia, 1978, JB Lippincott Co., p 65.
28. White AA, Panjabi MM, Posner I, et al.: *Spinal stability: evaluation and treatment*. In Murray DG, editor: *Instructional course lectures*, St. Louis, 1981, CV Mosby Co., p 457.

Chapter 95
Surgical Approaches to the Cervical Spine

William J. Richardson
Robert J. Spinner

Introduction

Posterior Approaches

    posterior approach to C3-C7

    posterior approach to the occiput and
      C1-C2

Anterior Approaches

    anteromedial (Smith-Peterson)
      approach

    anterior approaches to C1-C3

**Approach to the Cervicothoracic
Junction**

Summary

Introduction

The site of the primary pathologic condition usually dictates the type of surgical approach to the cervical spine. In general, the anterior approach provides the best access to vertebral bodies and intervertebral disc spaces; the posterior approach provides access to the spinous processes, laminae, and facets, as well as to the spinal cord, posterolateral corner of vertebral bodies, and the anulus fibrosus (for a lateral disc). Most commonly, the cervical spine can be exposed through the standard posterior midline or anteromedial approaches. However, on occasion, other surgical approaches must be used to visualize the less accessible, more vulnerable areas of the cervical spine. This chapter will discuss in detail the methods of approaching all areas of the cervical spine and will include illustrative case examples.

Posterior Approaches

Posterior Approach to C3-C7

The posterior approach is the most frequently used approach to the cervical spine. It provides safe access to the posterior elements, uses internervous planes, and is extensile, if needed. It can be used for posterior cervical fusions, decompressive laminectomies, discectomies, and foraminotomies.

The patient is placed in the prone position using a large chest pad for support with the head resting on a cerebellar frame or brace. The patient's neck is in a neutral position. Care is taken in positioning the patient to preclude intraoperative motion of the cervical spine, to maintain adequate ventilatory support, and to protect other parts of the body against pressure or traction injuries. Some spinal surgeons prefer to have the patient seated with the head in a brace; this position may decrease venous bleeding and assist in visualization as the blood drains from the wound, but it increases the risk of air embolism.

The area is widely prepped and draped sterilely. The bony landmarks, including the spinous processes of C2, C7, and T1, are palpated. The subdermal tissue may be infiltrated with a lidocaine/epinephrine solution. A generous midline posterior skin incision is made (Fig. 95-1) and the dissection is taken down through the subcutaneous tissue and fascia. Self-retaining retractors are useful in providing tissue tension to stay in the midline. The dissection continues through the nearly avascular plane, and any crossing veins are cauterized. The dissection is continued to the spinous processes through the ligamentum nuchae (Fig. 95-2, A-C).

A clamp or needle is placed on the spinous process and helps confirm location on a lateral radiograph. The paraspinal muscles and ligamentous attachments are stripped from the spinous process above and be-

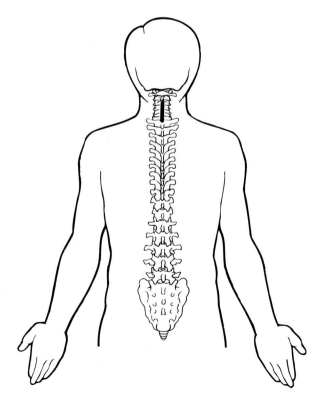

Fig. 95-1

Midline incision for a posterior approach to the lower cervical spine. (*Redrawn from Chan DPK, Whitesides TE Jr, Spetzler RF: Surgical approaches to the spine and bone grafts in spinal surgery. In Evarts CM, editor: Surgery of the musculoskeletal system, ed 2, New York, 1990, Churchill Livingstone.*)

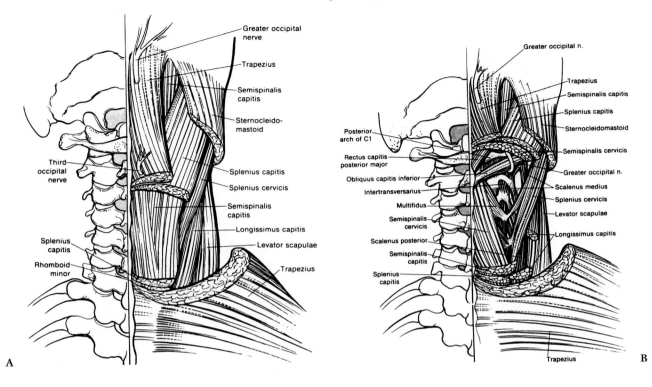

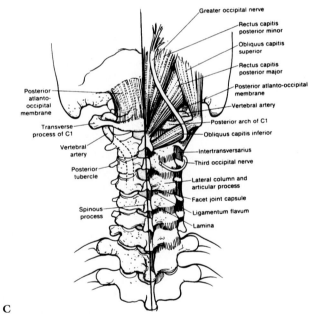

Fig. 95-2

Anatomy for a posterior approach to the cervical spine. **A,** Posterior cervical muscles. **B,** Superficial layer. **C,** Muscular attachments of the upper cervical spine. *(From Whitecloud TS III, Kelley LA: Anterior and posterior surgical approaches to the cervical spine. In Freymoyer JW, editor: The adult spine: principles and practice, New York, 1991, Raven Press.)*

low the space desired using the scalpel or electrocautery, and subperiosteal dissection is continued with a periosteal elevator (Fig. 95-3 and 95-4). The dissection is taken laterally at each level to expose the laminae to the lateral edge of the facet joints. Hemostasis of any venous bleeding or of the segmental bleeders is obtained using electrocautery. Sponges are packed at each level.

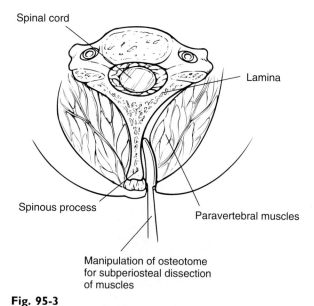

Spinal cord

Lamina

Spinous process

Paravertebral muscles

Manipulation of osteotome
for subperiosteal dissection
of muscles

Fig. 95-3

Method of subperiosteal dissection. *(Redrawn from Long DM, McAfee PC: Atlas of spinal surgery, Baltimore, 1992, Williams and Wilkins.)*

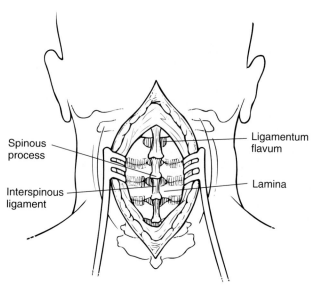

Spinous
process

Ligamentum
flavum

Interspinous
ligament

Lamina

Fig. 95-4

Posterior exposure of the cervical spine.

After the operation is performed, the incision is closed in layers, usually over a vacuum drain. Posterior cervical wounds do better with monofilament suture for skin closure.

Posterior Approach to the Occiput and C1-C2

Posterior approach to the occiput and upper cervical spine is similar to that previously discussed. It is

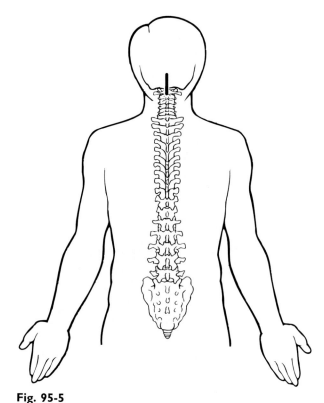

Fig. 95-5

Midline incision for a posterior approach to the upper cervical spine. *(Redrawn from Chan DPK, Whitesides TE Jr, Spetzler RF: Surgical approaches to the spine and bone grafts in spinal surgery. In Evarts C McC, editor: Surgery of the musculoskeletal system, ed 2, New York, 1990, Churchill Livingstone.)*

used for fusion or decompression. The patient is nasotracheally intubated. Somatosensory evoked cortical potentials are often used. The patient is most commonly repositioned prone and a radiograph is obtained. If there is instability of the occipitocervical region, the patient may be placed in a halo preoperatively. If the pathology allows, it is often helpful to flex the head slightly to open the space between the occiput and C1 ring. The head is secured in a well-padded head-holding device. The landmarks of the inion and the spinous processes of C2, C7, and T1 are identified. Countertraction may be achieved with adhesive tape over the trapezius.

An approximately 10-cm midline incision is made starting at the inion stretching inferiorly to the spinous process of C3 (Fig. 95-5). With the use of self-retaining retractors, the dissection is continued midline through the fascia and ligamentum nuchae directly onto the spinous process of C2. The bifid tips of C2 and C3 may be useful in identifying the relationship to the occiput and the more anterior position of the posterior tubercle of the atlas. The ligamentous and muscular attachments are removed using a scalpel. The retractors are repositioned at a

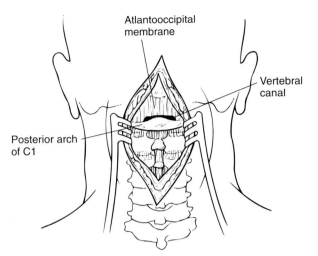

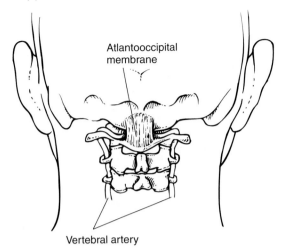

Fig. 95-6

Posterior exposure of the upper cervical spine.

deeper level. First the subperiosteal dissection with the periosteal elevator is performed at C2 in a medial to lateral direction, exposing the facet joints, leaving the capsular ligaments intact. Gentle subperiosteal dissection is then usually carried out at the base of the occiput before continuing at C1 (Fig. 95-6). Dissection at C1 may proceed laterally for 1.5 cm, taking special care to avoid injuring the vertebral artery (Fig. 95-7), large venous plexuses, or greater occipital nerve. The dissection may be extended to C3.

Anterior Approaches

Anteromedial (Smith-Peterson) Approach[14,15]

The Smith-Peterson approach allows anterior decompression of the spinal cord from C3 to T1. It is useful for disc excision, removal of osteophytes, vertebrectomy, and fusion. The patient is placed supine on the operating table with a folded towel between the scapulae. Head-halter traction is applied with 5 pounds of weight. The head is turned to the right. (The approach may be from the right or left. We prefer the left due to the lesser risk of injuring the recurrent laryngeal nerve.)

Palpable landmarks include the hyoid (C3), cricoid (C6), and thyroid cartilages (C4-C5); carotid tubercle (C6); carotid artery; and sternocleidomastoid muscle (Fig. 95-8). A transverse incision is made above the left clavicle at the appropriate level (Fig. 95-9). Such an incision can give

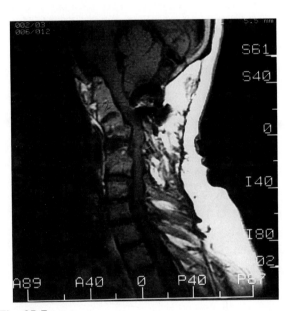

Fig. 95-7

The relationship of the upper cervical spine. *(Redrawn from Whitecloud TS III, Kelley LA: Anterior and posterior surgical approaches to the cervical spine. In Freymoyer JW, editor: The adult spine: principles and practice, New York, 1991, Raven Press.)*

access to three vertebral bodies; an oblique incision close to the anterior border of the sternocleidomastoid may give wider exposure. The dissection is taken down through the subcutaneous tissue to the platysma muscle, which is divided in line with the incision via electrocautery. The plane deep to the platysma is undermined to aid in mobilization. The fascia anterior to the sternocleidomastoid muscle is incised and the plane between it and the strap muscles is developed using sharp and blunt dissection through the pretracheal fascia. The carotid artery is identified and the dissection is carried down medial to it (Fig. 95-10a). The prever-

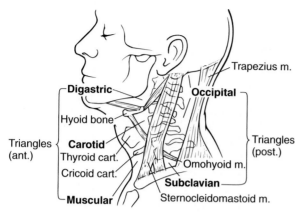

Fig. 95-8

The triangles of the neck. *(Redrawn from Whitecloud TS III, Kelley LA: Anterior and posterior surgical approaches to the cervical spine. In Freymoyer JW, editor: The adult spine: principles and practice, New York, 1991, Raven Press.)*

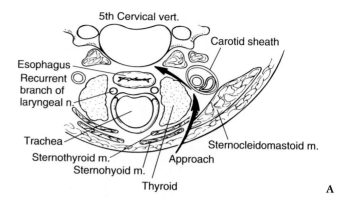

A

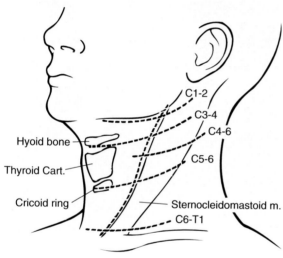

Fig. 95-9

The skin incisions for an anteromedial approach to the mid and lower cervical spine. The oblique incision along the medial border of the sternocleidomastoid muscle provides broader exposure than the transverse incision. *(Redrawn and modified from Whitecloud TS III, Kelley LA: Anterior and posterior surgical approaches to the cervical spine. In Freymoyer JW, editor: The adult spine: principles and practice, New York, 1991, Raven Press.)*

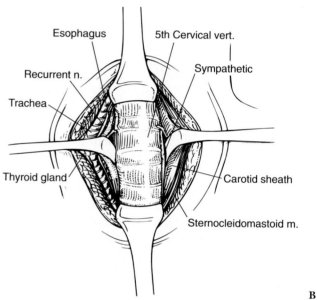

B

Fig. 95-10

Anteromedial approach to the mid and lower cervical spine. **A,** Direction of dissection. **B,** Exposure of vertebral bodies. *(Redrawn from Southwick WO, Robinson RA: Surgical approaches to the vertebral bodies in the cervical and lumbar regions, J Bone Joint Surg 39A:634, 1957.)*

tebral fascia is identified and divided longitudinally in the midline such as to avoid injury to the cervical sympathetic chain. The nasogastric tube within the esophagus and the vertebral bodies can then be palpated. The esophagus, trachea, thyroid gland, and recurrent laryngeal nerve are retracted medially with great care, and the sternocleidomastoid and carotid artery are retracted laterally, using thyroid retractors. The longus colli muscles are

then dissected laterally in a subperiosteal manner using a Kittner (Fig. 95-10b). A 25-gauge needle is inserted into the intervertebral disc and a tonsil clamp secures its position during a lateral radiograph to confirm the intraoperative position. Afterwards, dissection can be carried cephalad or caudad. Bovie and bipolar electrocautery may be used to coagulate venous vessels along the medial edge of the longus colli.

After the definitive procedure is performed, immaculate hemostasis should be attained. The incision is then closed in layers. A suction drain is placed deep to the platysma. The platysma and subcutaneous layers are closed. A subcuticular stitch with Steristrips provides a cosmetic closure.

Anterior Approaches to C1-C3

Over the past 60 years, different approaches to the anterior upper cervical region have been described. Each has its own set of risks and benefits. We currently use three anterior approaches to the upper cervical spine—transoral, anterior retropharyngeal, and anterolateral retropharyngeal—and have not used the techniques of temporomandibular joint dislocation[13] and tongue-splitting.[6] The transoral approach is the most direct and is useful particularly in certain pathologic conditions or physical states (no ability to extend the neck). Being transpalatal, it carries up to a 50% chance of perioperative infection. Thus, its use with bone grafts is not supported. The other two approaches are extramucosal and are therefore more amenable to bone grafting. The anterior retropharyngeal approach does allow wider exposure and an opportunity for strut grafting. The anterolateral retropharyngeal approach[19] does not provide as good an exposure to the basiocciput as the other two exposures. The approaches and constraints of the two retropharyngeal approaches place different anatomic structures at risk. Thus, the spinal surgeon must individualize each case.

Transoral Approach[5,8,16]

The transoral approach is infrequently used owing to its significant risks of infectious complications and its confined space; however, in selected cases, it may be useful, especially for basilar settling, congenital deformities, resecting the odontoid process, draining abscesses, or biopsying masses in the upper anterior cervical spine.

The patient is placed supine using the Mayfield head-holding device with the head in slight extension. Somatosensory cortical evoked potentials are useful in this procedure. An awake transoral intubation is performed and is converted to general anesthesia when the airway is established. The face and oropharynx are prepped. A Dingman retractor is used to provide good visualization of the oral activity. The soft palate and uvula may be kept out of the operative field with a red rubber catheter passed through each nostril and sutured to the uvula; gentle traction is applied to the sutures (Figs. 95-11 and 95-12).

The bony landmarks, including the anterior tubercle of C1 and the body of C2, can be palpated. Fluoroscopy or lateral radiographs may be helpful in defining the bony anatomy. The lateral retractors of the Dingman apparatus may be helpful. A midline longitudinal incision in the posterior pharyngeal wall is made and is undermined. A similar midline split

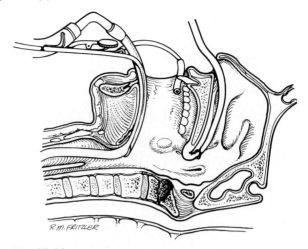

Fig. 95-11

Transoral approach to the upper cervical spine. *(Redrawn from Spetzler RF: Transoral approach to the upper cervical spine. In Evarts CM, editor: Surgery of the musculoskeletal system, New York, 1983, Churchill Livingstone.)*

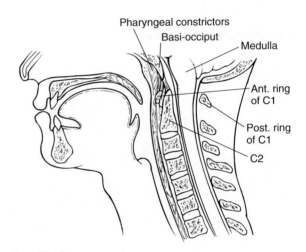

Fig. 95-12

Anatomic relationships of the transoral approach. *(Redrawn and modified from Whitecloud TS III, Kelley LA: Anterior and posterior surgical approaches to the cervical spine. In Freymoyer JW, editor: The adult spine: principles and practice, New York, 1991, Raven Press.)*

is made through the retropharyngeal area and in the anterior longitudinal ligament from C1 to C3. Care is taken to avoid injury to the pharyngeal mucosa. Hemostasis is achieved with bipolar electrocautery, though thermal necrosis may increase the risk of infection.

With a periosteal elevator the muscles are stripped laterally to the lateral masses. The flaps are preserved with traction stitches.

Once the definitive procedure is completed, the lateral wings of the Dingman retractor are removed. The pharyngeal and palatal incisions are closed in layers.

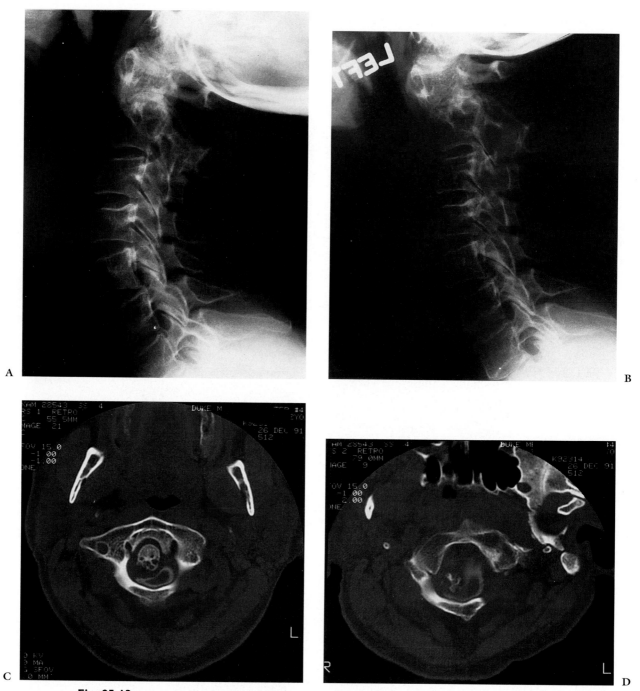

Fig. 95-13

Transoral approach for resection of the odontoid. **A,** Preoperative lateral radiograph in neutral demonstrates axial settling. **B,** Preoperative lateral radiograph in flexion demonstrates C1-C2 instability with widening of the predental space. **C,** Preoperative CT myelogram in neutral shows a deformed spinal cord. **D,** Preoperative CT myelogram in flexion shows further spinal-cord compromise.

Case Report A 52-year-old Caucasian female with a history of chronic seropositive rheumatoid arthritis, taking methotrexate and steroids, presented with a 1-year history of progressive neck and bilateral arm pain. She was found to have severe occiput-C2 instability (Fig. 95-13, *A* and *B*) with basilar settling and atlantoaxial subluxation. CT myelogram (Fig. 95-13, *C* and *D*) showed spinal impingement. MRI could not be used owing to cochlear implants.

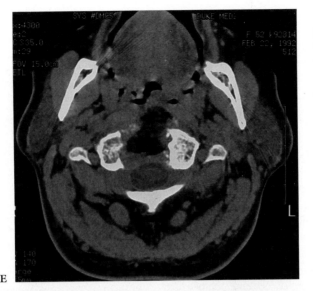

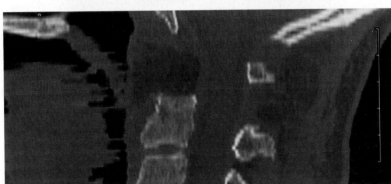

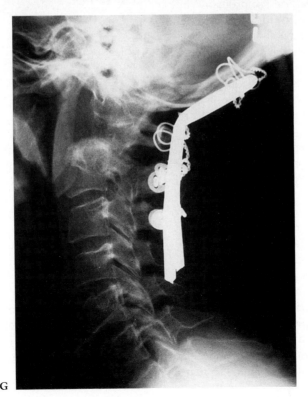

Fig. 95-13, cont'd

E, Postoperative axial CT scan after the resection of the odontoid shows a normal thecal sac. **F,** Postoperative CT scan with sagittal reconstruction shows the fat graft where the dens was. **G,** Postoperative lateral radiograph in neutral shows intact Luque instrumentation and fusion.

Traction was applied and serial radiographs showed slight improvement in alignment, but repeat CT myelogram showed continued but slightly improved spinal-cord compression. She underwent transoral resection of the odontoid. Two weeks later, she underwent occiput-C3 fusion using Luque rod instrumentation. A tracheostomy was performed to maintain her airway without disturbing the pharyngeal wound.

Postoperatively, she did well. Radiographs revealed good maintenance of the alignment (Figs. 13, E-G). She was placed in a Philadelphia collar and her halo was removed in the early postoperative period. She was placed in a soft collar 2 months later, which was removed several weeks later. At 1-year follow-up, she could flex her chin to four fingerbreadths from the chest, extend 10 degrees past neutral, and had 10 degrees of lateral rotation. Radiographs show good alignment with no motion in flexion or extension.

Anterior Retropharyngeal Approach9

The anterior retropharyngeal approach is useful for lesions from the clivus to C3, especially when bone grafting for fusion may be indicated. The patient is placed supine on the operating room table. Somatosensory evoked potentials are helpful in monitoring intraoperative neurologic changes. Skull tongs are used. The neck is extended maximally without inducing neurologic changes or symptoms. While awake, the patient is nasotracheally intubated and subsequently converted to general anesthesia. A T-shaped incision is made with the upper transverse submandibular incision made on the right side. The vertical limb is made, if necessary, for additional exposure (Fig. 95-14, A). The transverse incision is carried through the skin, subcutaneous tissue and the platysma. Subplatysmal flaps are raised. The retromandibular vein is identified, as is the marginal mandibular branch of the facial nerve with electric stimulation as it crosses the external facial artery and vein. These vessels are ligated. Care is taken to keep the exposure deep to the retromandibular vein to prevent injuring the facial nerve.

The anterior border of the sternocleidomastoid muscle is mobilized and the carotid pulse identified. The submandibular gland is resected by sharp and blunt dissection off of the mandible. The jugular and digastric lymph nodes are excised. The digastric and stylohyoid muscles are identified (see Fig. 95-14, B). The lingual nerve is identified beneath the mandible and is preserved. The hypoglossal nerve is dissected out throughout the length of the wound, so that it

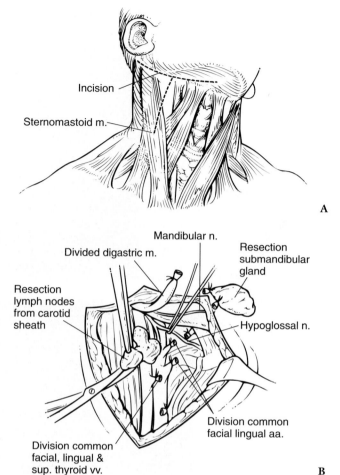

Fig. 95-14

Anterior retropharyngeal approach to the upper cervical spine via the submandibular incision. **A,** T-shaped incision. **B,** Exposure after vessels ligated and lymph/submandibular gland resected. *(Redrawn from McAfee PC and others: The anterior retropharyngeal approach to the upper part of the cervical spine, J Bone Joint Surg 69A:1371, 1987.)*

can be retracted superiorly. Inferiorly, the superior laryngeal nerve is preserved. The digastric muscle is divided. The hyoid and hypopharynx can then be mobilized medially, which avoids possible contamination from the nasopharynx, hypopharynx, and esophagus. Overzealous retraction can injure the neighboring cranial nerves.

The internal carotid artery, jugular vein, and vagus nerve are identified and the dissection is continued in the retropharyngeal space with the contents of the carotid sheath being retracted laterally and the larynx and pharynx, anteromedially. Branches of the carotid artery and the internal jugular vein are ligated in an inferior to superior manner to facilitate exposure (Fig. 95-15). The superior laryngeal nerve is protected. The alar and prevertebral fasciae are divided longitudinally and the longus colli

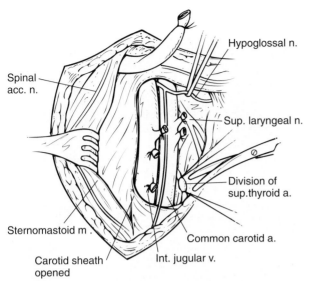

Hypoglossal n.

Spinal
acc. n.

Sup. laryngeal n.

Division of
sup. thyroid a.

Sternomastoid m.

Common carotid a.

Int. jugular v.

Carotid sheath
opened

Fig. 95-15

The relationship of the hypoglossal, spinal accessory, and superior laryngeal nerves to the deep dissection. *(Redrawn from McAfee PC and others: The anterior retropharyngeal approach to the upper part of the cervical spine, J Bone Joint Surg 69A:1371, 1987.)*

muscles are exposed. With the head in neutral position, the longus colli muscles are dissected subperiosteally from the anterior tubercle of the atlas and C2 body. Position may be confirmed by radiographs. The dissection is taken laterally, avoiding the vertebral arteries. The anterior longitudinal ligament may also be removed if necessary.

After the definitive procedure is performed (Fig. 95-16, *A* and *B*), hemostasis is achieved. The digastric tendon is repaired. Limbs of a suction drain are placed deep in the retropharyngeal and subcutaneous spaces. The platysma and subcutaneous layers are closed, and the skin is approximated.

Case Report A 56-year-old Caucasian male with longstanding rheumatoid arthritis status post posterior C1-C2 fusion 10 years earlier and C4-C5 anterior fusion 5 years earlier presented with a history of bilateral lower extremity sensory disturbances and weakness. One week prior to admission he had an acute exacerbation of his symptoms following a cough which led to his being unable to walk. Radiographs demonstrated his kyphosis and instability (Fig. 95-17, *A*); MRI revealed spinal-cord compression at C4-C5 (Fig. 95-17, *B*). He underwent anterior cervical multiple vertebrectomies with decompression from C3 to C7 using a fibular strut graft from C2 to T1 and distal plate fixation; he was maintained in a halo for 6 months (Fig. 95-17, *C*).

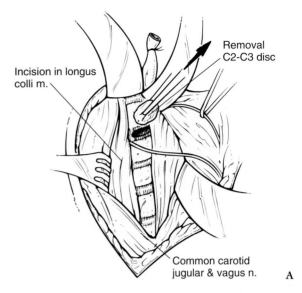

Incision in longus
colli m.

Removal
C2-C3 disc

Common carotid
jugular & vagus n.

A

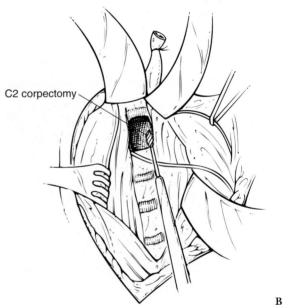

C2 corpectomy

B

Fig. 95-16

The exposure of the upper cervical vertebrae after the longus colli has been dissected laterally. **A,** C2-C3 discectomy. **B,** C2 corpectomy. *(Redrawn from McAfee PC and others: The anterior retropharyngeal approach to the upper part of the cervical spine, J Bone Joint Surg 69A:1371, 1987.)*

He is currently ambulating using a single forearm crutch.

Anterolateral Retropharyngeal (Whitesides-Henry) Approach[7,19]

The anterolateral approach is useful for C1-C2 fusions when the posterior ring of C1 is incompetent, thus avoiding occiput to C2 fusion. It may be replaced by Magerl's posterior screw fixation at C1-

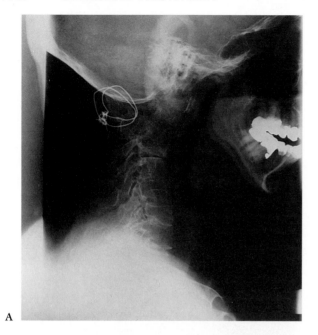

A

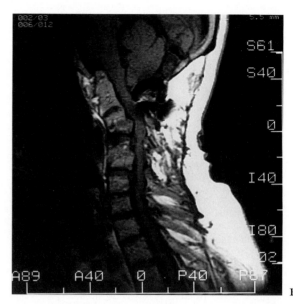

B

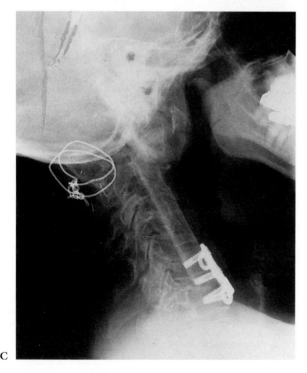

C

Fig. 95-17

Case example using the anterior retropharyngeal approach to the upper cervical spine. **A,** Preoperative lateral C-spine radiograph shows kyphosis and instability. **B,** Preoperative MRI demonstrates canal compromise and spinal-cord compression. **C,** Postoperative lateral C-spine radiograph shows the fibular graft and plate fixation.

C2. It has a high complication rate in patients with rheumatoid arthritis; hence, other approaches should be considered in these patients. The patient is placed supine. Fiberoptic nasotracheal intubation through the contralateral nostril is performed with the patient awake. When the airway is secured, general anesthesia is established. The mouth is kept closed. The neck is extended as far as possible and the head

is turned maximally. Skeletal traction with tongs or a halo device is used.

A hockey-stick incision along the anterior margin of the sternocleidomastoid muscle is made, superiorly veering across the proximal sternocleidomastoid, crossing the base of the temporal bone (Fig. 95-18). The external jugular vein is ligated and divided as it crosses the sternocleidomastoid. Posterior to it, the

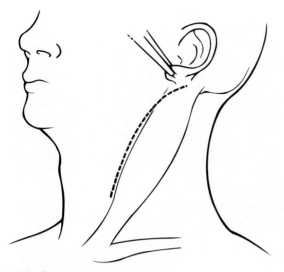

Fig. 95-18

Hockey-stick–shaped incision for the lateral retropharyngeal approach. *(Redrawn and modified from Whitecloud TS III, Kelley LA: Anterior and posterior surgical approaches to the cervical spine. In Freymoyer JW, editor: The adult spine: principles and practice, New York, 1991, Raven Press.)*

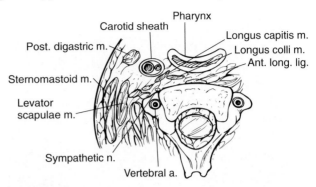

Fig. 95-19

The anterolateral approach to the upper cervical spine is posterior to the carotid sheath. *(Redrawn and modified from Johnson RM, Murphy MJ, Southwick WO: Surgical approaches to the spine. In Rothman RH, Simeone FA, editors: The spine, ed 3, Philadelphia, 1992, W.B. Saunders.)*

great auricular nerve is identified and preserved. The sternocleidomastoid is divided transversely below the mastoid process and the splenius capitis may be partially divided. The sternocleidomastoid muscle is then mobilized and everted. Using sharp and blunt dissection, the spinal accessory nerve is identified. The occipital artery is ligated. Lymph nodes can be excised to enhance visualization.

Dissection then continues in the retropharyngeal space laterally and posteriorly to the carotid sheath (Fig. 95-19). The sternocleidomastoid and spinal accessory nerve are retracted posteriorly, and the carotid sheath and its associated cranial nerves are gently retracted anteriorly. The transverse processes of the cervical spine become palpable. The plane between the alar and prevertebral fasciae is developed using finger dissection toward the anterior aspect of the vertebral bodies. The bony prominences of the anterior tubercle of C1 and the body of C2 become palpable. The anterior longitudinal ligament is incised in its midline and the ligaments and overlying muscles are dissected subperiosteally and laterally. The procedure is then repeated on the opposite side.

When the definitive procedure is finished, the wound is thoroughly irrigated and hemostasis is achieved. The sternocleidomastoid is repaired. The limbs of a suction drain are placed in the retropharyngeal and subcutaneous spaces. The platysma and subcutaneous tissue are closed in layers and the skin edges are reapproximated.

Case Report

A 45-year-old Caucasian male with an os odontoideum had undergone two prior attempts at posterior cervical fusion at C1-C2. He presented with pseudarthrosis with motion on flexion/extension as well as breakage of the wires (Figs. 95-20, *A* and *B*). CT scan revealed incompetence of the posterior ring of C1 (Fig. 95-20, *C*). He underwent anterior fusion with 3.5-mm Herbert screws at C1-C2 to preserve occiput-C1 motion (Fig. 95-20, *D*). Postoperatively, he has had good relief of his pain and can flex his chin within 2 fingerbreadths of his chest.

Approach to the Cervicothoracic Junction

The anterior cervicothoracic junction has historically been a difficult region for surgical exposure. Different exposures have been described, including lower anterior cervical,[12] sternal-splitting,[3,17] posterior thoracotomy,[18] costotransversectomy,[2] transverse supraclavicular,[11] excision of clavicle and manubrium,[4] and combined anterior cervical with third-rib thoracotomy.[10]

We prefer the approach described by Birch and colleagues.[1] The patient is placed in the deckchair position. Either side may be approached with the head turned slightly toward the contralateral side. A T-shaped incision is made with the transverse arm being 2 cm above the clavicle, and the midline vertical arm extending several centimeters down the sternum (Fig. 95-21, *A*). The incision is taken down to the platysma and flaps are elevated deep to it (Fig.

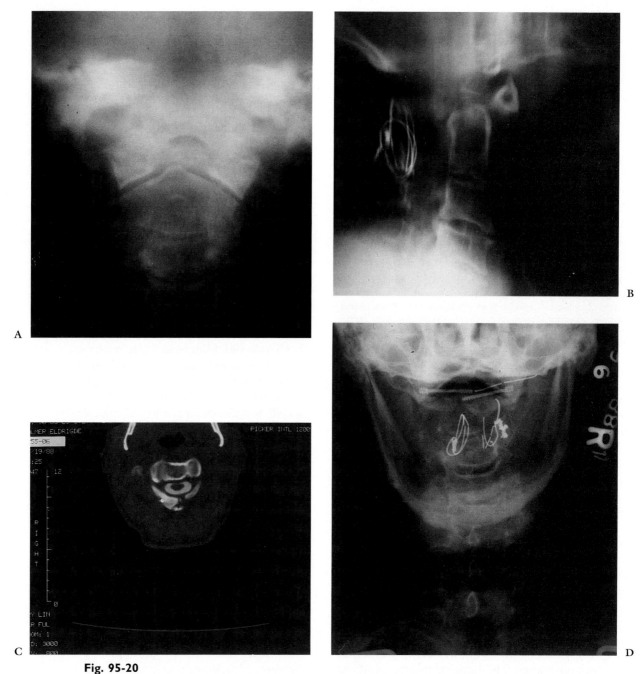

Fig. 95-20

Anterolateral approach to the os odontoideum. **A,** Preoperative anteroposterior tomogram shows the sclerotic margins of the os odontoideum. **B,** Preoperative lateral tomogram shows the broken posterior wire. **C,** Preoperative CT scan demonstrates the incompetent posterior ring of C1. **D,** Postoperative anteroposterior C-spine radiograph demonstrates the Herbert screw fixation.

95-21, *B*). The supraclavicular and accessory nerves are identified and preserved. The sternocleidomastoid muscle is defined. The pectoralis muscle is taken down from its clavicular insertion and the clavicle is freed to the sternoclavicular joint and the manubrium sterni. The omohyoid is divided. The upper outer corner of the manubrium, the first costal cartilage, and the medial half of the clavicle are divided. The bony flap can be elevated on its muscular pedicle (Fig. 95-21, *C*). In addition to the exposure of the great vessels and the lower roots of the brachial plexus (Fig. 95-21, *D*), a medial approach to the carotid artery can be used for ample exposure to the cervicothoracic junction with access to C3 through T4.

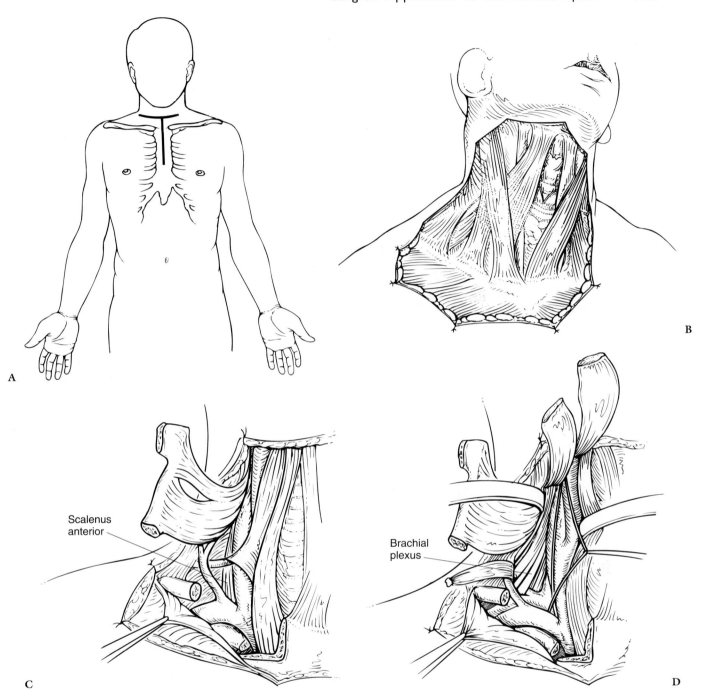

Fig. 95-21

Approach to the cervicothoracic spine. *(Redrawn from Birch R, Bonney G, Marshall RW: A surgical approach to the cervicothoracic spine, J Bone Joint Surg (Br) 72B:904, 1990.)* **A,** T-shaped incision. **B,** Subplatysmal flaps have been elevated. **C,** The bony flap is elevated on the pedicle of the sternocleidomastoid muscle. **D,** Exposure to the brachial plexus is obtained after the scalenus anterior and omohyoid are divided.

Scalenus
anterior

Brachial
plexus

Subsequently, the osseomuscular flap may be returned to its anatomic position. The clavicle may be fixated with plate and screws, and the manubrium reattached with wires. The wound is then closed in layers over a vacuum drain.

Summary

In summary, we have discussed surgical approaches to the entire cervical spine. The decision by the spinal surgeon in choosing a particular approach or a combination of approaches demands detailed knowledge of the anatomy and pathologic processes as well as the potential risks and benefits of each approach for each individual patient. A team approach composed of an orthopedist; neurosurgeon; and head and neck, and thoracic surgeon may be helpful in certain instances to provide the safest and best exposure.

References

1. Birch R, Boney G, Marshall RW: A surgical approach to the cervicothoracic spine, *J Bone Joint Surg* 72B:904, 1990.
2. Capener N: The evolution of lateral rachotomy, *J Bone Joint Surg* 36B:173, 1954.
3. Cauchoix J, Binet JP: Anterior surgical approaches to the spine, *Ann R Coll Surg* 21:237, 1957.
4. Charles R, Govender S: Anterior approach to the upper thoracic vertebrae, *J Bone Joint Surg* 71B:81, 1989.
5. Fang HSY, Ong GB: Direct anterior approach to the upper cervical spine, *J Bone Joint Surg* 44A:1588, 1962.
6. Hall JE, Denis F, Murray J: Exposure of the upper cervical spine for spinal decompression by a mandible and tongue-splitting approach: case report, *J Bone Joint Surg* 59A:121, 1977.
7. Henry AK: *Extensile exposures*, ed 2, Edinburgh, 1957, Livingstone, p 53.
8. Hodgson AR, and others: Anterior spinal fusion: the operative approach and pathological findings in 412 patients with Pott's disease of the spine, *Br J Surg* 48:172, 1960.
9. McAfee PC and others: The anterior retropharyngeal approach to the upper part of the cervical spine, *J Bone Joint Surg* 69A:1371, 1987.
10. Micheli LJ, Hood RW: Anterior exposure of the cervicothoracic spine using a combined cervical and thoracic approach, *J Bone Joint Surg* 65A:992, 1983.
11. Nanson EM: The anterior approach to upper dorsal sympathectomy, *Surg Gynecol Obstet* 104:118, 1957.
12. Perry J: Surgical approaches to the spine. In Pierce DS, Nickel VH, editors: *The total care of spinal cord injuries*, Boston, 1977, Little, Brown, p 53.
13. Riley LH Jr: Surgical approaches to the anterior structures of the cervical spine, *Clin Orthop* 91:16, 1973.
14. Smith GW, Robinson RA: The treatment of certain cervical-spine disorders by anterior removal of the intervertebral disc and interbody fusion, *J Bone Joint Surg* 40A:607, 1958.
15. Southwick WO, Robinson RA: Surgical approaches to the vertebral bodies in the cervical and lumbar regions, *J Bone Joint Surg* 39A:631, 1957.
16. Spetzler RF, Selman WR, Nash CL Jr: Transoral microsurgical odontoid resection and spinal cord monitoring, *Spine* 4:506, 1979.
17. Sundaresan N, Shah J, Feghali JG: A transsternal approach to the upper thoracic vertebrae, *Am J Surg* 148:473, 1984.
18. Turner PL, Webb JK: Surgical approach to the upper thoracic spine, *J Bone Joint Surg* 69B:542, 1987.
19. Whitesides TE Jr, Kelly RP: Lateral approach to the upper cervical spine for anterior fusion, *South Med J* 59:879, 1966.

Chapter 96

Degenerative Disc Disease of the Cervical Spine: Degenerative Cascade and the Anterior Approach

Steven C. Poletti

John A. Handal

Anatomy

Diagnosis

Pain Generators

Diagnostic Tests

Nonoperative Treatment

Operative Treatment

Anterior Approach

Summary

Anatomy

The term *cervical disc disease* implies that neck pathology exists as a result of disc degeneration. However, degenerative changes are often noted in the absence of clinical complaints. When cervical disc degeneration leads to osteophytic proliferation, it is commonly referred to as "spondylosis." In symptomatic spondylosis, the anterior, middle, and posterior columns can all be potential sources of pain. Thus, changes within the disc itself, osteophytic changes about the uncovertebral joints, facet degeneration, ligamentous hypertrophy, and instability can all contribute to pain.

It is well understood that degenerative changes can result in impingement on the neural elements, thus causing radiculopathy or myelopathy.[27] However, cervical and paracervical pain with disc degeneration is still poorly understood and accepted. Diagnosis of nonmyelopathic, nonradicular cervical spondylosis involves identification of the specific pain generators within a symptomatic segment.

Cervical disc disease is the result of a change in discal anatomy. In the earliest stages of development, a false joint develops between the convex surface of the inferior end plate in the superior vertebra (called the "enchancrue") and the bony projections on the concave superior end plate of the caudal vertebra (called the "uncus"). These uncovertebral joints are commonly called the "neurocentral joints" or the "joints of Luschka"[28] (Fig. 96-1, *A* and *B*). The presence of uncovertebral joints implies "normal" developmental changes of the disc with aging. These anatomic changes within the disc result in a biochemical change in the disc tissue, ultimately leading to disc dehydration. This disc dehydration kicks off the "degenerative cascade" that ultimately results in motion-segment alteration. Initially, biochemical changes result in increased spinal mobility at the affected level. Segmental instability can in turn lead to formation of osteophytic excrescences at the uncovertebral joints, at the intervertebral level, or at the level of the facet joints.

Diagnosis

Any comments on diagnosis of neck pain would not be complete without including mention of a neurologic examination and institution of appropriate conservative care. In the interest of brevity, we will assume that obvious cervical radiculopathy and myelopathy have been ruled out, and that differential diagnoses for cervical radiculopathy such as extraspinal tumors, focal entrapment syndromes,

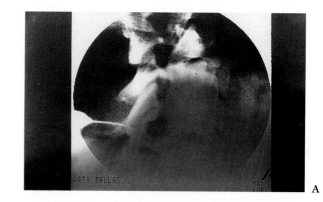

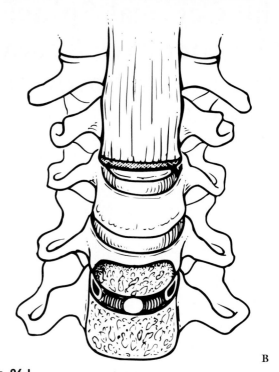

Fig. 96-1

Cross-sectional (**A**) and coronal (**B**) drawings of a normal adult cervical disc. The presence of the uncovertebral joint is a developmental change that occurs sometimes in the third decade of life.

brachial plexopathies, and shoulder disease have been explored. What we are focusing on, therefore, is the patient with persistent cervical and paracervical pain, posterior occipital pain, and nonspecific shoulder and interscapular pain. Imaging studies can be difficult to interpret in patients with nonradicular, nonmyelopathic neck pain. Age-related changes in disc morphology often cannot be differentiated from degenerative changes which cause symptoms. Cervical myelography demonstrated a 21% incidence of filling defects on asymptomatic subjects as studied by Hitsleberger and Witter.[21] More recently, Boden and colleagues[5] have noted that in asymptomtic patients who had undergone cervical MRI, 25% of those less than 40 years old had degenerative changes. Frank disc herniations were found in 10% of this group. Of those patients older than 40 years, 60% had degenerative disc changes and 20% had foraminal stenosis. Thus, the presence of degenerative changes on MRI or CT myelography is not enough to make a definitive diagnosis.[32]

Pain Generators

As McNab has stated, there are five sites of articulation between any two lower cervical vertebrae.[24] These are the disc anteriorly, the two uncovertebral joints centrally, and the two facet joints posteriorly. Each may contribute to symptoms seen in cervical disc degeneration.

The uncovertebral joints can form osteophytic ridges that can be readily appreciated on anteroposterior and oblique radiographs. Lateral osteophytes from the uncovertebral joints theoretically can cause vertebral artery compression, resulting in dizziness, intermittent visual changes, and retroocular pain. This is uncommon and poorly understood.[24]

More commonly, degenerative osteophytes from the uncovertebral joints extend posteriorly. In combination with osteophytic changes from the facet joints, nerve root or cord compression can occur.

Since the facet joints are diarthrodial, intrasynovial facet cysts can also occasionally form late in the degenerative cascade.[8,23] Vertebral body osteophytes have been described to cause dysphagia when anterior, or spinal stenosis posteriorly.[24]

Diagnosis of myelopathy or radiculopathy secondary to advanced localized osteophyte formation is well described and understood. However, in the early stages of cervical disc degeneration, one does not see classic nerve irritation or myelopathy. Symptoms are often neck pain associated with interscapular pain, posterior occipital headaches, and nonradicular shoulder pain. Many of these people are "written off" as having a soft-tissue etiology of their pain. However, in our opinion, longstanding pain demands a more specific pathoanatomic explanation.

The facet joint can be a potential source of longstanding cervical pain, as discussed by Aprill and Bogduk.[1,2,7] Provocative pain patterns have been reproduced with injections into different cervical facet levels in normal subjects.[14] In people with longstanding posterior cervical pain and interscapular pain, facet injection of Xylocaine and corticosteroid may provide relief, but this is unproven. Facet in-

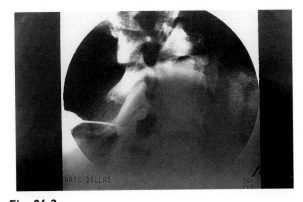

Fig. 96-2

Cervical facet injection. This commonly performed with the patient in a lateral position. In a well-performed injection, one should see contrast fill the facet articulation.

jections are more commonly thought to be diagnostic rather than therapeutic (Fig. 96-2).

Occasionally, patients can present with radiculopathy without an obvious sequestered disc herniation noted on scans. It is not readily apparent why patients can have cervical radicular pain without a sequestered disc herniation. In the lumbar spine, it has been postulated that "discogenic pain" can be associated with radicular leg pain. The etiology is unclear, but anular tears in the disc, with or without subligamentous central herniations, have been accepted by some as potential causes of longstanding low-back and leg pain. In that same vein, it is theoretically possible that a tear in the anulus of a cervical disc, with or without a subligamentous herniation, can contribute to radicular arm pain. However, asymptomatic disc bulges with subligamentous herniations are very common, especially in older patients. Thus, imaging studies are simply not enough to confirm this controversial diagnosis.

Diagnostic Tests

Careful differential diagnostic screening is necessary in patients with radiculopathy without a compressive disc herniation. If focal nerve entrapment and shoulder pathology have been ruled out, selective cervical nerve root injection may be helpful. To gain useful diagnostic information from a selective nerve root injection, it is important to use a small volume (less than 0.5 ml) of Xylocaine to ensure that only a single root is anesthetized. Like all subjective pain injection tests, the results should be viewed as "a piece in the puzzle" rather than an answer to the problem (Fig. 96-3). However, if a patient's arm pain is temporarily relieved by numbing a single nerve root,

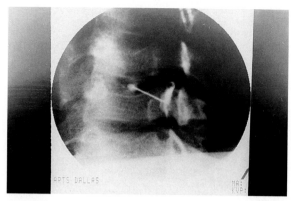

Fig. 96-3

Cervical selective nerve root injection. The patient is placed supine oblique. The needle should be directed toward the posterior aspect of the foramen to avoid the vertebral artery. Often, a patient's concordant arm pain is reproduced with contrast injection.

then it is reasonable to pursue a workup involving the motion segment associated with that nerve root.

Cervical discography as a means of diagnosing longstanding neck pain is as controversial as any subject in spinal medicine. Our experience with cervical discography is extensive. The technique of cervical discography is well described in this text. We have developed a classification system based on the anatomic compartments in and around the cervical disc (Fig. 96-4, *A–D*).

Most cervical discs that are morphologically abnormal reproduce concordant neck pain with contrast injection. In general, the greater the degree of degeneration, the higher the percentage of concordant neck pain with injection.

Therefore, when evaluating the results of cervical discography, it is very important to remember that it is very unusual to have a single symptomatic cervical disc noted on discography. In our study of 200 patients, only 10% had single-level involvement.[18] Multilevel involvement is the norm, with 78% having two or more symptomatic levels. Cervical discography should therefore be seen as a tool to diagnose the cause of neck pain rather than "to rule a patient in for surgery." In our experience, discography "rules out" more than it "rules in."

If a patient happens to have a single symptomatic degenerative level noted on discography, then it is our recommendation that he or she be considered for provocative cervical zygoapophyseal joint injections at that level. If the test is positive it can be assumed that this single motion segment is the patient's pain generator. This patient could be considered for a surgical disectomy and fusion, although psychometric evaluation and screening for secondary gain issues would be necessary.

Nonoperative Treatment

Virtually all patients with nonmyelopathic neck pain should have an initial trial of conservative therapy. Immobilization and antiinflammatory drugs are widely accepted. Boden and Wiesel advocate continuous soft-collar immobilization initially, and trigger point injections at 3 to 5 weeks post injury, although this is an admittedly empiric recommendation.[6] Cervical traction has been advocated by many and condemned by others.[20] Patients with severe posterior occipital headaches may benefit from occipital nerve blocks, but this too is unproven. Acute-modalities therapy and muscle relaxants may be useful for the initial 7 to 10 days post injury, after which isometric exercises can be instituted. Cervical epidural steroid injections can also occasionally be used in conjunction with a therapy program (see Chapter 22).

In general, results of nonoperative therapy are good.[16] Time may be the best therapy. De Palma and associates reported on 68 patients with neck pain considered to be treatment failures at 1 year post injury.[11] Five years later, 45% had satisfactory pain relief without treatment. However, patients with longstanding complaints of greater than 6 months often present for a diagnostic work–up, and diagnostic spinal injections can often be helpful in evaluating this difficult patient population.

Some patients with facet-mediated pain and nonprovocative discography may be candidates for cervical facet rhizotomy. We have no experience with this controversial procedure, and there are no long-term follow-up studies on its efficacy. Scheurer reported a 50% success rate at 15-months' follow-up in a series of 50 patients with chronic cervical pain,[30] and Ouderhoven reported 83% of 279 patients had good to excellent results at 26 months' follow-up.[26]

Operative Treatment

As has often been stated, cervical disc disease is divided into three subgroups: (1) cervical spondylitic myelopathy; (2) cervical spondylitic radiculopathy; and (3) nonradicular nonmyelopathic neck pain. Surgical approaches can be anterior or posterior.

In general, posterior approaches to the neck are reserved for multilevel myelopathic or radicular disorders. Far lateral disc herniations with unilateral radiculopathy may also be well served by a posterior approach. Posterior fusion has been described as an effective means of addressing pseudarthrosis after anterior fusion.[15] Increased popularity of posterior cervical instrumentation systems has raised questions as to the role of posterior fusion in treating symptomatic disc degeneration. In our opinion, this disc is

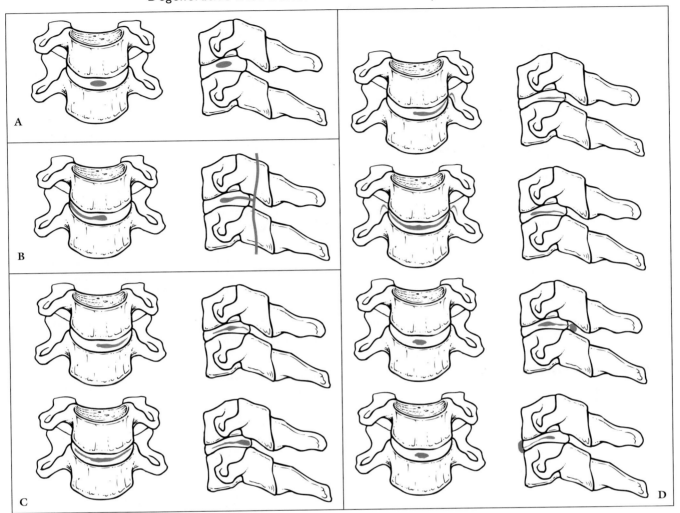

Fig. 96-4

Cervical discography: classification. **A,** Drawings of AP and lateral images of a normal cervical discogram. Contrast is confined to the central nucleus and does not extend beyond the anulus. **B,** Drawings of a type I cervical discogram show contrast extending through the anulus, but not beyond the outer anular fibers. Contrast may also extend into one or both uncovertebral joints. **C,** Drawings of AP and lateral images of a type II cervical discogram show contrast extending beyond the outer anulus. Posteriorly, contrast does not extend beyond the posterior longitudinal ligament. Anteriorly, a similar image can be seen with contrast contained by the anterior longitudinal ligament. **D,** Drawings of AP and lateral images of type III cervical discogram with contrast extending posteriorly into the epidural space. The contrast typically flows rapidly into the epidural space and is not confined. A type III cervical discogram is best seen on lateral fluoroscopic image during injection.

often the offending pain generator and must be addressed anteriorly.

Anterior cervical discectomy and interbody fusion is the most common choice to address cervical radiculopathy or myelopathy.[4,17,22,27] Removal of compressive osteophytes seems reasonable.[9] Those who claim that fusion without osteophytectomy will result in eventual absorption of the spurs have no scientific basis for that claim.

Discectomy without interbody fusion is advocated by many.[13,25,29] Spontaneous fusion occurs in 70% of patients,[25] and postoperative kyphotic angulation is surprisingly minimal (4.8 degrees average in one

study).[13] However, in one series, six of 10 patients who underwent discectomy without fusion developed arm pain postoperatively.[34] For patients with a large sequestered disc fragment without bone spurs, discectomy alone may be sufficient. However, if a large amount of osteophyte is removed, then discectomy with interbody fusion is probably the best choice.

In the rare patient with single-level discogenic neck pain, anterior cervical discectomy and fusion is the preferred surgical approach. In a well-quoted study, Whitecloud and Seago reported a 72% good-to-excellent result using anterior cervical discectomy and fusion in patients with cervical discogenic pain proven by discography.[33] Dohn has also reported a 62% good-to-excellent result in anterior discectomy and fusion for discogenic pain.[12] We believe that long-segment fusion (i.e., greater than two levels) is not a reasonable treatment option for cervical discogenic pain.

Anterior Approach

Patient positioning is important. We prefer a supine position with a bolster placed longitudinally between the scapulae. Typically, the shoulders are pulled caudally and held with benzoin-enforced athletic tape. The ulnar nerves should be well padded at the elbows. Slight extension of the neck can increase lordosis, which facilitates exposure.

A preincision lateral radiograph with a needle marker ensures proper incision level. Although there are individual differences, an incision one fingerbreadth above the clavicle should suffice for C6-C7 exposure, two fingerbreadths above the clavicle for C5-C6, and so on. Generally, it is preferable to be "too low" rather than "too high" with the incision, as superior dissection is easier.

Classically, the incision is described as being placed over the anterior border of the sternocleidomastoid. In our opinion, the incision should be just off of the midline, which lessens the amount of medial retraction necessary. In general, if a patient has left-side symptoms, the incision should be on the right side, and vice versa, because the neural foramen opposite the side of the incision is easier to decompress laterally. Although some contend that recurrent laryngeal nerve injury is more common with right-side exposure, we have not found this to be the case. In fact, many right-handed surgeons find a right-sided incision to be much easier.

The platysma is readily visible subcutaneously. We prefer to split the platysma longitudinally medial to the carotid pulse. Blunt dissection medial to the carotid pulse and lateral to the esophagus easily leads to the perivertebral fascia over the cervical spine. A nasogastric tube often aids in esophageal palpation. Sometimes strap muscles are in the way and need to be dissected. This can usually be accomplished bluntly with a Kittner ("peanut gauze") on the back of a curved snap. The longus coli muscles on either end of the spine should be retracted laterally. Bipolar cautery and a mini-periosteal elevator are used for this. We prefer self-retaining retraction, but have no use for the sharp-toothed retractor blades available with most systems.

Disc removal near and beyond the posterior longitudinal ligament demands magnification and illumination. With a sequestered disc herniation, it is necessary to take down the posterior longitudinal ligament and visualize the dura. A blunt nerve hook can often help to tease a fragment out of the neural foramen. In degenerative conditions, it is often necessary to remove a portion of the uncovertebral joint and decompress the foramen laterally. One may encounter the vertebral artery with wide inferior/anterior foraminal expansion.

In terms of discectomy/fusion technique, we believe that the distraction that is possible with vertebral body pin/retractor systems is superior to that possible with head-halter traction. Distraction is not in issue with soft disc herniations, but is very important when dealing with degenerative cervical disc disease.

In terms of the fusion techniques in the cervical spine, all surgeons should be familiar with the Cloward and Smith–Robinson techniques. In our opinion, the Smith–Robinson technique is preferred over the Cloward technique because of the anterior wedging and kyphotic angulation that can be seen with recession of the Cloward bone graft into cancellous vertebral bone.

However, graft settling is not uncommon even with a well performed Smith–Robinson technique.[3,10] In fact, there is no statistical superiority reported with either technique.

Some surgeons prefer to burr a slot into one or both of the vertebral bodies and fashion the interbody graft so that it interlocks into the vertebrae. This is done in an effort to prevent graft antero/retropulsion. In our opinion, preservation of subchondral vertebral bone and use of an ample, strong interbody graft are the keys to successful fusion. We prefer to distract the disc space to its normal height, but are mindful that overdistraction can cause facet compression, and possible postoperative shoulder/interscapular pain.

It is our empiric recommendation that allograft is preferable to autograft iliac crest. Cadaver fibula may have the advantage of resisting compressive forces and thus maintaining disc-space height.[19] However, although fibula may be stronger, its cortical boundaries may take longer to incorporate.

Anterior cervical plating has the theoretical advantage of maintaining disc-space distraction,[31] and this may warrant consideration in a two-level fusion, especially in a smoker. However, at the present time, the risks, expense, and increased time associated with anterior cervical plating do not justify its routine use in surgical management of cervical disc disease. Although discectomy without fusion may ultimately result in autofusion, it has the theoretic disadvantage of leading to further segmental hypermobility, and is thus probably not the best choice for addressing cervical discogenic pain.

Summary

Nonradicular nonmyelopathic neck pain is one of the most common, most frustrating problems that all clinicians who deal with spinal medicine encounter. A well-supervised conservative treatment plan should suffice for the vast majority of these patients. However, those with longstanding complaints deserve a workup. In our opinion, a workup often involves a cervical MRI scan, electrodiagnostics, and provocative spinal injections based on the patient's symptoms and corresponding abnormalities noted on scans. Preoperative psychometric screening is often useful, especially in patients with compensation issues.

Patients with longstanding neck pain often have their complaints heard with a veil of skepticism, especially when complicated by some type of compensation claim. By addressing the anatomic structures about the cervical vertebrae, we are attempting to explain and address these difficult complaints rather than dismiss them.

References

1. Aprill CA, Bogduk, N: The prevalence of cervical zygoapophyseal joint pain, *Spine* 17:744, 1990.
2. Aprill C, Dwyer A, Bogduk N: Cervical zygoapophyseal joint pain patterns II: a clinical evaluation, *Spine* 15:458, 1990.
3. Aronson N, Filtzer DL, Bagan M: Anterior cervical fusion by the Smith–Robinson approach, *J Neurosurg* 29:397, 1968.
4. Bernard TN Jr, Whitecloud TS III: Cervical spondylitic myelopathy and myeloradiculopathy: anterior decompression and stabilization with autogenous fibula strut graft, *Clin Orthop* 221:149, 1987.
5. Boden SD, McCowin PR, David DO: Abnormal magnetic-resonance scans of the cervical spine in symptomatic subjects, *J Bone Joint Surg* 72A:1178, 1990.
6. Boden SD, Wiesel SN: Conservative treatment for cervical disc disease, *Semin Spine Surg* 1:229, 1989.
7. Bogduk N, Marshland A: The cervical zygoapophyseal joints as a source of neck pain, *Spine* 13:610, 1988.
8. Cartwright MJ and others: Synovial cyst of a cervical facet joint, *Neurosurgery* 16:850, 1985.
9. Clifton AG and others: Identifiable causes for poor outcome in surgery for cervical spondylosis, *J Neuroradiol* 32(6):450, 1990.
10. Cloward RB: The anterior approach for removal of ruptured cervical discs, *J Neurosurg* 15:602, 1958.
11. De Palma AF, Rothman RH, Levit RL: The natural history of severe cervical disc degeneration, *Acta Orthop Scand* 43:392, 1972.
12. Dohn DF: Anterior interbody fusion for treatment of cervical disc condition, *JAMA* 197:897, 1977.
13. Dunsker SB: Anterior cervical discectomy with and without fusion, *Clin Neurosurg* 25:217, 1977.
14. Dwyer A, Aprill C, Bodduk N: Cervical zygoapophyseal joint pain patterns I: a study in normal volunteers, *Spine* 15:453, 1990.
15. Fairey ID and others: Pseudoarthrosis of the cervical spine after anterior arthrodesis, *J Bone Joint Surg* 72A:1171, 1990.
16. Gore DR, Septic SB, Garner GM: Neck pain: a long-term follow-up study of 205 patients, *Spine* 12:1, 1987.
17. Hanaik G, Fujiyoshi F, Kamei K: Subtotal vertebrectomy and spinal fusion for cervical spondylitic myelopathy, *Spine* 11(4):310, 1986.
18. Handal J, Poletti SC: *Cervical discography classification and morphology,* Presented at the North American Spine Society, Boston, MA, 1992.
19. Hanley EN and others: Use of allograft bone in cervical spine surgery, *Semin Spine Surg* 1:262, 1989.
20. Harris W: Cervical traction: review of the literature and treatment guidelines, *Phys Ther* 57:, 1977.
21. Hitsleberger WF, Witten RW: Abnormal myelograms in asymptomatic patients, *J Neurosurg* 28:204, 1968.
22. Kadoya A, Nakamura T, Kwak R: A microsurgical anterior osteophytectomy of cervical spondylitic myelopathy, *Spine* 9:437, 1984.
23. Kao CC, Winkler SS, Turner JH: Synovial cyst of spinal facet. *J Neurosurg* 41:372, 1974.
24. McNab I: *Symptoms in cervical disc degeneration in the cervical spine, ed 2,* Philadelphia, 1989, J.B. Lippincott, p 559.
25. Murphy MG, Gadow M: Anterior cervical discectomy without interbody graft, *J Neurosurg* 37:71, 1972.
26. Ouderhoven RC: The role of laminectomy, facet rhizotomy, and epidural steroids, *Spine* 4:145, 1979.
27. Parke W: Correlative anatomy of cervical spondylitic myelopathy, *Spine* 13:831, 1988.
28. Parke W, Sherk H: *Normal adult in the cervical spine, ed 2,* Philadelphia, 1989, J.B. Lippincott, p 11.
29. Rosenorn JR, Hansen E, Rosenor M: Anterior cervical discectomy with and without fusion, *J Neurosurg* 59:252, 1983.
30. Schaeurer JP: Radiofrequency facet rhizotomy in the treatment of chronic neck and low back pain, *Int Surg* 63:53, 1978.
31. Suh PB, Kostuik JP: Anterior cervical plate fixation with the titanium hollow screw plate system: a preliminary report, *Spine* 15(10):1079, 1990.
32. Teresi LM, Lufkin RB, Reicher MA: Asymptomatic degenerative disc disease and spondylosis at the cervical spine, *MR Imag Radiol* 164(1):83, 1987.
33. Whitecloud TS, Seago RA: Cervical discogenic syndrome: results of operative intervention in patients with positive discography, *Spine* 12:313, 1987.
34. Yamamoto I, Ikeda A: Clinical long-term results of anterior discectomy without interbody fusion for cervical disc disease, *Spine* 16(3):272, 1991.

Chapter 97

Degenerative Disc Disease of the Cervical Spine: Posterior Approach

F. Todd Wetzel

Laminotomy/Discectomy

    technique
    results
    complications

Cervical Laminectomy

    technique
    complications

Cervical Laminaplasty

    technique (after Hirabayashi and Herkowitz)
    complications

Summary

The radiographic changes of cervical spondylosis are quite variable, and frequently do not correlate precisely with a patient's symptoms. From a clinical perspective, degenerative cervical pathology may be classified according to production of axial or referred symptoms. Ducker and Zeidman[11] note four clinical categories: discogenic arthritic disruption and "quasi-radiculitis," radiculopathy, myeloradiculopathy, and myelopathy. For the purposes of this discussion, the following generalization correlating radiographic and clinical information will be made: spondylotic or discogenic pain syndromes result predominantly in axial pain complaints or nonradicular referred pain syndromes (the "quasi-radiculopathies" of Ducker and Zeidman); extremity pain and frank radiculopathy are not constant features of these processes.[10,13,52] Radiculopathy implies extremity pain in the distribution of a particular root or roots. Myelopathy connotes the presence of long-tract signs, including difficulty walking, wide-based gait, and balance problems. Patients may also report a loss of dexterity and nonspecific weakness.[6,46]

In those states in which axial and radicular pain are prominent features, conservative care has a significant role. In myelopathic processes, conservative care may be helpful if instituted early in the course.[2] In this case, axial pain and mild referred symptoms, usually of the upper extremity, are being treated. However, in the patient in whom long-tract signs are already present, conservative care has a very limited role.

In the absence of myelopathy, spondylotic and radicular complaints should, initially, be treated conservatively.[33,35,44] Orthotic supports and repositioning of pillows for sleep may be beneficial. The role of physical therapy is becoming increasingly clear, with isometric and active motion exercises. The utility of cervical traction in the treatment of radiculopathy is controversial. Some authors have reported response rates as high as 92%.[26] If any effect results from the traction method, it should be seen acutely. Overall, results of conservative treatment for spondylosis and radiculopathy are reported to be successful in 80% to 90% of patients. However, studies of the natural history reveal that as many as 55% of patients who initially obtain no relief from conservative treatment may remain symptomatic over the long term. Even with a satisfactory outcome from conservative treatment, as many as 25% of patients may be unable to return to their former occupations.[37,38,50]

In the patient who has failed conservative therapy and surgical intervention is contemplated, the surgeon must take into account several factors. The choice of approach is, obviously, critical. Many disease processes in the cervical spine can be approached either anteriorly or posteriorly. Chestnut and associates compared the results of anterior and posterior root decompression, and concluded that one approach is not clearly superior to the other.[9] Simeone recommends that the posterior approach be used for unilateral radiculopathy at one or more levels, cervical myelopathy with three-level compression, spinal cord compression secondary to degenerative subluxation, and spinal cord compression secondary to congenital or acquired stenosis from posterior compression.[47] Raynor studied the anterior and posterior approaches to root decompression on cadaver spines, and attempted to define the anatomic limits of each.[42] Posteriorly, 3 to 5 mm of root was routinely exposed after one third of the facet joint was removed. The anterior approach necessitated lateral disc and bone resection. Despite this, it was often difficult to visualize any length of root anteriorly.[9]

Prior to any surgical intervention, it is obviously incumbent upon the operating physician to pinpoint the pathologic entity responsible for the pain syndrome. As stated above, certain pathologic findings with concordant clinical symptoms may be more amenable to a posterior surgical approach. There are three basic posterior surgical approaches for degenerative cervical pathology: laminotomy-foramenotomy (with or with discectomy), laminectomy, and laminaplasty. Each of these techniques will be discussed individually in the sections that follow.

Laminotomy/Discectomy

The operative approach to nonosteophytic (so-called "soft") cervical disc herniations remains controversial. A variety of series comparing anterior and posterior approaches have reported similar results.[9,51] Herkowitz and colleagues, in a prospective study, compared patients undergoing anterior cervical discectomy and fusion with those undergoing posterior decompression for soft disc herniation.[23] While there was no statistically significant difference between the two groups, it was suggested that the anterior group had a superior long term outcome. Additional prospective studies are necessary to resolve this issue, despite the implication that the utility of the posterior approach for single segment pathology may be limited. Nonetheless, keeping in mind the guidelines of Simeone,[47] posterior decompression may be efficacious in certain instances, such as posterior or intraforaminal cervical disc herniation and posterior osteophytic compression.

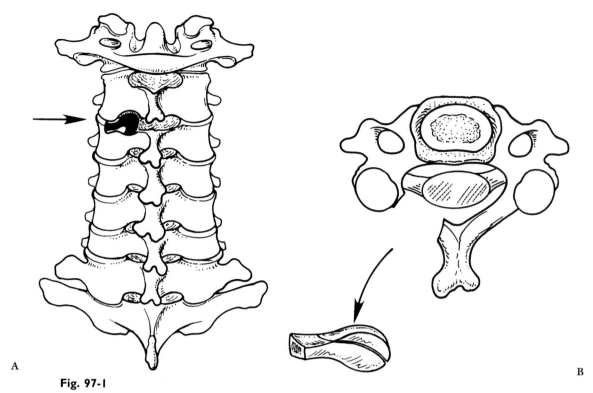

Fig. 97-1

Laminotomy/discectomy. Note the medial-lateral and cranial-caudal extent of the decompression. The nerve root is retracted cranially after the vascular cuff is cauterized and an appropriate foramenotomy performed. This allows discectomy if necessary. **A**, Anteroposterior view. Note partial facetectomy. **B**, Axial view. *(Redrawn from Simeone FA:* Cervial radiculopathy: posterior approach. *In Rothman RA, Simeone FA, editors:* The spine, *ed 3, Philadelphia, 1992, W.B. Saunders, p 609.)*

Technique

In performing a posterior laminotomy and foraminotomy, with or without disc resection, the patient may be positioned in the prone, seated, or "park bench" position.[28] Advantages and disadvantages are associated with each position. The prone position may cause engorgement of the epidural veins and soft tissue compression.[8] The sitting position leads to less venous engorgement; blood drains away from the surgical site. There is, however, an increased risk of cardiovascular instability and air embolization in the sitting position.[36] Theoretically, the park bench position combines many advantages of the sitting position, but diminishes the risk of cardiovascular maloccurrence.

Predominantly due to the exposure allowed, it is my preference to use the prone position. The patient is placed face down into a horseshoe headrest, or in a Mayfield headrest. Appropriate traction so as to flex the occiput is employed, via either a halter or Gardner-Wells apparatus. Ideally, the occiput should be flexed sufficiently to move the occipital prominence away from the surgical field. The cervical spine should be flexed so that it parallels the floor without placing the patient in undue reverse Trendelenburg positioning. All bony prominences must be padded, and the shoulders retracted to permit lateral x-ray visualization.

Appropriate radiographic confirmation of levels may be performed before the skin incision or after the spinous processes have been exposed. The incision, ordinarily 3 to 4 cm long, covers two spinous processes and spans the interspace to be opened. After subperiosteal stripping and retraction of the paraspinous muscles, the ligamentum flavum is raised with a small curette. A small Kerrison rongeur is inserted into the interlaminar space and a laminotomy performed, taking equal proportions of both cranial and caudal laminae (Fig. 97-1). Alternatively, laminae can be thinned with a high-speed burr prior to resection. Magnification in the form of either 3× loupes or an operating microscope may prove helpful.

The pedicles are situated sufficiently cranially and caudally that the laminotomy defect may be extended to the facet border. As Raynor[42] has noted, one third of the facet may be removed without compromising stability, permitting nearly full visualization of the nerve root. The lateral extent of foraminotomy may be determined by passing a small nerve hook or elevator between the nerve root and the facet. If the instrument can comfortably be passed around the nerve root, then sufficient decompression has been performed. If resistance is felt, a wider foraminotomy is indicated.

At this point, preparation is made for visualizing the soft disc if discectomy is desired. The steps for this include removal of the epidural venous plexus that cover the nerve root, to mobilize it, and gentle nerve root retraction to facilitate disc exposure. Following bipolar cauterization of the vascular cuff, the nerve root is visualized. The root may be retracted cranially. After the root has been retracted, a small 90° blunt nerve hook may be passed beneath the nerve root, lateral to the thecal sac. Any herniated disk fragments may thus be palpated. If a contained fragment is present with continued entrapment anterior to the posterior longitudinal ligament, the posterolateral aspect of the ligament should be incised. This can safely be done while retraction is maintained on the root. The root must be carefully protected at all times, and the cutting edge of the knife should face laterally, or away from the thecal sac, during this procedure. Following incision of the posterior longitudinal ligament, typically a fragment of disc is extruded. This can usually be removed quite easily with a small forceps or a pituitary rongeur. If, following incision of the posterior longitudinal ligament, an osteophyte is encountered, this may be addressed using a small diamond-tipped burr.

Following decompressive maneuvers, a small, blunt nerve hook should be passed circumferentially around the root to ensure that decompression is complete. After hemostasis with bipolar electrocautery, the laminotomy defect may be sealed with a small portion of thrombin-soaked Gelfoam or fat. The paraspinous muscles are then reapproximated using an absorbable suture. This reconstitutes the ligamentum nuchae. A drain is placed superficial to this, and subcutaneous tissue and skin are closed in separate layers.

Results

Overall, the results of this procedure are quite good. The series of Henderson and associates is illustrative. In this series of 846 patients who underwent posterior decompression, 96% obtained satisfactory results.[18] In examining this report and others, however, it is very difficult to separate the results of dis-cectomy from discectomy and foraminotomy. The key to a successful surgical procedure is full decompression of the involved root with resection of all discal or bony pathology, a point echoed by others.[34,39,45,49]

Complications

The overall complication rate for posterior discectomy and foraminotomy is approximately 3%.[18,45] Reported complications have ranged from wound infection to neurologic deficit. Characteristically, deficits are mild, with radicular symptoms that are transient. A syndrome similar to upper extremity autonomic dysfunction has been reported by Murphey and associates.[39] This, however, was a problem in fewer than 1% of the 648 patients reviewed. Abramovitz[1] has noted that patients with myelopathy are more likely to worsen intraoperatively, and speculated that this may be related to positioning in excessive flexion or extension. A comprehensive summary of reported complications noted in posterior and anterior surgery appears in Table 97-1.

As noted above, the approach to the cervical soft disc remains somewhat controversial. Additional prospective studies to determine the desirability of one approach are clearly needed. Certainly, at the current time, however, the posterior approach remains a safe method whereby root compression may be addressed.

Table 97-1
Complications associated with cervical disc surgery*†

	Posterior	Anterior
Neurologic		
Root	< 1%	
Cord	Rare	Total 0.3%
Air embolism	< 3%	Not reported
Infection	Not reported	0.4%–2%
Instability	Uncommon	?
Recurrent laryngeal nerve palsy	Not reported	2%
Esophageal injury	Not reported	< 0.1%
Stroke	Not reported	Rare, < 0.1%

*Percentages given only where experience permits accurate statement; descriptive terms used otherwise.
†From Abramovitz JN: Complications of surgery for discogenic disease of the spine, *Neurosurg Clin North Am* 4(1):167, 1993.

Cervical Laminectomy

To treat multilevel cervical stenosis with resultant myelopathy, the surgeon has two options from the posterior approach. One involves laminectomy with resection of all compressive structures, and the other involves laminaplasty, to expand canal dimensions.

Cervical spondylotic myelopathy results from a combination of factors. These include compressive forces on the spinal cord, resulting from canal narrowing, and dynamic forces, owing to the kinematic characteristics of the cervical spinal column.[4,12,14,43] Thus, any treatment must address both these issues—namely, decompression and stabilization. For that reason, in any extensive laminectomy, a posterior fusion, as discussed elsewhere in the text, is recommended.

The natural history of myelopathy is incompletely understood. In a recent review, LaRocca concluded that insufficient information was available for surgeons to predict accurately when surgical intervention would be beneficial.[31] The timing of surgical intervention is thus controversial. Additionally, follow-up of surgical patients has demonstrated that predicting the degree of postoperative improvement is difficult as well.[16,34] Thus, while a patient may be counseled to expect that surgical intervention will prevent further progression, assurance as to neurologic improvement cannot be reliably rendered.

The selection of an anterior or posterior approach for multilevel cervical stenosis is likewise controversial. Numerous studies have compared the results of anterior and posterior treatment. Gorter compared anterior fusion with total laminectomy and laminectomy-durotomy.[15] Overall, anterior surgery provided the best results, with the more extensive laminectomy-durotomy providing the worst results. Hukuda and associates compared three posterior procedures with three different anterior procedures.[27] A total of 191 patients were reviewed. The authors found that posterior procedures performed in severely myelopathic patients yielded neurologic recovery levels equivalent to anterior procedures performed in patients with milder disease. Herkowitz reviewed a series of patients with multilevel spondylotic radiculopathy treated with anterior decompression and fusion, laminectomy, or laminaplasty.[21] Overall, the results were best in the anterior group and worst in the laminectomy group. A telling complication—postoperative kyphosis—was noted in three patients in the laminectomy group. Zeidman and Ducker compared groups of patients undergoing anterior and posterior decompression for spondylotic myelopathy.[53] In this study the authors

performed more extensive procedures (greater than three levels) from a posterior approach. Good results were obtained with both approaches. This, in fact, reflects the consensus in the literature, preferring laminectomy in multiple level cases. At the present time, however, there is no prospective report comparing anterior and posterior approaches for equivalent pathology (e.g., all one- or two-level diseases). Hence, all these studies must be viewed with the realization that the definite superiority of one approach to address compression of a given extent has not yet been demonstrated.

Technique

The patient is positioned prone, in a manner similar to that described for laminotomy. The midline posterior incision is more extensive, usually owing to the number of levels to be decompressed. Lamina should not be removed until the levels have been localized with an appropriate lateral radiograph.

Following exposure, soft tissue, including supraspinous and intraspinous ligaments to be resected, is removed with a large rongeur. Spinous processes may also be removed at this point. A laminectomy may be performed by one of two approaches. In the first, the central intralaminar space is freed of ligamentum flavum with a small curved curette, and a Kerrison rongeur is used to perform the decompression. Alternatively, lamina may be abraded with a high-speed burr, until thin plates remain, along with associated ligamentum flavum. These may then be removed as the flavum is resected sharply.[48] Magnification in the form of loupes or operating microscope may be used at the discretion of the surgeon. Decompression is then carried laterally to the facets. Hemostasis is obtained with bipolar cautery. Considerable bleeding may be encountered from lateral epidural veins; these may require packing as well. Foramenotomies may be performed at levels where appropriate (Fig. 97-2).

Whether substantial additional benefit occurs from sectioning the dentate ligaments is not known (Fig. 97-3). Benzel and co-workers compared outcomes in patients undergoing laminectomy, laminectomy plus dentate ligament sectioning, and anterior cervical decompression and fusion.[5] These data suggest that patients with cervical kyphosis are treated most effectively with an anterior procedure, while those with normal cervical lordosis are best treated posteriorly. While the theoretical benefit from dentate ligament sectioning is evident, the practical utility remains to be proven.[5] Finally, depending on the extent of the decompression, consideration should

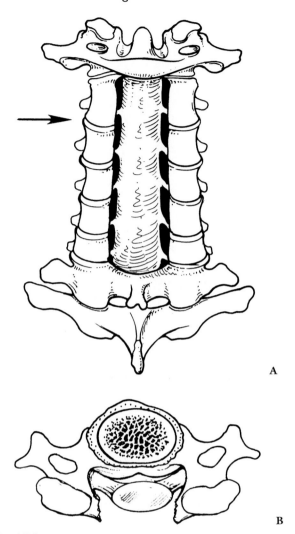

Fig. 97-2

Cervical laminectomy. After removing posterior elements, including the ligmentum flavum, foraminotomies may be performed as needed. **A,** Anteroposterior view. **B,** Axial view. *(Redrawn from Simeone FA, Dillin WH: Surgical management of cervical myelopathy: laminectomy. In Rothman RA, Simeone FA, editors: The Spine, ed 3, Philadelphia, 1992, W.B. Saunders, p 625.)*

be given to posterior fusion. Most techniques of posterior cervical arthrodesis are applicable, and are discussed elsewhere in the text.

Following the procedure, the soft tissue is closed tightly. The paraspinous muscles are approximated in the midline at the ligamentum nuchae. A closed drainage system is placed superficial to this. Subcutaneous tissue is closed in a separate layer. Postoperatively, the patient's neurologic status is monitored carefully for 24 to 48 hours. Any evidence of uncontrolled bleeding or expanding hematoma should be promptly addressed with appropriate diagnostic studies and, where appropriate, drainage.

Complications

Complications related to laminectomy are similar to those discussed for laminotomy. Motor deficits occur in fewer than 1% of cases.[7,17] No case of spinal cord injury has been reported, excepting the paper of Raaf,[41] who noted that one patient of 205 suffered cord injury secondary to a hematoma.

Cervical Laminaplasty

Laminaplasty, the procedure whereby canal dimensions are increased, has been described extensively by Hirabayashi and colleagues.[24,25] Indications for this procedure are cervical myelopathy secondary to cervical spinal stenosis, multilevel ossification of the posterior longitudinal ligament (OPLL), and spondylotic change of at least four segments.[24,25] The canal dimensions are enlarged by laminaplasty, while bony architecture is largely preserved. This may obviate the need for posterior arthrodesis and prevent the development of kyphosis. In an in vitro biomechanical study, Nowinski and associates compared laminectomy with laminaplasty.[40] Laminaplasty specimens were found to be stiffer than any laminectomy specimens; this was most noticeable in axial rotation.

In reviewing four currently available procedures for the surgical treatment of myelopathy—anterior cervical discectomy and fusion, anterior cervical corpectomy and fusion, posterior laminectomy, and laminaplasty—Kurz and Herkowitz concluded that laminaplasty was well suited to the patient with three-level disease contributing to myeloradiculopathic symptoms.[30] They also noted that "mild" instability may be addressed by performing arthrodesis on the hinged side. Laminaplasty was also believed to be advantageous in myeloradiculopathy with "developmental" cervical stenosis, anterior pseudarthrosis, or previously operated patients.[22]

Technique (after Hirabayashi and Herkowitz)

The patient is positioned in the prone position, and a midline incision is made following appropriate radiographic localization of levels.[19,41] Posterior spinous musculature is then stripped bilaterally. In the naturally occurring trough just medial to the facet joint and pedicle, gutters are created on either side of the spine using a high-speed burr. Based on preoperative imaging studies, the side exhibiting the greatest narrowing is the side of resection, with the hinge on the

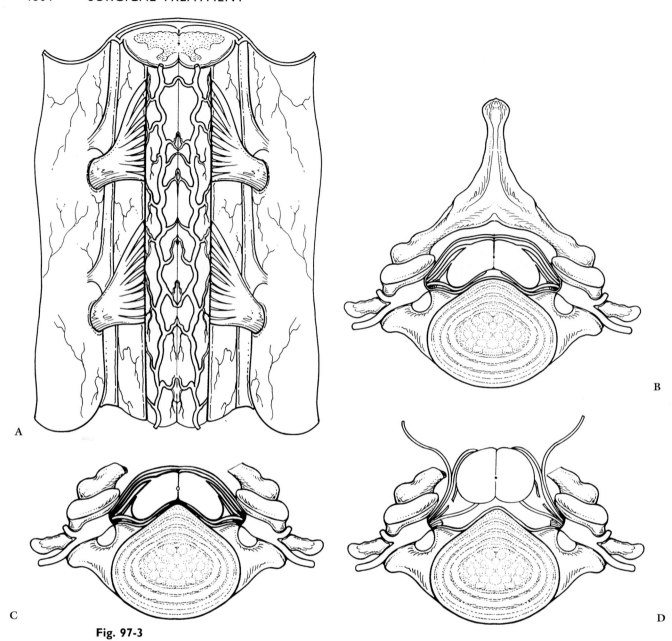

Fig. 97-3

Sectioning of the dentate ligaments following cervical laminectomy. **A**, Note ventral tethering of the dentate ligaments, which **B**, causes continued ventral compression. **C**, Following laminectomy, any dorsal compression is removed. **D**, Sectioning of the dentate ligaments theoretically allows posterior migration of the cord, thus facilitating decompression. *(Redrawn from Benzel EC and others: Cervical laminectomy and dentate ligament section for cervical spondylotic myelopathy, J Spinal Dis 4(3):286, 1991.)*

contralateral side (Fig. 97-4). Care should be taken to burr only one cortex on the side where the hinge is to be placed. On the expanded side, the canal may be entered after appropriate thinning with the burr, and gentle removal of the ligamentum flavum with a curved curette. A small Kerrison punch is used to thin the inner cortex along the levels to be elevated. Foraminotomies may be performed at each level according to the techniques noted above.

Nonabsorbable sutures are then passed through the base of the spinous processes at each segment to be elevated. Herkowitz recommends removing the tips of the spinous processes and placing them in the hinge site for additional reinforcement.[19]

Next, the hinge is lifted and the lamina swung open. An elevator should be gently passed on the anterior aspect of each lamina to be certain no adhesions are causing undue traction on the uncovered

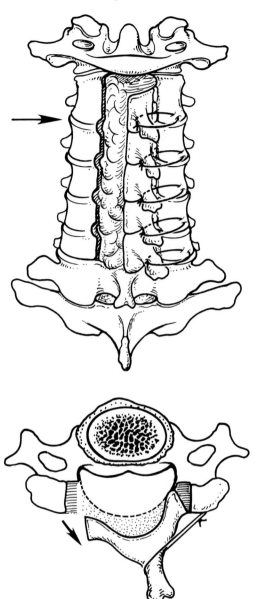

Fig. 97-4

Cervical laminaplasty. The hinge is cut on the most spacious side, and the lamina are open to perform canal expansion. Spinous processes are secured by a nonabsorbable suture or wire to the facet capsules or placed through the joint. **A,** Anteroposterior view, sutures placed on the hinge side. **B,** Axial view. Note expansion of canal dimensions, comparable to laminectomy. *(Redrawn from Herkowitz HN: Cervical laminaplasty: its role in the treatment of cervical radiculopathy,* J Spinal Dis *1:179, 1988.)*

dura. Once the expansion is performed, the nonabsorbable sutures within the spinous processes are sutured to the facet capsules at each level, or placed through a hole drilled in the cranial facet after the manner of Johnson and associates.[29] In general, laminar elevation should be 10 to 15 mm. This will expand the canal by the desired 5 mm.

A thin layer of fat or thrombin-soaked Gelfoam is placed over the exposed dura. Muscles are then returned to the midline, and the ligamentum nuchae is closed over the laminaplasty. A drain is placed cranial to this, and subcutaneous and cutaneous tissues are closed in separate layers. Postoperatively, it is recommended that the patient be placed in a Minerva orthosis for 6 to 8 weeks.

Complications

Complications from laminaplasty usually relate to closure of the hinge.[24,25] Herkowitz reported complications in two of 16 patients who underwent laminaplasty for radiculopathy.[20] In both these patients canal closure was noted with long-term follow-up. This resulted in recurrence of preoperative symptoms. This complication may be avoided by suturing the lamina to the facet.[19] This is of critical importance, as Hirabayashi has correlated clinical recovery rate with the amount of canal enlargement. His group demonstrated optimum results (an 81% recovery rate) with canal expansion of 5 mm.[24,25]

Summary

Overall, the posterior approaches described may be performed with a high expectation of success and low complication rate in the properly selected patient. While the accepted treatment of multilevel cervical stenosis is laminectomy—with arthrodesis as needed—laminaplasty is certainly a viable option in carefully selected patients. Overall, the posterior approaches described obviate the complications commonly encountered in anterior decompression and fusion. These include pseudarthrosis, donor site problems, hoarseness, tracheoesophageal tears, injury to recurrent laryngeal nerve and carotid artery, dysphagia, graft fracture, and dislodgement.[1] Arguably, it is possible to perform a wider canal decompression with a greater degree of safety from the posterior approach. These are some of the factors that must be borne in mind when selecting the correct operative approach to degenerative cervical disc disease. However, the absolute desirability of anterior versus posterior approaches in specific cases has not been definitely resolved. Additional prospective studies comparing similar patients are required.

References

1. Abramovitz JN: Complications of surgery for discogenic disease of the spine, *Neurosurg Clin North Am* 4(1):167, 1993.

2. Arnasson O and others: Surgical and conservative treatment of cervical spondylitic radiculopathy and myelopathy, *ACTA Neurochir (Wien)* 84:48, 1987.

3. Bailey R, Bagley C: Stabilization of the cervical spine by anterior fusion, *J Bone Joint Surg* 42A:565, 1960.

4. Barnes MP, Saunders M: The effect of cervical mobility on the natural history of cervical spondylotic myelopathy, *J Neurol Nursing Psychiatry* 47:17, 1984.

5. Benzel EC et al: Cervical laminectomy and dentate ligament section for cervical spondylotic myelopathy, *J Spinal Dis* 4(3):286, 1991.

6. Bernhardt M et al: Current concepts review: cervical spondylotic myelopathy, *J Bone Joint Surg* 75A:119, 1993.

7. Brain WR, Northfield P, Wilkinson M: The neurological manifestations of cervical spondylosis, *Brain* 75:187, 1952.

8. Brodsky A: *Management of cervical radiculopathy secondary to acute cervical disc degeneration and spondylosis by the posterior approach.* In CSRS, editor: *The cervical spine,* Philadelphia, 1983, J.B. Lippincott, p 395.

9. Chestnut RM, Abitbol JJ, Garfin SD: Surgical management of the cervical radiculopathy, *Orthop Clin North Am* 23(3):461, 1992.

10. Crock HV: Internal disc disruption: a challenge to disc prolapse fifty years on. The Presidential Address: International Society for the Study of the Lumbar Spine, *Spine* 11:650, 1986.

11. Ducker TB, Zeidman SM: The posterior operative approach for cervical radiculopathy, *Neurosurg Clin North Am* 4(1):61, 1993.

12. Epstein JA, Epstein BS, Lavine LS: Cervical spondylotic myelopathy, *Arch Neurosurg* 8:307, 1963.

13. The Executive Committee of the North American Spine Society: Position statement on discography, *Spine* 13:1343, 1988.

14. Gonzalez-Feria L: The effect of surgical immobilization after laminectomy in the treatment of advanced cases of cervical spondylotic myelopathy, *ACTA Neurosurg (Wien)* 31: 185, 1975.

15. Gorter K: Influence of laminectomy in the course of cervical myelopathy, *ACTA Neurochir* 33:265, 1976.

16. Gregorus FK, Estrin T, Crandall EH: Cervical spondylotic radiculopathy and myelopathy: a long term follow-up study, *Arch Neurol* 33:618, 1976.

17. Haft H, Shenkin H: Surgical end result of cervical ridge and disc problems, *JAMA* 186:312, 1963.

18. Henderson C and others: Posterior-lateral foramenotomy as an exclusive operative technique for cervical radiculopathy: a review of 856 consecutively operated cases, *Neurosurgery* 23:504, 1983.

19. Herkowitz HN: *Cervical laminaplasty,* In Rothman RA, Simeone FA, editors: *The spine,* Philadelphia 1992, W.B. Saunders, p 631.

20. Herkowitz HN: Cervical laminaplasty: its role in the treatment of cervical radiculopathy, *J Spinal Dis* 1:179, 1988.

21. Herkowitz HN: A comparison of anterior cervical fusion, cervical laminectomy, cervical laminaplasty for the surgical management of multiple level spondylitic radiculopathy, *Spine* 13:774, 1988.

22. Herkowitz HN: The surgical management of cervical spondylotic radiculopathy and myelopathy, *Clin Orthop* 239:94, 1989.

23. Herkowitz HN, Kurz LT, Overholt DP: Surgical management of cervical soft disc herniation: a comparison between the anterior and posterior approach, *Spine* 15:1026, 1990.

24. Hirabayashi K and others: Expansive open-door laminoplasty for cervical spinal stenotic myelopathy, *Spine* 8:693, 1983.

25. Hirabayashi K and others: Operative results and post-operative progression of ossification among patients with ossification of cervical posterior longitudinal ligaments, *Spine* 6:354, 1981.

26. Honet JC, Puri K: Cervical radiculitis: treatment and results in 82 patients, *Arch Phys Med Rehab* 57:12, 1976.

27. Hukuda S and others: Operations for cervical spondylotic myelopathy: the comparison of the results of anterior and posterior procedures, *J Bone Joint Surg* 67B:609, 1985.

28. Hunt WE, Miller CA: Management of cervical radiculopathy, *Clin Neurosurg* 33:485, 1986.

29. Johnson RM, Murphy JJ, Southwick WO: *Surgical approaches to the spine.* In Rothman RM, Simeone, FA, editors: *The spine,* ed 3, Philadelphia, 1992, W.B. Sanders, p 1689.

30. Kurz LT, Herkowitz HN: Surgical management of myelopathy, *Orthop Clin North Am* 23(3):495, 1992.

31. LaRocca H: Cervical spondylotic myelopathy: natural history, *Spine* 13:854, 1988.

32. LaRocca H: *Survey of current concepts in the evaluation and treatment common cervical spine disorders.* H. Andrew Wissinger, Chairman, editor: *Instructional course lectures,* A.A.O.S., vol 27, St. Louis, 1978, Mosby, p 144.

33. MacNab I: Cervical spondylosis, *Clin Orthop* 109:69, 1975.

34. Manabe S, Tateishi A: Epidural migration of extruded cervical disc and the surgical treatment, *Spine* 11:873, 1986.

35. Martin GM, Corbin KB: Evaluation of conservative treatment for patients with cervical disc syndrome, *Arch Phys Med Rehab* 35:87, 1954.

36. Matjasko J, Petrozza P, Cohen M: Anesthesia and surgery in the seated position: analysis of 554 cases, *Neurosurgery* 17:695, 1985.

37. McKenzie RA: *The cervical and thoracic spine,* Upper Hutt, NZ, 1990, Wright and Carman.

38. McLaurin RL: *Diagnosis and course of cervical radiculopathy.* In Dunkster SB, editor: *Seminars in neurological surgery: cervical spondylosis,* New York, 1981, Raven Press, p 104.

39. Murphey F, Simmons JC, Brunson B: Surgical treatment of laterally ruptured cervical disc: review of 648 cases, 1939 to 1972, *J Neurosurg* 38:679, 1973.

40. Nowinski GP and others: *A biomechanical comparison of cervical laminectomy and cervical laminaplasty.* Presented at the Annual Meeting of the Cervical Spine Research Society, Palm Desert, CA, 1992, p 3.

41. Raaf JE: Surgical treatment of patients with cervical disc lesions, *J Trauma* 9:327, 1969.

42. Raynor RB: Anterior or posterior approach to the cervical spine: an anatomic and radiographic evaluation and comparison, *Neurosurgery* 12:7, 1983.

43. Robinson R and others: Cervical spondylotic myelopathy, *Spine* 2:89. 1977.

44. Rubin D: Cervical radiculitis: diagnosis and treatment, *Arch Phys Med Rehab* 41:50, 1960.

45. Scoville WB, Dohrmann GJ, Corkhill G: Late results of cervical disc surgery, *J Neurosurg* 45:203, 1976.

46. Simeone FA: *Cervical disc disease.* In Rothman RH, Simeone RA, editors: *The spine,* ed 2, Philadelphia, 1992, W.B. Saunders, p 440.

47. Simeone FA: *Cervical radiculopathy: posterior approach.* In Rothman RA, Simeone FA, editors: *The spine,* ed 3, Philadelphia, 1992, W.B. Saunders, p 609.

48. Simeone FA, Dillin WH: *Surgical management of cervical myelopathy: laminectomy.* In Rothman RA, Simeone FA, editors: *The spine,* ed 2, Philadelphia, 1992, W.B. Saunders, p 625.

49. Stookey B: Compression of spinal cord and nerve roots by herniation of the nucleus pulposus in the cervical region, *Arch Surg* 40:417, 1940.

50. Verbiest H: The management of cervical spondylosis, *Clin Neurosurg* 20:262, 1973.

51. White A III and others: Relief of pain by anterior cervical spine fusion for spondylosis, *J Bone Joint Surg* 55A:525, 1973.

52. Whitecloud TS III, Seago RA: Cervical discogenic syndrome: results of operative intervention in patients with positive discography, *Spine* 12(4):313, 1987.

53. Zeidman SM, Ducker TB: *Cervical spondylotic myelopathy: comparison of the anterior and posterior approaches.* Presented at the Annual Meeting of the Cervical Spine Research Society, Palm Desert, CA, December 3–5, 1992.

Chapter 98

Cervical Spondylotic Radiculopathy and Myelopathy: Anterior Approach and Pathology

Sanford E. Emery

Pathology

Diagnostic Evaluation

Preoperative Planning

Surgical Options

     anterior cervical discectomy and fusion
     anterior vertebrectomy and fusion

Complications

     intraoperative
     postoperative
     graft-related

Literature Review

The Future

The anterior approach to the cervical spine was developed independently by Robinson,[22] Cloward,[8] Bailey and Badgley[1] in the 1950s. Over the past decade this approach has become the procedure of choice for many spine surgeons in the treatment of cervical myelopathy. The surgical techniques continue to become more refined as a better understanding of the pathology responsible for nerve root and spinal cord compression becomes evident. The most significant advancements have been made in neuroradiologic imaging, including water-soluble contrast agents and CT and MRI scanning. These studies allow excellent preoperative analysis of the pathoanatomy.

Disc material, uncovertebral osteophytes, osteophytic ridges at the anulus, and ossification of the posterior longitudinal ligament (OPLL), alone or in combination, can cause cervical root or spinal cord impingement.[5] This compressive pathology exists anterior to the cervical canal—thus, the anterior approach offers the most direct method of cervical decompression. Arthrodesis is always recommended after anterior decompression in this patient population to stabilize the involved segments, and correct kyphosis if present. Arthrodesis also halts the progression of further spondylotic changes over the involved segments, which could cause recurrent canal compromise.

As the population ages and longevity increases, degenerative conditions of the spine and their treatment will be of increasing importance in our healthcare system. Cervical myelopathy from disc herniations, OPLL, or a congenitally narrow canal is seen in all age groups. However, in this country cervical spondylosis is the most common cause of cervical myelopathy and largely occurs in the older population. The problem is certainly not endemic to North America, however, and much can be learned from centers around the world regarding the evaluation and treatment of this condition.

Pathology

The pathophysiology of cervical spondylosis is based on degeneration of the intervertebral discs.[5] With age comes loss of water content and proteoglycan changes involving the ratio of keratin to chondroitin sulfate. With subsequent loss of height and anular bulging comes cartilage fibrillation and fissuring. The uncovertebral and zygoapophyseal joints as well as vertebral end plates respond over time to this altered biomechanical motion segment by forming chondro-osseous spurs. These spurs are the radiographic hallmark of cervical spondylosis. Depending on their size and location, and on spinal-canal diameter, these osteophytes can compress the spinal cord and/or the nerve roots. Instability with dynamic neural compression may also occur.

Spinal cord impingement initially results in compromise of the blood supply as well as axoplasmic flow of the neural tissue. It is unknown and difficult to determine whether one mechanism is more significant than the other in clinical situations; both probably play important roles. Vascular compromise is believed to occur most readily in the small intramedullary arterioles of the gray matter.[6,9,19] Continued compression leads to demyelinization of the white matter, which is probably still a recoverable lesion.[15,17] Subsequent changes of gray matter infarction and gliosis become irreversible. In many patients with slow chronic compression from cervical spondylosis, it is surprising the degree of compression the spinal cord can tolerate and still function (Fig. 98-1).

Diagnostic Evaluation

The diagnosis of cervical spondylosis and radiculopathy or myelopathy can largely be made by history and physical examination. Nerve root compression presents as arm pain, usually in conjunction with paresthesias or weakness. Gait or balance complaints, tingling or numbness of the hands, and/or subjective weakness in the upper or lower extremities may be early symptoms of myelopathy. Neck pain with referral to the interscapular or shoulder regions is common, but some patients with myelopathy have no neck pain at all. Concomitant radicular signs and symptoms may be present. Physical examination will show hyperreflexia with long tract signs and may show weakness, spasticity, decreased or painful neck motion, and even a Lhermitte's sign. Atrophy may be present, particularly in the intrinsics, with focal hyporeflexia for a given nerve root if radicular compression exists or if there is anterior horn cell loss from severe spinal cord compression. Sphincter disturbance is a late sign indicating severe disease.

The diagnostic evaluation includes plain films with flexion and extension views, MRI and/or cervical myelography, and CT myelography. Electromyographic nerve conduction velocity studies are of little or no use. Currently at our institution we seldom rely on MRI alone and prefer the better resolution of myelography and CT myelography, particularly for evaluating the offending bony pathology. C1-C2 punctures using biplanar radiography result in superior dye concentration for cervical myelographic studies. These should be done by individuals fully trained in the technique, usually a neuroradiologist. If the diagnosis is not clear, a neurology consultation is indicated to consider the differential diagnostic entities

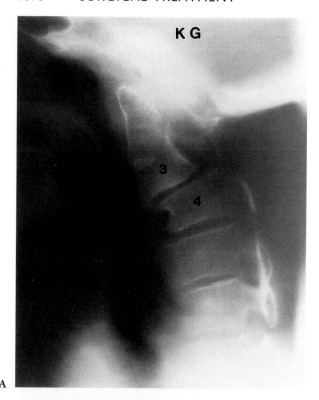

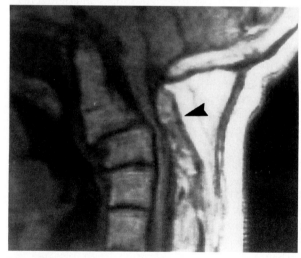

Fig. 98-1

A 40-year-old Caucasian male had complaints of gait difficulty with upper- and lower-extremity weakness of 1 year's duration. He was ambulatory but required a walker. Examination showed obvious long tract signs with bilateral upper- and lower-extremity weakness. A lateral tomogram (**A**) shows a Klippel-Feil deformity with a fixed subluxation of C3 on C4. A sagittal MRI (**B**) shows severe spinal cord compression at the level of the subluxation. The patient underwent anterior cervical vertebrectomy of C4 and fibular strut fusion followed by halo vest placement. The immediate postoperative period was uneventful but 1 week postoperatively the patient died of a myocardial infarction.

of demyelinating diseases, intracranial pathology, or metabolic disorders that might be responsible for the patient's findings.

Preoperative Planning

The usual indications for surgical treatment of radiculopathy is pain unresponsive to conservative measures or significant neurologic deficit. Once the diagnosis of cervical myelopathy has been established, surgical treatment is usually indicated. The natural history of myelopathy is slow deterioration, often in a stepwise fashion with periods of stable function followed by progression to a lower level.[7] Severe medical problems may preclude general anesthesia and surgical intervention, but generally even elderly patients will tolerate anterior decompression and fusion procedures quite well and ultimately benefit from the neurologic improvement. Progressive loss of neurologic function over hours or days requires urgent hospitalization, stabilization with a collar or traction, and prompt surgical decompression. This is uncommon, however, and most patients can be maintained in a soft cervical collar while the outpatient work-up and preoperative planning are undertaken.

The location, size, and extent of anterior compressive pathology will determine whether an anterior cervical discectomy and fusion or a subtotal vertebrectomy and fusion is indicated. To help make this decision, clear preoperative neuroradiologic studies are essential, as are dynamic flexion and extension plain films to identify compensatory subluxation. If the compressive pathology is limited to the disc spaces with small osteophytic changes present, a Robinson-type anterior cervical discectomy and fusion at the appropriate levels will suffice (Fig. 98-2). Generally, at our institution we will do up to three levels with this procedure if needed, but if four levels need decompression, vertebrectomies with a long strut fusion is recommended. Larger osteophytic ridges behind the vertebral body, OPLL, or stenosis from a congenitally narrow canal require hemi- or subtotal vertebrectomy and strut grafting rather than the simple discectomy and fusion (Fig. 98-3). For one-level vertebrectomy, an iliac crest graft is used unless severe osteopenia raises concern regarding graft strength. A fibula strut graft is used for three-level vertebrectomy procedures, with either iliac or fibular struts being quite satisfactory for two-level procedures. Though some have reported success with allograft, basic science and clinical studies indicate superior healing of autograft bone.[16]

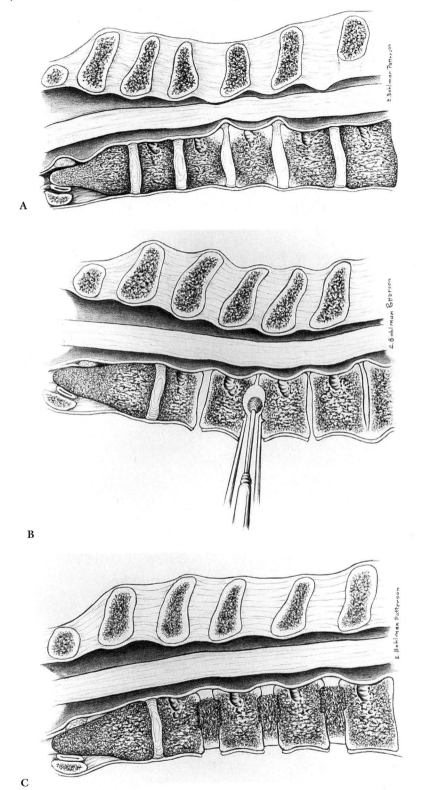

Fig. 98-2

A, A cervical spondylotic spine demonstrating a narrow canal, decreased height of the disc spaces, posterior osteophytes, and disc protrusions with buckled posterior longitudinal ligament and ligamentum flavum. **B,** Technique of removing posterior aspect of sclerotic end plates with a power burr. **C,** Bone blocks in place and properly countersunk. The entire disc has been removed at each level without violating the posterior longitudinal ligament. Distraction straightens the redundant posterior longitudinal ligament and ligamentum flavum, and immediate stability is achieved. *(From Bohlman HH: Cervical spondylosis with moderate to severe myelopathy: a report of 17 cases treated by Robinson anterior cervical discectomy and fusion, Spine 2:151, 1977.)*

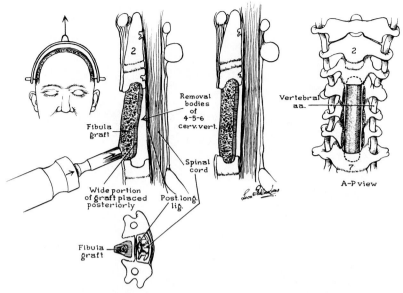

Fig. 98-3

The steps of the procedure that are performed after anterior corpectomy and decompression. Skeletal traction is carefully increased to reduce the kyphosis. The end plates are flattened with anterior and posterior lips fashioned to prevent graft migration. The graft is impacted into place, and decreasing the traction locks it home. *(From Zdeblick TA and Bohlman HH: Cervical kyphosis and myelopathy. Treatment by anterior corpectomy and strut-grafting.* J Bone Joint Surg 71(2):170-82, Feb., 1989.)

Surgical Options

Other techniques for surgical management of cervical spondylosis with radiculopathy or myelopathy include anterior and posterior approaches. For discectomy and fusion procedures, Cloward developed a dowel-type of bone graft plug harvested from the iliac crest.[8] This type of graft has been shown to be biomechanically inferior to Robinson-type grafts,[26] and we have seen problematic kyphosis from dowel grafts in our referral practice. Even with burring the vertebral end plates, segments grafted with tricortical iliac crest will on average increase in kyphosis only 3° and lose only 2 mm in height during the postoperative period.[12]

For more extensive disease, alternatives to anterior decompression and fusion include laminectomy and laminoplasty techniques. These are decompression procedures and do not stabilize the spinal segments. Multilevel laminectomy, particularly with foraminotomies or partial facetectomies, is destabilizing to some degree and late kyphosis can develop. Since the pathologic compression is usually anterior, any preoperative or subsequent cervical kyphosis can worsen rather than relieve cord impingement. Laminoplasty has been developed in an attempt to avoid postoperative instability associated with laminectomy. Normal cervical lordosis must be present preoperatively if one hopes to effect a decompression with this technique. More experience and long term follow-up with laminoplasty in spondylotic patients is needed before its risks and benefits are fully established.

Anterior Cervical Discectomy and Fusion

Anesthesia considerations are extremely important for patients with cervical radiculopathy and especially myelopathy. Any neck extension can be dangerous, and fiberoptic intubation is recommended. A standard Smith-Robinson approach to the cervical spine is used, beginning with a transverse incision, which is cosmetically quite acceptable.[4] A left-sided approach is generally used because of the more consistent course of the recurrent laryngeal nerve. Incision of the prevertebral fascia exposes the vertebrae and disc spaces. Cautery is used along the edges of longus colli bilaterally to avoid venous bleeding. A roentgenograph is obtained to ensure the appropriate level. Removal of the disc is then performed using a knife, small curettes, and pituitary rongeurs. Headlight and loupe magnification (preferably 3.5 × power or higher) are essential, and with this combination we have not found it necessary to use the operating microscope. All disc material is removed back to the posterior longitudinal ligament and out laterally to the uncovertebral joints. Gentle distraction of a disc space with Cloward-type lamina spreaders or Casper screw-post distractors facilitates safe and complete removal of compressive pathology. If the posterior longitudinal ligament is soft, it is left in place. If osteophytes are large enough to be causing cord or root compression, they should be removed with a diamond burr. Reaching behind osteophytes with curettes in an already tight canal with a compromised spinal cord is risky and unnecessary given the power instruments available today.

After adequate decompression, light burring of the vertebral body end plates is performed to expose bleeding subchondral bone (see Fig. 98-2). This will reduce the pseudarthrosis rate and results in minimal settling of the bone graft. Care is taken to leave a posterior lip on the superior and inferior vertebrae, which will prevent possible displacement of the graft posteriorly toward the canal. A small anterior lip is also fashioned that will discourage anterior displacement when the graft is countersunk. A tricortical iliac crest graft is harvested and trimmed to the appropriate size. Casper screw-post distractors allow easy placement of the bone graft. An intraoperative roentgenogram is obtained to document satisfactory position of the graft. A Penrose drain is placed along the vertebrae and the platysma, and subcutaneous and skin layers are closed. After a dressing is applied, a head–cervical–thoracic orthosis (i.e., a two- or four-poster type brace) is placed. The patient is maintained with the head of the bed elevated 30°. Mobilization of the patient can begin that day or certainly the following day. Duration of hospitalization largely depends on the severity of the myelopathy, with 3- to 5-day stay being typical.

In cases of discectomy and fusion, the brace is maintained for 6 weeks postoperatively. A soft collar can then be used as a step-down, for comfort as needed. Graft incorporation is usually evident radiographically within 6 to 12 weeks postoperatively.

Anterior Vertebrectomy and Fusion

Vertebrectomy procedures are much more demanding from a technical and postoperative standpoint, and should be performed by those experienced in anterior cervical spine surgery. Facility with power burrs is essential, and spinal cord monitoring as well as intensive care unit facilities are recommended.

As mentioned earlier, fiberoptic intubation with avoidance of neck extension is often necessary in patients with myelopathy. For vertebrectomy procedures, we routinely use cervical traction with Gardner Wells tongs or a halo ring. Low weight (e.g., 5 to 15 pounds) should be used, however, as the compromised spinal cord can be very sensitive to dis-

traction. Spinal cord monitoring should be functioning during the set-up when traction is initially applied.

A transverse incision can be used for multilevel vertebrectomy procedures. The deep cervical fascia must be incised longitudinally to allow mobilization of retractors for adequate exposure. After radiographic identification of location, discectomies are performed at the appropriate levels. It is helpful to identify the posterior longitudinal ligament at the disc spaces, as this reveals the depth of burring that will be required. The center portion of the vertebral bodies are then sequentially removed. Air-driven burrs are used initially to remove bone back to the posterior cortex. A diamond burr is then used to further thin and eventually create islands of the posterior cortical shell. These thin islands as well as residual disc material and thinned osteophytes can gently be pulled up off the posterior longitudinal ligament using tiny pituitary rongeurs and angled curettes. Care is taken to maintain midline orientation using the longus colli and uncovertebral joints for landmarks. If the posterior longitudinal ligament is soft it is not removed. The dura/posterior longitudinal ligament should slowly reexpand after decompression. Bleeding from cancellous bone and epidural veins can be vigorous at times, and preoperative autologous blood donation and even blood retrieval systems are recommended for multilevel procedures.

After decompression of the appropriate levels the traction may be slightly increased from the initial 5 to 10 pounds usually up to 15 or 20 pounds, depending on the level of the surgery. This should be done slowly, with spinal cord monitoring in attendance. The end plates of the vertebra are then prepared with a burr for the graft. Posterior cortical lips are fashioned to protect against posterior graft migration. Cup-like impressions are made in the body so as to lock in the graft (see Fig. 98-3). We do not place notched grafts on the anterior edge of the bodies, as this risks fracturing the anterior lip with resultant dislodgement, and also provides less surface area for graft–body contact. After seating of the graft, the traction is decreased and x-ray studies obtained to check the position. A full-thickness iliac crest strut is used for single-level vertebrectomies, either iliac crest or fibula for two-level procedures, and fibula struts for three or more level procedures (see Fig. 98-4).

For patients undergoing multilevel vertebrectomy a halo vest is often used for postoperative immobilization. This is routinely placed in the operating room at the end of the procedure. In patients with good bone stock, we have safely used a rigid

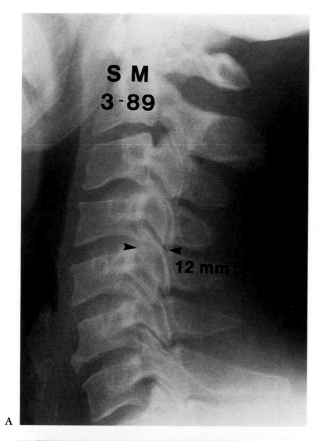

A

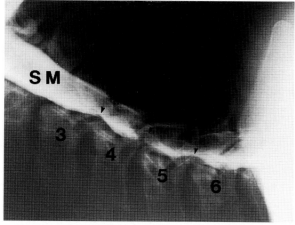

B

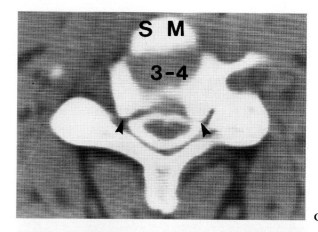

C

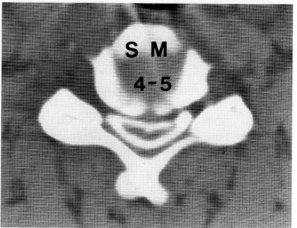

D

Fig. 98-4

A, Lateral roentgenogram of a 43-year-old man with complaints of left shoulder pain, gait abnormality, and leg weakness. He had mild spondylotic changes and a congenitally narrow cervical canal (12 mm). **B,** Lateral myelogram showing significant extradural defects at C3-C4, C4-C5 and C5-C6. **C,** CT myelogram shows large uncovertebral spurs (arrows) plus soft disc material protruding at C3-C4. **D,** Severe spinal cord flattening at C4-C5 from disc and osteophytic ridge.

head–cervical–thoracic orthosis. Duration of immobilization for these patients is generally 8 to 12 weeks, depending on radiographic confirmation of progression of healing.

In patients undergoing vertebrectomy we maintain the endotracheal tube for 24 to 72 hours postoperatively in an intensive care unit setting to allow upper airway swelling to subside.[11] After this, the patient may be mobilized as tolerated. Patients with severe myelopathy usually require physical therapy assistance and even rehabilitation center placement as they recover neurologically.

Complications

Complications of anterior surgery for cervical myelopathy can generally be grouped into intraoperative, postoperative, and graft-related categories.

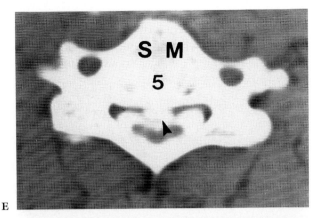

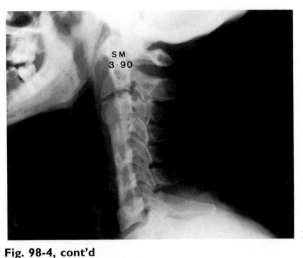

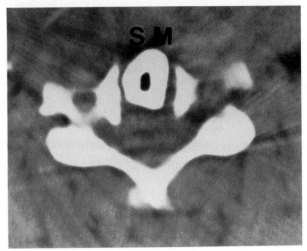

Fig. 98-4, cont'd

E, Ossification of the posterior longitudinal ligament (arrow) behind the body of C5 with spinal cord compression. F, The patient underwent a three-level corpectomy and fibular strut fusion from C3 to C7. G, Postoperative CT scan shows decompression of the cord and the strut in cross section. *(From Moskowitz RW and others:* Osteoarthritis: diagnosis and management, *Philadelphia, 1992, W.B. Saunders.)*

Intraoperative

Intraoperative complications with the anterior approach are well known and include carotid or vertebral artery laceration, esophageal tears, recurrent laryngeal nerve injury, and spinal cord injury. Knowledge of the anatomy and tissue planes is essential to minimize risks from the approach itself. We prefer a left-sided incision, given the more consistent path of the left recurrent laryngeal nerve. Awareness of the midline is critical when using a burr for vertebrectomies, as this is when the vertebral artery is most vulnerable. We usually use smooth retractors in the neck and have not seen esophageal injuries from their use. Errant use of the burr is more likely to injure the esophagus, and if there is any question, methylene blue may be placed down the nasogastric tube by the anesthesiologist to help identify a tear.

Meticulous technique with adequate visualization and magnification, as well as use of appropriate instruments, are essential in avoiding spinal cord injury. Patients with severe cord compression may be very sensitive to intraoperative traction, and judicious use of weights is recommended. Spinal cord monitoring, preferably with an experienced technician, is necessary for these procedures. If neural deficit is noted postoperatively, a roentgenograph should be obtained emergently to check graft position. Myelography or MRI is indicated to rule out other reversible causes of compression such as a hematoma. Reexploration may be indicated. Fortunately, neurologic and other intraoperative complications are rare, given appropriate attention to detail.

Atrophic or absent dura may present a problem, particularly in patients with severe OPLL. Treatment of the cerebrospinal fluid (CSF) leak is generally successful with fascial patching, fibrin glue, and a lumbar drain for 3 to 5 days to decrease CSF pressure.[25] Persistent leaking may require reexploration.

Postoperative

Postoperative problems include upper airway difficulties from edema,[11] as well as hematoma formation. All neck wounds should be drained, although this does not preclude the possibility of hematoma formation. The patient with a hematoma may be asymptomatic or may experience swallowing and/or respiratory difficulties. Evacuation of the clot is required emergently if respiratory symptoms are present. Severe swallowing limitations will also require drainage. Mild swallowing difficulties secondary to a hematoma usually resolve spontaneously and can be observed.

Dysphagia, unrelated to a hematoma, can occur after anterior cervical spine surgery. Occasionally this lasts longer than 1 or 2 days postoperatively. Our patients with dysphagia have all resolved spontaneously within 1 to 3 months postoperatively. Postoperative infection is rare in anterior cervical procedures, with or without the use of preoperative antibiotics. Infection should be considered, however, if pain or neurologic status worsens rather than improves several days or even weeks postoperatively. Halo or brace complications are generally minor. Close observation with early intervention can usually prevent halo pin problems or temporal mandibular joint symptoms from a cervical orthosis.

Graft-Related

Graft-related complications include dislodgement, collapse, and pseudarthrosis. Donor-site complications can also occur and include infection, hematoma, fracture, lateral femoral cutaneous nerve injury, and chronic pain. The technique of fashioning anterior and posterior lips on the vertebra with countersinking of the Robinson graft or a strut graft helps avoid graft displacement. Halo vest immobilization is not fail-safe but does help prevent fracture of the graft or the vertebral bodies, particularly in vertebrectomy patients with osteoporotic bone. We do not routinely use anterior plates in discectomy or vertebrectomy cases. Their use carries some risk of late esophageal injury from screw or plate migration.

Other graft complications include settling of the graft. Very little of this occurs with the Robinson-type graft, even when the end plates are burred to subchondral bone. Deeper burring through the end plate into pure cancellous bone is usually required for long strut graft placement, as hemicorpectomies are often required for adequate decompression. On occasion I have noticed some telescoping of the strut further into the body cephalad or caudad; however, to date this has not caused clinical symptoms or significant kyphosis in these patients.

Pseudarthrosis is more common with multilevel Robinson grafts than with single-level or long strut grafts.[10] This is probably related to the number of interfaces that must heal and also perhaps to biomechanical factors present at the interfaces. Burring of the end plates and achieving a congruent fit of the graft will minimize the risks of pseudarthrosis.[12] Patients with symptomatic pseudarthroses are studied with myelography and CT myelography to evaluate any new or recurrent neural compression. Revision surgery can then be performed either anteriorly or posteriorly. From an anterior approach, the pseudarthro-

sis can be removed with curettes and burrs as necessary, followed by repeat bone grafting. Posterior wiring and fusion with or without foraminotomies, depending on the pathology present, has also been shown to provide satisfactory results.[13]

Literature Review

Anterior cervical decompression and fusion with a Robinson type of bone graft was initially described for patients with neck pain.[23] This approach has since evolved to treat patients with radiculopathy[10] and myelopathy. Bohlman reported in 1977 on 17 patients with moderate to severe myelopathy treated with the Robinson-type anterior cervical discectomy and fusion.[3] Pantopaque myelography was used preoperatively to evaluate the areas of pathologic compression. Three patients were bedridden and 14 required ambulatory aids preoperatively. Postoperatively, 14 patients became ambulatory without aids, two could walk with a walker, and one patient was unchanged. For most patients, ambulatory improvement occurred within 6 months postoperatively. Signs and symptoms of nerve root compression also resolved in the vast majority of patients. Complications included a graft extrusion, one nonunion, and one collapsed graft; there were no neurologic complications.

As neuroradiologic evaluation of this patient population improved and the pathology was better appreciated, more aggressive decompressions with partial and subtotal corpectomies evolved. Hukuda and associates compared anterior and posterior procedures for the treatment of spondylotic myelopathy.[20] The anterior group comprised mostly Cloward-type procedures (156), but also had 46 Smith-Robinson and 12 subtotal corpectomy patients. All patients in the anterior and posterior groups showed improvement without one technique being clearly superior. It should be noted that anterior procedures were performed for pathology at less than three levels whereas posterior procedures were chosen for pathology at three or more levels, so direct comparison of the two groups should be made with caution. The authors believed that severity of myelopathy and duration of compression were significant variables affecting outcome. Yonenobu and colleagues[27] reviewed 95 patients, also a mix of posterior decompression (laminectomy) and Cloward, Smith-Robinson, and subtotal vertebrectomy procedures. For multisegmental disease they believed subtotal vertebrectomy was safer than the interbody fusion techniques because of better visualization. Laminectomy resulted in instability in some patients,

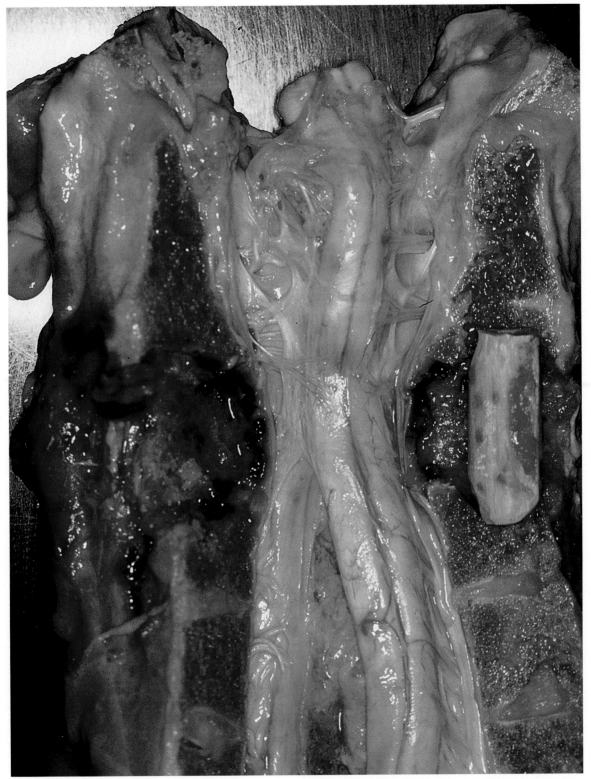

Plate VI-1

A, Gross pathologic examination of the spinal cord illustrates the area of indentation where the chronic anterior compression had been.

Plate VI-1 continued

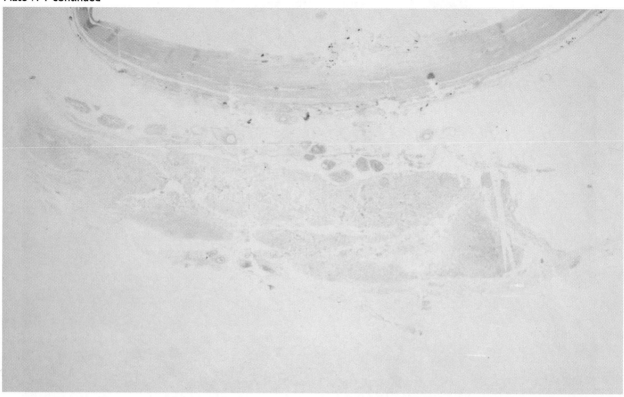

B, Histology shows severe flattening of the cord with distorted architecture.

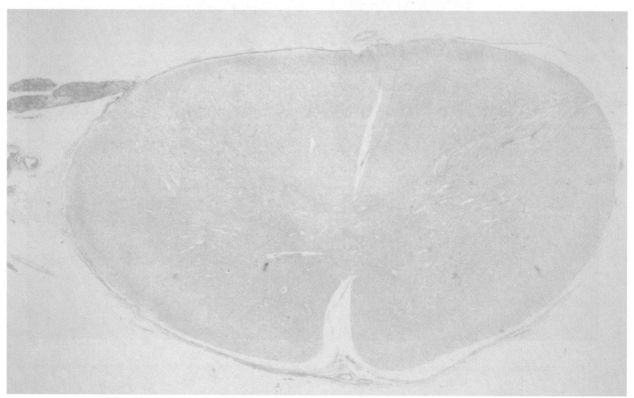

C, Section from the C1 level shows normal cord histology for comparison.

and the anterior procedures gave better results with respect to neurologic outcome.

Hanai and colleagues[18] reported on multilevel subtotal vertebrectomy and strut fusion in 30 patients. All patients showed improvement using the Japanese Orthopaedic Association scoring system. There were no neurologic complications or nonunions. Follow-up was from 1 to 6 years, with an average of 3 years. A similar patient group was reported by Bernard and Whitecloud,[2] on 21 patients with follow-up from 12 to 89 months (average, 32 months). Using the Nurick classification of myelopathy, 16 patients improved one grade or more, two deteriorated 1 year postoperatively after initial improvement, and three stabilized neurologically but did not improve. These authors used a notched fibular graft seated on the anterior lip of the vertebrae, not the technique described in this chapter, but had no pseudarthroses.

Saunders and associates[24] recently reported on 40 patients undergoing subtotal vertebrectomy and strut fusion for myelopathy. They noted significant improvement in 85% of their patients; three patients with severe deficits preoperatively had minimal improvement and three patients regressed after initial recovery. A high complication rate of 47.5% was reported. Though most of these were minor, 12.5% of patients still had long-term sequelae from a complication. Most recently, Okada and colleagues[21] reported on 37 patients who underwent a wider subtotal vertebrectomy (from pedicle to pedicle) followed by strut fusion. Thirty-six patients improved in ambulation, and one reverted to preoperative baseline after initial improvement. Three patients still showed continuing neurologic improvement more than 2 years postoperatively, while three had deteriorated relative to their maximum recovery. This decrease in function was believed to be secondary to increasing spondylotic changes at the adjacent level above the fusion. Variables related to outcome included severity of the myelopathy, duration of the symptoms, number of levels involved, and degree of cord atrophy. This last factor is consistent with the study by Fujiwara and associates relating the preoperative transverse area of the cord to surgical outcome.[14]

The Future

Success can be achieved with several different techniques for the surgical treatment of cervical radiculopathy and myelopathy. The best results for any given patient will depend on the specifics of that individual's anatomy and pathology. Anterior decompression and fusion has been shown to be safe and effective treatment for degenerative disorders of the cervical spine. The finer points of patient selection for anterior versus posterior procedures have yet to be worked out and will require long-term follow-up studies. All these procedures are technically demanding in a relatively high-risk population. Selection of a procedure will also depend on the surgeon's training, skill, and ability to manage potential complications.

References

1. Bailey R, Badgley C: Stabilization of the cervical spine by anterior fusion, *J Bone Joint Surg* 42A:565, 1960.
2. Bernard TN Jr, Whitecloud TS III: Cervical spondylotic myelopathy and myeloradiculopathy: anterior decompression and stabilization with autogenous fibula strut graft, *Clin Orthop* 221:149, 1987.
3. Bohlman HH: Cervical spondylosis with moderate to severe myelopathy: a report of 17 cases treated by Robinson anterior cervical discectomy and fusion, *Spine* 2:151, 1977.
4. Bohlman HH: *The neck.* In D'Ambrosia RD, editor: *Musculoskeletal disorders, regional examination and differential diagnosis,* Philadelphia, 1977, J.B. Lippincott, p. 178.
5. Bohlman HH, Emery SE: The pathophysiology of cervical spondylosis and myelopathy, *Spine* 13:843, 1988.
6. Breig A, Turnbull IM, Hassler O: Effects of mechanical stresses on the spinal cord in cervical spondylosis: a study of fresh cadaver material, *J Neurosurg* 25:45, 1966.
7. Clarke E, Robinson P: Cervical myelopathy: a complication of cervical spondylosis, *Brain* 79:483, 1956.
8. Cloward R: The anterior approach for removal of ruptured cervical disks, *J Neurosurg* 15:602, 1958.
9. Doppman JL: The mechanism of ischemia in anteroposterior compression of the spinal cord, *Invest Radiol* 10:543, 1975.
10. Bohlman HH, Emery SE, Goodfellow DB, Jones PK: Robinson anterior cervical discectomy and fusion for cervical radiculopathy: long term follow-up of 122 patients, *J. Bone Joint Surg* (9) 75-A: 1298, 1993.
11. Emery SE, Smith MD, Bohlman HH: Upper-airway obstruction after multilevel cervical corpectomy, *J Bone Joint Surg* 73A:544, 1991.
12. Emery SE, Bolesla MJ, Banks MA, Jones PK: Robinson anterior cervical fusion: comparison of standard and modified techniques, *Spine* 19:660, 1994.
13. Farey ID and others: Pseudarthrosis of the cervical spine after anterior arthrodesis: treatment by posterior nerve root decompression, stabilization and arthrodesis, *J Bone Joint Surg* 72A(8):1171, 1990.
14. Fujiwara K and others: The prognosis of surgery for cervical compression myelopathy, *J Bone Joint Surg* 71B(3):393, 1989.

15. Gledhill RF, Harrison BM, McDonald NI: Demyelination and remyelination after acute spinal cord compression, *Exp Neurol* 38:472, 1973.

16. Goldberg VM, Stevenson SS: Natural history of autografts and allografts, *Clin Orthop Rel Res* 225:7, 1987.

17. Gooding MR, Wilson CB, Hoff JT: Experimental cervical myelopathy: effect of ischemia and compression of the canine cervical spinal cord, *J Neurosurg* 43:9, 1975.

18. Hanai K, Fujiyoshi F, Kamei K: Subtotal vertebrectomy and spinal fusion for cervical spondylotic myelopathy, *Spine* 11:310, 1986.

19. Hukuda D, Wilson C: Experimental cervical myelopathy: effects of compression and ischemia on the canine cervical cord, *J Neurosurg* 37:631, 1972.

20. Hukuda S and others: Operations for cervical spondylotic myelopathy, *J Bone Joint Surg* 67B:609, 1985.

21. Okada K and others: Treatment of cervical spondylotic myelopathy by enlargement of the spinal canal anteriorly, followed by arthrodesis, *J Bone Joint Surg* 73A(3):352, 1991.

22. Robinson RA, Smith GW: Anterolateral cervical disc removal and interbody fusion for cervical disc syndrome, *Bull Johns Hopkins Hosp* 96:223, 1955.

23. Robinson RA and others: The results of anterior interbody fusion of the cervical spine, *J Bone Joint Surg* 44A(8):1569, 1962.

24. Saunders RL and others: Central corpectomy for cervical spondylotic myelopathy: a consecutive series with long-term follow-up evaluation, *J Neurosurg* 74:163, 1991.

25. Smith MD and others: Postoperative cerebrospinal fluid fistula associated with erosion of the dura: findings after anterior resection of ossification of the posterior longitudinal ligament in the cervical spine, *J Bone Joint Surg* 74A:270, 1992.

26. White AA, Hirsch C: An experimental study of the immediate load bearing capacity of some commonly used iliac bone grafts, *Acta Orthop Scand* 42:482, 1971.

27. Yonenobu K and others: Choice of surgical treatment for multisegmental cervical spondylotic myelopathy, *Spine* 10:710, 1985.

Chapter 99

Cervical Spondylotic Radiculopathy and Myelopathy: Posterior Approach

Richard S. Brower

Harry N. Herkowitz

Introduction

Natural History of Cervical Spondylotic Radiculopathy

Natural History of Cervical Spondylotic Myelopathy

Anatomy

Indications for Surgery

    cervical spondylotic radiculopathy
    cervical spondylotic myelopathy

Surgical Procedure

Surgical Technique

    laminotomy and foraminotomy
    laminectomy
    laminaplasty

Results

    radiculopathy
    myelopathy

Introduction

Cervical spondylosis as a radiographic diagnosis is prevalent in virtually any individual over 55 years old.[21] These degenerative changes, characterized by disc-space narrowing and facet arthrosis, tend to be global in nature, affecting multiple cervical motion segments (Fig. 99-1). Although controversy abounds regarding the clinical significance of these anatomic changes, it is readily apparent that problems arise when the local neurologic structures are affected. Both the nerve roots and the spinal cord may be vulnerable to irritation from these spondylotic changes. The main task in evaluating individuals with neck and radicular pain is to identify the exact area of nerve compromise.

Every effort must be made to match the clinical situation to the appropriate radiographic studies. History has demonstrated poor results of surgery for axial pain. Many individuals will have radiographic abnormalities even if their cervical spine is completely asymptomatic, particularly with the very sensitive MRI scan. Boden and associates reported a series of cervical MRI scans on 63 asymptomatic volunteers.[4] The studies demonstrated an abnormality in 14% of subjects younger than 40 years and in 28% of those over 40. Evidence of a degenerated disc was seen in 25% of the younger group and 60% of the older subjects. Their conclusion was that abnormal MR images are increasingly common with increasing age. They also emphasized the danger of making diagnostic decisions without careful matching of the clinical situation to the radiographic studies.[4] Failure to match these abnormalities with the clinical situation will result in less than optimal surgical results.

Natural History of Cervical Spondylotic Radiculopathy

The natural history of cervical spondylotic radiculopathy (CSR) is not well defined. Lees and Turner followed 51 patients with cervical spondylosis for 2 to 19 years. They reported that 25% had persistent symptoms, 30% had intermittent symptoms, and 45% had just one episode of pain.[37] Gore and associates followed patients with neck pain for 10 years.[22] The majority (79%) had less pain over time, with nearly half (43%) reporting no pain. However, 32% of the group continued to have severe or moderate pain. The author's conclusion was that individuals with worse discomfort had a poorer prognosis and that conservative treatment may be ineffective for many individuals.[22]

DePalma and colleagues reported on a series of 229 patients having symptomatic cervical spondylosis who were treated nonoperatively.[13] This group had no complaints consistent with radiculopathy. After 3 months, 29% had complete relief of pain, 49% had partial relief, and 22% had no relief. This last group (no relief) was followed for 1 year. Those patients refusing surgery were followed for 5 years, during which time 45% had a satisfactory outcome. Of the 55% having an unsatisfactory outcome, 25% were unable to resume their previous occupation. The authors concluded that cervical disc degeneration is a chronic disease that may be quite painful, resulting in long-term disability.[13]

Natural History of Cervical Spondylotic Myelopathy

Brain noted a difference in the clinical presentation of acute disc herniations and chronic spurring in 1948.[7] While acute protrusions were often linked to specific traumatic incidents and radiculopathy, chronic spondylotic spurs usually caused a myelopathy. His subsequent report in 1952 defined the syndrome of cervical spondylotic myelopathy (CSM).[8]

Brain also first emphasized the role of vascular impairment on the function of the cervical spinal cord.[6] Although there have been no definite reports of anterior spinal artery thrombosis, many studies have suggested that the sulcal and terminal vessels of the anterior spinal artery may be interrupted by direct spinal cord compression.*

The first examination of the natural history of CSM was by Clarke and Robinson.[10] They studied 120 patients, of whom 75% had episodic worsening of their clinical situation. Two thirds of these had continued deterioration between the acute episodes. The other one third stabilized between acute episodes of deterioration. Twenty percent of the original 120 patients demonstrated slow, steady deterioration, while five percent had rapid onset and progression of disease. They concluded that the overall prognosis of CSM was poor and that clinical improvement was rare. They found most lower-extremity problems to be motor in origin. Conversely, most upper extremities demonstrated sensory changes,[10] characterized by Ono and associates as "myelopathy hand."[43] These individuals complain of numb, clumsy hands.

The natural history of CSM was most famously discussed by Lees and Turner.[37] Of their 114 patients,

*References 9, 15, 18, 19, 31, and 50.

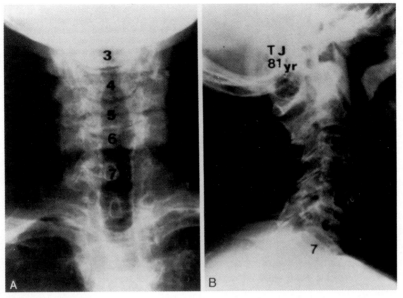

Fig. 99-1

Cervical spine radiograph demonstrating multilevel cervical spondylosis. *(From Rothman RH, Simeone FA: Cervical disc disease in the spine, ed 3, Philadelphia, 1992, W.B. Saunders.)*

64% did not exhibit progressive symptoms, while 26% worsened. Other authors have questioned their conclusion that conservative care should be the rule. Overall, the natural history seems to be one of stepwise progression of symptoms with variable-length plateaus, while occasional individuals will demonstrate rapid progression of their clinical picture.

The timing of surgery is an important issue in determining surgical outcome. Crandall and Gregorius demonstrated less optimal outcome for patients with symptoms longer than 12 months.[12] These patients were treated with either anterior cervical fusion or laminectomy. A tendency toward late deterioration in the laminectomy group was noted as late as 8 to 12 years after plateau. Guidetti and Fortuna reported 51% good or very good results of operative treatment in patients with less than 6 months of symptoms.[23] Their operative treatment consisted of either anterior cervical fusion with osteophytic resection or one of several variations in laminectomy technique. Only 16% of those with longer than 12 months' duration of symptoms demonstrated good or excellent results. Worse results were also seen in older individuals. They concluded that duration of symptoms was the more important factor in determining surgical outcome.[23]

Generally, CSM should not be considered a benign disease, as most patients will experience progression of their clinical situation. Surgical outcome can be expected to be less optimal both in

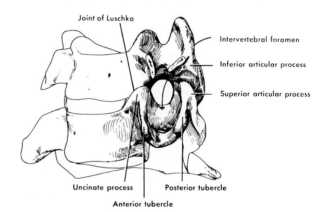

Fig. 99-2

Drawing indicating the boundaries of the cervical neuroforamen. *(From Rothman RH, Simeone FA: Cervical disc disease in the spine, ed 3, Philadelphia, 1992, W.B. Saunders.)*

older patients and in those with more than 1 year of symptoms. Surgery should not be withheld from these patients, but reasonable expectations of the prognosis must be understood by surgeon and patient alike.

Anatomy

The neurocanal is the most common site for nerve root compression in the cervical spine (Fig. 99-2). It is bounded by disc and uncovertebral joint anteriorly, facet and ligamentum flavum posteriorly, as well as the lateral edge of the lamina. Hypertrophy of any of these structures may cause nerve root compression. In the younger patient a posterolateral disc herniation is the most common cause of root compression. In older individuals, uncovertebral joint spur formation or hypertrophy of the facet is more common.

In the lumbar spine it is the traversing nerve root that is most commonly compressed by a disc herniation. In the cervical spine, the exiting root is usually compressed, for example, a C5-C6 disc herniation will entrap the C6 root. Epidural migration of a soft disc fragment may change the clinical picture, but this is far less common than in the lumbar spine. Additionally, a large central herniation may directly affect the spinal cord, creating a picture of myelopathy rather than radiculopathy. This is a rare occurrence.

The most prevalent concern in using the posterior approach to cervical spondylosis concerns postoperative instability (Fig. 99-3). Special attention must be paid to the integrity of the facet joint. Raynor and associates examined the effect of foraminotomy on facet strength in cadavers.[46] A 50% facetectomy was needed to expose 3 to 5 mm of nerve root, and a 70% facetectomy was needed to expose 8 to 10 mm of nerve root. They concluded that resection of more than 50% of the facet joint significantly compromised facet strength.[46]

More recently, an in vitro study by Zdeblick and colleagues reinforced the necessity of limited facetectomy.[58] They studied cadaver spines in several states; intact, after laminectomy, and after 25%, 50%, 75%, and 100% bilateral facetectomies. They concluded that segmental hypermobility of the cervical spine results if a foraminotomy involves resection of more than 50% of the facet.

The true incidence of postlaminectomy kyphosis is not well established in the literature. It is evident that the incidence is much higher in children than in adults.[38,42,51,54] The development of postlaminectomy kyphosis is troublesome for a number of reasons. First, it adversely alters the normal alignment and biomechanics of the cervical spine. Second, if the laminectomy was performed to relieve cord compression from anterior structures, lordosis is necessary to allow the cord to fall away from the impinging elements. Kyphosis effectively bowstrings the spinal cord over any anterior osteophytes that are present. Third, extensive surgical intervention is needed to salvage these unfortunate patients. Anterior strut grafting is required to reestablish normal alignment and provide decompression.

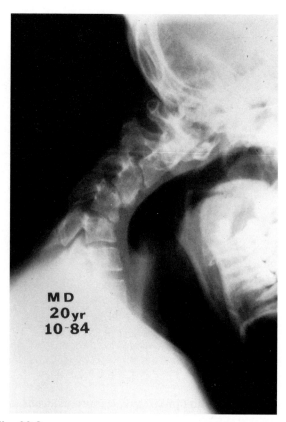

Fig. 99-3

Lateral radiograph demonstrating cervical kyphosis following an extensive cervical laminectomy. *(From Rothman RH, Simeone FA: Cervical disc disease in the spine, ed 3, Philadelphia, 1992, W.B. Saunders.)*

The anatomic differences between the anterior and posterior approach have been described by Raynor using cadaver cervical spines and plain radiography.[45] From the posterior approach, a quarter to a half of the facet had to be removed to visualize the root. Anterior osteophytes from the area of the uncovertebral joint were difficult to reach. In the clinical situation, this is made even more difficult by the presence of a venous plexus that frequently bleeds, obscuring visualization of the area. From the anterior approach, via a Cloward technique, Raynor found that the amount of root decompression obtained could easily be overestimated. Although uncovertebral spurs were easily reached, full root decompression required working beyond the area of direct visualization and was best performed with upbiting curettes. This study also demonstrated the unreliability of plain radiographs in determining the degree of root decompression achieved.[23] Since that time CT and MRI scanning have revolutionized visualization of the neurocanal.

Indications for Surgery

Cervical Spondylotic Radiculopathy

The indications for surgery are based on several factors: (1) duration and severity of radicular pain; (2) the presence of a neurologic deficit; and (3) a confirmatory radiographic study such as myelography, myelography combined with CT scan, or MRI correlating with the clinical findings.

The indications for surgery in cervical radiculopathy are as follows.

1. Persistent or recurrent arm pain not responsive to a 3-month trial of nonoperative treatment.

2. Progressive neurologic deficit.

3. Static neurologic deficit associated with radicular pain.

4. Any of the first three indications associated with a confirmatory imaging study (myelography with CT or an MRI).

Cervical Spondylotic Myelopathy

The indications for surgery in CSM are not as well defined as those for CSR. Since improvement with nonoperative care is unusual, operative treatment may be considered for any patient with myelopathy. Surgery should be performed in any patient demonstrating neurologic deterioration, in an attempt to halt progression of the disease process. Even patients with mild disease who have compromise of their daily activities are good candidates. Although older, more severely affected patients have a poor prognosis, they frequently have the most to gain from surgical intervention. The poor prognosis seen in patients with over 1 year of symptoms infers that early surgery may be more valuable.

This does not mean that all patients with myelopathy require surgical intervention. Patients who have a longstanding static neurologic situation may be observed. As well, some patients will have other medical problems making them poor risks for a surgical procedure. Patients with mild symptoms may not be limited enough in their normal activities to desire a surgical procedure.

Surgical Procedures

The most common posterior procedures used for cervical spondylosis are laminotomy with foraminotomy, laminectomy, and laminaplasty. All these procedures are done with the same positioning and basic surgical technique. They vary primarily in the amount of bone removed.

Laminotomy and foraminotomy require removal of just enough lamina to expose the lateral edge of the dura. The medial aspect of the facet is resected to visualize the exiting nerve root in its foramen. This technique is aimed at nerve-root compression within the foramen from disc material or uncovertebral or facet spurs. It does not decompress the spinal cord. Unilateral laminotomy and foraminotomy seems to have minimal effect on cervical stability.

Laminectomy requires the complete, bilateral removal of the lamina as well as the medial edge of the facet. Foraminotomies may be added at individual levels to decompress particular nerve roots. This requires sacrifice of the interspinous ligaments, ligamentum flavum, spinous processes, and the lamina. This combination of loss of attachment for the paraspinal muscles, facetectomy, and ligamentous sacrifice may have more serious effects on cervical stability. Laminectomy is used primarily in situations of myelopathy, with foraminotomies added for individual compressed nerve roots demonstrating radiculopathic symptoms.

The concept behind using laminectomy for myelopathy is that normal cervical lordosis will allow the cord to migrate from impinging anterior structures once the lamina are removed. The amount of migration achieved, if any, is highly unpredictable.[47] Without lordosis, any migration of the cord is impossible. For these reasons, as well as the risk of postlaminectomy kyphosis, patients without lordosis are not candidates for laminectomy. Preoperative evaluation of cervical alignment is vitally important prior to deciding to perform a laminectomy.[2]

Cervical laminaplasty was first described by Hattori in Japan, where ossification of the posterior longitudinal ligament (OPLL) is endemic.[29] The ossified mass consists of primarily lamellar bone with some woven bone. As the mass expands in size, narrowing of the spinal cord results in anterior spinal cord compression. Smith and associates recently described incorporation of the dura into the ossified mass, resulting in a dural defect after anterior decompression.[54]

Laminaplasty has been used for multilevel involvement of OPLL,[29] cervical myelopathy,[29,30,34,36] and radiculopathy.[26] The basic concept of laminaplasty is the hinging open of the posterior elements of the cervical spine, without removing them. Several variations have been described, all with the same goal—to avoid postlaminectomy kyphosis. Although originally described for use in myelopathy, this procedure has been shown to be successful in treating multilevel radiculopathy as well.[26]

Surgical Technique

Laminotomy and Foraminotomy

Indications

The primary indication for laminotomy and foraminotomy is a unilateral radiculopathy of one or more levels.

Procedure

The patient is first intubated and positioned on longitudinally placed rolls to allow abdominal decompression. The head is positioned with the neck in mild flexion and held with either a Mayfield pin-holder headrest or a horseshoe headrest. If the horseshoe headrest is used, special attention must be devoted to preventing pressure on the eyes. The operating table should be tilted so that the neck is parallel to the floor.

Radiographic localization of the operative level is important in performing a limited surgical exposure. A spinal needle may be placed down to a spinous process and a lateral roentgenograph taken. After the neck is prepped and draped, a midline incision is made between the spinous processes located above and below the intended operative level. Self-retaining retractors are placed after meticulous subperiosteal exposure of the lamina and facet are completed. A fine 1- or 2-mm Kerrison rongeur or burr may be used to remove bone above and below the interlaminar space, exposing the lateral edge of the dura (Fig. 99-4). The laminotomy should be directly over the junction of the nerve root and dura. Care must be taken to prevent excess sacrifice of the facet joint at this stage. Magnification and illumination in the form of a headlight and loupes or the operating microscope are mandatory to prevent neurologic injury.

The next step is to expose more of the nerve root with a high-speed burr. Burring is directed laterally, straddling the facet joint. The pedicles serve as the cranial and caudal limits of the decompression. Once the bone has been thinned, a combination of currettes and a fine Kerrison rongeur are used to complete the decompression of the nerve root (Fig. 99-5). Once a fine hockey stick–shaped probe passes out easily along the nerve root, the decompression is complete. For a hard disc or osteophyte impinging the nerve root, no further decompression is needed.

In the case of a soft disc herniation, palpation of the disc anterior to the nerve root is necessary. De-

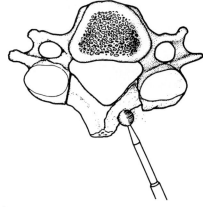

Fig. 99-4

Drawing demonstrating the opening made in the lamina using a 4-0 round burr. *(From Rothman RH, Simeone FA: Cervical disc disease in the spine, ed 3, Philadelphia, 1992, W.B. Saunders.)*

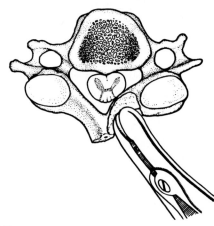

Fig. 99-5

Drawing demonstrating the thinned lamina prior to nerve-root exposure. *(From Rothman RH, Simeone FA: Cervical disc disease in the spine, ed 3, Philadelphia, 1992, W.B. Saunders.)*

pending on whether the major prominence of the disc is cephalad or caudad, the most direct route to the pathology should be taken, either over the shoulder of the root or through the axilla. The root may be gently retracted using a Penfield elevator, and the anulus incised. A fine pituitary rongeur is used for removal of the disc fragments, until the anulus is flat.

The wound should be thoroughly irrigated with saline solution, and a small free fat graft placed on the exposed nerve root. Fascia is closed with absorbable suture and staples or a running subcuticular closure of the skin is performed. The patient is discharged within 3 days and is provided with a soft cervical collar for comfort.

Laminectomy

Indications

Laminectomy may be considered in the patient with myelopathy secondary to spinal cord compression who may also have concurrent radiculopathic symptoms. Laminectomy is contraindicated in patients with preexistent cervical kyphosis or fractures, and in children unless fusion is also performed at the same time.

Procedure

The presence of myelopathy in patients about to undergo laminectomy necessitates awake fiberoptic intubation. Extension of the cervical spine is to be avoided as this markedly decreases the space available for the cord. Ideally, the patient should remain awake until positioning has been completed so that neurologic status may be checked prior to the induction of general anesthesia. Evoked potential monitoring, if available, should also be used. The patient is otherwise positioned as described for a laminotomy.

A midline incision is performed over the spinous processes of the levels to be decompressed. A meticulous, subperiosteal exposure of the posterior elements is next performed. Longitudinal troughs are created using a fine, high-speed burr, at the junction of the facets and the lamina (Fig. 99-6). Once the lamina have been thinned down to just remaining anterior cortex, a fine Kerrison rongeur is used to finish cutting the lamina. Using this technique, there is no need to place any instruments between the cord and the lamina, thus preventing iatrogenic cord injury. Once the troughs have been completed, the lamina are lifted off (Fig. 99-7). Residual ligamentum flavum may be released with a knife or currette. Once the lamina has been removed, foraminotomies may be performed at individual levels (Fig. 99-8). Again, the exposed dura is covered with a thin layer of fat or Gelfoam after wound irrigation. The fascia is closed in layers with absorbable suture. A Philadelphia collar is worn postoperatively for comfort, for no longer than 2 to 3 weeks.

Laminaplasty

Indications

The indications for laminaplasty, according to Hirabayashi and associates, are myelopathy due to (1) cervical stenosis; (2) continuous OPLL; or (3) multilevel spondylosis (four or more levels).[29]

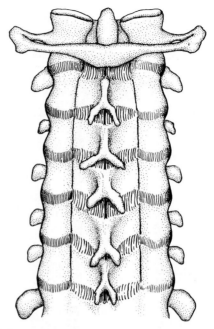

Fig. 99-6
Operative view of the cervical spine. The vertical lines indicate where the troughs are to be made in the lamina. *(From Rothman RH, Simeone FA: Cervical disc disease in the spine, ed 3, Philadelphia, 1992, W.B. Saunders.)*

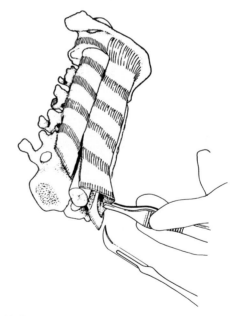

Fig. 99-7
After removal of the spinous processes, the lamina are elevated as a unit. Residual ligamentous attachments are incised with a scalpel. *(From Rothman RH, Simeone FA: Cervical disc disease in the spine, ed 3, Philadelphia, 1992, W.B. Saunders.)*

Laminaplasty may also be used in patients with multisegmental (three or more) cervical radiculopathy (Fig. 99-9).

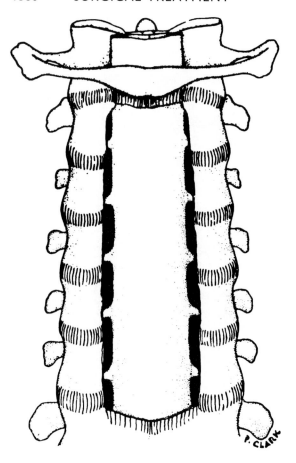

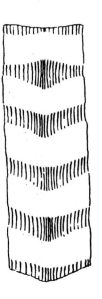

Fig. 99-8

View of the completed laminectomy. *(From Rothman RH, Simeone FA: Cervical disc disease in the spine, ed 3, Philadelphia, 1992, W.B. Saunders.)*

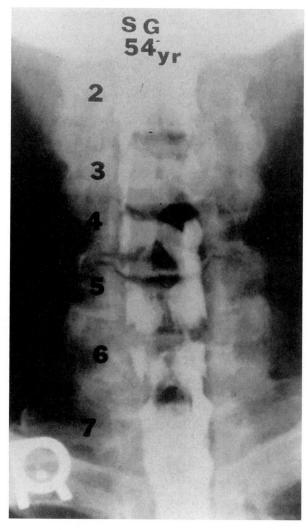

Fig. 99-9

Cervical myelogram of a 54-year-old male depicting multilevel cervical nerve root compression. *(From Rothman RH, Simeone FA: Cervical disc disease in the spine, ed 3, Philadelphia, 1992, W.B. Saunders.)*

Procedure

Step 1: The patient is positioned head down on a horseshoe head rest with the neck in a neutral or slightly flexed position.

Step 2: After exposure, two bony gutters are made with a high-speed burr from the upper to the lower vertebrae involved (Fig. 99-10). This should be performed just medial to the facet joint and pedicle (for example, with stenosis at C3-C4, C4-C5, and C5-C6, the bony gutter is developed through C3 superiorly and C6 inferiorly). On the side exhibiting the greatest narrowing or the side with the most significant radiculopathy, the burr should go to the inner cortex and break through at one segment. On the opposite side, the burr is used to go through the outer cortex. It may be necessary to burr to the inner cortex, but not through it. Next, a 1-mm Kerrison punch is used to remove the inner cortex from top to bottom on the side for which the lamina is to be elevated. In patients with significant radiculopathy, foraminotomies are performed at each segment (Fig. 99-11).

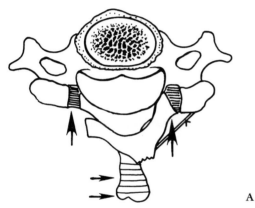

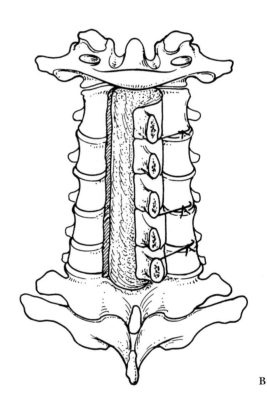

Fig. 99-10

Cross-section schematic demonstrating correct location of laminar troughs. *(Modified from Rothman RH, Simeone FA: Cervical disc disease in the spine, ed 3, Philadelphia, 1992, W.B. Saunders.)*

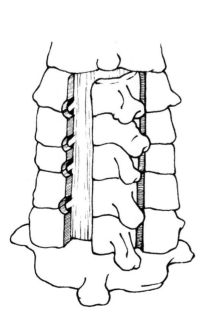

Fig. 99-11

Drawing depicting multilevel foraminotomies made on the patient's side with the greatest radicular compression. *(From Rothman RH, Simeone FA: Cervical disc disease in the spine, ed 3, Philadelphia, 1992, W.B. Saunders.)*

Step 3: Nonabsorbable sutures are passed through the base of the spinous processes at each segment. The tips of the spinous processes are removed at each level and fashioned into small strips for later use. Gently, pressure is placed along the spinous processes until the lamina begins to give way. It is essential to ensure that adhesions are not present between the dural sac and the undersurface of the lamina. A Penfield elevator is used to eliminate such adhesions. The amount of laminar elevation should be 10 to 15 mm. Kimura and associates showed that a laminar elevation of 10 mm

will expand the sagittal diameter of the spinal canal by 4 to 5 mm[36] (Fig. 99-12).

Step 4: Once the expansion is performed, the sutures within the spinous processes are secured into the facet capsules at each segment. The bone previously removed is placed in the trough on the hinged side. A thin layer of fat is removed from the subcutaneous tissue and placed over the exposed dura. If fat is not available, a Gelfoam pad is used (Fig. 99-13).

Step 5: The patient is maintained in a Minerva brace for 6 weeks postoperatively.

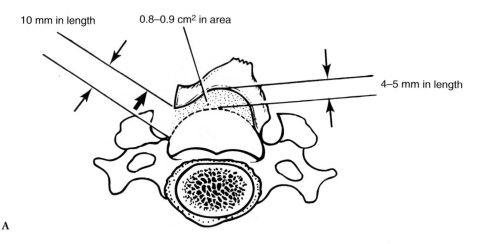

10 mm in length

0.8–0.9 cm² in area

4–5 mm in length

A

Widening of the Canal	Recovery Rate (%)
0.0–1.0 mm	34
1.0–2.0	62
2.0–3.0	65
3.0–4.0	72
4.0–5.0	81
5.0–6.0	60
6.0–7.0	62
7.0–8.0	57

B

Fig. 99-12

A and **B,** The distance that the lamina are elevated correlates with expansion of the bony canal and clinical recovery rate. *(Modified from Kimura I, Oh-Hama M, Shingo H: Cervical myelopathy treated by canal-expansive laminaplasty, J Bone Joint Surg 66A:914, 1984.)*

Fig. 99-13

Schematic depicting completed laminaplasty with sutures passed from spinous process to facet joint. Free fat placed over dural opening. *(From Rothman RH, Simeone FA: Cervical disc disease in the spine, ed 3, Philadelphia, 1992, W.B. Saunders.)*

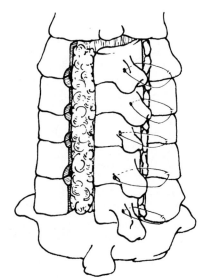

Results

The basic mechanisms between the anterior and posterior approaches are quite different. Anterior discectomy and fusion seeks to relieve nerve compression via several mechanisms. First, for soft disc herniations, the disc may be removed, even in the midline, an area inaccessible from the posterior approach. Second, anterior osteophytes may be directly removed if the surgeon feels this is necessary. The literature demonstrates that many of these hard bony ridges will resorb after a solid arthrodesis is attained.[5,48] However, not all osteophytes will resorb, as demonstrated by DePalma's series, in which only two thirds of posterior osteophytes resorbed.[13] Third, anterior bone grafting provides distraction between the vertebrae, thus enlarging and indirectly decompressing the neuroforamen. Fourth, solid fusion eliminates any effect that motion may have on irritating the nerve root. Lastly, anterior arthrodesis prevents the development of late instability and kyphosis.

The anterior approach has a number of disadvantages. Dissection is required between the carotid sheath and esophagus. Overenthusiastic retraction or injudicious technique may result in dire complications. Anterior techniques also depend on solid arthrodesis for an optimal result. If autograft is used, donor-site morbidity adds to the risk of the procedure. Allograft bone avoids this problem but is less likely to form a solid arthrodesis.[58] Graft dislodgement, an uncommon problem, may create the need for a repeat surgery if it occurs. The role of anterior plating procedures is not yet well defined.

The posterior approach to the cervical spine has a number of advantages. It is a direct surgical exposure, avoiding most vital structures of the anterior neck. Posterior techniques do not rely on obtaining solid arthrodesis to obtain a good clinical result. The nerve roots may be directly visualized and followed further laterally than is possible from the anterior approach.

The posterior approach does have several disadvantages. First, it does not allow the surgeon to address anterior compressing structures such as osteophytes. As discussed earlier, posterior movement of the cord away from anterior osteophytes is at best difficult to predict. Second, it requires at least partial resection of the facets to follow the nerve root laterally. This may result in clinical instability and the development of postlaminectomy instability (Fig. 99-14). Third, scar tissue will form over the exposed dura as part of the healing process. Fourth, the cord

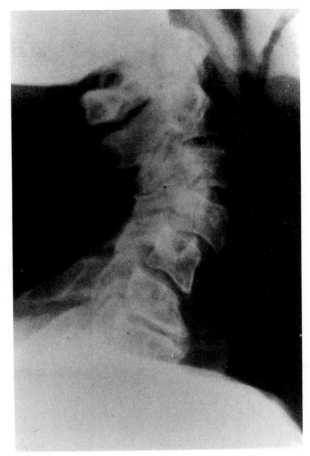

Fig. 99-14

Lateral radiograph showing the postlaminectomy instability that may occur after cervical laminectomy. *(From Rothman RH, Simeone FA: Cervical disc disease in the spine, ed 3, Philadelphia, 1992, W.B. Saunders.)*

may be injured due to direct manipulation, in an effort to resect anterior structures.

Radiculopathy

In general, the results of both anterior discectomy with fusion and laminotomy with foraminotomy have been quite good. Henderson and colleagues published a series of 846 consecutive patients undergoing foraminotomy for radiculopathy and reported a 96% success rate.[25] However, they also had a 14% reoperation rate for reasons not clearly defined. A report by Dillin and Simeone reported a success rate of 96%.[14]

Anterior discectomy with fusion has been shown to have excellent results for single-level radiculopathy. Aronson reported a series of 88 cases of soft cervical disc herniation treated by anterior cervical discectomy and fusion.[1] Although he did not document the criteria for success, his success rate was 100%. Gore and Sepic reported on 146 patients, 25% of whom had soft cervical disc herniations, with the rest having spondylotic spurs compressing the nerve roots.[20] They noted a 96% improvement rate using anterior cervical discectomy and fusion.

A recent study by Herkowitz and associates examined 44 consecutive patients with single-level cervical radiculopathy or myelopathy from soft disc herniations undergoing either anterior cervical discectomy and fusion or foraminotomy.[28] Good to excellent results were achieved in 94% of the anterior group and 75% of the foraminotomy group. Their conclusion was that either approach provided acceptable results, but the anterior fusion group had superior long-term outcomes.

In the setting of multilevel disease, patients undergoing anterior cervical discectomy with fusion (ACDF) demonstrate poorer results proportional to the number of levels fused. Robinson and associates reported satisfactory result rates of 94% for one-level, 73% for two-level, and 50% for three-level fusions.[49] Likewise, the nonunion rate rises with each additional level operated upon. The series by Connolly and associates reported a 15% pseudarthrosis rate for one- or two-level fusions and a 46% rate for three-level fusions.[11] An 80% union rate for one-level fusions was reported by White and colleagues, with a 66% union rate for multilevel fusions.[56] Review of the literature does suggest that bony union is not always necessary for a good result. DePalma and colleagues' series of 229 patients following ACDF showed no clinical difference between those patients with solid arthrodesis and those with a fibrous union.[13] A more recent study by Zdeblick and Ducker compared patients having ACDF with autograft or allograft.[57] In single-level fusions, both grafts produced a 5% nonunion rate, but autografts had an 8% incidence of delayed union versus 22% for allograft. In two-level procedures, autografts had a 17% nonunion rate compared with 63% for allografts. Graft collapse was six times (5% vs. 30%) more common after allograft procedures. Interestingly, there was no difference in relief of arm or neck pain.

Cervical laminaplasty, first designed for use in myelopathic patients, may have a role in treating cervical radiculopathy. A series by Herkowitz demonstrated an 87% good to excellent result in patients with multilevel radiculopathy.[27] This study used the technique of Hirabayashi[29,30] and Kimura[36] and their associates with several modifications: (1) the open side of the door was on the side of the predominant arm pain (if the arm pain was equal, the door was located on the side of greatest compression as determined by CT/myelogram); (2) foraminotomies were performed at symptomatic levels on the door side; (3) nonabsorbable suture was used to fix the spinous process to the facet capsule on the hinge side; (4) the hinge-side laminar bone trough was bone grafted with laminar bone from the door side and spinous process bone; (5) a thin autogenous free-fat graft was placed over the exposed dura; (6) somatosensory evoked potentials were monitored during the procedure; and (7) all patients were placed in a Philadelphia collar and mobilized on the day of surgery.[49]

In this series, patients with either unilateral or bilateral arm pain experienced relief. The fact that foraminotomies could not be performed on the hinge side did not affect the clinical outcome. Likewise, no patient experienced an exacerbation of symptoms on the hinge side. This suggests that opening the spinal canal obviates the need for a formal foraminotomy on the hinge side, although the exact mechanism of this phenomenon remains unknown.[49]

In summary, for the patient with radiculopathy, either an anterior or posterior approach may be used. Posterolateral soft disc herniations may be approached from either direction, but midline herniations should be approached anteriorly. In multilevel disease, the posterior approach may be advantageous, provided that limited resection of the facet is performed. Cervical laminaplasty may be used for patients with radiculopathy over many levels.

Author's Preference

The senior author (HNH) prefers anterior discectomy and fusion for one- or two-level cervical radiculopathy via the Robinson technique. Patients with three-level cervical radiculopathy undergo either anterior cervical discectomy and fusion or cervical laminaplasty, depending on their overall cervical alignment. For four or more level disease, cervical laminaplasty is performed as described above. Any patient with loss of normal lordosis is treated via an anterior approach.

Myelopathy

The presence of myelopathy with or without radiculopathy creates different concerns from the patient with only radiculopathy. In this setting, decompression of the spinal cord is necessary as well as nerve root decompression. Special attention must be paid to prevent iatrogenic damage to an already injured spinal cord.

Patients with myelopathy usually have disease at multiple levels, making postoperative stability an important issue. As the number of involved levels rises, individual discectomies and fusions are less attractive owing to the higher nonunion rate[49,58] and lower clinical success rate[49,52,55] seen with multilevel surgery. It is also much harder to predict surgical results for any procedure, as patients present with a wider range of symptoms.

Laminectomy for CSM allows the incorporation of foraminotomy at individual levels having radiculopathic symptoms with spinal cord decompression. Durotomy and resection of the dentate ligaments formerly was commonly included with laminectomy, but this practice has fallen into disfavor.[17,47] Reid demonstrated that dentate ligament resection did not allow increased mobility of the spinal cord in relation to the dura.[47] Dentate ligament resection has not been shown to have any advantage over simple laminectomy and foraminotomy by clinical trials.[23]

The anterior approach for myelopathy has more disadvantages as the number of involved levels increases. Longer decompressions require strut grafts and the use of a halo vest for immobilization to prevent graft dislodgement. The immediate postoperative period may be dangerous, as a report by Emery has described obstructive respiratory arrest in patients undergoing long anterior cervical fusions for cervical myelopathy.[16] In patients with OPLL, the dura may be incorporated into the calcified mass of the posterior longitudinal ligament, leading to large dural defects at the time of anterior decompression.[53]

Bohlman in 1977 reported a series of 17 patients treated for myelopathy with Robinson-type anterior cervical discectomy and fusion.[5] Fourteen patients required walking aids and three were bedridden. Five patients had single-level, seven had two-level, four had three-level, and one had four-level fusions. No attempt was made to resect posterior osteophytes. By the time of final follow-up, 15 patients were ambulatory without aid, one required a walker, and one remained bedridden. No patients demonstrated late deterioration.[5]

Hukuda and associates published a series of 269 patients operated on for myelopathy using several different surgical techniques.[33] One hundred fifty-six patients had Cloward type anterior discectomy and fusion, while 46 had Robinson-Smith technique. An additional 12 patients had vertebrectomy with strut grafting, and in all anterior procedures efforts were made to excise any anterior osteophytes. Of the 38 patients treated with posterior surgery, 14 had conventional laminectomy, seven had French window laminectomy, and 17 had French window laminaplasty. This was not a prospective study as the surgical technique was determined by radiographic studies. Patients with myelographic defects for one or two levels without canal stenosis received ACDF. For two- to three-level disease with stenosis, vertebrectomy was used. For three or more levels, barring preoperative instability, a posterior technique was performed. Their conclusion was that anterior discectomy and fusion should be recommended for one- or two-level disease. For patients with canal stenosis, vertebrectomy is preferable. Patients having disease at three or more levels should undergo a posterior procedure.[33]

Jenkins reported long-term follow-up of a group of five patients originally reviewed by Rogers.[35] All had had C1 to T1 laminectomy, durotomy, and dentate ligament resection 12 to 17 years earlier. All demonstrated neural improvement without any deterioration. He identified no incidence of postlaminectomy kyphosis.

Mikawa and associates noted a 36% incidence of altered cervical curvature in 64 patients treated by cervical laminectomy, with 14% having a deformity.[39] There were no neurologic changes attributed to these changes. Interestingly, deformity only developed in patients with OPLL. Postoperative loss of neurologic function has been documented by several authors. The incidence of this reported complication ranges from 19% to 53%.*

Careful examination of the patient's preoperative cervical alignment is vital in deciding upon the anterior or posterior approach. Recently, Benzel and associates reported a series of patients in whom the surgical approach was determined by sagittal alignment.[3] Patients with lordotic cervical spines underwent laminectomy while those with straight or kyphotic alignment underwent ACDF. Equal results were obtained from both surgical approaches.

For the patient about to undergo posterior decompression, the next decision regards whether laminectomy or laminaplasty should be performed. A number of variations of laminaplasty have been described, including Hirabayashi's open-door method[29] and Itoh and Tsuji's open door with bone graft method,[34] among others. All these procedures have common goals: (1) neural decompression, (2) maintenance of cervical stability, and (3) protection of the spinal cord from posterior trauma and dense scar proliferation. The value of laminaplasty over laminectomy is still being questioned. Series by Hukuda[32] and Nakano[41] and their associates have shown equal

*References 8, 10, 23, 24, 39, and 44.

results between laminectomy and laminaplasty. A series by Herkowitz evaluated the results of laminectomy, laminaplasty, and anterior fusion.[27] The success rate for laminectomy was only 66%, compared with 92% and 86% for anterior fusion and laminaplasty, respectively.

Herkowitz' series also noted that the greatest reduction of lateral flexion and rotation was seen in the laminaplasty group.[27] He also noted that three patients (out of 12) undergoing laminectomy developed postlaminectomy kyphosis. This is in direct disagreement with authors who believe that postlaminectomy kyphosis is a problem only in children.

Hirabayashi has correlated clinical recovery rate with the amount of widening of the sagittal diameter of the spinal canal.[29] For best results, a canal expansion of 4 to 5 mm is needed. This necessitates an open door of at least 10 mm. Either bone graft in the door side or nonabsorbable suture on the hinge side may be used to maintain the open door.

Author's Preference

The senior author prefers ACDF with resection of the osteophytes for patients with cervical myelopathy having one- or two-level disease. Generally, posterior osteophytes are resected to provide more immediate spinal cord compression. For patients with disease at three or more levels, open-door laminaplasty is performed.

References

1. Aronson N: The management of soft cervical disc protrusions using the Smith Robinson approach, *Clin Neurosurg* 20:253, 1973.
2. Batzdorf U, Batzdorff A: Analysis of cervical spine curvature in patients with cervical spondylosis, *Neurosurgery* 22(5):827, 1988.
3. Benzel EC and others: Cervical laminectomy and dentate ligament section for cervical spondylotic myelopathy, *J Spinal Disord* 4(3):286, 1991.
4. Boden SD and others: Abnormal magnetic-resonance scans of the cervical spine in asymptomatic subjects, *J Bone Joint Surg* 72A(8):1178, 1990.
5. Bohlman HH: Cervical spondylosis with moderate to severe myelopathy: a report of 17 cases treated by Robinson anterior cervical discectomy and fusion, *Spine* 2(2):151, 1977.
6. Brain WR: Cervical spondylosis, *Ann Intern Med* 41:439, 1954.
7. Brain WR: *Discussion on rupture of the intervertebral disc in the cervical region.* Proceedings of the Royal Society of Medicine XLI:509-516, March, 1948.
8. Brain WR, Northfield D, Wilkinson M: The neurological manifestations of cervical spondylosis, *Brain* 75:187, 1952.
9. Breig A, Turnbull IM, Hassler O: Effects of mechanical stresses on the spinal cord in cervical spondylosis: a study of fresh cadaver material, *J Neurosurg* 25:45, 1966.
10. Clarke E, Robinson PK: Cervical myelopathy: a complication of cervical spondylosis, *Brain* 79:483, 1956.
11. Connolly ES, Seymour RJ, Adams JE: Clinical evaluation of anterior cervical fusion for degenerative cervical disc disease, *J Neurosurg* 23:431, 1965.
12. Crandall PH, Gregorius FK: Long-term follow-up of surgical treatment of cervical spondylotic myelopathy, *Spine* 2(2):139, 1977.
13. DePalma A and others: Anterior interbody fusion for severe cervical disc degeneration, *Surg Gynecol Obstet* 134:755, 1972.
14. Dillin W, Simeone FA: Treatment of cervical disc disease: selection of operative approaches, *Contemp Neurosurg* 8:1, 1986.
15. Doppman JL: The mechanism of ischemia in anteroposterior compression of the spinal cord, *Invest Radiol* 10:543, 1975.
16. Emery SE, Smith MD, Bohlman HH: Upper airway obstruction after multi-level cervical corpectomy and myelopathy, *J Bone Joint Surg* 73A:544, 1991.
17. Epstein JA: The surgical management of cervical spinal stenosis, spondylosis, and myeloradiculopathy by means of the posterior approach, *Spine* 13:864, 1988.
18. Goodling MR: Pathogenesis of myelopathy in cervical spondylosis, *Lancet* 2:1180, 1974.
19. Goodling MR, Wilson CB, Hoff JT: Experimental cervical myelopathy: effect of ischemia and compression of the canine cervical spinal cord, *J Neurosurg* 43:9, 1975.
20. Gore DR, Sepic S: Anterior cervical fusion for degenerated or protruded discs, *Spine* 9:667, 1984.
21. Gore DR, Sepic SB, Gardner GM: Roentgenographic findings of the cervical spine in asymptomatic people, *Spine* 11(6):521, 1986.
22. Gore DR and others: Neck pain: long-term follow-up of 205 patients, *Spine* 12(1):1, 1987.
23. Guidetti B, Fortuna A: Long-term results of surgical treatment of myelopathy due to cervical spondylosis, *J Neurosurg* 30:714, 1969.
24. Haft H, Shenkin HA: Surgical end results of cervical ridge and disc problems, *JAMA* 186:312, 1963.
25. Henderson CM and others: Posterior-lateral foraminotomy as an exclusive operative technique for cervical radiculopathy: a review of 846 consecutively operated cases, *Neurosurgery* 13:5:504, 1983.
26. Herkowitz HN: Cervical laminaplasty: its role in the treatment of cervical radiculopathy, *J Spinal Disord* 1(3):179, 1988.
27. Herkowitz HN: A comparison of anterior cervical fusion, cervical laminectomy and cervical laminaplasty for the surgical management of multiple level spondylotic radiculopathy, *Spine* 13:774, 1988.
28. Herkowitz HN, Kurz LT, Overholt DP: The surgical management of cervical soft disc herniation: a comparison between the anterior and posterior approach, *Spine* 15:1026, 1990.
29. Hirabayshi K and others: Expansive open-door laminoplasty for cervical spinal stenotic myelopathy, *Spine* 8(7):693, 1983.

30. Hirabayshi K and others: Operative results and post-operative progression of ossification among patients with ossification of cervical posterior longitudinal ligaments, *Spine* 6:354, 1981.

31. Hukuda S, Wilson C: Experimental cervical myelopathy: effects of compression and ischemia on the canine cervical cord, *J Neurosurg* 37:631, 1972.

32. Hukuda S and others: Laminectomy versus laminoplasty for cervical myelopathy: a brief report, *J Bone Joint Surg [Br]* 70B:325, 1988.

33. Hukuda S and others: Operations for cervical spondylotic myelopathy, *J Bone Joint Surg* 67B:609, 1985.

34. Itoh T, Tsuji H: Technical improvements and results of laminoplasty for compression myelopathy in the cervical spine, *Spine* 10:729, 1985.

35. Jenkins DHR: Extensive cervical laminectomy: long-term results, *Br J Surg* 60:852, 1973.

36. Kumura I, Oh-Hama M, Shingo H: Cervical myelopathy treated by canal-expansive laminaplasty, *J Bone Joint Surg* 66:914, 1984.

37. Lees F, Turner JWA: Natural history and prognosis of cervical spondylosis, *Br Med J* 2:1607, 1963.

38. Lonstein J: *Post-laminectomy kyphosis, spinal deformities and neurologic dysfunction*, New York, 1978, Raven Press, p 53.

39. Mikawa Y, Shikata J, Yamamuro T: Spinal deformity and instability after multilevel cervical laminectomy, *Spine* 12:6, 1987.

40. Montgomery DM, Brower RS: Cervical spondylotic myelopathy: clinical syndrome and natural history, *Orthop Clin North Am* 23(3):487-93, July, 1992.

41. Nakano N, Nakano T, Nakano K: Comparison of the results of laminectomy and open-door laminoplasty for cervical spondylotic myeloradiculopathy and ossification of the posterior longitudinal ligament, *Spine* 13(7):792, 1988.

42. Oiwa T and others: Experimental study of post-laminectomy deterioration of cervical spondylotic myelopathy, *Spine* 10:717, 1985.

43. Ono K and others: Myelopathy hand: new clinical signs of cervical cord damage, *J Bone Joint Surg* 69B(2):215, 1987.

44. Phillips DG: Surgical treatment of myelopathy with cervical spondylosis, *J Neurol Neurosurg Psychiatry* 36:879, 1973.

45. Raynor RB: Anterior or posterior approach to the cervical spine: an anatomical and radiographic evaluation and comparison, *Neurosurgery* 12(1):7, 1983.

46. Raynor RB, Pugh J, Shapiro I: Cervical facetectomy and its effect on spine strength, *J Neurosurg* 63:278, 1985.

47. Reid JD: Effects of flexion-extension movements of the head and spine upon the spinal cord and nerve roots, *J Neurol Neurosurg Psychiatry* 23:214, 1960.

48. Robinson RA, Smith GW: Anterolateral cervical disc removal and interbody fusion for cervical disc syndrome, *Bull Johns Hopkins Hosp* 96:223, 1955.

49. Robinson R, Walker A, Ferlic D: The results of anterior interbody fusion of the cervical spine, *J Bone Joint Surg* 44A:1569, 1962.

50. Rothman RH, Simeone FA: *Cervical disc disease in the spine,* ed 3, Philadelphia, 1992, W.B. Saunders.

51. Shimomura Y, Hukuda S, Mizuno S: Experimental study of ischemic damage to the cervical spinal cord, *J Neurosurg* 28:565, 1968.

52. Sim FH and others: Swan-neck deformity following extensive cervical laminectomy: a review of 21 cases, *J Bone Joint Surg* 56A(3):564, 1974.

53. Simmons E, Bhalla S: Anterior cervical discectomy and fusion, *J Bone Joint Surg* 51B:225, 1969.

54. Smith MD and others: Postoperative cerebrospinal fluid fistula associated with erosion of the dura, *J Bone Joint Surg* 74A(2):270, 1992.

55. Tachdjian M, Matson D: Orthopedic aspects of intraspinal tumor in infants and children, *J Bone Joint Surg* 47A:223, 1965.

56. White A and others: Relief of pain by anterior cervical spine fusion for spondylosis, *J Bone Joint Surg* 55A:525, 1973.

57. Zdeblick TA, Ducker TB: The use of freeze-dried allograft bone for anterior cervical fusions, *Spine* 16(7):726, 1991.

58. Zdeblick TA and others: Cervical stability after foraminotomy, *J Bone Joint Surg* 74A(1):22, 1992.

Chapter 100

Cervical Fusions: Arthrodesis and Osteosynthesis of the Cervical Spine

Henrick Mike-Mayer
Howard B. Cotler
Stanley D. Gertzbein

History
Indications

    trauma
    tumors
    degenerative disc disease
    rheumatoid arthritis
    postoperative instability
    infection

Techniques

    upper cervical spine
    lower cervical spine

Complications
Results of Arthrodesis Without Instrumentation
Summary

History

The historical evolution of the concepts and techniques of cervical fusion has been covered in a previous chapter. This chapter will discuss the established techniques and their modifications as well as newer procedures and current trends. The techniques presented here are tried and true. The well-established techniques are primarily in reference to the bony fusions and wire internal fixation. New and controversial techniques for plate and screw fixation are evolving and may be useful in specific circumstances.

Indications

Indications for cervical spine fusion include conditions that produce pain or instability, such as trauma, tumors, degenerative disc disease, severe rheumatoid arthritis, postoperative instability, and infection. The definition of cervical spine stability as described by White and Panjabi[79] is the ability of the spine, under physiologic loads, to maintain a relationship between adjacent vertebrae in such a way that there is neither damage or subsequent irritation of the nerve roots, nor development of incapacitating pain or deformity secondary to structural deformation.

Trauma

Spinal fusion for injuries of the cervical spine decreases the length of hospitalization, prevents and/or corrects spinal deformities, and allows early mobilization and rehabilitation. It is indicated for unstable injuries or following decompression of the spinal canal.

Most Jefferson fractures do not require surgical stabilization unless there is 7 mm or more of combined lateral displacement of the lateral mass of C1 on open-mouth radiograph. This indicates a rupture of the transverse ligament and an unstable situation.[1]

Displaced odontoid fractures or unstable type II fractures are frequently associated with nonunion and require fusion. Type II fractures in older patients or patients with significant neurologic injury may benefit from fusion to assist in rehabilitation and nursing care. Established nonunions at 3 months that are symptomatic or unstable should also be fused. Several procedures have been described.* A fracture through one side of the posterior arch of C1 is not necessarily a deterrent to sublaminar wiring.[59]

*References 8, 21, 26, 32, 39, and 58.

Traumatic events to the subaxial cervical spine that create posterior instability or anterior fractures with excessive angulation or displacement should be fused posteriorly. In the presence of anterior compromise to the canal, or when there is evidence of a ruptured intervertebral disc, an anterior approach with disc excision followed by strut grafting and fusion is indicated. Anterior plate fixation[2,7,16] may be used to supplement the graft, or halo vest immobilization may be explored.

Reduced bilateral facet dislocations often do not undergo sufficient capsular healing to provide stability, and require fusion. Several techniques or their modifications that include the use of multilevel wires may be used.[58,64,67,68] In the absence of laminae or facet fractures, a Rogers fusion[67,68] is most often indicated. An oblique or facet wire technique is indicated if there is evidence of a facet fracture with subluxation or facet dislocation with recurrent subluxation.[59]

Tumors

Indications for surgical intervention in spine tumors include progressive neurologic deficit, instability, intractable pain, progressive deformity, and when total excision of the mass is possible. Relative contraindications include elderly and debilitated patients who would present unacceptable medical risks, when survival is expected to be less than 3 months, when high-dose therapeutic radiation would cause problems with tissue healing, or when the lesion is unresectable.

The most common cervical tumors are multiple myeloma and metastatic tumors,[72] which usually involve the anterior and middle columns. Anterior reconstruction with the use of cortical strut bone grafts, sometimes combined with posterior fixation, may be necessary. The use of methylmethacrylate[14] or special plates[27] may be required for additional stability. Halo stabilization can be used postoperatively.

If a single vertebral body is involved, it can be entirely excised with the adjacent discs through an anterolateral approach and stabilized with a graft, methylmethacrylate, or possibly metal struts. Involvement at multiple levels requires placement of anterior struts of rib or fibula and possibly the addition of a plate. Methylmethacrylate should be avoided if bone healing can be obtained and the prognosis for survival is good. Following anterior corpectomy and fusion, a posterior fusion may be necessary for additional stability.

Degenerative Disc Disease

Anterior arthrodesis in cervical disc disease offers a procedure with low morbidity and a high success rate.[47] Both the anterior and posterior approach have proponents.[36,44,53,54,66] Controversy exists whether to perform a simple fusion or a fusion and decompression, as some studies[19,66] indicate that osteophytes resorb in the presence of a solid fusion anteriorly.

Symptomatic motion segments may also be fused posteriorly after extensive foraminotomy.

Rheumatoid Arthritis

In patients with rheumatoid arthritis with upper cervical spine instability, a C1 to C2 fusion such as the Brooks may be done.[8] If atlantoaxial impaction is also present, the fusion should extend from the occiput to C2. Subaxial instability may likewise occur in rheumatoid arthritis secondary to erosion of the joints and may require posterior fusion for stabilization and prevention of further subluxation.

Postoperative Instability

Extensive laminectomies may destabilize the spine. Posterior fusion should be performed in conjunction with the posterior decompression if the amount of resection has rendered the spine unstable.

An anterior arthrodesis may be necessary in patients with a kyphotic deformity, as posterior procedures may not maintain the correction owing to lack of anterior support.

Infection

Persistent pain from instability or mechanical derangement following spinal infection can usually be addressed by standard posterior arthrodesis techniques. Unacceptable deformity or late-onset paraplegia secondary to infection may require anterior debridement, correction of the deformity, and fusion. Anterior debridement of the C1-C2 segment through an incision at the back of the pharynx can be performed and requires a tracheostomy and halo.[24] This approach may have a high morbidity but is useful when anterior decompression is required. Anterior approach for C1 and C2 lesions, although usually reported with a high incidence of infection,[17,24] has been shown to have a low infection rate and morbidity.[40]

Techniques

Upper Cervical Spine

Posterior Approaches and Fusions

The posterior approach is the most direct route to the spine. The posterior elements, including the spinous processes, laminae, and facets, offer a large surface area for fusion as well as cortical bone for secure fixation of instrumentation.

The main disadvantage of the posterior approach is that access to the anterior structures is not possible.

Preoperatively, patients are given prophylactic antibiotics in the immediate preoperative period. General endotracheal anesthesia is administered in the supine position on the carrier bed. Local anesthesia can be used for direct neurologic monitoring.[57] The patient is transferred to the prone position, maintaining the head-to-thorax relationship, and the patient is secured in a Mayfield headrest or a Gardner three-pin head holder (Fig. 100-1). Gardner–Wells tongs may be applied for traction prior to the procedure to provide stability and/or traction. If gross cervical instability is present the surgery may be done with the patient on a Stryker frame. A lateral radiograph is taken to assess the alignment of the spine.

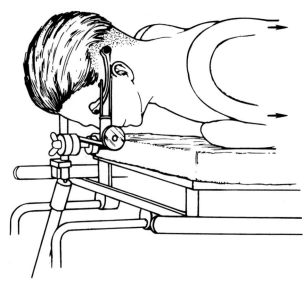

Fig. 100-1

Patient is turned onto operating room table with surgeon controlling head and neck by holding pin headrest. Surgeon places head and neck in desired position, and assistant secures frame to operating table. Countertraction is then applied to neck by taping shoulders to distal end of operating table. Lateral roentgenogram is obtained to verify that vertebrae are properly aligned. *(Redrawn from Griswold DM and others: Atlantoaxial fusion for instability, J Bone Joint Surg 60A:285, 1978.)*

Spinal cord monitoring should be routinely used if available, or else a wake-up test can be performed.

The back of the head is shaved and the entire posterior cervical region is scrubbed and painted with an antibacterial solution. Sterile drapes are applied exposing the area from the inion to the upper thoracic spine. Towel clips and/or adhesive drapes may be necessary to hold the drapes in place throughout the procedure.

Postoperatively, antibiotics are continued for 48 hours. External immobilization depends on the nature of the disorder, the procedure, and surgeon preference.

Occipitoatlantal Fusion Indications for occipitocervical fusion include instability, intractable pain, loss of bone substance, and occasionally severe rheumatoid arthritis that results in severe spinal cord compression at this level.

Various techniques of fixing the graft to the occiput to increase the union rate are described (Fig. 100-2). Wertheim and Bohlman[78] (Fig. 100-3) create a trough on either side of the external occipital protuberance making a midline ridge of bone. Using a towel clip or right-angle high-speed burr, a hole is placed through the outer table of the ridge of bone 2 cm above the rim of the foramen magnum. A wire is then passed through this hole. If a congenital anomaly of flattening of the occiput or basilar impression exists, it is helpful to use a high-speed burr and a rongeur to enlarge the posterior rim of the foramen magnum.[58] A drill hole is then placed through both tables of the occiput bilaterally, about 1 cm above the enlarged foramen magnum. A single strand of 18-gauge wire is then passed beneath the foramen and out the hole in the occiput on either side, the loop of wire lying beneath and just inferior to the inner cortex of the occiput.

A second 18-gauge wire loop is passed beneath the arch of C1 bilaterally. A third wire is passed through the base of the spinous process of C2. Alternatively, sublaminar wires may be passed beneath C2 and C3. Thus on each side of the midline there are four wires to secure the bone graft. The recipient bone should be decorticated with a high-speed burr.

Bone graft is obtained from the outer table of the iliac wing. The corticocancellous bone graft is split into two, each measuring 4 × 1 cm. Additional cancellous bone is placed medially and laterally to the graft. The wound is closed in layers.

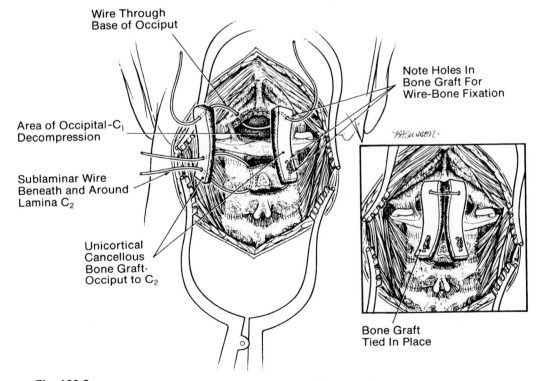

Fig. 100-2

Technique of occipitocervical fusion after enlargement of foramen magnum. *(Reprinted with permission from Meyer PR Jr, editor: Surgery of spine trauma, New York, 1989, Churchill Livingstone, p 489.)*

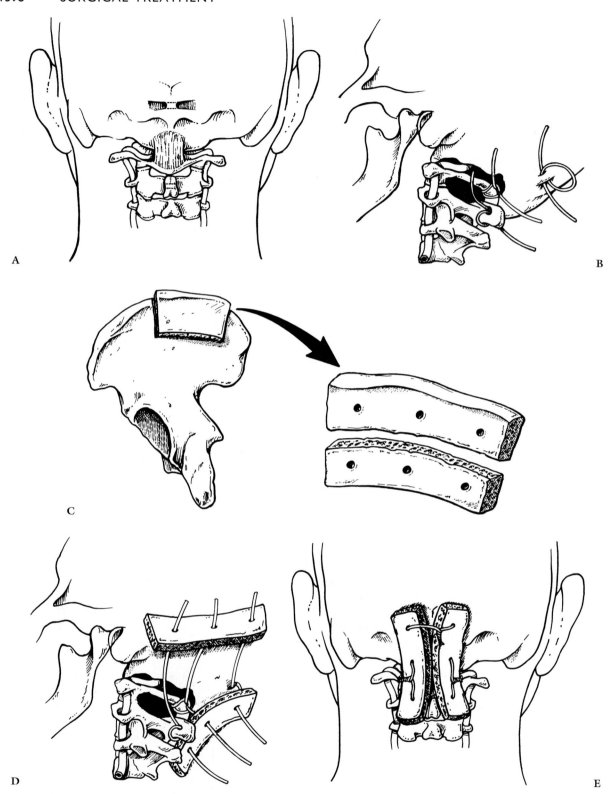

Fig. 100-3

Technique of occiptocervical fusion. **A,** Ridge is created on each side of external occipital protuberance using burr; hold is made in ridge. **B,** Wires are passed as illustrated. **C,** Corticocancellous graft is obtained from posterior iliac crest and horizontally divided; three holes are placed in each graft. **D,** Wires are passed through grafts. **E,** Wires are tightened to hold grafts in position. *(Redrawn from Wertheim SB, Bohlman HH: Occipitocervical fusion, J Bone Joint Surg 69A(6):834, 1987.)*

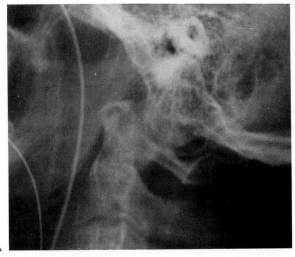

A

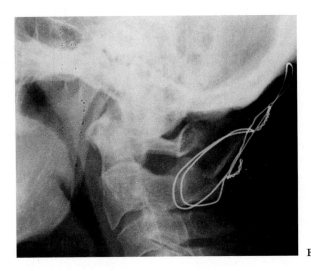

B

Fig. 100-4

A, Posterior occipitoatlantal dislocation. **B,** Due to C1 fracture, alternate wiring technique was performed to stabilize occipitoatlantal articulation. *(Reprinted with permission from Cotler JM, Cotler HB, editors:* Spinal fusion, *New York, 1990, Springer Verlag, p 207.)*

A halo is worn for 6 to 8 weeks, followed by a SOMI brace for 4 to 6 weeks, for a total of 3 months of bracing.

If the posterior ring of C1 is deficient, fractured, or removed surgically, an alternate procedure may be used (Fig. 100-4). Using the high-speed burr, a 4-cm transverse trough is formed 1.5 cm inferior to the external occipital protuberance. A transverse burr hole is then made through the protuberance through the outer table, and an 18-gauge wire is passed. Tricortical graft is harvested from the ileum with additional corticocancellous strips. Corticocancellous bone is split horizontally and the graft is fashioned into an H graft with one centrally located drill hole. The ligamentum flavum is stripped from the anterior surface of the C2 lamina using a Penfield dissector. An 18-gauge wire is passed superiorly beneath the lamina of C2. The looped wire is then passed through the central hole in the bone graft and the inferior wires are brought through the loop. Each leg of the H graft is allowed to straddle the spinous process of C2. The wires are tightened. Additional corticocancellous bone is then placed around the posterior elements of the occiput, C1, and C2.

Alternate Techniques Another useful technique is occipitocervical fusion using a Luque rectangle with fixation to the occiput with wire through the outer table of the calvarium and fixation to the cervical spine with sublaminar wires.[48] This is a difficult technique and is best left in the hands of experienced surgeons familiar with its particular indications and techniques.

C1-C2 Posterior Cervical Fusion

Brooks Technique[8,39] The Brooks technique provides more resistance to rotational movement and lateral bending than the Gallie fusion. It has a lower pseudoarthrosis rate than the Gallie fusion,[32] and is also better for fractures of the odontoid where posterior displacement is not as likely. A disadvantage is that two wires must be passed beneath the C2 lamina, increasing the potential for neurologic injury.

Modified Brooks Technique After the skin is prepped and draped, a midline skin incision is made from the inion to C3 following infiltration of the dermis with a 1:500,000 epinephrine solution for homeostasis. The incision is completed through skin and subcutaneous tissues. Dissection is in the avascular plane of the ligamentum nuchae to keep muscle bleeding to a minimum. An intraoperative radiograph may be taken but is not usually necessary as bony landmarks are visible (i.e., an absent C1 spinous process and a large bifid C2 spinous process). The lamina of C1 and C2 are exposed subperiosteally. At C1, dissecting medial to lateral prevents vertebral artery injury as it passes over and around the superior lateral surface of the posterior ring of C1. The vessel is approximately 2 cm from the midline and in danger if dissection is not kept subperiosteal. Below C1 the lateral limit of dissection is the medial edge of the foramen transversarium through which the vertebral artery passes.

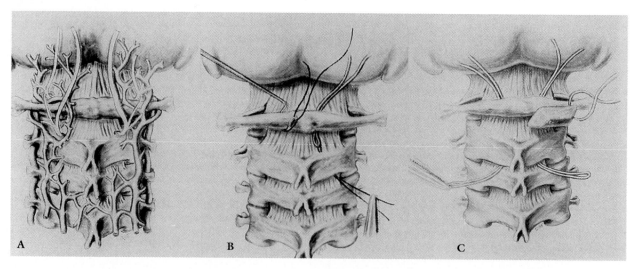

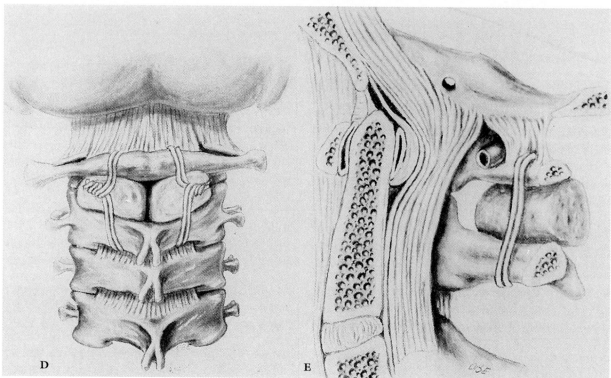

Fig. 100-5

Brooks fusion technique. **A,** Through midline approach, occipital nerves, which emerge from C1-C2 interlaminar space, and vertebral arteries are well protected by neck muscles. **B,** Sutures are passed under posterior arches of C1 and C2. Sutures are then used to guide wire under laminae of C1 and C2. **C,** After wires are passed, bone wedges are placed. **D** and **E,** Wires are tightened to secure bone graft and provide immediate stability. *(Reprinted with permission from Brooks AL, Jenkins EB: Atlantoaxial arthrodesis by the wedge compression method, J Bone Joint Surg 60A(3):279, 1978.)*

Once the initial exposure is completed (Fig. 100-5), subperiosteal dissection beneath C1 and C2 laminae is performed to create a channel for the passage of wires. Great care must be taken not to plunge anteriorly into the spinal canal. Two doubled 20-gauge wires are passed beneath C1 and C2 in the midline and then moved laterally. The wires must be pressed against the undersurface of the laminae to prevent anteriorly directed pressure against the posterior spinal cord (Fig. 100-6). A right-angle nerve-root hook can be used to hold the sublaminar wires against the posterior surface of the laminae to de-

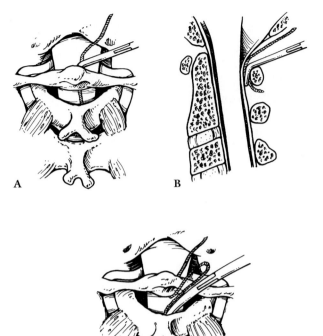

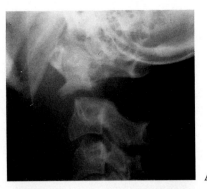

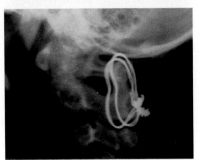

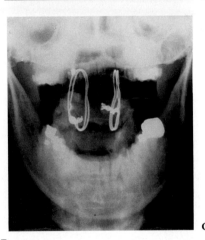

Fig. 100-6

A, B, and **C,** Two 24-gauge twisted wires are passed beneath the posterior atlantoaxial rings, two on each side of midline to hold grafts in place. (*Redrawn from Griswold DM and others: Atlantoaxial fusion for instability, J Bone Joint Surg 60A:285, 1978.*)

Fig. 100-7

A, Low type II fracture that could not be reduced by closed reduction. **B** and **C,** One year postoperatively, lateral and open-mouth roentgenograms show solid arthrodesis using Brooks technique. (*Reprinted with permission from Cotler JM, Cotler HB, editors: Spinal fusion, New York, 1990, Springer Verlag, p 207.*)

crease the chance of forward looping of the wire causing dural compression. Alternatively, using a curved ligature holder, a #1 Dermalon suture can be passed first to pull the wires through. Ensure that the wires are separated so they will not cross beneath the laminae. Bone grafts are then harvested from the posterior iliac crest and shaped into wedge-shaped blocks with an intact posterior cortex and an anterior wedge of cancellous bone. The rectangular pieces of bones should each be approximately 1 × 2.5 cm. Notches are created superiorly and inferiorly to improve the purchase of the wire, or holes may be placed in each end of the graft for the wires.

Next, the posterior cortices of C1 and C2 are decorticated with a high-speed burr. The bone blocks are positioned between the laminae of C1 and C2, with the cancellous side anterior. The looped ends of wire are cut, creating two wires for each graft. The wires are tightened individually and simultaneously to secure the grafts. (The modification includes placing a small segment of the bone graft between posterior elements of C1 and C2 and using only sublaminar wire for fixation.) Any traumatized muscle

tissue is debrided, and the wound is copiously irrigated and closed in layers (Fig. 100-7).

Gallie Technique[26,32] The Gallie technique is a simple, effective posterior fusion technique. It is useful for fractures of the odontoid with anterior displacement and other C1-C2 lesions.

The position and exposure are the same as described for the Brooks technique. A 1 × 3 × 1 cm corticocancellous graft is harvested from the posterior iliac crest. This is fashioned into an H shape

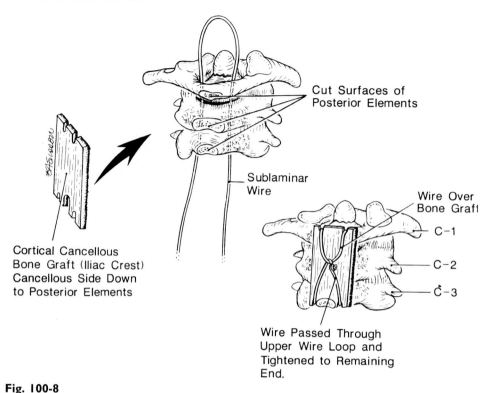

Cut Surfaces of
Posterior Elements

Sublaminar
Wire

Wire Over
Bone Graft

C-1

C-2

C-3

Cortical Cancellous
Bone Graft (Iliac Crest)
Cancellous Side Down
to Posterior Elements

Wire Passed Through
Upper Wire Loop and
Tightened to Remaining
End.

Fig. 100-8

Modified Gallie fusion technique for three-level stabilization. *(Reprinted with permission from Meyer PR Jr, editor:* Surgery of spine trauma, *New York, 1989, Churchill Livingstone, p 497.)*

with notches superiorly and inferiorly in the posterior cortical plate. A small notch is made in the superior surface of the base of the C2 posterior spinous process. A doubled 20-gauge wire is passed under the lamina of C1 in the inferior-to-superior direction. The free ends of the wire are then passed through the loop. The graft is placed between the inferior surface of the lamina of C1 and the superior surface of the lamina of C2. The wire is looped around and fitted into the notch created in the C2 spinous process and tightened (Fig. 100-8).

The construct is less intrinsically rigid, especially in osteopenic patients who may need a halo for 8 to 12 weeks until radiographic evidence of fusion is seen.

C1-C3 Posterior Cervical Fusion[59] In general, the use of sublaminar wires below C2 in the neurologically intact patient is contraindicated because of the risk of neurologic deterioration or injury. The following procedure may be useful in certain fractures of the ring of C2 (Hangman's fractures).

Technique One wire is passed beneath the lamina of C1 in routine fashion (Fig. 100-9). A second 20-gauge wire is passed through the base of the spin-

ous process of C3. The loop of wire above C1 is left intact, pulled inferiorly, and looped around the spinous process of C3. The rectangular bone graft is applied longitudinally over the posterior surface between C1 and C3. The inferior ends of the wire beneath C1 are passed through drill holes in the superior aspect of the rectangular bone graft. The ends of the inferior wire are passed through drill holes through the inferior aspect of the graft. The wires are then tightened.

Anterior Approaches and Fusions

Osteosynthesis of the Dens Internal fixation of the odontoid[4,49] may be performed in type II fractures to decrease the nonunion rate, especially in multiple trauma and noncompliant patients, in patients who have a fracture of the posterior arch of C1, or in patients who refuse halo treatment. A better range of motion is preserved compared with a posterior C1-C2 procedure by maintaining motion between C1 and C2. Screw fixation should not be used in established odontoid nonunions.

Technique This procedure is performed under anteroposterior (AP) and lateral imaging. If subopti-

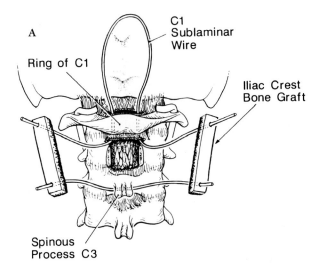

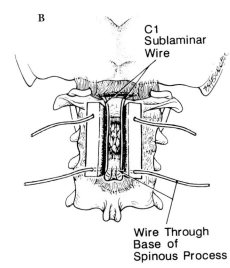

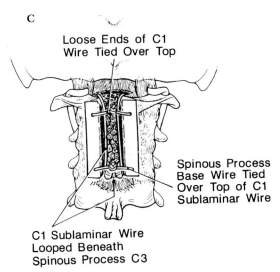

Fig. 100-9

C1-C3 fusion technique. (*Reprinted with permission from Cotler JM, Cotler HB, editors: Spinal fusion, New York, 1990, Springer Verlag, p 207.*)

mal visualization is present, the procedure must be abandoned. The patient is positioned supine, in traction. An anterolateral approach at the C4-C5 level and blunt dissection to the upper cervical spine is performed. Upon exposure of the base of the C2 vertebra, a 1.8-mm drill is directed from the base up into the dens. A screw is inserted to the tip of the dens. A second screw, parallel to the first, is added to provide rotational stability (Fig. 100-10). The screws developed by Knoringer[49] (Fig. 100-11) have threads of different pitch to apply compression to the fracture site, and can be recessed into the bone to prevent irritation of the surrounding tissues.

Posterior Atlantoaxial Screw Fixation[56]

The posterior elements of C1 and C2 are exposed. The facet joints are opened. About 5 mm of the posterior surface of the inferior articular process of C1 is exposed and K-wires are inserted into them (Fig. 100-12). The K-wires are used to retract the surrounding soft tissues, including the greater occipital nerve. A drill is placed at the lower edge of the inferior articular mass of C2, directed toward the facet joint just under the posterior cortex of C2, through the joint and into the lateral masses of C1. The appropriate length screw is inserted and checked radiographically. A posterior fusion is subsequently added (Fig. 100-13).

Lower Cervical Spine

Posterior Cervical Interspinous Fusions

Rogers Technique Originally described by William A. Rogers[67,68] and later modified by Zeigler and colleagues,[80] this technique is useful for flexion injuries with an intact anterior longitudinal ligament. It is also used for facet dislocations or subluxation injuries.

The patient is prone as for atlantoaxial fusion and the procedure may be done under local anesthesia to monitor the neurologic condition, or under general anesthesia with SSEP or wake-up test monitoring. A lateral radiograph is performed to check alignment.

The skin and subcutaneous tissues are incised to the spinous processes. At this point an intraoperative radiograph is obtained to check the correct levels for fusion. It is best to avoid subperiosteal stripping of any laminae not intended to be fused, to avoid incorporation into the fusion mass, especially in younger patients. The spinous processes, laminae, and facets are exposed at the appropriate levels.

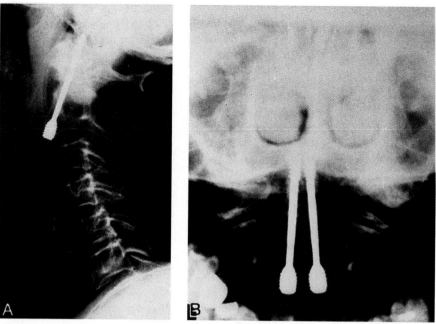

Fig. 100-10
Dens fracture, ventral dens fixation with two Knoringer screws.

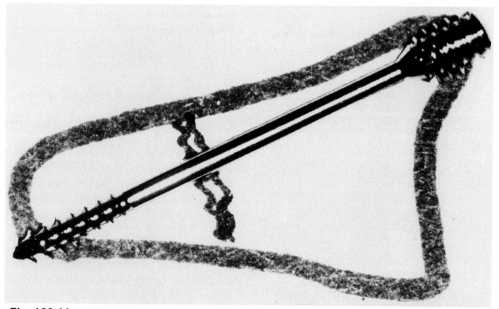

Fig. 100-11
Double-threaded compression screw developed by Knoringer. The caudal screw thread firmly anchored within the vertebral body of C2 does not irritate the C2-C3 segment. No threads lie within the fractured space. The dorsal cortex of the dens is utilized fully for anchorage.

An 18-gauge wire is passed through the base of the spinous process through a hole created by a towel clip, care being taken to avoid penetration of the spinal canal. The wire is then placed through a hole in the base of the inferior spinous process, as originally described by Rogers, or looped around the inferior spinous process. The wire is then tightened. Overtightening should be avoided. This could place the spine into hyperextension, and may compromise the space for the neurologic structures.

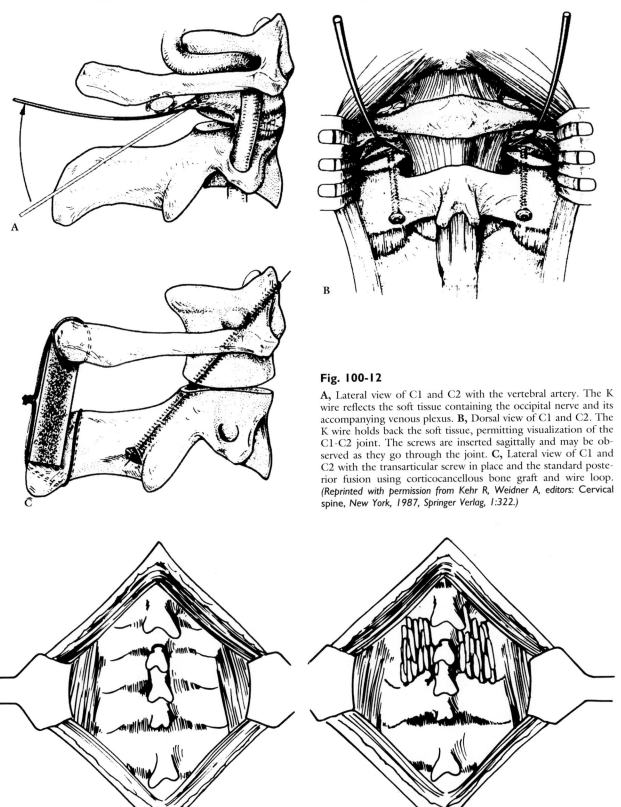

Fig. 100-12

A, Lateral view of C1 and C2 with the vertebral artery. The K wire reflects the soft tissue containing the occipital nerve and its accompanying venous plexus. **B,** Dorsal view of C1 and C2. The K wire holds back the soft tissue, permitting visualization of the C1-C2 joint. The screws are inserted sagittally and may be observed as they go through the joint. **C,** Lateral view of C1 and C2 with the transarticular screw in place and the standard posterior fusion using corticocancellous bone graft and wire loop. *(Reprinted with permission from Kehr R, Weidner A, editors:* Cervical spine, *New York, 1987, Springer Verlag, 1:322.)*

Fig. 100-13

Correct placement of matchstick is illustrated; cancellous grafts bridge adjacent laminae. *(Reproduced with permission from Rothman RH, Simeone FA:* The spine, *Philadelphia, 1982, W.B. Saunders, p 426.)*

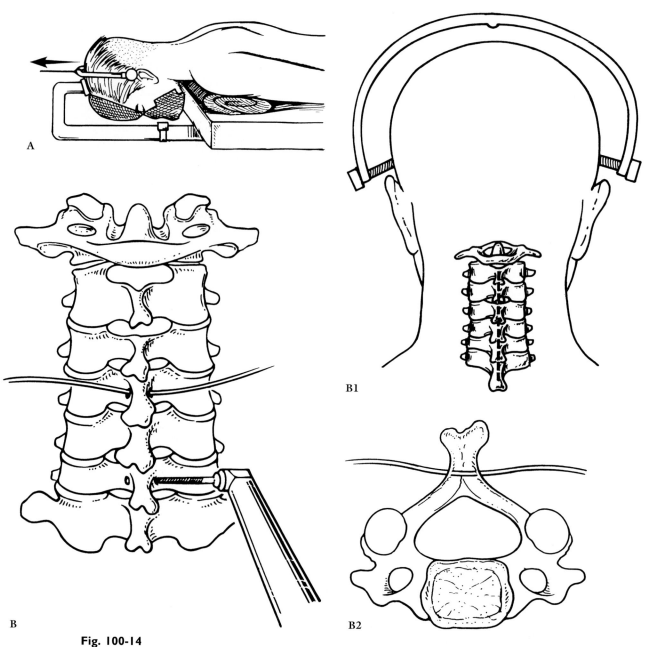

Fig. 100-14

Modified Rogers technique. **A,** Patient is positioned prone on wedge turning frame; midline posterior exposure is made. **B,** Drill holes are made in bases of spinous processes one level above and below injury level using right-angle burr.

Next, an iliac crest bone graft is harvested. Although Zeigler reports good incorporation of the graft without decortication, we prefer decortication of the posterior elements. Two bridging corticocancellous grafts are placed on either side with their edges beneath the wires to maintain their position. Surrounding the bone graft plates, bone chips or corticocancellous "matchsticks" are laid directly on the posterior cortices spanning the gap between the two laminae. The wound then is closed in layers. A hard collar is worn for 8 to 12 weeks or until radiographic evidence of consolidation is obtained.

Modified Rogers Technique There are numerous modifications of the Rogers technique (Fig. 100-14). The spine is exposed as for a Rogers fusion. Above and below the site of injury and intended fusion, a hole is created with a right-angle burr and

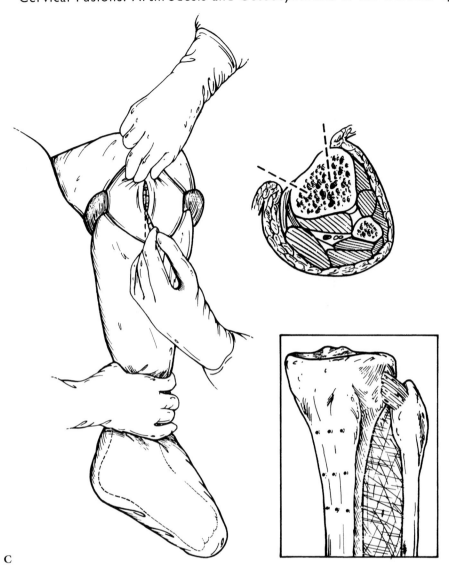

Fig. 100-14, cont'd

C, Technique for harvesting medial proximal tibial metaphyseal graft.

then enlarged with a towel clip at the juncture of lamina and posterior spinous process, and an 18-gauge wire is passed through the holes. Two strips of posterior ilium or tibial metaphysis are harvested. Oblique (45-degree) drill holes are placed through each end of the bone graft so the wires will converge over the center of the cortical surface of the graft. The superior and inferior wires are tightened simultaneously. As the wires are tightened, traction weights should be gradually removed so as to restore cervical lordosis. If there is obvious widening between one of the interspaces in the middle of the fusion, then the addition of a third wire is indicated. This wire is placed through the base of the middle spinous process, wrapped on one side under the next

inferior spinous process, and tightened. Radiographs are taken after all wires have been tightened.

Additional cancellous graft is placed in the gutters. For a single-level injury (i.e., bilateral facet joint dislocations), only a single-level fusion is required.

Oblique Wiring Technique Where instability of the facet joints remains after reduction, additional wiring of the facets may be used to stabilize the construct.

A Penfield dissector is placed between the inferior and superior facets at the level of instability, to open the joint. A drill hole is made through the center of the inferior facet with a right-angle drill. A 20-gauge stainless steel wire is passed through the hole and brought out through the facet joint. Using a

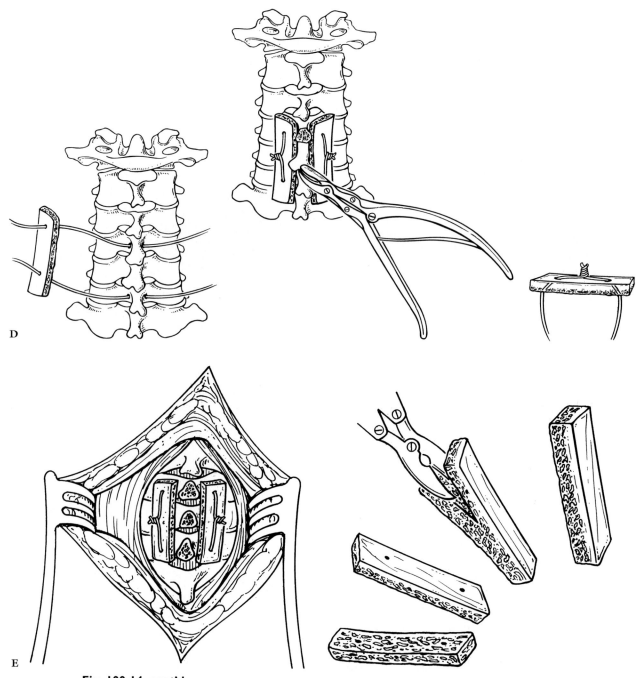

Fig. 100-14, cont'd

D, Wire is passed through bases of spinous processes. Oblique drill holes are made; wires are placed through bone plates and tightened. E, After wiring bone plates, graft is placed over posterior elements. *(Redrawn from Cotler JM, Cotler HB, editors: Spinal fusion, New York, 1990, Springer Verlag, p 207.)*

nerve hook, the wire is tightened around the next inferior intact spinous process. This is done bilaterally for bilateral facet joint instability. This technique is not used alone but in conjunction with the modified Rogers or triple-wire fusion technique (Fig. 100-15).

Posterolateral Facet Fusion

Callahan Technique[10] When there is a deficiency of the posterior elements such as after a wide decompressive laminectomy, the technique of Callahan[10] can be used. This is indicated after laminectomy in

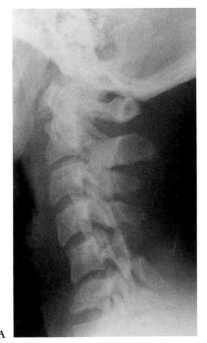
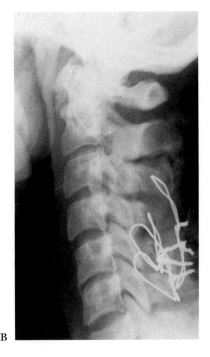
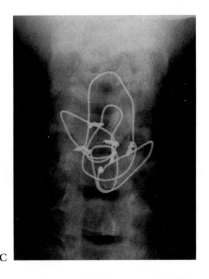

Fig. 100-15

A, C4-C5 and C5-C6 unilateral facet dislocations and C4-C5 laminae fractures in patient with incomplete quadriplegia. **B** and **C,** Anteroposterior and lateral postoperative roentgenograms show combined use of triple-wiring and oblique-wiring procedures. *(Reprinted with permission from Cotler JM, Cotler HB, editors: Spinal fusion, New York, 1990, Springer Verlag, p 207.)*

high-risk groups such as children and adults less than 25 years old. Recommendations to increase the success of the procedure include wiring the graft at each level to increase stability, extending the fusion one segment lower than the level of the laminectomy, ensuring that no structural deformities exist below the caudal end of the fusion, and obtaining the bone graft from the outer table of the iliac crest to provide two concave surfaces that fit into the cervical lordosis.

The capsules overlying the facet joints are debrided. A small flat instrument such as an elevator is placed into the facet joint and twisted to open the joint space. The articular cartilage is removed with a curette. A drill hole is made through the inferior facet at 90 degrees to the articular surface, with the elevator positioned in the joint to intervene between the tip of the drill or burr and the superior facet (Fig. 100-16). This will help protect the anterior structures such as the vertebral artery and nerve roots.

A 20-gauge wire is passed between adjacent ipsilateral facets and tightened. Alternatively, wires can be passed through each drill hole and used to anchor the bone graft. Two corticocancellous grafts from the iliac crest are obtained from the outer table (Fig. 100-17). The convex cancellous side of the graft is placed against the spine to help maintain cervical lordosis. The wires in each inferior facet are passed at each level around the graft. The bone graft is wired down to the facets, starting with the middle wire to snug the graft into the lordotic curve.

Other Techniques A modification by Garfin and associates[33] involves the use of Harrington compression rods to replace the corticocancellous struts. Autologous bone graft is then placed over the decorticated bone. This technique can be used if long struts are needed, and it provides increased strength.

Triple-Wire Technique[6,58] The Bohlman[6] or Garber-Meyer[58] triple-wire technique is similar to the Rogers technique[67,68] and can be used in degenerative spondylolisthesis. The patient is positioned and approached as in the Rogers technique. Holes are made through the bases of the transverse processes to be fused (Fig. 100-18). Wire is then passed between spinous processes through the holes. Additional wires are then passed through the holes to secure the corticocancellous bone graft on either side. The advantage of this fusion is the postoperative stability of the construct (Fig. 100-19). A Philadelphia collar or SOMI is worn postoperatively.

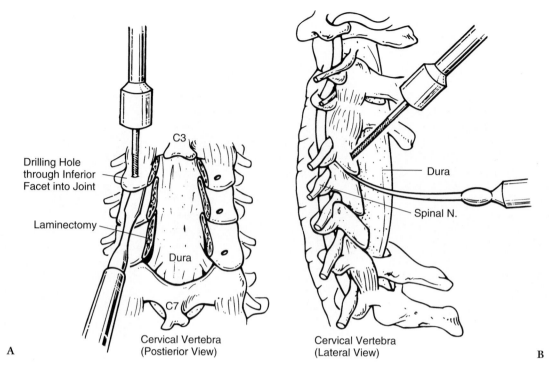

Fig. 100-16

A, Facet fusion: soft tissues and capsular ligaments are cleared from facets and posterior pillars, and facet joints are pried open using small curved elevator. Drill holes are made in posterior pillars, using 3-mm drill, at right angle to plane of facet joints. **B,** These holes are made eccentrically toward midline so that grafts ultimately may rest on large area of posterior pillar. During drilling, flat elevator is left between facets to protect facet below and vertebral artery and nerve roots to front. (*Redrawn from Callahan RA and others: Cervical facet fusion for control of instability following laminectomy, J Bone Joint Surg 59A:991, 1977.*)

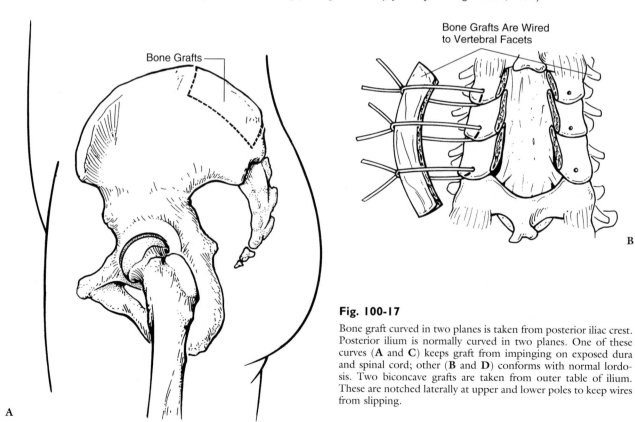

Fig. 100-17

Bone graft curved in two planes is taken from posterior iliac crest. Posterior ilium is normally curved in two planes. One of these curves (**A** and **C**) keeps graft from impinging on exposed dura and spinal cord; other (**B** and **D**) conforms with normal lordosis. Two biconcave grafts are taken from outer table of ilium. These are notched laterally at upper and lower poles to keep wires from slipping.

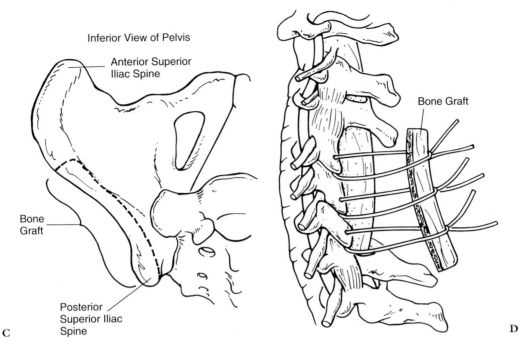

Fig. 100-17, cont'd

C and **D,** Twisted 24-gauge stainless-steel wire is then inserted into each hole, and tip of wires is grasped within joint space using fine, curbed clamp. Wires are placed at each level of intended fusion bilaterally. Grafts are then placed along posterior facet pillars, and wires are tightened and twisted around grafts. This is usually started at midpoint of fusion so that the graft will rest snugly against apex of lordotic curve. Wire that extends through hole in facet pillar is passed medially about graft (**C**); wire that emerges from facet joint is passed laterally. This prevents graft from drifting medially towards exposed spinal canal. *(Redrawn from Callahan RA and others: Cervical facet fusion for control of instability following laminectomy,* J Bone Joint Surg *59A:991, 1977.)*

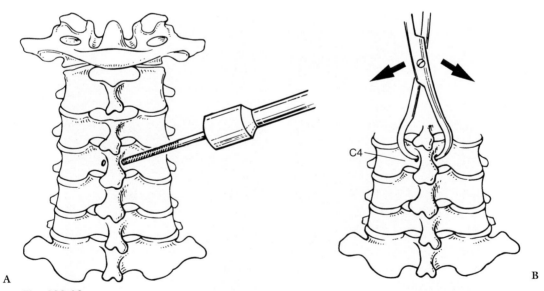

Fig. 100-18

Method of interspinous process wiring and fusion. **A,** Drill makes initial hole at base of spinous process. **B,** Towel clip used to enlarge hole should be "locked" in a superior–inferior direction to prevent additional contusion of neural elements. *(Reproduced with permission from Rothman RH, Simeone FA:* The Spine, *Philadelphia, 1982, W.B. Saunders, p 426.)*

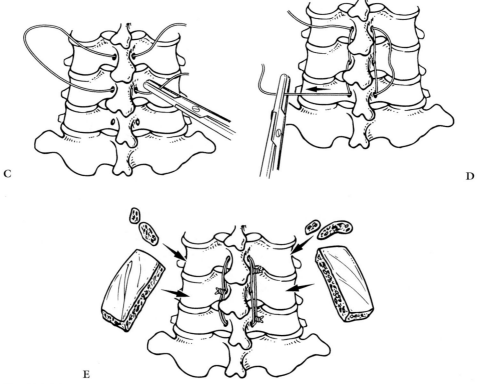

Fig. 100-18, cont'd

C, Wires passed between adjacent spinous processes. **D,** Secondary wires passed to "lock" whole construct together. **E,** Corticocancellous grafts positioned. Alternatively, holes can be created in grafts and secondary wire used to secure grafts on either side of spinous process, adding to strength of fusion. *(Redrawn from Rothman RH, Simeone FA: The spine, Philadelphia, 1982, W.B. Saunders, 1:135.)*

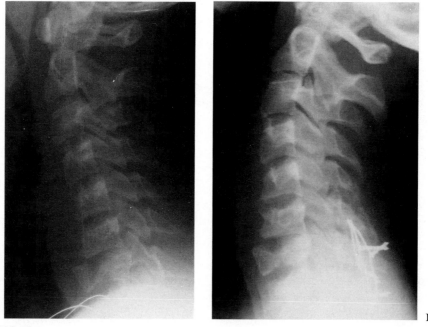

Fig. 100-19

A, C7 burst fracture in a neurologically intact patient. **B,** Lateral roentgenogram shows modified triplewiring technique.

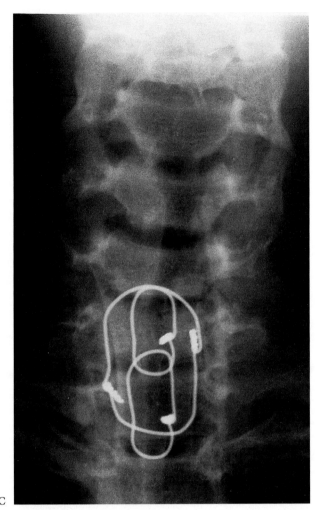

Fig. 100-19, cont'd

C, Anteroposterior roentgenogram shows addition of wire through base of superior spinous process to complement triple-wiring technique. (Reprinted with permission from Cotler JM, Cotler HB, editors: Spinal fusion, New York, 1990, Springer Verlag, p 207.)

The Dewar[11,12,18,71] procedure is another posterior wiring technique utilizing horizontal K-wires through the transverse processes wired together over bone blocks.

Posterior Plate Fixation Technique Internal fixation is often necessary for support of the unstable spine while healing is taking place. Rigid immobilization cannot be obtained with external immobilization. Internal fixation allows for immobilization of fewer levels and greater ease of nursing care and rehabilitation because of the immediate postoperative stability.

Posterior plate fixation is used most often in unstable cervical spine injuries with mainly posterior injury, including dislocation and fractures, or fracture-dislocations of the lateral masses. Plate fixation gives

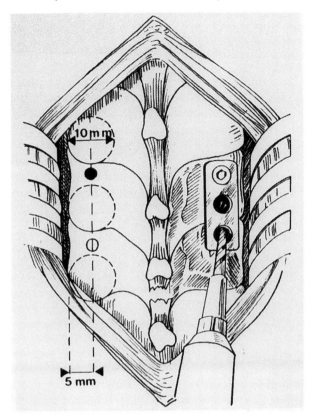

Fig. 100-20

The points of screw penetration are identified as follows: The projection of the articular surfaces on the vertebral arches is first identified by inscribing a 1-cm diameter circle beginning at the posteroinferior angle of the vertebral arches. The point of screw penetration lies halfway between two adjacent articular projections and 5 mm medial to the lateral margin of the articular pillars. (Reprinted with permission from Louis R: Posterior vertebral bone plates, Paris, 1982, Ceprime.)

increased stability over posterior spinous process wiring, especially in flexion stress. Studies show that in flexion stress, posterior wiring alone provides a 33% increase in stability. When the same wiring is done over a bone graft, there is a 55% increase, and an 88% increase when the wires pass through the articular masses. Fixation with a plate provides a 92% increase in stability.[77]

Various posterior plating techniques for the upper cervical spine and occiput are described.[51,55] Indications include tumors, congenital malformations, rheumatoid disease, and conditions causing cord compression.

Several plating systems and variations in technique are available for use in the lower cervical spine.[2,35,70]

Posterior Plating Technique The standard posterior approach is used and the spine is widely exposed. The entry points for the drill holes need to be selected (Fig. 100-20). Roy-Camille and associates[69] liken the posterior cervical spine to a hilly landscape. The valley is the area between the lamina and the facets, and the articular mass represents the hill. The vertebral artery is under the valley and the plates are placed on top of the hill, or the apex of the articular facets. Drilling is done with a measured drill bit with image intensification. The screws are drilled into the articular masses beginning at the apex and aiming from 0 to 10 degrees laterally to avoid the vertebral artery. Plates are bent into lordosis. Data suggest that spontaneous fusion of the bridged facets occurs without the need for bone graft, although we recommend bone grafting. The wound is closed routinely. A cervical collar is worn for 4 to 6 weeks.

A hook plate system designed by Magerl and colleagues[55] uses screw fixation of interlaminar hook plates (Fig. 100-21). These are used primarily in ligamentous injuries of the spine and provide a very biomechanically stable construct. The interlaminar or Halifax clamp provides a similar construct.[45]

Anterior Cervical Fusion

Robinson Technique[64-66] The patient is positioned supine in a Mayfield headrest after administration of general endotracheal anesthesia. If spinal instability is significant, Gardner-Wells tongs or halter traction at 4 kg initially may be used. The head is rotated slightly away from the side of the approach. The left side is usually chosen owing to the variability of the recurrent laryngeal nerve on the right.[74] Right-handed surgeons often prefer to approach from the right side because of decreased technical difficulty. SSEP for dorsal column and/or a wake-up test for anterior motor column monitoring is advocated.[52,80]

A transverse skin incision along Langer's lines improves cosmesis for one- or two-level fusions. An oblique incision along the anterior border of the sternocleidomastoid increases exposure when fusing multiple levels. A skin mark is made and subcutaneous tissue infiltration with epinephrine solution 1:500,000 is used for local hemostasis. The incision is completed through skin and subcutaneous tissues. The thin platysma muscle is defined and incised either along the anterior border of the sternocleidomastoid or in line with the muscle fibers. The carotid artery pulse is palpated within the carotid sheath. Fingers are used to bluntly dissect medial to the carotid sheath through the pretrachial fascia. The superior and inferior thyroid arteries may limit the exposure at this point. The superior thyroid artery may be ligated to increase exposure.

The recurrent laryngeal nerve is at risk during this exposure. It descends within the carotid sheath,

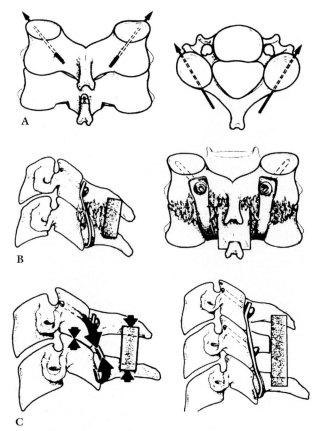

Fig. 100-21

A, Direction of the screws. The notches for the hooks in the lower lamina and for the H graft in the lower spinal process are shown. **B,** Hook plate fixation. The screws lie parallel to the articular surfaces. The plates are twisted to adapt to the bone surface. An H graft is placed between the spinal processes. Cancellous chips are applied. **C** (left), Biomechanics of the hook-plate fixation. Since the resulting force vector created by the plates lies within this triangle, the fusion is stable in all directions. **C** (right), Hook-plate fixation over two intervertebral segments (cancellous chips are not shown). *(Reprinted with permission from Kehr R, Weidner A, editors: Cervical spine, New York, 1987, Springer Verlag, 1:322.)*

loops around the arch of the aorta on the left side, and ascends between the trachea and esophagus to innervate the vocal cords. On the right side it loops around the subclavian artery before ascending. However, it can have different take-off points on the right side and its position is more variable, and thus there may be an increased risk of injury during the exposure. Excessive traction or improper placement of retractors can injure the recurrent laryngeal nerve and lead to postoperative hoarseness that can persist for several months.

After penetrating the pretracheal fascia, blunt dissection is directed medially underneath the esophagus. The anterior surface of the spine can be palpated and can be visualized with further retraction

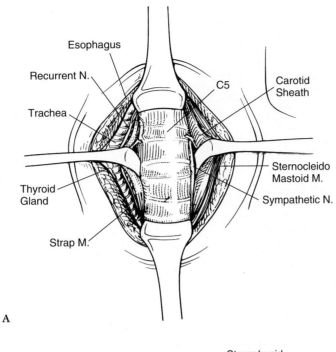

A

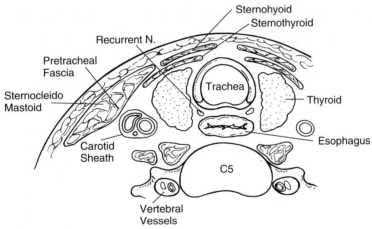

B

Fig. 100-22

Anterior approach to mid and lower cervical vertebrae, deep dissection. *(Redrawn with permission from South-wick, WO, Robinson RA: Surgical approaches to the vertebral bodies in the cervical and lumbar regions, J Bone Joint Surg 39A:634, 1957.)*

of the trachea and esophagus. The prevertebral fascia is well vascularized. Electrocautery or bipolar cautery should be used to incise the fascia and the anterior longitudinal ligament in the midline. The soft tissues can be elevated subperiosteally with an elevator. The longus colli and/or splenius capitus muscle attachments laterally are detached to expose the entire anterior surface of the vertebral bodies and discs. Care is taken not to injure the sympathetic chain, which runs anterior to the longus colli muscles. Be sure to place the retractor under fascia to avoid injury to the esophagus, sympathetic chain, or recurrent laryngeal nerve (Fig. 100-22). A needle,

with two 90-degree bends to prevent dural laceration from inadvertent advancement of the tip into the spinal canal, is inserted. A lateral radiograph is obtained to confirm the proper level (Fig. 100-23). The needle is placed as cephalad as possible to prevent obscuring of the needle by the shoulders.

During the procedure, the superficial temporal artery pulse is monitored to detect excessive retraction of the internal carotid artery. After the correct level has been determined, the annulus is incised and the disc is removed using pituitary rongeurs and curettes. The posterior longitudinal ligament is exposed but left intact if possible to protect the spinal

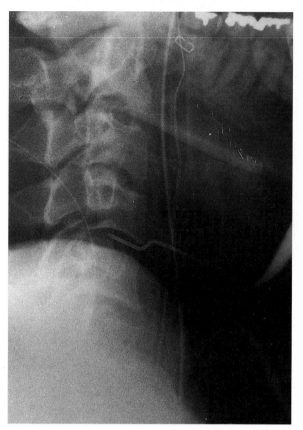

Fig. 100-23

Note 18-gauge spinal needle with two successive 90° bends used as intraoperative marker in the C3-C4 interspace. See text for additional discussion. *(Reprinted with permission from Cotler JM, Cotler HB, editors: Spinal fusion, New York, 1990, Springer Verlag, p 207.)*

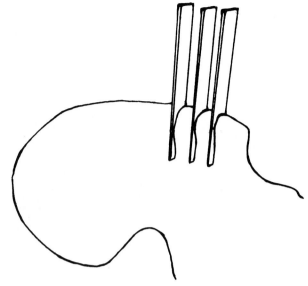

Fig. 100-24

Horseshoe-shaped corticocancellous bone graft is obtained from iliac crest using oscillating osteotomes positioned parallel to each other. Alternatively, an oscillating power saw may be used to harvest bone graft. Use of saw may create fewer "microfractures" in the graft. *(Reproduced with permission from White AA, Rothman RH, Ray CD, editors: Lumbar spine surgery: techniques and complications, St. Louis, 1987, Mosby, p 437.)*

cord. Loose fragments of disc material superiorly and inferiorly are identified and removed as indicated by preoperative studies. It is controversial whether or not the posterior osteophytes need to be removed, but this can be accomplished at this time if necessary.

A tricortical horseshoe-shaped graft approximately 1 cm in depth and 5 to 6 mm in width is harvested from the anterior iliac crest for each level to be fused (Fig. 100-24). The depth of the disc space is measured and the graft sized accordingly. The end plates are decorticated with a curette or a high-speed burr and a transverse groove is created in the superior and inferior end plates to help lock the graft into place after insertion. If the patient is in cervical traction, up to 15 kg of weight can be used to distract the interspaces for insertion of the graft. Alternatively, a Caspar[13] distractor can be used to obtain more localized distraction. The graft is tamped into place. The original Robinson technique places the cancellous side of the graft posteriorly (Fig. 100-25). Later modifications of the technique

place the cortical end posteriorly for increased strength and to prevent collapse (Fig. 100-26). The bone graft is recessed 1 to 2 mm to lock the graft into place. Care should be taken not to allow the graft to exert pressure on the anterior dural sac.

The cervical traction is discontinued or the Caspar retractor is removed. An anterior cervical plate can be used to ensure stability and prevent anterior extrusion of the bone graft if there is any doubt as to the stability of the construct or the postoperative compliance of the patient.

An intraoperative radiograph is obtained to check the depth of bone graft and alignment of the spine. The platysma is reapproximated with absorbable suture to help ensure a cosmetic result. The skin is closed with a subcuticular suture for cosmesis. A drain may be used if there is excessive bleeding from the bony bed during closure, and is removed in 24 to 48 hours. Postoperatively, a hard collar is worn for 6 to 8 weeks for a one-level, 8 to 10 weeks for a two-level, and 12 weeks for a three-level fusion. The collar is removed when there is radiographic evidence of trabecular bone formation across the fused segments.

Vertebral Body Reconstruction Technique[6] Anterior cervical procedures without instrumentation are contraindicated in the presence of simultaneous anterior and posterior instability. Anterior dissection

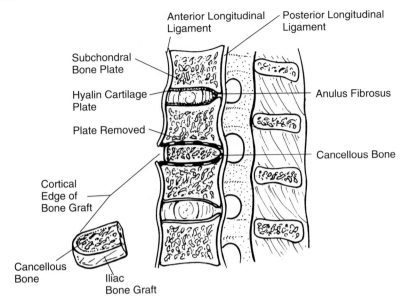

Fig. 100-25

Technique of Robinson and colleagues for anterior fusion of the cervical spine (see text). *(Reproduced with permission (modified) from Robinson RA and others: The results of anterior interbody fusion of the cervical spine, J Bone Joint Surg 44A:1569, 1962.)*

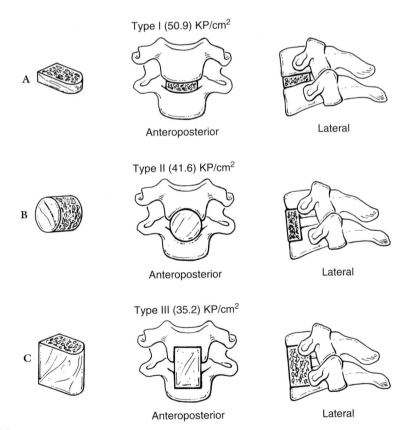

Fig. 100-26

Stability of several types of anterior cervical fusions to axial load. **A,** Smith-Robinson fusion. **B,** Cloward fusion. **C,** Bailey–Badgley fusion. *(Reproduced with permission from White AA III and others: Clin Orthop 91:22, 1973.)*

would further destabilize the spine and render the constructs unstable. Vertebral body reconstruction is necessary in cases with additional posterior instability. This approach is also indicated for surgical decompression of the anterior spinal cord, especially after extensive anterior debridement.

The patient is prepared and the spine is approached as for an anterior cervical fusion, as previously described. After the proper level is confirmed with a radiograph, the cephalad and caudad intervertebral discs are removed in toto. A #15-blade scalpel is used to incise the anulus, and the disc is removed with curettes and rongeurs or pituitary forceps. If the intervening vertebral body is fractured or retropulsed posteriorly into the canal, then the vertebral body is removed completely in its midportion using a Leksell or pituitary rongeur or pituitary forceps (Fig. 100-27). The posterior longitudinal ligament is left intact if possible to protect the spinal cord. The end plates superiorly and inferiorly are denuded of cartilage using a high-speed burr or curette. Holes are made in the superior and inferior end plates to accept the graft. The anterior vertebral borders are left intact to prevent expulsion of the graft. The space between the superior and inferior vertebrae is spanned with a T-shaped tricortical iliac crest bone graft. A fibular graft may be used instead to provide increased structural support. However, one disadvantage of using fibula is that it takes longer to incorporate. The bone graft should not be allowed to exert pressure posteriorly on the anterior dural sac. A modification of this technique involves creating channels in the cephalad and caudad vertebrae and inserting the bone graft with the three-sided cortical portion of the graft facing posteriorly (Fig. 100-28). Additional traction or a cervical distractor may be used to insert the bone graft in order to invaginate both ends. The traction may then be released to provide compression and lock the graft into place. A drain is placed and the wound is closed in layers.

An anterior vertebrectomy destabilizes the spine. If the posterior structures are intact or surgically stabilized, then a SOMI may be used postoperatively; otherwise, a halo is worn for 10 to 12 weeks.

In cases where there is instability after corpectomy and bone graft, cervical spine stability can be enhanced by using an anterior plate. In degenerative spines, areas of spondylosis at the ends of the vertebral end plates may need to be pared down to allow the plates to lay flush against the anterior vertebral bodies. A screw can be used to fix the bone graft to the plate. Traction should be removed before application of the plates and screws.

Anterior Plate Fixation Technique Most plates for anterior arthrodesis have two rows of screw holes for rotational stability. This provides more secure fixation and a decreased incidence of loosening. Even though biomechanical studies show that posterior fusions are more stable than anterior fusions,[77,79] clinical evaluation has demonstrated that anterior fusion with plate fixation produces satisfactory results.[4,13,15,34,43] The most rigid stabilization is provided by combining the two (Fig. 100-29).

The patient is positioned and the spine is approached as for an anterior cervical fusion. After addressing the pathology and placement of the bone graft, any traction used during the procedure is released. This allows for compression of the graft and proper sizing of the plate. The plate selected should not extend beyond the vertebral bodies to be fused.

The plate is positioned on the anterior surface of the spine in the midline. The longus colli muscles or the uncinate processes on either side both above and below the fusion site can help determine the exact midline when the vertebral bodies are no longer present.

Next, screw holes are drilled either with a stop drill or with the aid of an image intensifier to prevent penetration into the spinal canal and cord injury. The screws are then inserted with the plate seated flat against the bone to prevent motion between the plate and vertebra. The screws must penetrate the posterior cortex to ensure solid anchorage and prevent anterior screw migration. Specially designed plates and screws by Morscher (Synthes, Paoli, PA) can be used that obviate the need for posterior cortical purchase. After final tightening of the screws, the construct is checked in the AP and lateral planes radiographically (Fig. 100-30). The wound is copiously irrigated and closed in routine fashion.

Postoperatively, a hard cervical collar may be worn for 4 to 12 weeks depending on the number of levels fused and the stability of the construct.

Complications

Operating on the wrong level is one of the most common errors of spinal surgery. During the procedure an intraoperative radiograph helps confirm the correct level.

A retropharyngeal hematoma may develop, which may cause dysphagia. Meticulous hemostasis should be obtained prior to closure. If there is any doubt, or if excess bleeding from exposed raw cancellous bony surfaces is present, a drain should be placed. The drain is removed in 24 to 48 hours.

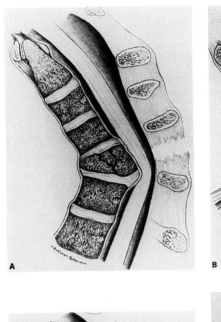
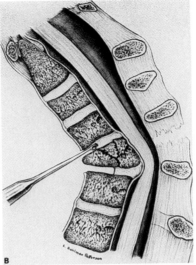
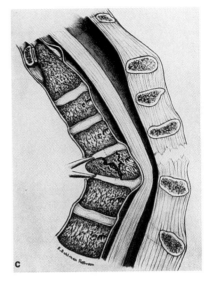

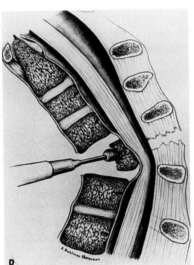
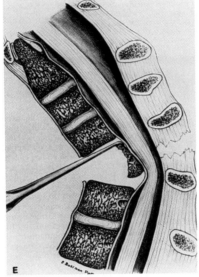
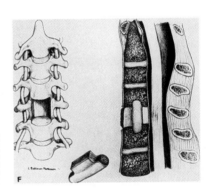

Fig. 100-27

A, Artist's drawing of a lateral view of a compression fracture of the C5 vertebra, showing typical compression fracture with protrusion of disc material and bone fragment and a kyphotic deformity causing compression of the anterior aspect of the spinal cord. **B,** Lateral view of the cervical spine showing initial removal of disc material on either side of the crushed vertebral body, which is used as a guide to identify the extent of the crushed bone superiorly and inferiorly, as well as posteriorly. **C,** Following initial disc removal on either side of the crushed vertebral body, hand ronguers were used to remove the first portion of the crushed vertebral body. **D,** The portion of the remaining crushed vertebral body is then removed with a power burr. All of the disc is removed back to the posterior longitudinal ligament to identify the extent of bony protrusion. **E,** The remaining posterior vertebral cortex is removed using a curette to peel the bone from the longitudinal ligament. **F** (left), Anterior view of the cervical spine showing the extent of vertebral body resection to the posterior longitudinal ligament, sparing the lateral cortices to protect the vertebral arteries. The posterior longitudinal ligament is not violated and no instruments enter the spinal canal. **F** (right), A full-thickness iliac crest graft is inserted to replace the resected vertebra. The cortical surface of the crest is placed posteriorly. This procedure corrects the kyphotic deformity and relieves the spinal cord compression. *(Reprinted with permission from Bohlman HH. J. Bone Joint Surg 61A:1119, 1979 (A and F); Rothman RH, Simeone FA: The Spine, Philadelphia, 1982, W.B. Saunders, 1:661 (B and C); and Bohlman HH, Eismont FJ: Clin Orthop 154:57, 1981 (D and E).)*

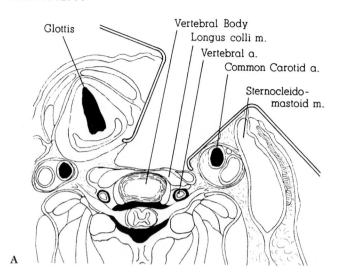

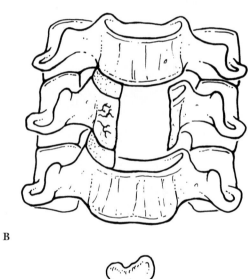

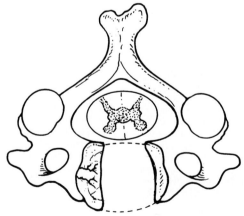

Fig. 100-28

Anterior cervical vertebral body reconstruction and fusion. **A,** Anterolateral approach is made. **B,** Anteroposterior and axial views of decompression.

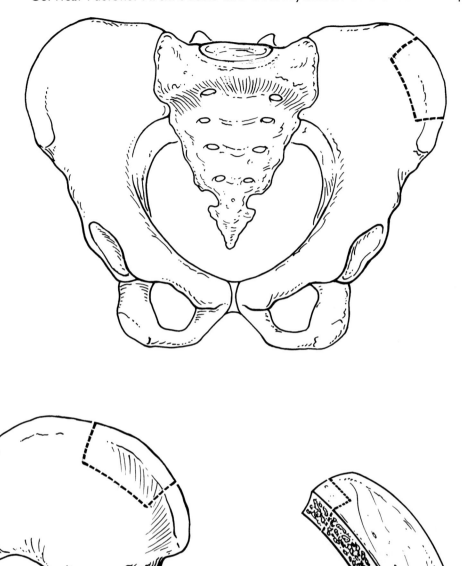

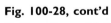

Fig. 100-28, cont'd

C, Harvesting and fashioning of tricortical graft.

Continued.

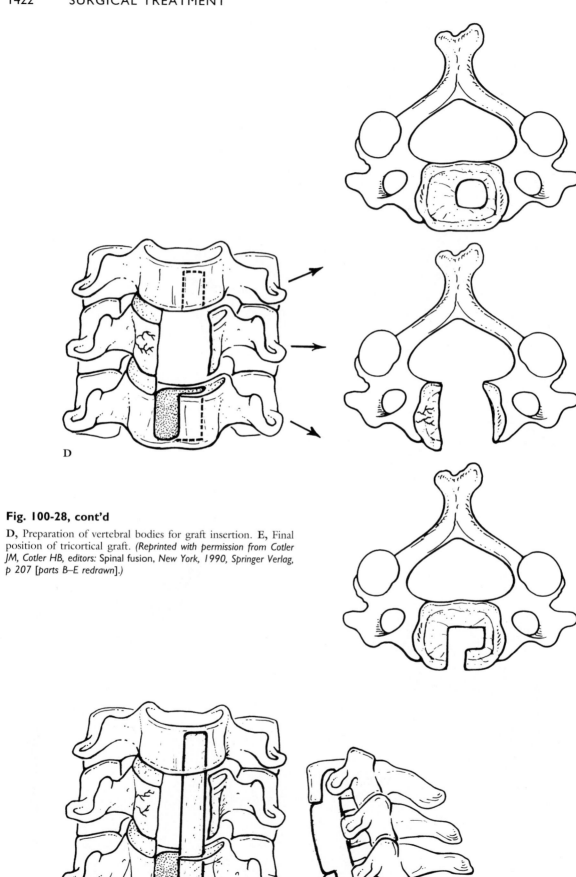

Fig. 100-28, cont'd

D, Preparation of vertebral bodies for graft insertion. **E,** Final position of tricortical graft. *(Reprinted with permission from Cotler JM, Cotler HB, editors: Spinal fusion, New York, 1990, Springer Verlag, p 207 [parts B–E redrawn].)*

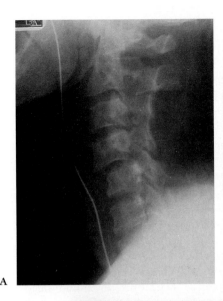

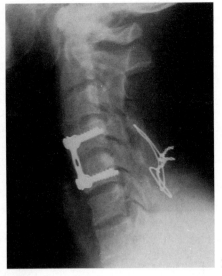

A

B

Fig. 100-29

A, C4-C5 unilateral facet dislocation in patient with incomplete quadriplegia. MRI demonstrated herniated disc. **B,** Anterior discectomy. Smith-Robinson fusion and stabilization followed by posterior open reduction and fusion using triple-wire technique. *(Reprinted with permission from Cotler JM, Cotler HB, editors: Spinal fusion, New York, 1990, Springer Verlag, p 207.)*

Fig. 100-30

A, C5 compressive flexion injury. **B,** Metrizamide-enhanced CT scan shows bilateral lamina fractures. **C,** MRI scan demonstrates anterior spinal-cord compression. **D** and **E,** Anteroposterior and lateral postoperative roentgenograms after C5 corpectomy, bone grafting, and stabilization with A-O plate. *(Reprinted with permission from Cotler JM, Cotler HB, editors: Spinal fusion, New York, 1990, Springer Verlag, p 207.)*

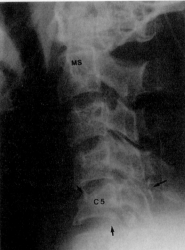

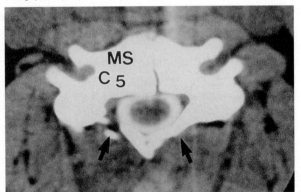

A

B

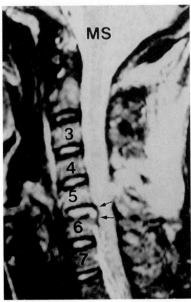

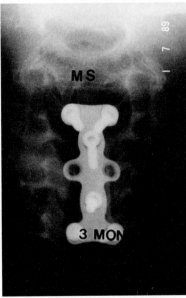

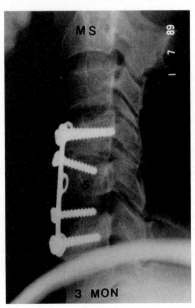

C

D

E

Anterior extrusion of the graft can occur and is more common in patients with posterior instability. If more than 50% of the graft is extruded or dysphagia is present, the patient should be taken back to the operating room for revision of the graft. Addition of anterior cervical plates will prevent extrusion of the graft.

Collapse of the vertebral body has been reported more often after the dowel technique. The construct may have to be revised if there is a significant angulation or a recurrence of symptoms.

Nonunion occurs infrequently in single-level anterior cervical fusions. As the number of levels fused increases, so does the nonunion rate. This occurs most often with three-level fusions. Successful treatment often requires the addition of a posterior fusion.

Neurologic injury to the spinal cord or nerve roots is a risk, especially when these structures are already compromised from acute trauma or chronic pressure from various causes.[28,29] The physiologic reserve to resist injury may already be depleted and a minor insult, such as from a surgical instrument, may cause or increase further damage. Quadriplegia has been reported following excision of a single-level lateral disc herniation.[31]

Degeneration of levels above and below the fused segments is more common after anterior surgery. Extension of the fusion mass beyond the intended levels of fusion is more often seen in the posterior approach.

Perforation of the pharynx, trachea, and esophagus can be avoided by placing retractor blades under the longus colli muscles and avoiding sharp blades. Some surgeons believe that using properly placed sharp retractor blades will prevent dislodgement of the retractor and possible traction injury to the surrounding structures. Temporary hoarseness and dysphagia is common following retraction against an in situ endotracheal tube. This is usually secondary to the resulting edema. More severe swelling may lead to tracheal obstruction.

Injury to the recurrent laryngeal or vagus nerve can result in vocal cord paresis and resultant hoarseness. This is usually a temporary condition. One study of 85 patients found an 11% incidence of voice changes, with three cases of permanent paralysis of the vocal cords.[42] The nerve is less prone to injury on the left side of the neck owing to its longer course and more protected position in the tracheoesophageal groove. Injury can be minimized by familiarity with the anatomy and approaches and use of meticulous technique, as well as being careful with retraction of the carotid sheath.

Injury to the cervical sympathetic chain can result in a Horners syndrome. Dissecting or placing retractors lateral to the longus colli muscles may injure the sympathetic chain.

Vascular injuries most commonly involve tears of the vertebral artery. The bleeding is difficult to control and usually necessitates exposure and direct visualization of the artery. The artery may be ligated if repair is not possible, but this may lead to symptoms if collateral circulation is not adequate. Much rarer are injuries to the carotid artery or jugular vein, which can bleed profusely or result in thrombosis of the vessel with resultant cerebral ischemia.

Dural tears can result in cerebrospinal fluid leakage and postoperative symptoms, including headaches. If leakage persists, complications such as pseudomeningoceles or draining fistulas may develop. This can lead to an increased risk of infection and meningitis. Intraoperative tears of the dura should be repaired with a water-tight closure using a fine nonabsorbable suture. The repair should be checked for leakage with a Valsalva maneuver.

Direct trauma to the spinal cord or nerve roots can occur, as well as indirect trauma such as injury to the anterior spinal artery. This arterial system has very little collateral circulation,[50] and disruption of flow can produce ischemic injury to the anterior cord.

Hematomas can cause pressure to the trachea, esophagus, and local neurovascular structures. This can usually be prevented by blunt dissection through avascular planes during the approach, meticulous hemostasis, and the use of a drain when necessary. Wound infections are uncommon and occur in about 1% of procedures.

Difficulties with instrumentation, including pull out of screws has been reported.

The risk of spinal cord injury after anterior cervical discectomy has been estimated as being less than 0.2%.[76] In a questionnaire study involving 528 replies representing 134,246 cases of anterior cervical discectomy and fusion, a 1.26% incidence of neurologic complications was noted.[28,29]

A 10-year review of the Robinson anterior fusion technique reported a 5% nonunion rate for single-level procedures, and a 15% rate for multiple level procedures.[6] A 13% incidence of graft displacement and 4.9% incidence of avascular necrosis of the vertebral body has been reported.[38]

Results of Arthrodesis without Instrumentation

Etter and associates[22] report their technique and results of 23 patients who underwent direct fixation of dens fractures with a cannulated screw system. A 92.3% union rate was obtained at an average of 5.5 months. However, there was a 17% major complication rate. Montesano and associates[60] reported union in 11 of 13 patients with no neurologic complications for type II odontoid fractures. Other authors[5,31,61] have used the technique with good results.

Cahill and associates[9] reported a stable fusion and excellent alignment in 18 patients who underwent dynamic studies at 3 to 4 months. Edwards and colleagues[20] reported on 27 patients in whom the oblique wire construct limited late deformity to an average of 0.2 mm translation and 1 degree of angulation. At 13 weeks all patients had solid fusion documented by dynamic studies.

Anderson and associates[2] in Seattle evaluated the efficacy of posterior arthrodesis of the cervical spine with AO reconstruction plates and autogenous bone graft in a prospective study. All 30 patients with unstable spines had solid fusions based on flexion and extension views at an average follow-up of 18 months. There were no neurologic or vascular complications, and all incomplete spinal cord injuries improved at least one Frankel grade level.

Ripa and colleagues[63] report on 92 patients who underwent a single anterior procedure involving appropriate anterior decompression, tricortical inlay bone grafting, and application of anteriorly applied cervical plates for treatment of acute lower cervical trauma. A 98.9% fusion rate at an average of 3.2 months postoperatively was obtained. There was a 2% incidence of complications directly related to the anterior hardware.

Bertalanfy and Eggert analyzed the complications of anterior discectomy without fusion of 450 consecutive patients treated surgically for degenerative disc disease. The most common complication was worsening of the preexisting myelopathy, occurring in 3.3% of patients. Wound infection developed in 1.6%. Additional radicular symptoms, recurrent nerve palsy, Horner's syndrome, respiratory insufficiency, epidural hematoma, and spinal instability each occurred in approximately 1% of patients. They report one case each (0.2% incidence) of a pharyngeal lesion, meningitis secondary to dural perforation, and epidural abscess, and two cases (0.4%) of nerve-root lesions. The overall complication rate has since been reduced owing to increased awareness and improved patient selection.

Summary

Arthrodesis of the cervical spine is a tried and true procedure that may benefit many patients, yet techniques continue to evolve. The surgeon must learn not to become too enamoured with glitzy new instrumentation and lose sight of the principle objective.

References

1. Allgower M, Perren SM, Matter P: A new plate for internal fixation—the dynamic compression plate (DCP), *Injury* 2(1): 1970.
2. Anderson PA and others: Posterior cervical arthrodesis with AO reconstruction plates and bone graft, *Spine* 16(3S):S72, 1991.
3. Barcena A and others: Spinal metastatic disease: analysis of factors determining functional prognosis and the choice of treatment, *Neurosurgery* 15:820, 1984.
4. Bohler J: Anterior fixation for acute fractures and non-unions of the dens, *J Bone Joint Surg* 64A:18, 1982.
5. Bohler J: Anterior stabilization of acute fractures and nonunions of the dens, *J Bone Joint Surg* 18, Jan. 1982.
6. Bohlman H: *Cervical spine and cord: trauma*. In *Operative techniques in orthopaedic knowledge update 2: home study syllabus*, Park Ridge, IL, 1987, American Academy of Orthopaedic Surgeons, p 275.
7. Bradford DS, Thompson RC: Fractures and dislocations of the spine: indications for surgical intervention, *Minn Med* 7:711, 1976.
8. Brooks AL, Jenkins EB: Atlantoaxial arthrodesis by the wedge compression method, *J Bone Joint Surg* 60A:279, 1978.
9. Cahill DW, Bellegarrigue R, Ducker TB: Bilateral facet to spinous process fusion: a new technique for posterior spinal fusion after trauma, *Neurosurgery* 13(1):1, 1983.
10. Callahan RA: Cervical facet fusion for control of instability following laminectomy, *J Bone Joint Surg* 59A:991, 1977.
11. Capicotto WN, Simmons EH, Graziano G: The Dewar fusion in traumatic injuries to the cervical spine, *Orthop Trans* 13:206, 1989.
12. Carl AL, Thomas S: *Posterior tension band wiring for unstable cervical spine injuries*, AAOS 58th Annual Meeting, Anaheim, CA, 1991.
13. Caspar W: *Anterior stabilization with the trapezial osteosynthetic plate technique in cervical spine injuries*. In Kehr P, Weidner A, editors: *Cervical spine I*, Wein–New York, 1987, Springer Verlag, p 198.
14. Clark CR, Keggi KJ, Panjabi MM: Methylmethacrylate stabilization of the cervical spine, *J Bone Joint Surg* 66A:40, 1984.

15. Correia Martins MA: *Anterior cervical fusion—indications and results.* In Kehr P, Weidner A, editors: *Cervical spine I,* Wein–New York, 1987, Springer Verlag, p 205.

16. Cotler HB and others: Closed reduction of cervical spine dislocations, *Clin Orthop Rel Res* 214:185, 1987.

17. Crockard HA: The Vui approach to the base of the brain and upper cervical cord, *Ann R Coll Surg* 67:321, 1985.

18. Davey JR and others: A technique of posterior cervical fusion for instability of the cervical spine, *Spine* 10(8):722, 1985.

19. DePalma A and others: Anterior interbody fusion for severe cervical disc degeneration, *Surg Gynecol Obstet* 134:755, 1972.

20. Edwards CC, Matz SO, Levine AM: The oblique wiring technique for rotational injuries of the cervical spine, *Orthop Trans* 10(3):455, 1986.

21. Edwards CC and others: *New techniques in spine stabilization,* Warsaw, IN, 1982, Zimmer.

22. Etter P and others: Direct anterior fixation of dens fractures with a cannulated screw system, *Spine* 16(3S):S25, 1991.

23. Fager CA: Failed neck syndrome: an ounce of prevention, *Clin Neurol* 27:450, 1980.

24. Fang HSY, Ong GB: Direct anterior approach to the upper cervical spine, *J Bone Joint Surg* 44A:1588, 1962.

25. Feilding JW, Hawkins RJ, Ratzan SA: Spine fusion for atlantoaxial instability, *J Bone Joint Surg* 58A:400, 1976.

26. Feilding JW and others: Tears of the transverse ligament of the atlas, *J Bone Joint Surg* 56A:1683, 1974.

27. Fidler MW: Pathologic fractures of the cervical spine: palliative surgical treatment, *J Bone Joint Surg* 67B:352, 1985.

28. Flynn TB: Neurological complications of anterior cervical discectomy in Louisiana, *J Louisiana St Med Soc* 136(7):6, 1984.

29. Flynn TB: Neurological complications of anterior cervical interbody fusion, *Spine* 7:536, 1982.

30. Frankel HL and others: The value of postural reduction in the initial management of closed injuries of the spine with paraplegia and tetraplegia, part I, *Paraplegia* 7:179, 1969.

31. Fujii E, Kobayashi K, Hirabayashi K: Treatment of fractures of the odontoid process, *Spine* 13:604, 1988.

32. Gallie WE: Fractures and dislocations of the cervical spine, *Am J Surg* 46:495, 1939.

33. Garfin SR, Moore MR, Marshall LF: A modified technique for cervical facet fusions, *Clin Orthop Rel Res* 230:149, 1988.

34. Gassman J, Seligson D: The anterior cervical plate, *Spine* 8:700, 1983.

35. Gill K and others: Posterior plating of the cervical spine: a biomechanical comparison of different fusion techniques, *Spine* 13(7):813, 1988.

36. Gore DR, Sepic SB: Anterior cervical fusion for degenerated or protruded discs: a review of one hundred forty-six patients, *Spine* 9:667, 1984.

37. Graham JJ: *Complications of cervical spine surgery.* In The Cervical Spine Research Society Editorial Committee, editors: *The cervical spine,* ed 2, Philadelphia, 1989, J.B. Lippincott.

38. Gregory CF: Complications of anterior cervical fusion, *J Bone Joint Surg* 46B:715, 1964.

39. Griswold PW and others: Atlantoaxial fusion for instability, *J Bone Joint Surg* 60A:285, 1978.

40. Harms XX: Personal communication.

41. Harrington KD: Current concepts review: metastatic disease of the spine, *J Bone Joint Surg* 68A:1110, 1986.

42. Heeneman H: Vocal cord paralysis following approaches to anterior cervical spine, *Laryngoscope* 83:17, 1973.

43. Herrman HD: Metal plate fixation after anterior fusion of unstable fracture dislocations of the cervical spine, *Acta Neurochir* 32:101, 1975.

44. Hodgson MB, Wong SK: A description of a technique and evaluation of results in anterior spinal fusion for deranged intervertebral disc and spondylolisthesis. *Clin Orthop Rel Res* 56:133, 1968.

45. Holness RO and others: Posterior stabilization with an interlaminar clamp in cervical injuries, *Neurosurgery* 14(3):318, 1984.

46. Jeanneret B and others: Posterior stabilization of the spine with hook plates, *Spine* 16(3S):S56, 1991.

47. Johnson RM and others: Immediate strength of certain cervical fusion techniques, *Orthop Trans* 4:42, 1980.

48. Jones AM, Rothman RH, Balderston RA: *Fusion techniques for degenerative disease.* In Cotler JM, Cotler HC, editors: *Spinal fusion: science and technique,* New York, 1990, Springer Verlag, p 189.

49. Knoringer P: *Double threaded compression screws in osteosynthesis of acute fractures of the odontoid process.* In Voth D, Glees O, editors: *Disease in the craniocervical junction,* Berlin–New York, 1987, de Gruyter, p 217.

50. Krauss DR, Stauffer ES: Spinal cord injury as a complication of elective anterior cervical fusion, *Clin Orthop Rel Res* 112, 1975.

51. Louis R: *Posterior vertebral bone plates,* Paris, 1982, Ceprime.

52. Lueders H and others: A new technique for intraoperative monitoring of spinal cord function: multichannel recording of spinal cord and subcortical evoked potentials, *Spine* 7:110, 1982.

53. Lunsford LD, Bissonette DJ, Zorub DS: Anterior surgery for cervical disc disease. Part 2: Treatment of cervical spondylotic myelopathy in 32 cases, *J Neurosurg* 53(1):1-11, July, 1980.

54. Lunsford LD and others: Anterior surgery for cervical disc disease. Part 1: Treatment of lateral cervical disc herniation in 253 cases, *J Neurosurg* 53:1, 1980.

55. Magerl F, Grob D, Seemann P: *Stable dorsal fusion of the cervical spine (C2-Th1) using book plates.* In Kehr P, Weidner A, editors: *Cervical spine,* Wein–New York, 1987, Springer Verlag, 1.

56. Magerl F, Seemann P: *Stable posterior fusion of the atlas and axis by transarticular screw fixation.* In Kehr P, Weidner A, editors: *Cervical spine,* Wein–New York, 1987, Springer Verlag, 1:322.

57. McAfee PC and others: The value of computed tomography in thoracolumbar fractures: an analysis of 100 consecutive fractures and a new classification, *J Bone Joint Surg* 65A:461, 1983.

58. Meyer PR Jr, editor: *Surgery of spine trauma,* New York, 1988, Churchill Livingstone.

59. Meyer PR, Cotler HB: *Fusion techniques for traumatic injuries.* In Cotler JM, Cotler HC, editors: *Spinal fusion: science and technique,* New York, 1990, Springer Verlag, p 189.

60. Montesano PX and others: Odontoid fractures treated by anterior odontoid screw fixation, *Spine* 16(3S):S33, 1991.

61. Nakanishi and others: *Orthop Trans* 6:176, 1982.

62. Rahn BA and others: Primary bone healing: an experimental study in the rabbit, *J Bone Joint Surg* 53A:783, 1971.

63. Ripa DR and others: Series of ninety-two traumatic cervical spine injuries stabilized with anterior ASIF plate fusion technique, *Spine* 16(3S):S46, 1991.

64. Robinson RA, Southwick WO: Indications and techniques for early stabilization of the neck in some fracture dislocations of the cervical spine, *South Med J* 53:565, 1960.

65. Robinson RA, Southwick WO: *Surgical approaches to the cervical spine.* In *AAOS: Instructional Course Lectures, vol XVII,* St. Louis, 1960, Mosby.

66. Robinson RA and others: The results of anterior interbody fusion of the cervical spine, *J Bone Joint Surg* 44A:1569, 1962.

67. Rogers WA: Fractures and dislocations of the cervical spine and end-result study, *J Bone Joint Surg* 39A:2, 1957.

68. Rogers WA: Treatment of fracture-dislocation of the cervical spine, *J Bone Joint Surg* 24A:254, 1942.

69. Roy-Camille R, Mazel C, Saillant G: *Treatment of cervical spine injuries by a posterior osteosynthesis with plates and screws.* In Kehr P, Weidner A, editors: *Cervical spine,* Wein–New York, 1987, Springer Verlag, 1:163.

70. Roy-Camille R and others: *Early management of spinal injuries.* In McKibbon B, editor: *Recent advances in orthopaedics,* Edinburgh, 1989, Churchill Livingstone.

71. Segal D and others: Tension band fixation of acute cervical spine fractures, *Clin Orthop Rel Res* 159:211, 1981.

72. Sim FH, Frassica FJ, Klassen RA: *Fusion techniques for tumors.* In Cotler JM, Cotler HC, editors: *Spinal fusion: science and technique,* New York, 1990, Springer Verlag, p 169.

73. Smith GW, Robinson RA: The treatment of certain cervical spine disorders by the anterior removal of the intervertebral disc and interbody fusion, *J Bone Joint Surg* 40A:607, 1958.

74. Southwick WO, Robinson RA: Surgical approaches to the vertebral bodies in the cervical and lumbar regions, *J Bone Joint Surg* 39A:631, 1957.

75. Stauffer ES: Wiring techniques of the posterior cervical spine for the treatment, *Orthopedics* 11:1543, 1988.

76. Sugar O: Spinal cord malfunction after anterior cervical discectomy, *Surg neurol* 53:12, 1980.

77. Ulrich C and others: *Comparative stability of anterior or posterior cervical spine fixation: in vitro investigation.* In Kehr P, Weidner A, editors: *Cervical spine, Wein–New York,* 1987, Springer Verlag, 1:65.

78. Wertheim SB, Bohlman HH: Occipitocervical fusion, *J Bone Joint Surg* 69A:833, 1987.

79. White AA, Panjabi MM: *Clinical biomechanics of the spine,* Philadelphia, 1990, J.B. Lippincott.

80. Zeigler J and others: Posterior cervical fusion with local anesthesia: the awake patient as the ultimate spinal cord monitor, *Spine* 12:206, 1987.

Chapter 101
Anterior Instrumentation of the Cervical Spine
Patrick J. Connolly

Hansen A. Yuan

Anterior Cervical Plate Fixation

indications for anterior cervical plate fixation

surgical approach

corpectomy

plate placement

titanium locking screw plate system

other plating systems

complications

summary

Anterior Screw Fixation

indications for odontoid screw fixation

contraindications

surgical technique

complications

summary

Anterior Cervical Plate Fixation

Since its introduction by Robinson and Smith in 1955,[38] anterior cervical spine fusion has become a well-accepted procedure. Its use in single-level degenerative disease is widespread, with a predictably good result.[3,14,19,38,40] Unfortunately, its use alone in tumor resection, fracture, and kyphotic deformity has led to an unacceptable rate of progressive deformity, instability, and graft extrusion.* For this reason, patients requiring anterior decompression for fractures, tumor, or kyphotic deformity often undergo a second posterior stabilization procedure and/or postoperative halo immobilization. To eliminate the need for a second surgical procedure after anterior corpectomy, the concept of anterior cervical plate fixation following graft placement was introduced.†

In 1980, Bohler[6] was the first to describe the use of a standard plate for anterior fixation of a cervical spine fracture. Orozco[34] introduced the H plate design in 1975. Since its introduction, the anterior cervical plate has not gained universal acceptance, largely because of the potential risks of spinalcord injury during screw placement or delayed soft tissue injury secondary to screw or plate migration.

Currently, three systems are in general use for anterior cervical plating.[9,26,29] The first is the stainless steel AO Orozco plate, which uses 3.5 AO screws and requires purchase of the dorsal cortex. The second system is the Caspar trapezoidal plate system. The third system is the titanium locking screw plate system (TLSP), which uses the Orozco H plate design. All the screws are 14 mm long and have expandable screw heads that lock the screw into the plate. The TLSP screws do not require dorsal cortex purchase.

Indications for Anterior Cervical Plate Fixation

Anterior cervical plate fixation should be considered when anterior decompression is necessary following burst fracture; fracture/dislocation associated with traumatic disc herniation; correction of cervical kyphosis; tumor resection; and multilevel anterior decompression and fusion for degenerative disease and other grossly unstable conditions of the cervical spine.* Anterior cervical plate fixation may eliminate the need for a secondary posterior procedure or post-

*References 2, 7, 22, 45, 46, 48, and 52.
†References 6, 8, 11, 16, 18, 21, 28, 31, 33, 34, 35, 37, 39, 41, 46, 47, and 51.
‡References 2, 3, 7, 27, 30, 37, 44, 47, and 51.

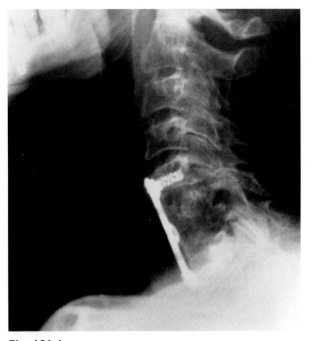

Fig. 101-1
Solid arthrodesis following two-level discectomy and fusion for degenerative disease.

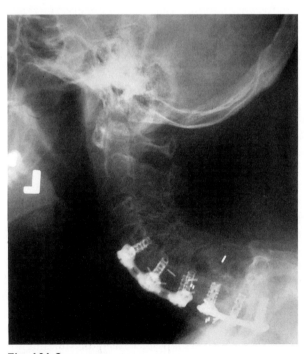

Fig. 101-2
Stable fixation following multilevel posterior laminectomy for meningioma.

operative halo immobilization. Anterior cervical plate fixation is probably not indicated for most single-level fusions performed for degenerative disk disease or disk herniation unless gross instability is present (Figs. 101-1 and 101-2).

Surgical Approach

If the spine is unstable, the patient is intubated and positioned in the supine position while awake. If skeletal traction is not used, the patient's head is secured to the operating table and the patient's shoulders are taped down to optimize the quality of intraoperative radiographs.

The surgical approach is from the left side when the required decompression is below C4. This is done to decrease the likelihood of injury to the recurrent laryngeal nerve. The sternal notch, anterior and medial borders of the thyroid cartilage, and the sternocleidomastoid (SCM) muscle are palpated. Either a transverse incision centered over the level of interest or a longitudinal incision just medial to the SCM muscle is performed. The epidermis is scored and the dermis is injected with a 1:500,000 mixture of epinephrine in saline. Sharp dissection is carried through the subcutaneous tissue and platysma, with care being taken to avoid injury to the branches of the anterior jugular vein. After meticulous hemostasis, the medial border of the SCM muscle is identified and the superficial cervical fascia is opened in a longitudinal fashion. The SCM muscle is retracted laterally. The interval between the SCM muscle and the strap muscles and sternohyoid is developed; the pulse of the carotid artery within the cervical sheath should be lateral.

The omohyoid muscle is identified as it crosses proximal–medial to distal–lateral at the C6 level, and divided. Blunt dissection is carried through the middle cervical fascia in a longitudinal fashion, with care being taken to avoid injury to the superior and inferior thyroid artery and vein. Next, the anterior cervical spine is palpated. In trauma, the deficit is often palpable. Blunt dissection is carried through the prevertebral fascia and the disc spaces above and below the level of corpectomy are identified. Once the confirmatory radiograph has been obtained, the extent of decompression and fusion are dictated by the preoperative assessment and diagnosis.

Corpectomy

The prevertebral fascia is incised in the midline at the level of decompression. The longus colli is subperiosteally dissected laterally on both sides of the midline to expose fully the vertebral body above and below the level of corpectomy. Initial attention is directed toward removing the discs above and below the level of corpectomy, using a #15 blade on a long handle. The anterior half of the disc is removed, as is subsequent disc material, using pituitary rongeurs

and small mastoid curettes. A high-speed burr is then used to remove the end plates and create a small recess for the graft in the vertebral bodies above and below the site of decompression. Following the removal of the discs above and below the level of corpectomy, a midline trough is made in the vertebral body and a rongeur is used to remove the large pieces of bone. The high-speed burr is then used again to remove bone down to the thin dorsal shell. Small Kerrison punches and angled curettes are carefully employed to remove the remaining bony shell and to complete exposure of the posterior longitudinal ligament. The end plates of the vertebral body above and below the site of decompression are now removed an appropriate site bicortical or tricortical graft is obtained and tapped into place.

Plate Placement

The anterior cervical plate is placed in the anterior midline of the cervical spine. A plate is chosen that spans the tricortical graft and allows the superior and inferior screws to secure the plate above and below the graft without penetrating the disc space. Available plating systems act as a tension band in extension and as a buttress in flexion.

Following successful application of the plate and screws, the wound is then irrigated and closed in layers over a drain. Postoperatively, the patient is immobilized in a Philadelphia collar for 6 to 12 weeks.

Titanium Locking Screw Plate System

The titanium locking screw plate system was developed primarily to prevent the migration or loosening of screws. A secondary advantage of the system is that it obviates the need to perforate the dorsal cortex to obtain excellent fixation. The plate is made of titanium. It is 2 mm thick and has a Orozco H plate design. In the initial design, the screws were made of hollow titanium plasma coated, with perforated cylinders that allowed for bony ingrowth.[36] These screws, however, have been withdrawn because of breakage secondary to fatigue, and the system now uses 14 mm solid titanium screws. The screw head is cross split just above the start of the threads and can be locked into the plate hole by means of an expansion bolt.

Surgical Technique

A plate size is selected that enables the superior and inferior screws to be placed in the upper region of the vertebral body above and below the graft site.

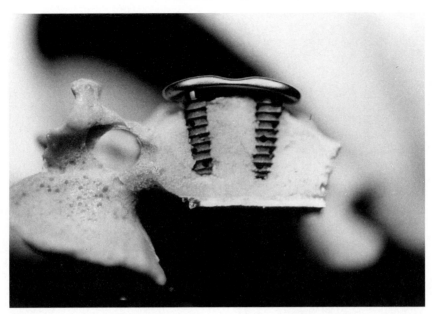

Fig. 101-3
The AO cervical spine locking plate system. Plates are 2 mm thick; length ranges from 24 mm to 92 mm.

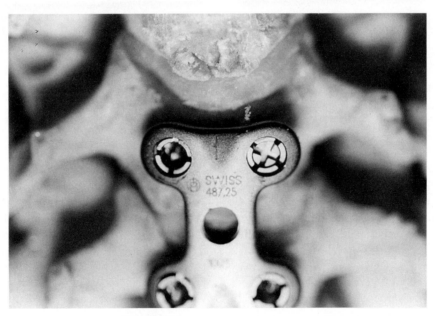

Fig. 101-4
Top right screw has locking screw in place.

To avoid perforation into the disc space, the surgeon must remember that the cervical discs are angled in a horizontal plane and that the alignment of the screw holes in relationship to the plate is relatively fixed at 90 degrees. Once the plate is properly aligned, it is held in place by an assistant while the surgeon drills the holes to a fixed depth of 14 mm. The hole is then tapped and the screws placed; at least two screws are placed above and below the graft. The screws are locked into the plate by insertion of the expansion bolt (Figs. 101-3, 101-4, and 101-5).

Other Plating Systems

The AO Orozco plate and the Caspar plate system both require that the screws purchase the dorsal vertebral body cortex, and unlike the TLSP system,

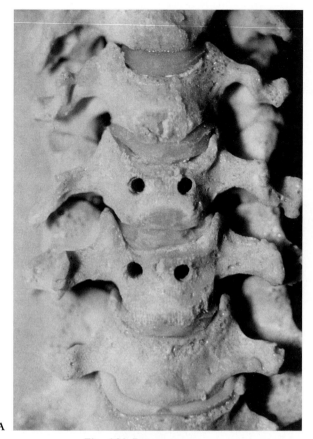

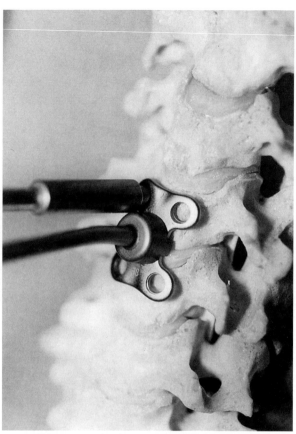

A

B

Fig. 101-5

A and **B,** Proper screw-hole placement in cranial portion of vertebral body. *(From Wetzel, FT, Normal Cervical Spine Morphomotry and Cervical Spinal Stenosus in Asumptomatic Professional Football Players, Spine 120 (65): 148-816, 1991)*

neither system has intrinsic stability between the screws and plates to lessen the chance of screw migration.

The AO Orozco plate is placed in the midline. The screw holes are drilled and tapped, and the screws are then placed in the superior aspect of the vertebral body above and below the graft site. It is essential to know the sagittal diameter of the vertebral body to prevent overpenetration into the spinal canal. Fluoroscopy is recommended for guiding screw placement, along with a special adjustable fixed drill guide. After drilling, the screw length is carefully measured with the depth gauge, and both cortices are tapped with a 3.5 mm tap. Two screws (four cortices) are placed in the vertebral bodies above and below the graft site. Postoperatively, patients are immobilized with a four-poster cervical orthosis for 6 to 12 weeks.

The Caspar trapezoidal plate system is similar to the AO Orozco plate in that the use of fluoroscopy is suggested because the screws are designed to purchase the dorsal cortex. The Caspar plate design is different in that the plate is trapezoidal and has two small spikes that are tapped into the vertebral bodies above and below the fusion prior to screw placement. Some of the screw holes are slots, which allow for a greater degree of freedom in screw placement. Postoperatively, patients are managed in fashion similar to patients who have been internally fixed with the Orozco or TLSP systems.

Complications

Most spine surgeons would agree that the most stable biomechanical technique for stabilization of the anterior column is an anterior cervical plate.[28,47] There is, however, hesitancy regarding the use of anterior plates because of longstanding concerns about their safety. The unique potential risks for anterior cervical plates are (1) spinal cord injury secondary to drilling or screw placement, and (2) early or delayed screw or plate loosening with subsequent injury to the soft tissues.

A number of recent reports have addressed these complications.[27,30,37,46,51] The incidence of hardware loosening is approximately 5%. There has been no reported spinal cord injury in any large series. Smith and Bolesta reported on two cases of esophageal erosion secondary to screw migration.[42] Neither case involved the screw plate locking design. In a recent report on the TLSP system,[27] two patients were noted to have hardware loosening; one of the patients required a second procedure to remove the loose screw/plate construct. Neither patient sustained a significant soft-tissue or esophageal injury. In both cases the caudal screws were placed in the disk space and were believed to be a technical error.

Summary

Anterior cervical plate fixation provides stable internal fixation for cervical spine injuries and multilevel decompressive procedures with a minimal complication rate.[27,30,37,46,51] Its use in the treatment of patients requiring anterior decompression for spinal-cord compression can eliminate the need for secondary posterior stabilization surgery and/or halo application. The use of anterior cervical plates as a means of early stabilization of cervical-spine injuries that predominantly involve the posterior column remains controversial. The use of anterior cervical plates following single-level anterior discectomy for degenerative disc disease is rarely indicated.

Anterior Screw Fixation

Although anterior interference screw fixation of cervical grafts has been reported in animal models, the clinical utility of anterior cervical screw fixation has found its greatest application in the treatment of odontoid fractures and nonunions.[49] Anterior screw fixation of the dens was originally performed by Nakanishi and associates in Japan.[32] Jeanneret and associates[22,23] and Bohler[4] have each reported the success of this operation in Europe, and most recently Geisler[17] and Esses[13] and their colleagues independently reported on two small series performed in North America. Each series varies in the number of screws used (one vs. two) for fixation as well as the type of screws used (cortical vs. cancellous; cannulated vs. noncannulated). Current opinion suggests that, where possible, two screws are better for rotational stability and that cannulated screws are perhaps safer and require less intraoperative imaging.

Indications for Odontoid Screw Fixation*

Anterior screw fixation of the odontoid is an alternative to halo immobilization or posterior C1-C2 fusion in treating odontoid fractures or nonunion. Type II odontoid fractures and "shallow" type III fractures have generally been listed as being amenable to dens screw fixation; in addition, concomitant dens fracture and C1 ring fracture have been heralded as ideal indications for dens screw fixation.

Although dens screw fixation has an esthetic appeal to most spine surgeons, the relative contraindications of dens screw fixation (for which there are many) must be reviewed.

Contraindications†

In North America anterior dens screw fixation has not gained universal acceptance and for this reason lack of experience with this technique may be considered a relative contraindication for its use. Pathologic fractures (including severe osteoporosis), which can lead to a significant rate of screw cut out, should be approached with caution and are often better treated by other means. Frontal oblique fractures tend to displace laterally with compression, and sagittal oblique type II or deep extension type III fractures often have little bone available to provide stable fixation. Additional contraindications are significant thoracic kyphosis and a large thoracic cavity, both of which make the surgical approach nearly impossible (Fig. 101-6).

*References 1, 4, 5, 10, 13, 15, 20, 22 to 25, and 30.
†References 1, 4, 5, 13, 22, 23, 25, and 30.

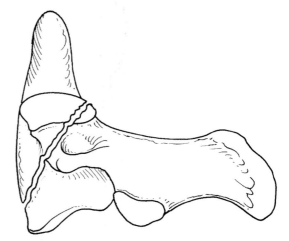

Fig. 101-6

An oblique type II dens fracture with fracture line running posterior–cranial to anterior–caudal is a contraindication to odontoid screw fixation.

Surgical Technique*

If possible, the patient is nasotracheally intubated and positioned while awake. The fracture should be reduced prior to incision. Biplanar fluoroscopy is used, as is spinal cord monitoring. Anteriorly displaced fractures are reduced by hyperextension and posterior displacement of the head, while posteriorly displaced fractures are reduced by hyperextension and anterior displacement of the head. A halo ring and posterior "roll towel" are helpful to obtain and maintain the reduction.

The anterior medial approach to C2 is used. The preference for a right- or left-sided approach is left up to the surgeon. The classic approach involves a transverse incision one fingerbreadth from the midline below the mandible and proceeding laterally, curving around the angle of the mandible posteriorly across the mastoid process. Bohler suggests using a transverse collar approach at the level of the cricoid cartilage[4]. The incision is 6 to 7 cm long,

*References 1, 4, 5, 13, 22, 23, 25, 30, and 50.

and its more caudal location allows the surgeon to avoid the superior laryngeal and hypoglossal nerves. The platysma is divided, the medial border of the SCM muscle is identified, and the carotid pulse is palpated. Blunt finger dissection allows identification of the retropharyngeal space and anterior longitudinal ligament. The anterior tubercle of C1 should be palpated and position verified via fluoroscopy. For adequate exposure it may be necessary to ligate the superior thyroid artery.

Placement of Holmann or right-angle retractors maintains the exposure of the C2-C3 disk space while a flexible guide wire is introduced at the anteroinferior portion of C2. Placement of this wire is guided by biplaner fluoroscopy; identifying the starting point for the guide wire is facilitated by resection of a small portion of the C2-C3 anulus and disk (Figs. 101-7 and 101-8).

Ideal fixation centers on the placement of two 3.5-mm screws. Unfortunately, this is not always possible and the surgeon may have to settle for one safe screw. Postoperatively the patient is maintained in a four-poster orthosis for 8 to 12 weeks.

Complications

To date there has been no reported spinal cord injury or death related to anterior dens screw placement. Screw breakage has largely been confined to

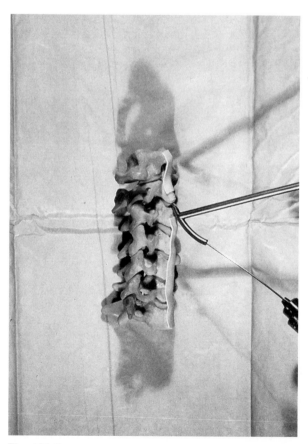

Fig. 101-7

Curved drill guide allows for accurate placement of guide wire for dens screw.

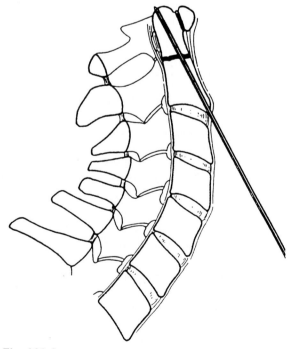

Fig. 101-8

Lateral view of ideal placement of odontoid screw guide wire.

single-screw placement and treatment of nonunion. A nonunion rate as high as 12% has been reported in the treatment of acute fractures.[1] Although screw malposition does not necessarily lead to clinical disaster,[13] this complication is reported in most series and highlights the importance of excellent biplanar fluoroscopic controlled screw placement.

Summary

Anterior screw fixation of the odontoid process has the advantage of decreasing the nonunion rate of type II dens fractures while preserving alantoaxial rotation. Although this technique was first used in the treatment of odontoid nonunions, its use today is in the treatment of type II and "shallow" type III dens fractures. The procedure has a number of relative contraindications, is technically demanding, and carries the risk of a number of serious potential complications. In the proper setting the dens screw allows for preservation of alantoaxial motion and an increased union rate. In an inappropriate setting this technique may have a catastrophic result.

References

1. Aebi M, Etter C, Coscia M: Fractures of the odontoid process: treatment with anterior screw fixation, *Spine* 14:1065, 1989.
2. Bell GD, Bailey SJ: Anterior cervical fusion for trauma, *Clin Orthop* 128:155, 1977.
3. Bernard TN, Whitecloud TS III: Cervical spondylotic myelopathy and myeloradiculopathy, *Clin Orthop* 221:149, 1987.
4. Bohler J: Anterior stabilization for acute fractures and non-unions of the dens, *J Bone Joint Surg* 64A:18, 1982.
5. Bohler J: Fracture of the odontoid process, *J Trauma* 5(3):386, 1965.
6. Bohler J, Gaudermak T: Anterior plate stabilization for fracture dislocations of the lower cervical spine, *J Trauma* 20:203, 1980.
7. Bohlman HH: Acute fractures and dislocations of the cervical spine, *J Bone Joint Surg* 61A:1119, 1979.
8. Brown JA and others: Cervical stabilization by plate and bone fusion, *Spine* 13:236, 1988.
9. Cabanella ME, Ebersold MJ: Anterior plate stabilization for bursting tear drop fracture of the cervical spine, *Spine* 13:888, 1988.
10. Clark CR, Charles R, White AA: Fractures of the dens: a multicentre study, *J Bone Joint Surg* 67A:1340, 1985.
11. DeOliveira J: Anterior plate fixation of traumatic lesions of the lower cervical spine, *Spine* 12:324, 1987.
12. Doherty BJ, Heggeness MH, Esses SI: A biomechanical study of odontoid fractures and fracture fixation, *Spine* 18(2):178, 1993.
13. Esses SI, Bednar DA: Screw fixation of odontoid fractures and nonunions, *Spine* 16S:483, 1991.
14. Farey ID and others: Pseudarthrosis of the cervical spine after anterior arthrodesis, *J Bone Joint Surg* 72A:1171, 1990.
15. Fuji E, Kobayashi K, Hirabayashi K: Treatment in fracture of the odontoid process, *Spine* 13:604, 1988.
16. Gassman J, Beligson D: The anterior cervical plate, *Spine* 6:700, 1981.
17. Geisler FH and others: Anterior screw fixation of posteriorly displaced type II odontoid fractures, *Neurosurgery* 25:30, 1989.
18. Goodman J, Seligson D: The anterior cervical plate, *Spine* 8:700, 1983.
19. Gore DR, Sepic SB: Anterior cervical fusion for degenerated or protruded discs: a review of one hundred forty-six patients, *Spine* 9:667, 1984.
20. Govender T, Haffee MR: Fractures of the dens: a clinical and anatomical study, *J Bone Joint Surg* 72B:337, 1990.
21. Herrmann HD: Metal plate fixation after anterior fusion of unstable fracture dislocation of the cervical spine, *Acta Neurochir (Wien)* 32:101, 1975.
22. Jeanneret B and others: *Anterior screw fixation of the dens fractures: results.* Presented at Socie'te' Internatonae de Chirugie Orthopedique et de Traumatologie. Montreal, Canada, September 10, 1990.
23. Jeanneret B and others: Atlantoaxial mobility after screw fixation of the odontois: a computed tomographic study, *J Spinal Dis* 4(2):203, 1991.
24. Kaplan SI, Tun CG, Sarkarati M: Odontoid fracture complicating ankylosing spondylitis, *Spine* 15:607, 1990.
25. Knoringer P: *Double threaded compression screws in osteosynthesis of acute fracture of the odontoid process.* In Voth D, Glees O, editors: *Disease in the craniocervical junction,* vol 217, Berlin, 1987, de Gruyter.
26. Kostuik JP, Connolly PJ: *Anterior cervical plate fixation.* In Garfin SR, Northup BE, editors: *Surgery for spinal cord injuries,* New York, 1993, Raven Press, p 163.
27. Kostuik JP and others: Anterior cervical plate fixation with the titanium hollow screw plate system (THSP), *Spine* 18:1273, 1993.
28. McAfee PC: *Cervical spine trauma.* In Frymoyer J, editor: *The adult spine,* New York, 1991, Raven Press, p 1099.
29. McAfee PC, Bohlman HH: One stage anterior cervical decompression and posterior stabilization with circumferential arthrodesis, *J Bone Joint Surg* 71A:78, 1989.
30. Meyer PR Jr, Rusin JJ, Haak MH: *Anterior instrumentation of the cervical spine.* In Cotler JM, An HS, editors: *Spinal instrumentation,* Baltimore, 1992, William & Wilkins, p 49.
31. Morscher E and others: Die Vordere Verplattung der halswirbelsaule mit dem hohischrauben plattensystem, *Der Chirurg* 57:702, 1986.
32. Nakanishi T and others: Internal fixation for the odontoid fracture, *Orthop Trans* 6:176, 1982.
33. Orozco R: Osteossintese en los lesiones traumaticos y degenecativos de los coluvos cervoca, *Rev Traumatol Cirurg Rehabil* 1:4252, 1971.
34. Orozco R, Liovet J: Osteosintesis en las fractures de raquis cervical, *Rev Ortop Traumatol* 14:285, 1977.

35. Orozco R, Liovet J: Osteosintesis en las lesiones traumaticas y degenerativas de la columna cervical. *Rev Traumatol Cirurg Rehabil* 1:45, 1971.

36. Raveh J and others: Use of tetanium coated hollow screw and reconstruction plate system in bridging of lower jaw defects, *J Oral Maxillofac Surg* 42:281, 1984.

37. Ripa DR and others: Series of ninety-two traumatic cervical spine injuries stabilized with anterior ASIF plate fusion technique, *Spine* 16:546, 1991.

38. Robinson RA, Smith GW: Anterolateral cervical disk removing and interbody fusion for cervical disk syndrome, *Bull Johns Hopkins Hosp* 96:223, 1955.

39. Schatzker J, Rorabeck CH, Wadell JP: Fractures of the dens: an analysis of thirty-seven cases, *J Bone Joint Surg* 53B(3):392, 1971.

40. Senegas J: Fractures et luxations recent du rachis cervical sans troubles neurologiques, *Rev Chir Orthop* 58:353, 1972.

41. Senegas J, Gauzere JM: Plaidoyer pour la chirugie anterieure dans le traitement des traumatismes graves des cinq dernieres vertebres cervicales, *Rev Chir Orthop* 62(suppl II):123, 1976.

42. Smith MD, Bolesta MJ: Esophageal perforation after anterior cervical plate fixation: a report of two cases, *J Spinal Dis* 5(3):357, 1992.

43. Southwick WO: Current concepts review: management of fractures of the dens (odontoid process), *J Bone Joint Surg* 62A:482, 1980.

44. Southwick WU, Robinson RN: Surgical approaches to the vertebrae bodies in the cervical and lumbar regions, *J Bone Joint Surg* 39A:631, 1959.

45. Stauffer S, Kelly EG: Fracture-dislocations of the cervical spine—instability and recurrent deformity following treatment by anterior interbody fusion, *J Bone Joint Surg* 59A(1):45, 1977.

46. Suh PB, Kostuik JP, Esses SI: Anterior cervical plate fixation with the titanium hollow screw plate system, *Spine* 15:1079, 1990.

47. Sutterlin IV and others: A biomechanical evaluation of cervical spinal stabilization methods on a bovine model, *Spine* 13:795, 1988.

48. Van Peteghem PK, Schweigel JF: The fractured cervical spine rendered unstable by anterior cervical fusion, *J Trauma* 19:110, 1979.

49. Vazquez-Seoane P and others: Interference screw fixation of cervical grafts: a combined in vitro biomechanical and in vivo animal study, *Spine* 18(8):946, 1993.

50. Watkins RG: *Surgical approaches to the spine*. New York, 1983, Springer Verlag, p 1.

51. Wolfhard C, Barbier DD, Klara PM: Anterior cervical fusion and caspar plate stabilization for cervical trauma, *Neurosurgery* 25(4):491, 1989.

52. Zdeblick TA, Bohlman HH: Cervical kyphosis and myelopathy—treatment by anterior corpectomy and strut-grafting, *J Bone Joint Surg* 71A:170, 1989.

Chapter 102
Sports Injuries of the Head and Cervical Spine

F. Todd Wetzel

Gregory A. Hanks

P. Dean Cummings

On-Field Examination

Transportation

Radiographic Evaluation

Sprains and Strains

Cervical Spine Fractures and Disc Injuries

    epidemiology
    biomechanics and kinematics
    cervical spine injuries in football
    cervical spine injuries in other sports

Neuropraxia of the Cervical Cord with Transient Quadriplegia

Brachial Plexus Neuropraxia

Criteria for Return to Sports Play

    absolute contraindications
    relative contraindications
    no contraindications

One of the most feared occurrences in sports is catastrophic injury of the cervical spine. Fortunately, most cervical spine injuries are simple sprains, but serious injuries do occur. Such injuries include fractures or dislocations, with or without neurologic injury, and neuropraxia of the spinal cord. Fatal injury to the head or neck, is, fortunately, rare. As expected, serious cervical spine injuries are most common in contact sports. In football, for example, 85% of reported fatalities are the result of intracranial or cervical spine injuries. Thus, the prompt and accurate diagnosis and treatment of the injured player is of more than casual interest to trainer, coach, and player alike.

In this chapter, the evaluation of the injured spine will be reviewed, followed by discussion of specific injuries and recommended treatment. Finally, a comprehensive approach toward determining return-to-play capacity will be proposed.

On-Field Examination

While rule changes and the modification of protective athletic equipment have decreased the risk of death and permanent injury during athletic participation, they have far from eliminated it.

In football, the institution of the recommendations of the National Operating Committee on Standards for Athletic Equipment regarding safety standards for football helmets[43] resulted in a dramatic reduction in both head and cervical spine fatalities between 1975 and 1984. The data show that the majority of head fatalities were secondary to subdural hematomas, and almost all the cervical spine fatalities were the result of fracture or dislocation. That this decline was related to rule changes and strict enforcement of these changes is far from conjectural. While fatalities decreased from 1960 to 1980, Torg and associates[90,93,97] reported that the incidence of nonfatal cervical spine injuries with permanent quadriplegia had increased. Helmet design was implicated; the development of a protective helmet–face mask system effectively protected the head but made the cervical spine vulnerable to injury when the head was used as a battering ram during tackling or blocking (so called "spear tackling"). A rule change was instituted, banning spearing and the use of the top of the helmet as the initial point of contact in making a tackle, and a marked decrease in nonfatal cervical spine injuries ensued. The occurrence of permanent cervical quadriplegia decreased from 34 known cases in 1976 to five in 1984. Thus, in some sense, the cervical spine may be more

vulnerable to injury owing to equipment rules specifically designed to offer increased cranial protection. As such, the probability of serious injury remains whenever athletes take the field. For this reason alone, awareness on the part of coaching and medical staff is critical. Four principles are important in the initial assessment of an athlete suspected of having a head or neck injury:

1. Evaluation—identification of conditions that are potentially life threatening or disabling.

2. Immobilization—use of proper techniques to secure the potentially unstable cervical spine.

3. Medical stabilization—provision of basic and advanced life support, if necessary.

4. Transportation—safe transfer of the athlete from the site of injury to a definitive-care site.

The head of the medical team is usually a physician or an athletic trainer with specialized training. The team physician is ultimately responsible for the evaluation and treatment of an injured athlete, and must maintain a high index of suspicion for head and cervical spine injuries. Familiarity with the sport, the rules of the game, and the protective equipment is necessary to understand common mechanisms of injury. A team physician must be more than a passive observer on the sidelines. He or she must be able to evaluate the performance of each athlete and observe subtle differences that may reveal an injury predisposing the athlete to a catastrophic head or neck injury. Assembling a knowledgeable medical support staff is important, as are discussions with the support staff in preparation for different emergency scenarios before each sporting event. It is the responsibility of the head of the team to ensure that the necessary medical equipment, such as a spine board, is available.

Sporting events that are considered to be "high risk," that is, contact sports, should have a medical team and qualified ambulance service in attendance. Low risk events should, at the very least, have an EMS on standby with a minimal response time. A constant line of communication must be available between the medical staff and the designated emergency facility. It is strongly recommended that the accepting medical care facility have an orthopaedic surgeon or neurosurgeon to meet the athlete upon arrival.[9]

When a suspected head or cervical spine injury occurs, the medical team should be promptly mobilized. If the patient has been rendered unconscious, the cervical spine should be treated as unstable until proven otherwise by examination after consciousness has been regained, or by appropriate ra-

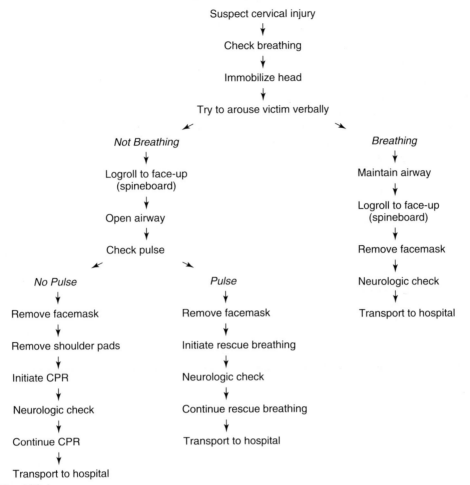

Fig. 102-1

Protocol for on-field evaluation of head and neck injuries. *(From Vegso JJ, Lehman RC:* Field evaluation and management of head and neck injuries. *In Torg JS, editor:* Athletic injuries to the head, neck and face, *Philadelphia, 1982, Lea & Febiger, with permission.)*

diologic studies. Adherence to the protocol can prevent a stable treatable injury from becoming a life-threatening catastrophe. Fig. 102-1 summarizes the protocol for evaluating the athlete suspected of having a head or neck injury.

The first priority of evaluation is the establishment of a preliminary level of consciousness and verification of spontaneous respiration. Mouth pieces should be removed; however, helmets should be left in place. The athlete is next positioned in the supine position using the log-roll technique. Use of a spine board is recommended. If breathing is labored or nonexistent, the head and neck should be secured and the face mask removed with a pair of bolt cutters or a utility knife, leaving the helmet in place. An airway is established using the chin lift maneuver, avoiding hyperextension or flexion. These deflections could cause additional neurologic injury in the

presence of an unstable spine. If the chin lift is not effective, the jaw thrust technique without the head tilt may be used. These maneuvers should not hyperextend the neck if performed correctly. If the airway is still compromised, the head may be gently tilted. Protection of airway patency is often necessary; this can be accomplished by placing an oropharyngeal or nasotracheal airway. If an airway cannot be maintained, advanced airway management, along with techniques of oxygenation and ventilation, should be instituted using the standards and guidelines for Cardiopulmonary Resuscitation (CPR) outlined by the American Heart Association.[6]

For athletes who are conscious and fully alert, the first step is reassurance; the patient should be kept calm and still. Dyspnea may be addressed by direct questioning. If the athlete is wearing a helmet, the chin strap should remain fastened in place. A history of past injuries of the neck is important. Albright and associates[3] report a 33% incidence of previous neck injury in high school seniors playing football. A follow-up study by Albright and associates[2] examined head and neck injuries in college football players over an 8-year period. The authors found that over their career, 29% of players had one or more head or neck injuries, and that once the first injury occurred, 42% suffered another head or neck injury.

The athlete should also be questioned for neck pain, numbness, tingling, burning of the extremities, or difficulty moving any limbs. If any of these symptoms are present, the cervical spine is presumptively unstable; immobilization and transportation for further evaluation is required.

In the athlete who is complaining only of neck pain, a standard cervical spine assessment is performed. The first step is palpation of the posterior neck for tenderness and/or deformity. If these are present, the patient should be immobilized and transported for evaluation for presumptive ligamentous injury or fracture. If negative, a detailed neurologic examination of the upper and lower extremities is performed. Any deficit should be treated as evidence of instability. If strength is fully intact, cervical range of motion may be assessed while questioning the athlete about pain, paresthesia, or dysesthesia. If the examination is entirely normal the athlete may then leave the field to be reevaluated in greater detail. It is important to maintain a high index of suspicion; if in doubt, immobilization and transportation for additional evaluation is strongly recommended. Proper immobilization and transportation of the injured athlete are crucial in preventing a therapeutic discontinuity.

Transportation

For effective resuscitation and transportation of an injured athlete, the athlete should be placed supine. This often requires movement of an athlete from an "injured" fetal or prone position. If the athlete must be moved, the head should be kept in axial alignment with the spinal column. One person must control the head while the athlete is rolled onto the spine board. This is easily performed by placing assistants at the shoulders, hips, and knees. The leader of the medical team, who controls the head, must explain each movement before it is carried out so the team can act in concert.

Following the transfer of the injured athlete onto a spinal board, immobilization of the head, neck, and the entire body is required to ensure that there is no movement about the cervical neuraxis. *Total* spinal immobilization is crucial. Immobilization of only the head and neck can result in excessive cervical motion. Placement of sand bags or foam pads alongside the athlete's head is helpful. The head and entire body should then be secured with straps (Fig. 102-2). Transfer off the field can be accomplished by placing two assistants on either side of the spinal board, with the leader ensuring stabilization of the neck and airway.

Prior to transfer by qualified emergency medical services personnel, a decision should be made to determine what type of care facility the injured athlete requires. The facility should provide trauma care and have an orthopedic surgeon or neurosurgeon in attendance to receive the athlete. While in transfer, a direct line of communication with the care facility should be maintained. If the athlete has sustained definite spinal cord injury, the intravenous administration of steroids should be given upon arrival at the medical-care facility. If given within 8 hours of injury, the administration of methylprednisolone has been found to improve neurologic outcome in some cases. Methylprednisolone is administered over a 24-hour period. An intravenous bolus dose of 20 mg/kg over 15 minutes is given initially, followed by a maintenance dose of 5.4 mg/kg/hr over the following 23 hours.[16]

At no time during the on-field evaluation, medical stabilization, immobilization, or transport of an athlete with suspected cervical spine injury should the helmet be removed. On arrival at the medical facility, the athlete's helmet may be removed while the athlete is completely immobilized. The technique for helmet removal requires two individuals. One faces the athlete and supports the posterolateral aspect of the neck. The other stands above the athlete and grasps the ear flaps, spreading and pulling the helmet off in an axial direction.

Radiographic Evaluation

An athlete who has sustained a neck injury based on the initial evaluation, or an unconscious athlete suspected of having a neck injury, should undergo a complete roentgenographic evaluation. Plain radiographs include the lateral, odontoid, and anteroposterior views. Visualization from the occiput to the superior portion of T1 is necessary on the lateral view. Oblique views are helpful if isolated nerve root symptoms are present. Further radiographic studies available include CT, bone scans, and MRI. An MRI should be obtained for any cord injuries or suspected disc abnormalities. Treatment for these injuries then proceeds along established pathways.

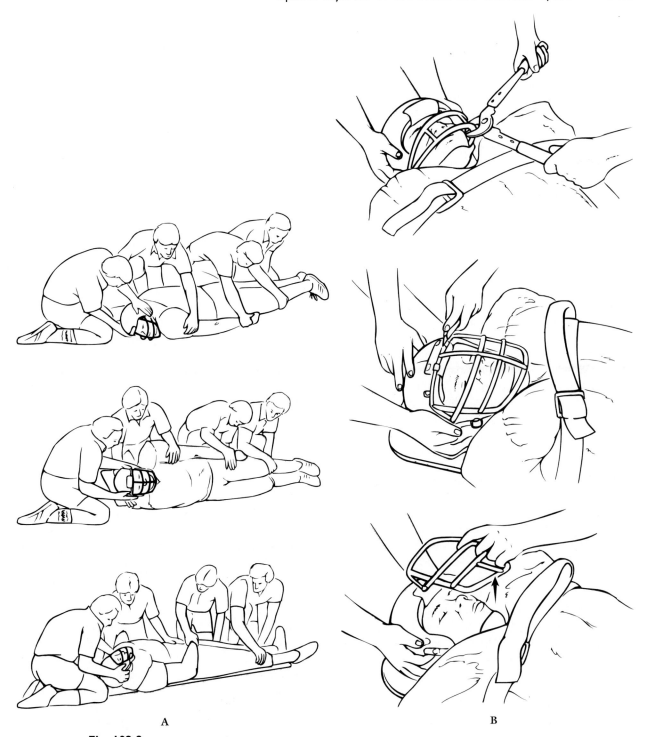

A   B

Fig. 102-2

Transfer and immobilization of the injured athlete. **A,** After it has been established that the athlete is breathing, the log roll onto the spine board is accomplished. This takes four people, to ensure that the transfer occurs with the cervical spine in normal axial alignment. **B,** The face mask is removed with either bolt cutters or a utility knife. The helmet is left in place and the athlete securely strapped to the board. *(From Vegso JJ, Lehman RC: Field evaluation and management of head and neck injuries, Clin Sports Med 6(1):1, 1987.)*

Sprains and Strains

As noted previously, most cervical-spine injuries are not fractures or cord injuries, but cervical sprains and muscle strains. An acute sprain is defined as an injury of the ligamentous structures, while a strain is an injury to the musculature. In the latter, there is no anatomic disruption to either ligament or muscle. Pain is localized to the cervical area, with limitation of end-range motion. Sprains and strains are thus minor, self-limiting injures that require only symptomatic treatment. It is, however, crucial to rule out the presence of a more serious underlying injury. All patients should undergo a thorough neurologic and range-of-motion examination. Any pain radiation, persistent pain, paresthesia, or weakness requires restriction of participation and subsequent evaluation by appropriate roentgenographic studies.

Treatment of the sprain is based on the degree of symptoms. Mild analgesics, antiinflammatory medicines, and ice are useful acutely. A soft cervical collar is helpful to reduce pain and cervical muscle spasm. Muscle strengthening exercises are instituted as soon as full, pain-free range of motion is attained. An athlete with a neck injury who has neck pain and limited range of motion, or neck pain and an abnormal neurologic examination, should have cervical spine x-ray studies, including flexion and extension views to rule out fractures and ligamentous disruption. If symptoms persist, further diagnostic studies, as noted above, are required.

Sideline evaluation of an athlete with a "minor" neck injury may be more complex than initially supposed. As with all neck injuries, the examiner must maintain a high index of suspicion for fracture and instability. Athletes often present with very nonspecific symptoms; this may add to the difficulty of differentiating between a routine cervical strain and an unstable cervical spine injury. Vegso and Lehman suggest that further investigation is warranted if any of the following findings or symptoms are present[102]:

1. Torticollis or wry neck posture
2. Painful cervical motion
3. Decreased range of cervical motion
4. Persistent paresthesia
5. Motor weakness

If any of these findings are present, a fracture should be ruled out. The athlete should immediately be immobilized and transported for roentgenographic evaluation.

If examination is entirely normal, return to activity is permitted. The athlete is prohibited from playing if the examination is abnormal. An examination that elicits numbness, tingling or weakness, pain, or limited neck mobility may indicate a more serious abnormality and immediate immobilization and further evaluation is recommended.

Cervical Spine Fractures and Disc Injuries

Injuries to the cervical spine during athletic endeavors constitute a major source of emotional and financial concern in the United States. The spectrum of cervical spine injuries range from the minor sprain to the catastrophic, or even fatal, lesion of dislocation with subsequent quadriplegia. The goal of this section is to review the pertinent data on these injuries, paying special attention to predisposing features and to rule changes instituted in an attempt to diminish the occurrence of injury.

The evaluation, treatment, injury mechanism, and immediate and long-term sequelae of cervical spine injuries have been widely studied.[*] A review of these data is beyond the scope of this section, and hence, only cervical injuries pertinent to the athlete will be addressed. It must, however, be borne in mind that any cervical injury may be encountered in the athlete[†], and that evaluation and treatment should proceed along conventional lines, regardless of etiology.

Epidemiology

As Torg has noted, head and neck injuries are the leading cause of direct fatalities in contact sports.[90] Hodgson, in a report of the National Operating Committee on Standards for Athletic Equipment in Football Helmet Certification program, noted that 18% of the fatalities incurred in football are due to neck injuries.[43] Torg and colleagues, reporting in the National Football Head and Neck Injury Register, suggested consideration of head and neck injury parameters. These included intracranial hemorrhage, intracranial hemorrhage resulting in death, cervical fractures, subluxations and dislocations, and cervical spine fractures with permanent quadriplegia.[97,98] The data concerning fracture, dislocation, and subluxation are of particular interest.

Schneider reported 78 cases of football injury occurring between 1959 and 1963.[72] He noted 56

---

[*]References 4, 10, 14, 18, 29, 33, 36, 48, 58, 59, 61, 63, 68, 69, 80, 107, and 108.
[†]References 2, 3, 5, 7, 11 to 13, 19-21, 24 to 26, 32, 34, 35, 37, 39, 45, 47, 49 to 51, 54, 55, 60, 62, 67, 70 to 78, 81, 83 to 86, 90 to 92, 99, 106, and 111.

fracture/dislocations below C4, with 30 complete spinal cord lesions. While numbers such as these are small, evidence suggests that factors predisposing to such injury, or indicative of subclinical injury, are more frequent. In reviewing recruits for the University of Iowa's football team, Albright and colleagues noted that 32% had roentgenographic evidence of prior cervical spine injury.[2] In the 104 high school football players surveyed by the same group, 16.3% admitted to a history of neck injury.[3]

A representative spectrum of cervical spine injury in football is provided by several authors.[34,75,77,90,94] In case reports of eight injuries incurred while playing tackle football, Torg and associates noted disc herniation, anterior subluxation on C3 with respect to C4, unilateral facet dislocation, and bilateral facet dislocation.[101] The clinical courses of these injuries are representative of the severity of underlying damage. One player who suffered a disc herniation at C3-C4 initially presented as a complete lesion.

Following successful anterior cervical discectomy and interbody fusion, complete recovery occurred. Two players who suffered C3-C4 subluxations remained neurologically intact. One healed uneventfully in an orthosis, and one underwent posterior cervical fusion. Two players with unilateral facet dislocations presented as complete quadriplegics, and subsequently improved to residual central-cord syndromes. The three players presenting with bilateral facet dislocations presented as complete lesions. Two of these players died, one 48 and one 72 hours following injury, and one remained a complete quadriplegic. It is of more than passing interest to analyze the mechanism of injury responsible for these injuries: all injuries were incurred as a result of spear tackling. In the case of subluxations and facet dislocations, attitudes of flexion and rotation were clearly evident as well. Marron and colleagues speculated that the mechanism of injury in most football injuries were forced cervical flexion.[52] He believed that these tended to be the most common and the most severe injuries. Marron also noted evidence of "spinal concussion," namely, transient quadriparesis, as a result of nonbony injuries.

Subsequent studies strongly suggest that this mechanism of injury—forced flexion—is incorrect, and that the principal deleterious mechanism is direct axial loading.* As such, in 1976, a rule change was instituted whereby spear tackling was prohibited. Review of epidemiologic data from the National Football Head and Neck Injury Register from 1976 to 1984 showed a diminution in the frequency of

*References 90, 94 to 96, 99, 101, and 105.

cervical injury rates following institution of this rule. In 1976, 34 cases were reported. This declined to five cases in 1984. At the high school level, 6.5 cervical spine injuries per 100,000 players were reported in 1975; this declined to 3.9 per 100,000 in 1984. At the collegiate level, 23.9 per 100,000 were reported in 1975, with 6.7 per 100,000 reported in 1984. The statistics on quadriplegia following institution of the rule prohibiting spear tackling are similarly encouraging. Again, at the high-school level in 1975, 2.2 cases per 100,000 were reported. This declined to 0.043 case per 100,000 in 1984. At the collegiate level, the data are even more encouraging, with a decline from 8.4 per 100,000 in 1975 to 0 per 100,000 in 1984. It remains somewhat problematic that players in positions to make open-field tackles are more prone to suffer significant cervical spine injury, with the defensive back being the player at the greatest risk.[96]

Biomechanics and Kinematics

The biomechanical data that support the wisdom of the rule banning spear tackling are no less impressive than the statistics demonstrating its efficacy. Roaf, in a classic biomechanical study of injury production mechanisms in the functional spine unit (FSU), concluded that hyperflexion of the cervical spine *never* produced a pure hyperflexion injury in an intact spine.[69] Hence, it was unlikely that extremes of flexion or extension were responsible for significant injury in football. Additionally, other mechanisms in which the face mask was used as a lever to force the posterior aspect of the helmet onto the cervical spine in an attitude of hyperextension (the so-called "guillotine mechanism") were invalidated. For the helmet to act as a "guillotine," the posterior aspect of the rim must contact the posterior aspect of the neck while the head is being forcibly hyperextended. The hypothesis underlying this mechanism of injury necessitated that the helmet functionally immobilize the caudal aspect of the neck, while, by hyperextension, the cranial aspect of the neck rotated around this pivot point. When the physiologic limits of extension were exceeded, injury theoretically occurred. Virgin studied 16 patients with a cineradiographic technique to determine whether or not the helmet was capable of producing a guillotine injury.[105] His subjects included seven members of the hospital staff, four professional football players, and five high school football players. Sixteen-millimeter film was used to record kinematics of the cervical spine, loaded at extremes of flexion and extension. No contact was noted between

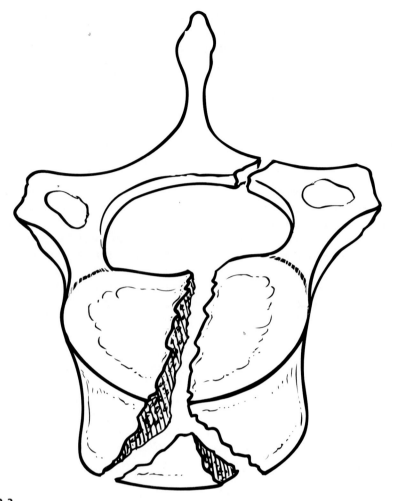

Fig. 102-3

The three-part two-plane fracture. This fracture results from axial loading, and is associated with a high incidence of neurologic compromise. *(From Torg JS and others:* **The axial load teardrop fracture,** Am J Sports Med *19(4):355, 1991.)*

the posterior aspect of the cervical spine and the helmet in any of five helmet designs.

The fractures produced by axial loading in different regions of the cervical spine have been identified. Torg and colleagues noted two distinct fracture patterns; teardrop, and three-part two-plane (Fig. 102-3).[94] In the former, neurologic integrity was the rule, while in the latter, permanent neurologic sequelae occurred. These may appear similar on plain films; obviously, the resultant instability of the two-plane fracture makes specific identification of paramount importance. In a study of 156 patients from the National Football League Head and Neck Injury Register, 55 patients with these fracture patterns were identified. In 35 of 48 patients, the injury-producing activity was known; this was spear tackling. Three types of collisions were identified. In direct collisions, two players in motion struck head-on, or

two players collided head-on with one moving and the other stationary. Additionally, there were oblique injuries with both individuals moving. Analysis of game films in all three circumstances confirm the presence of the helmet crown striking the opponent and producing an axial injury. With the cervical spine flexed 20 to 30 degrees, the impact of the crown produced straightening, or extension, of the spine. The spine was, thus, functionally in neutral at the time of impact. An axial load was applied owing to abrupt deceleration of the head and continuing momentum of the body (or, deceleration of the head with continuing inertia of the body). The cervical spine was crushed between the head and the body. Three groups were identified by appropriate radiographs: isolated teardrop fractures; three-part, two-plane fractures; and the third group where a lateral x-ray film alone was available, thus making differentiation between the two fracture patterns impossible. Forty-five of the fifty-five patients were permanently quadriplegic. In the three-part fracture, 27 of the 31 (87%) remained permanently quadriplegic, with the most frequent level of injury occurring at C4-C5 (74%). Additionally, facet disruption occurred in 89% of the cases. On radiographic study, sagittal fractures were noted, along with widening on the interpedicular space and asymmetry of the lateral borders.[96]

Cervical Spine Injuries in Football

From the above data, one may infer that axial loading can be expected to produce different injuries in different regions of the spine, based on regional kinematics. As noted above,[94] the predominance of injuries resulting in catastrophic neurologic events occurred at C4-C5. Again, from the National Football League Head and Neck Injury Register, information on injury response to axial loading in different regions of the cervical spine is available. Twenty-five cases of C3-C4 injuries, the so-called middle cervical spinal segment, were reported.[95] C3-C4 injuries were found to be unique, owing to the infrequency of fracture at this level, the difficulty of maintaining reduction, and the relatively favorable prognosis associated with aggressive intervention. Five categories of lesions were isolated in the upper cervical spine. These included herniated nucleus pulposus, subluxation, unilateral facet dislocation, bilateral facet dislocation, and vertebral body fracture. The presence of fracture at this level was relatively rare (four of 25 cases). Most acute herniated discs presented as transient quadriparesis. Regarding subluxation, the C3-C4 subluxation was easily reduced, but very difficult to maintain. Unilateral facet dislocations were found to be difficult to reduce in traction, and frequently required general anesthesia and closed reduction. Bilateral facet dislocations invariably required open reduction. The most favorable outcome, in terms of neurologic recovery, occurred with immediate reduction of facet dislocation. In the two cases of unilateral facet dislocation, reduction within 3 hours resulted in significant neurologic recovery. In the four cases of bilateral facet dislocation, no neurologic recovery occurred, regardless of treatment. Norton reported four C3-C4 injuries in a series of 88 patients.[59] Burke and Berryman reported two unilateral facet jumps in their series of 76 patients.[17] In Bohlman's classic series, only six of 300 cases occurred at C3-C4.[14] Likewise, O'Brien and co-workers noted only two cases in their series of 34.[61] Overall, in the National Football Head and Neck Injury

Register, 1062 cervical-spine injuries were reported in the 17-year period between 1971 and 1988. Only 25, or 2.4%, involved C3-C4.

In patients in whom a herniated disc was encountered, the outcome was uniformly good following anterior cervical discectomy and fusion. Subluxations were associated with neurologic integrity, but difficult to reduce and hold nonoperatively. Unilateral facet dislocation, reduced within 3 hours of injury, showed the most significant neurologic recovery, with two of six patients, all of whom presented as quadriplegics, resolving to central-cord syndromes. Bilateral C3-C4 facet dislocations fared poorly regardless of the outcome. Seven patients with this lesion all were quadriplegic at presentation, and all died as a result of their injuries.

In the lower cervical spine, catastrophic injury is comparatively rare. Clay shoveler's fractures have been reported in football players,[60] with avulsion of the spinous process secondary to the force transmitted throughout interspinous and supraspinous ligaments following an axial load. This would be likely under circumstances in which musculature is contracted to retract the scapula in preparation for contact. The treatment of these injuries is, as a rule, nonoperative, but on rare occasion excision of the un-united fragment may be required.

Cervical Spine Injuries in Other Sports

Cervical spine injuries have also been reported in connection with rugby. Sovio and colleagues reviewed the records of a British Columbia spinal cord injury unit from 1975 to 1982.[78] Of the 390 patients admitted, nine were injured while playing rugby. These injuries included a C1 fracture, a C3 compression fracture, two bilateral facet subluxations, a C4-C5 unilateral facet subluxation, a C6-C7 subluxation, a C2 fracture, a C4-C5 subluxation, and an apparently intact spine associated with transient numbness of the upper extremities. The spectrum of neurologic deficit ranged from none to fatal quadriplegia. Regarding mechanism of injury, again, axial loading in an attitude of neck flexion was implicated. The authors believed that players at the highest risk were those in the front row of the scrum, who had their upper extremities locked and necks flexed. The scrum is an ordered formation in which two sets of forwards pack themselves together with heads down in an attempt to push the opposing team off the ball. The axial loading and relatively flexed position of the cervical spine of multiple players make this a high-risk activity.[78] McCoy and associates corroborated this in a report of rugby injuries in school boys.[54] They noted seven injuries in 7 years—all subluxations. These occurred at C5-C6, C6-C7, and C7-T1.

Axial load appears to be the injurious mechanism in cervical spine injuries in hockey players as well. In Toronto, the incidence of cervical fractures in hockey players increased dramatically between 1974 and 1985.[83] Before 1973, no cervical spine injuries were reported at the Sunnybrooke Hospital. Between 1974 and 1980, one injury was reported, with five injuries reported from 1980 to 1981. Overall, 42 injuries were reported—from all of Canada—from 1976 to 1983. Twenty-eight of the forty-two patients suffered a spinal cord injury, and seventeen patients had complete lesions. Most injuries were suffered when the players were struck from behind, or collided with the boards with their head in a flexed position. The most frequent level of injury was C5-C6, with fracture/dislocations and fractures reported with a frequency similar to that in football. Interestingly, the frequency of injury was highest in organized leagues.[83,84]

Cervical spine fractures are apparently quite rare in wrestling. At the University of Iowa, over an 8-year period, wrestlers reported 104 neck injuries, representing 12.3% of total injuries incurred in wrestling. The most common cervical injuries were neurogenic pain syndromes ("burners") and cervical strain. The mechanisms of neurogenic pain were believed to be either transient foraminal encroachment resulting in nerve compression or stretch injuries. The former mechanism appears to be most common in wrestling. This is plausible, as attitudes of forced lateral flexion or extension are the position of the takedown. Disc herniation was rare.[111]

The use of the trampoline as a training device or recreational device in gymnastics has also received considerable notoriety regarding cervical spine injury. Rapp and Nicely reported 34 cases of quadriplegia and three deaths from trampoline-related injuries.[67] In 1975, Clarke, in a retrospective study of sports-related spinal cord injuries, distributed a large volume of questionnaires to various athletic centers.[23] In all, 18,805 high-school programs, 683 2-year college programs, and 1125 4-year college programs were polled. Eight sports accounted for all cervical spine injuries. Football was the most common cause of injury in 54%, with gymnastics second in 26%. In the 15 gymnastic injuries for which an apparatus was specified, eight occurred on a trampoline. In a comprehensive review of 25 years of literature, Torg reported 114 case of catastrophic cervical injuries (quadriplegia) associated with trampoline use.[88] In 1977, the American Academy of Pediatrics condemned trampoline use, except in the cases of supervised settings or in training elite athletes.[5]

Another sporting activity in which cervical spine injury has been addressed is diving. As Torg commented,[88] the true incidence of cervical spine injury secondary to shallow-water diving is unknown. In a review of 358 spinal cord injuries admitted to two Toronto hospitals, 11% were found to be secondary to diving accidents.[85] In an effort to explain this, Albrand and Walton constructed deceleration curves for dives of various heights into various depths of water.[1] These data indicated that a proper vertical entry with the hands in front of the cervical spine resulted in a maximum dissipation of velocity. The authors also discovered that velocity of entry is not dissipated until the diver reaches a depth of 10 to 12 feet, thus underscoring the primacy of adequate depth whenever diving activity is contemplated.

Other, less catastrophic, cervical spine injuries have been reported in athletic activities. Clay-shoveler's fractures have been reported to occur in power lifters[37] owing to the violent muscular contraction and the attitude of pure extension. In one case, an athlete was injured when a barbell fell back onto the squat rack. In addition, long-term unrecognized injury of the cervical spine has been dubbed "high jumper's neck" by Paley and Gillespie.[62] In this case report, the authors hypothesized that incorrect landing caused cervical subluxation and the resulting transient quadriparesis. Again, the deleterious mechanism here was axial loading, followed by forced cervical flexion.

Overall, with increasing supervision and appropriate athletic rule changes, the frequency of cervical fracture, dislocation, disc herniation, and resulting neurologic injury has declined. The role of axial loading in the production of serious cervical-spine injury cannot be overemphasized; appropriate rules prohibiting high-risk activities, such as spear tackling in football, have demonstrated their utility and should be strictly enforced.

Neuropraxia of the Cervical Cord with Transient Quadriplegia

The syndrome of neuropraxia of the cervical cord with transient quadriplegia has been well described by Torg and associates.[99] In this syndrome, the injured athlete experiences sensory changes, including burning paresthesia and numbness with variable motor changes. These episodes are by definition transient, and usually last 10 to 15 minutes. Complaints of neck pain are rare. In the initial study, the authors found statistically significant spinal stenosis in all the patients in whom this quadriplegia occurred. In an attempt to determine the long-term significance of such stenosis, the authors reviewed data collected from a survey of 503 schools participating in National Collegiate Athletics Association (NCAA) football. They concluded that little evidence existed to suggest that the occurrence of neuropraxia predisposed an individual to permanent neurologic injury. In a smaller companion report of two cases, Ladd and Scranton reported a similar syndrome recurring in two players with cervical spinal stenosis proven by myelography.[46] However, these authors suggested that athletes who exhibited these changes should be precluded from further participation in sports. Marron described the case of two high school football players who experienced painful and burning dysethesias in both hands following spear tackling.[52] Subsequent myelography revealed cord edema; the clinic syndrome lasted 18 to 24 hours. Marron termed this the "burning hand syndrome," and believed that the pathology was due to a central-cord lesion quite distinct from the transient neuropraxia described by Torg and associates.[97] In this injury, a lesion of the spinothalamic tract, in which the most medial fibers are those to the fingers and hands, resulted in the burning paresthesia. Whether or not the "burning hands syndrome" represents a specific entity is, however, a matter of some debate. As Raynor and Complik noted, the central-cord syndrome may represent a continuum of spinal cord injuries, rather than a distinct lesion.[68] Whether or not the final common end point of the spectrum would be transient or complete quadriparesis is likewise a matter of some speculation.

Given the potential severity of this entity, the determination of spinal stenosis or factors predisposing to it are of paramount importance. Several authors have attempted to quantify stenotic changes in a more reproducible manner.[64,65,99] On a lateral cervical radiograph, the dimension from the posterior aspect of the body to the spinal laminar line has been dubbed the "preexisting sagittal diameter."[109] This average sagittal diameter varies, however, when determined with lateral x-ray studies only. Mean diameters of 18.5 mm (range, 14.2 to 23 mm) and 17 mm (range, 13.9 to 20.3 mm) have been reported from C3 to C6, for a target distance of 5 feet from column to cassette.[15,41] At a target distance of 6 feet, a mean cervical sagittal diameter of 17.0 ± 5 mm has been reported.[57,66,110] It has been suggested that severe stenosis exists when cervical spinal canal sagittal dimensions are ≤ 13 to 14 mm.[30,31] In a study of myelopathic patients, the projected canal area was markedly smaller than the projected vertebral body area (85%).[37]

In an effort to determine the most accurate method for radiographic diagnosis of spinal stenosis, Pavlov and colleagues studied 97 patients.[65] The control group consisted of 74 asymptomatic patients and the experimental group of 23 athletes with evidence of transient neuropraxia, as described by Torg and associates.[99] Canal dimensions were measured by two methods. In one, sagittal diameter was measured from plain radiographs. A measurement of less than 14 mm was believed to represent a stenotic canal. The second method used was a ratio of sagittal canal diameter to sagittal vertebral body width (Fig. 102-4). Data were analyzed by use of the Mann-Whitney U test and relative operating characteristic curves. Using the sagittal measurement technique, 65% of the canals subsequently determined to be stenotic were designated normal, and 1% of normal canals were interpreted as stenotic. Using the ratio technique, 98.5% of the stenotic canals were detected using a ratio of 0.75, and 96.3% were detected using a ratio of 0.8. Using a cutoff ratio of 0.82, only 8% of stenotic canals were interpreted as normal, and 6% of normal canals interpreted as stenotic.

The clinical significance of this has, however, remained unclear. It is a particularly germane issue when the physician is faced with the decision of prohibiting an athlete from further participation in sports activities because of an episode of transient quadriplegia. This problem was addressed in a recent study by Torg and colleagues.[100] The study compared spinal-canal vertebral body ratios at C3, C4, C5, and C6 in four groups of football players. These groups included asymptomatic college football players, asymptomatic professional football players, players of various levels who had been rendered quadriplegic, and players with documented episodes of cervical-cord neuropraxia. No mean difference in canal cerebral body ratios was detected between the asymptomatic and quadriplegic group. However, the group in which transient neuropraxia occurred did have significantly smaller ratios than either the patients rendered permanently quadriplegic or the patients who were asymptomatic. On this basis, the authors concluded that the presence of stenosis and cord neuropraxia should not be used to prohibit participation in sporting events.

While additional study in this area is required, Herzog and associates recently introduced the concept of "functional reserve" in evaluating the cervical spine for the presence of significant stenosis.[40] Eighty professional football players were studied us-

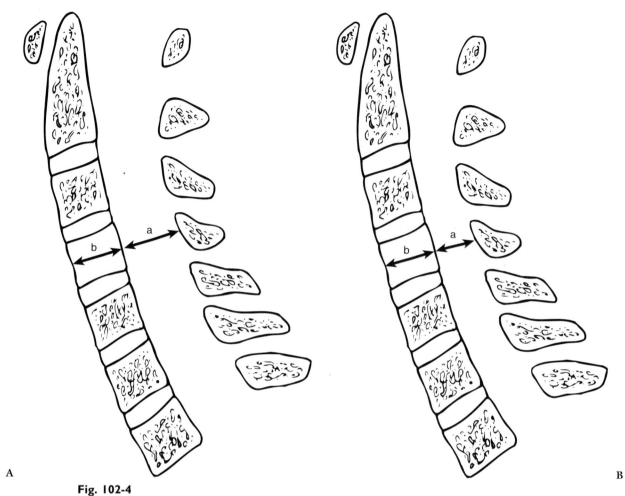

A   B

Fig. 102-4

Assessment of canal stenosis via the ratio method. These measurements are obtained from a lateral cervical spine film. *a* is measured from the posterior surface of the vertebral body to the most posterior laminar surface, while *b* is measured from the anterior to posterior surface of the vertebral body. The ratio of *a* to *b* is the measure then used to determine canal stenosis. Normal ratio is approximately 1.00. **A** illustrates a normal canal; **B** illustrates a congenitally stenotic canal with a ratio of approximately 0.5. *(From Pavolov H and others: Cervical spinal stenosis: determination with vertebral body ratio method, Radiology 164:771, 1987.)*

ing plain radiographs, CT, and MRI. Normal values were established for spinal morphology and segmental motion, and an attempt was made to detect the most accurate method to screen for spinal stenosis. Several measurements of sagittal diameter were analyzed, as noted in Fig. 102-5. These were then compared with the ratio method described earlier.[99] A ratio of less than 0.8 was found in 100 of the 454 levels studies, with 49% of the athletes demonstrating an abnormal ratio at one or more levels. The developmental sagittal diameter in athletes was found to be minimally larger than in normal subjects. Optimal dimensions for assessment using plain radiographs included D and II in neutral, and DI in extension. Given the predominance of a myelopathy in

a canal with a sagittal diameter less than 12.5 mm, the authors recommended MRI in cases where canal dimensions were lower than this value. The normal sagittal diameter of the cord and the canal was dubbed the "functional reserve." While the authors do not define normal functional reserve, they do point out the fact that this is apparently the primary determinant of whether significant spinal cord injury can occur. In a very real sense, this appears to be a critical determinant of the risk of spinal cord injury and will, with further investigations, probably supplant or augment plain radiographic techniques. In the algorithm proposed by Herzog and colleagues, the final determinant of significant stenosis would be the MRI.[40] While it is quite tempting to conclude

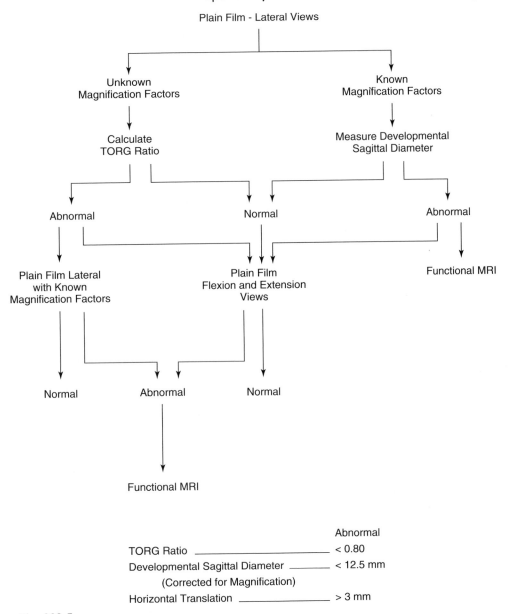

Fig. 102-5

Alternative measurements. Determination of the functional reserve capacity of the cervical spine. The measurements described are a diagrammatic description of measurement parameters with the cervical spine in the neutral and extension positions. These same parameters measured on a sagittal cervical-spine x-ray film. *(From Herzog RJ and others: Normal cervical spine morphometry and cervical spinal stenosis in asymptomatic professional football players, Spine 16(6S):178, 1991.)*

that a small functional reserve (1 to 2 cm) is indicative of higher risk for permanent injury, additional long-term clinical studies are needed to either validate or refute this concept.

Brachial Plexus Neuropraxia

The "burner" is a common injury in football and other sports. This injury has also been called "pinched nerve," "stinger," "zinger," or "brachial plexopathy." It represents transient dysfunction of the brachial plexus after a blow to the side of the head, neck, or shoulder.

There are two common mechanisms of injury. The most common etiology for a burner is a transient stretch of the brachial plexus, resulting from either a combination of lateral flexion of the cervical spine to the asymptomatic side with concomitant depression of the involved shoulder, or pure forced shoulder depression. Another, less common, mechanism is lateral rotation and extension of the spine toward the symptomatic side, causing a transient compression of the nerves. Other reported mechanisms are a direct blow or contusion and hyperextension stretch injuries.[104]

Symptoms consist of a sudden sharp or burning pain in the shoulder with paresthesia or dysesthesias radiating into the arm. There is often an associated unilateral sensory and motor loss. The numbness and burning often involve the entire extremity, with complete transient paralysis of the arm with a sensory loss over two or more dermatomes. Examination may reveal tenderness to palpation over the brachial plexus, in the absence of posterior neck tenderness. Symptoms may be increased with passive movement of the head and neck to the opposite side.*

The severity of the injury has been classified by Clancy, using clinical and electromyography (EMG) criteria.[22] In Grade I injuries, EMG/NCV are normal. These are, by far, the most common; complete recovery within 2 weeks is the rule. Most Grade I injuries recover within seconds. There may be tenderness in the upper and middle trapezius area for several days. Neck pain or tenderness is not present, and its presence should alert one to the possibility of a more serious neck injury. Grade II injuries are associated with significant weakness. Electromyograms show evidence of an axonal injury. As a rule, the deficiency persists for longer than 2 weeks. Although this appears to represent an axonotmesis, the recovery may be complete within 6 weeks. The most severe, and fortunately the rarest type, are the Grade III injuries. These produce significant weakness with poor recovery. Little improvement occurs for at least 1 year. Electromyography reveals axonal injury; this is true neurotmesis.

Most burners involve the upper trunk on the brachial plexus with resultant weakness of the deltoid, infraspinatus, supraspinatus, and biceps muscles. Burners are surprisingly frequent. Chrisman and associates reported an incidence of 565 per year in football players.[21] Vereschagin and colleagues reported a 10% incidence per year,[104] and Clancy reported that 49% of players experience at least one burner over the course of a collegiate football career.[22] Football participation accounts for the vast majority of reported burners, but they also occur in wrestlers. In football, burners occur among both offensive and defensive players, but substantially more are sustained by defensive players. Approximately 74% of burners occur during tackling, 21% during blocking, and 5% during other activities.

Differential diagnosis is important. Shoulder dislocation, rotator cuff injury, fracture, nerve root injury, and brachial neuritis should be considered. Careful physical examination will localize the lesion and determine whether a patient can return to athletic participation. Electromyographic and radiologic evaluation is indicated for patients with persistent symptoms, or those with any other suspected pathology.

The mainstay of treatment is rest. The athlete should be protected from trauma until symptoms resolve. Return to sports is permitted when:

1. Full, painless active range of motion of the neck is demonstrated.

2. Full return of strength of neck movement (painless manual resistance) is apparent.

3. Restoration of range of motion and strength of the shoulder musculature has occurred. This includes shrugs, abduction, forward flexion, elbow flexion/extension, wrist flexion/extension, and grip strength.

4. Normal sensation is present over all dermatomes.

Repeat examinations are important for all patients. Even those with a mild, transient burner should be reexamined at the end of the contest, the next day, and 1 week later because weakness can develop hours or days after the initial injury.

Initial treatment of the burner is symptomatic. Ice, rest, and antiinflammatory medication are prescribed. Strengthening exercises of the involved musculature are initiated as soon as symptoms permit. Those with severe plexus (Grade II and Grade III) injuries who have significant disability and no recovery after 1 year may benefit from surgical treatment. Such patients *might* be candidates for neurolysis, nerve repair or grafting, tendon transfer, or shoulder arthrodesis. Injuries requiring surgical treatment are extremely rare.

It appears that burners are common among football players. Rule changes prohibiting spear tackling have dramatically reduced the incidence of severe head and neck injuries. However, new tackling rules may have increased the incidence of brachial plexus neuropathies. Further studies are required to determine whether preventive exercises, alterations of tackling technique, or protective collars will reduce the incidence of this injury.

There are no well-established guidelines for treatment or return-to-play recommendations for patients who sustain multiple burners. It is not known which of these athletes are at risk for more serious

*References 8, 9, 28, 38, 42, 44, 53, 56, 79, 82, 103, and 104.

permanent plexus injuries if athletic participation is continued.

Criteria for Return to Sports Play

Determining whether an athlete can safely return to a high-risk sport after sustaining a cervical spine injury is often a difficult decision. Until recently, criteria that outlined specific guidelines restricting athletes from participating in sports that place them at risk for a catastrophic event had not been well established. Torg[89] attributes this to two factors:

1. Our litigieous society (meaning "no" is the easiest response).

2. A dearth of credible data pertaining to postinjury risk factors.

In addition, the competitive spirit and personality of the athletes who nearly universally desire to return to sports tend to cloud the decision-making process.

As previously noted, the risk of catastrophic injury to the athlete is extremely low. The question remains: Which injury predisposes an athlete to a catastrophic event? White and associates provided biomechanical data on the stability of the adult cervical spine. Based on these data, the cervical spine is unstable or on the brink of instability if any of the following are present:

1. All the anterior or all the posterior elements are destroyed or unable to function.

2. More than 3.5 mm of horizontal displacement of one vertebra in relation to an adjacent caudal vertebrae is present.

3. More than 11 degrees of rotational difference between adjacent motion segments, cranial and caudal, is present.[108]

Torg and Glasgow have compiled criteria to serve as guidelines for athletes who have either sustained a cervical injury or have evidence of cervical-spine abnormalities.[87] These criteria may be used in their broadest form to determine whether an athlete should return to a high-risk sporting activity.

Absolute Contraindications

Congenital anomalies constitute a source of serious concern, particularly in the cranial cervical spine. Odontoid anomalies, such as odontoid agenesis, and atlantooccipital fusion fall into this category. A Type I Klippel-Feil lesion, entailing fusion of C2 to C3 with occipitalization of the atlas, is an absolute contraindication to participation. As the patient matures, the odontoid may become hypermobile, thus narrowing the spinal canal at this critical diameter. The Type II pattern, a long fusion with an abnormal occipital cervical junction, is also a contraindication. The poorly developed arch of C1 in this syndrome is frequently a source of symptoms as patients age; any acute stress could be catastrophic.

Developmental stenosis, as noted above, is no contraindication per se, even with documented episodes of neuropraxia. However, as Torg and Glasgow[87] note, the combination of development stenosis (vertebral body:canal ratio ≤ 0.08) and ligamentous instability, intervertebral disc disease, MRI evidence of cord defects or swelling, or positive neurologic findings, is a source of some concern. In this case, particularly with any suspicion of instability,[107,108] the athlete should not be permitted to play.

Relative Contraindications

Developmental stenosis with symptoms with a canal:vertebral ratio ≤ 0.08, and three episodes of neuropraxia or symptoms lasting 36 hours, should alert the physician to the possibility of significant cord injury.[42,87] Under these circumstances cervical MRI is recommended with determination of the functional reserve capacity, as noted above.

In the patient who has had previous trauma, the situation is less clear. Healed fractures of the odontoid, Type I and II, fall into this category, as do healed lateral mass fractures of C2 and the caudal cervical spine. In the case of the healed nondisplaced Jefferson fracture no firm recommendation can be made; the decision must be individualized. Likewise, a stable two- or three-level cervical fusion is not an absolute contraindication to play. However, keeping in mind the increased risk of injury to the segments cranial to the fusion, caution is advised when the proximal extent of the fusion involves C3 or C4.

No Contraindications

Spina bifida occulta, as well as developmental stenosis in the asymptomatic patient, are incidental findings at best. Stable compression fractures of the vertebral body without evidence of ligamentous instability by the criteria of White and associates[107,108] are likewise no contraindication to return to play once the fracture is healed. Additional fractures falling into this category are end-plate fractures without involvement of posterior ligamentous structures and healed clay-shoveler's fractures.

Healed intervertebral disc injury or healed anterior cervical discectomy and fusion at a single level are not contraindications. A stable single-level posterior fusion is likewise no contraindication to participation.

It must be emphasized, as noted above,[87] that these are guidelines. It is a particularly challenging decision for the physician to evaluate patients with relative contraindications. In these cases the goals and expectations of the athlete and pertinent family members must be assessed, as well as the potential of catastrophic injury should participation be resumed. Unfortunately, much of the information available on the natural history of these conditions is imprecise; in certain congenital conditions in which the natural history is known (such as Type II Klippel-Feil), the decision can be made with greater objective corroboration.

References

1. Albrand WO, Walton J: Underwater deceleration curves in relation to injuries from diving, *Surg Neurol* 4:461, 1975.
2. Albright JB and others: Head and neck injuries in college football: an eight-year analysis, *Am J Sports Med* 12(3):147, 1985.
3. Albright JB and others: Nonfatal cervical spine injuries in interscholastic football, *JAMA* 236:1243, 1976.
4. Allen BL and others: A mechanistic classification of closed, indirect fractures, and dislocations of the lower cervical spine, *Spine* 7:1, 1982.
5. The American Academy of Pediatrics: The Committee on Accident and Poison Prevention and Committee on Pediatric Aspects of Physical Fitness, Recreation, and Sports: trampoline II, *Pediatrics* 67:438, 1951.
6. The American Heart Association standards and guidelines for cardiopulmonary resuscitation and emergency care, *JAMA* 255:2841, 1986.
7. Andrish JT and others: A method for the management of cervical injuries in football: a preliminary report, *Am J Sports Med* 5(2):89, 1977.
8. Barnes R: Traction injuries of the brachial plexus in adults, *J Bone Joint Surg* 31B:10, 1949.
9. Bateman JE: Nerve injuries about the shoulder in sports, *J Bone Joint Surg* 49A:785, 1967.
10. Bauze RJ, Ardran GM: Experimental production of forward dislocation the human cervical spine, *J Bone Joint Surg* 60B:239, 1978.
11. Bixby-Hammett D, Brooxs WX: Common injuries in horseback riding: a review of United States Pony Clubs, Inc., *Sports Med* 9(1):36, 1990.
12. Bluce DA, Schut L, Sutton LM: Brain and cervical spine injuries occurring during organized sports activities in children and adolescents, *Primary Care* 11(1):175, 1984.
13. Blyth C, Arnold D: *The Forty-Seventh annual football fatality report*, Chapel Hill, NC, 1979, The American Football Coaches Association.
14. Bohlman, HH: Acute fractures and dislocations of the cervical spine: an analysis of three-hundred hospitalized patients and review of the literature, *J Bone Joint Surg* 61A:1119, 1979.
15. Boijsen E: Cervical spinal canal in intraspinal expansive processes, *Acta Radiol* 42:101, 1954.
16. Bracren MD and others: A randomized, controlled trial of methylprednisolone or raloxone in the treatment of acute spine cord injury, *N Engl J Med* 322:1405, 1990.
17. Burke DC, Berryman D: The place of closed manipulation in the management of flexion rotation dislocations of the cervical spine, *J Bone Joint Surg* 53B:165, 1971.
18. Burnstein AJ, Otis JC, Torg JS: *Mechanisms and pathomechanics of athletic injuries to the cervical spine.* In Torg JS, editor: *Athletic injuries to the head, neck, and face,* Philadelphia, 1982, Lea & Febiger, p 139.
19. Cantu RC: Head and spine injuries in the young athlete, *Clin Sports Med* 7(3):459, 1988.
20. Carter DR, Frankel VH: Biomechanics of hyperextension injuries to the cervical spine in football, *Am J Sports Med* 8:302, 1980.
21. Chrisman OD and others: Lateral-flexion neck injuries in athletic competition, *JAMA* 192(7):117, 1965.
22. Clancy WG: *Brachial plexus and upper extremity peripheral nerve injuries.* Reprint from *Athletic injuries to the head, neck, and face,* Philadelphia, 1982, Lea & Febiger, p 215.
23. Clarke KS: A study of sports-related spinal cord injuries in schools and colleges, 1973-1975, *J Safety Res* 9:140, 1977.
24. Clarke K: Survey of spinal cord injuries in schools and college sports, 1973-1975, *J Safety Res* 9:140, 1977.
25. Clarke K, Braslow A: Football fatalities in actuarial perspective, *Med Sci Sports* 10:94, 1979.
26. Clarke K, Powell J: Football helmets and neurotrauma—an epidemiological overview of three seasons, *Med Sci Sports* 11:138, 1979.
27. Crispin AR, Lees F: The spinal canal in cervical spondylosis, *J Neurol Neurosurg Psychiatry* 26:166, 1963.
28. Dillian L and others: Brachial neuritis, *J Bone Joint Surg* 67A:878, 1985.
29. Ducker TB and others: Timing of operative care in cervical spine cord injury, *Spine* 9:525, 1984.
30. Epstein JA and others: Myelopathy in cervical spondylosis with vertebral subluxation and hyperlordosis, *J Neurosurg* 32:421, 1970.
31. Epstein VS, Epstein JA, Jones MD: Cervical spinal stenosis, *Radiol Clin North Am* 15:215, 1977.
32. Fielding JW, Fietti VG, Mardam-Bey TH: Athletic injuries to the atlantoaxial articulation, *Am J Sports Med* 6(5):226, 1978.
33. Fielding JW and others: Tears of the transverse ligament of the atlas: a clinical and biomedical study, *J Bone Joint Surg* 56A:1683, 1974.
34. Funk FJ Jr, Wells RE: Injuries of the cervical spine in football, *Clin Orthop* 50, 1975.
35. Gerberich SG and others: An epidemiological study of high school ice hockey injuries, *Childs Nerv Syst* 3(2):59, 1987.

36. Herkowitz MD, Rothman RH: *Subacute instability of the cervical spine.* Presented at the Tenth Annual Meeting of the Cervical Spine Research Society, New York, December 1-4, 1982.

37. Herrick RT: Clay shoveler's fracture in power lifting, *Am J Sports Med* 9(1):29, 1981.

38. Hershman EB, Wilbourn AJ, Bergfeld JA: Acute brachial neuropathy in athletes, *Am J Sports Med* 17(5):655, 1989.

39. Herzog R: *Symposium on neck injuries in the athlete.* Presented at the Annual Meeting of the American College of Sports Medicine, Salt Lake City, 1980.

40. Herzog RJ and others: Normal cervical spine morphometry and cervical spinal stenosis in asymptomatic professional football players, *Spine* 16(6S): 178, 1991.

41. Hinck VS, Hopkins CE, Savara BS: Sagittal diameter of the cervical spinal canal in children, *Radiology* 79:97, 1962.

42. Hirasawa Y, Sakakida K: Sports and peripheral nerve injury, *Am J Sports Med* 11(6):420, 1983.

43. Hodgson VR: National Operating Committee on Standards for Athletic Equipment: football helmet certification program, *Med Sci Sports* 7:225, 1975.

44. Kawai H and others: Nerve repairs for traumatic brachial plexus palsy with root avulsion, *Clin Orthop* 237:75, 1988.

45. Kewalramani LS, Kraus JF: Acute spinal cord lesions from diving: epidemiological and clinical features, *West J Med* 126(5):353, 1977.

46. Ladd AL, Sacranton PE: Congenital cervical stenosis presenting as transient quadriplegia in athletes, *J Bone Joint Surg* 68A(9):1371, 1986.

47. Lehman LR, Ravich SJ: Closed head injuries in athletes, *Clin Sports Med* 9(2):247, 1990.

48. Levine AM: Cervical spine trauma, *AAOS Orthopaedic Knowledge Update 3,* 1990, p 395.

49. Lorentzon R, Wedren H, Pietila T: Incidence, nature and causes of ice hockey injuries: a three-year prospective study of a Swedish elite ice hockey team, *Am J Sports Med* 16(4):392, 1988.

50. Lorentzon R and others: Injuries in international ice hockey: a prospective, comparative study of injury incidence and injury types in international and Swedish elite ice hockey, *Am J Sports Med* 16(4):389, 1988.

51. Marks MR, Bell GR, Boumphrey FRS: Cervical spine fractures in athletes, *Clin Sports Med* 9:13, 1990.

52. Marron JC, Steele PB, Berlin R: Football head and neck injuries—an update, *Clin Neurosurg* 27:414, 1980.

53. McCann PD, Bindelglass DF: The brachial plexus, *Orthop Rev* 20(5):413, 1991.

54. McCoy GF and others: Injuries of the cervical spine in schoolboy rugby football, *J Bone Joint Surg* 66B(4):500, 1984.

55. McElhaney J and others: *Biomechanical analysis of swimming pool neck injuries.* In *The human neck: Anatomy, injury mechanisms, and biomechanics,* Warrendale, PA 1979, Society of Automotive Engineers, p 47.

56. Millesi H: Brachial plexus lesions, *Operative Orthop* 2:1417, 1988.

57. Moiel RH, Raso E, Waltz TA: Central cord syndrome resulting from congenital narrowing of the cervical spinal canal, *J Trauma* 10:502, 1970.

58. Norrel H: Treatment of unstable spinal fractures and dislocations, *Clin Neurosurg* 25:193, 1970.

59. Norton WL: Fractures and dislocations of the cervical spine, *J Bone Joint Surg* 44A:115, 1962.

60. Nuber GW, Shaffer MF: Clay shoveler's injuries, *Am J Sports Med* 15(2):182, 1987.

61. O'Brien PJ, Schweigel JF, Thompson WJ: Dislocations of the lower cervical spine, *J Trauma* 22:710, 1982.

62. Paley D, Gillespie G: Chronic repetitive unrecognized flexion injury of the cervical spine (high jumpers' neck), *Am J Sports Med* 14(1):92, 1986.

63. Panjabi MM and others: Multidirectional instability of traumatic cervical spine injuries in porcine model, *Spine* 14:1111, 1989.

64. Pavlov H, Torg JS: Roentgen examination of cervical spine injuries in athletes, *Clin Sports Med* 6(4):751, 1987.

65. Pavlov H and others: Cervical spinal stenosis: determination with vertebral body ratio method, *Radiology* 164:771, 1987.

66. Payne EE, Spillane JD: The cervical spine: an anatomico-pathological study of seventy specimens with particular reference to the problems of cervical spondylosis, *Brain* 80:571, 1957.

67. Rapp GF, Nicely PG: Trampoline injuries, *Am J Sports Med* 6:269, 1978.

68. Raynor RB, Complik B: Cervical cord trauma: the relationship between clinical syndromes and force of injury, *Spine* 10(3):193, 1985.

69. Roaf R: A study of the mechanics of spinal injuries, *J Bone Joint Surg* 42B:810, 1960.

70. Sches AT: Rugby injuries of the spine and spinal cord, *Clin Sports Med* 6(1):87, 1987.

71. Sches AT: Verlex impact and cervical dislocation in rugby players, *S Afr Med J* 59:227, 1981.

72. Schneider R: Serious and fatal neurosurgical football injuries, *Clin Neurosurg* 12:226, 1965.

73. Schenider RC, Kriss FC: Decisions concerning cervical concussions in football players, *Med Sci Sports* 1:115, 1969.

74. Schenider RC and others: Vascular insufficiency and differential distortion of brain and cervical caused by cervicomedullary football injuries, *J Neurosurg* 33:363, 1970.

75. Schenider RD and others: Serious football injuries involving the head and spinal cord, *JAMA* 177:362, 1961.

76. Shields C, Fox J, Stauffer E: Cervical cord injuries in sports, *Phys Sports Med* 6:21, 1978.

77. Snook GA: Head and neck injuries in contact sports, *Med Sci Sports* 1:117, 1969.

78. Sovio OM, Van Peteghem PK, Schweigel JF: Cervical spine injuries in rugby players, *Can Med Assoc J* 130:735, 1984.

79. Speer KP, Bassett FH: The prolonged burner syndrome, *Am J Sports Med* 18(6):591, 1990.

80. Spence DF, Becker S, Sell KW: Bursting atlantal fracture associated with rupture of the transverse ligament, *J Bone Joint Surg* 52A:543, 1970.

81. Steinbruck K, Paeslack V: Analysis of 139 spinal cord injuries due to accidents in water sports, *Paraplegia* 18(2):86, 1980.

82. Sugioka H: Evoked potentials in the investigation of traumatic lesions of the peripheral nerve and the brachial plexus, *Clin Orthop* 184:85, 1984.

83. Tator CH: National survey of spinal injuries in hockey players, *Can Med Assoc J* 130:875, 1984.

84. Tator CH: Neck injuries in ice hockey: a recent unresolved problem with many contributing factors, *Clin Sports Med* 6:101, 1987.

85. Tator CH, Edmunds VE, New ML: Diving: a frequent and potentially preventable cause of spinal cord injury, *Can Med Assoc J* 124:1323, 1981.

86. Taylor TK, Coolican MR: Spinal cord injuries in Australian football, 1960-1985, *Med J Aust* 147(3):112, 116:118, 1987.

87. Torg JS, editor: *Athletic injuries to the head, neck and face,* St. Louis, 1991, Mosby, p 589.

88. Torg JS: Epidemiology, pathomechanics, and prevention of athletic injuries to the cervical spine, *Med Sci Sports Exer* 17(3):295, 1985.

89. Torg JS: Management guidelines for athletic injuries to the cervical spine, *Clin Sports Med* 6:53, 1987.

90. Torg JS: Severe and catastrophic neck injuries resulting from tackle football, *College Health* 25:224, 1977.

91. Torg JS: Trampoline-induced quadriplegia, *Clin Sports Med* 6:73, 1987.

92. Torg JS, Das M: Trampoline-related quadriplegia: review of the literature and reflections on the American Academy of Pediatrics position statement, *Pediatrics* 74(5):804, 1984.

93. Torg JS, Gennarelli TA: *Head and neck injury.* In Grana W, Kalenak A, editors: *Clinical sports medicine,* Philadelphia, 1991, W.B. Saunders.

94. Torg JS and others: The axial load teardrop fracture, *Am J Sports Med* 19(4):355, 1991.

95. Torg JS and others: Axial loading injuries to the middle cervical spine segment, *Am J Sports Med* 19(1):6, 1991.

96. Torg JS and others: The National Football Head and Neck Injury Registry, *JAMA* 254(24):3439, 1985.

97. Torg JS and others: National Football Head and Neck Injury Registry: Report on Cervical Quadriplegia, 1971-1975, *Am J Sports Med* 7:127, 1979.

98. Torg JS and others: The National Football Head and Neck Injury Registry—Report and Conclusions, 1978, *JAMA* 241:1477, 1979.

99. Torg JS and others: Neuropraxia of the cervical spinal cord with transient quadriplegia, *J Bone Joint Surg* 68A(9):1354, 1986.

100. Torg JS and others: *The relationship of cervical spinal canal narrowing to permanent neurologic injury to the athlete: an epidemiologic survey.* Presented at the Seventeenth Annual Meeting of Cervical Spine Research Society, December, 1989.

101. Torg JS and others: Spinal injury at the level of the third and fourth cervical vertebra from football, *J Bone Joint Surg* 19A:1015, 1977.

102. Vegso JJ, Lehman RC: Field evaluation and management of head and neck injuries, *Clin Sports Med* 6(1):1, 1987.

103. Vegso JJ and others: Rehabilitation of cervical spine brachial plexus and peripheral nerve injuries, *Clin Sports Med* 6(1):135, 1987.

104. Vereschagin KS and others: Burners—don't overlook or underestimate them, *Phys Sports Med* 19(9):96, 1991.

105. Virgin H: Cineradiographic study of football helmets and the cervical spine, *Am J Sports Med* 8(5):310, 1980.

106. Watkins RG: Neck injuries in football players, *Clin Sports Med* 5(2):215, 1986.

107. White AA, Panjabi MM: Update on the evaluation of instability of the lower cervical spine, *AAOS, ICLV* 36:513, 1987.

108. White AA and others: Biomechanical analysis of clinical stability in the cervical spine, *Clin Orthop* 109:85, 1975.

109. Wilkinson HA, LeMay ML, Ferriss EJ: Roentgenographic correlation in cervical spondylosis, *Am J Radiol* 105:380, 1969.

110. Wolf BS, Khilnani M, Malis L: Sagittal diameter of the bony cervical canal and significant in cervical spondylosis, *J Mt Sinai Hosp* 23:283, 1956.

111. Wroble RR, Albright JP: Neck and low back injuries in wrestling, *Clin Sports Med* 5(2):295, 1986.

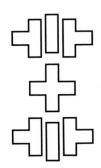

PART VII

Tumor, Trauma, Infection, Deformity, and Other Conditions

Section 1
Tumors

103   Surgical Treatment of Spinal Tumors

P. James Nugent

Chapter 103
Surgical Treatment of Spinal Tumors

P. James Nugent

History

benign primary bone tumors
malignant primary bone tumors
metastatic bone tumors

Presentation

investigations

Diagnostic Decision Making

Technique

biopsy
general surgical principles and
    recommendations
anterior cervical spine
posterior cervical spine
anterior thoracic spine
posterior thoracic spine
anterior lumbar spine
posterior lumbar spine
anterior sacral spine
posterior sacrum

Complications and Alternatives

Future Considerations

History

Surgical treatment of spinal tumors has seen significant advances over the past 40 years. Previously, spine tumors were considered unresectable and surgical goals were limited to posterior decompression of the neural elements. There was significant morbidity with anterior approaches, and the results of surgical intervention for spinal tumors was disappointing.*

However, current imaging techniques such as high-resolution MRI and CT reconstructions today allow surgeons to discern the precise location and amount of destruction. This allows rational decisions regarding the approach that would allow greater exposure for debridement or resection of the tumor and reconstruction of the spine. Rigid anterior and posterior spinal instrumentation allows reconstruction of a variety of complex spinal conditions. Along with increased knowledge of spinal biomechanics, the spinal surgeon of the 1990s has an opportunity to intercede beneficially in most patients with spinal tumors.

There also have been significant advances in oncology. Seventy percent of patients with primary malignancies will develop skeletal metastasis. Effective chemotherapy and radiation therapy to both systemic and local disease allow many more patients with spine tumors to be considered for spinal surgery. Because of the oncologist's ability to prolong life, surgical relief of pain, correction or prevention of deformity, and decompression of the neural elements may prove more fruitful for selected individuals than ever before.

En bloc resection of primary tumors of the spine with effective oncologic management may offer surgical cures of otherwise lethal conditions. Aggressive surgical treatment in patients with neural compression has been shown to result in marked neurologic improvement in 71% to 93% of patients with surgical decompression.[20,22,25] The recognition of improvement in neural function following decompression has stimulated a new wave of aggressive surgical treatment of spinal tumors.

Tumors of the spine are classified as primary—originating in the spine, or secondary—originating elsewhere in the body and metastasizing to the spine (see box). Primary tumors may be benign or malignant. Secondary, or metastatic, tumors are malignant by virtue of their spread to the spine from a distant source.

* References 1, 4, 13, 18, 19, 25, 27, 28, 41 and 42.

Tumors of the Spine

Benign Primary Bone Tumors

Osteochondroma

Osteoid osteoma

Osteoblastoma

Aneurysmal bone cyst

Hemangioma

Giant-cell tumor

Eosinophilic granuloma

Lipoma

Malignant Primary Bone Tumors

Multiple myeloma

Osteosarcoma

Ewing's sarcoma

Chordoma

Chondrosarcoma

Metastatic Bone Tumors

Breast

Lung

Lymph system

Prostate

Kidney

Thyroid

Gastrointestinal tract

Benign Primary Bone Tumors

Primary bone tumors of the spine are rare, accounting for 0.04% of all tumors.[8] Approximately 7% of patients with *osteochondromas* will have involvement of the spine, and 80% of these are located in the cervical and upper thoracic region.[6,17,24,34] The bony contour of the lesion may be visualized with plain radiographs, tomography, or CT scans, but the growing cartilaginous cap is best demonstrated with MRI or myelography. The lesions are slow growing and most remain asymptomatic. Neural compression is rare,[23] but because of the location in the spine and slow progressive compression on the cervical or thoracic cord, this benign tumor may have catastrophic effects if left untreated. Excision of the tumor leads to good neurologic recovery in nearly 90% of patients with impairment.[24]

Twenty-five percent of patients with *osteoid osteoma* and 41% of patients with *osteoblastoma* will have spinal involvement. Both of these lesions usually involve the posterior elements. Patients present in their second or third decade of life with complaints of back pain unrelated to activity, more noticeable at night, and typically relieved with aspirin. The distinction between these two entities is their size. By definition an osteoid osteoma is less than 2 cm in diameter. The smaller osteoid osteoma may not be apparent on plain radiographs, whereas a large osteoblastoma may show considerable expansile mass. Typically, there is an expansion of cortical bone and a thin rim of reactive bone interposed between the lesion and soft tissue. Technetium-99 MDP scans are a sensitive method of localizing the lesion. Thin-cut high-resolution CT imaging demonstrates the lesion very well.

Aneurysmal bone cysts involve the posterior elements in 60% of cases and are typically found in the lumbar spine. The name is taken from its radiographic appearance—an aneurysmal expansion with an osteolytic cavity. Treatment consists of excision if possible. Curretage alone results in a 13% recurrence rate, but recurrences can be treated appropriately with a second curretage.[16]

Hemangiomas of the spine are common. Approximately 10% of the population have hemangiomas of the spine. They typically involve the anterior vertebral body. They are benign vascular lesions of rare clinical significance. The diagnosis is usually made incidentally on plain radiographs. Classically, vertical striations are noted secondary to abnormally thickened trabeculae. In the rare cases where treatment is necessary for relief of pain or neural compression, most lesions respond to radiotherapy alone. If surgical intervention is contemplated a preoperative embolization should be performed to decrease blood loss during surgery.

Giant-cell tumors are slow-growing neoplasms that typically occur in the anterior vertebral body when they involve the spine.[43] They cause considerable morbidity by their locally aggressive nature and preponderance to recur if not totally excised. Radiographically there is a region of lysis that may thin and expand through the cortex. CT and MRI scans demonstrate the amount of bone destruction and degree of soft-tissue involvement, respectively. En bloc resection is the best procedure. This entails an anterior approach and vertebrectomy (possibly two or three consecutive vertebrectomies if necessary) to appropriately extricate all the tumor cells. Curretage and local chemolysis of cryolysis is frought with recurrence.[9,40] Appropriate reconstruction of the spine is required after the vertebrectomies to pro-

vide stability and allow postoperative mobilization. Different reconstructive procedures are described later in this chapter.

Malignant Primary Bone Tumors

Multiple myeloma is the most common primary malignant neoplasm of bone. The incidence is between 2 to 3 cases per 100,000 people. Historically the prognosis for multiple myeloma was poor, with a 5-year survival rate of 18%. Aggressive chemotherapy may improve the prognosis today. Plasmacytoma may be considered a solitary region of myeloma and carries an improved prognosis. Radiation is the procedure of choice for painful lesions without evidence of spinal-cord compression or instability. Surgical decompression and reconstruction are indicated when there is significant neural compression or instability. The surgical technique is described later in this chapter.

Osteosarcoma of the spine is rare. Involvement of the spine accounts for 2% of all osteogenic sarcomas. Osteosarcoma may be associated with Paget's disease or prior radiation of a different tumor. Delay in diagnosis and inability to perform en bloc resection leads to a poor prognosis. The median survival ranges between 6 and 10 months.[2,31] Cure of these lesions relies on aggressive wide surgical excision and associated radiotherapy and chemotherapy.[36,49] There are no long-term reports on aggressive treatment of these lesions.

Ewing's sarcoma of the spine is usually found in the sacrum but occasionally in the anterior vertebral bodies. The prognosis is generally poor. Multiagent chemotherapy and radiotherapy are the treatments of choice. Surgical decompression and stabilization are indicated if there is significant neural compression or instability.

Chordoma is a rare, slow-growing tumor. It is locally invasive and rarely metastasizes. It arises in the midline of the spine from remnants of the notochord, most commonly in the sacrum. Cure of the lesion depends on surgical en bloc extirpation. Complete sacrococcyxectomy with sacrifice of the sacral nerve roots is typically necessary. If the S2 nerve roots can be spared there is surprisingly little morbidity. Recurrence is a poor prognostic sign and survival is related to local control of recurrence.

Chondrosarcomas are slow-growing malignant tumors that involve the spine 10% of the time. Radiographically, they are radiolucent lesions with calcifications of the soft-tissue mass. CT and MRI scans are necessary to determine the extent of the lesion. They are resistant to radiotherapy and chemotherapy. A complete surgical excision is necessary for cure.[35] Reconstruction is necessary to provide adequate stability. Local recurrence is a poor prognostic sign.

Metastatic Bone Tumors

Metastatic disease is the most common tumor encountered in the spine. There are approximately one million new cases of cancer each year, and it is estimated that 50% of these patients will develop spinal metastasis.[12] As with the appendicular skeleton, the usual sources of primary tumors are breast, lung, lymph system, prostate, kidney, thyroid, and gastrointestinal tract. The vertebral body is most commonly involved. A careful history corroborated by a thorough physical examination often leads to a diagnosis of the primary lesion.

There are two routes that the cancerous emboli may metastasize to reach the spine. First, the tumor cells may be spread hematogenously, and after filtering through the lung will be distributed throughout the arterial system. The rich vascular network of the cancellous vertebral body acts as a filter and enlodgement is possible. Second, the tumor cells may traverse the paravertebral venous plexus directly. Batson is credited with describing this venous plexus, which has been shown to have bidirectional blood flow dependent on the intraabdominal pressure.[3] Cells from the breast may be carried directly into the thoracic vertebrae and cells from the prostate or lower gastrointestinal tract may pass directly to the lumbar vertebrae. Because of the rich nutrient supply the vertebral body appears to accommodate metastatic tumors and this may explain their predominance for sites of metastatic disease.

The approach and reconstructive procedure are based on the location of the tumor, extent of involvement, presence of neural compression, and associated systemic or localized metabolic bone disease (typically osteoporosis). Not at issue is whether the tumor is benign or malignant, or primary or metastatic.

The primary goals of surgical treatment of spinal tumors are to relieve pain; to decompress the neural elements, if necessary; and to prevent or correct deformity. These goals are palliative in diffuse metastatic disease. En bloc resection may provide surgical cure in well-localized benign or malignant lesions of the spine.[37]

Rigid stabilization allows immediate postoperative mobilization and reduces the risk of postoperative complications. Rigid stabilization will significantly relieve pain in most patients affected with spinal tumors. However, patients with metastatic disease may continue to have pain from other areas of involvement and may require high dose narcotics for pain relief.[22]

Kostuik and Errico have conceptualized the stability of the spine affected with tumor by dividing the spine, via CT scans, into six columns.[22] Instability is defined as involvement of three or more of these columns. Surgical reconstruction is then recommended.

Presentation

Patients may present with back pain (85%), radicular pain symptoms (20%), or cord or cauda equina compression (8-14%)[14,32,33] or they may be asymptomatic (2.5%).[39] The latter are usually noted on a bone scan during metastatic work-up.

The etiology of the pain varies and may result as one of the following: an expansion of the tumor perforating the cortex and irritating the periosteum; pain from secondary compression fractures; deformity with associated mascular spasm; or acute or chronic neural compression. Localized back pain is the most common presenting symptom in patients with neoplasias of the spine. Pain at rest and night pain are common.

Generally, patients under the age of 21 will have benign lesions of the spine and patients over 21 will have malignant lesions.[39] Also, typically, posterior lesions are benign and anterior lesions are malignant.[39]

Investigations

Plain radiographs give considerable information. Although 30% to 50% of the bone must be destroyed before plain radiographs are sensitive, certain radiographic features help distinguish the character of the tumor. Slow-growing benign tumors typically have a response from the surrounding bone such as a sclerotic rim (Fig. 103-1). Aggressive malignant tumors appear moth-eaten or show permeative destruction (Fig. 103-2). The loss of one pedicle on the anteroposterior (AP) view of the spine is termed the "winking owl" sign and indicates significant bony destruction of the pedicle, typically from an anterior mass that has spread into the pedicle (Fig. 103-3). Vertebral collapse with longstanding destruction of the body also is common. A presumptive diagnosis of lesions such as hemangioma, aneurysmal bone cyst, osteoblastoma, or giant-cell tumor may be made on plain radiographs.

Technetium 99 bone scans are sensitive but not specific for neoplastic disease. The extent of dissem-

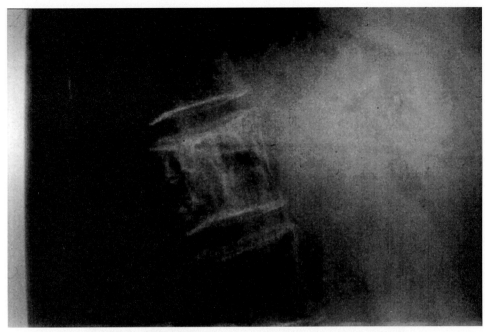

Fig. 103-1
Benign hemangioma of the thoracic spine.

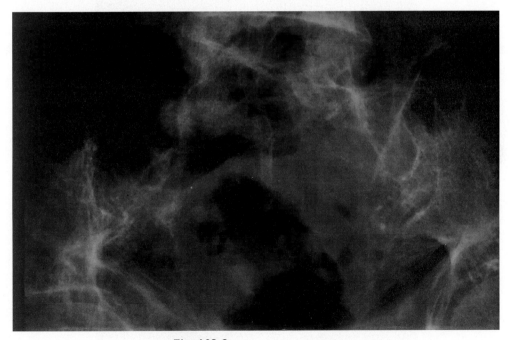

Fig. 103-2
Malignant lymphoma of the sacrum.

ination is easily recognized but isolated lesions may be overread. Fracture, infection, or any inflammatory process will create a focal uptake of the nucleotide.

CT scans are very specific for changes in bone mineralization. They demonstrate bony involvement, both trabecular and cortical, earlier than plain radiographs (Fig. 103-4). Because CT and radiog-

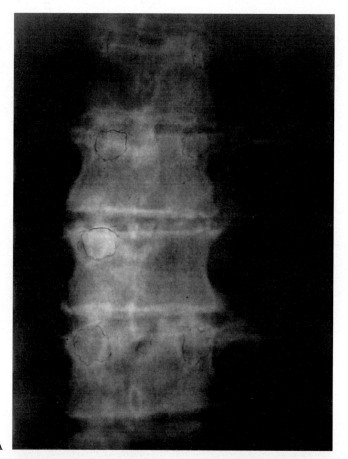

A

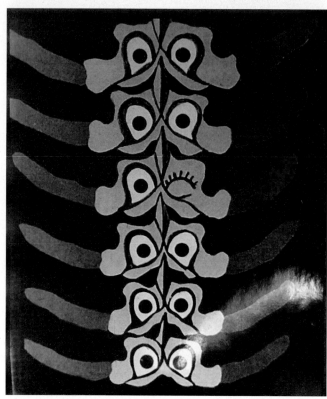

B

Fig. 103-3

A and **B,** The tumor has destroyed the pedicle and the radiographic finding resembles a "winking owl," as shown in **B.**

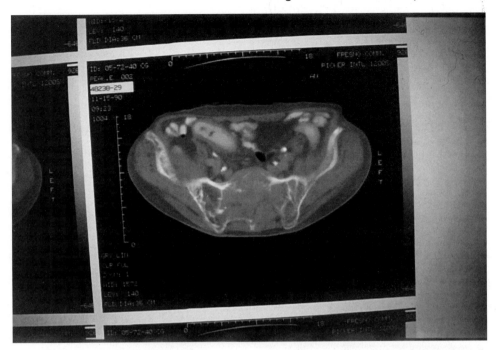

Fig. 103-4

CT image of sacrum destroyed by lymphoma.

raphy image the bone, they are superior to other modalities for demonstrating the degree of bony destruction and assessing spinal stability. CT reconstructions may be of value in assessing the degree of destruction.

MRI scans are now standard for tumor evaluation in the spine. Imaging of the soft tissues is possible with MRI; therefore, the extent of tumor involvement can be assessed (Fig. 103-5). However, it must be recognized that MRI scans underestimate the degree of bony involvement. Therefore, CT and MRI scans complement each other in the evaluation of spinal tumors. The degree of neural compromise and extent of compression is best visualized with sagittal MRI scans. Myelogram followed by CT is another good way of evaluating the degree of neural compression.

Differential white blood cell count, eryththrocyte sedimentation rate, liver function tests, and coagulation times are essential to rule out infection and evaluate the liver for altered function.

Angiography and embolization are recommended for vascular tumors such as metastatic renal cell (Fig. 103-6). In our experience surgeries for renal cell carcinoma that were not embolized had to be terminated prematurely because of bleeding. Following appropriate embolization, a second decompressive and stabilization procedure was completed successfully.[21]

Diagnostic Decision Making

The decision to provide surgical treatment to patients with tumors of the spine should always be individualized to each patient. Generally, patients with 6 weeks of expected longevity will benefit from surgical treatment. Relief of pain from debulking the tumor and stabilizing the spine is a foremost indication. It is worthwhile in any patient who will medically tolerate the surgical morbidity. Decompression of the neural elements in the face of neurologic demise is also an indication. Evidence of instability or impending pathologic fracture is also an indication for surgery.

Although all patients with metastatic disease to the spine will die, to die paraparetic, especially with loss of visceral control, is to die without dignity.

An expeditious work-up with radiographs, CT reconstructions, and MRI scans will enable the surgeon to identify the area of the vertebral column involved. Surgical intervention should primarily address the area involved with tumor. For example, when the tumor is located in the anterior body, as it is in 66% of spinal tumors,[38] then the surgical approach, debulking, decompression, and reconstruction should be from the front. Conversely, when the tumor is primarily in the posterior elements, then the approach, debulking, decompression, and reconstruction should be from the back.

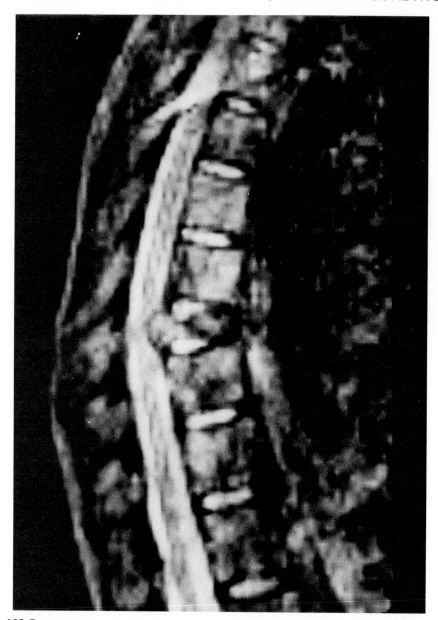

Fig. 103-5

MR image of anterior spinal tumor. (*From Kostuik JP, Weinstein JN:* Differential diagnosis and surgical treatment of metastatic spine tumors. *In Frymoyer JW, editor:* The adult spine: principles and practice, *New York, 1991, Raven Press.*)

A circumferential reconstruction, either at the same setting or delayed, may be indicated if there is evidence of instability after reconstruction from only one side.

The decision to reconstruct the spine with metal-reinforced polymethylmethacrylate (PMMA) or bone graft is not controversial at the present time. Benign tumors with confident surgical excision may be reconstructed with bone graft. Autogenous bone graft is always preferable to allograft bone. Contrarily, metal-reinforced PMMA is the construct of choice in all other cases. PMMA alone does not withstand the forces of the spine under physiologic loads and has been noted to fail in the early and late follow-up periods.[26] As a cement that resists compression, PMMA has poor torsional and tensile properties. However, reinforcing the cement with metal rods strengthens the composite in all planes of force.

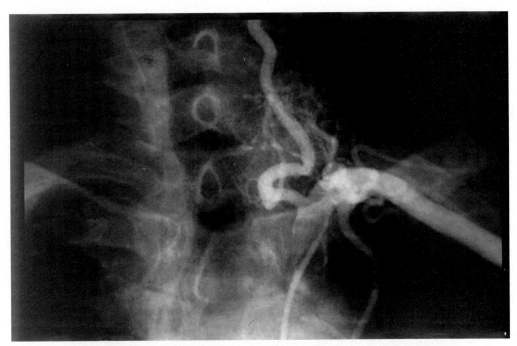

Fig. 103-6

Metastatic renal-cell carcinoma of the upper thoracic spine is extremely vascular.

This construct is quick, so that the surgical time is decreased (no need for autogenous bone graft harvesting), as is blood loss. The cement fills in the cavities of the cancellous bone and decreases blood loss as well. The construct is immediately stable and allows patients to become mobile immediately.

The composite can be used in the cervical, thoracic, and lumbar spines through an anterior approach (Figs. 103-7, 103-8, and 103-9). This approach decreases the risk of postoperative complications. There are several reports of reconstruction with PMMA of the spine anteriorly.* Iliac bone graft augmentation has been recommended for long-term stability.[26] Because the average longevity in a series of 100 patients with metastatic spine disease was 11 months, and ranged between 1 and 48 months,[20] augmentation has not been necessary in my experience.

Significant return of neurologic function is increased with the use of an anterior approach when the offending tumor is anterior and causing anterior compression.[22] Seventy-one percent of patients had meaningful return of neurologic function following anterior decompression in my experience.[22]

*References 5, 7, 11, 15, and 29 to 30.

Technique

Biopsy

Percutaneous biopsy of tumors at all levels of the spine may be performed effectively with fluoroscopic assistance. Obtaining adequate tissue may be a problem with this technique, and definitive open biopsy with simultaneous debulking and reconstruction may be a better alternative. The procedure is performed in the operating room, which encourages sterile technique, and allows for assistance and the opportunity to deal with complications expeditiously if necessary. Intravenous access is obtained in each patient for sedation if necessary.

Odontoid lesions may be biopsied transorally. The procedure is identical to the transoral approach described later. Lesions of the C2 body may be biopsied directly anterior through the midline of the pharynx. Anterior lesions of the lower cervical spine are biopsied from the common anterior lateral direction.

For anterior cervical lesions the patient is placed supine. A surgical roll is placed between the upper scapulae, and the neck is prepped in a sterile fashion. Local anesthetic is infiltrated into the skin and soft tissues. The landmarks are identified, but the

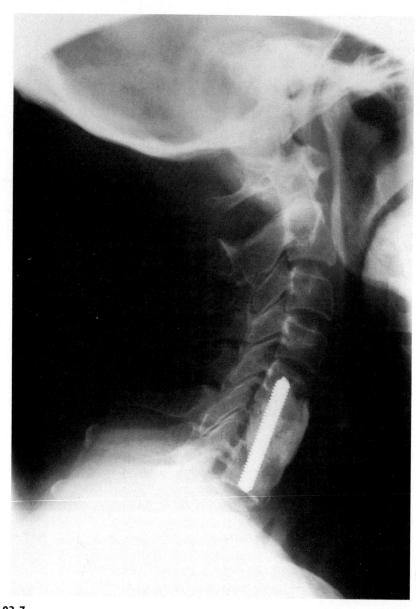

Fig. 103-7

PMMA reconstruction of cervical region. (*From Kostuik JP, Weinstein JN:* Differential diagnosis and surgical treatment of metastatic spine tumors. *In Frymoyer JW, editor:* The adult spine: principles and practice, *New York, 1991, Raven Press.*)

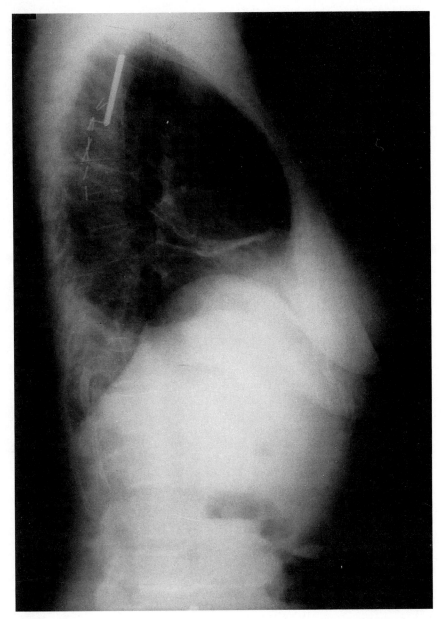

Fig. 103-8

PMMA reconstruction of thoracic region. (*From Kostuik JP, Weinstein JN:* Differential diagnosis and surgical treatment of metastatic spine tumors. *In Frymoyer JW, editor:* The adult spine: principles and practice, *New York, 1991, Raven Press.*)

level is verified with intraoperative fluoroscopy. A large-bore 16-gauge needle is used to reach the body. A smooth Steinman pin is directed into the body to be biopsied in the lower cervical spine, and after fluoroscopic confirmation, a cutting hollow cylinder, such as a Craig needle, is passed over the Steinman pin and into the lesion (Fig. 103-10).

Anterior lesions of the thoracic and lumbar spine are biopsied from a posterolateral portal on the left side. With the patient in the lateral decubitus position, the skin is anesthetized 8 to 10 cm (a handbreadth) from the midline and a Seinman pin is directed at a 60 degree angle into the vertebral body of interest. A toothed trochar, such as a Craig needle, is introduced over the Steinman pin into the body. Multiple specimens may be obtained in this fashion. Intravenous sedation is helpful but not necessary. Neurologic status can be assessed during the procedure while it is performed under local anesthesia. Chest radiographs should be obtained after the procedure when thoracic levels are biopsied. Small pneumothoraces are not uncommon. A 16-gauge angiocath may be introduced into the fifth intercostal space anteriorly and the free air removed. If there is a persistent air leak, a chest tube is necessary.

Biopsy of anterior sacral lesions also can be performed from a posterolateral direction. The patient may be in the lateral or prone position. Oblique orientation of the fluoroscopic C-arm will identify the sacral foramina to be avoided.

Posterior lesions of the cervical, thoracic, lumbar, sacral, and coccygeal spine can be biopsied directly posteriorly with fluoroscopic guidance.

General Surgical Principles and Recommendations

The surgical approaches to the cervical, thoracic, lumbar, and sacral regions are diagrammed in Figs. 103-11, 103-12, 103-13, and 103-14. Several aspects of surgery are applicable to all regions and are addressed here. Incisions should be ample. Consideration for exposure should outweigh cosmesis. Systematic meticulous exposure aids in visualization, reduces blood loss, and allows easier debulking and reconstruction. There is no substitute for excellent assistant surgeons during the procedure. Competent surgical nurses with knowledge of the procedure, instruments, and hardware are essential. Red-blood-cell saving devices are not used because of the risk of spreading tumor cells throughout the body. Spinal cord monitoring is recommended in all procedures in which the cord or nerve roots are to be exposed or manipulated.

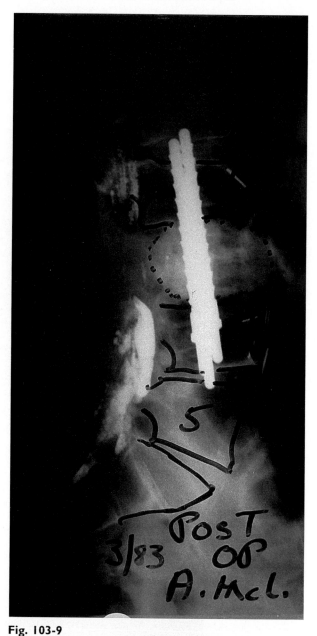

Fig. 103-9

PMMA reconstruction of lumbar region. (*From Kostuik JP, Weinstein JN:* Differential diagnosis and surgical treatment of metastatic spine tumors. *In Freymoyer JW, editor:* The adult spine: principles and practice, *New York, 1991, Raven Press.*)

Preoperative angiography and embolization are recommended in vascular tumors such as metastatic renal cell carcinoma. This will also identify the artery of Adamkawitz in lower thoracic lesions. The artery of Adamkawitz is credited with supplying the watershed of the thoracic spine. For practical purposes, it is of no consequence and its sacrifice may be necessary for exposure. In my experience this has not lead to untoward neurologic complications.

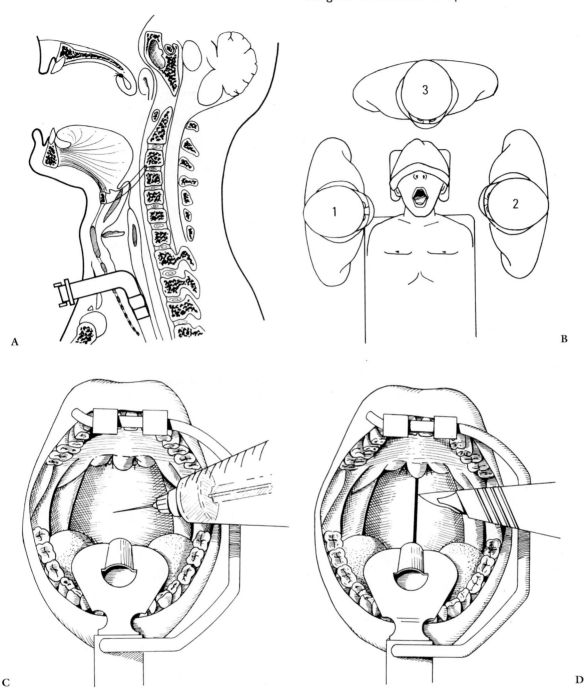

Fig. 103-10

Transoral approach to C1 and odontoid. **A,** Anatomical study in the sagittal plane. The position of the upper cervical spine in relation to the pharynx is shown. The depth of the transoral approach is obvious, as is the need to retract the uvula during the approach. A tracheostomy has been made. **B,** The anesthetic machines are situated at the feet of the patient, thus freeing the whole of the operative field. The operator (1) is at the right side of the patient. The first assistant (2) is at the left. A possible second assistant is at the head of the patient (3). **C,** The mouth is held open by a self-retaining retractor with a tongue depressor. The soft palate can either be retracted by a retractor or by suturing its free border along with the uvula to the palate. The posterior wall of the pharynx is then infiltrated with local anesthetic combined with adrenaline. **D,** The incision in the posterior pharyngeal wall is made with a scalpel from the tubercle of the atlas to the prominence of the C2-C3 disc.

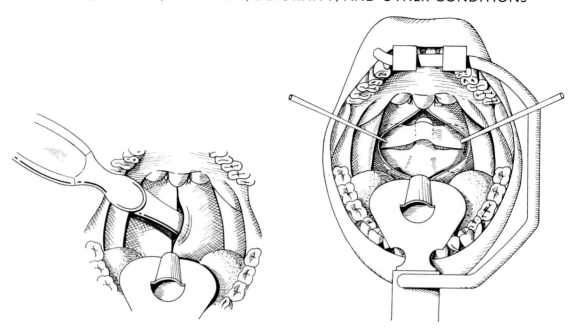

E   F

Fig. 103-10, cont'd

E, The anterior surfaces of the atlas and axis are dissected laterally using an elevator. **F,** The margins of the incision are retracted laterally by Kirschner pins placed in the lateral masses of the atlas and axis. The approach is direct, deep, and narrow. *(From Roy-Camille R, Mazel C: Surgical exposures and procedures. In Laurin CA, Riley LH Jr, Roy-Camille R, editors:* Atlas of orthopaedic surgery, *vol 1, General principles and spine, Masson, 1989, Paris.)*

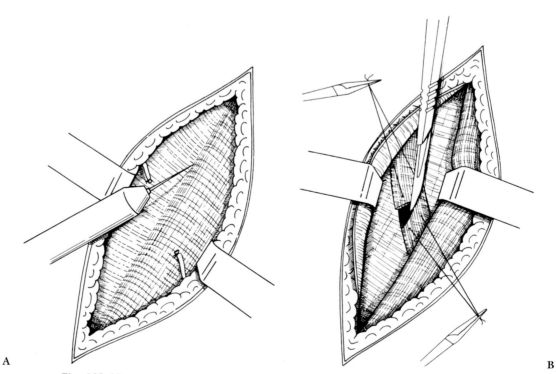

A   B

Fig. 103-11

Anterior approach to the sternomastoid spine. **A,** The skin and platysma are incised. **B,** Division of the omohyoid muscle is only needed in approaches to C5, C6, and C7. The anterior border of the sternomastoid is the guide to the dissection.

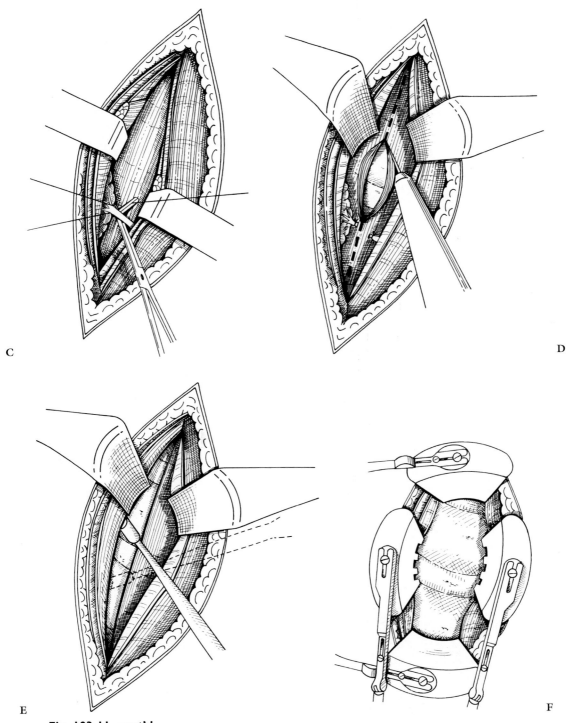

C

D

E

F

Fig. 103-11, cont'd

C, Ligation of the inferior thyroid vessels. **D,** Incision of the anterior longitudinal ligament with cutting diathermy between the longus colli muscles. **E,** Subperiosteal dissection is easy on the anterior and lateral surfaces of the vertebral bodies but is more difficult over the discs. **F,** A Cloward self-retaining retractor has been positioned. (*From Roy-Camille R, Mazel C: Surgical exposures and procedures. In Laurin CA, Riley LH Jr, Roy-Camille R, editors: Atlas of orthopaedic surgery, vol 1, General principles and spine, Masson, 1989, Paris.*)

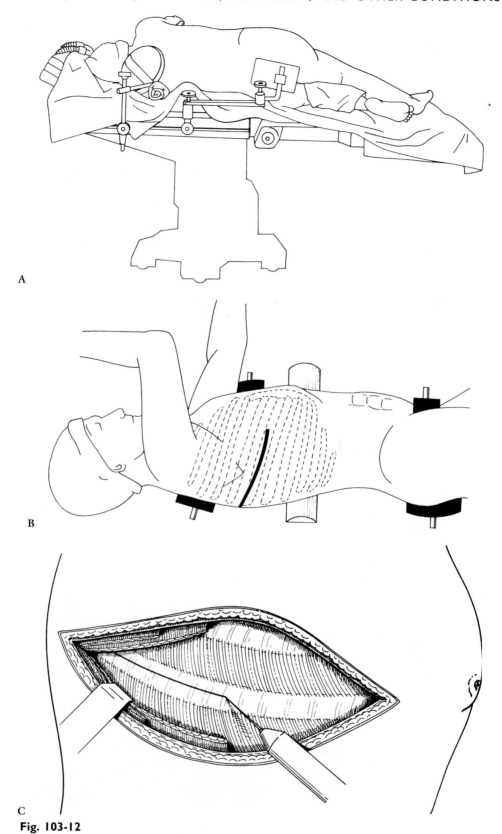

Fig. 103-12

Transpleural thoracotomy approach to the anterior thoracic spine. **A,** Lateral position of the patient on the table. **B,** Incision made along the rib that lies two levels above the vertebra to be reached. **C,** Division of muscle and periosteum with cutting diathermy.

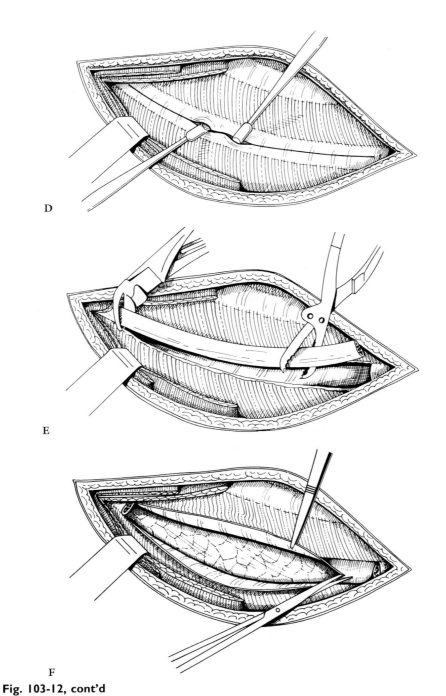

Fig. 103-12, cont'd

D, The rib is dissected subperiosteally. **E,** Resection of the rib is not essential but is mandatory in adults with a rigid thorax. **F,** Opening of the pleura is made in the bed of the rib.

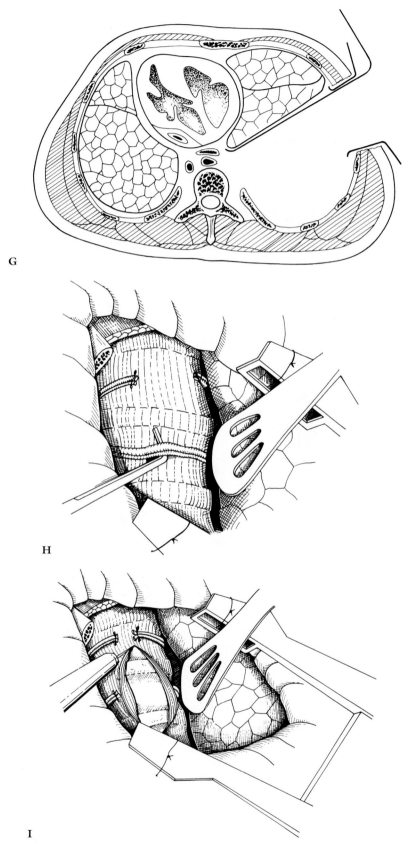

Fig. 103-12, cont'd

G, With the lung retracted, the spine is visualized. H, Ligation of the vascular pedicles. I, The periosteum is incised with cutting diathermy after ligation of the vascular pedicles.

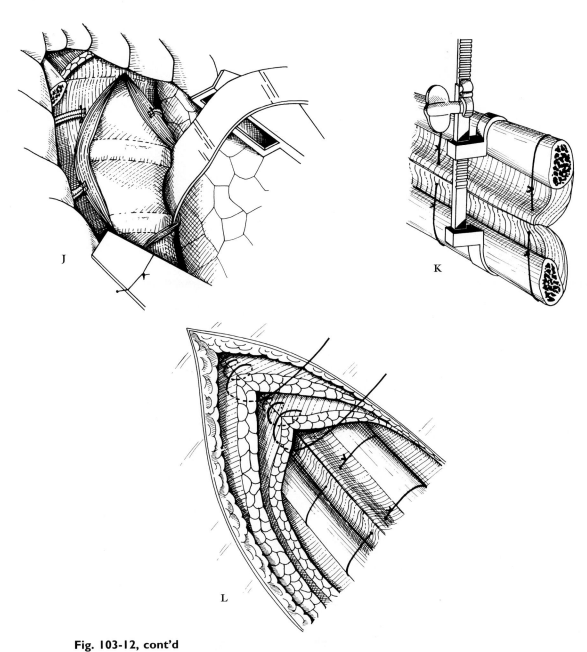

Fig. 103-12, cont'd

J, A malleable retractor with a reversed curve is placed on the opposite side of the vertebral body. **K,** Use of the rib approximator to facilitate closure. **L,** Airtight closure of successive layers. (*From Roy-Camille R, Mazel C: Surgical exposures and procedures. In Laurin CA, Riley LH Jr, Roy-Camille R, editors:* Atlas of orthopaedic surgery, *vol 1, General principles and spine, Masson, 1989, Paris.*)

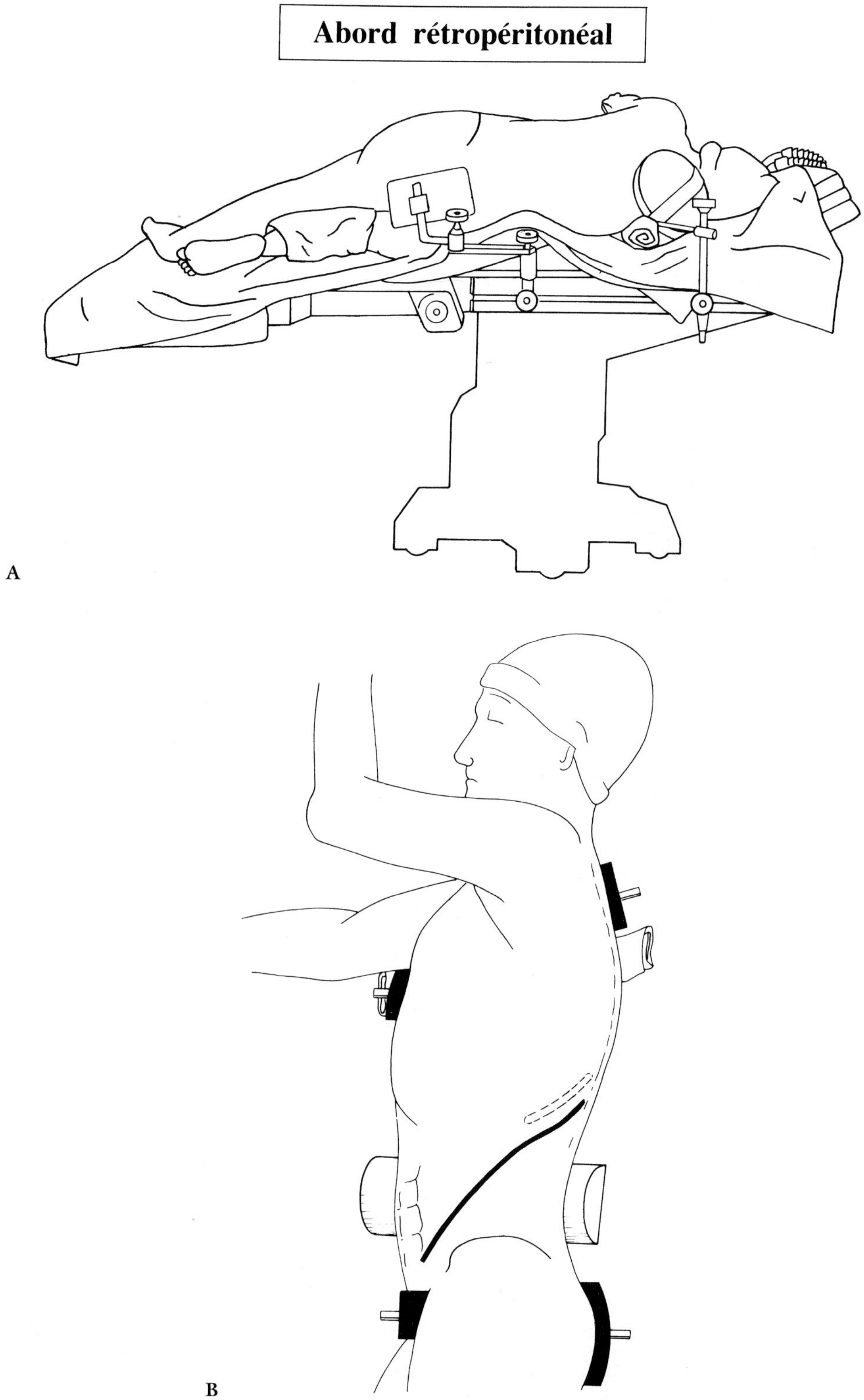

Abord rétropéritonéal

A

B

Fig. 103-13

Retroperitoneal approach to the lumbar region. **A,** Lateral position on an ordinary table. A pad of adjustable height is placed at the level of the vertebra to be reached to "break" the patient. **B,** The skin incision, running obliquely downward and forward, is made between the tip of the twelfth rib and the anterior superior iliac spine. It starts posteriorly at the edge of the paravertebral muscles and ends at the lateral margin of the rectus abdominis.

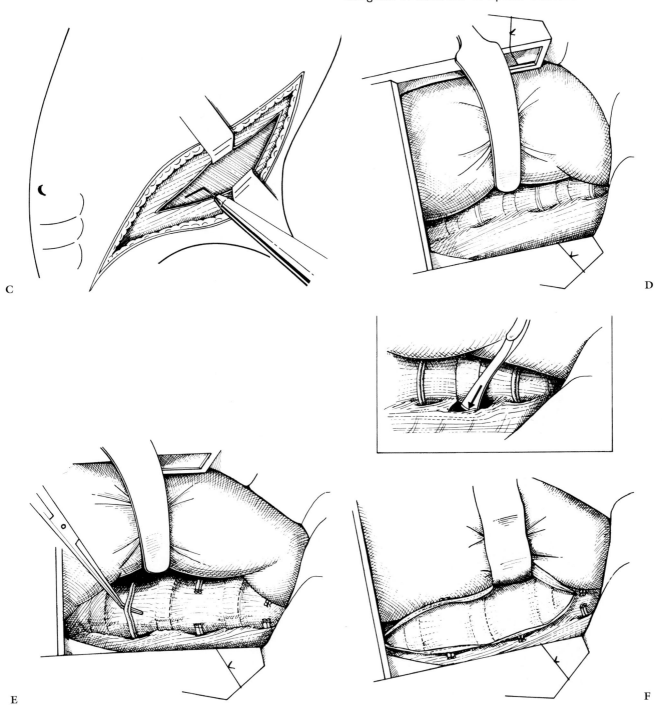

C   D

E   F

Fig. 103-13, cont'd

C, The external oblique, internal oblique, and transversus abdominis muscles are split with cutting diathermy. The peritoneal sac is retracted anteriorly. **D,** Retraction of the peritoneal sac from the psoas exposes the vessels in front of the spine. They are carefully dissected with a swab mounted on a stick. (Inset: The attachments of origin of the psoas are dissected laterally and posteriorly. The intervertebral foramina are thus exposed.) **E,** Ligature of the fragile lumbar vessels is essential. It allows the aorta and the inferior vena cava to be retracted anteriorly and medially. **F,** After incision and retraction of the periosteum, the anterior and lateral aspects of the vertebral bodies are exposed. A malleable retractor on the opposite side of the vertebral bodies retracts the peritoneal sac and the vessels. (*From Roy-Camille R, Mazel C: Surgical exposures and procedures. In Laurin CA, Riley LH Jr, Roy-Camille R, editors: Atlas of orthopaedic surgery, vol 1, General principles and spine, Masson, 1989, Paris.*)

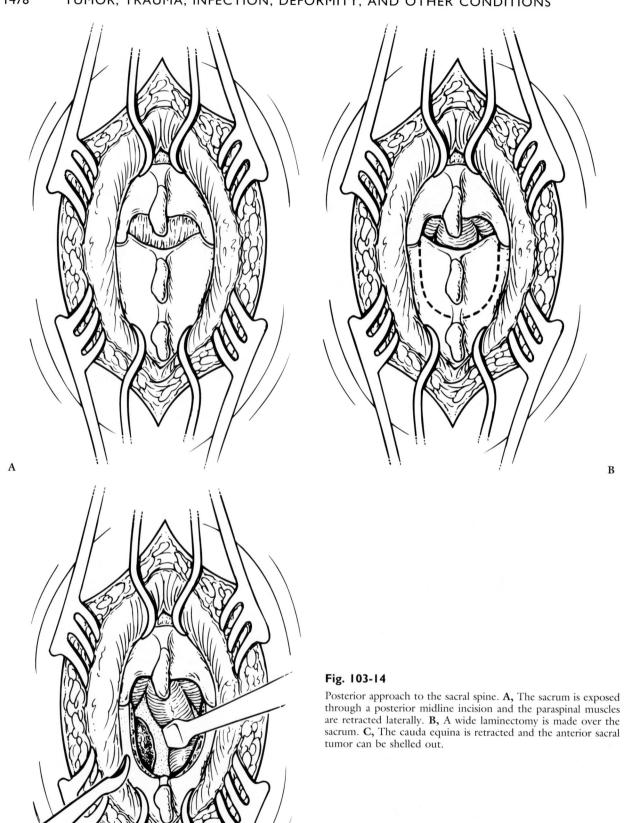

A

B

C

Fig. 103-14

Posterior approach to the sacral spine. **A,** The sacrum is exposed through a posterior midline incision and the paraspinal muscles are retracted laterally. **B,** A wide laminectomy is made over the sacrum. **C,** The cauda equina is retracted and the anterior sacral tumor can be shelled out.

Anterior Cervical Spine

Lesions of the odontoid process can be approached transorally or from an anterolateral direction. For the transoral approach, the patient is positioned supine, and intubation is performed with a small endotracheal tube, which is securely fastened. Awake intubation may be necessary if the spine is unstable. If the patient's mouth does not allow adequate space for an endotracheal tube within the operating field, an elective tracheostomy should be performed. Hydrogen peroxide is used to sterilize the mouth and pharynx. Intravenous cephalosporin and penicillin are administered prophylactically. A glossal retractor affords exposure of the pharynx; the use of a headlight is recommended. Biopsy of the odontoid can be performed through the pharynx. Incising the posterior pharynx leads directly to the transverse ligament of the atlas. Dissecting this off the odontoid allows exposure to the odontoid. The tumor can be excised with small angled curettes in an eggshell technique. Stabilization is then performed from a posterior approach with occiput-C2 fusion. In most instances the posterior occiput-C2 stabilization may be performed first. This contributes stability to the spine during positioning for the second procedure. In addition, it will prevent contamination of the posterior wound with tumor cells.

The anterior approach to C2 through C7 (less the odontoid) is made in the standard anterolateral fashion. The left side is preferred because the recurrent laryngeal nerve lies along the trachea and there is less risk of injury during the approach. With the patient supine, a waterbag is placed between the shoulder blades to extend the neck and aid in exposure. Large longitudinal or transverse incisions are centered over the vertebrae of interest. The platysma is sectioned in line with the skin incision and then the sternocleidomastoid muscle and carotid sheath are swept laterally. The tracheoesophygeal complex is carefully retracted medially. Blunt retractors are preferred to the tracheoesophygeal complex to prevent perforation. In the inferior cervical region the omohyoid muscle is sectioned for additional exposure. The longimus colli muscles are reflected from the midline. The anterior longitudinal ligament lies beneath this, covering the anterior vertebral bodies and discs. Hemostasis is achieved with electrocautery and thrombin-soaked Gelfoam and paddies. Intraoperative radiographs may be necessary for localization of the tumor. Rongeurs and curettes are used to evacuate the tumor. A tumor extending posteriorly must be removed. Often the tumor can be removed easily along a plane of the dura, but occasionally the tumor may be scarred into the dura. The superior and inferior discs are removed and the spinal cord inspected for adequate decompression. Often there is a noticeable indentation of the dura after the tumor is removed. The adjacent vertebral bodies are then addressed. In cases of localized disease, when a confident excision and surgical cure are anticipated, the reconstruction should consist of autogenous bone graft and AO plate instrumentation. If the procedure is palliative for widespread disease or there is need for prolonged radiation and/or chemotherapy of localized disease, then a metal-reinforced PMMA construct is advisable.

The preferred metal-reinforced PMMA reconstruction is performed as follows. Craters are created with angled currettes in the end plates of each vertebral body. Bone from the center of each body is removed. Heavy Harrington compression rods are then cut to a length to span the defect and the two adjoining vertebral bodies. These are impaled into one vertebral body and then angled into the other and impacted into position. Occasionally a trough must be made to allow insertion of the rods. PMMA is then used to reconstruct the region of the vertebrectomy. Care should be taken to protect the dura from the expanding exothermic PMMA. This construct is inherently stable. It affords immediate mobilization without the need for orthoses. If multiple levels are addressed, stability may not be sufficient and posterior stabilization may be necessary. The stability of the construct is greatest at the time of the operation and may gradually weaken with time. The purpose is to provide a construct that will provide stability for the remainder of the patient's life.

Reconstruction with bone graft is performed in the following manner. Tricortical iliac crest bone graft (ICBG) is preferred; however, fibula may be necessary in unusual multilevel vertebrectomies. Craters are sculptured into the adjacent intact vertebral end plates and a piece of tricortical ICBG is fashioned to fill in the void and lodge securely in the superior and inferior craters of the adjacent vertebrae. Occasionally, a trough must be made in the inferior vertebrae to allow insertion of the bone graft. The graft is oriented with the cortex anterior. This allows secure fixation with AO cervical plates and screws that span from the intact vertebrae to the graft (Fig. 103-15).

Posterior Cervical Spine

The hair should be shaved well above the occiput, and an ample region prepped and draped. A longitudinal midline incision is centered over the verte-

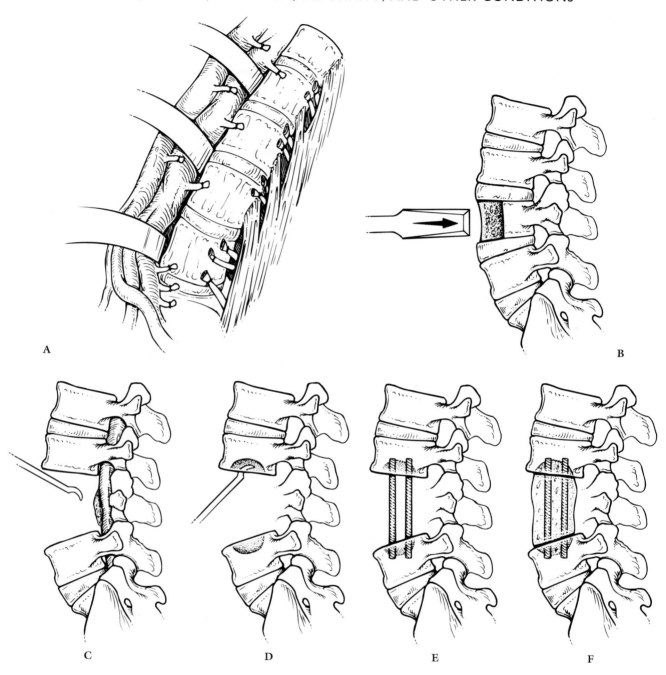

Fig. 103-15

Anterior PMMA steel rod reconstruction of anterior spine. **A,** Ligation of segmental vessels above and below allows retraction of great vessels. **B,** Systematic removal of vertebral body with handed chisel. **C,** Small curette dissecting tumor off of dura. **D,** Curette used to create 2-cm diameter craters in adjacent vertebral bodies. **E,** Threaded steel rod secured to adjacent vertebral bodies with PMMA. **F,** Additional cement used to construct vertebral body and secure to steel rods.

brae of interest. The occipital ridge must be exposed for occipital fusions. The paraspinal muscles are reflected laterally through a midline bloodless plane. The affected posterior elements are excised, and neural decompression is performed. Spinous process

wiring or lateral mass plates with extension to the occiput, if necessary, provide adequate internal fixation. Struts of autogenous ICBG are secured into the region with hardware. In metastatic disease, PMMA is preferred to supplement the fixation. Either wires secured to threaded Steinman pins enlodged in the spinous processes or Luque rectangles with sublaminar wires reinforced with PMMA provide a good construct. No postoperative immobilization is required.

Anterior Thoracic Spine

The anterior thoracic spine is accessed through a thoracotomy. I prefer the transpleural approach. However, when there has been prior surgery, radiation, or other causes of pleural adhesions, an extrapleural approach may be preferred. The entire thoracic spine and C7 may be approached through a thoracotomy. I do not believe that a sternotomy is necessary; the associated morbidity is unwarranted. In the upper thoracic vertebrae exposure is aided by including the left arm in the operative field. The approach is easier if the thoracotomy is made one or two levels above the vertebrae of interest. The upper thoracic vertebrae can be adequately approached through the fourth rib.

The left-side-up position is preferred because it is easier to mobilize the aorta than the vena cava. It is also easier to repair the aorta than it is the vena cava, should a vascular injury occur. The rib removed may be used as bone graft if a fusion is to be performed. The pleura is dissected off the lateral spine in the area of interest. Segmental vessels are ligated two levels above and below the region to be resected. This allows retraction of the great vessels. The resection is performed by piecemeal removal of the affected bodies and adjacent discs with handled chisels. Tumor extruded posteriorly must be peeled off the dura. If complete excision of the tumor is obtained and no radiation or chemotherapy is anticipated (usually with a benign tumor), the deficit may be reconstructed with autogenous bone. Tricortical ICBG fashioned to the defect may be wedged into position and the region rigidly stabilized with internal fixation. The Kostuik–Harrington device works extremely well for this purpose.[20] If the lesion is malignant and the goal was debulking with or without neural decompression, then PMMA reinforced with one or two steel rods is preferred (see Fig. 103-8).

Posterior Thoracic Spine

The posterior approach to the spine is much more familiar to most surgeons and thus unfortunately leads to its use in inappropriate situations. The proposed incision is etched with a skin knife, and a 1:500,000 solution of epinephrine in saline is infused into the dermis and then along the paravertebral muscles to decrease bleeding. When the tumor is confined within the posterior elements and there is no cortical destruction, a subperiosteal dissection along the spinous process and lamina can be performed. If a total excision is attempted in lesions with cortical perforation, then an extraperiosteal dissection should be performed. An en bloc is optimal for primary malignancies and affords a surgical cure. Generous incisions will aid in retraction and visualization of the region to be debrided. An extended posterior approach is possible for tumors that involve the pedicle and lateral-posterior body as well. Circumferential debulking and stabilization will offer superior exposure in most cases. Internal fixation following debridement is best achieved with segmental fixation. Pedicle fixation may be necessary in cases of severe osteoporosis. Infusion of liquid PMMA into the pedicles to increase the screw's purchase may be necessary. Extrusion of the cement into the spinal canal must be avoided.

Luque rods fixed with sublaminar wires and reinforced with PMMA have provided stability. In my hands there has been minimal morbidity in cases of multilevel disease.

Anterior Lumbar Spine

The patient is placed in the right lateral decubitus position. The left-side-up position is preferred even when the majority of the tumor is on the right side of the vertebral body. This is because of the easier dissection and mobilization of the aorta as opposed to the vena cava. Repair of the aorta or its segmental branches is always easier than repair of the venous system.

The flank incision is made and a retroperitoneal dissection is carried down to the spine. A thoracoabdominal approach with sectioning of the diaphragm is necessary to reach L1. A paramedian incision is used to reach L5-sacral tumors. The segmental vessels are ligated two levels above and below the region of interest. This allows the necessary retraction of the great vessels for exposure of the anterior vertebral bodies.

The affected vertebral body is removed in a systematic fashion with handled chisels or rongeurs. The handles allow accurate positioning around the spine and afford more control of the instrument. Intervertebral discs above and below the body or bodies of interest are excised. The dissection is carried posterior to the dura and a meticulous removal of adherent tumor is performed with small curettes. Often there is a definite plane between the dura and the tumor. Other times the tumor is scarred into the dura and the surgeon must be prepared to repair any lacerations of the dura. Affected nerve roots are dissected free of tumor. Hemostasis is achieved with thrombin-soaked Gelfoam and bipolar electrocautery. The remaining superior and inferior intact vertebral bodies are then addressed.

There are generally three iliolumbar veins in the region of L5-sacrum that must be identified and ligated. These are not usually addressed in anatomy books and they deserve special mention. Reconstruction in the lumbar spine is similar to the thoracic region. Three metal rods with PMMA are preferred in the lumbar spine (see Fig. 103-9).

Posterior Lumbar Spine

The patient is positioned prone on a frame that allows the abdominal contents to be free, thereby reducing venous compression and decreasing blood loss during surgery. The hips should be extended to ensure lumbar lordosis if a reconstructive fusion is contemplated. A midline incision is carried down to the spinous processes and dissection is carried laterally to afford exposure of the posterior elements. Determination of the level may be made by visual inspection, defining the sacrum and counting cephalad; by intraoperative radiography; or by counting ribs. Thorough debridement and decompression of the neural elements is performed. Stabilization of the spine is then performed. Bone screws allow superior fixation. Osteoporotic bone may require PMMA augmentation inside the pedicle and body. Visual inspection of the neural elements should be made following any PMMA injection to ensure that none of the PMMA was forced into the spinal canal. If there is question as to the longevity of the patient it is wiser to reconstruct the spine with a PMMA-reinforced bone screw system, such as Cotrel–Dubousset. This allows immediate rigid stabilization and affords aggressive mobilization.

Anterior Sacral Spine

Tumors in the anterior sacrum are approached anteriorly through the pelvis when the tumor is to be resected. Partial or complete pelvectomy is associated with considerable morbidity. Decompression of the cauda equina for an anterior metastatic sacral lesion may be accomplished through a posterior approach. There is adequate room for retraction of the cauda equina laterally to allow visualization of the anterior sacrum and adequate debridement.

Posterior Sacrum

The sacrum can be decompressed effectively with a posterior approach. The cauda equina is retracted laterally, allowing ample space for debridement. Excision of the sacrum or hemisacrum can be performed in this manner. Reconstruction of the pelvis with fixation to the ileum is performed with plates and reinforced with acrylic.

Complications and Alternatives

Complications of spinal tumor surgery are listed in the box below. Complications can be either avoided or dealt with effectively by paying attention to detail. The history and physical examination will alert the surgeon to many otherwise unsuspected complications. A detailed physical examination is essential to document the results of surgery and the postoperative progress.

Iatrogenic kyphosis is not uncommon. It is a result of failure to understand the anatomy, biomechanics, and different approaches to the spine. The typical patient has a metastatic lesion to the bodies of two thoracic vertebrae with perhaps 20 degrees of kyphotic angulation at this level. A posterior laminectomy and attempts at decompression are performed. The anterior bodies are not addressed. The spinal cord remains tented over the anterior vertebral body tumor mass. Subsequently, the vertebral bodies continue to collapse, the kyphosis worsens, and the neural elements become further compressed. The patient is worse now than before surgery. This scenario can be avoided by addressing the area of the spine involved at the initial surgical treatment.

Complications of Spinal Tumor Surgery

Nonunion	0% to 8%
Pulmonary embolus	1%
Thrombophlebitis	1%
Iliac vein laceration	3%
Paraesthetic myalgia	3%
Postthoracotomy syndromes	3%
Infection	4%
Pain	4% to 20%
Temporary neurologic deficit	4%
Instrumentation failure	5%

In this case an anterior thoracotomy, corpectomies, and PMMA instrumentation would have sufficed.

Future Considerations

The goals of surgical treatment of spinal tumors will remain the same in the future. However, with improvements in oncology, including chemotherapy, radiation therapy, and immunochemotherapy, increasing numbers of patients will present with primary or metastatic tumors to the spine, with a greater likelihood of cure. Therefore, the treatment of these conditions will become even more important. The reconstructive technique will necessarily have to evolve to accommodate the greater longevity of these patients. The ability to reconstruct the spine with biocompatible components and agents that stimulate bone growth will eventually lead to discarding use of cement in the spine. However, these patients are different in that they may require additional chemotherapy or radiation treatment to the area to increase the chances of survival. Most likely this will encumber the reconstructive agents. The long-term results of these treatments must be addressed.

Eventually, the treatment of all tumors will be medical, with surgery reserved for advanced cases with existing neurologic compression or spinal instability.

An improved understanding of spinal mechanics, spinal cord physiology, anesthesia, critical-care units, and spinal-instrumentation devices now allows surgeons to approach the spine anteriorly, posteriorly, laterally, and circumferentially without the associated morbidity previously described.

Adequate debridement and decompression of the neural elements is most effectively performed through an approach that exposes directly the area of destruction. Therefore, tumors that affect the anterior vertebral body should be addressed through an anterior approach (Fig. 103-16). Conversely, tumors that involve the posterior elements should be approached from a posterior direction (Fig. 103-17). A circumferential procedure may be indicated if significant involvement of both columns indicates instability. More often than not it is the surgical debridement that creates the instability, and simply reconstructing the region debrided is all that is required.

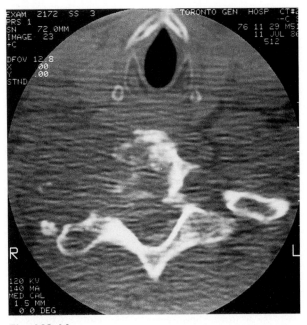

Fig. 103-16

Anterior involvement by tumor. (*From Kostuik JP, Weinstein JN: Differential diagnosis and surgical treatment of metastatic spine tumors. In Frymoyer JW, editor: The adult spine: principles and practice, New York, 1991, Raven Press.*)

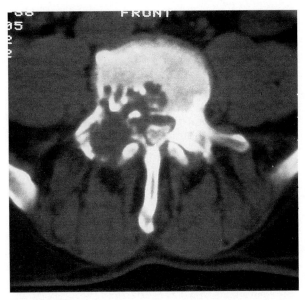

Fig. 103-17

Posterior involvement by tumor. (*From Kostuik JP, Weinstein JN: Differential diagnosis and surgical treatment of metastatic spine tumors. In Frymoyer JW, editor: The adult spine: principles and practice, New York, 1991, Raven Press.*)

References

1. Alexander E Jr, Davis CH Jr, Field CH: Metastatic lesions of the vertebral column causing cord compression, *Neurology* 6:103, 1956.

2. Barwick KW, Huvos AG, Smith J: Primary osteogenic sarcoma of the vertebral column: a clinicopathologic correlation of ten patients, *Cancer* 46:595, 1980.

3. Batson OV: The role of the vertebral veins in metastatic processes, *Ann Intern Med* 16:38, 1942.

4. Brice J, McKissock W: Surgical treatment of malignant extradual spinal tumours, *Br Med J [Clin Res]* 1(5446):1341, 1965.

5. Bucy PC: The treatment of malignant tumors of the spine: a review, *Neurology* 13:938, 1963.

6. Chiurco AA: Multiple exotoses of bone with fatal spinal cord compression: report of a case and brief review of the literature, *Neurology* 20:275, 1970.

7. Cross GO, White HL, White LP: Acrylic prosthesis of the fifth cervical vertebrae in multiple myeloma, *J Neurosurg* 35:112, 1971.

8. Dahlin DC: *Bone tumors: general aspects and data on 6,221 cases*, Springfield, OH, 1986, Charles C Thomas.

9. Di Lorenzo N and others: Giant-cell tumors of the spine: a clinical study of six cases, with emphasis on the radiological features, treatment, and follow-up, *Neurosurgery* 6(1):29, 1980.

10. Dubosset J: Strategy for the surgical treatment of primary bone tumors of the spine in children, *Chir Organi Mov* 75(suppl 1):89, 1990.

11. Dunn EJ: The role of methylmethacrylate in the stabilization and replacement of tumors of the cervical spine: a project of the Cervical Spine Research Society, *Spine* 2:15, 1977.

12. Fornasier VL, Horne JG: Metastasis to the vertebral column, *Cancer* 36:590, 1975.

13. Giannotta SI, Kindt GW: Metastatic spinal cord tumors, *Clin Neurosurg* 25:495, 1978.

14. Gilbert RW, Kim JH, Posner JB: Epidural spinal cord compression from metastatic tumor: diagnosis and treatment, *Ann Neurol* 3(1):40, 1978.

15. Hamdi FA: Prosthesis for an excised lumbar vertebra, *Can Med Assoc J* 100:576, 1969.

16. Hay MC, Paterson D, Taylor TK: Aneurysmal bone cysts of the spine, *J Bone Joint Surg [Br]* 60(3):406, 1978.

17. Kak VK and others: Solitary osteochondroma of spine causing spinal cord compression, *Clin Neurol Neurosurg* 87(2):135, 1985.

18. Kennady JC, Stern WE: Metastatic neoplasms of the vertebral column producing compression of the spinal cord, *Am J Surg* 104:155, 1962.

19. Kleinman WB, Kiernan HA, Michelsen WJ: Metastatic cancer of the spinal column, *Clin Orthop* 136:166, 1978.

20. Kostuik JP: Anterior spinal cord decompression for lesions of the thoracic and lumbar spine, techniques, new methods of internal fixation results, *Spine* 8:512, 1983.

21. Kostuik JP, Weinstein JN: *Differential diagnosis and surgical treatment of metastatic spine tumors.* In Frey-moyer JW, editor: *The adult spine: principles and practice,* New York, 1991, Raven Press.

22. Kostuik JP and others: Spinal stabilization of vertebral column tumors, *Spine* 13:250, 1988.

23. Loftus CM and others: Solitary osteochrondroma of T4 and thoracic cord compression, *Surg Neurol* 13:355, 1980.

24. Malat J, Virapongse C, Levine A: Solitary osteochondroma of the spine, *Spine* 11(6):625, 1986.

25. Manabe S and others: Surgical treatment of metastatic tumors of the spine, *Spine* 14(1):41, 1989.

26. McAfee PC and others: Failure of stabilization of the spine with methylmethacrylate: a retrospective analysis of twenty-four cases, *J Bone Joint Surg [Am]* 68(8):1145, 1986.

27. Mullan J, Evans JP: Neoplastic disease of the spinal extradural space, *Arch Surg* 74:900, 1957.

28. Nather A, Bose K: The results of decompression of cord or cauda equina compression from metastatic extradural tumors, *Clin Orthop* 169:103, 1982.

29. Ono K, Tada K: Metal Prosthesis of the cervical vertebrae, *J Neurosurg* 42:562, 1975.

30. Scoville WB and others: The use of acrylic plastic for vertebral replacement or fixation in metastatic disease of the spine, *J Neurosurg* 27:274, 1967.

31. Senning A, Weber G, Yasargil MG: Zur operativen Behandlung von Tumoren der Wirbelsaule, *Schweiz Med Wochenschr* 48:1574, 1962.

32. Shives TC and others: Osteosarcoma of the spine, *J Bone Joint Surg [Am]* 68(5):660, 1986.

33. Siegal T, Siegal T: Surgical decompression of anterior and posterior malignant epidural tumors compressing the spinal cord: a prospective study, *Neurosurgery* 17(3):424, 1985.

34. Siegal T, Tiqva P, Siegal T: Vertebral body resection for epidural compression by malignant tumors, *J Bone Joint Surg [Am]* 67:375, 1985.

35. Slepian A, Hamby WB: Neurologic complications associated with hereditary deforming chondrodysplasia: review of literature and report on 2 cases occurring in the same family, *J Neurosurg* 8:529, 1951.

36. Stener B: Total spondylectomy in chondrosarcoma arising from the seventh thoracic vertebra, *J Bone Joint Surg [Br]* 53(2):288, 1971.

37. Sundaresan N and others: Combined treatment of osteosarcoma of the spine, *Neurosurgery* 23(6):714, 1988.

38. Sundaresan and others: Spondylectomy for malignant tumors of the spine, *J Clin Oncol* 7(10):1485, 1989.

39. Weinstein JN: *Spinal tumors.* In Weinstein JN, Wiesel SW, editors: *The lumbar spine,* Philadelphia, 1990, W.B. Saunders.

40. Weinstein JN: Surgical approach to spine tumors, *Orthopedics* 12(6):897, 1989.

41. Weinstein JN, McLain RF: Primary tumors of the spine, *Spine* 12(9):843, 1987.

42. White WA, Patterson RH, Bergland RM: Role of surgery in the treatment of spinal cord compression by metastatic neoplasm, *Cancer* 27(3):558, 1971.

43. Yan SC, Xu QM, Lin JR: Diagnosis and treatment of giant cell tumor in the thoracic spine, *J Surg Oncol* 40(2):128, 1989.

Section 2
Trauma

104   Cervical Spine Fractures

Patrick J. Connolly
Hansen Yuan

105   Thoracolumbar Spine Fractures

John D. Schlegel
Hansen A. Yuan
Rand L. Schleusener

Chapter 104
Cervical Spine Fractures

Patrick J. Connolly

Hansen Yuan

Mechanism of Injury

Gunshot Wounds

Outline of Treatment for Cervical Spine Fractures

Upper Cervical Spine Injuries

    occipitoatlantal dislocations
    occipital condyle fractures
    C1 burst fractures
    C1-C2 dislocation
    odontoid fractures
    rotatory atlantoaxial subluxation
    pedicle fractures of C2

Lower Cervical Spine Injuries (C3-C7)

Fractures of the Vertebral Body

    anterior wedge compression fractures
    fractures of the vertebral body with canal
      compromise
    facet joint injuries
    fractures of the posterior elements
    lateral mass fracture
    posterior element fracture associated with
      vertebral body dislocation
    hyperextension injuries
    hyperextension fracture/dislocation

Surgical Technique

    lateral mass plate fixation
    Bohlman's triple wire fixation
    Dewar posterior cervical fusion
    anterior reduction of bilateral jumped facets

Outline of Stabilization Techniques for Cervical Spine Fractures

Selected Cases

Summary

The number of cervical spine injuries per year is over one million, while the reported incidence of spinal-cord injury is approximately 10,000 new cases per year. The vast majority of these injuries are secondary to motor vehicle accidents, falls, or athletic injuries. Recent reports however, indicate a disturbingly increased incidence of cervical spine injuries related to firearms.[12] Despite a heightened awareness of cervical spine injuries both in the field and in the emergency room, a number of cervical spine fractures still are missed in the emergency room. Bohlman[9] and others reported approximately 30% incidence of failure to diagnose cervical spine fractures in the emergency room. It cannot be overemphasized that a proper evaluation for cervical spine injury requires obtaining a history from the patient or from observers at the scene of the accident, examining the spine for areas of localized tenderness, as well as performing a neurologic evaluation. Obtaining cervical spine radiographs without examining the patient is an incomplete examination.

Although the use of high-dose steroids for spinal-cord injury has not been fully accepted by the orthopedic community in the past, recent reports by the NASCIS II study in the *New England Journal of Medicine* have demonstrated improvement in recovery of neurologic function following high-dose methylprednisolone. The current recommendation is for patients with spinal cord injury to receive a 30 mg/kg intravenous infusion of methylprednisolone over a 15-minute interval, followed 45 minutes later by a 23-hour infusion of methylprednisolone at 5.4 mg/kg per hour.[10]

Although it seems logical that fracture dislocations of the cervical spine should be reduced as soon as possible, recent reports of progressive neurologic deficit following reduction of cervical spine injuries raise the issue of whether every patient with a cervical spine fracture dislocation should have an MRI prior to attempts at reduction.[21,30,31] Currently at our institution, patients are initially stabilized in halo traction, and an urgent MRI is organized. An attempt at closed reduction with weights and frequent neurologic assessment is often performed while awaiting the cervical MRI. Patients are rarely, if ever, treated surgically prior to completion of the cervical MRI. In the odd case in which a patient is unable to undergo an MRI, a myelogram CT scan is performed before surgical intervention.

Previous concerns regarding postsurgical edema and progressive neurologic deficit often delayed surgical stabilization for up to 14 days.[39-41] In our experience, this has not been a problem; thus, our approach is one of early closed reduction via traction followed by early decompression and stabilization.

Mechanism of Injury

Most cervical spine fractures can be classified on the basis of the mechanism of injury. For this reason it is important to obtain as much information about the circumstances of the accident when evaluating the patient with a cervical spine fracture.* The forces and mechanism that produce the spine fracture vary according to the level of injury. A severe flexion or extension force is responsible for occipital atlas injuries. Axial loading is accountable for fractures of the ring of C1. Rotation and hyperflexion most often account for injury at the atlantoaxial level. Hyperextension and axial loading are believed to be the most common cause of spondylolisthesis of the axis (C2), and further injury may be associated with a second force of anterior flexion and compression. Injuries to the lower cervical spine may occur secondary to the forces of flexion, extension, lateral rotation, axial loading, or a combination of these forces.

Allen and associates,[1] in a retrospective review of 165 cases of cervical spine injury, developed a mechanistic classification of closed indirect fractures and dislocations of the lower cervical spine (see box). The authors divided the injuries into six groups, which they referred to as "phylogeny" to emphasize the orderly sequence of the injury mechanism. Each phylogeny was named according to the presumed attitude of the cervical spine at the time of failure and initial dominant mode of failure. The categories are compressive flexion, vertical compression, distractive flexion, compressive extension, distractive extension, and lateral flexion. In their classification, the probability of associated neurologic lesion was directly related to the type and severity of the cervical injury.

*References 1, 3, 7, 32, 33, 44, 45, 46, 49, and 51 to 53.

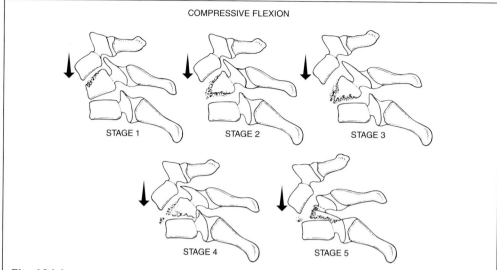

Fig. 104-1

Compressive Flexion Injury

STAGE 1: Blunting and rounding off of anterior superior vertebral margin.

STAGE 2: Loss of anterior height and beak-like appearance anterior inferiorly.

STAGE 3: Fracture line from anterior surface of vertebral body extending obliquely through subchondral plate and fracture of the beak.

STAGE 4: Some displacement (less than 3 mm.) of posterior inferior vertebral margin into neural canal.

STAGE 5: Displacement (greater than 3 mm.) of posterior part of body.

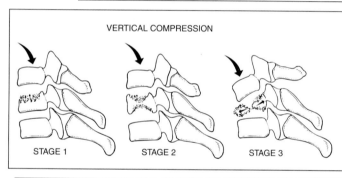

Fig. 104-2

Vertical Compression Injury

STAGE 1: Central cupping fracture of superior or inferior end plate.

STAGE 2: Similar to Stage I but fracture of both end plates.

STAGE 3: Fragmentation and displacement of vertebral body.

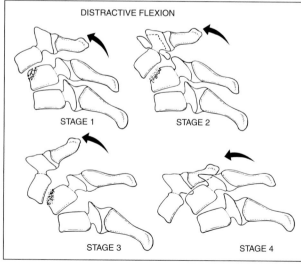

Fig. 104-3

Distractive Flexion Injury

STAGE 1: Facet subluxation in flexion and divergence of spinous process.

STAGE 2: Unilateral facet dislocation.

STAGE 3: Bilateral facet dislocation with fifty percent anterior vertebral body displacement.

STAGE 4: Full width vertebral body displacement.

COMPRESSIVE EXTENSION

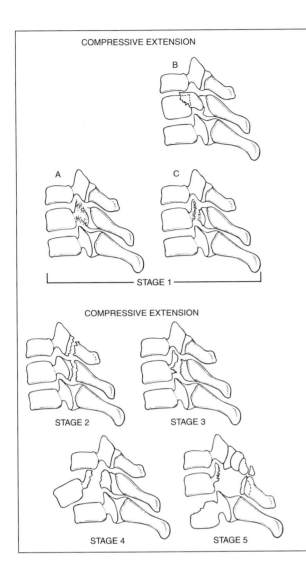

STAGE 1

COMPRESSIVE EXTENSION

STAGE 2   STAGE 3

STAGE 4   STAGE 5

Fig. 104-4
Compressive Extension Injury
STAGE 1: Unilateral vertebral arch fracture. Articular process (Stage 1-A), pedicle (Stage 1-B), or lamina (Stage 1-C).
STAGE 2: Bi-lamina fractures that may be at multiple contiguous levels.
STAGE 3: Hypothetical, characterized by bilateral fractures of vertebral arches and partial anterior vertebral body displacement.
STAGE 4: Further anterior vertebral body displacement.
STAGE 5: Full width anterior vertebral body displacement.

DISTRACTIVE EXTENSION

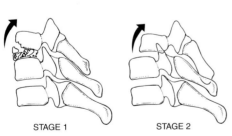

STAGE 1   STAGE 2

Fig. 104-5
Distractive Extension Injury
STAGE 1: Failure of anterior ligamentous complex. There may be widening of the disc space and/or anterior inferior teardrop avulsion fracture.
STAGE 2: Posterior displacement of upper vertebral body.

LATERAL FLEXION

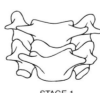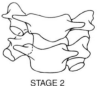

STAGE 1   STAGE 2

Fig. 104-6
Lateral Flexion Injury
STAGE 1: Asymmetric compression fracture of vertebral body with associated vertebral arch fracture, ipsolateral.
STAGE 2: Displacement of ipsolateral arch fracture.

Ultimately, each fracture has a "personality" of its own, and the major goal of any classification system is not necessarily to label every injury but rather to provide the treating physician with a better understanding of the mechanism of specific injuries and to determine the pathologic anatomy based on the bony injury and relative displacements seen on imaging studies.

Gunshot Wounds

The incidence of spinal cord injury related to gunshot wounds has increased significantly over the past 10 years. Capen recently reported an increased incidence of 25% of spinal cord injury related to gunshot wounds.[12] This data from 1991 reported that 52% of total admissions for spinal cord injury at their institution were related to gunshot wound trauma.

Spinal cord injuries related to gunshot wounds rarely cause sufficient bone or ligamentous injury to warrant surgical treatment. Immobilization with a halo vest or rigid cervical orthosis usually allows adequate healing and stability. The issue of removing a bullet from the spinal canal remains controversial. The argument for bullet removal falls around the prevention of CSF leak, meningitis, blood toxicity, pain, neurologic decline, and bullet fragment migration. The argument for a nonoperative approach is that retention of bullet fragments does not routinely lead to complications and that the risks of surgical intervention outweigh potential benefits of fragment removal.

Overall, these cases are never straightforward and need to be evaluated on a case-by-case basis. Certainly if the bullet fragment is representative of compressive pathology, its removal may benefit the patient. Likewise, bullet migration in the spinal canal or progression of neurologic deficit is an indication for surgical intervention.

A recent study by Richards evaluated the effects of bullet removal in spinal cord injury patients with pain. The conclusion of the study was that removal of the bullet did not affect the incidence of pain. Waters reported the effects of removal of bullet fragments retained in the spinal canal for injuries from T1 to L4[54]. The conclusion from this study is that bullet removal from the canal between T1 and T11 had no significant effect on motor recovery, but when bullets were removed from the cauda equina region patients did receive some benefit.

In conclusion, we do not routinely remove bullet fragments from the spinal canal; essentially, our indications for removal of bullet fragments are limited to progressive neurologic injury that can be accounted for by the mass effect of the missile fragment.

Outline of Treatment for Cervical Spine Fractures

Table 104-1 provides the reader with information on the type of fractures, mechanism of injury, the author's choice of treatment, and other treatment options.

Upper Cervical Spine Injuries

Occipitoatlantal Dislocations

Occipitoatlantal dislocation is a devastating injury; it is usually fatal and rarely presents for treatment. The vast majority of patients reported in the literature have an associated intercranial injury, and most cases result from high-speed accidents. Long-term survivors are unusual.[20,34]

These dislocations involve the ligaments that secure the cranium to the cervical spine. A variety of forces have been implicated, but hyperextension, rotation, and distraction are considered the most important mechanisms of injury. In a recent study by Dickman and associates,[20] occipitoatlantal dislocations were classified into three specific types. Type 1 injuries involved anterior displacement of the occiput; type 2, longitudinal distraction; type 3 injuries were posterior dislocations.

Radiographically, displacement was determined by Wackenheim's line (Fig. 104-7), which is a line that extends caudally along the posterior surface of the clivus. Normally, this line is tangential to the posterior tip of the dens. If the occiput is displaced anteriorly the line will intersect the dens. If the occiput is distracted or displaced posteriorly, the line will be separated from the tip of the dens.

Treatment

Dickman and colleagues[20] in their series stressed that traction was contraindicated and that a halo vest alone was inadequate treatment. Early operative intervention in the way of posterior occipital cervical fixation and fusion was reported as the treatment of choice.

Table 104-1

Outline of treatment for cervical spine fractures

Type of Fracture	Mechanism of Injury	Author's Choice of Treatment	Other Treatment Options
Occipital condyle	Type I, II—axial load Type III—rotation	Type I, II—rigid cervical orthosis Type III—halo vest	Halo vest
Occipitoatlantal dislocation	Hyperextension, rotation, distraction	Halo vest plus PSF* with plates O-C2	Halo vest
Bilateral posterior arch C1	Axial load with extension	Rigid cervical orthosis	Halo vest
Anteroposterior arch (Jefferson) C1	Axial load	< 7 mm—rigid cervical orthosis > 7 mm—halo vest	Halo vest
C1/C2 Subluxation	Flexion	PSF with Magerl screws and Gallie wire	Halo vest
Dens			
Type I		Rigid cervical orthosis	Halo vest
Type II	Flexion; rarely extension	Halo vest	Odontoid screw; PSF
Type III	Flexion; rarely extension	Halo vest	PSF
Bilateral pars interarticularis (hangman's)			
Type I	Hyperextension and axial load	Closed reduction and halo	Rigid cervical orthosis
Type II	Hyperextension and axial load	Closed reduction and halo	Anterior discectomy and C2-C3 fusion with anterior cervical plate
Type IIa	Flexion and posterior distraction	Closed reduction and halo	Anterior discectomy and C2-C3 fusion with anterior cervical plate
Type III	Flexion and posterior distraction	Closed reduction and halo	Anterior discectomy and C2-C3 fusion with anterior cervical plate
Atypical	Hyperextension and axial load	Closed reduction and halo	Halo traction
Combined C1 and C2 fractures	Axial load and flexion	Halo vest	Halo vest and odontoid screw
Wedge compression fractures	Compression and flexion	Rigid cervical orthosis	Halo vest
Vertebral body fractures without posterior element involvement (burst)	Compression and flexion or vertical compression	Neuro intact—reduction, halo vest Neuro deficit—corpectomy, fusion, AC* plate	Halo vest

Table 104-1, con't

Outline of treatment for cervical spine fractures (continued)

Type of Fracture	Mechanism of Injury	Author's Choice of Treatment	Other Treatment Options
Vertebral body fractures with posterior element involvement (burst)	Compression and flexion or vertical compression	Corpectomy, fusion, AC plate; PSF with fixation	Corpectomy, fusion, AC plate alone, or reduction and PSF with fixation alone
"Tear drop" fracture-dislocation	Compression and flexion	Corpectomy, fusion, AC plate; PSF with fixation	Corpectomy, fusion, AC plate alone, or reduction and PSF with fixation alone
Unilateral facet dislocations	Distractive flexion	Reduction and PSF with fixation	Closed reduction, halo vest
Bilateral facet dislocations	Distractive flexion	Reduction and PSF with fixation	Closed reduction, halo vest
Fractures and dislocation with acute disc herniation	Distractive flexion	Anterior cervical discectomy, fusion, AC plate	Awake closed reduction and PSF with fixation
Hyperextension fracture/dislocations	Compressive extension or distractive extension	Reduction, anterior cervical discectomy, fusion, AC plate	Reduction, halo
Articular process fractures	Compressive extension or distractive extension	Neuro intact—rigid cervical orthosis	Halo
		Radiculopathy—posterior foraminotomy, lateral mass plates, PSF	PSF with wire stabilization
Laminar	Compressive extension or distractive extension	Rigid cervical orthosis	Halo vest
Floating lateral mass	Lateral flexion or compressive extension or distractive extension	Rigid cervical orthosis With radiculopathy and/or listhesis— lateral mass plates and PSF	Halo vest
Pedicle	Compressive extension or distractive extension	Nondisplaced—rigid cervical orthosis Displaced—halo or PSF	Halo vest

*PSF = Posterior Spinal Fusion; AC = Anterior Cervical

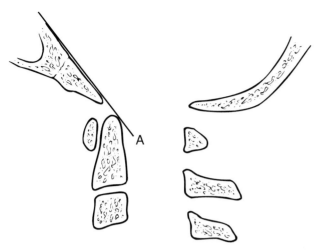

Fig. 104-7

Wackenheim's line is the line that extends caudally along the posterior surface of the clivus. Normally, this line should be tangential to the posterior tip of the dens. If the occiput is displaced anteriorly, the line will intersect the dens. If the occiput is distracted or displaced posteriorly, the line will be separated from the tip of the dens. *(Redrawn from Dickman CA, Douglas RA, Sonntag VKH: Occipitalocervical fusion: posterior stabilization of the craniovertebral junction and upper cervical spine. BNI Q6:2, 1990 [Barrow Neurological Institute, Phoenix, AZ].)*

Occipital Condyle Fractures

Occipital condyle fractures are uncommon. Their diagnosis requires a high index of suspicion. Clinically, the patients are often unconscious following a motor-vehicle accident or fall. Anderson and Montesano[4] classified these injuries into three types. The type 1 occipital condyle fracture (Fig. 104-8, *A*) is an impaction injury secondary to axial loading. The diagnosis is confirmed by CT scan that shows comminution of the occipital condyle with minimal node displacement of fragments into the foramen magnum. It is believed to be a stable injury and can be managed with a cervical collar. In type 2 injury (Fig. 104-8, *B*), the occipital condyle fracture occurs as part of a basilar skull fracture. It has a stable fracture pattern and can be treated with a Philadelphia collar. The type 3 occipital condyle fracture (Fig. 104-8, *C*) is an avulsion injury. The mechanism of injury is either a rotation or lateral bending moment that causes the ala ligaments to avulse a portion of the occipital condyle. This injury is potentially an unstable injury and requires halo immobilization.

C1 Burst Fractures

Fractures of the atlas generally are the result of an axial load injury. The C1 ring fracture may be iso-

lated to the anterior arch, which is believed to be secondary to an axial load with flexion force. Isolated posterior arch fractures are caused by an extension force combined with the axial load. The classic Jefferson fracture is a four-part atlas fracture that can potentially be unstable. Stability is determined by Spence's rule, which measures the spreading of the lateral masses on the AP radiograph of the odontoid process.[49] Normally at the atlantoaxial joint, the lateral borders of the lateral masses of the first cervical vertebra form a straight line with the lateral borders of the body of the second cervical vertebra. If the total excursion of the lateral masses is greater than 7 mm, the transverse ligament is most likely torn and the fractures deemed unstable (Fig. 104-9).

Treatment

Stable C1 fractures can be treated with a hard collar to allow bony healing. Unstable C1 fractures require initial treatment with halo vest immobilization for 8 weeks usually followed by an additional 4 weeks in a Philadelphia collar. Not all of these C1 fractures heal by osseous union but rather by a stable fibrous union that requires no further treatment. Occasionally the fracture in the ring of C1 goes through the facet joint; these patients are at a higher risk for chronic neck pain and spastic torticollis. Patients who remain symptomatic may require posterior C1-C2 arthrodesis for their chronic pain.

C1-C2 Dislocation[8,9]

Atlantoaxial dislocation without fracture is an uncommon injury. It is usually seen as anterior dislocation of the atlas on the axis, indicating complete disruption of the transverse ligament. Posterior atlantoaxial dislocation is extremely rare and indicates disruption of the apical and alar ligaments with maintenance of the transverse ligament. These are both unstable injuries.

Treatment

The anterior C1-C2 instability is treated by reduction and posterior C1-C2 fusion. The rare posterior C1-C2 dislocation requires axial skeletal traction for reduction, after which a posterior C1-C2 fusion should be performed.

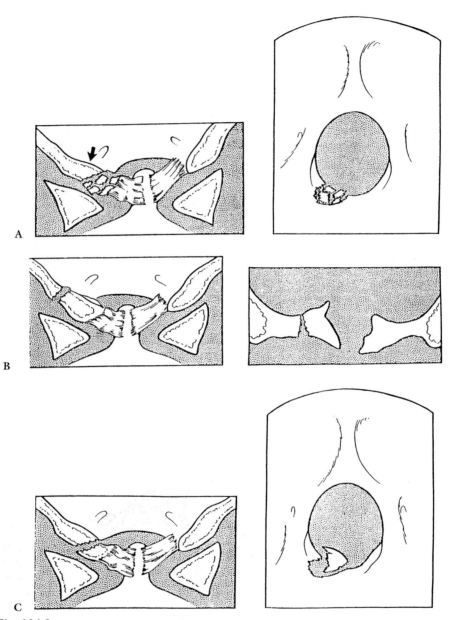

Fig. 104-8

Occipital condyle fracture. **A,** The type 1 occipital condyle is an impaction injury secondary to axial loading. It is believed to be a stable injury and can be managed with a cervical collar. **B,** The type 2 occipital condyle fracture occurs as part of a basilar skull fracture. It has a stable fracture pattern and can be treated with a Philadelphia collar. **C,** The type 3 occipital condyle fracture is an avulsion injury. This injury is potentially unstable and requires halo immobilization. *(From Anderson PA, Montesano PX: Morphology and treatment of occipital condyle fractures, Spine 13:731, 1988.)*

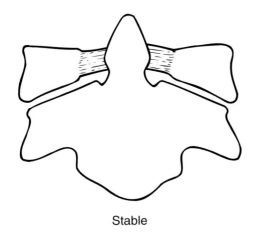

Stable

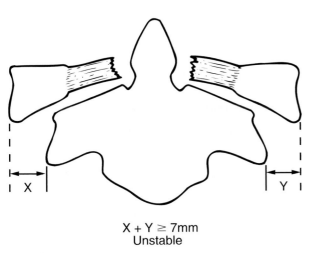

$$X + Y \geq 7mm$$
Unstable

Fig. 104-9

Spence's rule measures the spreading of the lateral masses on the AP x-ray study of the odontoid process. If the total excursion of the lateral masses is greater than 7 mm, the transverse ligament is most likely torn and the fractures deemed unstable. *(Redrawn from Spence KF, Decker MS, Sales KW: Bursting atlantal fractures associated with rupture of the transverse ligament, J Bone Joint Surg 52A:543, 1970.)*

Odontoid Fractures[*]

Fractures of the odontoid may occur with or without displacement. Fractures of the odontoid are most often caused by flexion injury causing anterior displacement of the odontoid process. Odontoid fractures with posterior displacement have a much higher incidence of neurologic injury and are caused by hyperextension force.

The classification of odontoid fractures is that of Anderson and D'Alorzo (Fig. 104-10). The type 1 injury is extremely uncommon and is an oblique fracture through the upper part of the odontoid process.

[*]References 3, 9, 13, 26, 27, 35, 36, 40, 43, 47, and 48.

This fracture probably represents an avulsion fracture in which the alar ligaments attach to the tip of the odontoid process. A type 2 fracture occurs at the junction of the odontoid process and the body of the second cervical vertebra. In the type 3, dens, fracture, the fracture line extends downward into the cancellous portion of the body.

The blood supply to the odontoid is received by cephalad and caudad vessels, and the midportion of the odontoid represents a watershed area. This watershed area explains the higher incidence of delayed union and nonunion of type 2 odontoid fractures.

Treatment

The importance of this classification system is that it enables us to predict outcomes of treatment. Type 1 fractures are extremely uncommon and can be safely treated with a Philadelphia collar for 6 to 8 weeks. Type 3 odontoid fractures have an 85% to 90% union rate and most often can be successfully treated with a halo vest for 12 weeks. These fractures, however, are not benign lesions and in some series have a high rate of malunion, so careful alignment in the halo vest is necessary.

Type 2 fractures have the highest rate of nonunion, with reports of up to 60%. Displacement and angulation contribute to the higher rate of nonunion. Care must be taken to obtain reduction prior to halo vest immobilization. Primary posterior C1-C2 fusion is a surgical option for treating type 2 fractures. In addition, anterior screw fixation is a reasonable surgical alternative for these troublesome fractures. It cannot be overemphasized that if you are able to obtain anatomic alignment and you avoid overdistraction in the halo vest, many of these fractures will go on to heal with halo vest immobilization.

Rotatory Atlantoaxial Subluxation[23]

Rotatory atlantoaxial subluxation is an uncommon injury in which a patient presents with painful torticollis following a traumatic event. It is believed that the injury is a result of a flexion rotation force. These patients present in the classic cock-robin position with the head laterally bent to one side and slightly rotated in the opposite direction. Anteroposterior radiographs are often difficult to obtain, and the lateral radiograph demonstrates the axis subluxed forward with the lateral mass visible anterior to the odontoid process. The injury is one of the capsule of the atlantoaxial joint. This injury often can be treated conservatively with rigid immobilization for

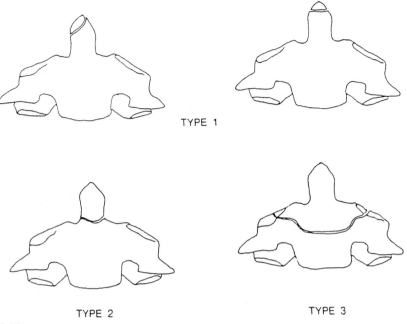

TYPE 1

TYPE 2

TYPE 3

Fig. 104-10

Odontoid fractures. The classification of odontoid fractures is that of Anderson and D'Alonzo. Type 1 injury is an oblique fracture through the upper part of the odontoid process. Type 2 fracture occurs at the junction of the odontoid process and the body of the second cervical vertebra. In type 3 fracture, the fracture line extends downward into the cancellous portion of the body. *(From Anderson LD, D'Alonzo RT: Fractures of the odontoid process of the axis, J Bone Joint Surg 56A:1663, 1974.)*

6 to 8 weeks, but occasionally it requires skeletal traction to reduce the subluxation. If rotatory subluxation is left untreated, it may go on to the rotatory fixation deformity described by Fieldings and Hawkins[23] and require posterior C1-C2 fusion.

Pedicle Fractures of C2[29,50]

Traumatic spondylolisthesis of the axis (C2) is commonly referred to as a hangman's fracture. This injury ordinarily occurs by a hyperextension force in which the occiput is forced into extension against the atlas, producing a fracture of the C2 pedicles. If a flexion component is added to the injury, there may be disruption of discs and ligaments, causing a forward subluxation of C2 on C3. Levine and Edwards have recently reported their classification of this injury. A type 1 (Fig. 104-11, *A*) injury is secondary to hyperextension and axial loading and includes all nondisplaced hangman fractures as well as all fractures that showed no angulation and less than 3 mm of displacement of C2 on C3. Type 2 hangman's fracture (Fig. 104-11, *B-D*) is a hyperextension and axial loading injury that shows significant angulation and translation. The type 2A hangman's fracture (Fig. 104-11, *E*) is believed to have a dif-

ferent mechanism of injury from the typical type 2; it is believed to be caused by flexion as well as posterior distraction force. Type 2A fractures show minimal anterior translation but have severe angulation and appear to be hinging from the anterior longitudinal ligament. Type 3 hangman's fracture (Fig. 104-11, *F*) is secondary to a flexion as well as posterior distraction force and shows both severe angulation and displacement along with unilateral or bilateral facet dislocation at the level of the C2-C3 facets.

At the C2-C3 level there is a relatively large amount of room for the spinal cord, and these injuries rarely result in neurologic deficit. Recently, Starr and Eismont reported the atypical hangman's fracture (Fig. 104-11, *G*), which, unlike the typical type 1 and type 2 hangman's fractures, occurs through the posterior aspect of the vertebral body.[50] Unlike the other forms of C2 traumatic spondylolisthesis, the atypical hangman's fracture produces canal compromise and is associated with a much higher rate of neurologic injury.

Treatment

The traumatic C2 spondylolisthesis can be successfully treated with initial traction for reduction and

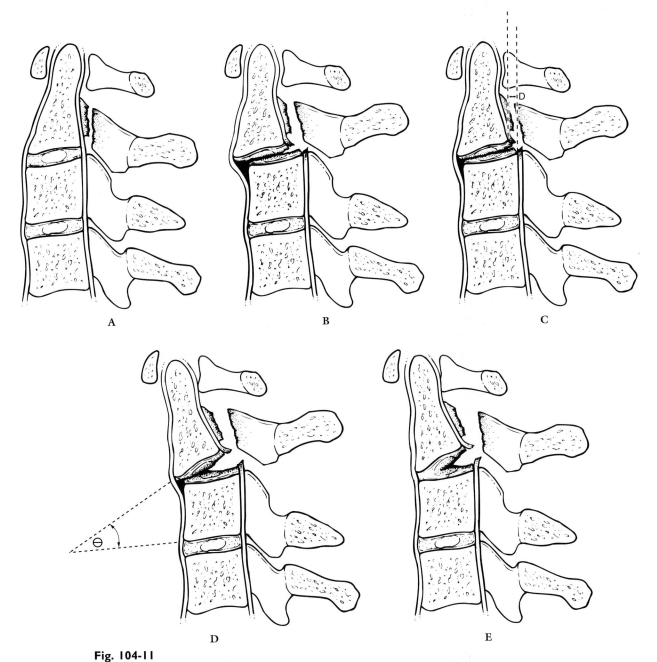

Fig. 104-11

Hangman's fracture. **A,** A type 1 injury is secondary to hyperextension and axial loading and includes all nondisplaced hangman's fractures as well as all fractures that show no angulation and less than 3 mm of displacement of C2 on C3. **B,** Type 2 hangman's (**B, C, D**) is a hyperextension and axial loading injury that shows angulation and greater than 3 mm of translation. **C,** Translation is measured from the posterior margins of the second and third vertebral body at the level of the disc space. **D,** Angulation is measured drawing lines along the inferior end plates of C2 and C3. **E,** The mechanism of injury of the type 2A hangman's fracture differs from the typical 2 injury. Type 2A fracture shows minimal anterior translation but has severe angulation and appears to be hinging on the anterior longitudinal ligament.

then halo immobilization. The type 2A hangman's fracture often has an increase in its deformity with traction and it is usually best treated with reduction under fluoroscopy with halo vest immobilization.

Type 3 hangman's fracture requires reduction of the unilateral and bilateral facet dislocation; this can often be done by halo traction. If reduction is not obtained, the treating physician is left with the choice

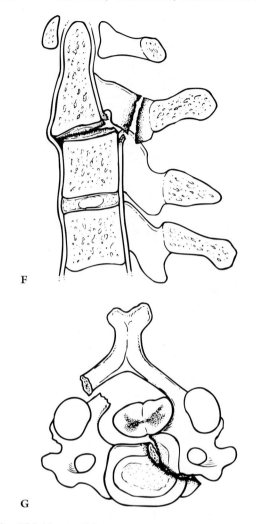

Fig. 104-11, cont'd

F, Type 3 injury is secondary to a flexion as well as posterior distraction force and shows both severe angulation and displacement along with unilateral or bilateral facet dislocation at the level of the C2-C3 facets. *(A-F redrawn from Levine AM, Edwards CC: The management of traumatic spondylolisthesis of the axis, J Bone Joint Surg 67A:217, 1985.)* **G,** The atypical hangman's fracture occurs through the posterior aspect of the vertebral body. Unlike the other forms of C2 traumatic spondylolisthesis, the atypical hangman's fracture produces canal compromise and is associated with a much higher rate of neurologic injury. *(Redrawn from Starr JK, Eismont FJ: Atypical hangman's fracture; Spine 18:1954, J.B. Lippincott, 1993.)*

of either an anterior C2-C3 discectomy and fusion with anterior plate fixation or a posterior reduction of the facet dislocation with posterior facet wiring and postoperative halo immobilization.

Lower Cervical Spine Injuries (C3-C7)

The Allen-Ferguson Classification of cervical spine injury[1] is extremely useful in understanding the mechanism of injury of cervical spine fractures, but because it is a mechanistic classification, its use in describing fractures from one physician to another is often cumbersome. For this reason, I prefer to discuss fractures in regard to their relationship to the injured anatomy.

Fractures of the Vertebral Body

Anterior Wedge Compression Fractures

The anterior wedge compression fractures are compression/flexion injuries that most often occur at the C4-C5 and C5-C6 level. The wedge is formed predominantly by depression of the superior end plate, and the degree of depression is dependent on the severity of the forces. At times, these injuries can be subtle, but if the anterior height of the vertebral body is 3 mm or greater than the posterior vertebral body height, a wedge fracture of the vertebral body is suspect. These fractures do not involve compromise of the spinal canal and, although there is a risk of later posttraumatic kyphotic deformity, the patient with this injury can be managed quite nicely with a rigid cervical orthosis for 8 to 12 weeks.

Fractures of the Vertebral Body with Canal Compromise

When fractures occur with marked anterior wedging of the vertebral body or comminution of the vertebral body, these fractures are often associated with canal compromise and neurologic injury. It is in this group of fractures that I find the work of Allen and Ferguson most useful.[1] Essentially, these injuries are caused by compression/flexion or vertical compression forces. It is in this group where we have our "burst fractures," "teardrop fractures of Schneider and Kahn," and "three-column injury."[17]

In treating these fractures, the information necessary for decision making is (1) What is the patient's neurologic status?, (2) What is the status of the canal compromise?, and (3) What is the status of the posterior elements?

Patients with neurologic deficit require anterior corpectomy and anterior strut graft reconstruction. If the patient has no disruption of the posterior elements, then I believe an anterior strut graft along with anterior cervical plate alone is usually sufficient. If the patient has posterior element injury, then he or she requires supplemental posterior fusion and instrumentation. Treating patients with "cervical burst fractures" with anterior strut graft alone without supplemental posterior stabilization and fusion or anterior cervical plate fixation runs the risk of graft displacement or late kyphotic deformity.

Facet Joint Injuries

Injuries to the facet joints of the cervical spine are among the most common injury patterns seen in patients with cervical spine injury. They are often associated with motor-vehicle accidents or falls from heights, and the injury level is usually the C5-C6 or C6-C7 level.[1,9,40,43] The mechanism is that of distractive flexion, and the injuries include facet joint subluxation, perched facets, unilateral facet dislocation, bilateral facet dislocation, and facet subluxation/dislocation associated with facet fracture. These injuries are often associated with neurologic deficit, in the form of nerve root and/or spinal cord injury. Ideally, these injuries are best treated with closed reduction via halo skeletal traction followed by posterior stabilization and fusion.[14–16]

Recent reports of catastrophic neurologic damage following closed reductions have questioned this classic approach to the treatment of this injury.[21,24,31,42] This injury pattern almost always involves some injury to the disc, and the issue of whether all patients should have an MRI prior to attempt at reduction has not been totally resolved. Currently at our institution, the patients are placed in traction and an MRI is ordered. If the patient is awake and alert, attempts at closed reduction are made while awaiting the MRI. If the patient is obtunded and an interval neurologic assessment cannot be performed, then attempt at reduction is not made prior to MRI of the cervical spine. Prior to the patient going to the operating room, an MRI is obtained and, if a large disc is noted, an anterior approach to discectomy, reduction, and stabilization is performed.

Treatment of Facet Dislocation

Following reduction of facet dislocation, our method of choice is posterior stabilization and fusion using wiring technique or posterior cervical plates. These injuries can be successfully treated with halo immobilization without surgical intervention but run the risk of upwards of 60% loss of reduction as well as potential long-term instability and pain.[5,28,55] Associated facet fractures must be addressed at the time of surgery, and often they require a limited foraminotomy for removal of bony fragments. It is important not to ignore these facet fragments, to avoid chronic nerve root irritation.

Fractures of the Posterior Elements

Fractures of the posterior elements include fractures of the lamina, pedicle, and articular process. These injuries occur most often from motor-vehicle accidents or falls and are often associated with injuries to the upper cervical spine. The mechanism of injury is most often a compressive extension injury or a distractive extension injury, and one or more levels may be involved.

Although these injuries can often be treated with 8 to 12 weeks of rigid cervical immobilization via cervical orthosis or halo, the more severe injuries involve injury to the disc and have a tendency toward delayed forward subluxation. For this reason, these injuries should be observed carefully when treating them nonoperatively.

Lateral Mass Fracture

The floating lateral mass fracture (Fig. 104-12) involves a pedicle fracture and ipsilateral lamina fracture causing a complete detachment of the entire lateral mass from the vertebral body. This fracture pattern may be isolated as a result of a lateral flexion type of injury or may be just a component of a more severe hyperextension injury.

These fractures will go on to heal with a rigid cervical orthosis for 8 to 12 weeks. If there is an associated disc injury or anterior column disruption, there is a tendency for forward subluxation and surgical stabilization may be required.

The presence of nerve root compression may necessitate a posterior fusion with a limited posterior foraminotomy and lateral mass plates.

Posterior Element Fracture Associated with Vertebral Body Dislocation

This is the most severe form of the compressive extension injuries and should not be confused with fracture/dislocation associated with facet dislocation. This injury involves fracture of the vertebral arch (articular process, pedicle, lamina) along with anterior displacement of the vertebral body. This injury is quite unstable and, in our experience, requires both anterior and posterior stabilization.

Hyperextension Injuries

Hyperextension injuries are most often associated with blows to the head and face secondary to motor-vehicle accidents or falls. The mechanism of in-

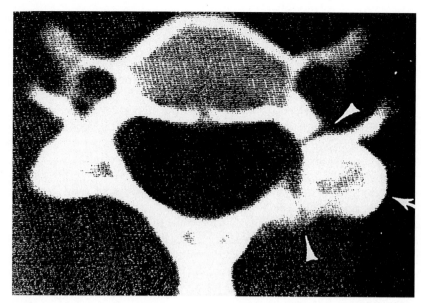

Fig. 104-12

The floating lateral mass fracture involves a pedicle fracture and ipsilateral lamina fracture, causing a complete detachment of the entire lateral mass from the vertebral body. *(From Esses SI: Fixation of the cervical spine, Curr Opin Orthop 78, 1993.)*

jury is one of distractive extension; the milder form is the "teardrop avulsion fracture," which is a small bony avulsion off the anterior inferior portion of the vertebral body. Patients with this injury can be treated with a rigid cervical orthosis for 8 weeks.

Hyperextension Fracture/Dislocation

If the injury force is severe enough, there can be a posterior dislocation of the vertebral body up to 25%. This injury should not be confused with a unilateral facet dislocation.

This is a very unstable injury that requires reduction and anterior cervical fusion with anterior plate stabilization.

Surgical Treatment

Lateral Mass Plate Fixation*

The procedure is performed through a posterior midline cervical incision (Fig. 104-13, *A*). The boundaries of the lateral mass are the respective facet joints inferiorly and superiorly; laterally, the far edge of the facet articulation; and medially, the junction of the lamina and facet. The structures to be avoided are the cord, which is medial to the lamina facet junction, the vertebral artery, which is directly anterior to the valley of the lamina facet junction, and the respective nerve root, which has an exit point at the

anterior lateral portion of the superior facet. The starting point (Fig. 104-13, *B*) is 1 mm medial to the center of the lateral mass and the screw is directed in a 30-degree lateral and 15-degree cephalad direction. Screw length should not be more than 18 mm; on average, a screw 14 mm long will allow for bicortical purchase.

Bohlman's Triple Wire Fixation[56]

The procedure is performed through a posterior midline cervical incision (Fig. 104-14). Towel clip or burr is used to make the hole base of the spinous process of the involved motion segment and allow for wire passage. Initial 20-gauge wire is passed through the hole at the base of the spinous process and looped around the superior portion of the superior spinous process and the inferior portion of the inferior spinous process. Thus, this wire is passed through the hole of each spinous process twice and then tightened down to maintain the reduction. Next, two separate 22-gauge wires are passed through the same respective holes; one wire superiorly and one wire inferiorly. These wires are then passed through separate holes in the cortical cancellous graft and are then tightened down on each other, stabilizing the construct.

*References 2, 6, 11, 22, 25, 37, and 38.

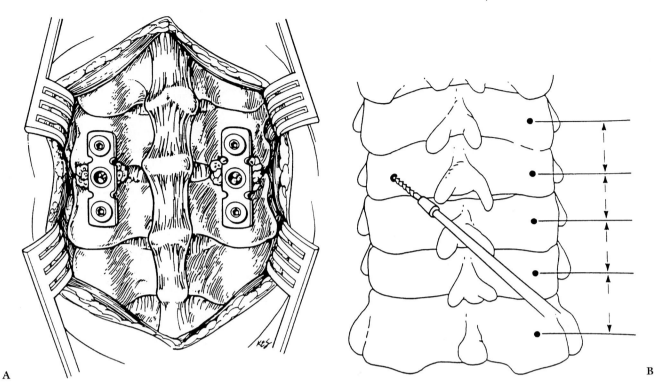

A

B

Fig. 104-13

Lateral mass plate fixation. **A,** The boundaries of the lateral mass are the respective facet joints inferiorly and superiorly. Laterally: the far edge of the facet articulation; medially: the junction of the lamina and facet *(From Anderson PA and others: Posterior cervical arthrodesis with AO reconstruction plates and bone graft, Spine 16(suppl):72, 1991.)* **B,** The starting point is a 1 mm medial to the center of the lateral mass and the screw is directed in a 30 degree lateral and 15 degree cephalad direction. Screw length should not be more than 18 mm; on average, a screw 14 mm long will allow for bicortical purchase *(From An H: Posterior instrumentation of the cervical spine. In An H, editor: Spinal instrumentation, Baltimore, 1992, Williams and Wilkins, Fig. 217.)*

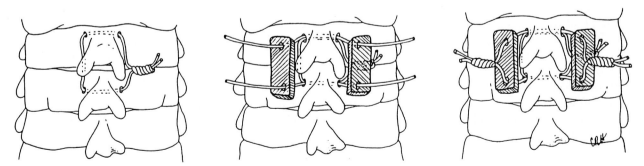

Fig. 104-14

Bohlman's triple-wire fixation. A towel clip is used to make the hole at the base of the spinous processes. Twenty-gauge wire is passed through the hole and looped around the superior portion of the superior spinous process and the inferior portion of the inferior spinous process. Thus, this wire is passed through the hole of each spinous process twice and then tightened down to maintain the reduction. Two separate 22-gauge wires are passed through the same respective holes: one wire superiorly and one wire inferiorly. These 22-gauge wires are then passed through holes in the cortical cancellous graft and tightened. *(From An H: Posterior instrumentation of the cervical spine. In An H, editor: Spinal instrumentation, Baltimore, 1992, Williams and Wilkins.)*

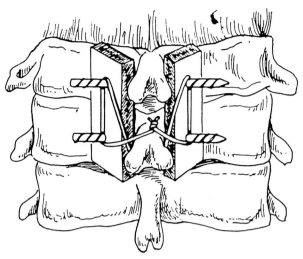

Fig. 104-15

Dewar posterior cervical fusion. Following reduction and decortication, two 2-mm K-wires are introduced percutaneously through the paraspinal muscles to enter and exit at the base of the spinous processes of the involved motion segment. The original technique required pin placement through predrilled cortical cancellous bone graft. Modification of this technique uses a slot in the bone graft that allows for the cortical cancellous strips to be placed after the K-wire has been drilled through the base of the spinous processes. An 18-gauge wire is passed around the two K-wires and looped around the distal spinous process in Gallie fashion. The wires are then tied in front of the distal spinous process. *(From Wilber RG, Peters JG, Likavec MJ: Surgical techniques in cervical spine surgery. In Errico TJ, Bauer RD, Waugh T, editors:* Spinal trauma, *Philadelphia, 1991, J.B. Lippincott.)*

Dewar Posterior Cervical Fusion[18]

Approach again is posterior cervical midline (Fig. 104-15). Following reduction and decortication, two K-wires (2 mm) are introduced percutaneously through the paraspinal muscles to enter and exit at the base of the spinous processes of the involved motion segment. The original technique required pin placement through predrilled cortical cancellous bone graft. Modification of this technique uses a slot in the bone graft that allows for the cortical cancellous strips to be placed after the K-wire has been drilled through the base of the spinous processes. An 18-gauge wire is passed around the two K-wires and looped around the distal spinous process in Gallie fashion. The wires are then tied in front of the distal spinous process.

Anterior Reduction of Bilateral Jumped Facets[19] (Fig. 104-16)

This technique is used if closed reduction has not been attained and MRI indicates a large disc herniation that may further compromise the patient's neurologic status. The patient is placed in a supine position on a turning frame, and a standard anterior Southwick

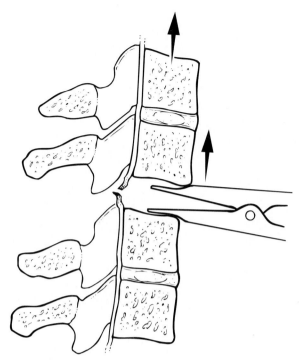

Fig. 104-16

Anterior reduction of bilateral facet dislocation. This technique is used if closed reduction has not been attained and MRI indicates a large disc herniation that may further compromise the patient's neurologic status. The disc at the injured level is completely removed and although at times it is necessary to perform a hemicorpectomy of the superior vertebral body, initially attempts are made to preserve the vertebral end plates. A Harrington distractor is placed into the intervertebral disc space. The disc space is distracted approximately 8 mm, allowing the tip of the lower facet of the upper body to now override the upper facet of the lower body. The upper vertebral body is then pushed posteriorly, reducing the dislocation. *(Redrawn from DeOliveira JC: Anterior reduction of interlocking facets in the lower cervical spine,* Spine *4:195, 1979.)*

Robinson approach to the spine is used. The disc at the injured level is completely removed and although at time it is necessary to perform a hemicorpectomy of the superior vertebral body, initially, attempts are made to preserve the vertebral end plates.

Following complete discectomy, a distractor similar to a Harrington distractor is placed into the intervertebral disc space. It is important to place the distractor deep enough into the disc space so that you avoid just distracting the anterior portion of the vertebral bodies. The disc space is distracted approximately 8 mm, allowing the tip of the lower facet of the upper body to now override the upper facet of the lower body. The upper vertebral body is then pushed posteriorly, reducing the dislocation. Interoperative radiographs are then taken to confirm reduction, followed by standard anterior fusion and plate fixation.

Outline of Stabilization Techniques for Cervical Spine Fractures

The following table provides the reader with information on the type of procedure, indications, degree of difficulty, and the advantages and disadvantages of several stabilization techniques (Table 104-2).

Table 104-2

Outline of stabilization techniques for cervical spine fractures

Procedure	Indication	Degree of Difficulty*	Advantages	Disadvantages
Dens screw	Type II odontoid fracture	3–4	Immediate stable fixation with the potential of preserving motion segment	Preoperative and interoperative fluoroscopy set up is time consuming; potential for disaster if screw malpositioned at this level
Anterior cervical plate	(1) Three-column fracture	3	Immediate stable fixation when utilizing anterior approach; decreases anterior graft complications	Potential for soft-tissue injury immediate or delayed
	(2) Disc herniation associated with lower cervical fracture/dislocation	4		
	(3) Unstable hangman's fracture associated with C2-C3 disc disruption	5		
	(4) Anterior column fracture requiring decompression and fusion	2		
Magerl Screws	C1-C2 fusion for transverse ligament rupture or primary posterior fusion for odontoid fracture	4	Rigid posterior C1-C2 fixation	Technically demanding; disaster potential with poor screw placement or anomalous vertebral artery
Posterior Rogers wire	(1) Unilateral or bilateral facet dislocation	1	Simple to use, safe, time-tested technique	Not as strong as other posterior fixation techniques; rotational stability is dependent on status of posterior elements
	(2) Lower cervical fracture/dislocation	2		
	(3) Posterior fixation for three-column injury	2		
Triple wire	(1) Unilateral or bilateral facet dislocation	2	Safe, time-tested technique	Requires intact spinous process; all the wires can be cumbersome

Table 104-2

Outline of stabilization techniques for cervical spine fractures (continued)

Procedure	Indication	Degree of Difficulty*	Advantages	Disadvantages
Triple wire	(2) Lower cervical fracture/dislocation	2		
	(3) Posterior fixation for three-column injury	2		
Dewar wire	(1) Unilateral or bilateral facet dislocation	2	Safe, time-tested technique with superior rigidity and rotational control than simple Rogers wire	K-wires require separate stab incisions; spinous process must be intact
	(2) Lower cervical fracture/dislocation	2		
	(3) Posterior fixation for three-column injury	2		
Sublaminar wires	C1-C2 fusion for transverse ligament rupture or primary posterior fusion for odontoid fracture	3	Simple construct construct with acceptable fusion rate	Initial stability dependent on quality of bone graft; postoperative halo vest immobilization is usually required
Hook/plate systems	(1) Unilateral or bilateral facet dislocation	2	Avoids C7 lateral mass screw in C6-C7 injury	Stability dependent on hook purchase
	(2) Lower cervical fracture/dislocation	2		
	(3) Posterior fixation for three-column injury	2		
Posterior plates and lateral mass screws	(1) Unilateral or bilateral facet dislocation	2	Immediate stable fixation with rotational control regardless of status of posterior elements	Potential for vertebral artery or nerve-root injury with poor screw placement
	(2) Lower cervical fracture/dislocation	3		
	(3) Posterior fixation for three-column injury	3		
Facet wires	Rheumatoid arthritis, soft osteoporotic bone	3	Does not require spinous process to be intact; provides reasonable fixation in osteoporotic bone	Not as strong as other posterior fixation techniques
Halifax clamp	(1) Unilateral or bilateral facet dislocation	2	No distinct advantage	
	(2) Lower cervical fracture/dislocation	3		
	(3) Posterior fixation for three-column injury	3		

*1 = easy; 5 = most difficult

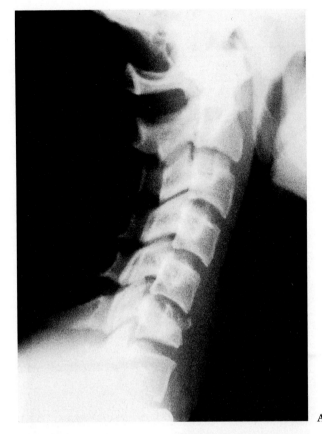

A

Selected Cases

Case 1 (Fig. 104-17)

Eighteen-year-old football linebacker with 9-month history of chronic neck pain following a tackle during the last game of the season. This C6 compression fracture was noted to have a posttraumatic kyphotic deformity (**A**) as well as instability on flexion/extension radiograph (**B, C**).

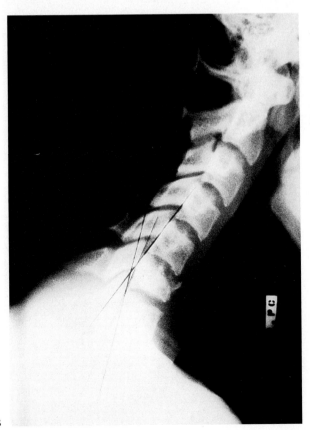

B

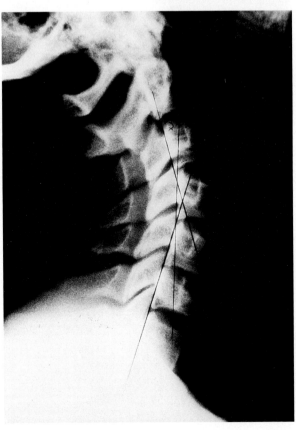

C

Case 1 cont'd

He underwent C6 corpectomy, fusion, and anterior cervical plating (**D, E**). Patient was asymptomatic at follow-up.

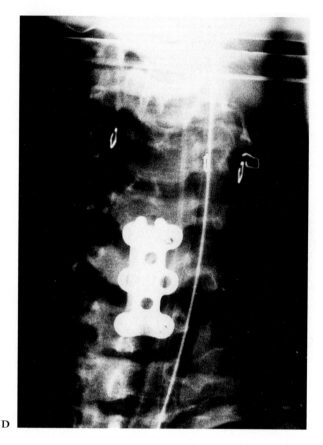

D

E

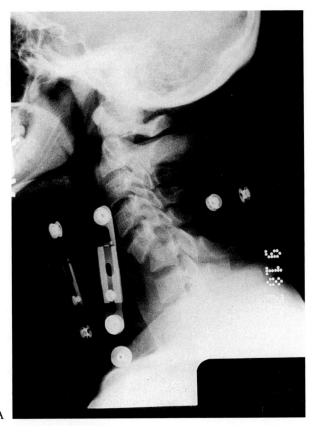

A

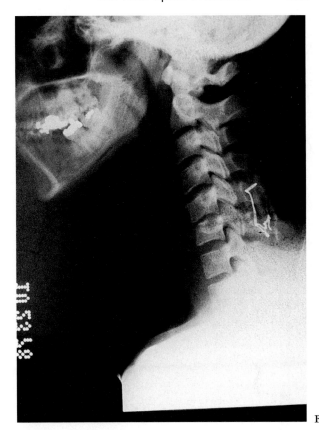

B

Case 2 (Fig. 104-18)

Young male in his twenties sustained a bilateral facet dislocation treated with closed reduction, posterior Roger's wire, and fusion. **A,** bilateral facet dislocation C5-C6. **B,** patient fused following closed reduction and posterior Roger's wire fixation.

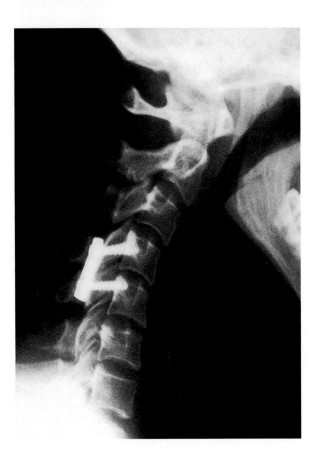

Case 3 (Fig. 104-19)
Young male in his thirties sustained a bilateral facet dislocation treated with closed reduction, single-level lateral mass plating, and fusion.

Summary

The treatment of cervical spine injuries remains a challenge to the spine surgeon. Although our armamentarium has increased significantly over the past 10 years, our goals of early stabilization and maximizing neurologic recovery remain the same.

Upper cervical cord injuries have not been shown to benefit from anterior decompression; therefore, the most important aspect of treatment of patients with upper cervical spine fractures is immobilization and stabilization of the spine. In the treatment of lower cervical spine injuries, the concern is not only to obtain stabilization but also to address decompression of the spinal cord and/or nerve roots. For this reason the neurologic status of the patient plays a greater role in determining the choice of treatment in these patients.

Cervical fractures each have their own personality, and the choice of treatment should be based on the personality of the fracture and the abilities of the surgeon.

References

1. Allen BL and others: Mechanistic classification of closed indirect fractures and dislocations of the lower cervical spine, *Spine* 7:1, 1982.
2. An HS, Gordin R, Renner K: Anatomic considerations for plate-screw fixation of the cervical spine, *Spine* 16(suppl):548, 1991.
3. Anderson LD, D'Alonzo AT: Fractures of the odontoid process of the axis, *J Bone Joint Surg* 56A:1663, 1974.
4. Anderson PA, Montesano PX: Morphology and treatment of occipital condyle fractures, *Spine* 13:731, 1988.
5. Anderson PA and others: Failure of halo vest to prevent in vivo motion to patients with injured cervical spines, *Spine* 16(suppl):501, 1991.
6. Anderson PA and others: Posterior cervical arthrodesis with AO reconstruction plates and bone graft, *Spine* 16(suppl):72, 1991.
7. Bauze RJ, Ardran JM: Experimental production of forward dislocation in a human cervical spine, *J Bone Joint Surg* 60B:239, 1978.
8. Beatson TR: Fractures and dislocations of the cervical spine, *J Bone Joint Surg* 65B:21, 1963.
9. Bohlman HH: Acute fractures and dislocations of the cervical spine, *J Bone Joint Surg* 61A:1119, 1979.
10. Bracken MD and others: A randomized controlled trial of methylprednisolone or naloxone in the treatment of acute spinal cord injury, *N Engl J Med* 322:1405, 1990.
11. Camille RR and others: Treatment of lower cervical spine injuries C3-C7, *Spine* 17S:442, 1992.
12. Capen DA and others: Spinal cord injury from civilian gunshot wounds: the Rancho experience 1980–1988, *J Spinal Dis* 4:306, 1991.
13. Clark CR, White AA: Fractures of the dens, *J Bone Joint Surg* 67A:1340, 1985.
14. Cotler HB and others: Closed reduction of cervical spine dislocation, *COOR* 214:185, 1987.
15. Cotler HB and others: The medical and economic impact of closed cervical spine dislocations, *Spine* 15:448, 1990.
16. Cotler JM and others: Closed reduction of traumatic cervical spine dislocation using traction weights up to 140 pounds, *Spine* 18:386, 1993.
17. Cybulski GR and others: Complications in three column cervical spine injuries requiring anterior-posterior stabilization, *Spine* 17:253, 1992.
18. Davey JR and others: Technique of posterior cervical fusion for instability of the cervical spine, *Spine* 10:1722, 1985.
19. DeOliveira JC: Anterior reduction of interlocking facets in the lower cervical spine, *Spine* 4:195, 1979.
20. Dickman CA and others: Traumatic occipitoatlantal dislocations, *J Spinal Dis* 6:300, 1993.
21. Eismont FJ, Arena MJ, Green BA: Extrusion on an intravertebral disc associated with traumatic subluxation or dislocation of cervical facets, *J Bone Joint Surg* 73A:1555, 1991.
22. Esses SI: Fixation of the cervical spine, *Curr Opin Orthop*:89, 1993.
23. Fielding JW, Hawkins RJ: Atlantoaxial rotatory fixation, *J Bone Joint Surg* 56A:1681, 1974.
24. Harrington JF, Likavec MJ, Smith AS: Disc herniation in cervical fracture subluxation, *Neurosurgery* 29:374, 1991.
25. Heller JG and others: Anatomic comparisons of the Roy Camille and Mageral techniques for screw placement in the lower cervical spine, *Spine* 16(suppl):552, 1991.
26. Jeanneret B, Mageral F: Primary posterior fusions C1/C2 in odontoid fractures: indications, technique, and results of transarticular fixation, *J Spinal Dis* 5:464, 1992.
27. Jonsson H and others: Hidden cervical spine injuries in traffic accident victims with skull fractures, *J Spinal Dis* 4:251, 1991.
28. Koch RA, Nichol VL: The halo vest, *Spine* 3:103, 1978.
29. Levine AM, Edwards CC: The management of traumatic spondylolisthesis of the axis, *J Bone Joint Surg* 67A:217, 1985.
30. Lintner DM, Knight RQ, Cullen JP: The neurologic sequelae of cervical spine facet injuries, *Spine* 18:725, 1993.
31. Mahale WJ, Silver JR, Henderson NJ: Neurologic complications of the reduction of cervical spine dislocations, *J Bone Joint Surg* 75B:403, 1993.
32. Marar BC: Hyperextension injuries of the cervical spine, *J Bone Joint Surg* 56A:1655, 1974.
33. Marar BC: The pattern of neurologic damage as an eighth of the diagnosis of the mechanism in cervical spine injuries, *J Bone Joint Surg* 56A:1648, 1974.
34. Montaine I, Eismont FJ, Green BA: Traumatic occipitoatlanto dislocation, *Spine* 16:112, 1991.
35. Montesano PX and others: Odontoid fractures treated by anterior odontoid screw fixation, *Spine* 16(suppl):33, 1991.
36. Moskovich R, Crockard HA: Atlantoaxial arthrodesis using interlamina clamps, *Spine* 17:261, 1992.

37. Nazaraine SM, Louis RP: Posterior internal fixation with screw plates in traumatic lesions of the cervical spine, *Spine* 16(suppl):64, 1991.

38. Raynor RB, Carter FW: Cervical spine strength after facet injury in spine plate application, *Spine* 16(10)(suppl):558, 1991.

39. Raynor RB, Koplik B: Cervical cord trauma, *Spine* 10:193, 1985.

40. Reich SM, Cottler JM: Mechanisms and patterns of spine and spinal cord injuries, *Trauma Quart* 9:7, 1993.

41. Ripa DR and others: Series of 92 traumatic cervical spine injuries stabilized with anterior ASIF place fusion technique, *Spine* 16(suppl):46, 1991.

42. Rizzolo SJ and others: Intervertebral disc injury complicating cervical spine trauma, *Spine* 16(suppl):187, 1991.

43. Rizzulo SR, Cotler JM: Unstable cervical spine injuries: specific treatment approaches, *J Am Acad Orthop Surg* 1:57, 1993.

44. Roaf R: Lateral flexion injuries of the cervical spine, *J Bone Joint Surg* 45B:36, 1963.

45. Roaf R: A study of the mechanics of spinal injuries, *J Bone Joint Surg* 42B:810, 1960.

46. Ryan MD, Taylor TK: Odontoid fractures in the elderly, *J Spinal Dis* 6:397, 1993.

47. Sasso R and others: Biomechanics of Odontoid fracture fixation, *Spine* 18:1950, 1993.

48. Southwick WO: Management of fractures of the dens, *J Bone Joint Surg* 62A:482, 1980.

49. Spence KF, Decker MS, Sales KW: Bursting atlantal fractures associated with rupture of the transverse ligament, *J Bone Joint Surg* 52A:543, 1970.

50. Starr JK, Eismont FJ: Atypical hangman's fracture, *Spine* 18:1954, 1993.

51. Taylor AR: The mechanism of injury to the spinal cord and neck without damage to the vertebral column, *J Bone Joint Surg* 33B:543, 1951.

52. Taylor AR, Blackwood W: Paraplegia in hyperextension cervical injuries with normal radiographic appearances, *J Bone Joint Surg* 30B:245, 1948.

53. Taylor JR, Twomy LT: Acute injuries to the cervical joints, *Spine* 18:1115, 1993.

54. Waters RL, Adkins RH: The effects of removal of bullet fragments retained in the spinal canal, *Spine* 16:934, 1991.

55. Whitehill R, Richmond JA, Glasser JA: Failure of immobilization of the cervical spine by the halo vest, *J Bone Joint Surg* 68A:326, 1986.

56. Wiland DJ, McAfee PC: Posterior cervical fusion with triple wire strut technique: 100 consecutive patients, *J Spinal Dis* 4:15, 1991.

Additional Readings

Alberque F and others: Frequency of interabdominal injury in cases of blunt trauma to the cervical spinal cord, *J Spinal Dis* 5:476, 1992.

Bohler J, Gaudernak T: Anterior plate stabilization for fracture dislocations of the lower cervical spine, *J Trauma* 20:203, 1980.

Cheng CLY and others: Bodysurfing accidents resulting in cervical spine injuries, *Spine* 17:257, 1992.

Epstein JA and others: Cervical myelopathy caused by developmental stenosis of the spinal canal, *J Neurosurg* 51:362, 1979.

Grob D and others: Posterior occipital cervical fusion, *Spine* 16(3)(suppl):17, 1991.

Hajek PD and others: Biomechanical study of C1/C2 posterior arthrodesis techniques, *Spine* 18:173, 1993.

Hanley EN, Harvell JC: Immediate post-operative stability of atlantoaxial articulation: a biomechanical study comparing simple mid-line wiring in the Gallie and Brooks procedures, *J Spinal Dis* 5:306, 1992.

Hanson PB and others: Anatomic and biomechanical assessment of transarticular screw fixation for atlantoaxial instability, *Spine* 16:1141, 1991.

Jeanneret B and others: Posterior stabilization of the cervical spine with hook plates, *Spine* 16(3)(suppl):56, 1991.

Kuhn JE, Graziano GP: Airway compromise as a result of retropharyngeal hematoma following cervical spine injury, *J Spinal Dis* 4:264, 1991.

Lundqvist C and others: Spinal cord injuries, *Spine* 16:78, 1991.

MacMillan M, Stauffer ES: Traumatic instability in the previously fused cervical spine, *J Spinal Dis* 4:449, 1991.

Matsuura P and others: Comparison of computerized tomography parameters of the cervical spine: normal control subjects and spinal cord injury patients, *J Bone Joint Surg* 71A:183, 1989.

Montesano PX and others: Biomechanics of cervical spine internal fixation, *Spine* 16(suppl):10, 1991.

Myers BS and others: A role of torsion cervical spine trauma, *Spine* 16:870, 1991.

Odor JM and others: Incidence of cervical spinal stenosis in professional and rookie football players, *Am J Sports Med* 18:507, 1990.

Pelker RR, Duranceau JS, Panjabi MM: Cervical spine stabilization: a three-dimensional biomechanical evaluation of rotational stability, strength, and failure mechanisms, *Spine* 16:117, 1991.

Podolsky S and others: Efficacy of cervical spine immobilization methods, *J Trauma* 23:461, 1983.

Rodrigues FA, Hodgson BF, Craig JB: Posterior atlantoaxial arthrodesis, *Spine* 16:878, 1991.

Schneider RC: Chronic neurologic sequelae of acute trauma to the spine and spinal cord, *J Bone Joint Surg* 38A:985, 1956.

Schneider RC, Kahn EA: Chronic neurologic sequelae of acute trauma to the spine and spinal cord, *J Bone Joint Surg* 41A:449, 1969.

Star AM and others: Immediate closed reduction of cervical spine dislocations using traction, *Spine* 15:1068, 1990.

Sutterlin CE and others: Biomechanical evaluation of cervical spine stabilization methods in bovine model, *Spine* 13:795, 1988.

Torg JS and others: National Football Head and Neck Injury Registry: report of cervical quadraplegia, 1971-1975, *Am J Sports Med* 7:127, 1979.

Torg JS and others: Neuropraxia of the cervical spinal cord with transient quadraplegia, *J Bone Joint Surg* 69A:1354, 1986.

Urlich C and others: Biomechanics of fixation systems to the cervical spine, *Spine* 16(suppl):4, 1991.

Vaccaro AR and others: Noncontiguous injuries of the spine, *J Spinal Dis* 5:320, 1992.

Yablon IG and others: Nerve root recovery in complete injuries of the cervical spine, *Spine* 16(suppl):518, 1991.

Chapter 105

Thoracolumbar Spine Fractures

John D. Schlegel
Hansen A. Yuan
Rand L. Schleusener

Introduction

History

Initial Patient Management

Neurological Status

    normal neurologic examination
    complete neurologic injury
    incomplete neurologic injury

**Spinal Stability and Classification
  of Injury**

    simple unicolumn injuries
    compression fractures
    flexion/distraction injuries
    fracture dislocations
    burst fractures

Other Issues

Summary

Introduction

Injury to the thoracic and lumbar spine is not uncommon in this country. Each year an estimated 200,000 Americans sustain a fracture of the vertebral column. A small percentage of these are associated with neurologic injury.

In 1970, the United States Congress identified the need to develop specialized units to care for patients who had been devastated by spinal cord injury. The designation of these regional units allowed them to build a patient base adequate to develop expertise in the acute care and rehabilitation of patients with spinal cord injury. It also allowed the development of various treatment protocols, which led to the accumulation of statistically meaningful research data. The results of this research have led to many important advances in the care of patients with spinal cord injury.

Precise epidemiologic data regarding the incidence of spinal cord injury in the United States is not available. However, estimates report the incidence rate at approximately 35 per million per year. The four leading causes of spinal cord injury are (in order of prevalence) motor vehicle accidents, gunshot wounds, falls, and diving. This chapter will emphasize the management, classification, treatment, and outcome data associated with thoracolumbar spine fractures.

History

Five thousand years ago, the Egyptians described findings consistent with spinal cord injury. These case reports were graphically detailed. They were viewed as problems not to be treated. This attitude persisted for several thousand years afterward.

In the past century, our approaches to the thoracolumbar spine have changed. In the early 1900s, patients with neurologic deficit usually died secondary to sepsis, uremia, pulmonary disease, or pressure sores. Beohler of Austria advocated treatment of these injuries via postural reduction. In the 1940s, the availability of antibiotics as well as the advance of medical treatment allowed for more sophisticated treatment of thoracolumbar injury.

This chapter will evaluate the issues and advances that have led to the development of our present understanding.

Initial Patient Management

A patient suffering an injury to the thoracolumbar spine has had a major traumatic insult. The most common causes of thoracolumbar injury are motor vehicle accidents, significant falls, and gunshot wounds. The patient is usually immobilized at the accident scene on a standard frame or backboard by emergency medical personnel. Basic neurologic evaluation is performed after life-support systems are identified and stabilized. The patient is then transferred to a medical facility and physician involvement is activated.

The principles surrounding management of traumatized patients obviously are beyond the scope of this text. Vital signs are stabilized, an appropriate airway is established, venous access is obtained, and screening laboratory evaluation carried out. This initial management is usually done by a trauma or general surgeon who involves the appropriate subspecialists at the time of patient arrival. Though the spinal physician is usually not actively involved in treatment of disorders of the internal organs, it is important that the extent and scope of such injuries be recognized, as studies document the importance of early and expeditious stabilization of some spinal injuries in the patient with multiple traumas.[55]

After the patient is appropriately stabilized, a meticulous spinal evaluation is mandatory. This includes the history and mechanism of injury. If the patient is mentally alert, information can be obtained regarding localization of pain and numbness or weakness in the lower extremities. Simple palpation over the thoracolumbar spine is very important. It is crucial to recognize any palpable defect between the spinous processes. If the patient is mentally impaired, he or she should be assumed to have injury until proven otherwise.

A good neurologic evaluation of the extremities is extremely valuable. This is well known to most, but should include excellent documentation of motor, sensory, and reflex changes. A rectal examination and bulbocavernosus response must be included.

After the appropriate initial history and physical examination is performed and documented, imaging studies are performed. The most important imaging studies are simple anteroposterior (AP) and lateral radiographs of the thoracic and lumbar spine.[41] Since the most common area of injury in the thoracolumbar spine is the thoracolumbar junction, it is important to visualize this area specifically. Simple radiographs of the thoracic and lumbar spine often show the thoracolumbar junction at the film periphery, making documentation of injury in this common area more difficult. Basic radiographic evaluation will usually isolate most injuries and fractures. If a fracture or dislocation is present, some type of scanning technology is then performed.

CT scanning has been a mainstay in spinal injuries.[46] It shows bony detail to an excellent degree, specifying not only the fracture type but also canal compromise, associated adjacent fractures, lamina fractures, cord impingement, and other significant findings. There is a 10% likelihood that a fracture can occur in a contiguous region, making scanning and evaluation regarding these injuries crucial.

Variants of a conventional CT scan may be beneficial, depending on the situation. CT myelography gives excellent information regarding spinal canal compromise and the integrity of the neural sheath. In addition, sagittal or coronal reformations may give information regarding translational or rotational injuries that are a little more occult in the axial plain.

Magnetic resonance imaging is an adjunct to, not a replacement for, CT scanning. It is a relatively new technology that is excellent in showing soft tissue structures. It can show not only ligamentous injuries and avulsions but also intradiscal pathology. Fracture dislocations can be associated with discal injury and this information can be important during the treatment phase.[52,56]

In summary, radiographic techniques are crucial in patient evaluation and will help guide treatment protocol. The specific treatment and assessment of patients with spinal cord injury involve (1) the patient's neurological status, and (2) the classification and inherent stability of the spinal fracture. These two entities dictate the treatment and prognosis for thoracolumbar spinal injury.

Neurologic Status

The documentation of neurologic status is as important as the actual examination itself. The management of the patient depends on the neurologic status; thus, status should be documented initially as well as at subsequent examinations. It is important to be alert for perianal dysfunction, rectal tone, and bulbocavernosus reflex.

In the early course of spinal injury, "spinal shock" may be present. This is manifest by the absence of bulbocavernosus reflex and usually resolves within the first 12 to 24 hours. The bulbocavernosus reflex is elicited by placing a finger in the rectum and subsequently pulling on the Foley catheter. A reflex contraction of the anal sphincter denotes a positive response.

Numerous classification systems exist that document neurologic status.[26] The hallmark classification system was developed by Frankel and associates[20] and divided neurologic dysfunction into five groups (see box). The Frankel Classification has stood the

Frankel Classification of Neurologic Status

> A. Complete neurologic injury
>
> B. Incomplete: preserved sensation only
>
> C. Incomplete: nonfunctional motor
>
> D. Incomplete: functional motor
>
> E. Complete recovery (may have abnormal reflexes)

test of time and is a commonly used indicator of neurologic function.

Modifications of the Frankel Classification have been developed. The Sunnybrook Cord Injury Scale and the Motor Index Score adapted for the American Spinal Injury Association (ASIA) are offshoots of the Frankel Classification. The ASIA Index is given in Table 105-1 and is commonly accepted as a neurologic functional evaluation. Unfortunately, many of these classifications become cumbersome and difficult to memorize; also, they are not universally accepted and therefore are subject to some scrutiny and disrepute.

Treatment of specific neurologic patterns will be discussed.

Normal Neurologic Examination

If the patient is neurologically intact, the inherent stability of the fracture pattern needs to be assessed

Table 105-1

Motor Index Score adapted for ASIA

Grade on Right	Muscle	Grade on Left
0–5	C5	0–5
0–5	C6	0–5
0–5	C7	0–5
0–5	C8	0–5
0–5	T1	0–5
0–5	L2	0–5
0–5	L3	0–5
0–5	L4	0–5
0–5	L5	0–5
0–5	S1	0–5
50	Total score: 100	50

to delineate active treatment guidelines. As a general rule, most of these injuries can be treated conservatively with either simple mobilization or bracing. If the fracture is unstable, then even in the face of a normal neurologic evaluation, surgical intervention may be required.

The treatment and management of neurologically intact patients with burst fractures is often controversial. Many studies document that conservative management in the large preponderance of these cases is reasonable and efficacious.* In a patient with a neurologically intact lesion, careful observation is carried out for 24 hours. Expeditious mobilization is initiated and neurologic status watched carefully.

Complete Neurologic Injury

Patients with immediate and complete paraplegia have devastating injuries and problems. The annual financial cost for such patients can be up to $100,000. These patients require early mobilization and rehabilitation to attain optimum function. Often, injuries to the thoracic spine are inherently stable and the patient is mobilized in a Thoraco-Lumbar-Sacral Orthosis (TLSO). Many fractures require early surgical intervention for stabilization, reducing morbidity and escalating entrance into rehabilitation.

Incomplete Neurologic Injury

In patients with a Frankel Classification of B, C, or D, treatment is crucial. Initial management usually consists of careful observation and immobilization with bed rest or preferably on a rotokinetic bed. In 1990, Bracken and colleagues performed a study published in the *New England Journal of Medicine* that showed efficacious usage of methylprednisolone in patients with spinal cord injuries if given within 8 hours of injury.[5] The initial dose is 30 mg/kg and it is then continued at 5.4 mg/kg per hour over a 24-hour period. Improvement in neurologic function was obtained under this protocol and is the present standard of care in this particular patient group. Bracken and colleagues stated "Although the completeness of injury is strongly related to the degree of neurologic recovery, both patients with complete injuries and those with in complete injuries improved more after treatment with methylprednisolone than after placebo."[5] There are no studies documenting the effectiveness of high dose steroid usage in root or cauda equina level injuries.

In a patient with incomplete neurologic lesion, careful monitoring is continued for 24 to 48 hours. Operative intervention is often necessary. Early decompression and stabilization is beneficial, especially in the patient with bony or discal encroachment on the spinal canal, or in the patient with neurologic worsening. If the patient is improving neurologically, then observation can be maintained for a period of time prior to surgical stabilization. The details of the surgical approach depend on fracture stability and will be discussed below.

Scientific data are somewhat inconsistent in reference to treatment of this particular patient subgroup. Frankel, in his original description of postural reduction, obtained one Frankel Grade of improvement with this methodology alone.[20] This appears to be a reasonable expectation and has not been significantly improved on in other large series. Dickson and colleagues obtained comparable neurologic improvement with indirect reduction via posterior instrumentation.[15] Dunn, in the early 1980s, reported almost two Frankel Grade improvements in patients undergoing anterior decompression, debridement, and instrumentation.[16] In many respects, though, the "jury is out" and the approach (anterior or posterior) and timing do not appear to be directly related to a significant difference in improvement.[55] The fracture type probably plays more of a role in defining surgical approach than the optimism regarding neurologic improvement.

Spinal Stability and Classification of Injury

The inherent stability, or lack of same, is crucial to our understanding of spinal disease. Multiple definitions and arguments rage over this topic.*

The American Academy of Orthopaedic Surgeons defines instability as an abnormal response to applied loads characterized by movement in the motion segment beyond normal constraints.[18] Similarly, White and Panjabi have defined spinal stability as the ability of the spine, under physiologic loads, to limit patterns of displacement so as to preclude damage or irritation to the neural elements, and to prevent incapacitating deformity or pain due to structural changes.[61]

Specific guidelines for the evaluation of spinal instability based on biomechanical and clinical experience have been suggested.* Noteworthy from the biomechanical perspective are proposed instability

---

*References 1, 2, 6, 39, 47, 48, 53, and 60.

*References 10, 18, 22, 28, 30, 31, 50, 51, 61, and 65.
*References 9, 10, 18, 22, 28, 30, 31, 50, 51, and 65.

ranking systems. These guidelines stemmed largely from in vitro experimental protocols seeking to determine the relative importance of the various spinal structures to stability by way of sequential transection of the soft-tissue components of the functional spinal unit.

In reference to basic fractures, our understanding of stability was addressed initially by Sir Frank Holdsworth.[30] He divided fracture classifications into flexion, flexion rotation, extension, and compression. He developed a two column theory of the spine, with a heavy emphasis on the posterior ligamentous column for stability. His classification system was simple and directed treatment for at least 20 years.

In 1983, Frances Denis made great changes and advances in our understanding of the spinal column.[10] He believed that the posterior column had been overemphasized and that the two column theory did not adequately explain some fractures, including the flexion/distraction injury. Based on this, he developed a three column mechanism with an anterior, middle, and posterior column of the thoracolumbar spine. The anterior column consists of the anterior half of the vertebral body as well as the adjacent disc. The middle column consists of the posterior half of the vertebral body, the adjacent disc, and the posterior longitudinal ligament. The posterior column is formed by all structures posterior to the middle column. Inherent instability was manifest by injury to the middle column or by injury to at least two of the three columns. Based on this classification, he divided spinal fractures into four types: compression fractures, burst fractures, flexion/distraction injuries, and fracture dislocations. The compression fracture does not involve the middle column and therefore is stable. The burst fracture involves at least the anterior and middle column, and the injury is unstable. The flexion/distraction and fracture dislocation injuries are multicolumn injuries and obviously are unstable.

Recent research by James and associates has modified this concept somewhat.[31] Nevertheless, the Denis concept formulates the active classification system that we use for spine fractures. The confusion stemming from the Denis information involves the burst fracture. A multitude of articles exist supporting that many burst fractures do well with conservative management and are possibly not inherently unstable.* Contrary to this, other data document late posttraumatic problems (kyphosis).[43,54,57,62] Based on that, a laboratory study was conducted by James and

associates using cadaveric models.[31] In summary, sequential disruption of the anterior, then anterior and middle, and then anterior, middle, and posterior columns were performed in cadaveric L1 samples (Fig. 105-1). The anterior and middle column disruption was done with osteotomes producing a burst fracture model. The posterior column disruption was carried out via resection of the intraspinous and capsular ligaments. Using spectrophotometric measurement, insignificant added instability was produced by destruction of the middle column over pure anterior column disruption. When the posterior column was subsequently disrupted, statistically significant changes were noted. These data support the theory that the inherent burst fracture with just anterior and middle column disruption is most likely not an unstable injury and does not require surgical intervention in the face of a normal neurologic evaluation. Those patients that have added posterior column ligamentous disruption do develop posttraumatic kyphosis and are at risk. A series of 20 conservatively treated patients with burst fracture at the University of Utah have been followed over the past 3 years, and support this theory. In addition, serial and subsequent CT evaluations on many of these two column injuries reveal canal resorption, as has been described by Krompinger and Weinstein and their associates.[19,39,60]

In summary, we believe that a patient with a neurologically intact burst fracture should undergo the routine initial management described above. If the patient has anterior and middle column deficit only, and is neurologically intact, he or she is fitted and treated in an orthosis. If widening is noted between the spinous processes on AP evaluation in the upright position, or if significant tenderness is appreciated on palpation of the intraspinous ligaments, then posterior ligamentous disruption is possible and surgical intervention may need to be considered. An example is the patient described in Fig. 105-2. He is a 28-year-old man who was treated with initial conservative management. He had posterior ligamentous disruption and developed posttraumatic kyphosis. He went on to anterior/posterior osteotomy with good realignment of his spinal canal (Fig. 105-2). In contradistinction, Fig. 105-3 shows a patient without posterior instability after conservative management.

The treatment, evaluation and classification of certain individual fracture-types will now be discussed. These are divided into (1) simple unicolumn injuries; (2) compression fractures; (3) flexion/distraction injuries; (4) fracture dislocations; and (5) burst fractures.[17]

---

*References 1, 2, 6, 39, 47, 48, 53, and 60.

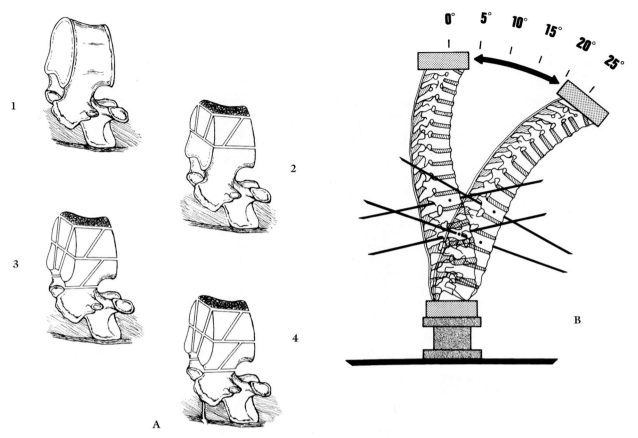

Fig. 105-1

A, Sequential L1 cadaveric model showing intact (*1*), anterior column disruption (*2*), anterior and middle column disruption (*3*), and full three column disruption (*4*) prior to biomechanical testing. **B,** Testing apparatus used for testing the floor models in **A.**

Simple Unicolumn Injuries

Simple avulsion injuries and minimally displaced, nonfocal lesions can occur around the thoracolumbar spine. These include transverse process fractures, facet fractures, lamina fractures, and spinous process fractures. Obviously, the inherent stability of the fracture is important to recognize so that soft tissue ligamentous injury is not overlooked. In most of these cases the treatment is simple and supportive. After a very limited period of bed rest, the patient is mobilized with either a light support or no orthosis at all. Muscular and ligmentous pain can be significant for up to 4 to 6 weeks. Nevertheless, active mobilization is important and crucial in the long-term prognosis of these patients. Usually these injuries heal without problem and are not associated with long-term impairment.

Compression Fractures

Compression fractures are axial-loading fractures in the thoracolumbar spine. They usually involve acute compression of the anterior column. There is minimal if any middle column disruption, and no posterior injury, instability, or clinical tenderness. These injuries also are inherently stable, as described by Denis. Their treatment, as with the first group, is usually supportive.[17] Some physicians prefer to place these patients in an orthosis, either lightweight or custom made. In many respects, this may be overtreatment, as the injury is inherently stable. Since the vertebral body consists of cancellous bone, there is almost always some degree of settling. This is true

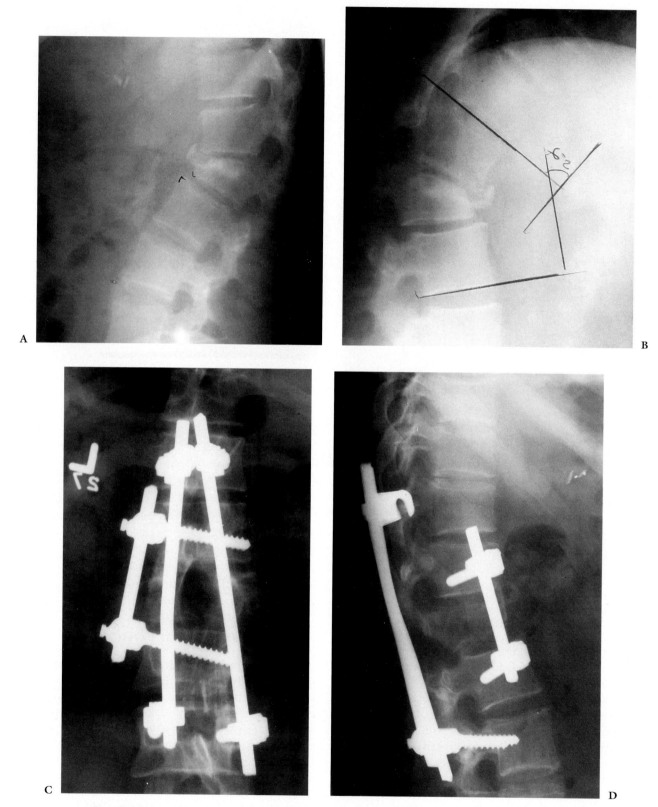

Fig. 105-2

A 28-year-old male with posttraumatic kyphosis. He had posterior ligamentous disruption leading to kyphosis deformity and pain. **A** and **B,** Preoperative radiograph showing the overall sagittal alignment and the degree of kyphotic angulation in this patient. **C** and **D,** AP and lateral radiograph after anteroposterior osteotomy and reduction.

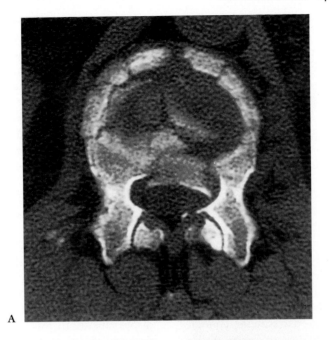

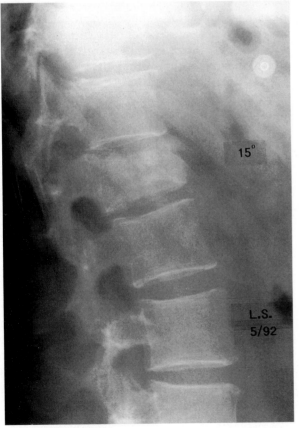

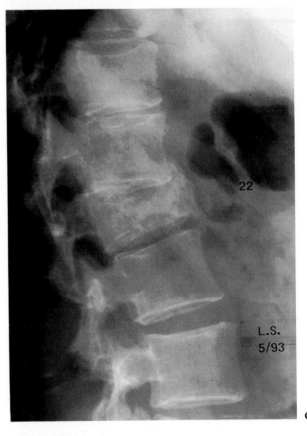

Fig. 105-3

A through **C,** The patient LS with a neurologically intact burst fracture and 50% canal compromise on CT scan (**A**). Routine upright radiographs showed no spinous process widening. He healed uneventfully and regained full function. Slight "settling" of the cancellous vertebral body is shown, and in the absence of posterior ligamentous injury is of no clinical significance.

not only for compression fractures but for burst fractures. Treatment does not alter this settling and should be discussed with the individual patient at the time of injury. These injuries usually heal without untoward consequences and are not associated with any long-term dysfunction (see Fig. 105-3).

Flexion/Distraction Injuries

The classic flexion/distraction injury was initially characterized by Chance, a radiologist, in the 1940s.[7] Also known as seat belt injuries, they have subsequently been described as "Chance-fractures." These injuries occur commonly at the thoracolumbar junction or slightly below. They represent flexion and distraction mechanisms with the fulcrum of force far anterior to the spinal column. Because of this, associated intraabdominal injuries are possible.[40]

This fracture pattern is usually obvious on clinical evaluation and radiographic assessment. Tenderness of the intraspinous ligaments or the posterior structures is evident as well as splaying of the spinous processes.

Management of this injury must be done carefully. Obviously the fracture is unstable, as it involves all columns of the spine. It is important to assess the neurologic status, which may affect the overall treatment plan. Two types of flexion/distraction fractures occur: (1) an injury that occurs through the bony column; and (2) an injury that occurs largely through the ligamentous column. The flexion/distraction mechanism that occurs through the bony column usually goes through the vertebral body, through the pedicle, and out the posterior bony structures (many times this also includes the transverse processes bilaterally). Kyphosis is evident and the posterior soft tissues are often disrupted to the point that dura or ligamentum flavum are evident quite readily on surgical exposure. The second type of fracture involves the soft-tissue structures—it has similar mechanisms but the forces are applied through the disc space, ligamentous structures, and the intraspinous ligaments posteriorly. The bony injury can usually be treated conservatively. The patient is usually placed in a hyperextended position and molded for either a hyperextension TLSO or a hyperextension body cast. Roentgenograms are obtained to assess reduction, but assuming the bony structures are approximated, the patient will usually heal without untoward consequence. Obviously the neurologic status may affect any decision making in reference to treatment. If the patient is neurologically compromised and has intracanal pathology,

surgery may be contemplated separate from the usual conservative treatment.

On the contrary, the ligamentous injury is usually more difficult to stabilize conservatively. A few surgeons will recommend attempted conservative management, but most believe that operative intervention is required. The ligamentous structures do not always stabilize and the patient is at risk for future flexion injuries and kyphotic deformity. In this situation, some type of posterior procedure is the treatment of choice. Posterior exposure and approach is made to the injured area and some type of compressive force placed via instrumentation across the posterior elements. The mainstay in treatment for this has been the Harrington compression system. Today, numerous hook-and-bone screw systems exist. It is important to realize the mechanism of injury and reproduce this mechanism during reduction, opposing those forces that caused the initial displacement. In this situation, flexion and distraction are the major deforming forces, therefore extension and posterior compression are the treatment guidelines.

A representative case is shown in Fig. 105-4. This is a 22-year-old man involved in a significant motor vehicle accident suffering a flexion/distraction injury at L1. This patient had jumped facets with an open facet noted on CT scan. Compression instrumentation was placed posteriorly via bone screws—in this case the AO Fixateur Interne.[13,14] The patient healed, was neurologically intact, and had no long-term dysfunction associated with his injury. Most unstable injuries in our hands are treated with a minimum of 3 months in a TLSO, not only for comfort but to supply external immobilization in addition to the internal fixation.

Fracture Dislocations

Fracture dislocations of the thoracolumbar spine are high kinetic energy injuries. These injuries can be subtyped into flexion, extension, flexion/rotation, distraction, or translational injuries.[11,35] Any injury causing a fracture and dislocation, in any plane, is grossly unstable. All three columns must be disrupted for this to occur. These injuries can occur in the thoracic or lumbar spine. They commonly occur at the thoracolumbar junction at the base of the stabilizing rib cage. All these injuries represent forcible impact and are often associated with neurologic deficit, many times a complete deficit.

Though the subtypes differ, the treatment principles remain the same. The subtypes (flexion, ex-

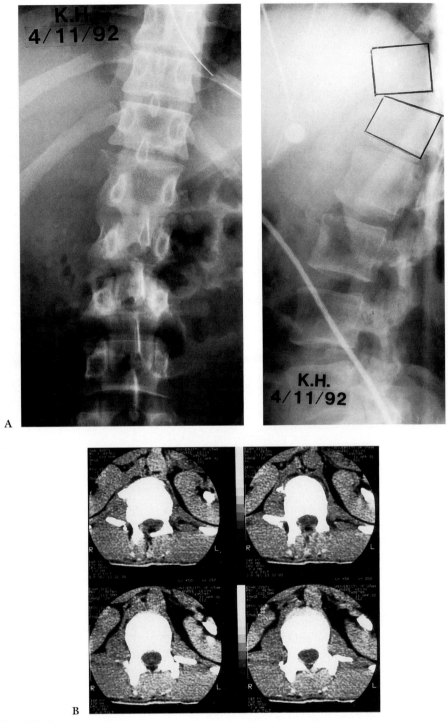

Fig. 105-4

A, AP and lateral of ligamentous chance fracture L1. **B,** CT scan showing "open facets."

tension, translational, sheer, or flexion/rotation) are important to recognize as they help in the assessment and reduction of the fracture.

Based on the inherent instability of these injuries, operative intervention is usually required. Many of

these patients have complete paraplegia. They are best served by early stabilization allowing for mobilization, functional recovery, and placement in active rehabilitation. Almost all these injuries are best approached posteriorly. Reduction is carried out by

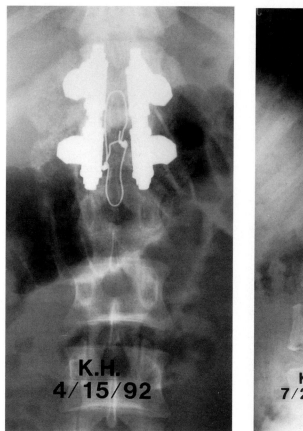
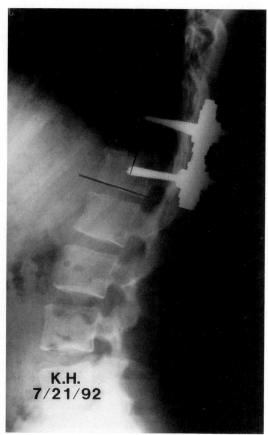

C

Fig. 105-4, cont'd

C, Postoperative AP and lateral reduction films.

recreation of the initial deformity and reversal of the deforming forces.[34] A multitude of instrumentation systems are available. Most surgeons prefer some type of hook/rod construct. The gold standard has been the Harrington rod, which has recently been supplemented with either spinous process wiring or sublaminar wiring. Based on the instability of the lesion, we usually like to engage at least three intact lamina above and below the injury. If the patient has a complete neurologic lesion, the preservation of motion segments is not as important in the decision-making process. Use of pedicular instrumentation is somewhat more tenuous in this situation, as it may not provide the inherent stability necessary to maintain alignment in these grossly unstable individuals. In summary, we usually prefer some type of modification of the original Harrington instrumentation. If the patient is neurologically intact, we will usually reinforce the Harrington instrumentation with spinous process wiring (Drummond). If the patient is neurologically completely paraplegic, then we will usually perform segmental sublaminar stabilization over the Harrington instrumentation via the technique by Luque. Many other systems exist, including TSRH, CD, Modulock, Isola, and so on, and all can be quite easily used to maintain alignment and stability in these injuries.

Burst Fractures

The burst fracture is the more controversial and most common of the major fracture types.[12,23,45,48,64] It is produced by an axial loading mechanism, often in combination with a flexion or rotational component. Denis has divided the burst fractures into five types: superior end-plate injuries, inferior end-plate injuries, both end-plate injuries, rotational injuries, and lateral flexion injuries.

The treatment is based on the neurologic status of the patient and the inherent stability of the fracture pattern. Four basic treatment approaches are available for management of burst fractures.

Conservative Management

Conservative management of burst fractures is well supported throughout the literature and represents the mainstay treatment of the neurologically intact burst fracture.* Although some individuals support prolonged bed rest in the initial management of this injury,[48,60] we prefer fairly rapid mobilization.[6] If the patient is neurologically intact, he or she is fit with a TLSO and mobilized within 24 to 48 hours of hospitalization, assuming there are no other contraindications. Upright AP and lateral radiographs are crucial. As mentioned, if there is posterior intraspinous widening or evidence of posterior ligamentous disruption, the patient is at risk for posttraumatic kyphosis. In those individuals, we recommend surgical intervention. In our hands, this entails posterior instrumentation and fusion.

The remainder of the neurologically intact burst fractures are treated conservatively. The issue of canal compromise is the controversial area surrounding these individuals. We accept canal compromise up to 60% and even 70% if the patient is neurologically intact and understands the prognosis regarding the injury. With canal compromise greater than 60%, we usually give the patient the option of surgical versus nonsurgical management. We are presently carrying out a prospective study evaluating the risk factors associated with the neurologically intact patient. Data exist that even with significant canal compromise, the patient can resorb the canal and function in essentially a normal fashion without long-term impairment.[19,39,48,60] In summary, conservative management is the treatment of choice in most neurologically intact patients.

Posterior Indirect Reduction

Reduction of burst fractures via the posterior indirect method has been used for at least 30 years. Dickson and associates, in their series performed in the 1970s, noted relief of neurologic function with simple distraction and Harrington instrumentation.[15] The key to debridement of the canal is restoration of the initial anatomy.[68] The emphasis should be not only on distraction, but also on correction of the kyphotic deformity; this can be carried out with hook and rod systems. The Edward rod sleeves have been used to help correct inherent kyphosis. Bending or contouring of the rods also may be useful in this management. A variety of other pedicular instrumentation systems, including the AO Fixateur Interne and the RF system, directly and easily allow for distraction as well as reduction of kyphosis.[33]

*References 1, 2, 6, 39, 47, 48, 53, and 60.

In 1992, Fredricksen and associates won the Volvo Award for showing the anatomic basis for indirect reduction.[21] Sequential cuts were carried out in cadaveric burst fracture segments. These cuts showed that the posterior longitudinal ligament played a role, yet not the most major role, in reduction of these fragments. The anulus fibrosus appeared to be a significant contributor to reduction of the fracture pattern. Therefore, distraction not only of the posterior ligamentous structures but also of the anterior and middle column anular structures is quite important in pulling this impacted cancellous bone out of the canal.

Clinically, indirect reduction does appear to debride the canal to some degree.* Gertzbein and co-workers reported moderate improvement in canal compromise in their series of patients undergoing indirect reduction.[24] With today's more modern technical hardware, reduction may be more readily possible. Almost all authors agree that indirect reduction within 72 hours is important, as the fracture gets "sticky" quickly and indirect techniques become less useful with time.

In our hands, indirect reduction is a mainstay in patients who are neurologically intact but require surgical stabilization. In a patient with a very minor neurologic lesion—Frankel D or better—posterior indirect reduction is a reasonable alternative. In patients with more severe neurologic deficits, in which the pathology is largely anterior, we strongly prefer an anterior approach including debridement, vertebrectomy, and stabilization.

A representative case of indirect reduction is shown in Fig. 105-5. This represents a 44-year-old

*References 34, 42, 58, 59, 63, 64, and 68.

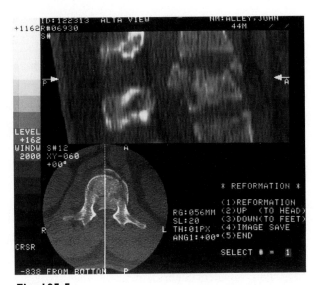

Fig. 105-5

A, Preoperative scan of neurologically intact burst fracture.

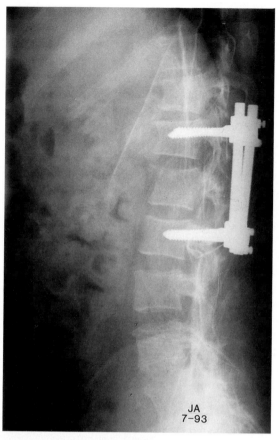

B

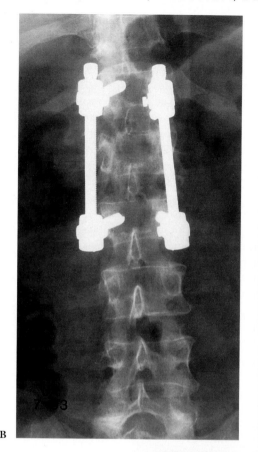

C

Fig. 105-5, cont'd

B, Postoperative AP and lateral x-ray studies showing reduction with the RF system. **C,** Postoperative CT scan showing indirect reduction.

male who had an axial loading injury with 80% canal compromise. Posterior pedicular instrumentation with restoration of anatomy was performed. The patient had excellent debridement of the canal, as shown in the postoperative CT scans. Nevertheless, maintenance of reduction is quite difficult. Pedicular instrumentation has had some untoward late consequences, including screw breakage with reproduction of mild deformity. Myllynen and associates had recreation of deformity even after removal of Harrington rods in fracture situations.[49] The overriding factor is that the vertebral body is largely cancellous bone with large venous lakes and insufficient structural support to maintain long-term healing and maintenance of anatomic restoration.

Direct Decompression via the Posterolateral Technique

Some authors believe that posterolateral decompression is effective in patients with vertebral burst fractures.[29] This is done either through a costotransversectomy approach or via pedicular decompression. It certainly has efficacious usage in certain situations in which a posterior approach is required, such as flexion/distraction injuries. Nevertheless, our experience and feeling regarding this approach for burst fractures (when the pathology is largely anterior to the spinal column) is that it can be somewhat risky and does not always debride the spinal canal consistently. In addition, often some type of laminectomy or decompression procedure is usually performed at the time of posterolateral decompression. This destabilizes the posterior elements, and can lead to late instability and posttraumatic kyphosis. Though many respectable and outstanding surgeons use this technique, in our hands it has limitations and very rare indications.

Anterior Approach

In patients with burst fractures and anterior canal compromise, we believe the anterior approach with debridement and decompression is the most favorable approach. This is the only way the canal can be appropriately decompressed and improvement in neurologic status optimized.*

The anterior approach to the spinal column is not difficult. The approach will not be detailed here, but is described in other chapters. In summary, for an L1 burst fracture a left-sided approach through the tenth rib is performed. The diaphragm is taken down and segmental vessels ligated, exposing the left spinal column from T12 to L2.

Anterior vertebrectomy is performed at this time. Anatomic landmarks are identified. A #15 blade is used to resect the disc between T12-L1 and L1-L2. After this is done, pituitary rongeurs are used to evacuate the disc totally. A burr or osteotomes are then used to remove the middle portion of the ver-

tebral body of L1. We prefer to try to preserve the very anterior aspect of the body as well as the anterior longitudinal ligament, to help provide stability. Certain points need to be emphasized at this juncture: if the patient has an old fracture, if there is significant canal stenosis, or if there is kyphosis greater than 20 degrees, then it is very important to remove a significant aspect of the mid and anterior vertebral bodies prior to canal debridement. We prefer to take an anterior and middle trough resected down to the opposing cortex of the body. If the dural sheath is exposed on the side of surgical entry or if a wide trough is not cut, then the dura can button-hole through this entry point, migrate anteriorly, and make surgical decompression of the remainder of the canal essentially impossible. This point cannot be overemphasized. We prefer to cut a deep trough while doing a vertebrectomy and to approach the dural tube at either its middle or opposite aspect. After that, we burr back to the posterior cortical margin and use a curette or small Kerrison rongeur to try to remove the posterior wafer of the vertebral cortex.

After the spinal decompression is complete, fixation of the spine may be necessary. Anterior strut fusion has a basic biomechanical advantage over posterior fusion, as the bone graft is under compression. Posterior fusions, especially in kyphotic situations, are more likely to resorb or progress to pseudarthrosis, as the graft is under tension. Even with the biomechanical advantage of compression, strut grafting alone in certain pathologic conditions is insufficient without supplemental internal fixation. At the thoracolumbar junction stresses on the vertebral body can approach three times body weight. Bone-graft material is a nonphysiologic entity that has to revascularize and heal. This is excessive force to be placed on graft material, and augmentation with instrumentation is necessary.

The technique for bone grafting is simple, yet important. A slot is fashioned in the vertebral bodies above and below. A slot would be cut on the undersurface of the T12 vertebral body, as well as the superior surface of the L2 vertebral body. This slot should be cut directly left to right with no migration, either toward the spinal canal or anterior toward the vascular structures. We actually prefer to start the slot slightly posterior to the midportion of the body of the associated vertebrae and carry it slightly anteriorly as we go across the body. This helps prevent graft migration or dislodgment. The graft should be stable, it should not be allowed to move, and it should be in anatomic position. Anteroposterior and lateral radiographs are performed at this time.

---

*References 4, 8, 16, 25, 27, 32, 36 to 38, 44, 66, and 67.

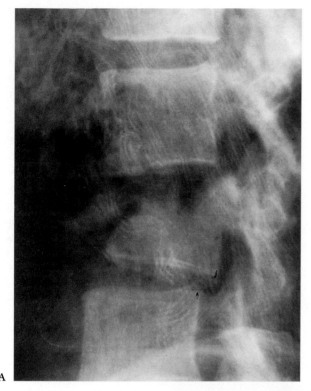

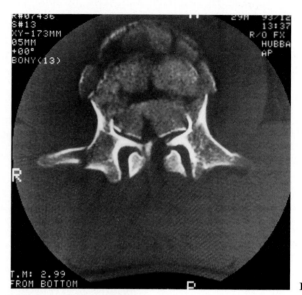

Fig. 105-6

A 28-year-old male with L3 burst fracture and incomplete neurological picture. **A,** Lateral radiograph showing fracture pattern. **B,** Preoperative CT scan: the patient underwent anterior vertebrectomy, instrumentation, and fusion. **C,** Postoperative CT scan.

From a technical standpoint, instrumentation associated with bony fusion is not a new concept. It is routinely used almost without exception in injuries to upper and lower extremities. Acceptance in spinal problems has been much slower. Obviously, potential complications play a role in that. But acceptance of intervertebral fixation for cervical procedures as well as more recently for thoracolumbar procedures appears to be gaining popularity.

The technique for anterior instrumentation is quite simple. A subperiosteal exposure of the entire vertebral body above and below is necessary. Most

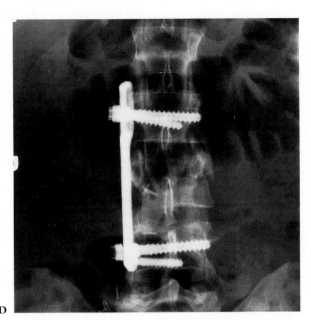

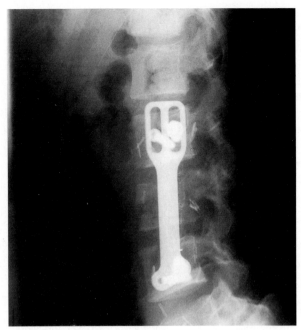

D

Fig. 105-6, cont'd

D, AP and lateral x-ray studies showing instrumentation and reduction.

anterior systems require some type of screw placement into the vertebral body above and below the injured levels. Some require fixation of the opposing cortex, though this needs to be done carefully. It is important for wide exposure to be obtained, and this necessitates the entire body of T12 and L2 to be exposed in this particular situation. It is important to try to reduce the kyphosis and restore the spinal column to as normal an anatomic alignment as possible. After this is done, the device is secured to the T12 and L2 bodies and anatomic reduction is restored. A representative case is shown Fig. 105-6.

In summary, in patients with vertebral burst fractures, and especially in those with neurologic insults, we believe strongly that timely anterior vertebrectomy, fusion, and instrumentation is the most appropriate way to proceed. Dunn in 1984 reported two Frankel Grade improvements with this technique, using the Zimmer anterior fixation device.[16] We believe it is the safest and best way to provide optimal canal debridement and give the patient the best chance for neurologic improvement and recovery.

Other Issues

We have defined basic principles in reference to thoracolumbar fractures. Other issues also play a role in management of these patients. In children and adolescents, neurologic deficit or insult can occur in up to 20% of patients with no definable lesion on radi-

ographic study.[3] The mechanism for this is somewhat obscure but may be related to a vascular etiology. Patients with osteoporosis, ankylosing spondylitis, or other major metabolic disorders have special problems associated with thoracic and lumbar fractures that are inherent to their disease and somewhat beyond the scope of this text.

Early management and intervention is quite important in patients with multiple traumatic injuries. Evaluation was carried out in the Syracuse Medical Center reviewing 138 spinal fractures.[55] Spinal fractures in multiple traumatized patients (injury severity score > 18) were divided into two groups—spinal surgery less than 72 hours or later than 72 hours after injury. Patients with isolated thoracolumbar fracture also had their surgery either before 72 hours or after 72 hours. Multiple-trauma patients with spinal fractures undergoing early surgery had statistically significant less morbidity and shorter hospital stays compared with the late surgery group (Table 105-2). In summary, it is our strong belief that in patients with injuries of severity score greater than 18, early surgical intervention is important to provide the patient appropriate resuscitation of other vital organ systems. This is well researched in the extremity trauma literature and is becoming more evident in spine trauma. Patients who had isolated thoracolumbar injuries did not appear to be as time-dependent in their surgical intervention when it was required.

Table 105-2

Patients with multiple traumatic injuries (ISS > 18)

	Surgery < 72°	Surgery > 72°
Number	35	25
Average ISS	27.5	28.4
COMPLICATION		
Pulmonary	3 (8.5%)	12 (48%)
DVT	0	2 (8%)
Pressure sore	2 (5.7%)	7 (28%)
UTI	8 (22.8%)	8 (32%)
Wound infection	0	2 (8%)
Hospital days	682 (19.5/patient)	875 (35/patient)
ICU days	151 (4.3/patient)	391 (15.6/patient)
Ventilator days	51 (1.5/patient)	281 (11.3/patient)
Hospital cost per patient	$6700	$22,490

Summary

We have given an overview of basic principles involving care of thoracolumbar fractures. Many factors are involved in decisions associated with these injuries. The issue of treatment specifically revolves around fracture stability type and neurologic status. we have emphasized those types of injuries that can be problematic and described treatment basics and alternatives.

Salient summary points include

1. Use of methylprednisolone in patients with acute spinal cord injury.

2. Conservative management of most neurologically by intact burst fractures.

3. Emphasis on the posterior ligamentous column in identifying "unstable burst fractures."

4. Aggressive early surgical stabilization in indicated spinal injuries in multiply traumatized patients.

References

1. An HS and others: Low lumbar burst fractures: comparison among body cast, Harrington rod, Luque rod, and Steffee plate, *Spine* 16(S8):440, 1991.

2. An HS and others: Low lumbar burst fractures: comparison between conservative and surgical treatments, *Spine* 16(8): pp 440–444, 1991.

3. Bohlman HH: Current concepts review: treatment of fractures and dislocations of the thoracic and lumbar spine, *J Bone Joint Surg* 67A(1):165, 1985.

4. Bohlman HH, Freehafer A, Dejak J: The results of treatment of acute injuries of the upper thoracic spine with paralysis, *J Bone Joint Surg* 67A(3):360, 1985.

5. Bracken MB and others: A randomized, controlled trial of methylprednisolone or naloxone in the treatment of acute spinal cord injury: results of the Second National Acute Spinal Cord Injury Study, *N Engl J Med* 332(20):1405, 1990.

6. Cantor JB and others: Nonoperative management of stable thoracolumbar burst fractures with early ambulation and bracing, *Spine* 18(8):971, 1993.

7. Chance GQ: Note on a type of flexion fracture of the spine, *Br J Radiol* 21:452, 1948.

8. Clohisy JC and others: Neurologic recovery associated with anterior decompression of spine fractures at the thoracolumbar junction (T12-L1), *Spine* 17(8S):325, 1992.

9. Cotterill PC and others: Production of a reproducible spinal burst fracture for use in biomechanical testing, *J Orthop Res* 5(3):462, 1987.

10. Denis F: The three column spine and its significance in the classification of acute thoracolumbar spinal injuries, *Spine* 8(8):817, 1983.

11. Denis F, Burkus JK: Shear fracture-dislocations of the thoracic and lumbar spine associated with forceful hyperextension (lumberjack paraplegia), *Spine* 17(2):156, 1992.

12. Denis F and others: Acute thoracolumbar burst fractures in the absence of neurologic deficit: a comparison between operative and non-operative treatment, *Clin Orthop* 189:142, 1984.

13. Dick W: The "Fixateur Interne" as a versatile implant for spine surgery, *Spine* 12(9):882, 1987.

14. Dick W and others: A new device for internal fixation of thoracolumbar and lumbar spine fractures: the "Fixateur Interne," *Paraplegia* 23:225, 1985.

15. Dickson JH, Harrington PR, Erwin WD: Results of reduction and stabilization of the severely fractured thoracic and lumbar spine, *J Bone Joint Surg* 60A:799, 1978.

16. Dunn HK: Anterior stabilization of thoracolumbar injuries, *Clin Orthop Rel Res* 189:116, 1984.

17. Esses SI: The placement and treatment of thoracolumbar spine fractures: an algorithmic approach, *Orthop Rev* 17(6):571, 1988.

18. Farfan HF, Gracovetsky S: The nature of instability, *Spine* 9:714, 1984.

19. Fidler MW: Remodelling of the spinal canal after burst fracture: a prospective study of two cases, *J Bone Joint Surg* [Br] 70B:730, 1988.

20. Frankel HL and others: The value of postural reduction in the initial management of closed injuries to the spine with paraplegia and tetraplegia, *Paraplegia* 7:179, 1969.

21. Fredricksen BE and others: Vertebral burst fractures: an experimental, morphologic, and radiographic study, *Spine* 17:1012, 1992.

22. Frymoyer JW, Selby DK: Segmental instability: rationale for treatment, *Spine* 10:280, 1985.

23. Gertzbein SD: Scoliosis Research Society: Multicenter Spine Fracture Study, *Spine* 17:528, 1992.

24. Gertzbein SD and others: Canal clearance in burst fractures using the AO Fixateur Interne, *Spine* 17(5):558, 1992.

25. Gertzbein SD and others: Decompression and circumferential stabilization of unstable spinal fractures, *Spine* 13(8):892, 1988.

26. Green BA and others: Acute spinal cord injury: current concepts, *Clin Orthop Rel Res* 154:125, 1981.

27. Grootboom MJ, Govender S, Charles RW: Anterior decompression of burst fractures with neurological deficit, *Injury* 21:389, 1990.

28. Haher TR and others: The contribution of the three columns of the spine to rotational stability: a biomechanical model, *Spine* 14(7):663, 1989.

29. Hardaker WT and others: Bilateral transpedicular decompression and Harrington rod stabilization in the management of severe thoracolumbar burst fractures, *Spine* 17(2):162, 1992.

30. Holdsworth F: Review article: fractures, dislocations, and fracture-dislocations of the spine, *J Bone Joint Surg* 52A(8):1534, 1970.

31. James KS and others: Biomechanical evaluation of the stability of thoracolumbar burst fractures, *Spine* 1993, in press.

32. Kaneda K, Abumi K, Fujiya M: Burst fractures with neurologic deficits of the thoracolumbar-lumbar spine, *Spine* 9(8):788, 1984.

33. Karlstrom G, Olerud S, Sjostrom L: Transpedicular fixation of thoracolumbar fractures, *Contemp Orthop* 20(3):285, 1990.

34. Keene JS and others: Compression-distraction instrumentation of unstable thoracolumbar fractures: anatomic results obtained with each type of injury and method of instrumentation, *Spine* 11(9):895, 1986.

35. Kelly RP, Whitesides TE: Treatment of lumbodorsal fracture-dislocations, *Ann Surg* 167:705, 1968.

36. Kostuik JP: Anterior fixation for burst fractures of the thoracic and lumbar spine with or without neurologic involvement, *Spine* 13(3):286, 1988.

37. Kostuik JP: Anterior fixation for fractures of the thoracic and lumbar spine with or without neurologic involvement, *Clin Orthop Rel Res* 189:103, 1984.

38. Kostuik JP: Anterior stabilization, instrumentation and decompression for post-traumatic kyphosis, *Spine* 14(4):379, 1989.

39. Krompinger WJ and others: Conservative treatment of fractures of the thoracic and lumbar spine, *Orthop Clin North Am* 17(1):161, 1986.

40. LeGay DA, Petrie DP, Alexander DI: Flexion-distraction injuries of the lumbar spine and associated abdominal trauma, *J Trauma* 30(4):436, 1990.

41. Lin RM, Panjabi MM, Oxland TR: Functional radiographs of acute thoracolumbar burst fractures: a biomechanical study, *Spine* 18(16):2431, 1993.

42. Lindahl JW, Irstam L, Nordwall A: Unstable thoracolumbar fractures: a study by CT and conventional roentgenology of the reduction effect of Harrington instrumentation, *Spine* 9(2):214, 1984.

43. Malcolm BW and others: Post-traumatic kyphosis: a review of forty-eight surgically treated patients, *J Bone Joint Surg* 63A:891, 1981.

44. McAfee PC, Bohlman HH, Yuan HA: Anterior decompression of traumatic thoracolumbar fractures with incomplete neurological deficit using a retroperitoneal approach, *J Bone Joint Surg* 67A(1):89, 1985.

45. McAfee PC, Yuan HA, Lasda NA: The unstable burst fracture, *Spine* 7(4):366, 1982.

46. McAfee PC and others: The value of computed tomography in thoracolumbar fractures, *J Bone Joint Surg* 65A(4):461, 1983.

47. Mick CA and others: Burst fractures of the fifth lumbar vertebra, *Spine* 18(13):1878, 1993.

48. Mumford J and others: Thoracolumbar burst fractures: the clinical efficacy and outcome of nonoperative management, *Spine* 18(8):955, 1993.

49. Myllynen P, Bostman O, Riska E: Recurrence of deformity after removal of Harrington's fixation of spine fracture, *Acta Orthop Scand* 59(5):497, 1988.

50. Oxland TE and others: An anatomic basis for spinal instability: a porcine trauma model, *J Orthop Res* 9:452, 1991.

51. Posner I, Edwards WT, Hayes WC: A biomechanical analysis of the clinical stability of the lumbar and lumbosacral spine, *Spine* 7:374, 1982.

52. Pratt ES, Green DA, Spengler DM: Herniated intervertebral discs associated with unstable spinal injuries, *Spine* 15(7):662, 1990.

53. Reid DC and others: The nonoperative treatment of burst fractures of the thoracolumbar junction, *J Trauma* 28(8):1188, 1988.

54. Roberson JR, Whitesides TE: Surgical reconstruction of late post-traumatic thoracolumbar kyphosis, *Spine* 10(4):307, 1985.

55. Schlegel J and others: Timing of surgical stabilization and fusion in acute spinal fractures, 1993, in press.

56. Shirado O and others: Influence of disc degeneration on mechanism of thoracolumbar burst fractures, *Spine* 17(3):286, 1992.

57. Shufflebarger HL, Clark CE: Thoracolumbar osteotomy for postsurgical sagittal imbalance, *Spine* 17(8S):287, 1992.

58. Starr JK, Hanley EN: Junctional burst fractures, *Spine* 17:551, 1992.

59. Wang GJ and others: The treatment of fracture dislocations of the thoracolumbar spine with halofemoral traction and Harrington rod instrumentation, *Clin Orthop Rel Res* 142:168, 1979.

60. Weinstein JN, Collalto P, Lehmann TR: Thoracolumbar "burst" fractures treated conservatively: a long-term follow-up, *Spine* 13(1):33, 1988.

61. White AA, Panjabi MM: *Clinical biomechanics of the spine*. Philadelphia, 1978, J.B. Lippincott.

62. Whitesides TE: Traumatic kyphosis of the thoracolumbar spine, *Clin Orthop Rel Res* 128:78, 1977.

63. Willen JAG, Gaekwad UH, Kakulas BA: Burst fractures in the thoracic and lumbar spine: a clinico-neuropathologic analysis, *Spine* 14(12):1316, 1989.

64. Willen J, Lindahl S, Nordwall A: Unstable thoracolumbar fractures: a comparative clinical study of conservative treatment and Harrington instrumentation, *Spine* 10(2):111, 1985.

65. Wittenberg RH and others: A biomechanical study of the fatigue characteristics of thoracolumbar fixation implants in a calf spine model, *Spine* 17(6S):121, 1992.

66. Young B, Brooks WH, Tibbs PA: Anterior decompression and fusion for thoracolumbar fractures with neurological deficits, *Acta Neurochir* 57:287, 1981.

67. Yuan HA and others: Early clinical experience with the Syracuse I-plate: an anterior spinal fixation device, *Spine* 13(3):278, 1988.

68. Zou D and others: Mechanics of anatomic reduction of thoracolumbar burst fractures, *Spine* 18(2):195, 1993.

Chapter 106
Management of the Spinal Cord–Injured Patient

E. Shannon Stauffer

Physical Examination

    spinal shock
    Browne–Sequard syndrome
    central cord lesion

Prognosis for Recovery of Complete Lesions

Determination of Injury by Imaging Techniques

    ct scans
    mri scans

Preventing Medical Complications

    urinary and bowel complications
    cardiac complications
    autonomic dysreflexia
    pulmonary complications
    skin ulcers
    joint and muscle contractures
    deep venous thrombosis
    sexual dysfunction

Nutritional Support

Pain Management

Late Complications

    sitting pressure sores
    fracture of the long bones

Rehabilitation and Activities of Daily Living

Adjunct to Independent Living

    orthotics
    standing
    ambulation

Surgical Reconstruction of the Quadriplegic Hand

    specific transfers for specific levels

Community Reentry

Life Expectancy

Summary

The rehabilitation of a patient with a spinal cord injury begins with the recognition of the injury. Plans must be formulated in the emergency room to prevent medical complications and to predict a general prognosis that can be presented to the family to prepare their coping with this devastating injury. It is important to document the severity of the injury, the level of the injury, and the amount of preservation of voluntary neurologic function below the zone of the cord lesion.

It is important to document the history of the injury. Persons involved with high-velocity injuries are more likely to suffer complete a spinal cord lesion. Those who are injured with low-velocity impact are more likely to have an incomplete cord injury. The observation by the patient and others as to the function observed after the injury is important to ascertain whether the patient has lost additional neurologic function during the interval between the injury and your examination. The age of the patient must be taken into consideration. Young adults between the ages of 15 and 35 have a resilient spine, and it takes a significant amount of energy to disrupt the spine by fracture or dislocation. This energy is impacted into the spinal cord and frequently causes complete neurologic lesions. Middle-aged people from 35 to 55 have stiffer spines that may fracture with less trauma, and impart less injury to the spinal cord, producing spinal cord injuries of moderate severity. Patients over 55 years of age have decreased elasticity, bulging of the intervertebral discs, and the formation of vertebral osteophytes.

This, coupled with the hypertrophy, thickening, and decreased elasticity of the dorsal ligaments, provide an atmosphere for an impact on the spinal cord associated with minor dorsal element fractures or with no radiologic evidence of fracture at all and can cause severe spinal cord injury, usually of an incomplete nature, with some distal sparing of voluntary neurologic function.

Physical Examination

The physical examination for documentation of spinal cord function or loss thereof is performed in a systematic fashion beginning with the area of the body under volitional control. During conversation the examiner is able to observe the spontaneous voluntary motions of the face, head, and neck. A motor examination is then performed to document the muscles that are under active control and those which are paralyzed. If the patient is breathing voluntarily, this indicates that there is voluntary function from the brain down through the brainstem to the upper four cervical nerves. The phrenic nerve, which controls the diaphragm, gets innervation from C3, C4, and C5 with a greater portion coming from C4. The patient is then asked to shrug his shoulders. Active power in the trapezius documents the spinal accessory nerve (cranial nerve 11) and indicates the patient's understanding of the motor examination. Next the patient is asked to take a deep breath and cough. The rise of the abdomen indicates active diaphragm contraction. The rise or paradoxical fall of the rib cage documents the presence or absence of intercostal muscles. Palpating the abdomen while having the patient cough will document the presence or absence of abdominal muscles.

Attention is next turned to the upper extremity. Cervical 5 nerve root function is documented by active contraction of the deltoid and biceps muscle. Cervical 6 is documented by active extensor, carpiradialis longus, and brevis. Cervical 7 is documented by active finger extensors and triceps. Cervical 8 is documented by active finger flexors. Thoracic 1 is documented by active intrinsic function.

Attention is then turned to the lower extremities. Lumbar 1 nerve function is documented by hip flexion; L2 by hip adduction; L3 by quadriceps function; L4 by anterior tib function; L5 by extensor hallucis longus function; and S1 by toe flexors and gastrosoleus function. Sacral 2, 3, and 4 function is documented by voluntary sphincter contraction during the rectal examination. When the selected muscles are documented as being present or absent, one then determines the muscle grade of the intact muscles. It can be done in a unilateral fashion, examining the right upper extremity, then the left upper extremity, then the right lower extremity, then the left lower extremity. By examining one extremity at a time no dangerous stresses are placed on the injured spinal column. Following the muscle examination a sensory examination is performed. The patient should have sensibility over the face, which is supplied by cranial nerve 5 and be able to discriminate between the sharp and dull end of a pin. Cervical 2 is documented by the skin on the back of the head; C3 by the skin down over the neck; and C4 by the cape of skin down over the supraclavicular area. Cervical 5 is documented by the skin over the deltoid and biceps down into the radial side of the forearm. Cervical 6 is documented by perception of sensibility over the thumb, index, and long finger; C7 by better sensation over the long and ring finger; and C8 by better sensation over the ring and additionally the small finger. Thoracic 1 is documented by the sensation along the ulnar side of the hand and arm.

If the person appears to be a complete-lesion quadriplegic with no voluntary muscle function and no sensibility in the muscles and skin supplied by the spinal cord below the zone of injury, one must document the complete absence of muscle power and sensation before the diagnosis of complete quadriplegia can be made. This is accomplished by the rectal examination. If the person appears to have complete paralysis below the zone of injury and there is no voluntary function of the toe flexors, and the rectal examination demonstrates no voluntary contraction of the anal sphincter, and there is no sensation either within the rectum or the perianal area, then the patient can be diagnosed as a complete-lesion quadriplegic.

Spinal Shock

Following a severe injury to the spinal cord, which may be complete or incomplete, the spinal cord distal to the zone of injury suddenly becomes areflexic. During this period of spinal shock, which may last 6 to 48 hours, a complete lesion cannot be verified since the patient may appear to have a complete lesion, but is in spinal shock. As the patient comes out of the spinal shock, he or she may show signs of progressive neurologic recovery, indicating an incomplete spinal cord injury.

While performing the rectal examination, if the anus is patulous and there is no voluntary contraction, a tug on the catheter or squeeze of the glans penis or tap on the mons pubis normally will cause a reflex contraction of the anal sphincter. If this is absent, the patient is still in spinal shock, and a definite diagnosis of complete lesion cannot be made. If however, the reflex is present and the patient is out of spinal shock, in the absence of any sensibility of motor power below the level of the lesion, he or she can be diagnosed as having a complete spinal-cord lesion, which has a poor prognosis for any functional recovery.

To predict the probability of recovery and compare results with published data, the severity of the injury should be documented according to the standards described by the American Spinal Injury Association. The severity of the spinal cord injury is categorized by the classification described by Frankel:

A. Complete lesion, no sensibility and no voluntary muscle power distal to the zone of injury.

B. Sensory sparing only, no voluntary motor function.

C. Sensory sparing plus "useless" motor function in the lower extremities (muscle grades 1-2).

D. Sensory sparing plus "useful" motor power (3-4).

E. Normal sensation plus normal motor power (5/5).

By using the specific muscles described above, the examiner can assign a quantitative motor index to document the severity of the injury. Five muscles in each upper extremity (biceps, extensor carpi radialis longus, finger extensors, finger flexors, intrinsics) and five muscles of each lower extremity (iliopsoas, quadriceps, anterior tib, extensor hallucis longus, gastrosoleus) are considered. Each of the 20 muscles is graded 0 to 5 on the manual muscle test scale, for a possible total of 100, indicating normal muscle strength. This documentation provides a baseline upon which recovery of strength can be documented.

If the paralysis is found to be incomplete (voluntary muscle control), with recognition of sensibility, especially sacral sparing sensibility, the diagnosis will be an incomplete spinal cord lesion (Frankel B, C, or D) and should further be documented as to the most likely anatomic area of the spinal cord to be injured. It is rare that patients have a pure documentable anatomic lesion, but for prognostic reasons it is important to place the patient in the most closely identified category by physical examination. Labeling the patient "mixed lesion" does not help in the prognosis of recovery or in the recognition of recovery patterns on follow-up examination.

Browne–Sequard Syndrome

If the patient has a greater weakness on one side of the body and greater sensory loss on the contralateral side, this indicates a partial injury to the spinal cord on the side of the greatest motor loss. This incomplete syndrome has the best prognosis for recovery. Ninety percent of these patients will demonstrate enough recovery to have voluntary bowel and bladder control and be able to ambulate even though they may need an orthosis on the weaker leg and crutches for stability and balance.

Central Cord Lesion

Central cord lesion is the most common incomplete spinal cord syndrome. Clinical examination will demonstrate the presence of sensibility in the area supplied by the sacral nerve roots, particularly in the perianal area on the rectal examination, and possibly over the toes and plantar surface of the foot. This "sacral sparing" is enough to make the diagnosis of central cord syndrome with or without the addition of voluntary sphincter control or voluntary toe flexor muscles. Recovery can be expected to occur to varying degrees, usually beginning with distal muscles first; that is, toe flexors, toe extensors, ankle, knee, and hip. Approximately 50% to 60% of patients will make enough recovery to be functional ambulators, as the central part of the spinal cord (gray matter and central tracks to upper extremities and trunk) is most injured and the peripheral white matter (long track to sacral, lumbar, and lower trunk muscles) is least injured. Recovery of hand function is less likely than recovery of the lower-extremity muscles. This patient usually is left with residuals of varying amounts of lower extremity muscle function, complicated by spasticity, which may prevent functional ambulation. The upper extremities have little recovery owing to gray matter damage, and usually are left with a weak, flaccid paralysis. Approximately 50% to 60% of these people have functional recovery.

Prognosis for Recovery of Complete Lesions

If the patient has suffered a spinal cord injury and is documented to have no voluntary muscle power or sensibility below the zone of the lesion for 24 hours, and if the bulbocavernosus reflex has returned without perianal sensory perception, no distal functional recovery can be anticipated.

The injury not only injures the spinal cord at the level of the fracture, it also injures the nerve roots that emanate from the spinal cord above the zone of injury and exit the foramen at the level of injury. This nerve root can be expected to demonstrate recovery of an additional level of muscle power in the upper extremity in approximately 66% of patients. Injuries of the cervical spine at C4-C5 producing a "high quadriplegia" will demonstrate recovery of the C5 nerve root in only 25% to 30% of patients. However, injuries one level lower, at C5-C6 will demonstrate a 60% to 70% recovery of one nerve root level, and injuries at C6-C7, 80% to 90% of patients will have recovery of at least one nerve root level function. The prediction of this nerve root function helps determine rehabilitation goals.

Most nerve root level recovery occurs within 6 to 12 weeks, and may continue to get stronger for 12 to 18 months. Beyond 18 months no further recovery or increase in strength can be anticipated. About 10% of patients who have documented complete lesions will be found to recovery some scattered distal leg or trunk sensation and some trace muscle power as long as 3 to 6 months following the injury, but this recovery will not be of any functional value.

Determination of Injury by Imaging Techniques

It is difficult to predict the amount of spinal cord injury from x-ray images. There are some guidelines, however. Injuries to the upper cervical spine (C3-C4 and C4-C5), even with relatively mild displacement, are more frequently associated with complete spinal cord injuries than injuries in the lower cervical spine. At C6-C7, patients may have severe fractures or dislocations and have little or no neurologic loss. In general, however, the most common injuries, the C6 burst fracture with retropulsion of bone into the canal and the C5-C6 complete bilateral facet dislocations, are more likely to be associated with severe spinal cord injuries.

CT Scans

CT scans demonstrating greater canal compromise correlate with a greater degree of spinal cord injury in the cervical spine.

Fracture in the midthoracic area (T2-T7) has a higher frequency of spinal cord lesions owing to the small diameter of the spinal canal housing the small spinal cord, which does not tolerate forces in the translation or compression. The further down the spine one goes the more tolerance the spinal cord has to injury without suffering severe paralysis. In the lumbar spine large amounts of translation and canal compromise can be sustained without significant injury to the cauda equina. The amount of canal compromise on the CT scan can be an indication of the amount of injury to the conus and the cauda equina in the upper lumbar spine. Less than 30% compromise usually does not correlate with severe spinal cord injury. Greater than 60% compromise has a higher incidence of spinal cord and nerve root injury. The CT evidence of bone compression between 30% and 60% canal compromise does not correlate with a specific amount of spinal cord or nerve root damage to a significant degree. Therefore, the severity of the fracture, level of the fracture, and amount of canal compromise on the CT scan may be an indication of the severity of the spinal cord injury but must be correlated with the clinical findings on history and physical examination.

MRI Scans

Recent advances in magnetic resonance scanning has helped identify spinal cord lesions. A review by Bondurant and Cotler (*Spine* 15:161, 1990) identified three MRI types of imaging that indicate the amount of damage to the cord and aid in prognosis.

Type 1 was an area of decreased signal, indicating intraspinal hemorrhage, conferring the poorer prognosis with no increase in Frankel classification and minimal improvement of motor index from 32 to 42.

Type 2 images were those with hyperintensity or a bright signal consistent with cord edema. This was the most common image found. These patients had the least amount of initial injury and the best prognosis. They increased at least one Frankel grade and their motor trauma index went from 71 to 92.

Type 3 images were a dark hypointense center surrounded by a bright hyperintense periphery indicating hemorrhage in the center with edema surrounding it. These patients also improved at least one Frankel grade; however, their injuries were more severe, improving from an initial motor trauma index of 37 to a recovery of 76. It is of note that 20% of their patients (8/37) had significant spinal cord injuries clinically, but normal images on the MRI scan.

Preventing Medical Complications

When a patient is diagnosed as having a spinal cord injury and the amount of recovery has been predicted, the next step is to plan the rehabilitation and prevent the medical complications that may delay or prevent the rehabilitation or may be fatal if not recognized. During the initial acute stage of treatment, the complications that are common to each organ system of the body must be anticipated, prevented, recognized if they occur, and treated appropriately.

Urinary and Bowel Complications

The first complication to be addressed is the paralysis of bladder function. A Foley catheter is introduced into the bladder and precise urinary outputs are monitored each hour for the first 48 to 72 hours, to prevent fluid overload. During the period of spinal shock, which may be the first 24 to 48 hours following the injury, the body undergoes a "relative sympathectomy." There is flaccid paralysis of the voluntary musculature; dilation of the arterial capillary bed, producing an expanded intravascular space; and decreased peripheral resistance to the cardiovascular system, which results in a decreased systemic blood pressure in the patient. It is important not to overload the cardiovascular system with fluids during this period. When the period of spinal shock is over, peripheral resistance returns. The kidneys may not be able to eliminate the overload of fluid and car-

diopulmonary complications may occur (see below). Therefore, the Foley catheter is introduced until the intake and output has stabilized and the cardiovascular system has regained its tone. Following this the patient is placed on intermittent catheterization, initially every 4 hours. The patient's fluid intake is carefully measured as well as the urinary output. If the bladder does not fill more than 500 ml at each catheterization, the interval can be extended to intermittent catheterization every 6 hours during the rehabilitation. Later in the rehabilitation time, this can be adjusted to convenient times for the patient according to his or her oral intake, as long as the bladder does not get distended more than 600 ml at one time. If the bladder is allowed to overdistend, small tears in the mucous membrane can occur, which will allow any bacteria that may be in the urine to enter the bloodstream and cause septicemia.

Urinary tract infections will frequently occur during the initial hospitalization, particularly if a catheter is left in place for longer than 48 hours. Bacteria may be introduced by faulty intermittent catheterization techniques. The presence of bacteria in the urine itself is not an indication for active treatment. Many patients do have colonization of their bladder without inflammation and without symptoms. If, however, the person develops systemic reaction such as fever or if the urine becomes very cloudy, a urinalysis should be performed for bacterial count. Bacterial counts of over 100,000 colonies per milliliter indicate active treatment with appropriate antibiotics for the eradication of the bacteria. Occasionally the patient will need suppressive antibacterial treatment such as Macrodantin or Septra on a long-term basis, but it is best to use antibiotics only for the acute infectious episodes, if practical.

Bowel management consists of the introduction of a nasogastric (NG) tube in the early acute phase to prevent the ileus that frequently accompanies fractures of the spine. Development of distension of the stomach or bowel will compromise diaphragm function and decrease inspiratory volume. Patients will frequently develop bleeding from the gastric mucosa following a spinal cord injury. This may be accentuated by the administration of steroids, which are used to decrease the severity of the incomplete spinal cord injury. Gastrointestinal bleeding that occurs about the end of the first week can be severe. It is usually not from an ulcer but from a hemorrhagic gastritis. This can be prevented by the use of the H_2-receptor antagonist, Cimetidine, which is administrated intravenously and then orally in decreasing doses after removal of the NG tube. The reflex emptying of the bowel during the period of rehabilitation is accomplished by appropriate manipulation of the diet, stimulant suppository on a daily or every-other-day basis, and the administration of oral stool softeners (Doxinate), which are adjusted to maintain a soft consistency of the stool.

Cardiac Complications

When a person first suffers a severe injury to the cervical spinal cord, he or she develops a low blood pressure (usually 90-95/50-60). As long as this maintains urinary output, attempts to increase the blood pressure with excessive amounts of fluids should be prevented. Cardiopressors are sometimes used to increase the blood pressure in the theory that the decreased blood pressure may increase the cord injury and the blood pressure should be maintained to provide profusion of the swollen spinal cord. Cardiopressors rarely are effective in maintaining the blood pressure over 100, and fluid overload is more dangerous than beneficial, and may be fatal. During the first several days the patient may also have various cardiac arrhythmias. These must be monitored closely to detect episodes of bradycardia which may lead to a sudden cardiac arrest and to provide sufficient resuscitation should cardiac arrest occur. After the first several days, the rhythm stabilizes to normal and the blood pressure gradually rises to approximately 100-110/60-70, which is a typical blood pressure for a chronic quadriplegic.

Autonomic Dysreflexia

As the period of spinal shock dissipates, the voluntary musculature and the sympathetic nervous system gradually develop a state of hyperreflexia. Without the inhibitory influence of the brain and cerebellum reflex centers, the spinal reflexes are more easily set into motion. The deep-tendon reflexes of the lower extremities become hyperactive and may develop clonus. The sympathetic nervous system also becomes hyperactive, and any noxious stimuli may cause an overreaction of the sympathetic nervous system. This causes constriction of the peripheral vascular tree, which results in hypertension. The hypertension then stimulates the baroreceptors in the carotid sinuses, which send impulses into the brain to inhibit the hypertension. Since the impulse cannot be carried down the spinal cord to inhibit the sympathetic nervous system, it can only be carried down through the vagus nerve to decrease the heart rate. Therefore, as long as the noxious stimulus continues to stimulate the sympathetic nervous system in the spinal cord, the blood pressure remains high

and the pulse decreases. Blood pressure may go as high as 220/150 and the patient, even if young, may suffer a cerebral hemorrhage. Therefore, it is imperative, if the young spinal cord patient presents with increasing hypertension, to look for and remove any noxious stimuli. The first treatment is to check the catheter and make sure it is flowing. If it is not flowing, the catheter should be changed for a new one. If it is open, it can be irrigated with a solution of 10 ml of 1% Zylocaine diluted to 30 ml and slowly introduced into the bladder to assure free flow of the catheter and also to anesthetize the bladder mucosa. If this does not bring down the blood pressure, a rectal examination with Nupercainal ointment on a gloved finger should be performed to make sure there is no fecal impaction. The patient should be sitting in an upright position to decrease the pressure to the brain. An IV should be started and the following medication may be injected slowly: dioxide (Hyperstat) 5 mg/kg (usually a 150-300 mg bolus is injected slowly as a single bolus). This usually works rapidly and there is no hypotensive overshoot. If this is not sufficient, hydralazine (Apresoline) may be injected, but this must be injected very slowly over 30 to 60 minutes since the action of this drug may cause the patient to precipitously become hypotensive.

If a patient is subject to autonomic dysreflexia on a repetitive basis, B & O suppositories (belladonna and opium alkaloids) may be kept on hand to insert into the rectum to alleviate the pounding headache and increasing blood pressure.

Pulmonary Complications

Pulmonary complications are the most significant life-threatening conditions during the first week following an injury. If they are anticipated and understood, they are preventable.

With an injury to the cervical spinal cord that causes paralysis in the trunk, the only muscles available for respiratory function are the diaphragm and the cervical accessory muscles, which help elevate the clavicle and the upper ribs. The intercostal muscles that help with forced inspiration and expiration are paralyzed. The abdominal muscles, which provide forced exhalation, are also paralyzed. The amount of diaphragm function remaining depends on the level of the spinal cord injury. At the typical fracture dislocation at the C5-C6 level, the C4 nerve root is intact and will provide for continued diaphragm function. As the diaphragm contracts, inhalation occurs, but this only amounts to the patient's normal tidal volume. The patient does not have any inspiratory reserve and therefore inhales only approximately 20% of normal vital capacity (1000/5000). Expiration occurs only by relaxation of the diaphragm and 1000 ml will escape passively. Without the inspiratory reserve of the intercostals and the expiratory reserve of the forced expiration of the abdominals, the patient cannot fully expand all the alveoli and cannot cough or expel the mucous secretions that occur in the tracheobronchial tree. This leads to increased retention of pulmonary secretions, which leads to atelectasis rapidly complicated by pneumonia. If these complications are not anticipated and prevented, the patient may expire, usually on the fifth to seventh day post injury. It is important to begin aggressive pulmonary toilet immediately following the injury, encouraging breathing as deeply as possible, assisting exhaling and coughing with manual pressure over the abdomen. If the patient has difficulty removing secretions, bronchoscopic cleanout may be necessary several times during the first several weeks. With aggressive pulmonary therapy, physical therapy, and suctioning and bronchoscopy, tracheostomy is rarely needed. If, however, the patient develops fatigue in breathing, or retained secretions cannot be removed satisfactorily, a tracheostomy should be performed to assist in decreasing dead space and ease the suctioning of secretions. Tracheostomy is usually temporary; after several weeks, the problem of secretions decreases.

If, during the first 2 to 3 days, the patient is given a fluid overload as described previously, in an attempt to elevate blood pressure, and the vascular tree contracts after spinal shock is over, the kidneys may not be able to eliminate the excess volume of fluid overload. Pulmonary edema may occur, which will complicate the atelectasis/pneumonia problem. Therefore, accurate fluid replacement to replace only those fluids secreted, and aggressive respiratory therapy, can prevent the pulmonary complications that in the past have been the greatest cause of death in quadriplegic patients.

Skin Ulcers

During the first several days or weeks after injury, the severity of the acute problems of paralysis, bladder, and pulmonary management in the intensive-care unit quickly overshadow the thoughts of maintaining skin integrity. One to 2 hours on a hard x-ray table or 4 to 5 hours in one position in the ICU bed may cause ischemia to the skin and underlying tissues over bony prominences, which will slowly develop into pressure ulcers on the skin. It is important that all team members treating the patient, including nurses, therapists, and x-ray technicians, appreciate the pressure mechanics causing skin necrosis. Areas over bony prominences, particularly the sacrum and trochanters, must be examined each nursing shift and appropriately supported with pillows and positioning to avoid prolonged pressure. Pressure ulcers are the most common delay of rehabilitation and cause for rehospitalization to the acute hospital from the rehabilitation unit. All areas of redness must be carefully observed and kept free of pressure until the redness disappears.

Joint and Muscle Contractures

It is important to prevent contractures of the upper-extremity joints and to maintain flexibility of the muscles for future rehabilitation. Daily passive range-of-motion exercises of all joints is important during the first several weeks following traumatic quadriplegia. It is important not to stretch out the muscles but allow them to develop myelostatic contractures. This will allow reflex gross grasp and prehension to develop in the paralyzed hand during rehabilitation, which will be discussed under Rehabilitation and Activities of Daily Living. During the acute period it is important to provide passive hand splints to maintain position of function of all upper-extremity joints.

Deep Venous Thrombosis

Owing to the muscle paralysis, recumbent position, and cardiovascular dynamics associated with quadriplegia, these patients have a high incidence of deep venous thrombosis (DVT), which may lead to a pulmonary embolism and death. As soon as the initial hemorrhagic period is over and there is minimal chance of bleeding into the fractured spine or injured spinal cord area, the patient should be placed on prophylactic low-dose Coumadin to keep the prothrombin time between 1.2 and 1.5 control. The patient should wear sequential positive pressure lower-extremity boots while in bed and antiembolism stockings while sitting in the wheelchair. Daily range-of-motion exercises with elevation and straight-leg raising of the lower extremities, and stretching of the hamstring muscles should be used to prevent stasis in the veins of the lower extremity, which can lead to DVT and pulmonary embolism. Since the patient does not have protective sensation of the lower extremities, the physical signs must be appreciated to make the diagnosis of DVT. The first physical sign to look for is mild elevation of temperature of unknown etiology. If the pulmonary system and the urinary system have been investigated and are free of infection, one must suspect a DVT. The second sign is unilateral swelling of the lower extremities. If DVT is suspected, formal anticoagulation with therapeutic doses of anticoagulant is indicated to prevent propagation of a blood clot. The patient should be kept at bed rest with elevation during the active phases of the phlebitis, but as soon as the inflammation decreases, the patient may be mobilized again to the wheelchair with antiembolism stockings.

Sexual Dysfunction

The complication of sexual dysfunction should be addressed early in the course of the hospitalization by the physician and the medical psychologist, to help the patient and family understand the prognosis for sexual function, methods of achieving sexual function, and prognosis for bearing children. Female patients usually have no physiologic abnormalities with sexual function. The limitations are secondary to the anesthesia and the muscle paralysis accompanying the quadriplegia. Male patients, however, have serious dysfunction. They cannot achieve psychogenic erections, but can get reflex erections with stimulus to the penis and perineal area. The patients are usually not able to experience a sexual climax, and ejaculation of seminal fluid may occur anytime during or after coitus. Following a complete spinal cord injury, sperm formation is usually faulty and sparse and patients rarely can father children in a long-term quadriplegic state.

Nutritional Support

During the initial hospitalization following a quadriplegia, patients undergo a significant negative nitrogen balance. They rapidly lose muscle mass. It is important to maintain good nutrition. A high protein–high fiber diet is necessary. It is best not to use a high intake of dairy products to provide protein, since the patient is also in a negative calcium balance and putting out large amounts of calcium through the urine. This has a tendency to increase the development of urinary calculi. Carbohydrate intake should be tailored to the needs of the patient to maintain ideal body weight. If the patient is normal body weight, a high protein–high carbohydrate diet is indicated. If the patient has an excess of body adipose tissue, the carbohydrates should be curtailed.

Pain Management

Most patients with paralysis and loss of sensibility in the trunk and lower extremities will complain of "pain." This is very difficult for the patient to describe. Usually it is a dysesthesia type of pain. There may be some pins and needles feeling, and there may be some shooting pains in the extremities, but it rarely is a severe pain and it is best treated with less than narcotic medication. If the patient understands that the pain is not coming from the extremity itself, but instead from the inflammation and healing at the level of the injury of the spinal cord, from which it is being transmitted to the brain, they are more able to understand and tolerate the unusual and bizarre sensations that they are getting. Since the patient does not have adequate terminology to describe these sensations, he or she calls them pain. Therefore, this frequently results in administration of narcotic medication to relieve the "pain." Obviously a narcotic is only going to relieve it temporarily, and the patient is in great danger of becoming dependent on the narcotic medication. Therefore, it is important to use nonnarcotic medications to help the patient with discomfort while he or she is learning to live with it.

Late Complications

Other complications to be anticipated and prevented during the first year following spinal cord injury are discussed here.

Sitting Pressure Sores

Sitting pressure sores are pressure sores over the ischial tuberosity and the coccyx from sitting in a wheelchair. Once the patient is out of bed, he or she is not immune to pressure sores, and careful attention must be paid to the fitting of the wheelchair and the pressure measurements of the wheelchair cushion, over the sacrum, coccyx, ischial tuberosity, trochanters, and posterior thighs to distribute pressure and prevent pressure sores in these areas. Definite periodic follow-up at least semiannually is necessary to monitor skin integrity.

Fracture of the Long Bones

After the first year following a spinal cord injury, osteoporosis of the long bones of the lower extremities is sufficient to set the stage for pathologic fractures from relatively trivial trauma. If the patient has a lot of spasticity, osteoporosis is less. If the patient has a flaccid paralysis, the osteoporosis is greater. Range of motion of tight joints as well as falls or minor accidents may cause fractures of the long bones. These usually occur in the metaphyseal areas. The distal femur is the most common, approximal tibia is second most common, neck of femur third most common, and distal tibia fourth. These fractures are usually minimally or moderately displaced and will heal with external immobilization. It is not recommended to use a circular plaster cast or open reduction and internal fixation for these chronic pathologic osteoporotic fractures. Open reduction and internal fixation usually results in a failure of fixation and loss of stability and the stripping of blood supply may lead to nonunion. Immobilization with large soft pillow splints for the initial period until the swelling goes down, followed by well-padded bivalve plaster splints with the leg extended for sleeping position and the knee flexed for sitting in the wheelchair will provide satisfactory stability for the healing of the fracture. Minimal to moderate amounts of angulation or rotation are not significant in the quadriplegic patient confined to a wheelchair. Spasticity of the lower extremities usually increases during the first 6 weeks. It plateaus at about 6 months to 1 year following the injury. Recommendations for management of spasticity are the use of various medications for the first year. If spasticity persists at the end of 1 year, then surgical procedures can be recommended to weaken the muscles and decrease the spasticity. The patient must realize, however, that the surgical procedures will make the muscles weaker and they may cause some atrophy of the muscles. The first surgical procedure usually necessary is an adductor tenotomy and anterior obturator neurectomy. This will usually decrease the adductor-flexor spasticity of the hips, and generally decrease the spasticity in the lower extremities. If this is not sufficient, a percutaneous three-step cut, tendo Achilles lengthening will decrease the clonus and spasticity of the ankle, which will tend to decrease the spontaneous spasticity of the rest of the lower extremity. Rarely, a patient will need an intrapelvic release of the iliopsoas to relieve hip flexor spasticity.

Heterotopic ossification is a condition that occurs in spinal cord and head injured patients. It is an increased accumulation of intermuscular calcification followed by ossification around the hip and knee joint. It occurs most commonly about the hip joint along the anterior aspect, extracapsular, and extends from the anterior superior iliac spine down to the lesser trochanter. This may progressively become more mature until the patient has complete ankylosis of the hip. If this is managed with early physical therapy and aggressive range-of-motion exercises, it may keep breaking up the bone as it forms and result in a functional range of motion of the hip. If it becomes ankylosed one must wait until at least 1

year has elapsed and the serum alkaline phosphatase is normal, after which the bony bar can be resected with good results. If the procedure is performed too early, there are frequent complications of excess bleeding, followed by wound hematoma, infection, and even recurrence of the heterotopic ossification. At the first sign of heterotopic ossification and during the postoperative period, therapeutic amounts of Didronel may be used to decrease the severity of the heterotopic ossification.

Rehabilitation and Activities of Daily Living

Rehabilitation goals for a person with quadriplegia include reintegration into family and community life, and vocational readjustment commensurate with the patient's abilities. This begins with mobilization into the wheelchair, learning transfer techniques, dressing upper extremity and lower extremity techniques. Activities of daily living include preparing and eating meals and personal hygiene such as shaving, brushing teeth, and bathing. The amount of physical mobility is directly dependent on the level of nerve root muscle function.

If the patient has a permanent neurologic deficit above the C4 level, he or she will be respirator-dependent. He can be mobilized to the wheelchair by passive lifting. His respiration can be supported in a wheelchair via a portable respirator attached to the wheelchair, and he can control the propulsion and direction of the wheelchair with micro switches positioned to be controlled by his tongue or by his chin. He will have no voluntary upper extremity function and will require constant attendant help 24 hours a day in case of respirator failure or falling out of the wheelchair. Persons with very high cervical lesions such as C1 and C2 can be treated with phrenic nerve stimulator implants to provide electronic impulses for diaphragm contraction and breathing. These phrenic pacers frequently can be used only part-time during the day to prevent nerve and diaphragm fatigue; the patient is usually placed on a volume respirator at night while sleeping.

The C4 functional level is a person who is breathing on his or her own but has zero upper-extremity muscle function. He is able to be passively lifted into a power wheelchair and can control the wheelchair with tongue, chin, or head control switches. He will require attendant care approximately 20 hours per day for activities of daily living, bathing, feeding, and bowel and bladder management. He can, however, be left for an hour or so during the day, or during the night while sleeping, with little danger.

The C5 functional-level patient will have active shoulder flexion, and abduction and active elbow flexion, but will not have any wrist or hand function and will therefore require passive lift into a power chair. He will be able to control the power chair with either head control or customized hand controls on the wheelchair arm. He will need external powered hand splints for prehension function but should be able to feed himself, provide part of his activities for daily living for personal hygiene (washing, brushing teeth, shaving, etc.) with the use of externally powered hand splints and mobile arm supports on the wheelchair. This patient needs attendant help approximately 16 hours per day. He needs help getting into the wheelchair, bathing, with bowel and bladder management, and getting back out of the wheelchair and into bed.

The C6 functional-level patient should be able to transfer himself into a regular wheelchair and propel the wheelchair on level surfaces. He will need wrist extensor-driven flexor hinge hand splints for prehension activities such as eating, writing, and using typing sticks. Depending on his age he will need from 4 to 8 hours a day assistant help with getting dressed and undressed, household cleaning activities, and help with meal preparation. This level patient should, however, be able to transport himself in and out of a car, drive a car with hand controls, and may be employed in a sedentary job.

The next level is the C7 level. This patient has additional muscle power in the finger extensors and triceps and wrist flexors. He is much more able to transfer independently and propel a wheelchair up and down inclines and curbs. He still, however, has no finger flexors for grip on prehension between the thumb and index finger and needs a flexor hinge hand splint for prehension activities. This patient is also a candidate for tendon transfers, which will be discussed later. His needs for attendant care are between zero and 4 hours per day for housekeeping activities and help with shopping and putting away groceries and other heavy objects, and he may need help with bowel and bladder management as well as some lower-extremity dressing.

The C8 functional-level patient has finger flexors in addition to the rest of the upper extremity muscles. His only deficit is intrinsic weakness, and he can do very well with transfer activities, propelling his wheelchair up and down inclines and curbs, and with the use of an opponens hand splint can manage eating utensils and typing sticks quite well. This patient will need perhaps zero to 2 hours per day attendant help for housekeeping and meal preparation.

If the patient has all the nerve roots intact down to and including T1, he or she has full innervation of the upper extremities and is classified as a paraplegic. These patients should be able to be fully independent, should not need any hand splints, and perhaps need attendant help several hours a week for housekeeping and meal preparation.

It is necessary to define these goals early in the patient's hospitalization, to estimate the functional gains anticipated and to estimate the length of stay. With spinal stability the patient's hospitalization usually lasts 4 to 5 months before the patient has reached maximum hospital benefits and is able to be discharged to home and followed with outpatient therapy.

Adjunct to Independent Living

Orthotics

The most important prescription for spinal-cord injured patients' function is the wheelchair. If the person has active wrist extensors and elbow flexors, he or she should be able to propel a manual wheelchair fitted to individual specifications. If the person is a C5 and does not have wrist extensors, he or she will need an electric-powered wheelchair for mobilization and electric hand splints for prehension. There are varieties of prehension hand splints that can be fabricated for the C6 and C7 patient with active wrist extensors. They each have in common a mechanism to provide prehension through active wrist extension.

Standing

Several centers advocate the patient standing upright with supports at least once daily for a short period of time. The benefits are purported to be less osteoporosis, less muscle atrophy, better urinary tract drainage, better pulmonary toilet, and a better feeling of well being. These have not been supported in literature. In fact, the person has to be upright on his feet at least 8 hours a day to prevent the deterioration effects of recumbency on the muscles and bones for the lower extremities. There is no question that standing will make the patient feel better emotionally; in addition, contractures cannot occur if he or she is indeed able to stand daily with the hips and knees extended.

Ambulation

All patients are hopeful to be able to walk. Computerized ambulation with electronic stimulation of nerves and muscles has been investigated for at least 20 years, and although there are examples of patients who can use electronic stimulation to provide muscle contraction, these have not been clinically successfully applied at present. These are still in the experimental, evaluational stage.

Surgical Reconstruction of the Quadriplegic Hand

Surgical procedures to improve upper-extremity function of the traumatic quadriplegic patient can be considered after the patient has made maximum functional recovery and completed a successful rehabilitation program to meet the maximum functional goals for his level of function. Surgical reconstruction is usually not recommended until 1 year has elapsed since the injury. By that time the person has learned what he can do independently in activities of daily living and when he needs assistance, and will have reasonable expectations of the goals to be achieved by tendon transfers. It is important during this first year that the joints of the hand remain free of contracture. Contractures are prevented by daily range-of-motion exercises by the patient or attendant. It is also important that the finger flexor and extensor muscles be allowed to develop a myostatic contracture, so the fingers will extend at the MP joints when the wrist is flexed and flex into a grasp when the wrist is extended by the tenodesis effect of the myostatic contracture. Finger flexors and particularly the thumb flexors should not be stretched with the wrist in extension. Tightness of thumb flexor and thenar eminence muscles will help develop the gross key pinch grasp useful for the quadriplegic. The patient's current independence status, particularly in dressing, transferring, and wheelchair propulsion, must be carefully considered prior to recommending tendon transfer. Tendon transfers and tenodesis and joint stabilizations will frequently limit the range of motion of the wrist and fingers and may prohibit the patient from performing his previously independent transfer activity. Most quadriplegic patients learn to use their tenodesis gross grasps and occasionally use an orthosis for prehension for writing or typing, but are able to do quite well without tendon transfers. The specific improvement to be expected by the tendon transfer must be clearly understood by the patient. So too should the possible disadvantages of decrease in power of the transferred muscles. It is important to ensure that no independent transfer, dressing, wheelchair propulsion, or driving capability is lost.

The principal of surgically improving upper-extremity function is to identify the lowest functioning muscle whose function can be sacrificed by tendon transfer to provide the function that would be provided by the next lower nerve root level.

Specific Transfers for Specific Levels

The patient with a C5 functional level who has weak deltoid and biceps function will not have any muscles that can be sacrificed for transfer. The C5 level patient who has a strong biceps will usually have a grade 4/5 brachioradialis. The brachioradialis may be transferred to the extensor carpiradialis brevus to provide active wrist extension. The brachioradialis must be 4/5 in strength. Since it has a short excursion, the patient may have limited wrist flexion and have a small opening for grasp. The brachioradialis transfer works best for the patient who is a C6 level with a weak extensor carpiradialis longus. In this case the strong brachioradialis improves wrist extension both in power and direction by transferring its power into the extensor carpiradialis brevis.

The patient with a C6 functional level who has extensor carpiradialis longus as the lower muscle and who develops a gross "tenodesis" grasp may have this function improved by pin stabilization of the IP joint and a tenodesis of the flexor pallius longus to provide a tenodesis pinch. If the brachioradialis is of sufficient strength, this can be transferred to the flexor pollius longus to provide an active key pinch with wrist extension. The extensor pollius longus can be tenodised to the dorsum of the wrist to provide passive opening of the grasp with wrist flexion.

The C7 quadriplegic who has a strong extensor carpiradialis brevus can sacrifice the extensor carpiradialis longus to be transferred to the finger flexors. The brachioradialis can also be transferred in this patient to the thumb flexor. This will give the patient active finger and thumb flexion and extension.

The low quadriplegic (C8 quadriplegic) who lacks only intrinsics can have intrinsoplasties performed using the Zancolli capsular advancement or intrinsic tenodesis procedures. It usually is not satisfactory to sacrifice the sublimus for active intrinsoplasty.

Community Reentry

It is important in the very beginning of the patient's hospitalization to involve the family in the diagnosis, prognosis, and rehabilitation plan. All during the rehabilitation the family learns what the patient can do for himself and what he needs help to do. As soon as spinal stability permits and the patient and family understand the essentials of careful transfer techniques and are able to manage the bladder program, the patient is encouraged to go on a day pass. This gets the patient out of the hospital, back into his home for the day, and he learns some of the difficulties he is going to have when he goes home permanently. As soon as the family is able, overnight weekend passes are encouraged to further ascertain the problems the patient is going to face when he goes home. Early in the rehabilitation program, housing arrangements must be addressed. Living arrangements should be visited by the occupational therapist and physical therapist to identify any architectural barriers and any remodeling that will be necessary to accommodate the patient's wheelchair and other needs.

Patient transportation is managed easiest by a van. Hydraulic lifts can be placed on the side of the van and the patient can be lifted into the van, wheelchair and all, strapped into the wheelchair supports and be safely transported. He may be able to drive with hand controls if he is a C6 level or better. Low quadriplegics are able to transfer in and out of a regular two-door sedan and fold their wheelchair in behind the seat. The minimum requirements for driving with hand controls are strong shoulder flexor, elbow flexor, and wrist extensor muscles. The patient must have pectoralis muscles to adduct the arm across the chest and sufficient elbow and wrist strength to operate hand controls safely.

Vocational issues are addressed early in the hospitalization. Occupational therapists and a social worker review the patient's occupational history and begin to suggest appropriate changes or modifications of the job site. The best results in getting patients back to work occur in patients who formerly had sedentary desk-type work. Frequently, these patients can go back to their former job with job-site modification. If the patient has been a laborer or required physical use of the lower extremities and hand function, he will need to be retrained for a sedentary type occupation. There is usually no injury to the mentality or the intelligence of these patients, and therefore they are good candidates for retraining and vocational support for school. Very frequently they can be overeducated. It is easier to remain in school than it is to compete in the workforce; thus, they become overqualified for positions that they can not realistically expect to obtain.

Life Expectancy

The life expectancy of persons with a cervical spinal cord injury depends on the age at injury and the

Table 106-1

Estimate of life expectancy*

Age	General Population	Paraplegic Inc.	Paraplegic Comp.	Quadriplegic Inc.	Quadriplegic Comp.
20 Male	50	48	34	41	22
Female	56	54	42	49	30
40 Male	32	30	19	24	10
Female	37	35	24	30	14
60 Male	16	15	07	11	03
Female	20	19	11	15	05

*From DeVivo MJ and others: Prevalence of spinal cord injury: a reestimation employing life table techniques, *Arch Neurol* 37:707, 1980.

severity of the injury. The review of DeVivo estimates the life expectancy as shown in Table 106-1.

These figures are only estimates; they are based on past experience, and each year the life expectancy of the spinal cord-injured patient gets greater with better care and prevention of complications. The main cause of death secondary to the quadriplegia over the years continues to be pulmonary complications. Suicide continues to be a major cause of death, either volitionally or accidentally.

Summary

Management of the spinal cord-injured patient is a complex multidisciplinary effort. To be successful it requires close coordination between many subspecialists. No one professional has all the knowledge or tools to handle the entire problem. A well-trained managing specialist can oversee and coordinate the entire effort to obtain the smoothest and most complete return of the patient to a productive life.

Additional Readings

1. Comarr AE, Hutchinson RH, Bors E: Extremity fractures of patients with spinal cord injuries, *Am J Surg* 103:732, 1962.
2. DeVivo MJ and others: Prevalence of spinal cord injury: a reestimation employing life table techniques. *Arch Neurol* 37:707, 1980.
3. Eichenholtz SN: Management of long bone fractures in paraplegic patients, *J Bone Joint Surg (Am)* 45:299, 1963.
4. Frankel HL: The value of postural reduction in the initial management of closed injuries of the spine, *Paraplegia* 7:179, 1969.
5. Frankel HL and others: Value of postural reduction in the initial management of closed injuries of the spine with paraplegia and tetraplegia, *Paraplegia* 7:179, 1969.

6. Grulia UF: Prevention of thromboembolic complications in paraplegia, *Paraplegia* 23:124, 1969.

7. Lamb DW, Chan KM: Surgical reconstruction of the upper limb in traumatic paraplegia: a review of 41 patients, *J Bone Joint Surg* 8B:119, 1983.

8. Moberg E: Surgical treatment for absent single-hand grip and elbow extension in quadriplegia, *J Bone Joint Surg* 57A:196, 1975.

9. Moberg E: The present state of surgical reconstruction of the upper limb in tetraplegia, *Paraplegia* 25:351, 1987.

10. Smith R: *Tendon transfers for quadriplegia*. In *Tendon transfers of the hand and forearm*, Boston, 1987, Little, Brown.

11. Stauffer ES: Neurologic recovery following injuries to the cervical spinal cord and nerve roots, *Spine* 9:532, 1984.

12. Weingarten SI: Fever and thromboembolic disease in acute spinal cord injury, *Paraplegia* 26:35, 1988.

13. Wharton GW, Morgan TH: Ankylosis in the paralyzed patient, *J Bone Joint Surg (Am)* 52:105, 1970.

14. Zancoli E: *Structural and dynamic basis of hand surgery*, Philadelphia, 1979, J.B. Lippincott.

Section 3
Infection

107   Spinal Infection
      Matthew F. Gornet

Chapter 107
Spinal Infection
Matthew F. Gornet

Pathophysiology

Microbiology

Laboratory Analysis

Radiographic Analysis

> plain film
> nuclear medicine scans
> computed tomography
> magnetic resonance imaging

Pyogenic Vertebral Osteomyelitis

Spinal Epidural Abscess

> clinical presentation
> radiographic analysis

Granulomatous Disease of the Spine

Nonoperative Treatment

Operative Treatment

Summary

This chapter deals with the spectrum of spinal infections. Each spinal infection possesses a pathophysiology that is unique to the organism and route of inoculation. To make better sense of this topic, we will attempt to consolidate diagnostic tests and treatments that all infections have in common and work toward variations that depend on the infecting organism.

Pathophysiology

Many confusing terms are used in an attempt to categorize and define infections of the spine. This is because controversy still exists regarding the vascular route of hematogenous infection. Why, for instance, do children afflicted with discitis tend to improve spontaneously, often without antibiotics, while adults usually go on to significant destruction of the intervertebral disc and adjacent bony end plates? The answer to this question might be found in Pasteur's simple words, "the organism is nothing, the environment is everything."

The environment where infection begins, and the host's ability to neutralize bacteria at that site, are paramount. The vascular environment of the vertebral body and disc is unique; which makes the spine more susceptible to infection than other areas of the body. In fact, it has been shown that the spine is the number one site of hematogenous osteomyelitis in adults and the third most common site of osteomyelitis for all age groups.[47] Therefore, the key to understanding the pathophysiology of spinal infection is understanding the unique blood supply of the vertebral body.

Excluding direct iatrogenic inoculation, which we will discuss later, the vascular system is the route of inoculation that is believed to precipitate most spinal infections. Batson postulated that infection spread to the spine by a special venous system.[2] This venous system, which Batson first described, now bears his name. In the Batson system, venous blood leaves the pelvis and abdomen and flows through the vertebral bodies into the thorax. Because Batson's system is valveless, the direction of flow varies with respiration, coughing, and straining. The vertebral plexus receives blood directly from the pelvis; Batson believed that this might explain why infections of the urinary tract and perineum were often found to be the precipitating cause of vertebral osteomyelitis. This explanation also seemed to correlate well with metastatic spread of certain tumors, such as prostrate cancer.

Wiley and Trueta[51] refuted Batson's hypothesis and postulated that bacteria spread through the arterial system (rather than the venous) was the likely culprit responsible for most cases of vertebral osteomyelitis. Indeed, the rich blood supply along the anterior vertebral body correlates with the most common sites of vertebral osteomyelitis[52] (Fig. 107-1).

A brief note is required concerning the vascular supply of the intravertebral disc in children. During infancy and childhood, blood vessels penetrate the end plate of the vertebal body and terminate in the disc.[10,25,42,49] This provides a rich vascular supply to the intervertebral disc and a relatively good ability to clear potential bacterial infection. However, the vascular supply of the vertebral body and intervertebral disc changes in adulthood. Vessels that previously penetrated the vertebral end plate now pass close to the end plate, turn 180 degrees, and return back to the metaphysis. This vascular system is similar to the vascular system of the metaphysis of long bones just adjacent to the growth plate. It is theorized that bacteria may have greater potential to dislodge at this point.

Microbiology

Staphylococcus aureus is the most common organism implicated in both primary and postoperative vertebral osteomyelitis.[4,17,53]

Gram-negative infections appear to be increasing in frequency, the most common of these being *Escherichia coli*. This is often the direct result of seeding from the urinary tract. Gram-negative infections as a whole are opportunistic, often striking diabetics and the elderly.[39] They tend to have a more virulent course. Cahill and his colleagues[7] have shown that even in the elderly these infections can be treated successfully. While there are multiple reports of many offending gram-negative organisms, special mention must be made concerning *Pseudomonas aeruginosa*. This particular organism, along with tuberculosis, is seen in increasing frequency among inner-city IV drug users (IVDA). One must always be on guard for an unusual organism in any immunocompromised host. It is our experience, as well as that of others,[15] that even in this population, *Staph. aureus* still is the most frequently identified offending bacteria.

Laboratory Analysis

On initial evaluation, all patients suspected of having vertebral osteomyelitis should undergo blood cultures, especially during any spike in fever. This may provide the only information available as to the source of the offending bacteria. Most series show only 50% of initial blood cultures grow the causative

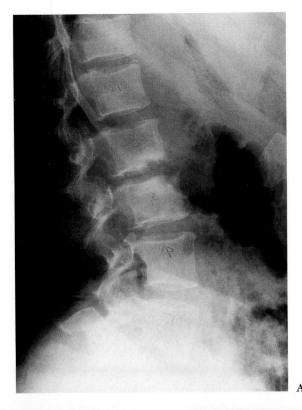

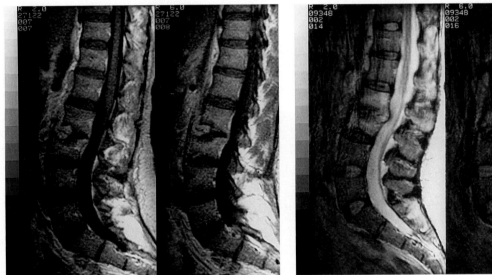

Fig. 107-1

A, Lateral lumbar spine demonstrates early changes in the anterior metaphysis at L2-L3 under the anterior longitudinal ligament. Typical of pyogenic osteomyelitis of the spine. **B,** The suspected infection is confirmed on MRI. **C,** Late changes with collapse and neurological changes.

organism.[17,35] In addition, urine and any other potential source of infection should be cultured.

A standard hematologic screen with measurement of the white blood count is of less diagnostic value. In fact, the majority of patients present with a white blood count in the normal range.[48] The most valu-able laboratory test for assessing the presence of spinal infection and gauging the impact of therapy is the erythrocyte sedimentation rate (ESR).[12,37,44,53] While this test is very nonspecific, it correlates quite well with the presence of active disease, with the exception of the early postoperative period.[27]

Radiographic Analysis

Plain Film

Plain radiographs reveal the classic manifestations seen in any bone infection. These include areas of bone lysis in combination with bony sclerosis. Early, one typically sees vertebral end-plate sclerosis with lysis of overlying subchondral bone (Fig. 107-2). A paravertebral abscess may or may not be present.

As duration of the infection lengthens, disc height is lost and an increase in bony destruction is noted. This bony destruction may be in conjunction with signs of instability (kyphosis, translation, etc.).

Nuclear Medicine Scans

Nuclear medicine scans may show abnormalities even before changes are seen in plain radiographs.[28] Technetium-^{99m} (T-^{99}) is a radioactively labeled hydroxydiphosphonate. This tracer tends to be absorbed by any area of bone that is undergoing increased turnover. A new variation of the T-^{99} bone scan is to couple the radioisotope with human immunoglobulin. Combining T-^{99} with human immunoglobulin may even offer increased sensitivity compared with T-^{99} alone when evaluating chronic osteomyelitis,[40] although this claim is refuted by others.[26,36]

An indium-^{111}-labeled white blood cell scan is an additional test used to identify sites of infection. The principle behind indium-^{111} is that labeled white blood cells will congregate in areas of infection. Indium-^{111} used in combination with T-^{99} may be more sensitive in localization of infection.[32] Whalen and associates have questioned indium-^{111} sensitivity in identifying infection in patients undergoing antibiotic therapy. Whalen believes that because of decreased sensitivity, only those patients not previously treated with antibiotics should be tested.[50]

Computed Tomography

Computed tomography (CT) occupies the central point in the diagnosis of osteomyelitis.[4,5] CT with sagittal reconstruction allows accurate demonstration of bony destruction. This can be measured

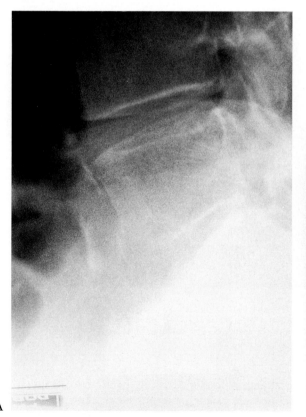
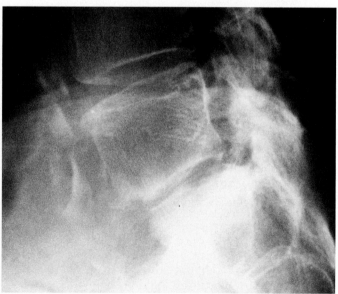

A   B

Fig. 107-2

A, Early metaphyseal erosion, with blurring of the end plate definition. **B,** Six weeks later, loss of disc height is noted, with end plate sclerosis.

against future CT scans to assess the success of treatment. A CT scan may also be used diagnostically as an aid in guiding needle biopsies of individual vertebra.[19,34]

CT scans can also accurately identify any accompanying soft-tissue abscess, such as paravertebral or psoas infections.

Magnetic Resonance Imaging

Magnetic resonance imaging (MRI) has recently emerged as a leader in early detection of vertebral osteomyelitis.[6,30] MRI used for diagnosing spinal infections only dates to 1984.[29,31] The findings on MRI for vertebral osteomyelitis are as follows.

T_1—Decreased signal or "darkening" around the area of infection. The borders between the intervertebral disc end plate and vertebral body are blurred.

T_2—Increased signal intensity or "brightness" around the area of the infection (disc and end plate).

Overall, the accuracy of MRI in properly identifying osteomyelitis of the spine was found to be 94%.[30] MRI was found to be superior to CT in identifying osteomyelitis of the spine.[6] Currently, we reserve MRI for early identification of a suspected spinal infection in the postoperative patient. We also use MRI's capabilities to image the spinal canal in patients with suspected infection and neurologic deficit (Fig. 107-3).

Pyogenic Vertebral Osteomyelitis

The hallmark of all pyogenic spine infections is pain. Several studies have confirmed that more than 90% of patients afflicted with vertebral osteomyelitis present with pain.[33,38] The patient may state that the pain developed in an acute or chronic fashion. The presentation is largely dependent on the virulence of the organism in relation to the host's defenses. Often times the initial symptoms are nonspecific, and diagnosis can be delayed for up to 3 months.[13,46] Pain from vertebral osteomyelitis can often be separated from other causes of back pain, such as regional backache and degenerative disc disease, because the pain from vertebral osteomyelitis is usually not relieved with rest.

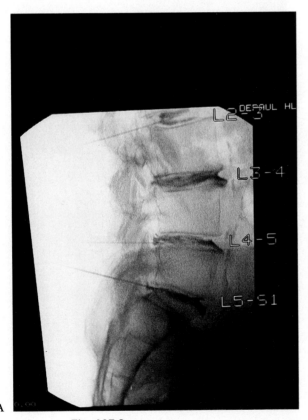
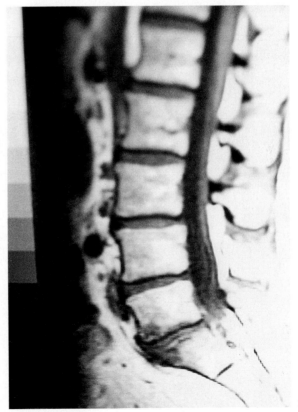

Fig. 107-3

A, Discogram at L5-S1 as the precipitating cause of infection. **B,** Changes on T1-weighted MRI 9 days after discogram. No plain radiographic changes were seen at this time.

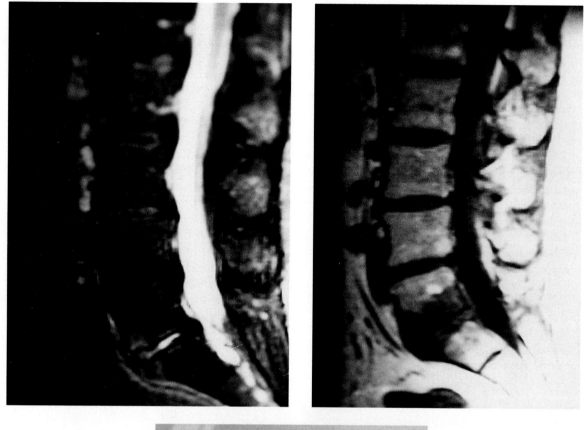

C

D

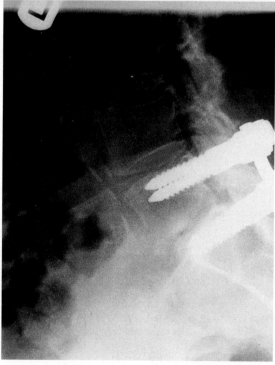

E

Fig. 107-3, cont'd

C, Changes on T2-weighted MRI 9 days after discogram. **D,** Changes of T1 and T2 MRI 6 weeks after discogram. **E,** Three months after anterior and posterior spinal fusion with solid union.

Neurologic examination may encompass a spectrum from normal to complete paralysis. With the exception of vertebral osteomyelitis with concomitant spinal epidural abscess, neurologic symptoms usually present late in the disease process, if at all. Several groups of patients are deemed at high risk for neurologic progression: those with diabetes, rheumatoid arthritis, or urinary tract infection; the elderly; and any immunocompromised host.[14] Patients rarely present with signs of sepsis or bacteremia (fever, chills). In fact, according to Garcia,[17] only one third of patients present with fever greater than 100°F, and fewer than 5% of patients have fever greater than 102°F.

The lumbar spine is most often infected, followed by the thoracic spine. The cervical spine is least affected. Males tend to be more commonly affected than females in all large studies by at least a 2:1 ratio.

Spinal Epidural Abscess

Spinal epidural abscess remains an uncommon clinical entity. The incidence has been estimated at approximately 1 per 10,000 admissions.[22] In contrast to vertebral osteomyelitis, the majority of patients with spinal epidural abscess present with fever and elevated white blood cell count.[11] *Staph. aureus* remains the predominant infectious agent in 60% of cases. In Darouiche's series,[11] infection other than *Staph. aureus* was associated with IV drug abuse, decubitus ulcers, urinary tract infection, and recent spine surgery. Granulomatous epidural abscesses such as *Mycobacterium tuberculosis* are generally less common.[52]

Clinical Presentation

Clinical symptoms encompass a spectrum from back pain to paralysis.[21] Most often, patients present with back pain and mild radicular symptoms, and therein lies the challene of obtaining a proper diagnosis. Operative intervention should be based on any progression of neurologic deterioration, continued failure to respond to antibiotics, an ESR that does not decrease, and continued progressive radiologic changes of bone destruction. Initial treatment consists of parenteral antibiotics and close serial neurologic examinations. Surgical treatment for epidural abscess usually consists of laminectomy. The outcome does not seem to be affected by age, gender, source of infection, or infecting organism.[47] The most important prognostic factor for successful outcome seems to be prompt, early diagnosis and treatment.

Radiographic Analysis

The most useful imaging study for diagnosing epidural abscesses is often debated. MRI and CT myelography have been found to be equally sensitive.[22] MRI with T_1- and T_2-weighted images, enhanced with gadolinium contrast, offers a more definitive interpretation of any process causing thecal displacement. The advantages of using CT myelography are the additional information one gains as an adjunct to this procedure. CT myelography allows better interpretation of bone destruction in adjacent vertebral osteomyelitis and may give additional diagnostic help through interpretation of cerebrospinal fluid analysis. It is this author's opinion that MRI is so sensitive that patients with vertebral osteomyelitis are often overdiagnosed as having concomitant epidural abscess secondary to intense inflammatory response adjacent to the osteomyelitis.

Granulomatous Disease of the Spine

This discussion of spinal infections has deliberately been placed last. A disproportionate amount of hospital and colleague interest is always generated by the admission of patients with granulomatous infection of the spine, because these infections are so rare.[54] Granulomatous disease refers to any agent that promotes granuloma formation via the host's immunologic response. By far the number one agent causing granulomatous infections of the spine is *M. turberculosis*. Other agents include *Brucella aspergillus* and *Cryptococcus neoformans*.

In tuberculosis of the spine (Pott's disease), infection is the result of hematogenous spread. The seeding focus of infection may be active or latent and is often difficult to locate. Vertebral involvement may be central, paradiscal, or anterior. Typically one sees infection spread to the anterior vertebral body and eventually eroding into the disc space. The infection usually tracks along bone, elevating the anterior and posterior longitudinal ligaments and periosteum. This causes further necrosis of bone via devascularization. The process is slow, and typically multiple vertebral bodies are involved at presentation.[23,24] The abscess may invade paravertebral tissues anteriorly or track posteriorly across the dura. Morbidity is directly dependent on early diagnosis and treatment (see the section below on Operative Treatment). The hallmark of medical treatment is isoniazid 10-15 mg/kg (adults)[46] in conjunction with rifampicin 10 mg/kg. Combination chemotherapy is used because there has been a new alarming rise of drug-resistant TB within inner cities, especially among HIV-positive patients.[9,43]

Nonoperative Treatment

After the diagnostic evaluation of vertebral osteomyelitis is complete, nonoperative management may begin on those patients believed not to warrant operative intervention. This treatment includes rest, appropriate intravenous antibiotics, and an orthosis. A neurologic examination is initially monitored daily, as changes in the baseline examination may indicate that operative intervention is needed. An ESR is drawn every week. Any decline in the value of the ESR is correlated with the patient's clinical response. The patient may progress in his or her level of ambulation when the pain decreases to an acceptable level; this usually requires 7 to 10 days on antibiotics. Patients are treated with a minimum of 3 weeks of IV antibiotics depending on the organism and duration of infection prior to presentation. A 6-week course of antibiotics is usually required. One of the most important aspects of nonoperative management is monitoring the patient's long-term response to treatment for signs of vertebral collapse, instability, disease progression, and neurologic changes. Any of these conditions necessitate operative intervention. Most infections responding to treatment will go on to obliterate the disc space and spontaneous fusion of adjacent vertebra.

Operative Treatment

The goals of operative intervention are the same for tuberculous and pyogenic vertebral osteomyelitis. Namely, drainage of any abscess, debridement of infected tissue, and stabilization of any segment of the spine that may have lost structural integrity. In granulomatous disease of the spine, the general consensus among authors is that the spine should be approached in an anterior fashion with radical debridement of necrotic tissue and anterior fusion.[1,14,16,18,41] While laminectomy may appear easier and less risky for neurologic decompression, it may lead to loss of structural integrity, increased deformity, and neurologic deterioration.[3] Still others advocate that posterior spinal fusion must be added to anterior spinal fusion for best results.[45] This may be true in children, in whom continued posterior growth in the presence of anterior fusion may contribute to an increase in kyphotic deformities. Recent reports have shown that even patients with

draining sinuses and confirmed abscesses can be treated with medical chemotherapy if followed closely.[8]

In pyogenic vertebral osteomyelitis, debridement remains the hallmark of operative treatment. Diagnostic consideration should be given to paravertebral and psoas abscesses so that treatment can be rendered at the time of intervention. An interbody graft should be placed if a significant bony defect results after debridement. Allograft or bone substitutes should not be used. If more than one interspace is involved, if the spine will be subjected to large forces such as obesity, or if the vertebral body is felt to be osteoporotic, the surgeon may consider supplementing anterior fusion with posterior spinal fusion and instrumentation. This provides added stability for those patients with weak bone and helps hold anterior grafts in position.

Postoperative spine infections are unique in that the infectious agent is often resistant to standard therapy. Rates of postoperative infection range from 0.7% to 12%,[18] depending on the operation. Spinal instrumentation within a wound acts as a foreign body and makes eradication of infection more difficult. The balance of hardware removal must be made in conjunction with potential pseudarthrosis. Delayed primary closure may be necessary, as well as healing by secondary intention.

Summary

The subject of spinal infections is very complex. For this chapter the emphasis has intentionally been placed on "classic" spine vertebral osteomyelitis, with less focus on the more uncommon fungal and granulomatous infections. Spinal epidural abscess has been discussed briefly. Clinical presentations and laboratory and radiologic workups that are common to all spinal infections have been grouped together. In addition, general principles of operative and nonoperative treatment of spinal infections have been discussed.

References

1. Bailey HL and others: Tuberculosis of the spine in children, *J Bone Joint Surg [Am]* 54:1633, 1972.
2. Batson OV: The function of the vertebral veins and their role in the spread of metastasis, *Ann Surg* 112:138, 1940.
3. Bohlman HH, Freehafer AA, Dejak J: The results of treatment of acute injuries of the upper thoracic spine with paralysis, *J Bone Joint Surg [Am]* 67:360, 1985.
4. Brant-Zawardzki M, Burke BD, Jeffery RB: CT in the evaluation of spine infection, *Spine* 8:358, 1983.

5. Burke DR, Brant-Zawardzki M: CT of pyogenic spine infection, *Neuroradiology* 27:131, 1985.

6. Chandnani VP and others: Acute experimental osteomyelitis and abscesses: detection with MR imaging versus CT, *Radiology* 174:233, 1990.

7. Chen CW and others: Gas-forming vertebral osteomyelitis in diabetic patients, *Scand J Infect Dis* 23(2):263, 1991.

8. Controlled trial of short-course regimens of chemotherapy in the ambulatory treatment of spinal tuberculosis: results at three years of a study in Korea. 12th Report of the Medical Research Council Working Party on Tuberculosis of the Spine, *J Bone Joint Surg [Br]* 75(2):240, 1993.

9. Coronado VG and others: Transmission of multidrug-resistance *mycobacterium tuberculosis* among persons with human immunodeficiency virus infection in an urban hospital: epidemiologic and restriction fragment length polymorphism analysis, *J Infect Dis* 168(4):1052, 1993.

10. Coventry MBM, Ghormley RK, Kernohan JW: The intravertebral disc: its microscopic anatomy and pathology. 1: Anatomy, development and physiology, *J Bone Joint Surg* 27(A):105, 1945.

11. Darouiche RO and others: Bacterial spinal epidural abscess: review of 43 cases and literature survey, *Medicine (Balt)* 71(6):369, 1992.

12. Devereaux MD, Hazelton RA: Pyogenic spinal osteomyelitis—its clinical and radiologic presentation, *J Rheumatol* 10(3):491, 1983.

13. Digby JM, Kersley JB: Pyogenic non-tuberculous spinal infection, *J Bone Joint Surg [Br]* 61:47, 1979.

14. Eismont FJ and others: Pyogenic and fungal vertebral osteomyelitis with paralysis, *J Bone Joint Surg [Am]* 65:19, 1983.

15. Engress C and others: Cervical osteomyelitis due to IV heroin use: radiologic findings in fourteen patients, *Am J Roentgenol* 155(2):333, 1990.

16. Fourth Report of the Medical Research Council Working Party on Tuberculosis of the Spine: A controlled trial of anterior spinal fusion and debridement in the surgical management of tuberculosis of the spine in patients on the standard chemotherapy: a study in Hong Kong, *Br J Surg* 61:853, 1974.

17. Garcia A Jr, Granthan SA: Hemotogenous pyogenic vertebral osteomyelitis, *J Bone Joint Surg [Am]* 42:429, 1960.

18. Gepstein R, Eismont FI: *Post-operative spine infection.* In Weinstein JN, Weisel SW, editors: *The lumbar spine,* Philadelphia, 1990, W.B. Saunders.

19. Ghelman B and others: Percutaneous computed-tomography-guided biopsy of the thoracic and lumbar spine, *Spine* 16(7):736. 1991.

20. Gorse GJ and others: Tuberculous spondylitis, *Medicine* 62:178, 1983.

21. Heusner AP: Non-tuberculosis spinal epidural infections, *N Engl J Med* 239:845, 1948.

22. Hlavin ML and others: Spinal epidural abscess: a ten year prospective, *Neurosurgery* 27:177, 1990.

23. Hodgson AR, Stock FE: Anterior spine fusion for the treatment of tuberculosis of the spine, *J Bone Joint Surg [Am]* 42:295, 1960.

24. Hodgson AR, Wong W, Yau A: *X-ray appearances in tuberculosis of the spine,* Springfield, Mo., 1969, Charles C Thomas.

25. Holm S: Nutrition of the intravertebral disc—transport and metabolism, *Connect Tissue Res* 8:101, 1981.

26. Hotze AL and others: Technetium-99M-labeled antigranulocyte in antibodies in suspected bone infections, *J Nucl Med* 33(4):526, 1992.

27. Jonsson B, Soderholm R, Stromqvist B: Erythrocyte sedimentation rate after lumbar spine surgery, *Spine* 16(9):1049, 1991.

28. Kern RZ, Houpt JB: Pyogenic vertebral osteomyelitis: diagnosis and management, *Can Med Assoc J* 130(8):1025, 1984.

29. Modic MT, Pavlicek W, Weinstein MA: Magnetic resonance imaging of intervertebral disc disease: clinical and pulse sequence considerations, *Radiology* 152:103, 1984.

30. Modic MT and others: Magnetic resonance imaging of musculoskeletal infections, *Radiol Clin North Am* 24:247, 1986.

31. Modic MT and others: Vertebral osteomyelitis: assessment using MR, *Radiology* 157:157, 1985.

32. Mountford PJ and others: Dual radionucleotide subtraction imaging of vertebral disc infection using an 111IN-labeled leucocute scan and an 99MTC tin caloid scan, *Eur J Nucl Med* 8 (12):557, 1983.

33. Muscher DM and others: Vertebral osteomyelitis still a diagnostic pitfall, *Arch Intern Med* 136:105, 1976.

34. Odendaal T, Lemmer LB: The value of percutaneous trephine biopsy in the diagnosis of lesions of the vertebral column, *S Afr Med J* 79(1):21, 1991.

35. Patzakis MJ and others: Analysis of 61 cases of vertebral osteomyelitis, *Clin Orthop* 264:178, 1991.

36. Reuland P and others: Detection of infection in postoperative orthopedic patients with technetium-99M-labeled monoclonal antibodies against granulocytes, *J Nucl Med* 32(12):2209, 1991.

37. Ros PM, Fleming JL: Vertebral body osteomyelitis, *Clin Orthop* 118:190, 1976.

38. Sapico FL, Montgomery JZ: Pyogenic vertebral osteomyelitis: report of nine cases and review of the literature, *Rev Infect Dis* 1:754, 1979.

39. Sapico FL, Montgomery JZ: Vertebral osteomyelitis, *Infect Dis Clin North Am* 4(3):539, 1990.

40. Sciuk J and others: Comparison of technetium 99M polyclonal immunoglobulin and technetium 99M monoclonal antibodies for imaging chronic osteomyelitis, *Eur J Nucl Med* 18(6):401, 1991.

41. Sixth Report of the Medical Research Council Working Party on Tuberculosis of the Spine: 5-year as-

sessments of controlled trials of ambulatory treatment, debridement and anterior spinal fusion in the management of tuberculosis of the spine: studies in Bulawayo (Rhodesia) and Hong Kong, *J Bone Joint Surg [Br]* 60:163, 1978.

42. Smith NR: The intravertebral disc, *Br J Surg* 18:358, 1931.

43. Snider DE Jr, Dooley SW: Nosocomial tuberculosis in the AIDS era with an emphasis on multidrug-resistant disease, *Heart Lung* 22(4):365, 1993.

44. Stone DB, Bonfiglio M: Pyogenic vertebral osteomyelitis: a diagnostic pitfall for the internist, *Arch Intern Med* 112: 491, 1963.

45. Tuberculosis of the spine: a review of 236 operative cases in underdeveloped regions from 1954–1964, *J Spinal Disord* 5(3):286, 1992.

46. Vincent KA, Benson DR, Voegeli TL: Factors in the diagnosis of adult pyogenic vertebral osteomyelitis, *Orthop Trans* 12:523, 1988.

47. Waldvogel FA, Medoff G, Swartz MN: Osteomyelitis: a review of clinical features, therapeutic considera-

tions and unusual aspects (3 parts), *N Engl J Med* 282:198, 260, 316, 1970.

48. Waldvogel RA, Vasey H: Osteomyelitis: the past decade, *N Engl J Med* 303:360, 1980.

49. Wenger DR, Bobechko WP, Gilday DL: Spectrum of the intravertebral disc space infection in children, *J Bone Joint Surg* 60(A): 100, 1978.

50. Whalen JL and others: Limitations of Indium leucocyte imaging for the diagnosis of spine infections, *Spine* 16(2):193, 1991.

51. Wiley AM, Trueta J: The vascular anatomy of the spine and its relationship to pyogenic vertebral osteomyelitis, *J Bone Joint Surg [Br]* 41:796, 1959.

52. Willis TA: Nutrient arteries of the vertebral bodies, *J Bone Joint Surg [Am]* 31:538, 1949.

53. Wisneski RJ: Infectious disease of the lumbar spine: diagnostic and treatment considerations, *Orthop Clin North Am* 22(3):491, 1991.

54. Wood GW, Edmonson AS: Osteomyelitis of the spine, *Spine State Art Rev* 3:461, 1989.

Section 4
Deformity

108 Congenital Spinal Deformity

Thomas S. Renshaw

109 Spinal Deformity in Children,
     Adolescents, and Young Adults

Robert W. Gaines, Jr.

110 Adult Scoliosis

John G. Finkenberg

111 Clinical Cervical Deformity and
     Postlaminectomy Kyphosis

Edward D. Simmons
Peter N. Capicotto

Chapter 108
Congenital Spinal Deformity
Thomas S. Renshaw

CONGENITAL SCOLIOSIS

Embryology Specific to Congenital Scoliosis

Etiology

Classification of Congenital Spinal Deformities

    failure of formation
    failure of segmentation

Natural History

Evaluation of the Patient

Other Abnormalities Associated with Congenital Scoliosis

    spinal abnormalities
    genitourinary abnormalities
    cardiac abnormalities
    other abnormalities

Radiographic Evaluation
Treatment

    observation
    orthotic treatment
    surgical treatment

Problems with and Complications of Surgical Treatment

CONGENITAL KYPHOSIS

Evaluation of the Patient

Classification

    failure of formation
    failure of segmentation

OTHER CONGENITAL DEFORMITIES

Congenital Kyphoscoliosis

Congenital Lordosis

CONGENITAL SCOLIOSIS

Congenital scoliosis results from abnormal development of one or more vertebrae. It should be differentiated from other types of scoliosis, such as the infantile idiopathic type, wherein an abnormal spinal curvature may be present at birth, but not as the result of anomalous vertebral development.

The significance of congenital scoliosis lies in its potential for producing progressive, severe deformity that can lead to pulmonary compromise, cor pulmonale, cosmetic disfigurement, back pain, and much less often, paralysis. Congenital scoliosis is the third most prevalent type of scoliosis, after idiopathic scoliosis and deformity associated with neuromuscular diseases.

Embryology Specific to Congenital Scoliosis

Congenital scoliosis cannot be understood without a knowledge of the development of the human spine. This has been well described in Chapter 59, which covers embryology. Nevertheless, some brief specific review will be helpful.

Paired mesodermal somites have developed by the twentieth gestational day. The inner part of each somite becomes the sclerotome, which is the precursor to the vertebra, after the thirtieth day. Each bilaterally paired sclerotome block has loose cells at the cephalic end and more dense cells at the caudal end. A transverse cleft then develops between these two cellular halves, and some of the dense cells adjacent to this cleft migrate cranially to surround the notochord as the precursor of the intervertebral disk. The remaining dense cells fuse with the loose cells of the caudally adjacent sclerotome to become an individual vertebral body. Induction of the vertebral body is mediated by the neural tube and the notochord, but the neural crest cells induce the development of the posterior neural arch. This is consistent with congenital spine anomalies involving only the anterior vertebral elements, only the posterior vertebral elements, or various combinations. Since each vertebral body is formed from the fusion of a pair of bilateral sclerotomes by the fortieth day, unilateral defects are also possible.

Neural arches form after the vertebral bodies have nearly completed their segmentation. In approximately 10% of the population, the paired neural arches fail to fuse in the posterior midline, producing spina bifida occulta. When this defect occurs in the lumbosacral region, spondylolysis and spondylolisthesis are more likely to develop. With more-substantial defects of the neural arch, maldevelopment and exposure of the neurologic tissue (a myelomeningocele) may occur. This severe condition most likely reflects the failure of neural tube closure.

The notochord gradually regresses, disappearing in the vertebral bodies, but becoming the mucoid nucleus pulposus of the intervertebral disk. It is possible that persistent remnants of notochordal tissue in the cervical or sacrococcygeal regions can develop into the tumors known as cordomas.

Etiology

The disturbances in the normal development of the spine that result in congenital spinal anomalies may be caused by teratologic agents or can be on a genetic basis. Several agents potentially can damage the normal developmental process of the embryonic spine. These include hypoxia, drugs, radiation, and perhaps viruses.

The genetic aspects of congenital scoliosis have been studied by several authors. Wynne-Davies reported on 337 patients.[31] She noted that when multiple anomalies occur, there is a 5% to 10% risk of similar abnormalities occurring in subsequent offspring. She did not find an increased risk if the anomaly was an isolated lesion, such as a single hemivertebra. Winter, however, found only two children of 1250 studied who had siblings with multiple anomalies. He reports a 1% likelihood of finding an isolated anomaly in a first-degree relative.[25] Sporadic anomalies, some similar and some not, have been reported in cousins. When congenital scoliosis is reported in one twin, the cotwin usually has no anomaly. Rarely have the spines of both twins been involved.[2]

Classification of Congenital Spinal Deformities

A classification system for congenital spinal deformities is important in order to predict natural history, to aid in treatment planning, and for research purposes. Anomalies are commonly classified by their pathoanatomic type and their location in the spine. It is believed that all vertebral malformations are discernible during the mesenchymal stage prior to the formation of cartilage and bone.[20] Congenital spinal anomalies result from either failure of formation, failure of segmentation, or a combination of abnormalities of the anlage of the vertebral column.

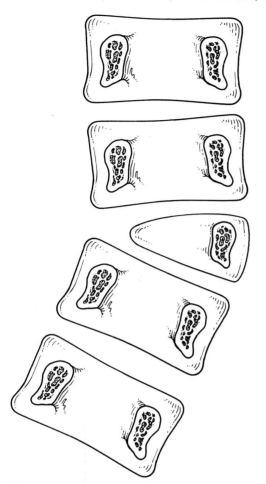

Fig. 108-1

Hemivertebra producing congenital scoliosis and caused by unilateral failure of sclerotomal formation. *(From Winter RB: Congenital deformities of the spine, New York, 1983, Thieme-Stratton, Inc.)*

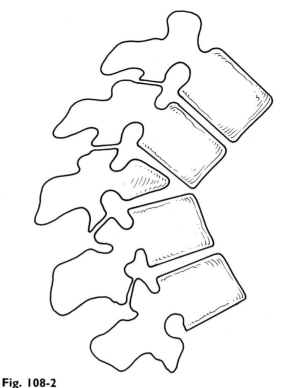

Fig. 108-2

Congenital kyphosis caused by failure of anterior vertebral body development. *(From Winter RB: Congenital deformities of the spine, New York, 1983, Thieme-Stratton, Inc.)*

Failure of Formation

Problems of formation are the result of absence of the induction or development of the appropriate embryonic cells. If the defect is bilateral, an entire vertebra may be absent or be hypoplastic in the anterior vertebral body, the posterior arch, or both. A unilateral defect of sclerotomal formation results in a hemivertebra on the opposite side (Fig. 108-1). This also may occur anteriorly (Fig. 108-2), posteriorly, or both. Multiple hemivertebrae may occur sequentially or be separated by normal or abnormal interval vertebrae and occur on ipsilateral or contralateral sides of the spine (Fig. 108-3).

Most defects of formation are asymmetrical, resulting in hemivertebrae or wedge-shaped vertebrae. The classic hemivertebra does not cross the midline and most likely results from failure of de-

velopment of its contralateral paired somite block. About two thirds of hemivertebrae are fully segmented, with growth potential at each end and disc material separating it from the vertebrae above and below. Approximately one fifth are semisegmented with one growth plate open and an adjacent disc. The remainder are unsegmented, being fused to the vertebrae above and below (Fig. 108-4). Hemivertebrae may be incarcerated (tucked into the spine) and cause no deformity since the vertebrae above and below are able to compensate for the malformation, or nonincarcerated and at the apex of a scoliosis (Fig. 108-5).[25] Approximately 90% are nonincarcerated.

It is more common for a hemivertebra to be more deficient anteriorly than posteriorly, and this can lead to kyphoscoliosis. Wedge-shaped vertebrae result from partial unilateral maldevelopment, but there is usually an entire disk above and/or below. The fifth lumbar vertebra is probably the most common site of this deformity. If the defect formation is symmetrical, several lesions are possible, including complete aplasia of the vertebra, aplasia of the vertebral body, or aplasia of the posterior elements. Complete or in-

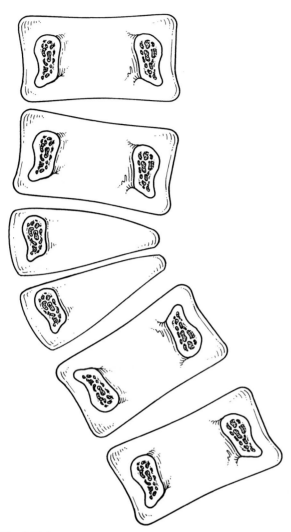

Fig. 108-3
Congenital scoliosis caused by multiple hemivertebrae. This has a worse prognosis than a single hemivertebra. *(From Winter RB: Congenital deformities of the spine, New York, 1983, Thieme-Stratton, Inc.)*

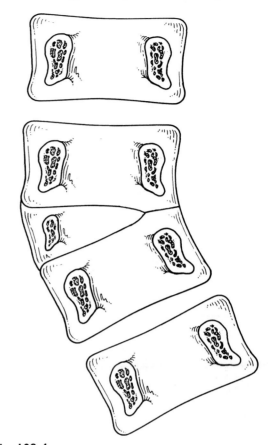

Fig. 108-4
Congenital scoliosis produced by a completely unsegmented hemivertebra. *(From Winter RB: Congenital deformities of the spine, New York, 1983, Thieme-Stratton, Inc.)*

complete failure of midline fusions of the paired somites can result in butterfly vertebrae (Fig. 108-6).

Failure of Segmentation

Defective segmentation of the vertebrae can be symmetrical or asymmetrical. If a sclerotomal cleft fails to develop, fused vertebral bodies result. This may be unilateral, leading to an anterolateral bar (Fig. 108-7), or bilateral, producing two blocked vertebrae (Fig. 108-8). The blocked vertebrae do not produce deformity, but if several of these occur in succession, substantial failure of longitudinal growth of the spine will result and pulmonary compromise may result. Posterior defects of segmentation, when sym-

metrical, are rare, but can result in severe progressive lordosis (Fig. 108-9). More common are anterior symmetrical defects of segmentation, caused by failure of the mesoderm to cleft into somites and producing a congenital kyphosis (Fig. 108-10). Asymmetrical segmentation defects produce unilateral unsegmented bars and scoliosis. These may involve the anterior or posterior elements or both, and the resultant congenital scoliosis is usually rapidly progressive to severe deformity.

It is not uncommon for defects of formation and segmentation to occur in the same spine (Fig. 108-11). These can be unilateral or bilateral, anterior or posterior or both, and produce progressive and nonprogressive curves. With regard to frequency, unilateral unsegmented bars and hemivertebrae are the two most common defects, followed by multiple anomalies, block vertebrae, and wedge-shaped vertebrae. Some congenital vertebral anomalies are so complex and difficult to define as to be virtually un-

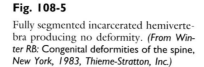

Fig. 108-5

Fully segmented incarcerated hemiverte-bra producing no deformity. *(From Winter RB:* Congenital deformities of the spine, *New York, 1983, Thieme-Stratton, Inc.)*

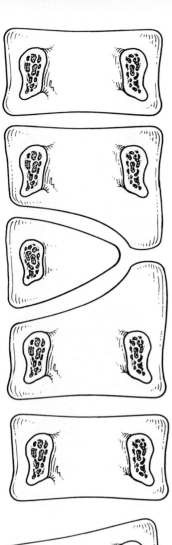

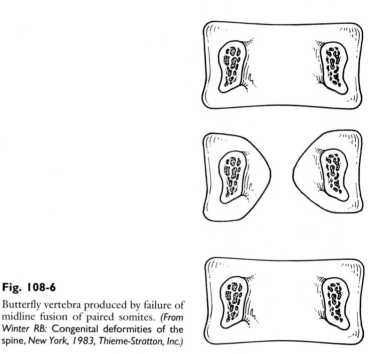

Fig. 108-6

Butterfly vertebra produced by failure of midline fusion of paired somites. *(From Winter RB:* Congenital deformities of the spine, *New York, 1983, Thieme-Stratton, Inc.)*

Fig. 108-7

Congenital scoliosis resulting from uni-lateral unsegmented bar. This is pro-duced by failure of sclerotomal clefting. *(From Winter RB:* Congenital deformities of the spine, *New York, 1983, Thieme-Stratton, Inc.)*

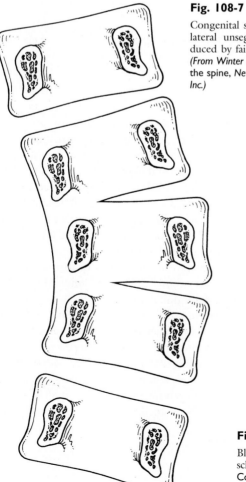

Fig. 108-8

Blocked vertebrae caused by complete sclerotomal cleft failure. *(From Winter RB:* Congenital deformities of the spine, *New York, 1983, Thieme-Stratton, Inc.)*

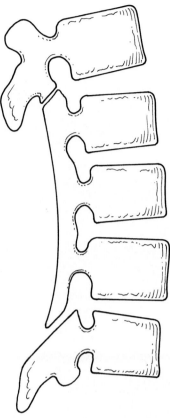

Fig. 108-9

Congenital lordosis produced by rare failure of posterior segmentation. *(From Winter RB: Congenital deformities of the spine, New York, 1983, Thieme-Stratton, Inc.)*

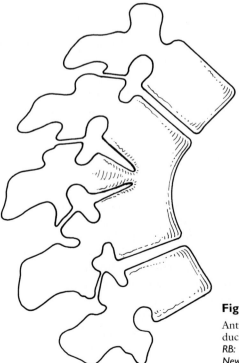

Fig. 108-10

Anterior failure of segmentation producing congenital kyphosis. *(From Winter RB: Congenital deformities of the spine, New York, 1983, Thieme-Stratton, Inc.)*

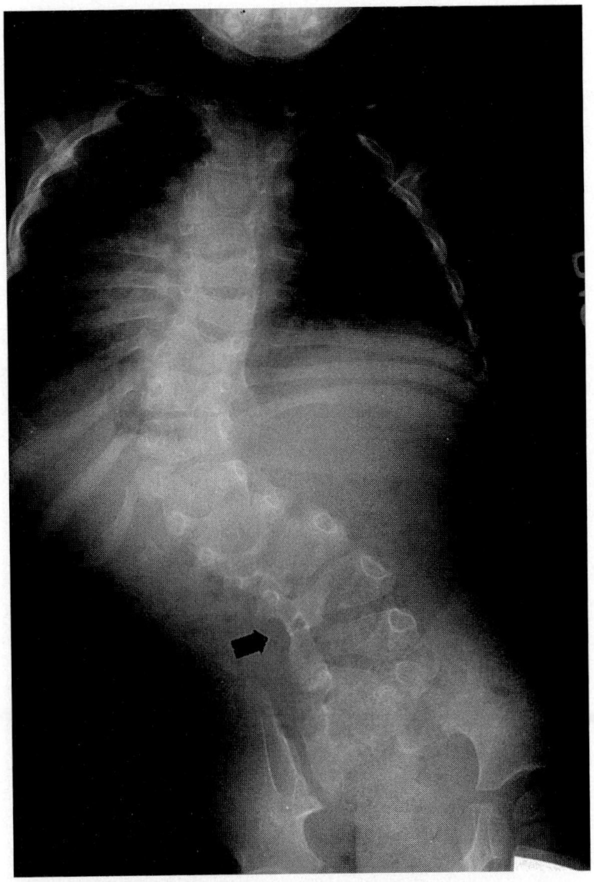

Fig. 108-11

Congenital curves caused by different anomalies. Arrow points to unilateral bar producing right lumbar curve. Note two low thoracic hemivertebrae producing left thoracolumbar curve.

classifiable. An uncommon, but severe anomaly is spondylothoracic dysplasia, also known as the Jarcho-Levin syndrome, wherein most or all of the thoracic vertebrae are involved[12,13] (Fig. 108-12). Severe stunting of trunk growth results, often with resultant severe pulmonary compromise. It is clear that careful individualized follow-up with radiographic documentation and study is necessary for the successful treatment of the patient with congenital scoliosis.

Occipitocervical malformations occur at the occiput or C1 and can include basilar impression, anomalies of the odontoid, failure of segmentation of the occiput and atlas, and defects of formation or segmentation of C1 and C2 (Fig. 108-13). Cervical anomalies from C2 to C6 include synostoses,

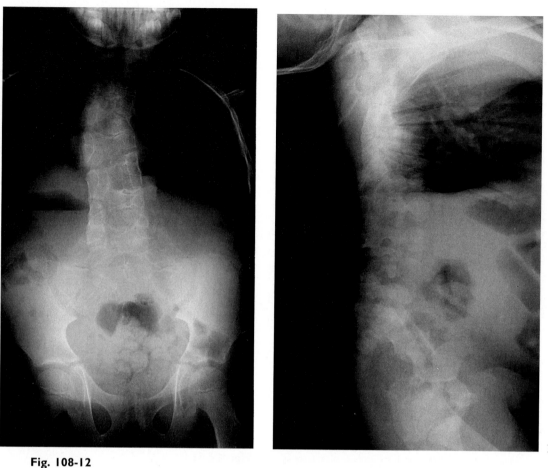

Fig. 108-12

A, Posteroanterior radiograph of spondylothoracic dysplasia. Note anomalies throughout entire thoracic and lumbar spine. **B,** Lateral view of the same patient.

hemivertebrae, and mixed anomalies such as the Klippel-Feil syndrome. Cervicothoracic anomalies occur at C7 or T1 and may be associated with upper extremity malformations including Sprengel deformity, cervical ribs, or cervical anomalies.

The thoracic spine, from T2 to T11, is the most common site for multiple and mixed lesions. Additional malformations of the ribs are often present (Fig. 108-14). Thoracolumbar malformations occur at T12 or L1. Hemivertebrae are frequently seen in this location, often with anterior deficiency such that kyphoscoliosis results. The lumbar anomalies occur from L2 to L4. In this region, single anomalies are more common than multiple. The lumbosacral junction, L5 and S1, can be the site of several abnormalities. Failure of fusion of the posterior elements results in spina bifida, defects of formation or segmentation can result in an oblique lumbosacral take-off (Fig. 108-15), and severe spinal decompensation, and other lesions such as lumbarization of S1 or sacralization of L5, either unilaterally or bilaterally, are frequent findings.

Natural History

The natural history or risk for progression of congenital scoliosis is very often impossible to predict accurately. It may be helpful to attempt to analyze the potential growth available on one side of the spine in comparison to the other. For example, unilateral unsegmented bars virtually always cause progression or worsening of a curve (Fig. 108-16). Curves caused by fully segmented hemivertebrae and multiple hemivertebrae on the same side are usually progressive (Fig. 108-17). Thoracic curves are more likely to progress than those in other regions. Curves tend to be more progressive at the time of the infantile and adolescent growth spurts than during the slow steady growth of the juvenile period. Nevertheless, each patient must be carefully followed and good-quality radiograms studied.

Many studies have been done to assess the risk of progression of congenital scoliosis and, overall, most have concluded that at least 50% of all congenital scoliosis deformities will progress substantially, to

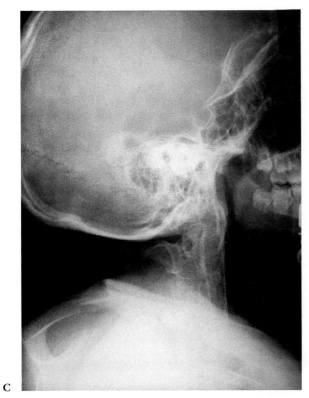

C

Fig. 108-12, cont'd

C, Lateral view of cervical spine of same patient. Note complete failure of segmentation.

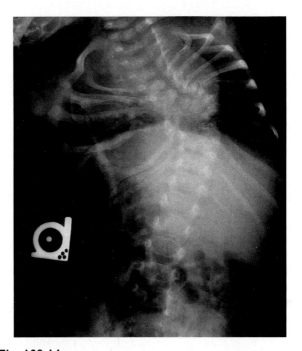

Fig. 108-14

Multiple thoracic rib anomalies associated with severe congenital scoliosis in midthoracic region.

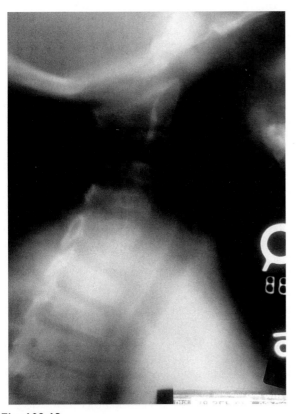

Fig. 108-13

Cervical anomalies, including posterior fusion of C1-C2 and C5-C6.

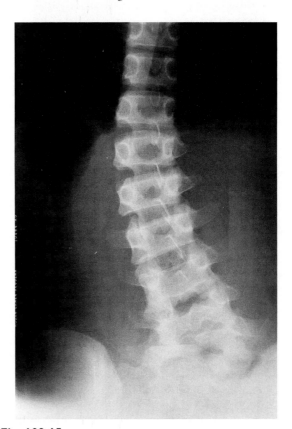

Fig. 108-15

Right hemivertebra at S1 producing right lumbosacral curve with compensatory left thoracolumbar curve and spinal decompensation.

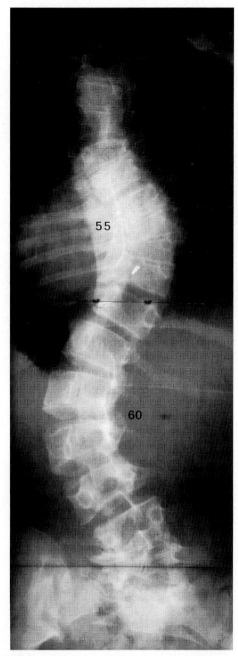

Fig. 108-16

Progressive right thoracic scoliosis caused by left unilateral bar spanning four segments. In this case involved area was fused in early childhood. Note that left thoracolumbar compensatory curve continued to progress and exceeds congenital curve in magnitude.

the point at which surgical treatment will be required.[15,30] About 10% to 15% will be completely nonprogressive, and the remaining 35% to 40% will progress either minimally or at least not enough that surgery will be necessary.[29]

Scoliosis caused by abnormalities of segmentation have the worst prognosis. These are most common

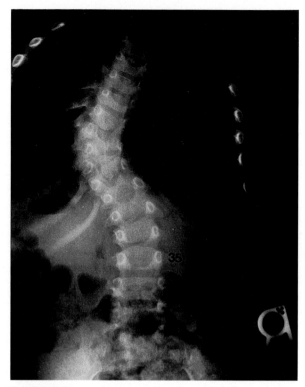

Fig. 108-17

Progressive 60-degree left thoracic congenital scoliosis caused by two left hemivertebrae at T8 and T10.

in the thoracic spine and least common in the cervical spine. Curves caused by unilateral unsegmented bars are almost always progressive, and the more segments involved by the bar, the worse the prognosis. In rare instances, the contralateral side will also be abnormal, with distorted anatomy, rudimentary disks, and probable radiolucent fibrocartilaginous tethers that limit the potential progression of the curve. Nevertheless, most surgeons think that the presence of a unilateral unsegmented bar is an indication for surgery without the necessity to document curve progression.

Hemivertebrae are less predictable with regard to curve progression. Some hemivertebrae are well incarcerated or incorporated into the spine and are not associated with any deformity whatsoever. Others may appear innocuous, but relentlessly progress to severe deformity. A hemivertebra that is not incarcerated and is fully segmented on each end has at least two more growth plates than the contralateral vertebral area and is much more likely to cause a progressive deformity. Although a hemivertebra that is completely unsegmented and, therefore, fused to both neighbors should be less likely to progress, one must remember that it may simply be the apex of a longer curve, and the nonanomalous vertebrae that make up the rest of the curve can participate in progression without change across the specific pathologic apex. One would be correct in expecting multiple hemivertebrae on the same side, particularly if they are close together, to have a bad prognosis. If there are multiple hemivertebrae on both sides of the spine, there are several possibilities, including maintenance of spinal balance without deformity, progression of one curve with nonprogression of others, or double progressive curves on opposite sides of the spine.

Mixed anomalies are almost always unpredictable and require documentation of progression prior to recommending surgical stabilization. Nevertheless, it is classically recognized that perhaps the worst possible situation is a unilateral unsegmented bar on the opposite side of the spine from one or more fully segmented hemivertebrae. This situation is a clear indication for surgical stabilization without waiting for the inevitable progression (Fig. 108-18). Spines with extensive involvement with mixed anomalies over multiple levels are most often balanced and their curves are usually, but not always, nonprogressive. Often the major problems with these lesions are that they result in substantial shortening of the trunk and that they are very difficult to classify and analyze.

It is most important to continually be cognizant of the behavior of the compensatory curves and the larger curve of which the structural abnormality is a part, as well as the behavior of the congenital anomaly itself. Continued monitoring of any sagittal-plane deformity is also essential.

Evaluation of the Patient

Evaluation of the patient with congenital scoliosis includes a basic history and physical examination, a careful and thorough neurologic examination, a radiologic study of the spinal column, and a search for associated abnormalities in other tissues or systems. In addition to the general medical history, the history of the pregnancy is important, and events such as maternal trauma, illness, or exposure to drugs or toxins should be documented and related to the stage of the pregnancy. The family history is important regarding other first-degree relatives or antecedents with spinal deformity, vertebral malformations, or lesions such as myelomeningocele. A history of maternal diabetes is noted in approximately 20% of patients with the lumbosacral anomaly sacral agenesis.[10] The patient's developmental history, including motor milestones and sphincter function, is important, as is a more detailed neurologic history of

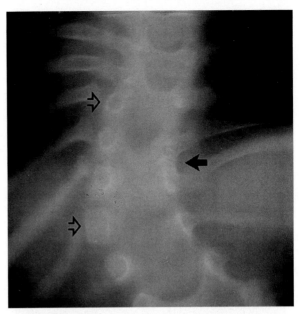

Fig. 108-18

Tomogram showing two left thoracic hemivertebrae *(open arrows)* opposite single right interpedicular bar *(solid arrow)*. This situation is certain to produce rapid curve progression.

any weakness, sensory abnormalities, or gait disturbances.

In addition to the general physical examination, specific attention to the spine, trunk, lower extremities, and neurologic examination is essential. A short neck, low-set ears, torticollis, and/or Sprengel deformity may be associated with anomalies of the cervical and upper thoracic spine. Chest examination should include rib and sternal evaluation, a search for scars indicating prior cardiac or pulmonary surgery, and auscultation for cardiac murmurs. Testing for superficial abdominal reflexes is important since these are frequently absent in spinal cord lesions such as syringomyelia. Observation of the back from behind and from the side is important for noting asymmetry in the standing and forward bending positions and the overall height of the trunk in comparison with the general body proportions. Pelvic obliquity should be noted in both standing and sitting positions and spinal balance or compensation should be assessed. The skin over the spine is observed for clues to underlying pathology such as hypertrichosis and hemangiomas or other nevi; subcutaneous masses such as lipomas, tumors, or cysts; dimples or sinus tracts; and scars from previous surgery. Spinal mobility and the presence or absence of paraspinal muscle spasm or tenderness should be noted. The lower-extremity examination includes evidence of limb-length inequality, thigh or calf atro-

Other Abnormalities Associated with Congenital Scoliosis

Questions regarding other spinal conditions and problems in other systems and physical examination for other congenital anomalies in these systems should not be omitted.

Spinal Abnormalities

Malformations of the spine, spinal cord, and spinal canal occur in 10% to 20% of patients with congenital spinal abnormalities.[4,16] These range from the innocuous spina bifida occulta to the severe myelomeningocele and anencephaly and include such defects as Klippel-Feil syndrome, diastematomyelia, diplomyelia, tethering of the spinal cord, the Arnold-Chiari malformation, syringomyelia, dermoid cysts, other types of cysts, and lipomas (Fig. 108-19). Because association of these lesions with congenital spinal deformity is relatively common, any patient who is scheduled to undergo correction of a congenital spinal deformity should have evaluation of the entire spine, the spinal cord, and the spinal canal by appropriate means, such as MRI, prior to undergoing surgery.

Genitourinary Abnormalities

Anomalies in other systems are frequently associated with congenital scoliosis. The genitourinary tract is the most common site, where a prevalence of anomalies ranging from 18% to 37% has been reported.[6,14] The association of renal anomalies with congenital scoliosis may be partially explained by the fact that the urinary system differentiates from the same general mesodermal region from which the vertebral column develops. The most frequent structural urologic anomalies are a solitary kidney, renal duplication, renal ectopia, and horseshoe kidney, in decreasing order of occurrence. Other problems such as ureteral reflux, obstructive uropathy, and neurogenic bladder have also been reported.[6] Of note, there is no relationship between the presence of a renal malformation and the magnitude or location of the spinal anomaly.

Cardiac Abnormalities

The next most common extraspinal anomalies are cardiac, occurring in 5% to 10% of the patients with congenital scoliosis. Of note, a reported series of patients with congenital heart disease had a higher

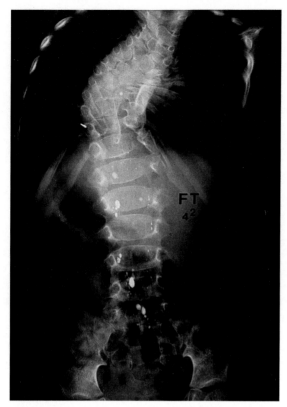

Fig. 108-19

Multiple thoracic anomalies, including diastematomyelia at T12 and open thoracolumbar myelomenigocele, unilateral bar on right in midthoracic region, and multiple left hemivertebrae.

phy, foot deformity or difference in foot size, and joint contractures. Of critical importance is a thorough neurologic evaluation, looking for signs of motor or sensory disturbance, deep-tendon reflex asymmetry, pathologic reflexes, and abnormal sphincter tone.

It is extremely important to consider the entire spine from several perspectives when evaluating congenital scoliosis. One must consider at least four separate spinal configurations: The anomalous region or regions are usually readily apparent and are often the sole focus of the inexperienced physician. They are most often located at the apex of the curvature, but can be found throughout the deformed region. Also important is the entire curve, of which the structurally abnormal segment may be only a small part. It is possible for the anomalous segment to be a nonprogressive part of an increasing, longer curvature. The third consideration is the compensatory curve that develops in normal spine segments cephalad and caudal to the congenital scoliosis. Fourth, one must always consider the sagittal plane alignment of the spine when planning any management of a congenital curve.

prevalence of congenital scoliosis than the general population.[9] Many types of congenital heart defects have been reported; such lesions occur more frequently in children with spinal anomalies of the thoracic region.

Other Abnormalities

Chest-wall deformities and anomalies are often associated with congenital scoliosis, particularly the more severe spinal deformities. These include rib distortion from spinal rotation, absence of one or more ribs, and fusion of adjacent ribs.

Pulmonary malformations, including partial or total unilateral absence of a lung, are more common in congenital scoliosis than in the general population. Gastrointestinal abnormalities include tracheoesophageal fistula and imperforate anus. The VATER association of vertebral anomalies, imperforate anus, tracheoesophageal fistula, anomalies of the radial side of the forearm and hand, and renal anomalies is well recognized. Abnormalities of the head and neck, particularly malformations of the ear, facial bones, and cleft lip or palate have also been noted in association with congenital scoliosis.

Associated anomalies of the upper extremity include Sprengel deformity, which is the most common, followed by variants of radial hemimelia ranging from absent or hypoplastic thumb to radial clubhand. In the lower limbs, the results of neurologic deficit are often seen, including cavovarus foot; clubfoot; hypoplasia of a limb; muscle atrophy; and motor, sensory, or reflex changes. Congenital limb deficiencies such as proximal focal femoral deficiency, fibular hemimelia, and tibial hemimelia can occur.

Many other relatively rare syndromes have been reported in association with congenital scoliosis. These include Aarskog syndrome, caudal regression, Goldenhar syndrome, Holt-Oram syndrome, Klippel-Feil syndrome, multiple pterygium syndrome, and Jarcho-Levin syndrome.[25]

Radiographic Evaluation

Radiographic evaluation is of paramount importance in the diagnosis, documentation, follow-up, and management of congenital scoliosis. At the initial visit, anteroposterior and lateral plain radiograms are obtained as base-line measurements. Since anomalies may be multiple and occur anywhere in the spine, it is essential that the entire spine, from occiput to coccyx, be imaged. Standing films are routinely obtained, although with lower-extremity contractures or limb-length inequality, a sitting film will be appropriate. Once the pathologic lesion has been identified, a supine anteroposterior film will show improved bone detail for better definition of the anomaly. If this is still not adequate, plain tomography in the coronal and/or sagittal projection will usually clarify the lesion. CT scanning with three-dimensional reconstructions may also be of value. Films taken to show flexibility or correctability of the scoliosis are not routinely obtained unless surgery is to be performed. Then supine anteroposterior maximal bending films and traction films are valuable in selecting fusion levels and planning instrumentation techniques.

At routine follow-up visits, curve progression, or lack thereof, is best documented on a plain erect film, the curve being measured by the method of Cobb. Curve measurement in congenital scoliosis is often quite difficult. It is very important to use the same technique of patient positioning and radiographic parameters in obtaining each radiogram at follow-up visits. Often vertebral end plates are poorly defined, in which case the pedicles may be a more accurate point of reference on successive films. If pedicles are not clearly seen, one must be creative, but the same landmarks on the same vertebrae should be used every time in order to detect true progression. It is important not to "overmeasure" a deformity, particularly in cases of hemivertebrae, in which angulated end plates may be well incarcerated within the spine. In such cases, drawing perpendiculars to the lateral border or general longitudinal contour of the spine is more valid. Curves measured should include the anomalous segment, the longer curve of which this is often a part, compensatory curves cranial and caudal, and the sagittal spinal contours.

CT scans are indicated to define the bony anatomy of the spinal canal, particularly in cases of bifid posterior elements and diastematomyelia. In the latter condition a midline bony, cartilaginous, or fibrous spur partially or completely divides the canal in the sagittal plane. These lesions may be single or multiple and may occur at any level, although they are most common in the thoracic spine. A bony stem may sometimes be seen on a plain radiogram. This lesion is usually associated with localized widening of the interpedicular distance and spina bifida occulta at the same level. Diplomyelia occurs at the level of the lesion and may extend the caudal length of the spinal cord. The value of CT scans is enhanced with contrast material when one is assessing the status of the spinal cord and nerve roots. MRI is also of great value for this purpose.

Myelography with injectable contrast material, of great value in the past, has been largely supplanted by MRI. Whereas such studies are not necessary for every patient with congenital scoliosis, they are indicated in instances of neurologic deficit, rapid progression of deformity when there is other evidence of potential intraspinal pathology, and when any surgical correction of the deformity is contemplated. Lateral images in both flexion and extension are particularly useful to assess the relationship between the bony spine and the neural elements in cases of suspected instability.

The current imaging technique of choice for detecting and evaluating malformations of the urinary tract is ultrasonography. This technology has evolved to the point at which precise definition of even subtle abnormalities such as mild obstruction can be detected. If high-quality ultrasonography is not available, then a plain radiographic study with an intravenous contrast agent is the classic method of evaluating the urinary tract.

Treatment

The options for treatment of congenital scoliosis are periodic observation with documentation, treatment with an orthosis, or surgical treatment. No other method of "treatment" has any effect on the natural history of congenital scoliosis.

Observation

Periodic observation with radiographic documentation is appropriate for curves that are small (less than 30 degrees) and curves that have proven to be nonprogressive, unless, even though they are nonprogressive, their magnitude is such that surgery is indicated to improve spinal imbalance or to decrease severe magnitude. The frequency of follow-up visits for curves being observed varies with the age of the patient and the type, magnitude, and location of the malformation. Infants should be seen at least every 3 to 6 months during the first few years of life because of their rapid growth and risk of curve progression. During the juvenile period of relatively less rapid growth, annual follow-up of nonprogressive curves is satisfactory, particularly if the curve has a natural history that would be expected to be stable or if the curve is of small magnitude. The risk of curve progression increases at the time of the onset of the adolescent growth spurt, and most curves should be followed every 6 months from that time until growth is complete. It is usually wise to continue to monitor congenital scoliosis in adults every 5 years.

Orthotic Treatment

Treatment by a spinal orthosis will not have any effect on the structural anomaly. Orthoses can, however, often control compensatory curves above or below the congenitally abnormal curve and can sometimes halt, or at least delay, the progression of a long, flexible curve of which the anomalous area is only a part.[22] In this latter situation, slowing of curve progression can allow beneficial growth prior to the time of definitive spinal fusion. Again, it must be strongly stated that an orthosis will have no beneficial effect on a structurally abnormal, progressing, congenital segment. In this instance, prompt surgery is mandatory to halt curve progression. Although the Milwaukee brace is the benchmark for orthotic treatment in congenital scoliosis, successful control of appropriate curves in the lower thoracic and lumbar spine can sometimes be achieved with low-profile orthoses.

Surgical Treatment

Surgical treatment is indicated for progressive congenital scoliosis; for small curves that are certain to progress, such as those caused by unilateral unsegmented bars, with or without contralateral hemivertebrae; and for curves of severe magnitude or with substantial decompensation even though they may not be progressing. Several technical options are available for the arthrodesis of congenital scoliosis. These include posterior in situ fusion, anterior and posterior in situ fusion, anterior hemiepiphysiodesis with posterior hemiarthrodesis, hemivertebra excision, and the use of corrective implanted instrumentation with any of these techniques. With any method, it may be wise to use autologous bone graft, if possible, which in at least one study has been shown to be superior to allograft bone.[1] A large amount of bone graft is necessary to develop a large fusion mass in order to counteract the forces of unopposed growth. Prior to the use of any corrective instrumentation, imaging evaluation of the entire spinal cord is mandatory to assess the 10% to 20% likelihood of an intraspinal anomaly and avoid disastrous consequences, such as paraplegia, if damage to the spinal cord occurs by disturbing an unrecognized lesion. Unless internal spinal fixation is deemed to be very adequate, it is wise to provide 6 months of postoperative cast or orthosis external support for spinal fusions in congenital scoliosis patients. Noninstrumented fusions extending into the cervical spine should be treated postoperatively with a halo cast or vest.

An issue that frequently arises is the tethering effect of a spinal fusion, done at a very young age, on the further growth of the spine in the fusion area. A progressing congenital deformity will produce only a shorter and more deformed vertebral column, so that although a solid arthrodesis of the spine does not grow in length in any useful manner, a timely arthrodesis will prevent the deformed area from becoming even more deformed and shortened.

Length of the Fusion

The length of the fusion in congenital scoliosis depends on the number of involved segments, the length of the entire curve containing the anomaly, and the age of the patient. In older children, the rules of spinal balance apply and the entire curve, from the cephalad stable vertebra to the caudad stable vertebra, is usually included in the fusion. In younger children it is sometimes preferable simply to fuse the anomalous segment, with or without postoperative orthotic treatment of the normal vertebrae remaining in the curve, or of compensatory curves, in order to gain further beneficial growth of the spine. This is often done with full knowledge that "adding on" or progression of the curve is likely and that further surgery may be necessary when the child is older.

Posterior in Situ Fusion

Posterior in situ fusion is most appropriate for short rigid curves that are not correctable (for example, those caused by short unilateral unsegmented bars) or short progressive curves of mild degree caused by hemivertebrae in patients in mid or later childhood. Such fusions should include one normal vertebra cephalad and caudad to the anomaly. It is necessary to support the fusion with a postoperative cast or brace in order to decrease the risk of pseudarthrosis and perhaps obtain some correctability or improve balance in short curves with some flexibility. Patients with posterior in situ fusions must be followed throughout the growth period. If "adding on" occurs in the flexible, nonanomalous segments above and/or below the curve, then an orthosis or extension of the fusion should be considered.

If bending of the fusion mass increases the scoliosis or if the rotational "crankshaft" phenomenon occurs, producing the further deformity of lordoscoliosis because of continued anterior growth, then an anterior fusion should be done as well as consideration given to reexploring the posterior fusion mass.[8] Terek et al. noted that the rotation that developed was always associated with curve progression and that no curve that had anterior and posterior hemiarthrodesis had the "crankshaft" phenomenon.[21] The safety and value of posterior in situ fusion has been well documented by Winter et al.[26] In their series of 163 patients, there were no neurologic complications and only one case of iatrogenic thoracic lordosis, and with a mean follow-up of 7 years, only 14% of the patients had the "crankshaft" phenomenon or bending of the fusion mass.

Posterior Fusion with Internal Fixation

Posterior fusion with implanted corrective instrumentation is indicated to achieve correction in curves with flexibility, to correct spine imbalance, or to stabilize long rigid curves as an augmentation to the arthrodesis. It is imperative to rule out intraspinal anomalies, usually by means of MRI, prior to attempting instrumented correction. The magnitude of curves treated with posterior fusion and instrumentation should be moderate. For severe rigid curves, an anterior procedure to obtain correctability, such as osteotomies or multiple discectomies, is required. The choice of instrumentation includes rod systems with multiple hooks, rod systems with sublaminar or intraspinous wires, and the augmentation of either technique, if indicated, with bone-screw fixation. If correction by internal fixation is carried out, monitoring of spinal cord function may be extremely important. Such monitoring can be done by means of the wake-up test and the immediate postoperative clonus test and may be usefully augmented with intraoperative monitoring techniques for somatosensory and/or motor evoked potentials.[17]

Combined Anterior and Posterior Fusion

Combined anterior and posterior surgery, usually done during the same operation, can be extremely useful in congenital scoliosis. The advantages of anterior fusion combined with posterior fusion are that correctability is improved (Fig. 108-20), the pseudarthrosis rate should be less, and future bending or torquing of the fusion mass is prevented. The morbidity from an anterior fusion added to a posterior fusion is small. Fusing only the convex side of a curve that has growth potential on the concave side can result in some correction as the child grows.[23] This is particularly useful with a single hemivertebra or adjacent hemivertebrae in young patients. For the convex anterior/posterior surgery to be worthwhile, there must be adequate growth time remaining. The fusion should extend to a normal vertebra above and

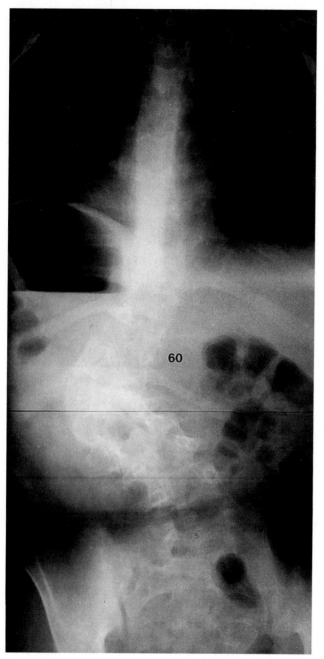

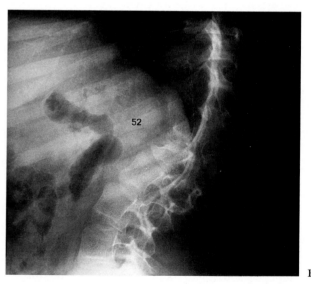

Fig. 108-20

A, Posteroanterior radiographs showing short angular left thoracolumbar curve caused by a posterolateral hemivertebra. **B,** Lateral view of same patient demonstrating kyphosis.

below the defective segments. In situations in which there is a need for fusion over several segments and the child is young and has substantial potential growth remaining on the convex side, but not on the concave side (e.g., an unsegmented bar), then a complete bilateral anterior and posterior fusion should be done to prevent bending or "crankshafting" of the fusion with time and growth. According to Winter et al., the operation of anterior hemiepiphysiodesis and posterior hemiarthrodesis is best suited to the child under age 6 years with pure scoliosis, no sagittal plane deformity, and a progressive curve of less than 70 degrees spanning five segments or less.[29] The curve should be in the thoracic or lumbar spine.

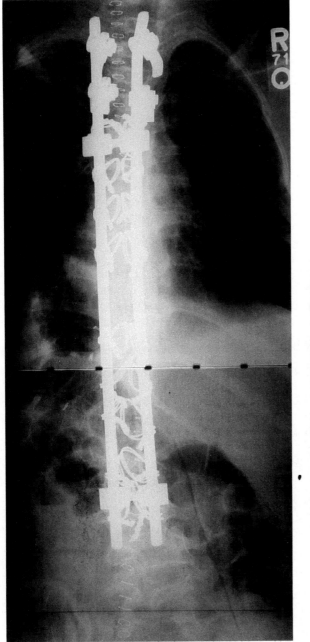

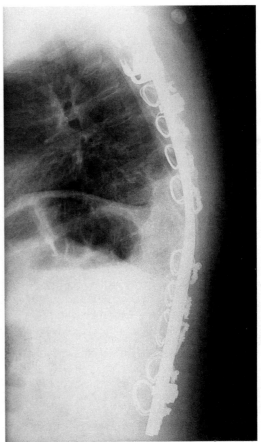

Fig. 108-20, cont'd

C and D, Postoperative radiographs of same patient following excision of hemivertebra and correction of kyphoscoliosis with segmental instrumentation.

Hemivertebra Excision and Fusion

Hemivertebrae may be excised in order to obtain substantial correctability of scoliosis or spinal decompensation, particularly in the lumbar and lumbosacral regions. This technique usually involves the anterior excision of the hemivertebra and the adjacent disks above and below, plus the addition of anterior autogenous bone graft. It is most often followed directly, but may be staged, with a posterior fusion, excising any remnant of the hemivertebra posteriorly, adding abundant autogenous bone graft, and often using internal fixation and/or corrective postoperative cast immobilization. This technique has proven to be reasonably safe at the lumbosacral junction and in the lumbar spine.[3]

Some surgeons prefer to excise the anterior hemivertebra via a posterior transpedicular approach—the so-called eggshell vertebrectomy. The risk of neurologic damage increases if hemivertebra excision is carried out in the thoracic or cervical spine. The problems with hemivertebra excision surgery in these areas include the production of instability, which can result in damage to the spinal cord, and/or the compromise of the vascular supply to the cord itself. The younger the patient who is an appropriate candidate for hemivertebra excision, the better the result, because of increased flexibility of compensatory curves. It may also be helpful to perform convex anterior hemiepiphysiodesis and posterior hemiarthrodesis at the cephalad and caudad disk space to gain further correction from growth. Hemivertebra excision is a closing wedge procedure. The concave ligaments should be left intact as a "periosteal hinge" to prevent instability. When hemivertebra excision is done, internal fixation with instrumentation is almost always necessary to stabilize the spine at the level of the excision and improve correctability. As always, when internal fixation is used, preoperative evaluation of the spinal canal is appropriate. In addition to hemivertebrectomy, complete vertebrectomy is possible at the apex of curves in order to obtain substantial correction, but at the cost of increased neurologic risk from gross instability. If a severe truncal imbalance deformity is not correctable by anterior and posterior surgery, one may consider double osteotomy of the pelvis, lengthening the ilium on one side and shortening it on the other, to improve the decompensation.

Reexploration of the Fusion

In the past, some surgeons have recommended reexploration of posterior fusions in congenital scoliosis at 6 months postoperatively in order to detect and repair pseudarthroses or add bone graft to areas where there was little apparent fusion. Now, with standard techniques of facet fusion, decortication, and the use of large amounts of autogenous bone graft, routine reexploration is not generally practiced. In children over 5 or 6 years of age who require more than one- or two-level fusions, most surgeons deem it advisable to add internal fixation in further attempts to avoid pseudarthrosis occurrence.

Abnormalities in the Spinal Canal

Abnormalities in the spinal canal, caudal tethering of the spinal cord, or cephalad anomalies such as the Arnold-Chiari malformation and syringomyelia, should be controlled or relieved by appropriate neurosurgical intervention prior to or concomitant with the treatment of the scoliosis. In cases of diastematomyelia, the indications for excision of the stem are debatable. Many neurosurgeons prefer simply to follow asymptomatic lesions. If, however, surgical treatment of congenital scoliosis is to be carried out, then it is wise to remove the diastematomyelia at the same time, in order to avoid the possibility of having to approach it at a later date through substantial scar tissue and/or a fusion mass.

Severe Chest-Wall Malformations

One technique for correction of severe chest wall malformations associated with congenital scoliosis has been reported by Campbell et al.[5] This involves implantation of an expandable vertical rib prosthesis to increase thoracic volume and afford some curve correction. This technique is still in its investigational stages and shows promise for selected patients.

Role of Traction

The role of traction in the surgical treatment of congenital scoliosis is reserved for the occasional patient with severe, rigid deformity wherein the surgeon feels that the safest course may be slow, gradual correction with the patient awake. In such cases, traction can be used postoperatively, prior to cast application, if the surgery did not include internal fixation. In other cases it may be desirable to do a preliminary surgical osteotomy or discectomy procedure and then use a period of traction prior to a second-stage operation with corrective instrumentation. Since traction may stretch the spinal cord over the apex of a rigid deformity, it must be used with great caution, and frequent monitoring of the neurologic status of the patient (at least every 8 hours) must be carried out.

Problems with and Complications of Surgical Treatment

Potential problems with and complications of surgery for congenital scoliosis include death, paralysis, failure of the fusion (pseudarthrosis), instrumentation failure, infection, and syndrome of inappropriate antidiuretic hormone (SIADH) elaboration, as well as other well-recognized situations. According to Hall, death during or after surgery is more frequent in congenital scoliosis than in idiopathic scoliosis.[11] It is most often the result of complications of respiratory insufficiency associated with severe thoracic deformity. Paraplegia may occur because of mechanical overdistraction of the spinal cord, particularly if there is an intraspinal lesion; because of instability with translational impingement on the cord; or because of vascular compromise to the cord. Preoperative assessment with appropriate imaging techniques such as MRI, intraoperative spinal cord monitoring, and gradual corrections help lower the risk of paralysis. Nevertheless, this risk cannot be reduced to zero.

Pseudarthrosis is best avoided by a meticulous fusion technique with facet excision, laminar decortication, and the use of abundant local and other autogenous bone graft. Children over 3 years of age usually have enough iliac donor bone, although it may be necessary to use both ilia as donor sites. Augmentation with allograft should be used if an adequate volume of autogenous bone is lacking. Failure of instrumentation is best avoided by obtaining a solid fusion, by using good judgment with regard to the size and strength of the spine vis-à-vis the internal fixation device and appropriate tempering of the amount of force applied to the spine through the implant. In children with concomitant congenital heart lesions or compromised pulmonary function, one should minimize SIADH elaboration by replacing fluid loss with colloid and limited crystalloid, as advocated by Flynn et al.[10]

CONGENITAL KYPHOSIS

Congenital kyphosis is not as common as congenital scoliosis and is defined as a posterior angulation of the spine in the sagittal plane, caused by a congenital structural defect of a vertebra or vertebrae. The deformity may be an isolated phenomenon or can occur with other defects such as myelomeningocele and bone dysplasias that have spinal involvement. These latter associated conditions will not be discussed in this section. Congenital kyphosis has the potential to produce substantial deformity, pulmonary compromise, cor pulmonale, and paraparesis or paraplegia. Early diagnosis and often treatment, therefore, is a necessity.

The deformity is almost always caused by either failure of segmentation or failure of formation of a vertebral segment or segments. A much less common occurrence, congenital rotatory dislocation with kyphosis, has been described by Dubousset.[7]

The indications for surgery in congenital kyphosis are documented progression of the kyphosis, the presence of any neurologic deficit, intractable discomfort, and progressing or significant pulmonary compromise.

Evaluation of the Patient

The work-up prior to surgical treatment of congenital kyphosis should include renal ultrasonography to assess the status of the urinary tract, since patients with congenital spinal deformities are at greater risk for such anomalies, assessment of pulmonary status and pulmonary function studies if indicated, adequate radiographic documentation that may require plain or computerized tomography to define the spinal anomaly precisely, and an MRI to define the status of the spinal canal and spinal cord. Patients with severe pulmonary compromise benefit from an aggressive respiratory therapy program prior to surgery and may have their pulmonary functions improved by a period of preliminary halo-gravity traction. Traction can be of benefit in improving pulmonary function, but carries a high risk of spinal cord injury by stretching the more flexible spinal cord and vertebrae above and below the rigid kyphos over the apex of the kyphos. If traction is considered, it should be gradually applied and carefully monitored by thorough neurologic evaluation at least every 8 hours. The maximum benefit of traction should be obtained within 10 to 14 days.

Classification

Failure of Formation

General Principles and Assessment

Defects of formation are more common than defects of segmentation and are capable of producing deformities of far greater magnitude that can lead to paraplegia. Failure of formation occurs in the anterior vertebral body or bodies and results in one or more posterior hemivertebra (Fig. 108-21). With failure of formation the defect can be variable, from minimal wedging in one vertebra to complete absence of more than one vertebral body. The magnitude and risk of progression of the deformity as well as the likelihood of back pain and pulmonary compromise are directly proportional to the magnitude of the vertebral deficit.[25] If the defect is anterolateral, kyphoscoliosis will result.

The natural history of congenital kyphosis caused by defects of formation is almost always continuous progression. The more acutely angled the kyphosis, the greater the risk of anterior spinal cord compression and paraplegia. The rate of progression of this type of congenital kyphosis is variable, but usually varies from 2 to 10 degrees per year and is accelerated by the infantile and adolescent growth spurts.

Dubousset importantly calls attention to the fact that the spinal canal may or may not be well aligned in cases of this type of congenital kyphosis.[7] When there is a step-off or subluxation of the spine, the spinal cord is at much greater risk, particularly with any injury to the vertebral column at the level of the defect. The subluxation is evident by a step-off noted in the contour of the posterior wall of the vertebral bodies as seen on a lateral plain radiogram, plain tomogram, or CT scan. This is a particularly unstable situation and demands prompt surgical stabilization. A similar risk can occur when there is complete failure of formation of a vertebral body and posterior elements. MRI and/or CT scanning, with three-dimensional reconstructions if necessary, may be required to precisely define the pathologic anatomy of this type of congenital kyphosis.

Treatment

Because of their poor prognosis, defects of formation require early diagnosis and prompt surgical treatment. Again, there is no nonoperative treatment that affects the natural history of this problem.[30]

In the best situation, the diagnosis is made in infancy or early childhood, and successful treatment can be obtained by posterior spinal fusion as soon as any instability is detected or progression of the kyphosis is documented. Preoperative hyperextension lateral radiography or MRI study is helpful in determining the amount of nonossified soft tissue that fills the anterior formation defect. If this space is large, then the likelihood of pseudarthrosis is higher, and an anterior procedure should be done to remove the fibrous or fibrocartilaginous tissue and replace it with either bone chips or a strut graft. If the space is not large anteriorly, the kyphotic deformity is not large (less than 75 degrees), and the patient is an infant or young child (less than 5 years old), a posterior fusion is done, incorporating one level above and one below the abnormal vertebra. Abundant autogenous bone is used and may be augmented with allograft if necessary. The patient is then placed in a hyperextension cast for 6 months followed by an extension orthosis for at least an additional 6 months and sometimes longer if the entire curve is long. Some surgeons elect to explore the posterior fusion mass routinely at 4 to 6 months postoperatively to reinforce it with more bone graft in an attempt to reduce the likelihood of bending of

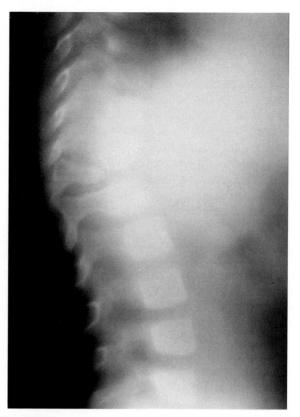

Fig. 108-21
Lateral tomogram showing congenital kyphosis caused by anterior failure of formation.

the fusion or pseudarthrosis formation.[7] About two thirds of patients treated in this manner will show some beneficial correction of the kyphosis because of continued growth from the anterior open growth plates opposite the fused posterior segment.[24] In children older than 5 years in whom the kyphosis is less than 55 to 65 degrees, posterior fusion by itself with or without instrumentation is usually successful.[28] On the other hand, regardless of the age of the patient or the magnitude of the anterior "empty space," an anterior fusion should routinely be done if the angular kyphosis is greater than 65 to 70 degrees. After skeletal maturity, for all patients anterior and posterior arthrodesis combined with posterior instrumentation is necessary to stop progression, gain correction, and produce a solid arthrodesis in this type of congenital kyphosis.

As previously mentioned, traction is dangerous in congenital kyphosis because the likely result is simply stretching of the spinal cord across the rigid, anterior kyphotic bony segment. This can result in a substantial risk of paraplegia.[27]

As is the case in the treatment of congenital scoliosis, if one is contemplating active correction of congenital kyphosis it is important to visualize the spinal canal and the spinal cord by means of a preoperative MRI study to rule out intraspinal pathology such as a tethered spinal cord, diastematomyelia, syringomyelia, or other congenital lesions.

An important consideration in the surgical treatment of congenital kyphosis is sagittal plane spinal balance. It is wise to assess the flexibility of the cephalad and caudal compensatory lordoses with appropriate preoperative bending radiograms in order to determine the correct fusion limits precisely. It is particularly important for the lumbar spine to have sufficient mobility and lordosis to balance a kyphotic deformity cephalad to it.

Anterior Fusion The technique of anterior surgery should result in a solid anterior load path from the top to the bottom of the curve. The specific technique will depend on the magnitude of the curve, but will include release of the soft-tissue tether, including the anterior longitudinal ligament; all components of the disk back to the posterior annulus fibrosis and posterior longitudinal ligament, which are left intact; and any abnormal fibrous or fibrocartilaginous material that may exist in place of the absent portion of the vertebral body. Small curves can be managed by such excision and grafting with multiple chips of autogenous rib. Large deformities require vertical strut grafts, the most anterior of which may be at a distance of several centimeters from the anterior apex of the kyphosis. In such cases, all the space between the anteriormost strut and the apex should be filled with smaller struts. Autogenous fibula or a rib graft, often on its vascular pedicle, are appropriate sources of anterior struts. When using anterior strut grafts, maximum correction should be obtained at the time of graft placement so that further posterior correction does not dislodge the grafts. This is done by using temporary mechanical distraction devices to obtain maximum correction at the time of graft insertion and then removing the device.[18]

Length of the Fusion The length of the anterior fusion should extend, as a minimum, from the normal vertebral body above to the normal vertebral body below the anomalous region. Whether the fusion should extend beyond these limits depends on the flexibility of the compensatory lordoses as assessed preoperatively on a hyperextension, lateral radiogram. The length of the posterior fusion must extend to the central gravity line of the body superiorly and inferiorly.[25]

Severe Kyphoses in Older Patients Severe rigid congenital kyphoses in older patients can be treated by posterior closing wedge osteotomy with anterior release and strut grafting. Posterior fixation is obtained with a dual-rod, multiple-hook compression type of tension-band system. Great care must be exercised in decompressing nerve roots and preventing displacement of the spinal canal or any soft-tissue impingement on the spinal cord during these procedures.

Stabilization may then be obtained either by single or multiple strong anterior bony strut grafts, such a fibula, or, if strong enough, free or vascularized pedicle rib struts, or by using small fragments of the autogenous rib to pack the empty disk spaces and then accomplish posterior internal fixation, either a multiple hook and rod system, or one-fourth-inch diameter Luque rods with sublaminar wires.

Anterior Decompression of the Spinal Cord If the kyphosis is of large magnitude and/or rigid, with any evidence of spinal cord compression anteriorly, then it is necessary to decompress the spinal cord from in front and perform an anterior fusion. This is combined with a posterior fusion with internal fixation. When anterior decompression is accomplished by resecting enough bone from the vertebral body to decompress the spinal cord completely, then strut grafting is essential. It needs to be emphasized that the spinal cord compression in congenital kyphosis is always anterior and never posterior. Posterior laminectomy, therefore, is contraindicated since it will simply result in further instability, progression of the deformity, and further spinal cord compression.

Anterior decompression is accomplished by beginning cephalad and caudal to the apex and progressively removing bone toward the apex from either end. The spinal cord should never be retracted posteriorly and the decompression should not start at the apex since the risk of further neurologic deficit is greater. Anterior decompression and strut grafting is always followed, either at the same time or within 2 weeks, by posterior internal fixation and fusion. This technique can give dramatic correction, but carries a risk of paralysis because of potential temporary instability at the time of surgery or interruption of the blood supply to the spinal cord, since many times the lesion is in the watershed area of the thoracic spine. The length of the posterior fusion following anterior surgery must include all the vertebrae in the kyphotic area (defined by maximum Cobb measurement) and at least one normal vertebra above and below the area.

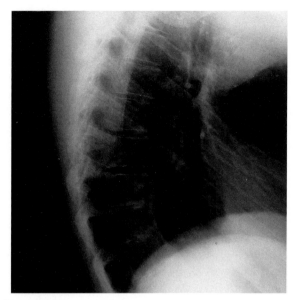

Fig. 108-22

Congenital kyphosis caused by failure of anterior segmentation.

Decompression without Bony Resection In cases of relatively flexible congenital kyphosis and neurologic deficit of recent onset, success has been reported in some instances by using preoperative external correction by means of hyperextension casts and recumbency to provide "decompression" followed by anterior and posterior fusion without anterior decompression.[7] This technique avoids the risk of surgical decompression of the spinal cord. However, it is not suitable for a congenital kyphosis with a rigid apex.

Failure of Segmentation

General Principles and Assessment

This is the more "benign" type of congenital kyphosis (Fig. 108-22). It is neither as deforming nor as progressive as kyphosis caused by defects of formation. Defects of segmentation may not be apparent in infants and young children because in some instances they exist as a cartilaginous anlage of the unsegmented bar and do not ossify until mid or later childhood.

Failure of segmentation is most likely to occur in the low thoracic region or thoracolumbar junction and rarely, if ever, causes paraplegia. It may, however, be associated with substantial compensatory hyperlordosis in the lumbar region, and this compensatory deformity may become symptomatic.[28] Back pain in older patients with congenital kyphosis is usually localized to the compensatory hyperlordosis caused to the kyphotic deformity. Pain is more likely to develop when the hyperlordosis extends over fewer segments, for example, when the kyphotic apex is in the low thoracic or thoracolumbar region. It is extremely unusual for the kyphotic region itself to produce discomfort.

The defect of segmentation is usually present as a pure anterior bar so that only kyphosis results. If the failure of segmentation is anterolateral, kyphoscoliosis develops. The failure of segmentation may occur at one or many levels. In the latter case, the deformity will usually be much larger than when segmentation fails to occur at a single level. In the single-level situation, there is more room for compensatory lordotic compensation cephalad and caudal to the defect.

Failure of segmentation results in an anterior tether, and with unopposed posterior growth, progressive kyphosis ensues. The deformity rarely, if ever, becomes severe enough to produce anterior compression of the spinal cord and subsequent neurologic deficit. The magnitude of congenital kyphosis is measured by the method of Cobb on an upright lateral radiograph. In most cases, the first normal end plates above and below the congenital defect are used as the upper and lower limits of the curve. In some cases, however, the apical defect will be part of a larger curve and in these situations it is wise to measure both the apical defect and the limits of the larger curve that describe the greatest amount of deformity. Radiography in the coronal plane is always necessary, at least at the time of initial diagnosis, to rule out the concomitant existence of congenital scoliosis. Unlike congenital scoliosis caused by defects of segmentation, when such defects cause pure congenital kyphosis they are much less of a problem.

Treatment

There is no effective nonoperative treatment for this condition. No type of orthotic treatment of physical therapy or other type of mechanical treatment has any effect on the natural history of this condition. The treatment for progressive deformity is surgery.

For small progressive deformities, particularly those detected early, the treatment is posterior spinal fusion extending from one level above to one level below the segmentation defect. Most surgeons elect to use a compression hook and rod system and autogenous bone graft. Fusions of this type have a high success rate (greater than 95%), but do not produce correction of the deformity. In cases with failure of segmentation extending over several levels or with severe deformity, correction is possible by producing anterior

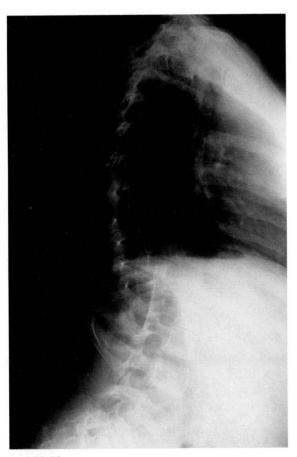

Fig. 108-23
Congenital lordosis caused by failure of segmentation of posterior arch structures.

osteotomies with bone resection at the level of the absent disc spaces and adding autogenous bone graft to the anterior osteotomies. This is then followed, usually at the same operative setting, by posterior compression instrumentation and fusion to stabilize the spine and provide correction of the deformity.

OTHER CONGENITAL DEFORMITIES

Congenital Kyphoscoliosis

Kyphoscoliosis is treated in a very individualized manner, using principles applied to both scoliosis and kyphosis. This means that often both anterior and posterior fusions will be necessary. When anterior surgery is done, the approach should be from the convex side of the scoliosis. Anterior and posterior surgery is also necessary in young patients with kyphoscoliosis to obtain correction and prevent the crankshaft phenomenon.[7]

Congenital Lordosis

Congenital lordosis is exceedingly rare and is essentially always caused by failure of segmentation of the posterior arch structures (Fig. 108-23). This produces a tethering effect on the spine which, since anterior vertebral body growth proceeds "normally," results in a relentlessly progressive lordotic segment. Unabated, this deformity can severely compromise pulmonary function by markedly limiting intrathoracic volume. The failure of segmentation more often is slightly posterolateral, producing lordoscoliosis rather than strictly lordosis.

Although there is very little information in the literature regarding congenital lordosis,[25] it is probably more common in the thoracic region than in the lumbar spine.

The treatment of congenital lordoscoliosis is surgical. Orthotics cannot control this deformity. Anterior vertebral body growth must be stopped by arthrodesis, combined with posterior fusion as well. The fusion should include at least one level cephalad and caudal to the unsegmented area. Correction may be obtained in more severe deformities by performing osteotomies of the posterior bar and adding posterior segmental internal fixation. When the posterior column is lengthened during correction, the anterior column should be shortened by disc and wedge osteotomies to lessen the risk of a neurologic injury.

Congenital lordosis, without scoliosis, is treated by an anterior fusion alone if correction is not necessary in mild deformities. For more severe involvement, anterior and posterior correction and fusion should be considered. This is done by performing disc excisions and anteriorly based wedge osteotomies of the anterior spine and osteotomizing the posterior bar, then obtaining careful safe correction by means of segmentally applied internal fixation (again, anterior shortening with posterior lengthening).

References

1. Abdu WA, Hoffinger S, Renshaw TS: *The fate of posterior spinal fusions in congenital scoliosis,* Presented at the Scoliosis Research Society 25th annual meeting, Honolulu, Hawaii, September, 1990.
2. Akbarnia B, Moe JH: Familial congenital scoliosis with unilateral unsegmented bar: case report of two siblings, *J Bone Joint Surg* 60A:259, 1978.
3. Bradford DS, Boachi-Adjei O: One stage anterior and posterior hemivertebral resection and arthrodesis for congenital scoliosis, *J Bone Joint Surg* 72:536, 1990.

4. Bradford DS, Heithoff KB, Cohen M: Intraspinal abnormalities in congenital spine deformities: a radiographic and MRI study, *J Pediatr Orthop* 11:36, 1991.

5. Campbell RM, Smith MD, Pinero R: Treatment of severe chest wall malformations associated with scoliosis by vertical, expandable prosthetic ribs: a preliminary report, *Orthop Trans* 15:118, 1991.

6. Drvaric DM, et al.: Congenital scoliosis and urinary tract abnormalities: are intravenous pyelograms necessary? *J Pediatr Orthop* 7:441, 1987.

7. Dubousset J: Congenital kyphosis. In Bradford DS, Hensinger RM, editors: *The pediatric spine,* New York, 1985, Thieme, Inc.

8. Dubousset J, Herring JA, Shufflebarger H: The crank shaft phenomenon, *J Pediatr Orthop* 9:541, 1989.

9. Farley FA, et al.: Natural history of scoliosis in congenital heart disease, *J Pediatr Orthop* 11:42, 1991.

10. Flynn JC, Kendra J, Price CT: *The protocol to modify the inappropriate antidiuretic hormone syndrome in the scoliosis surgery patient,* Presented at the Scoliosis Research Society 26th annual meeting, Minneapolis, September 24–27, 1991.

11. Hall JE: Congenital scoliosis, In Bradford DS, Hensinger RM, editors: *The pediatric spine,* New York, 1985, Thieme, Inc.

12. Heilbronner D, Renshaw TS: Spondylothoracic dysplasia, *J Bone Joint Surg* 66A:302, 1984.

13. Jarcho S, Levin PM: *Hereditary malformations of the vertebral bodies,* Bull Johns Hopkins Hosp 62:216, 1938.

14. MacEwen GD, Winter RB, Hardy JH: Evaluation of kidney anomalies in congenital scoliosis, *J Bone Joint Surg* 54A:1451, 1972.

15. McMaster MJ, Ohtsuka K: The natural history of congenital scoliosis: a study of 251 patients, *J Bone Joint Surg* 64A:1128, 1982.

16. McMaster MJ: Occult intraspinal anomalies in congenital scoliosis, *J Bone Joint Surg* 66A:588, 1984.

17. Owen JH, et al.: The clinical application of neurogenic motor evoked potentials to monitor spinal cord function during surgery, *Spine* 16(Suppl):385, 1991.

18. Pinto WC, Avanzi O, Winter RB: An anterior distractor for the intraoperative correction of angular kyphosis, *Spine* 3:309, 1978.

19. Renshaw TS: Sacral agenesis: a classification and review of 23 cases, *J Bone Joint Surg* 60A:373, 1978.

20. Stagnara P: *Spinal deformity,* Paris, 1988, Butterworth & Co.

21. Terek RM, Wehner J, Lubicky JP: Crank shaft phenomenon in congenital scoliosis: a preliminary report, *J Pediatr Orthop* 11:527, 1991.

22. Winter RB, et al.: The Milwaukee brace in the nonoperative treatment of congenital scoliosis, *Spine* 1:85, 1976.

23. Winter RB: Convex anterior and posterior hemiarthrodesis and hemiepiphyseodesis in young children with progressive congenital scoliosis, *J Pediatr Orthop,* 1:361, 1981.

24. Winter RB, Moe JH: Arthrodesis for congenital spine deformity in children prior to age five years, *J Bone Joint Surg* 64A:419, 1982.

25. Winter RB, *Congenital deformities of the spine,* New York, 1983, Thieme-Stratton, Inc.

26. Winter RB, Moe JH, Lonstein JE: Posterior spinal arthrodesis for congenital scoliosis, *J Bone Joint Surg* 66A:1188, 1984.

27. Winter RB, Moe JH, Lonstein JE: The surgical treatment of congenital kyphosis: a review of 94 patients, age five years or older, with two years or more follow-up in 77 patients, *Spine* 10:224, 1985.

28. Winter RB: *Congenital spine deformity,* In Bradford DS, et al.: *Moe's textbook of scoliosis and other spinal deformities,* ed 2, Philadelphia, 1987, W.B. Saunders Co.

29. Winter RB, et al.: Convex growth arrest for progressive congenital scoliosis due to hemivertebra, *J Pediatr Orthop* 8:633, 1988.

30. Winter RB: Spinal problems in pediatric orthopaedics. In Morrissy RT: *Lovell and Winter's pediatric orthopaedics,* ed 3, Philadelphia, 1990, J.B. Lippincott Co.

31. Wynne-Davies R: Congenital vertebral anomalies: etiology and relationship to spina bifida cystica, *J Med Genet* 12:280, 1975.

Chapter 109
Spinal Deformity in Children, Adolescents, and Young Adults
Robert W. Gaines, Jr.

IDIOPATHIC SCOLIOSIS
Etiology and Natural History

 infantile idiopathic scoliosis
 juvenile idiopathic scoliosis
 adolescent idiopathic scoliosis

Pathogenesis

Terminology

 rotational prominence
 spinal balance (decompensation)
 spinal curvature flexibility
 stable zone
 tilt angle
 cobb angle
 perdriolle method
 primary and compensatory curves

Physical Examination

 curve patterns
 flexibility
 neurologic examination
 cardiopulmonary function
 quantitation of structural changes

Nonoperative Treatment

Surgical Treatment

 indications and choice of procedure
 single-stage instrumentation and fusion
 internal fixation
 staged reconstruction and fusion

**Indications for Instrumentation
 of the Pelvis**

**Indications for Operative Treatment
 of Adults**

Operative Results

**PARALYTIC (NEUROMUSCULAR)
SCOLIOSIS**

Natural History

Comprehensive Care

Physical Examination

Nonoperative Treatment

Surgical Treatment

**Complications and Results of Surgical
Treatment**

**JUVENILE KYPHOSIS
(SCHEUERMANN DISEASE)**

**Histologic, Radiographic, and Physical
Examination**

Nonoperative Treatment

Surgical Treatment

**NEUROFIBROMATOSIS AND
SCOLIOSIS**

Etiology and Natural History

Classification

Radiographic Evaluation

Treatment

IDIOPATHIC SCOLIOSIS

Idiopathic scoliosis is the lateral spinal curvature that occurs because of impaired spinal column development. The spinal column of a patient with idiopathic scoliosis is normal at birth. During early or late childhood or adolescence the lateral curve develops. Many patients with idiopathic scoliosis have a positive family history, but some do not.[9]

Etiology and Natural History

Three distinct types of idiopathic scoliosis are clearly identifiable: infantile, juvenile, and adolescent. These are discussed below.

Infantile Idiopathic Scoliosis

Infantile idiopathic scoliosis exists mostly in Britain or in British descendants. The spinal curvature appears in infancy and is associated with plagiocephaly. Two curve types are seen—a rapidly progressive type that leads to extremely severe curves despite treatment and a resolving type in which the curve tends to resolve by 1 or 2 years of age with or without treatment. The etiology is unknown for both types. Sex incidence is equal.

Juvenile Idiopathic Scoliosis

Children 4 to 8 years of age show their curves following 3 to 6 years of straight spinal growth. These children first show flattening of their normal thoracic kyphosis and subsequently demonstrate spinal rotation, and a lateral curvature develops. Their family history may or may not be positive. Sex incidence is equal. It is not seen in blacks. Without successful treatment, severe deformity and pulmonary compromise usually occur.

Adolescent Idiopathic Scoliosis

This is the most common type of idiopathic scoliosis seen in North America. Normal spinal development occurs up to age 9 or 10. Then curvature develops during the adolescent growth spurt (Fig. 109-1). While minor observable differences in spinal contour exist equally in screened populations of girls and boys, the incidence of development of curves over 30 degrees occurs seven times more frequently for the girls. A positive family history exists in about 50% of patients (Fig. 109-2). The curves seen in untreated patients are generally smaller than in patients with the juvenile type or the progressive-type infan-

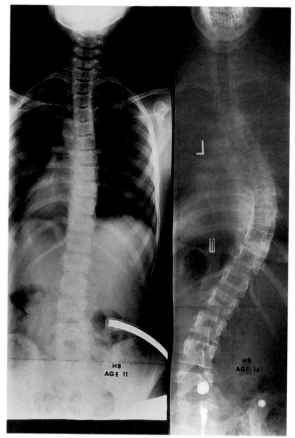

Fig. 109-1

Curve progression over 5 years (age 11 and age 16).

tile curvatures. However, without treatment, many patients' curvatures progress to 90 to 100 degrees and cause pulmonary and spinal column dysfunction as well as disfigurement. Premature death from severe idiopathic scoliosis is not as common as it is from severe paralytic or congenital scoliosis.

While the beginnings and major progression of spinal curves of patients with adolescent idiopathic scoliosis occur during the adolescent growth spurt, many of those that reach 35 to 40 degrees by the end of skeletal growth continue to increase at variable rates throughout adult life.

Pathogenesis

While patients with smaller curves may have normal sagittal curve alignment, most severely progressive curves, particularly in the thoracic spine, are associated with a loss of thoracic kyphosis. The loss of thoracic lordosis precedes or accompanies the development of the lateral curve. If spinal stiffening seems to accompany the loss of kyphosis, in a preadolescent

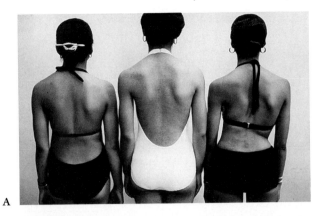

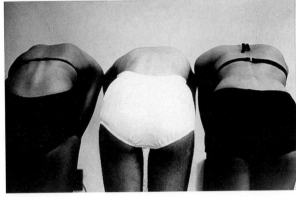

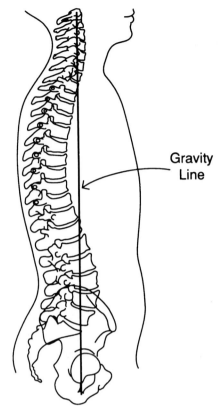

Fig. 109-2

A, Three sisters with scoliosis. **B,** Rib humps on "the bend" test.

Fig. 109-3

Normal sagittal plane alignment.

girl, the likelihood of severe curve development is likely, according to most experts. This fact strongly supports alterations in biochemical and biomechanical dysfunction of the intervertebral disc with secondarily-induced abnormalities of vertebral growth as a mechanism for the development of the curve in scoliosis patients. Studies of disc components by Ponseti did not show distinct differences from controls. However, histologic analysis of surgically excised facet joints from surgical patients suggested that the posterior element changes were secondary alterations and muscle biopsies in idiopathic scoliosis have been normal. The ribs and sternum become progressively more distorted in size and shape.* The predictors of curve severity in patients are poorly understood.

Terminology

Rotational Prominence

The physical evidence of spinal curvature is earliest seen in most patients on the "bend test." Minor unevennesses in thoracic or lumbar paravertebral areas,

*References 4, 10, 13, 14, 16, and 17.

due to spinal rotation, appear as "rib humps" or "lumbar humps."

Spinal Balance (Decompensation)

Coronal Plane

A plumb line dropped from the occiput normally falls between the buttocks and bisects the S1 spinous process. As more-severe curvatures develop, progressive loss of balance (spinal decompensation) may occur. This occurs more regularly and in greater severity in congenital and neuromuscular scoliosis than in idiopathic scoliosis. (It almost never becomes worse than 3 cm in idiopathic scoliosis.)

Sagittal Plane

Normal humans show a normal cervical lordosis, thoracic kyphosis and lumbar lordosis. A plumb line dropped from the tip of the odontoid in a normal population usually drops 1 cm anterior to the S1 vertebral body. Abnormalities in spinal growth and development or in treatment of developed curves can alter this normal balance (Fig. 109-3).

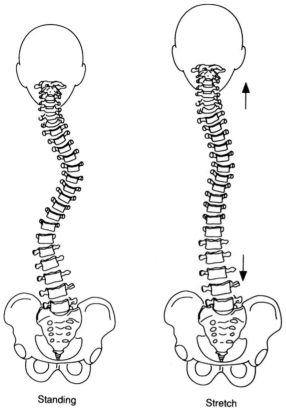

Standing   Stretch

Fig. 109-4

Anteroposterior standing and stretch x-ray films demonstrate curve severity and flexibility.

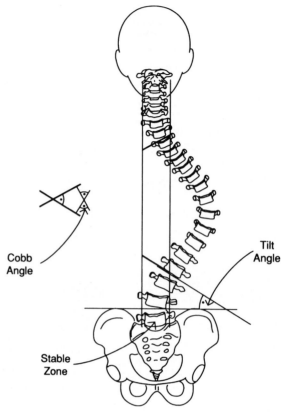

Fig. 109-5

Technique of measurement of the Cobb angle, the tilt angle and the "stable zone" for scoliosis patients.

Spinal Curvature Flexibility

Spinal curvature flexibility describes the ability of a spinal curvature to be straightened. This can be assessed by either lateral bending or traction, clinically or on x-ray films. Along with curve etiology and curve severity, curve flexibility is a fundamentally important determinant of curve prognosis and response to treatment. Its relevance to these issues cannot be overemphasized (Fig. 109-4).

Stable Zone

The stable zone is the region of the spinal column that exists between two parallel lines erected through the S1 articular processes perpendicular to a line across the top of the pelvis (Fig. 109-5).

Tilt Angle

The tilt angle is the angle between the most tilted lumbar vertebral body and the line across the top of the pelvis (Fig. 109-5).

Cobb Angle

The Cobb angle is the internationally accepted method for measuring coronal plane magnitude of spinal curvatures (Fig. 109-5).

Perdriolle Method

The Perdriolle method is the accepted standard for measuring the rotational deformity of vertebrae involved in a scoliotic curvature.

Primary and Compensatory Curves

The pneumonic WARP describes curve characteristics that differentiate primary from compensatory curves. Primary curves show greater Wedging, Angulation (higher Cobb angles), and more Rotation (by Perdriolle method) and more often lead to a loss of Position (lead to spinal decompensation). Compensatory curves show less structural change in patients with smaller primary curves and more structural change in patients with primary curves over 60 to 70 degrees.

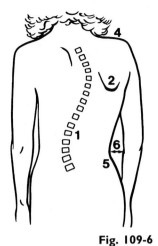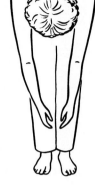

Note:

1. Shape of spine
2. Prominent shoulder blade
3. Rib hump
4. Shoulder level
5. Hip level
6. Distance between body and arms

Fig. 109-6

Scoliosis—physical findings on clinical examination.

Curve flexibility on traction x-rays also provides a useful indicator of curve correctability (see Fig. 110-4). Even intraoperative use of the image intensifier to judge the response of a compensatory curve to correction of the primary curve is quite useful. Bending films generally show slightly greater curve correction than stretch films. However, since the goal of curve correction is maximum curve correction, while restoring spinal balance, curve flexibility achieved on stretch films provides a more clinically useful measure of curve flexibility.

Physical Examination

The earliest manifestation of a developing scoliosis is a rotational prominence with or without an accompanying loss of thoracic kyphosis (Fig. 109-6). A large rotational prominence in the thoracic region is called a "rib hump." Uneven flanks are called "lumbar humps." A particularly large and angular rib hump is called a "razorback."

Curve Patterns

Manifestations of scoliosis depend on the spinal region where the curve or curves develop. Adolescent idiopathic scoliosis can be divided into five curve patterns, as described below.

Thoracic

The spinal curvature is entirely contained in the thoracic spine (usually between T4 or T5 and T11-T12), and 80% of the time it is convex to the right. Right ribs are prominent posteriorly and recede an-

teriorly. Left ribs decline posteriorly and are prominent anteriorly (Fig. 109-7).

Double Thoracic Major

There are two curves in the thoracic spine—the upper one, T1-T4, generally is convex to the left; the lower one, T5-T11-T12, is convex to the right. Rib deformities are similar to the single thoracic curve, but the high thoracic curve gives rise to a high left shoulder and an uneven neckline.

Thoracolumbar

The primary curve occurs across the thoracolumbar junction. Decompensation occurs even in curves of 20 to 30 degrees, and it develops toward the convex side of the curve. Rib distortion may occur but is mild. Waistline unevenness and apparent difference in iliac crest height are the most prominent findings (Fig. 109-8).

Lumbar

Curve entirely confined to the lumbar spine. No rib deformity. Waistline asymmetry, "apparent" leg length discrepancy, and spinal decompensation (90% to the left) are characteristic features (Fig. 109-9).

Double Primary Curve

Two curves of approximately equal severity and flexibility exist—one in the thoracic spine (usually convex to the right) and one in the lumbar or thoracolumbar spine (usually convex to the left). Findings

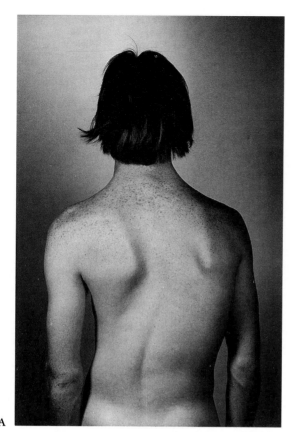
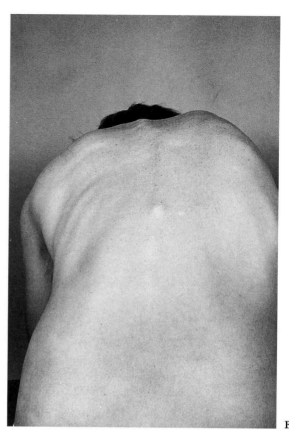

A

B

Fig. 109-7

A, Thoracic scoliosis. **B,** Same patient during "bend" test.

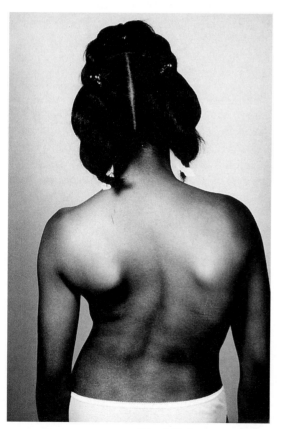
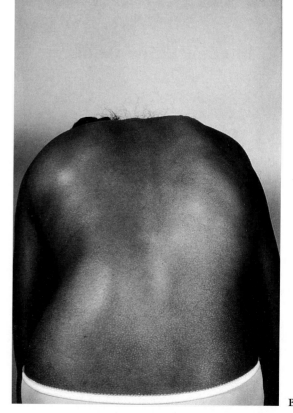

A

B

Fig. 109-8

A, Thoracolumbar scoliosis. **B,** Same patient during "bend" test.

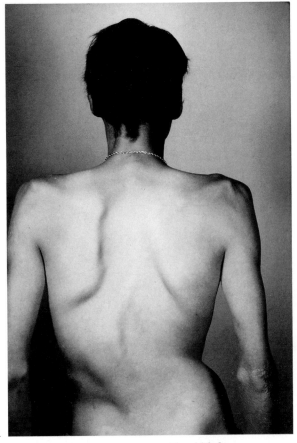

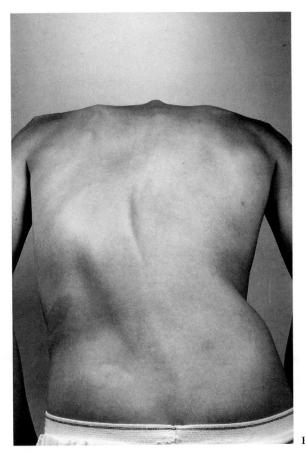

Fig. 109-9

A, Lumbar scoliosis. **B,** Same patient during "bend" test.

typical of primary thoracic or lumbar curves occur but with little spinal decompensation (Figs. 109-10 and 109-11).

Flexibility

Clinical assessment is easiest to make on prone examination by lateral bending and spinal distraction. Quantitation of correction by x-ray study is useful.

Neurologic Examination

Routine clinical neurologic examination of patients with idiopathic scoliosis is usually normal. Recent documentation of a 20% incidence of clinically silent syringomyelia on MRI in patients with juvenile idiopathic scoliosis makes the routine use of abdominal reflexes an essential part of routine neurologic examination of patients with idiopathic scoliosis. Patients with idiopathic scoliosis who have unusual curve patterns or stiff curves should undergo preoperative myelography or MRI.[3] All patients with

congenital disease who require an operation need preoperative MRI.

Cardiopulmonary Function

Most patients with idiopathic scoliosis who have curves under 40 degrees have normal pulmonary functions. Patients with curvature greater than 45 degrees should have formal quantitation of their pulmonary function with measurements of arterial blood gas levels and an electrocardiogram as baseline studies.

Quantitation of Structural Changes

Uniqueness of rib cage structure can be measured and recorded by a straight-edge ruler, by scoliometer, by Moire photography, or by various computer-based light reflection techniques (ISIS).

Quantitation of vertebral rotation can be made only by radiographic techniques—that is, either by the Perdriolle method or by axial CT (AARO). Ax-

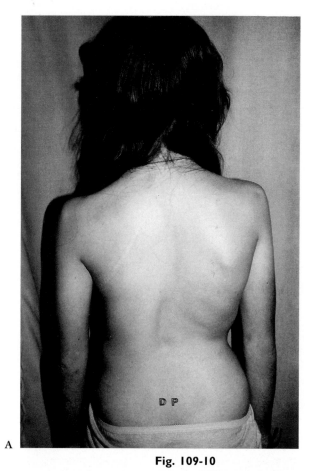
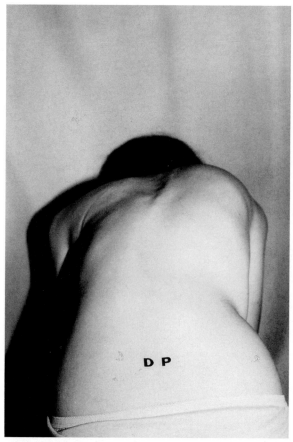

Fig. 109-10

A, Mild double primary curve. **B,** Same patient during "bend" test.

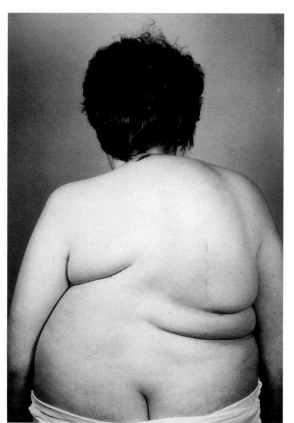
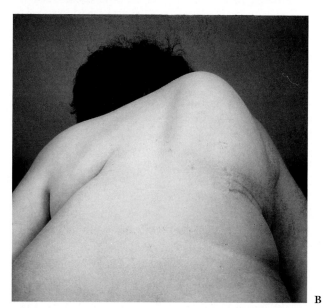

Fig. 109-11

A, Very severe double primary curve in adult. **B,** Same patient during "bend" test.

ial CT scanning can be also used to measure the thoracic deformity.

Standard x-ray assessment of spinal curvatures includes standing anteroposterior and lateral 36-in. film of the entire spine T1-S1. These permit measurement of both primary and secondary curves and of the presence or absence and amount of spinal decompensation.

Flexibility x-ray studies by stretching or bending are essential before determining treatment of any curvature.

Nonoperative Treatment

Use of bracing to control the development of progressive curves in growing children is an established treatment technique for idiopathic scoliosis. However, effective bracing has limited application. Only children who have supportive families, growth remaining, and curves less than 35 degrees are candidates. Thus, most candidates are discovered in societies with effective early-detection programs[19] (like the school screening programs prevalent in the United States).

Bracing a scoliotic curve stabilizes it and prevents the worsening of the curve that normally occurs during a growth spurt. A few younger children may gain some permanent spinal straightening. A few children have curves that progress despite bracing. Most of them have more severe and stiffer curves with reduced thoracic kyphosis, or curves which don't correct when the brace is applied. (Fig. 109-12). Bracing is used from the age when the curve is identified until the end of skeletal growth. For this reason, the length of treatment is measured in years—not weeks or months.

Surgical Treatment

Indications and Choice of Procedure

Surgical stabilization of a spinal curvature improves the patient's spinal balance to improve spinal efficiency, prevents further deterioration of the curva-

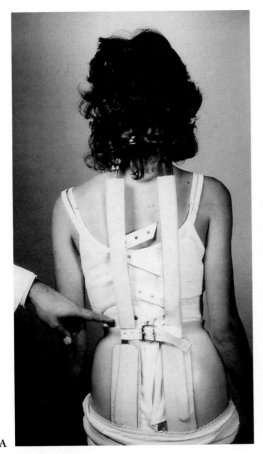

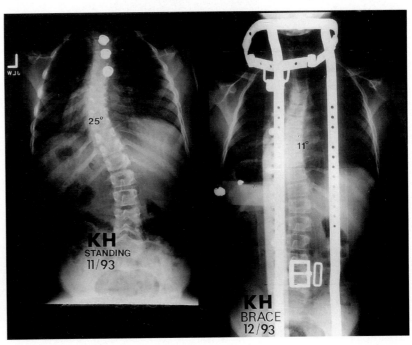

Fig. 109-12

A, Milwaukee brace for nonoperative treatment of scoliosis. **B,** Curve correction in brace is necessary for successful treatment.

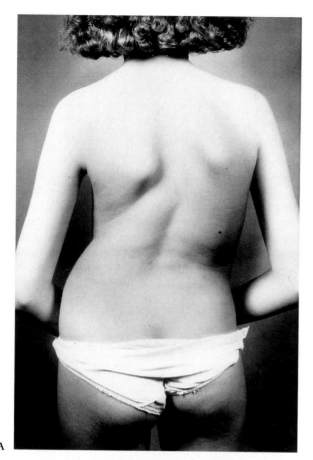

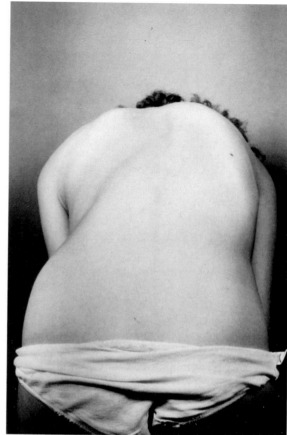

A

B

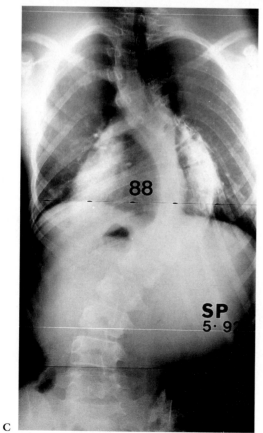

C

Fig. 109-13

A, Preoperative photograph of 13-year-old girl with right thoracolumbar curve with significant and mildly structural high thoracic compensatory curve. **B,** Forward-bending photographs of same patient. **C,** Standing films demonstrate severe curve.

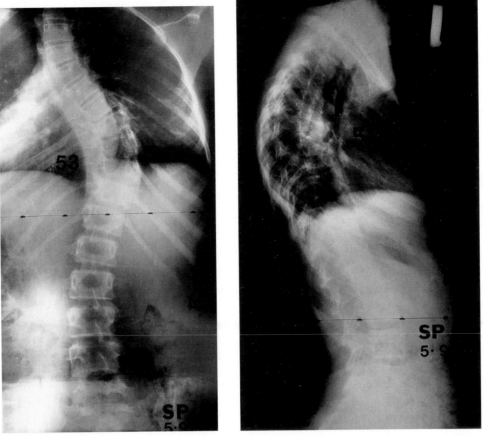

Fig. 109-13, cont'd

D, Stretch films shows flexibility of both curves in distraction. E, Sagittal plane balance is demonstrated.

ture to prevent further spinal imbalance and cardiopulmonary and lumbar spinal deterioration, and improves the patient's appearance to prevent the development of a potentially psychologically crippling deformity (Fig. 109-13). Surgery is needed when the curvature of a patient with idiopathic scoliosis progresses beyond 45 degrees by the Cobb angle, when the tilt angle increases beyond 20 degrees, or when spinal decompensation extends beyond 3 cm. Preliminary stretch and/or bending films are used to assess the correctability of the curves.

Surgical goals are to reduce the curvature to the maximum degree that spinal cord safety permits, restore anteroposterior and sagittal plane spinal balance, restore the tilt angle to less than 10 degrees, leave the fusion mass in the "stable zone" of Harrington, and fuse as few segments as possible while obtaining goals 1 to 4 (see Fig. 109-5). The preoperative curve severity and flexibility are the guides to selection of the surgical procedure of choice. If the curve is relatively small (40 to 70 degrees) and flexible (≥ 50% correction on the stretch film), a sin-

gle-stage spine instrumentation and fusion is carried out. The treatment of larger or stiffer curves may require staged reconstruction using preliminary discectomy and/or apical vertebrectomy and second staged posterior instrumentation and fusion.

Single-Stage Instrumentation and Fusion

Preoperative preparation

The operating nurse must be familiar with spinal surgery and Isola spinal implants. The anesthesiologist should be capable of providing hypotensive anesthesia. The operating table must accommodate the prone patient and have the capability for biplane imaging. An operating image intensifier and a qualified operator must be available.

Exposure and Fusion-Bed Preparation

After sterile preparation and draping and induction of hypotensive anesthesia, routine subperiosteal exposure of the primary curve is achieved. Preoperative review of standing and stretch x-ray films generally makes a preoperative plan possible. However, if the flexibility of compensatory curves makes a firm decision regarding whether to instrument and fuse compensatory curves uncertain, a final decision can be deferred until exposure and instrumentation of the primary curve has been accomplished. At that time, assessment of spinal compensation, curve correction, the tilt angle, and the stable zone can be performed. If the goals of surgery are achieved, the compensatory curve can be left unexposed and uninstrumented. If the spine is unbalanced, then the compensatory curve needs exposure, instrumentation, and fusion.

Before placing implants, the spinous processes in the fusion area are carefully cleaned and then excised at their bases. The transverse processes on the concave side are similarly cleaned and decorticated. Both the spinous processes and superficial cortex of the concave transverse processes are saved as bone graft.

The capsules of the concave facet joints are then excised. The caudal edge of each inferior facet in the primary curve is squared off to accept an open Isola hook. A monolevel or bilevel claw is placed at the top level of the instrumented segment. Pedicle screws are placed at the lower levels, if the pedicles are large enough.

Intraoperative curve flexibility is then assessed by the operator and the surgical assistant. The assistant pushes on the convex ribs to gain lateral and rotational correction while the operator maintains counterpressure on the left lumbar spine and the high left thoracic area to maintain spinal balance. The image intensifier can be used to assess both the primary and secondary curves before firm decision about fusion levels is made.

Internal Fixation

For straightforward primary thoracic or thoracolumbar primary curves, the end vertebra of the fusion mass is the level that restores spinal balance and realigns the tilt angle and puts the fusion mass in the stable zone. It is generally between T12 and L3. Pedicle screws are used at as many levels as possible. The diameter of the pedicles obviously determines which levels can accommodate screws. Screws provide much more positive three-dimensional vertebral maneuverability than hooks can provide. The appropriate pedicles are probed and proper placement is confirmed by C arm. Appropriate diameter and length screws are then applied and appropriate

position again confirmed by C arm (Fig. 109-14). The concave apex of the curve is then identified. An 8-mm open or closed hook is then placed securely into the facet joint. A hook holder is applied and the spinal column is lifted upward toward the ceiling of the operating room, attempting to derotate the major curvature and to correct loss of thoracic kyphosis. The amount of derotation and restoration of thoracic kyphosis is clinically assessed, and plans are made for achieving as much correction as these components of the primary curve as the inherent flexibility of the primary curve will permit. While the derotation and sagittal and coronal plane corrections are manually held, estimates regarding rod contouring and hook size and position are made. The variable hook throat height of the Isola hooks permits accommodation of varying amounts of residual thoracic lordosis on the rod. Appropriate bending of the rod accomodates the patient's final corrected saggital plane contour.

Two rods are used. Generally a one-fourth-inch rod on the concave side and a three-sixteenths-inch rod on the convex side are used. In patients lighter than 75 lb 2 three-sixteenths-inch rods are used. In patients over 200 lb, 2 one-fourth-inch rods are necessary. When the appropriate-diameter rods have been selected, they are cut to span the fusion area and bent to accommodate the residual deformity.

If major residual lateral plane deformity remains at the apex of the curve, the use of sublaminar wires at the apex rather than hooks makes instrumentation simpler. Surgeons unfamiliar with sublaminar wiring faced with such a situation may choose not to instrument these apical levels and may bypass them. Open hooks are then applied at each level on the major curve and the claw applied at the top level. Throat heights are chosen to accommodate the rod.

Slotted connectors are chosen and positioned on the rod to permit easy rod application. The concave rod is then dropped into the open hooks and the slotted connectors drop onto the bone screws at the lower end of the curve. Nesting nuts are added onto the slotted connectors to obtain preliminary purchase. The rod is positioned in the slot in all the open hooks before any caps are applied. Starting on the easiest and the most available hook, the caps are sequentially applied and advanced with the cap approximator.

Once all the caps are fully locked on the rod, and the slotted connectors have been firmly secured on the screws by the nesting nuts, curve correction is performed. Segmental correction of the concave

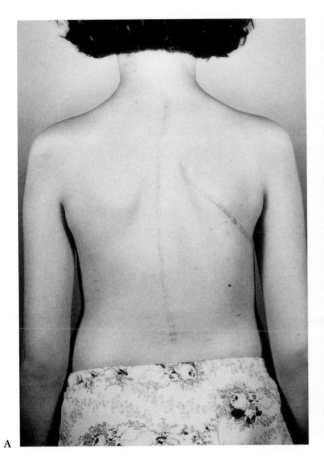

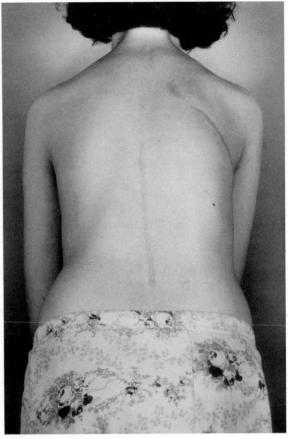

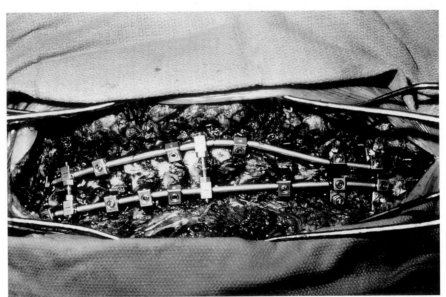

Fig. 109-14

A, Thoracolumbar scoliosis, anteroposterior view. **B,** Same patient during stretch x-ray study. **C,** Anteroposterior view after curve correction.

Continues.

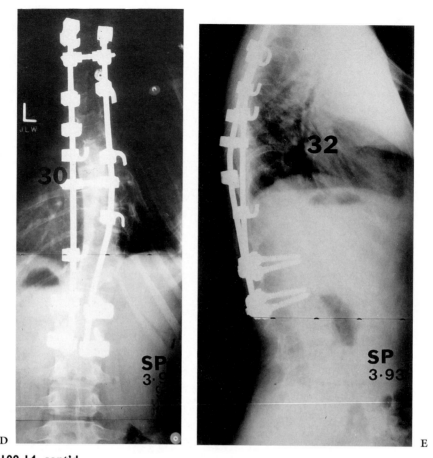

D   E

Fig. 109-14, cont'd

D, Sagittal view after curve correction. **E,** Instrumentation in place. Excellent curve correction as well as balance in coronal and saggital plane and tilt angle correction achieved.

side is performed moving levels above the apex cephalad along the rod and moving levels caudal to the apex away from the apex. Junctional levels (the end of primary and beginning of compensatory curves) are adjusted to correct the tilt angle and restore spinal balance.

Once curve correction is optimal, the set screws on the hooks and slotted correctors are finally turned onto the rod forcing the rod into the V groove inside the anchors. After satisfactory position is accomplished, transverse process hooks of proper throat height are applied to the convex side. The three-sixteenths-inch rod is dropped into the hooks and the slotted correctors are applied in a similar way to the concave side. Correction is achieved and the set screws are set (Fig. 109-15).

The iliac crest is exposed. An iliac graft is obtained and the bone mixed with local bone. The laminae involved in the fusion area are decorticated and the graft applied to areas around the implants. The intertransverse area receives a disproportionate amount of graft

on the concave side, particularly if there is more than 20 degrees of remaining residual curvature.

Routine closure is accomplished over a drain after copious antibiotic irrigation is performed. The patient is carefully nursed and ambulated in a TLSO (thoracolumbar spinal orthosis) when postoperative soreness permits. Standing postoperative films are made prior to discharge from the hospital.

Postoperative bracing and activity restrictions are guided by the patient's age, residual curve, and radiographic confirmation of fusion maturation. Some limitations are maintained in all patients for at least 4 months, and bracing is maintained in all patients for 2 to 4 months.

Staged Reconstruction and Fusion

Curves over 70 degrees in Cobb measurement with less than 50% flexibility or curves in young children with more than 3 to 4 years of additional growth (in whom crank-shafting is a likelihood) are candidates for staged reconstruction. The first-stage procedure

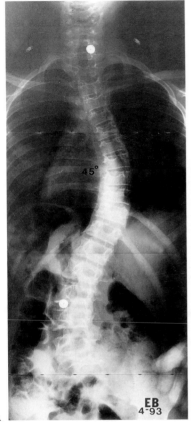

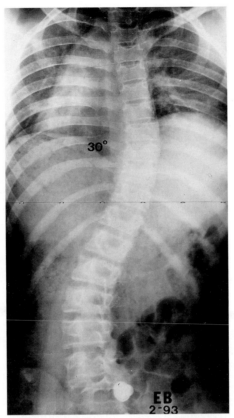

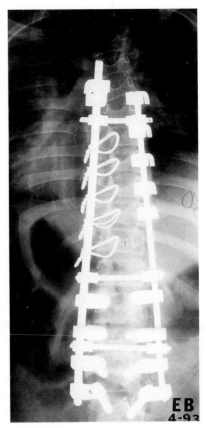

A

B

C

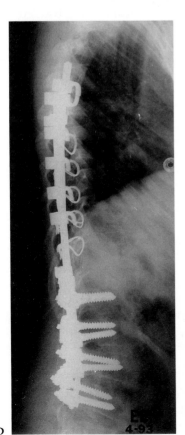

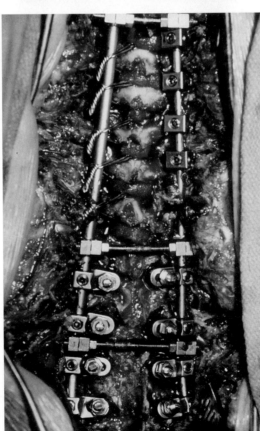

D

E

Fig. 109-15

A, Postsurgical correction following two-stage instrumentation and fusion. Preliminary stage was six apical discectomies. Second stage was Isola posterior instrumentation. **B,** Forward-bending photographs of same patient. **C,** Isola instrumentation in place. **D,** Instrumentation demonstrates excellent spinal balance in instrumentation of both major lower thoracic curve and upper structural compensatory curve. Distraction forces and compression forces were used on both rods, on opposite sides of curve, to balance spine. **E,** Sagittal-plane balance 10 months postoperatively is excellent.

removes the intervertebral discs at the most rigid segments of the major curve (the apical segments) to improve the correction that can be achieved from a posterior approach alone. The posterior instrumentation and fusion is performed exactly the same as the first-stage procedure. Somatosensory evoked potential monitoring is mandatory, however. The second-stage posterior instrumentation can be performed either during the same anesthetic as the first stage or may be delayed a week or two.

Following a staged reconstruction, a period of 3 to 4 weeks of bed rest in a TLSO is usually routine to permit preliminary healing before ambulation. TLSO is used for 3 to 4 months, until radiographic confirmation is confirmed.

Indications for Instrumentation of the Pelvis

Spinal-pelvic fixation is used to correct severe spinal decompensation (to restore severely disordered spinal balance) in the coronal plane. Since idiopathic scoliosis, by virtue of the development of compensatory curves, virtually never causes the spine to decompensate more than 3 cm, spinal-pelvic instrumentation is only rarely necessary in patients with idiopathic scoliosis. Neuromuscular scoliosis, on the other hand, commonly causes severe spinal decompensation. Such patients represent the majority of patients requiring rebalancing by instrumentation into the pelvis.

Indications for Operative Treatment of Adults

The fundamentals of surgical treatment of scoliosis of adults are generally the same as for adolescents. Judgments about staged surgery are more difficult, since the curves are generally a bit more severe and less flexible and the morbidity of staged reconstruction is a bit higher in adults. In the fifth, sixth, and seventh decades, scoliosis and spinal stenosis commonly coexist. Patients generally have known about their scoliosis for years and are brought for treatment because of inability to perform their activities of daily living due to leg pain and weakness. For these patients, decompression at the same time as posterior instrumentation and fusion relieves their symptoms and restores spinal balance.

Staged procedures are rarely necessary in older adults with stenosis. The severe disc degeneration that generally permits the progressive increase in lateral curvature generally does not stiffen lumbar or thoracolumbar curves enough to prevent reestablishing spinal balance in a single stage.

Older adults presenting with stenosis generally have neglected thoracolumbar curves with fairly severe spinal decompensation and gross apical disc degeneration. For such patients, surgical treatment should be based on restoring spinal compensation, decompressing the canal to relieve cauda equina pressure, and gaining spinal stabilization and fusion to maintain spinal compensation. Emphasis on curve correction in both the coronal and sagittal plane is counterproductive in most older adults with scoliosis and spinal stenosis. Such efforts, particularly successful efforts, are very destructive to load-sharing between the spinal column and the spinal implant used for spinal rebalancing. Since the discs in these patients have generally lost almost all their tissue, excellent curve correction, and, particularly, excellent correction of the sagittal plane, causes a total loss of anterior column vertebral apposition without the normal disc tissue of the adolescent to maintain anterior column load transfer. Thus, excellent curve and sagittal plant correction for adults with stenosis should be attempted only if a second-stage anterior discectomy and interbody grafting with autograft-filled carbon cages is accomplished.

Postoperative treatment is similar to that provided for adolescents. Most older adults with stenosis who need spinal-pelvic fixation require spinal screws into the S1 level. They wear a TLSO with an added leg extension for 2 months after the surgery to protect the lumbosacral instrumentation and fusion.

Operative Results

Several reports exist regarding the results of more than 20 years of surgical reconstruction done for idiopathic scoliosis. Each documents long-lasting well-maintained spinal alignment and maintenance of activities of daily living at almost normal levels. Fertility of female patients is unaffected and employment options are good.[11,22,23,25] Late deterioration of spines that were inadequately rebalanced is common. The reoperations necessary to reinstrument and regraft patients with pseudarthrosis documents the importance of care of both the initial choice of instrumentation and fusion level and performance of the fusion.

Complications in adolescent idiopathic scoliosis are quite rare. Infection occurs in less than 1% of patients with conventional prophylactic antibiotics and antibiotic wound irrigation. Implant displacement is rare so long as careful application is performed and postoperative patient compliance is good. Paraplegia, if it ever occurs in idiopathic scoliosis, is due either to overzealous attempts at corrections; attempting surgical correction on a patient with an unrecognized intra spinal syrinx, tether, diastematomyelia or cord tumor; or an iatrogenic technical problem. Spinal cord monitoring can help monitor cord function and is quite sensitive. It does not replace good preoperative work-up, care in surgical correction, or good surgical technique, however.

Pseudarthrosis occurs in about one fourth of 1% of patients surgically treated for adolescent idiopathic scoliosis. The rate in adults is a little higher. This is explained by their generally more difficult curves and less vigorous healing response.

Operative correction of the preoperative curve is based on the flexibility of the curve, the type of surgical implant system used (segmental or non-segmental), and the way the system is used. Each human spine curvature has an inherent elastic limit, which can best be defined only in the operating room once the spinal muscles, capsules, and ligaments are removed. Thus, the residual fixed deformity in the intervertebral disc and facets and costovertebral joints limits correction in both the coronal and sagittal planes unless they have been excised. Implants merely "take the slack out" of the curvature and bring the spinal column to its elastic limit. Implant systems that use segmental fixation (e.g., Luque SSI, CD, TSRH or Isola) generally do a better job of obtaining correction of the multiplanar scoliotic deformity than implant systems that use only end purchase (Harrington distraction rods) or cast correction. A certain amount of successful correction of the coronal and sagittal deformity is due to operator application of the implants. Even most modern implants can be ineffective in achieving three-dimensional curve correction if three-dimensional correction is not attempted.

As a general rule, 50% to 70% of Cobb angle correction and 30% to 50% of rib deformity can be expected. Great variation exists, however, as explained above.

PARALYTIC (NEUROMUSCULAR) SCOLIOSIS

Paralytic scoliosis is caused by diseases that cause muscle imbalance in the spinal column. The Scoliosis Research Society has classified paralytic disorders as follows:

A. Neuropathic
  1. Upper motor neuron
      a. Cerebral palsy
      b. Spinocerebellar degeneration
          1) Friedreich's ataxia
          2) Charcot-Marie-Tooth
          3) Roussy-Levy
      c. Syringomyelia
      d. Spinal cord tumor
      e. Spinal cord trauma
  2. Lower-motor neuron
      a. Poliomyelitis
      b. Other viral myelitides
      c. Traumatic
      d. Spinal muscular atrophy
          1) Werding-Hoffman
          2) Kugelberg-Welander
      e. Dysautonomia (Riley-Day)
B. Myopathic
  1. Arthrogryposis
  2. Muscular dystrophy
      a. Duchenne (pseudohypertrophic)
      b. Limb-girdle
      c. Facioscapulohumeral
  3. Fiber-type disproportion
  4. Congenital hypotonia
  5. Myotonia dystrophica

Natural History

The natural history of scoliosis in patients with paralytic scoliosis depends directly on the natural history of the underlying disease. Patients with progressive conditions show greater progression of their curves as the weakness increases. Static disease processes that produce paralytic scoliosis (i.e., cerebral palsy, spinal cord tumor, spinal cord trauma, or poliomyelitis) produce scoliosis that may be mild, if the primary disease is mild, or may be quite severe, if the primary disease is severe[5] (Figs. 109-16 and 109-17).

The natural history of curve development in paralytic scoliosis is different than in idiopathic scoliosis. Paralytic curves generally involve six or more segments. The curvatures are generally 8-10 segments when they develop and are very, very flexible. They generally show rapid progression during times of clinical neurologic or muscular deterioration or rapid growth (Fig. 109-18). Compensatory curves do not develop as commonly as they do in idiopathic scoliosis. For this reason, spinal decompensation develops quite commonly and quite early in many patients with paralytic scoliosis. In idiopathic scoliosis,

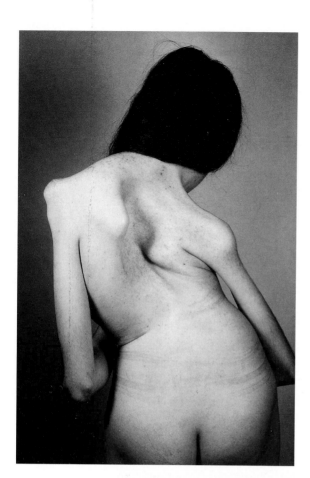

Fig. 109-16

Striking paralytic scoliosis due to poliomyelitis

Fig. 109-17

A, Severe thoracic scoliosis due to traumatic paraplegia secondary to spinal cord infarct at age 2. **B,** Radiographic documentation (anteroposterior view) in same patient.

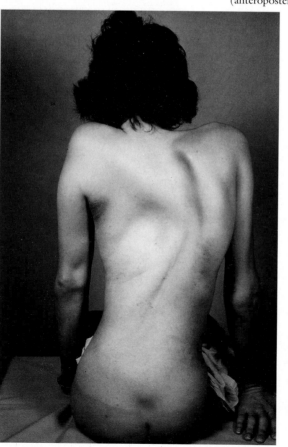

A

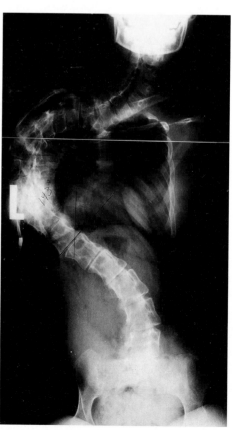

B

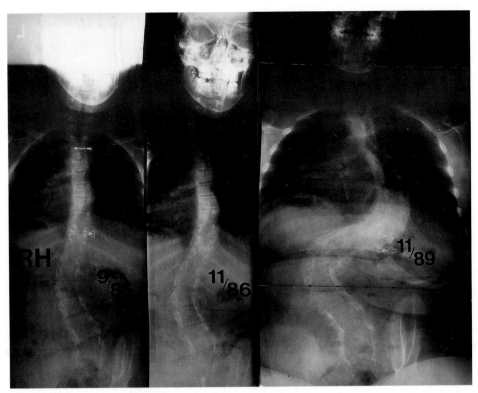

Fig. 109-18

Rapid progression of paralytic scoliosis over 3 years.

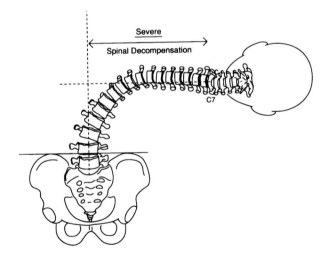

Fig. 109-19

Illustration and measurement of spinal decompensation.

the development of severe spinal decompensation is almost never seen (Figs. 109-19, 109-20, and 109-21).

Paralytic disorders commonly lead to sagittal plane imbalance (Fig. 109-22). In addition, curvatures of paralytic patients commonly progress after skeletal maturity if the primary disease progresses.

Lower-extremity contractures and pelvic obliquity are commonly seen in most paralytic disorders but are not seen in patients with idiopathic scoliosis. The development of these lower-extremity contractures may or may not contribute to the spinal deformity. Long curves that extend into the pelvis are commonly seen in neuromuscular patients.

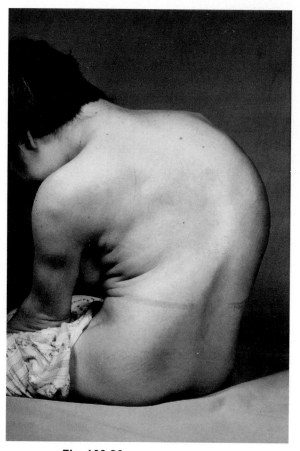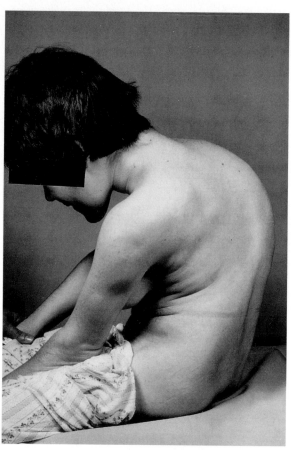

A   B

Fig. 109-20

A, Severe spinal decompensation associated with cerebral palsy. **B,** Same patient showing sagittal plane decompensation.

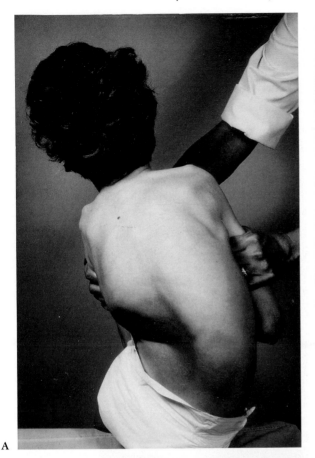

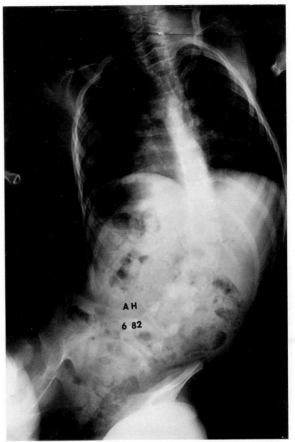

Fig. 109-21

A, Lack of development of a compensatory curve leads to severe spinal decompensation in this patient with cerebral palsy. **B,** Radiographic documentation of spinal decompensation. **C,** More-striking decompensation.

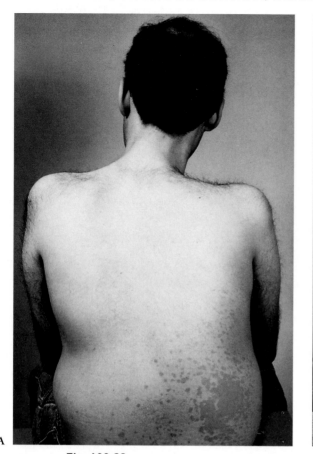
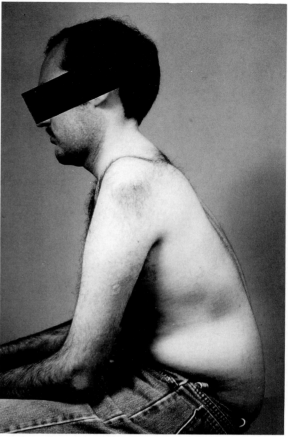

Fig. 109-22

A, Posteroanterior view of a patient with Kugelberg-Welander disease with severe sagittal plane imbalance due to lumbar kyphosis. **B,** Same patient on lateral view.

Comprehensive Care

Comprehensive care of paralytic patients is essential to make sure the treatment of the spinal deformity is carried on in a coordinated manner that improves the patient's functional outcome. Scoliosis care must include input from pediatricians, neurologists, and rehabilitationists who understand the patient's primary diagnosis and prognosis. Seizures; hydrocephalus; deteriorating cardiac, pulmonary, and/or genitourinary function; and emotional, psychiatric, and occupational dysfunctions all complicate the treatment of spinal disorders in paralytic patients. All must be carefully handled to optimize the patient's independence. Ancillary consultants may document deficiencies in other organ systems as necessary to document a patient's organ system performance completely.

Physical Examination

Spinal curvature is examined in the sitting position in wheelchair-bound patients or the standing position for ambulatory patients. Particular attention must be paid to documenting the extent of spinal decompensation since spinal imbalance is the most serious functional handicap for patients with paralytic scoliosis. Sagittal plane assessment is essential as well. Flexibility assessment by gentle distraction or lateral bending is essential to document the flexibility of the curvature. Radiographic confirmation of the information achieved by physical examination helps determine fusion levels (Fig. 109-23, *A* and *B*).

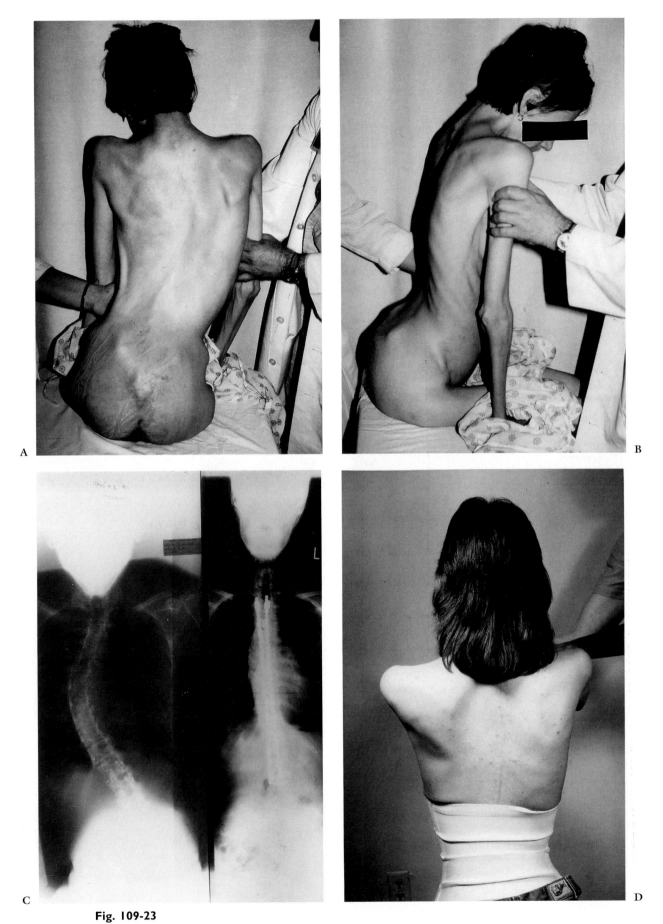

Fig. 109-23

A, Paralytic scoliosis due to traumatic quadriplegia—physical examination. **B,** Same patient—sagittal plane view. **C,** Radiographic outcome of surgical treatment. **D,** Clinical outcome.

Nonoperative Treatment

While spinal bracing represents an important nonoperative treatment technique for patients with idiopathic scoliosis, it is much less effective in paralytic patients. Bracing represents a reasonable treatment selection only in patients with static paralytic disorders (like very mild cerebral palsy or for patients with resected spinal tumors in childhood). Bracing to prevent curve development in patients with progressively deteriorating neurologic or myopathic disorders is unrealistic and has proven to be ineffective. The use of specially developed wheelchair backs can be partially effective in maintaining spinal compensation in wheelchair-bound patients. However, they will not prevent progression or provide permanent spinal realignment for patients whose curves reach greater than 30 to 40 degrees.

Surgical Treatment

For this reason, patients whose long-term severe medical condition and lifestyle warrant surgical consideration should undergo surgery as soon as curves reach 30 to 40 degrees and are shown to be progressive or to cause spinal decompensation. Even at 6 to 8 years of age, spinal fusion can be used to control the development of severe spinal decompensation and restore sitting balance rather than waiting for completion of skeletal growth and the development of a severe and more rigid curvature. Waiting for spinal growth to develop is unrealistic and inappropriate in patients with progressive paralytic scoliosis.

The fundamentals of treatment are to produce a level pelvis that is parallel to the wheelchair seat or to the floor, to restore the sagittal plane contour to as close to normal as possible, and to produce a spinal fusion that is contained within the stable zone with a tilt angle very close to zero. Spinal curvatures must be corrected virtually to straight if reconstruction is to be successful in restoring spinal compensation for patients with paralytic scoliosis. Sagittal plane restoration also must be close to normal (Fig. 109-23, *C* and *D*). For many patients with paralytic scoliosis, this type of surgical reconstruction means very long spinal fusions. For some of them, the entire

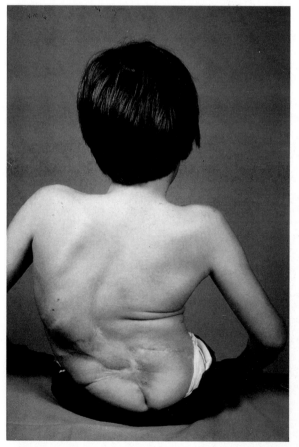
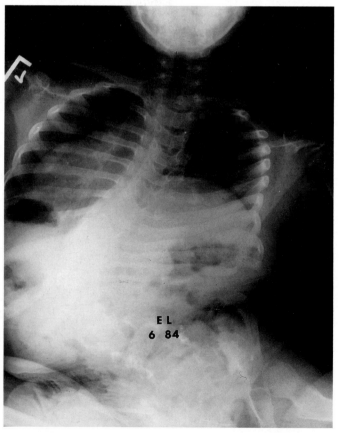

A   B

Fig. 109-24

A, Paralytic scoliosis associated with meningomyelocele. **B,** Same patient—radiographic finding.

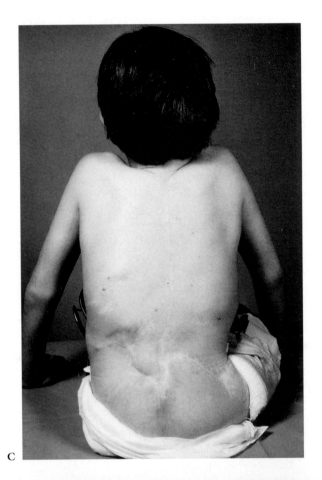

C

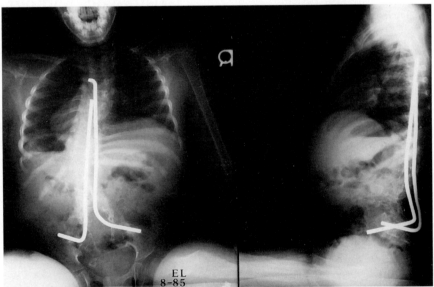

D

Fig. 109-24, cont'd
C, Postoperative clinical outcome. D, Long-segment fusion with rods and sublaminar Mersilene tapes.

spine from T1 to the pelvis must be instrumented and fused. The earlier this is done, the more straightforward the surgery is for the surgeon and for the patient and the fewer complications result. For this reason, an aggressive approach is clinically the most realistic one (Fig. 109-24).

While staged surgical reconstruction has been used for many patients with larger curves, early diagnosis and operative intervention when curvatures are flexible enough to permit single-stage posterior instrumentation and fusion without preoperative release makes surgery much easier on the patient. Segmental spinal instrumentation, particularly using bone screws, permits restoration of alignment and solid spinal fusion with minimal complications.[2,21,27]

Patients with lower-extremity contractures need release of those contractures whether at the foot, knee, or hip, either concomitantly with the surgical instrumentation or before or after, depending on the severity of the hip and spine deformities.

Complications and Results of Surgical Treatment

The complications associated with surgery for paralytic scoliosis depend on the progression of the primary disease, the severity and flexibility of the curvature and the general health of the patient. Patients with severe respiratory limitations need preoperative tracheostomy and ventilatory support. Patients who need extensive surgery and are poorly nourished preoperatively must be supplemented by either gastric (gastrostomy tube) or intravenous hyperalimentation. For this reason, many patients with progressive paralytic disorders are much better treated as soon as the curve becomes a clinical problem (30 to 40 degrees) rather than waiting until clinical deterioration occurs.

The development of bone-screw–based spinal instrumentation systems has revolutionized the surgical treatment of these unfortunate patients. Surgical reconstruction is now a very standard procedure in experienced hands.

When the spine can be corrected into normal alignment (in both the coronal and sagittal plane) and grafted with autograft, the results of surgery are almost always satisfying to the doctor, the parents, and the patient. When poorly nourished, debilitated patients undergo surgery without full correction of their decompensation, the results are not as gratifying to any of the participants.

JUVENILE KYPHOSIS (SCHEUERMANN DISEASE)

Juvenile kyphosis, or "Scheuermann disease," is a developmental deformity that causes painful kyphosis of the spine. It generally appears in 10- to 13-year-old children prior to the adolescent growth spurt and may progress during the completion of skeletal growth. As opposed to idiopathic scoliosis, it is quite frequently a painful problem. Patients are frequently referred for persistent back pain that is greater than nuisance grade and requires medication on a regular basis. Any patient with these symptoms should be promptly referred for assessment by a spinal surgeon. Fifty to sixty percent of the patients are overweight, some considerably so. Sex ratio is equal and 15% to 20% of the patients have a positive family history.[18]

Other than the overweight condition demonstrated by many patients, there are no commonly associated conditions. The disease does not give rise to spinal cord compression unless it is extraordinarily severe. For many with mild to moderate deformity, little functional deficit develops. For these reasons some surgeons consider the disease a benign problem. For most patients, however, the functional disability is considerable and the pain is a consistent, persistent clinical problem that warrants treatment.[8,20]

Histologic, Radiographic, and Physical Examination

Juvenile kyphosis develops secondary to damaged growth centers in the anterior portions of the vertebral bodies. Postmortem specimens demonstrate herniation of nuclear material through the vertebral end growth plates at several consecutive levels. This causes disc-space narrowing as well as damage to the anterior growth plate of the involved vertebrae. The combination of these two processes produces the characteristic kyphosis on physical examination and the radiographic appearance of Scheuermann disease—that is, disc-space narrowing, vertebral wedging, and vertebral end-plate irregularity. A very slight scoliosis may also exist in the area where the kyphotic deformity is maximal. Rarely, the changes associated with Scheuermann disease occur at isolated single levels. These radiographic oddities are referred to as "Schmorl nodes."

The diagnosis of Scheuermann disease requires the identification of three consecutive levels of 5 degree wedging or more (Fig. 109-25). For many sur-

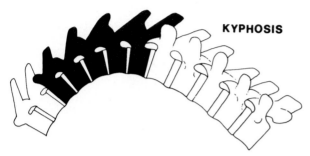

KYPHOSIS

Fig. 109-25

Loss of height of vertebral bodies and/or discs leads to kyphosis.

geons, the disease must exist in its full-blown state before treatment is begun. For the author, the occurrence of less severe changes associated with characteristic symptoms is perfectly adequate in an obese child to warrant treatment.

Nonoperative Treatment

Nonoperative treatment for all patients includes a combination of weight reduction (for obese patients), dorsal hyperextension exercises, and postural instructions to increase the patient's active control over the developing kyphotic deformity. Bracing is included for curves of 50 degrees in patients who are emotionally prepared to accept spinal bracing. Considerable permanent improvement in many patients can be achieved in postural control by Milwaukee bracing. Prompt symptomatic response to conservative care is characteristic of most patients. Radiographic demonstration of reconstruction of the anterior wedged portions of the apical vertebra is well documented in many series. The structural improvement of the vertebral anatomy provides permanent improvement in what could otherwise be a very unsightly kyphotic deformity.

Surgical Treatment

Operative treatment is offered to patients whose deformities or symptoms have not responded to conservative treatment. The symptoms must be functionally disabling and/or the kyphotic deformity must be greater than 60 degrees in patients who have achieved most of their skeletal growth. For such patients, surgical treatment is necessary and appropriate. The type of surgical reconstruction selected depends on the severity, rigidity, and location of the curvature. Hyperextension x-ray films demonstrate the flexibility of the curve. Curves between 55 and 80 degrees that correct 50% or more on hyperex-

tension are treated by a single-stage posterior approach from two vertebra above the apex to two vertebra below. Restoration of sagittal alignment is essential. Bone screws are used wherever the pedicles are large enough to accommodate a screw; a posterior fusion with autogenous bone graft is placed in the midline and in the intertransverse area. A very thick fusion is necessary (Fig. 109-26).

Patients with more severe or rigid kyphotic deformities who require treatment will require a staged approach. Preliminary discectomy through thoracotomy or a thoracolumbar approach will produce flexibility of the apical segments. Posterior instrumentation is then carried out, either as part of the same anesthetic procedure or at a second procedure a week later. Again, bone screws are used wherever the pedicles will accommodate them and a posterior and intertransverse fusion with autogenous bone graft is performed. Postoperative braces are used for 3 or 4 months until the fusion mass is obvious on x-ray films (Fig. 109-27).

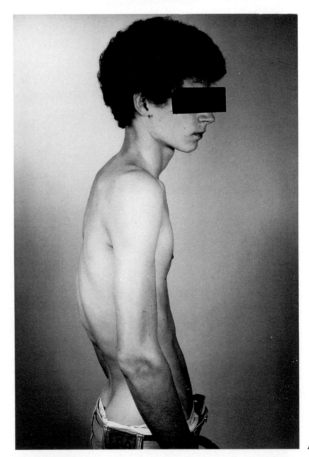

A

Fig. 109-26

A, Clinical appearance of patient with Scheuermann disease—sagittal plane.

Continues.

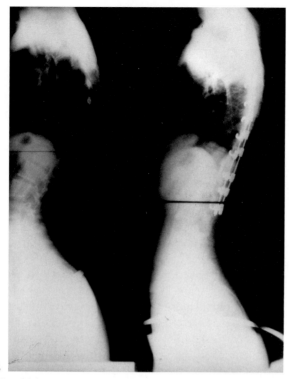

Fig. 109-26, cont'd

B, Radiographs showing sagittal correction of curve. **C,** Sagittal plane clinically after surgical correction.

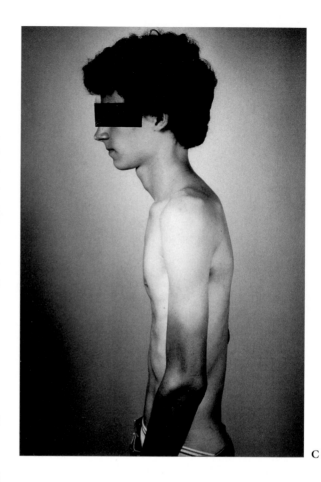

C

Fig. 109-27

A, Scheuermann disease—marked thoracolumbar kyphosis.

A

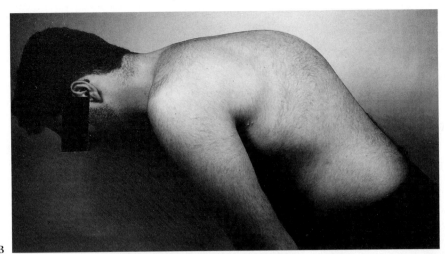

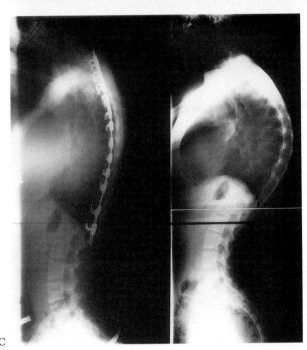

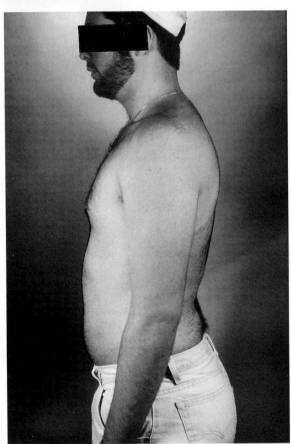

Fig. 109-27, cont'd
B, Bend test (from side) shows the "dome" characteristic of any kyphosis. **C,** Lateral radiographs showing achieved correction. **D,** Sagittal contour after correction.

Surgical treatment of patients with kyphosis produces people who function extremely well in the long run. Complications are minor in experienced hands, and pain relief and restoration of spinal anatomy are predictable. Nonunion occurs on 0.5% to 1% of patients. If symptomatic, a pseudarthrosis can be repaired by repeat autografting and spinal immobilization.

NEUROFIBROMATOSIS AND SCOLIOSIS

Etiology and Natural History

The bone changes in von Recklinghausen disease were described for the first time by Gould in 1918. According to different studies the incidence of scoliosis in neurofibromatosis is 0% to 20%. It is slightly more frequent in females than in males, and much more frequent in whites than blacks. Scoliosis presents, with decreasing frequency, in the thoracic spine, the thoracolumbar, and cervical spine[1,15] (Fig. 109-28).

While the scoliosis of neurofibromatosis can be caused by vertebral compression by neurofibromas, most cases, and all severe cases, are due to dysplastic vertebral growth. The severity of the scoliosis is related more to curve type than familial tendencies (Fig. 109-29).

Classification

Three types of curves are seen in patients with scoliosis who have neurofibromatosis. First, a dysplastic type may occur with a few severely rotated and deformed vertebrae (and pencilled ribs) that rapidly produce severe deformity (Fig. 109-30). There is also a nondysplastic type with characteristics identical to those of idiopathic scoliosis. The third type is intermediate between the dysplastic and nondysplastic types and shares characteristics of each. The curve prognosis depends on its type and on the

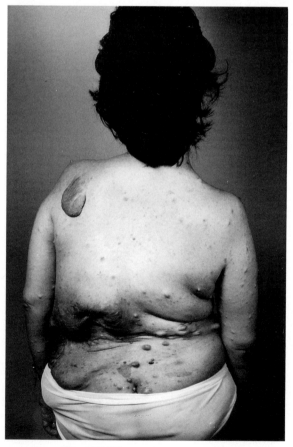
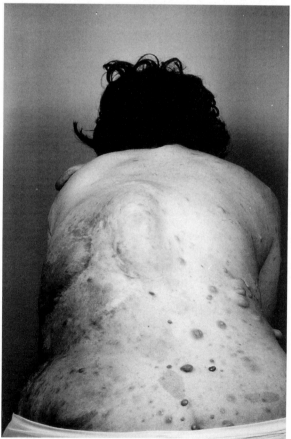

Fig. 109-28

A, Classic patient with severe thoracolumbar deformity and cutaneous neurofibromas and fibrous lesions.
B, Bend test—previous flank excision of malignant neurofibrosarcoma.

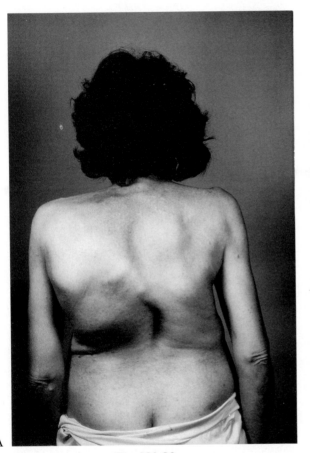

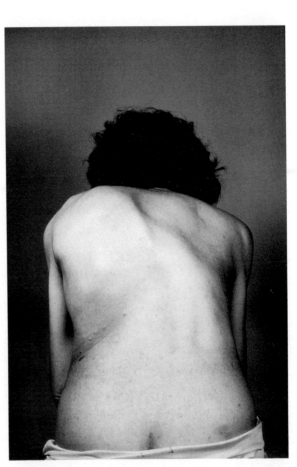

A   B

Fig. 109-29

A, Similarly severe kyphoscoliosis with less-classic cutaneous findings. **B,** Bend test.

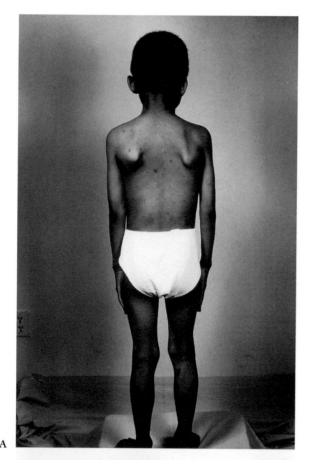

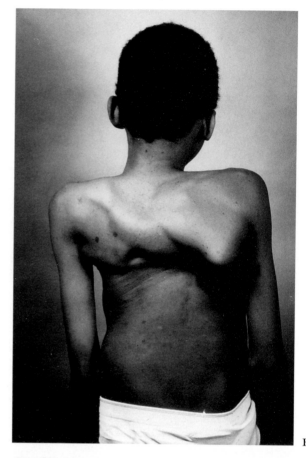

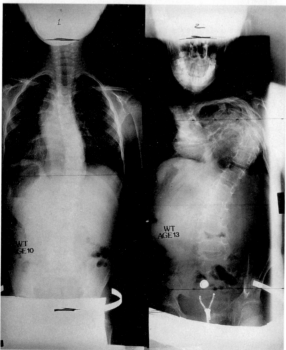

Fig. 109-30

A, 10-year-old with minor lateral curve but flat thoracic contour and café' au lait spots. **B,** Unfortunate lack of treatment leads to development of severe deformity in 3 years. **C,** X-ray films at ages 10 and 13 (same time as in Panels **A** and **B**).

amount of kyphotic deformity in the curve.[12] Nondysplastic curves progress in the same manner as idiopathic curves. Dysplastic curves are aggressively progressive—especially those with an exaggerated kyphotic component. In untreated dysplastic curves, paraparesis and paraplegia can develop because of the kyphotic deformity and spinal cord compression.

Cervical neurofibromas invading the spinal canal rarely occur. Though many of these patients are asymptomatic, dysphagia, torticollis, and neurologic deficit can be presenting symptoms. Sarcomatous degeneration of large neurofibromas can occur.

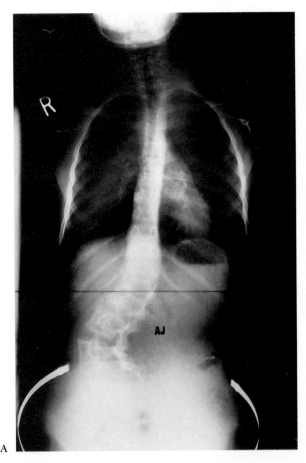

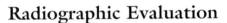

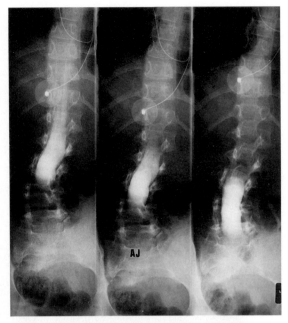

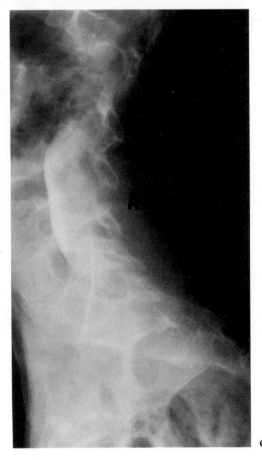

Fig. 109-31

A, Short sharp lumbar curve with scalloped vertebrae and severe rotational deformity. **B** and **C,** Marked dilatation of the dural sac in area of major vertebral deformity.

Radiographic Evaluation

Besides plain anteroposterior and lateral to x-ray films to define the deformity, it is important to evaluate the diameter of the spinal canal and the shape and size of the spinal cord preoperatively. Intraspinal meningoceles, and widened intervertebral foramina may occur due to saccular dilatation of the dura or the presence of intraspinal neurofibromata (dumbbell tumors) (Fig. 109-31). Neurofibromatosis patients with scoliosis can also have spondylolisthesis. A myelogram followed by CT scan seems to give the best data (Fig. 109-32). 3D magnetic resonance imaging (MRI) can be helpful. Somatosensory evoked potentials (SSEPs) are useful during all surgical procedures. Preoperative base-line SSEPs are important.

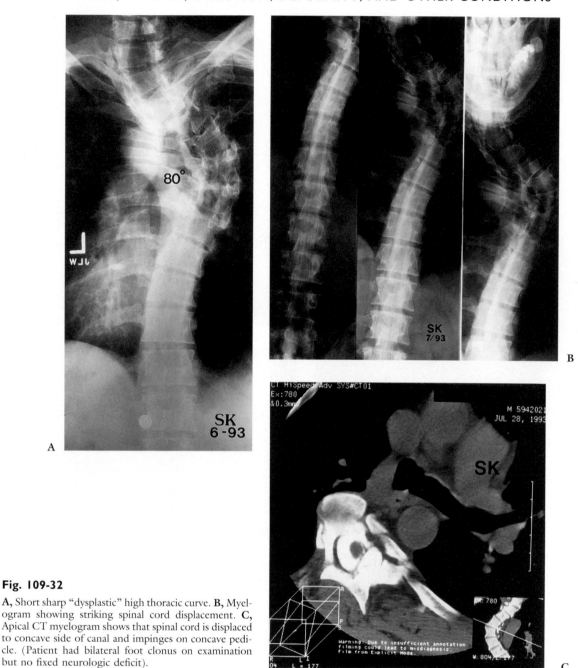

Fig. 109-32

A, Short sharp "dysplastic" high thoracic curve. **B,** Myelogram showing striking spinal cord displacement. **C,** Apical CT myelogram shows that spinal cord is displaced to concave side of canal and impinges on concave pedicle. (Patient had bilateral foot clonus on examination but no fixed neurologic deficit).

Treatment

The treatment of scoliosis in neurofibromatosis again depends on the curve type.[24] The treatment of nondysplastic curves is the same as in idiopathic scoliosis—bracing (Milwaukee or TLSO) for minor curves and surgical correction for cases with curve progression. Nonoperative treatment of dysplastic curves is ineffective. Surgery is indicated for curve progression or neurologic deficit. For moderate curves (40 to 60 degrees), posterior fusion is sufficient. Cases with kyphosis over 60 degrees need anterior and posterior spinal fusion. Carefully planned operative procedures are generally very successful. Nevertheless the treatment of severe, rigid curves in neurofibromatosis occasionally produces an outcome that may be esthetically less pleasing than planned, particularly when compared with the results of corrective procedures performed for patients with idiopathic scoliosis.

References

1. Akbarnia BA, Gabriel KR, Beckman E, Chalk D: Prevalence of scoliosis in neurofibromatosis, *Spine* 17 (Suppl 8):S224, 1992.

2. Ashkenaze D, Mudiyam R, Boachie-Adjei O, Gilbert C: Efficacy of spinal cord monitoring in neuromuscular scoliosis, *Spine* 18:1627, 1993.

3. Barnes PD, Brody JD, Jaramillo D, et al.: Atypical idiopathic scoliosis: MR imaging evaluation, *Radiology* 186:247, 1993.

4. Beauchamp M, Labelle H, Grimard G, et al.: Diurnal variation of Cobb angle measurement in adolescent idiopathic scoliosis, *Spine* 18:1581, 1993.

5. Bridwell KH, DeWald RL, editors: *The textbook of spinal surgery,* Philadelphia, 1991, J.B. Lippincott Co.

6. Carr W, Moe JH, Winter RB, Lonstein JE: Treatment of idiopathic scoliosis with Milwaukee brace, *J Bone Joint Surg* 62A:599, 1980.

7. Edelmann P: Brace treatment in idiopathic scoliosis, *Acta Orthop Belg* 58(Suppl 1):185, 1992.

8. Farsetti P, Tudisco C, Caterini R, Ippolito E: Juvenile and idiopathic kyphosis: long-term follow-up of 20 cases, *Arch Orthop Trauma Surg* 110:165, 1991.

9. Green NE: Adolescent idiopathic scoliosis, *Spine State Art Rev* 4(1):211, 1990.

10. Jacobs RR, editor: *Pathogenesis of idiopathic scoliosis:* Proceedings of an international conference, Chicago, 1984, Scoliosis Research Society.

11. Jeng CL, Sponseller PD, Tolo VT: Outcome of Wisconsin instrumentation in idiopathic scoliosis: minimum 5-year follow-up, *Spine* 18:1584, 1993.

12. Joseph KN, Bowen JR, MacEwen GD: Unusual orthopedic manifestations of neurofibromatosis, *Clin Ortho Relat Res* 278:17, 1992.

13. Karol LA, Johnston CE, Browne RH, Madison M: Progression of the curve in boys who have idiopathic scoliosis, *J Bone Joint Surg* 75A:1804, 1993.

14. Kearon C, Viviani GR, Killian KJ: Factors influencing work capacity in adolescent idiopathic thoracic scoliosis, *Am Rev Respir Dis* 148:295, 1993.

15. Landolt AM: Neurofibromatosis, meningomyelocele and scoliosis, *Dtsch Med Wochensch* 115(38):1452, September, 1990.

16. Machida M, Dubousset J, Imamura Y, et al.: An experimental study in chickens for the pathogenesis of idiopathic scoliosis, *Spine* 18:1609, 1993.

17. Maquire J, Madigan R, Wallace S, et al.: Intraoperative long-latency reflex activity in idiopathic scoliosis demonstrates abnormal central processing: a possible cause of idiopathic scoliosis, *Spine* 18:1621, 1993.

18. McKenzie L, Sillence D: Familial Scheuermann disease: a genetic and linkage study, *J Med Genet* 29:41, 1992.

19. Montgomery F, Willner S: Screening for idiopathic scoliosis: comparison of 90 cases shows less surgery by early diagnosis, *Acta Orthop Scand* 64:456, 1993.

20. Murray PM, Weinstein SL, Spratt KF: The natural history and long-term follow-up of Scheuermann kyphosis, *J Bone Joint Surg* 75A:236, 1993.

21. O'Brien T, Akmakjian J, Ogin G, Eilert R: Comparison of one-stage versus two-stage anterior/posterior spinal fusion for neuromuscular scoliosis, *J Pediatr Orthop* 12:610, 1992.

22. Sarwark JF, Loque E: Idiopathic scoliosis: new instrumentation for surgical management, *AAOS* 2:67, 1994.

23. Shaughnessy WJ: Management of adolescent idiopathic scoliosis, *Curr Opin Rheumatol* 5:301, 1993.

24. Sirois JL III, Drennan JC: Dystrophic spinal deformity in neurofibromatosis, *J Pediatr Orthop* 10:522, 1990.

25. Upadhyay SS, Ho EKW, Gunawardene WMS, et al.: Changes in residual volume relative to vital capacity and total lung capacity after arthrodesis of the spine in patients who have adolescent idiopathic scoliosis, *J Bone Joint Surg* 75A:46, 1993.

26. Willers U, Normelli H, Aaro S, et al.: Long-term results of Boston brace treatment on vertebral rotation in idiopathic scoliosis, *Spine* 18:432, 1993.

27. Williamson JB, Galasko CSB: Spinal cord monitoring during operative correction of neuromuscular scoliosis, *J Bone Joint Surg* 74B:870, 1992.

Chapter 110
Adult Scoliosis
John G. Finkenberg

History

Patient Evaluation and Selection

Multidisciplinary Evaluation

Nonoperative Care

Surgical Indications

Risks of Surgery

Surgical Planning

Surgical Techniques

     posterior fusion and instrumentation
     anterior fusion and instrumentation

Problems Specific to Adult Scoliosis

     paralytic curves
     scoliosis in the aged
     iatrogenic flat-back deformities
     degenerative adult scoliosis

Overview

Scoliosis diagnosed during skeletal immaturity is usually categorized as idiopathic, congenital, paralytic, or myopathic. In addition to these diagnoses, adult scoliosis may be secondary to degeneration, osteoporosis, and osteomalacia and may follow multilevel surgical decompression procedures. It is unusual for a patient to have idiopathic scoliosis diagnosed for the first time as an adult, except for lumbar curves, which because of aging changes and degeneration increase in adult life. However, patients with mild scoliosis and minimal symptoms will seek medical advice as adults.

The indications for treatment include pain, progression of deformity, and occasionally cosmetics. Neurologic dysfunction is unusual, but should be investigated in detail if the patient shows signs and symptoms of spinal stenosis, secondary to degenerative scoliosis with or without preexisting adolescent idiopathic scoliosis. Unfortunately, over the past 10 years more cases of postsurgical chronic low-back pain have been presented due to iatrogenic flat-back syndrome or accelerated degenerative changes at levels adjacent (usually distal) to the prior fusion or instrumentation. Due to a risk of neurologic damage, loss or correction, infection, pulmonary compromise, pseudarthrosis, and death, most surgeons were reluctant to attempt any surgical treatment for patients with adult scoliosis. These risks as well as our concern for the functional capacity of patients following surgery resulted in surgeons such as Nachemson recommending conservative management.[37]

Following the advent of Harrington rods in the 1960s, a more aggressive approach to treating adult spinal deformities was instituted.[17] Successes with the Harrington rod instrumentation system resulted in an explosion of spinal instrumentation, which includes that by Dwyer,[11,16,48] Luque,[19,32,33,46] Zielke,[24,49] and Cotrel-Dubousset.[8-10] Each of these systems was created to overcome the obstacles met with the Harrington instrumentation system. As time passes, the advantages, disadvantages, and indications for each of these systems has been well documented in the literature. The Isola and Rogozinski are two other instrumentation systems being used extensively. The improvement in preoperative evaluation and intraoperative patient care, which includes positioning frames, cell savers, spinal cord monitoring, and superior anesthesia monitoring machines has resulted in improving success with the surgical treatment of adult scoliosis.

Adult spinal deformities are often complex and require a team approach among experienced surgeons, medical internists, and therapists. It is common to find patients with concomitant medical problems that require thorough preoperative investigation as well as close postoperative monitoring. In this chapter, we will cover some of the history concerning the treatment of adult scoliosis, preoperative evaluation, patient selection, instrumentation selection, surgical procedure, postoperative management, and complications. An effort will be made to discuss the surgical procedures in a stepwise fashion with special emphasis being placed on circumferential surgical fusions and instrumentation. The complications and alternatives, as well as future considerations, regarding the treatment of adult scoliosis will also be reviewed.

History

Kostuik and Bentivoglio[27] found a prevalence rate of 3.9% of adult thoracolumbar or lumbar scoliosis on reviewing 5000 intravenous pyelogram x-ray films. These curves appeared to be structural and represented progression of deformities present in adolescents. Saands and Eisberg reviewed 194,060 chest radiograms and found that 1.9% of the population had a spinal deformity that was mild (10 to 19 degrees).[43] Weinstein and Ponsetti[47] attempted to define parameters that would assist doctors in determining which patients had increased likelihood of curve progression. They found that the progression was greatest if the curve involved the lumbar spine, the fifth lumbar vertebrae was not level with the sacrum, and the apical vertebrae had more than 33% rotation. Thoracic and thoracolumbar curves between 50 and 75 degrees progressed 30 and 22.3 degrees, respectively, over approximately 40 years. In agreement, Kostuik and Bentivoglio noted the worst prognosis for progressing deformity was in the thoracolumbar and lumbar curves that were imbalanced and extended down to the lumbosacral junction. Historically, imbalanced curves with the apex at L2-L3 or L3-L4 demonstrating grade 3 rotation are difficult to correct unless the surgical treatment is attempted at an early age.

Scoliotic curves greater than 45 degrees, truncal imbalance, and decreasing lumbar lordosis appear to result in increasing reports of pain. Approximately 60% of patients with lumbar and thoracolumbar scoliosis will report pain.[27] Thoracic curves do not appear to cause pain, but can result in some pulmonary dysfunction if the curve is hypolordotic. Despite reporting the same prevalence, Nachemson[35-37] and Nilsonne and Lunderen[39] found few cases of patients with clinically significant pain. It is not uncommon for the 42- to 60-year-old age group to demonstrate more reports of pain than the over 60-year-old age group as they are more active and often hold physically demanding jobs.

Resulting from dissatisfaction with the present fusion rates for patients with complex instabilities involving the anterior and posterior spine, circumferential spine surgery for adult scoliosis has become more popular. It is controversial when used as a primary procedure because it is usually reserved for patients in whom prior surgery has failed, who have difficult deformities, and who have tumors or trauma that involve all three columns of the spine. Hoover,[20] Goldner,[13] and O'Brien[40] have published papers regarding circumferential fusion. Each surgeon feels that this procedure has improved his rate of fusion as well as clinical results. Patient selection is difficult, but most authors agree that candidates should present with chronic pain and have failed all conservative treatments. The success of a spinal fusion depends on identifying the source of pain, selecting the appropriate patient, and having the surgical expertise as well as the necessary patient support during the immediate postoperative period.

Patient Evaluation and Selection

A thorough history and examination is necessary with any patient demonstrating a spinal disorder. The history should include questions concerning pain, curvature progression, neurologic dysfunction, and prior management of scoliosis. Occasionally patients will mention the change and degree of curvature, but often they report deformity progression by changes in clothing size, loss of height, or increase in their rib hump. If prior x-ray films are available, they should be reviewed and curves measured by the same observer. Attention should be given to measuring the curves from the same vertebral level on each x-ray film.

It is important to discuss with the patient how the curvature has affected activities of daily living as well as how he/she has coped with the deformity and discomfort.

Pain localization and magnitude should be documented. Occasionally, pain drawings can help a patient describe the discomfort. It is important to elicit from the patient how the pain affects activities at home and work, during social functions or recreation, and during sexual activities. A pain pattern such as paravertebral/axial versus radicular, sclerotomal versus nonanatomic, and progressive should be elicited from the patient in the initial history.

Neurologic dysfunction may be evidenced by weakness, abnormal reflexes, paresthesias, or bladder and bowel dysfunction. Remember that urinary stress incontinence may be secondary to spinal stenosis. Patients with adult scoliosis rarely present with paraparesis or paraplegia. Intercostal neuralgia may present at the apex of a thoracic or thoracolumbar curve. It is also necessary to separate mechanical pain from psychologic overlay.

Progression in a patient's scoliosis following skeletal maturity has been documented by several authors.[4,31,39] There appears to be a greater incidence of back pain with scoliotic curves greater than 45 degrees. In the thoracolumbar and lumbar spine, curves in excess of 45 degrees inevitably progress and pain develops. This would be in agreement with Weinstein and Ponsetti,[47] who showed that curves less than 30 degrees are unlikely to progress and those greater than 50 degrees progress at a rate of 0.75 degree to 1 degree per year. Most authors believe that this is due to escalated degeneration. In female patients, the secondary degenerative changes may produce a lumbar kyphoscoliosis. This often requires circumferential fusion for adequate surgical correction.

Cosmetic reasons are an uncommon indication for surgery with adult scoliosis with the exception of young adults who demonstrate significantly unbalanced curves. Kostuik et al.[31] noted in a long-term functional outcome study following surgery for an adult scoliosis that cosmetics play a significant role in patients' deciding to undergo surgery. Thoracoplasty can play an additional role in improving the cosmetic outcome. The rib humps develop with increases in rotatory deformity, which usually parallels scoliosis curve changes in the coronal plane.

A complete physical examination should rule out obvious causes for back and extremity pain that are not due to scoliosis. The following represents a list that would be included in every spine evaluation.

1. Visualization of the patient's back while standing to evaluate truncal balance, skin markings, rib hump location, gross deformity, thoracic kyphosis, lumbar lordosis, and prior surgical scars.

2. Range of motion testing to include flexion, extension, lateral flexion and rotation. Rib hump severity can be assessed with forward flexion to 90 degrees.

3. Palpation of spinal processes and paravertebral muscles.

4. Muscle testing with grading on a 0 to 5 scale.

5. Fine touch and pain sensation to include pinprick, light touch, and vibration.

6. Deep tendon reflexes at the biceps, brachial radialis, triceps, patella, and the ankle.

7. Straight leg raising in the seated as well as supine position.

8. Femoral stretch testing.

9. Bilateral hip examination.

10. Hip flexion, abduction, and external rotation (FABER) testing to evaluate the sacroiliac joint.

11. Rectal examination.

12. Gait analysis.

This examination represents an overview that would uncover any obvious abnormalities. A more detailed investigation may be necessary if the patient demonstrates subtle abnormal findings.

Radiography is necessary to determine the degree of scoliosis, etiology, progression, and flexibility. Standing posterior-anterior or lateral roentgenograms on 14-×-36-in. cassettes are standard. Side-bending views obtained in the supine position are beneficial for evaluating curve flexibility. A CT myelogram is indicated for patients demonstrating symptoms consistent with spinal stenosis. MRI is helpful if spinal cord pathology is suspected or any evaluation of the soft tissues is necessary. A technetium bone scan will help direct the investigation if the patient's pain pattern is not consistent with the degenerative changes seen on plain films. It is important to reemphasize that the degree of flexibility noted on the bending x-ray films do not demonstrate a high correlation with the degree of correction obtainable in surgery.[28]

Discography is helpful in localizing pain as well as in determining what levels must be included in the spinal fusion.[5,26,44] This is particularly true for lumbar and thoracolumbar curves. It is essential to request a discogram that includes an intervertebral disc morphology evaluation as well as a pain provocation test. Discography is best performed by the treating surgeon. The study is usually done under fluoroscopy, and permanent radiograms can be obtained to document needle placement. Discography should be performed at each vertebral level surrounding the spinal pathology in the cranial as well as caudal direction until provocation testing results in no back or lower-extremity discomfort.

Facet blocks have also been used to help localize pain. If discography produces pain or facet block relieves it, that spinal level should be incorporated in the fusion. If the discogram is negative and the facet block does not relieve the pain, then this vertebral level should not be incorporated in the fusion. The evaluations will also include selective nerve root injections for patients who have radicular pain. If pain relief occurs, a decompression at this level may be indicated.

Multidisciplinary Evaluation

Patients with adult scoliosis have undergone multiple operations and may present with drug dependencies secondary to chronic pain. In addition, they are taking myriad medications for illnesses that involve the cardiovascular or respiratory systems. An internist should conduct a thorough medical screen to determine if there are any nonmechanical reasons for their back discomfort. In addition, this examination should determine if the patient is capable of undergoing general anesthesia and a major surgical procedure. It is not uncommon for a patient to lose approximately 2000 ml of blood with an anterior abdominal approach to the spine and 3000 to 4000 ml with a posterior spinal approach. At this time, it is also possible to screen patients for hepatitis and human immunodeficiency virus (HIV) for their protection as well as that of the operating team.

The physicians at some institutions think that patients should undergo psychologic testing because they usually present with psychopathology secondary to chronic pain syndromes. Each institution should make an attempt to examine the patient in a systematic fashion. The MMPI and various pain questionnaires are often lengthy and cumbersome to review but may distinguish a subset of patients who will have a poor prognosis with regard to pain relief. Patients with behavioral problems and drug dependencies usually do not respond to surgery no matter which procedures are used. However, patients with documented psychiatric disorders appear to respond to surgery as well as the general population.

It is important for patients to understand the surgical objectives as well as long-term goals. In addition, patients should be aware of the risks, benefits, and alternatives to surgery. They should be aware of their chances for returning to their present occupations or for the need to enroll in a retraining program. Obviously, a patient's educational and work background as well as age and physical condition will determine which avenues will be pursued following the surgery. A return-to-work date is helpful in directing the patient with a postoperative rehabilitation program. The literature has shown that ongoing litigation and workers' compensation are negative influences with regard to becoming pain-free and returning to work.[35]

Every patient should undergo a preoperative educational session with nursing staff who are dedicated to spine care. This should include learning about the surgical procedure, the recovery process, and potential benefits and risks of the surgery. An appointment should be made for the patient to view a videotape about the surgical procedure and the recovery process. The videotape should discuss routines of the hospital, methods of analgesia, and the fact that all narcotics will be discontinued on discharge from the hospital. The patient should understand that he/she will be sent home with instructions on exercising as well as given nonsteroidal antiinflammatory medications as well as acetaminophen for analgesia. A portion of the tape should be dedicated to the physical therapist for introducing the exercise programs that the patient will participate in as an inpatient as well as at home. If patients understand how important exercise is to the healing process, they may be more cooperative following the surgery.

Nonoperative Care

Volumes of information have been written on nonoperative therapies for patients with chronic back pain. These treatment regimens range from complete bed rest to manipulation and traction. Sporadic testimonials of miraculous recoveries perpetuate these varied treatments. Disc degeneration is responsible for many reports of chronic back pain. The natural history of this disease is characterized by exacerbations and remissions with eventual plateauing of the patient's level of discomfort no matter what the treatment process. Rest for acute back pain is recommended less often because there is interest in keeping patients mobile and in good physical condition.

Numerous medications have been prescribed for back pain, but the trend appears to be away from strong narcotics, muscle relaxants, and outpatient treatment. Drug dependency and depression appear to be two factors that decrease the chances for a good outcome following any surgical procedure.

Patients should understand that exercises will not prevent or decrease curve progression, but should maintain flexibility. Low-impact aerobics, bicycling, speed walking, and swimming represent the best forms of exercise for patients with chronic back pain.

Judicious use of amitriptyline or other mood elevators may prove beneficial for the patient with chronic back pain who suffers from sleep disturbance and chronic anxiety.

It is rare for a patient with adult scoliosis to benefit from traction or the use of transcutaneous electrical nerve stimulation (TENS). Ultrasonography and diathermy are helpful only for patients who suffer with muscle spasms secondary to the scoliosis. Once again, the treatment methods appear to decrease discomfort on a temporary basis but do not change the progression of the disease or the incidence of pain recurrence.

The role of orthotics, braces, and corsets are unknown, as the literature does not support their use in the prevention of curve progression. Rarely is the support provided by these orthoses beneficial over the long term.

Surgical Indications

The indications for surgery in an adult with scoliosis are intractable pain not relieved by nonoperative treatments, to prevent further deformity, to manage neurologic dysfunction, and occasionally to improve cosmetic appearance. Pain continues to be the most common indication for surgery. Surgical outcome depends on localizing the pain, as this helps to determine the correct surgical procedure. Discograms have regained popularity as proponents of the test claim that it gives insight into the morphology of the disc in addition to evaluating the patient's pain response with provocation testing. Several authors feel that disc injection remains the sole procedure capable of correlating pathoanatomy and symptomatology. Ideally the test is done at every level suspected of causing pain, including at least one level cranially or caudally that is nonpainful and morphologically normal. It has been suggested that patients should be considered poor candidates for surgery if the typical pain is reproduced at multiple levels that appear morphologically normal. Degenerative scoliotic lumbar curves ending caudally at the L4-L5 or L5-S1 disc levels should undergo discogram testing of the lowest two intervertebral discs because they often are the contributor to this patient's low-back pain.

We feel that adults under 35 years old with progressively increasing curves should receive fusions for thoracolumbar or lumbar curves greater than 45 degrees, as inevitably the curve degenerates and results in pain. Patients who are immature, demonstrate truncal imbalance, and have curves greater than 40 degrees should receive a fusion. If the curve is rigid it may require a two-stage surgical procedure. The first stage would involve an anterior vertebral release and interbody bone grafting. A second procedure should be a posterior fusion and instrumentation. An adult patient with a flexibility curve and retained lumbar lordosis may be treated by Zielke instrumentation.[28]

Occasionally, patients with adult scoliosis, either degenerative or idiopathic with superimposed degenerative changes, present with clinical signs consistent with spinal stenosis. Neurologic deficits that accompany scoliosis represent added reasons for surgical correction. Unfortunately, patients with radicular pain arising from the compensatory curve are not usually relieved by fusion and instrumentation procedures of the primary curve.[21]

Unbalanced curves will often appear cosmetically worse than the more severe balanced scoliotic deformities. Kostuik et al.,[31] on questioning 100 adult patients who had undergone spinal fusion approximately 10 years after their surgery, found that cosmetics was an important factor in their deciding to have surgery. Few surgeons would consider performing surgery for cosmetic reasons alone. It should be approached as an additional benefit of surgery, rather than as an indication. Limited thoracoplasty can help diminish prominent rib humps.

Successful spine surgery will result if the correct procedure is matched with an appropriate candidate. This requires an ability to localize the pain source and to separate mechanical pain from psychologic overlay. Finally, the surgical team must be well versed in performing the procedure and dealing with inevitable intraoperative complications.

Risks of Surgery

An analysis of the risk:benefit ratio must be reviewed with every patient considering surgery for adult scoliosis. Obviously, the alternatives to surgery represent an important part of this decision. Unlike children, adults must consider a loss of earning ability, independence, sex life, and an ability to care for their family. In addition, there are risks of significant bleeding, infection, partial or complete neurologic loss, bowel or bladder dysfunction, pulmonary embolism, thromboembolism, and sexual dysfunction (i.e., retrograde ejaculation with anterior lumbosacral procedures). There are risks of pseudarthrosis, instrumentation failure, graft dislodging, residual pain, and death. The chances for a successful fusion to decrease pain and deformity appear to be inversely related to the number of surgical procedures attempted. There is no literature to support that all patients with thoracic curves over 50 degrees are guaranteed to lose pulmonary function, experience intractable pain, or progress to disfiguring levels. There are no alternatives to segmental spinal instrumental systems for patients with adult scoliosis who require posterior fusions and instrumentation procedures. Currently, we feel that the Cotrel-Dubousset instrumentation is the most versatile stabilizing form of instrumentation and offers the greatest potential for correction.

Surgical Planning

The decision regarding which vertebral levels require a fusion is determined by several methods. Few spine surgeons will argue that they need to incorporate vertebrae that demonstrate rotary subluxation, displacement with wedging, and severe degenerative arthritis. Hemisacralization and an oblique L5 vertebrae should indicate the need to include a fusion at the L5-S1 junction. It appears imperative to include all levels that are "pain generators." These levels are best identified by discography and facet blocks. Most adult patients with degenerative scoliosis suffer from concomitant spinal stenosis. The appropriate levels for decompression are best identified using CT myelography. We have not found that intraoperative somatosensory evoked potentials are useful in determining whether an adequate cord or root decompression has been accomplished. Thorough preoperative planning (history, clinical examination, x-ray films, and CT myelogram) to localize stenotic regions accompanied by direct visualization of these areas will ensure an adequate decompression. A postoperative CT myelogram may be helpful if a patient's neurologic exam worsens or if inadequate decompression is suspected.

When posterior fusion is required, segmental spinal instrumentation is preferred over rigid-plate systems as they are more versatile. Adult degenerative scoliosis often involves vertebrae that are rotated or resting in an oblique position due to severe degeneration. Segmental spinal instrumentation systems (SSI) will allow for pedicle fixation despite abnormal alignment. We are convinced that fusion rates are substantially improved when combined anterior/posterior fusions/instrumentation procedures are done for adult degenerative scoliosis requiring fusion to the sacrum. We have been performing an anterior interbody fusion at the L4-L5 and L5-S1 levels with Yuan I plates being placed between L4-L5 and two 6.5-mm AO cancellous screws being placed between L5 and S1. This procedure has been followed by a posterior fusion and instrumentation using the Cotrel-Dubousset system. An example of this procedure can be seen in Fig. 110-1, which depicts a 75-year-old woman with adult degenerative scoliosis and lumbar spinal stenosis. Her chief symptom was radiating pain into the left lower extremity. The patient began having "numbness and tingling" sensations in her left lower extremity, specifically from the knee to the top of her foot. Her leg pain and weakness became incapacitating after walking approximately three blocks. Medical management and physical therapy failed.

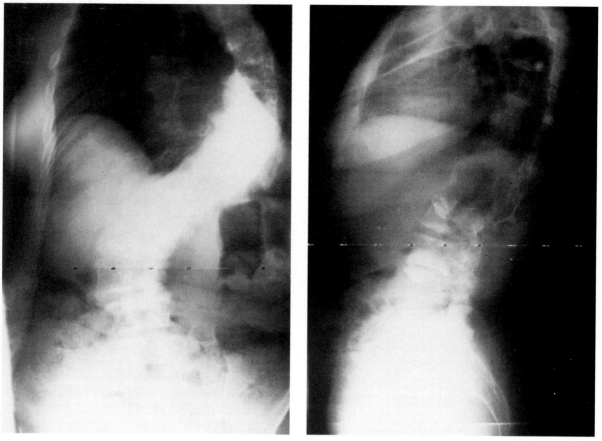

A   B

Fig. 110-1

A, Anteroposterior and **B**, lateral thoracolumbar x-ray films of 75-year-old woman with adult degenerative scoliosis and lumbar spinal stenosis.

On examination, she had diminished patella reflexes and absent ankle reflexes bilaterally. Muscle strength was slightly decreased in the bilateral quadriceps, with 1.5 cm of thigh atrophy on the left. Her fine touch and pain sensation were intact. Straight leg raising did not produce any back pain bilaterally.

Routine scoliosis x-rays demonstrated a 79-degree T4-T12 left thoracic and 47-degree T12 to L4 right lumbar scoliosis. There was marked imbalance in the scoliosis, with the C7 plum line resting 3.5 cm to the right. Bending x-ray films showed marked rigidity and a thoracolumbar scoliosis. A CT myelogram demonstrated a complete block of the dye at the L3 vertebral level (Fig. 110-2). A CT reconstruction (axial, sagittal view, and three-dimensional studies) show multiple regions of spinal stenosis between L2 and L4 (Fig. 110-3). Because of her reports of left-lower-extremity pain, denial of significant back pain, and requests for no surgical correction of her rigid thoracoscoliosis, we performed an L2-L4 spinal decompression/laminoplasty and fusion with instru-

mentation of these levels using the Cotrel-Dubousset system. The posterior bone elements (spinous process and lamina) were removed en bloc to expose the spinal column. The spondylitic bony formation was excised from the lateral aspects of the spinal column, and the neuroforamina were explored to ensure patency. After fully decompressing the spinal cord, the spinous process and lamina were replaced into their original positions using AO cortical screws through the spinous process and unilateral facet joints. These fixation screws used in the laminoplasty should be directed toward the base of the transverse process on the opposite facet joint. Fusion and instrumentation of the L2-L4 lumbar spine were performed to decrease the chances of postoperative scoliosis progression secondary to spinal instability created by the decompression procedure (Fig. 110-4).

Surgical Techniques

The Harrington posterior instrumentation system has been a mainstay for treatment of adult scoliosis,

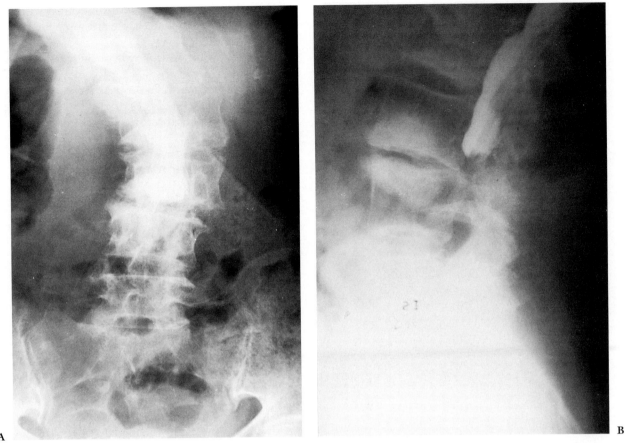

Fig. 110-2

A, Anteroposterior and **B,** lateral thoracolumbar CT/myelograms demonstrating complete block of metrizamide dye at L3.

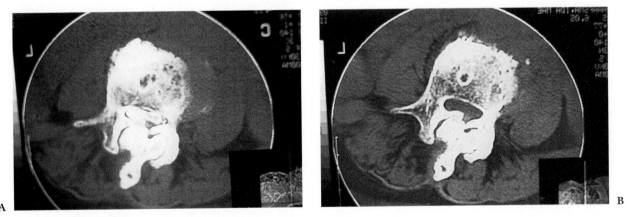

Fig. 110-3

CT scan axial reconstructions demonstrating central (**A**) and lateral (**B**) recess spinal canal lumbar stenosis.

but lacks the versatility and stability found in many of today's systems. In addition, it is not uncommon for the use of a Harrington system to result in loss of lumbar lordosis, which is inevitable with any distraction device. It is the lack of any lumbar or sacral

screw fixation that makes this system outdated. Fusion and instrumentation surgery for adult scoliosis can occur as an anterior,[24,34] posterior,[34] and a combined procedure.[6,22] The Zielke technique[34] is an excellent method of anterior fusion and instrumen-

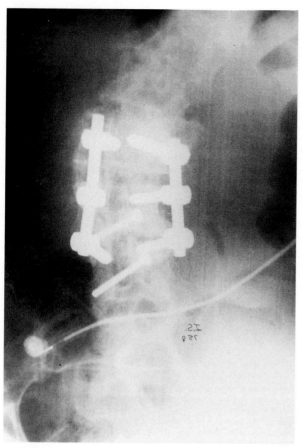

Fig. 110-4

Anteroposterior lumbar x-ray films demonstrating an L2-L4 lumbar posterior fusion and instrumentation with decompression laminoplasty.

tation for lumbar and thoracolumbar curves if no kyphotic deformities are present.

In addition, if the curve appears to be rigid, a two-stage procedure would be optimal. This involves an anterior approach, which consists of multiple-level discectomies, intervertebral bone grafting, and instrumentation. Appropriate devices would include Kostuik-Harrington or Kaneda instrumentation. At the same sitting or approximately 1 week post operatively, a posterior instrumentation and fusion procedure can be done using the Cotrel-Dubousset system.

If the patient presents with a mobile kyphoscoiosis, treatment should consist of a single-stage posterior fusion and instrumentation using the Cotrel-Dubousset system. Proponents of the system have demonstrated its ability not only to restore lumbar lordosis but to derotate the spine.[9,25] The Luque-rod system with the Galveston technique[7,15,18,23] has fallen from favor because of its increased risk of neu-

rologic damage associated with sublaminar wire passage and increased sacroiliac pain using the Galveston technique.

The following section will include information concerning patient positioning for the anterior and posterior approaches. A surgical technique section will be included on use of the Cotrel-Dubousset, Zielke, Kostuik-Harrington, and Kaneda systems.

Posterior Fusion and Instrumentation

Patient Positioning

Figure 110-5 shows the ideal patient position for a posterior spinal fusion and instrumentation. The trunk rests on a Hall-Recton frame, which allows the abdomen to hang free. This decreases the abdominal pressure and diminishes the distension of the epidural veins. The arms should be positioned comfortably toward the head of the table to minimize surgical interference and increase anesthesia access. The head should rest on a Mayfield "horseshoe" holder, and the lower extremities are placed on a foam rubber pad to allow the hips to be in slight hyperextension. This will maintain or increase the lumbar lordosis. The knees are padded and the toes are allowed to hang free over the end of the padding.

Posterior Approach (Cotrel-Dubousset)

An incision is made midline over the spinous processes (Fig. 110-6) to extend two levels above and below the intended levels of fusion.

Approximately 30 ml of 1:500,000 (1.0 ml of 1:1000 epinephrine in 500 ml of normal saline) epinephrine saline solution is injected at each vertebral level. The needle is placed subcutaneously and then on the posterior bony elements (lamina/transverse process) at each level involved in the fusion.

Once the posterior bony elements are exposed, the various lamina and pedicle hooks are introduced.

If sacral or lumbar screws are being used, they should be placed in the assigned position marked on the preoperative scoliosis x-ray films (3-ft standing, anteroposterior, and lateral films) (Fig. 110-7).

Screws are inserted at the confluence of the pars interarticularis and the transverse process. A 3.2-mm drill is directed medially and slightly cranially or caudally according to preoperative lateral x-ray films taken of the lumbar spine. We have found that the AO drill gives the surgeon the best control during drilling for the screws. A depth gauge is then introduced into the drilled hole to determine the length

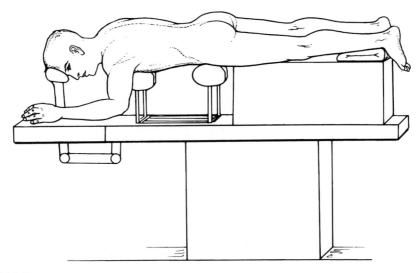

Fig. 110-5

Positioning of patient for posterior spinal fusion and instrumentation. Lumbar spine is kept in full extension to maintain normal lumbar lordosis.

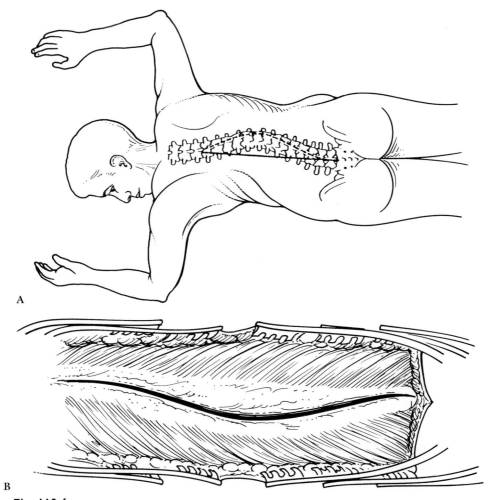

A

B

Fig. 110-6

A, Straight-line incision is made through skin followed by **B,** a curvilinear incision through the deep fascia overlying the spinous processes.

Fig. 110-7

Preassigned positions for lamina **A** and pedicle hooks **B** should
be marked on a preoperative scoliosis film.

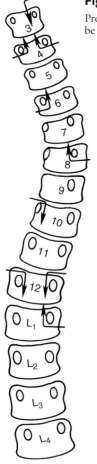

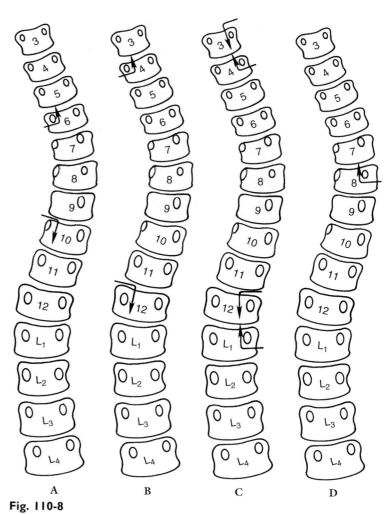

A   B   C   D

Fig. 110-8

Preassigned positions: **A** lamina hooks and **B** pedicle hooks.

of the screw and to determine if the pedicle walls are
intact. Approximately 80% penetration into the vertebral body is ideal. The pedicle cortex is drilled with
a 4.5-mm drill prior to introduction of the screw.
Short, smooth Steinman pins can be placed into the
pedicle holes for x-ray confirmation of the position
prior to introducing any of the screws.

Decisions regarding positioning of the hooks and
rods should follow the general guidelines below.

1. Place the appropriate (open) hooks (i.e., pedicle hook and laminar hook) on the pedicle above
and the lamina below, one to two vertebral levels
away from the curve apex on the "concave" side (Fig.
110-8, *A*).

2. A second set of divergent (closed) hooks should
be placed at the end of the "concave" curve on the vertebrae next to the neutral vertebrae (Fig. 110-8, *B*).

3. A claw configuration (i.e., downgoing closed
laminar hook and upgoing closed pedicle hook) are
placed either on the vertebrae at the end of the "convex" curve cranially or spanning over two vertebrae
at the upper end of the "convex" curve (Fig.
110-8, *C*).

4. The next open pedicle hook is placed at the
apex of the curve on the convex side in an upgoing
direction (Fig. 110-8, *D*).

5. The final closed pedicle hook is placed on the
vertebra at the end of the "convex" curve caudally.

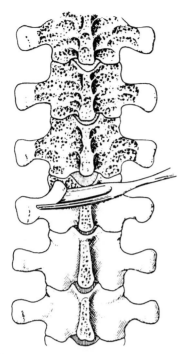

Fig. 110-9

Decortication of posterior bony elements is crucial to good fusion and should be done meticulously. Care should be taken not to fracture bone associated with hook positions. *(Courtesy of AMS, Hayward, CA.)*

6. The concave rod should be prebent to fit into the hooks as they lie on the spine. The curve of the rod should maintain or improve the normal thoracic kyphosis and lumbar lordosis once the rod is rotated 90 degrees.

7. Screws may be placed into the lumbar vertebrae for fixation if the posterior bony elements are osteoporotic or have been removed by prior surgery.

8. Blockers must be placed on the rod once it has been prebent. The blockers allow the rod to remain attached to the open hooks. Place the blockers on the side of the hook on which you plan to apply pressure when reducing the scoliotic curve.

9. The rod should never end at the apex of the thoracic kyphosis or the lumbar lordosis.

10. Prior to placing the concave rod into the appropriate hooks, the posterior bony element should be decorticated (Fig. 110-9).

11. The concave rod is inserted into the upper and then lower vertebrae closed hooks.

12. In situ bending iron are used to seat the rod into the remaining open hooks.

13. The rod is attached to the hooks by sliding the blockers into the open hook once the rod is seated.

14. C rings are placed on the rod up against the hooks to maintain the hooks in their position.

15. The rod is rotated to improve vertebral rotation and obtain improved thoracic kyphosis and lumbar lordosis.

16. The screws are then tightened to secure the hooks to the rods and to keep the rod from derotating.

17. The scoliotic curve is corrected with gradual distraction (concave side) and compression (convex side) maneuvers using a rod holder and spreader.

18. After decortication and instrumentation have been completed on the concave side, the same maneuvers are performed on the convex side of the curve with the exception of the rod rotation.

19. When the second rod is secure, the first rod is rechecked for satisfactory position.

20. The DDT (Dispositif de Traction Transversale) devices are placed between the rods (minimum of two).

21. The DDT device is secured to one of the rods using an open-ended wrench. The outside nut is tightened against the opposite rod until the DDT bar begins to bend anteriorly. Then the center claw is secured to the opposite rod.

22. The hexagonal set screws are broken off at every level. The wound is irrigated and closed over a small closed suction drain. The deep fascia is closed with a number one absorbable suture in figure-eight stitches. The skin edges are approximated with a running zero absorbable suture and closed with a running 3-0 absorbable undyed suture. If a wake-up test (stagnara) is planned, this should be done before breaking off any hexagonal set screw heads.

Alternative Procedures

There are many curve combinations possible, and each will require a slightly different construct. Rigid scoliotic curves may require anterior releases or even posterior releases if a prior fusion has been performed. The goal of treating certain rigid thoracolumbar and lumbar curves in a staged procedure is to reduce the high complication rate, reduce the rate of pseudarthrosis and poor curve correction, and improve on truncal imbalance and lumbar hypolordosis. Typically, patients with a rigid lumbar kyphoscoliosis will undergo an initial anterior release, accompanied by placing morsalized bone graft in the interspaces. This procedure is followed by a second-stage Cotrel-Dubousset instrumentation to derotate the curve and restore lumbar lordosis. We averaged a 63% curve correction with this procedure.

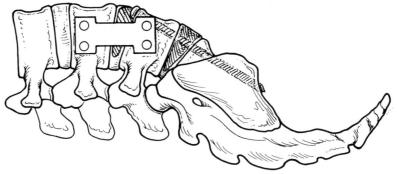

Fig. 110-10

Two AO cancellous screws are positioned from anterior superior portion of L5 vertebrae into sacrum. Yuan I plate is positioned between L4 and L5 vertebrae.

A second example of when a combined anterior and posterior fusion approach could be used is in a patient who demonstrates the need to extend the fusion to the sacrum due to painful degeneration associated with a rigid kyphoscoliosis. Our approach with these patients has been to perform an anterior release the entire length of the curve. This included an L4-L5 and L5-S1 interspace discectomy. These interspaces were then filled with a wedge-shaped bone graft from the iliac crest and augmented with two AO cancellous screws positioned from the anterior superior portion of the L5 vertebrae into the sacrum (Fig. 110-10). These screws usually measure approximately 60 to 70 mm in length and could be palpated on the anterior surface of the sacrum. Morsalized bone graft was placed between the above intervertebral bodies in which discectomies had been performed. One week later, a Cotrel-Dubousset instrumentation was placed on the patient extending down to and including the sacrum.

Complications

The rate of complications with use of the Cotrel-Dubousset system is significant. We have noted continued pain in approximately 16%, superficial wound infection, hemothorax, neuropraxia, prominent rods, hook pull-out, pseudarthrosis, and flat-back deformity. Based on this experience, we recommend that the supplemental distal lumbar fixation be achieved with bone screws. The failure in fixation of this system has been noted following the incorporation of bone screws. In two patients with osteoporotic bone, the screws were noted to pull out of their position on derotation of the rod. This complication was treated by placing polymethylmethacrylate (PMMA) acrylic into the pedicle prior to replacement of the screw. Special efforts must be

made not to force the methacrylate into the pedicle hole, as small openings of pedicle could result in PMMA being extruded into the canal. The PMMA is introduced into the drilled pedicle using the tube technique.

The Cotrel-Dubousset instrumentation system is versatile and provides an excellent means of correcting and stabilizing complex adult structural deformities. There is a steep learning curve to its proper use. More complicated deformities and degenerative conditions require a surgeon who has obtained advanced training. A significant number of complications encountered with this system will decrease with experience.

Anterior Fusion and Instrumentation

Patient Positioning and Anterior Approach

Positioning the patient for an anterior approach depends on the surgical procedure and the vertebral levels of interest. A one-level L5-S1 discectomy and interbody fusion can be performed through a midline or transverse Pfannenstiel incision with the patient supine (Fig. 110-11). The L1-L5 vertebrae can be approached through a left paramedian and cranial flank extension excision with the patient lying supine. A soft bump can be placed under the left hip. The T9-L5 vertebrae can be approached through a transpleural retroperitoneal incision that removes the rib two levels above the vertebrae of interest. This incision extends caudally into the paramedian incision over the abdomen. This approach is also done with the patient supine and a bump under the left hip and shoulder. If one or two levels must be exposed for debridement and fusion, a flank incision is used with the patient in a semilateral (45 degrees) right decubitus position. This position al-

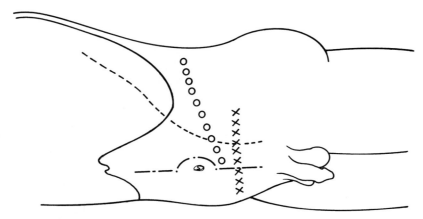

Fig. 110-11

Anterior/retroperitoneal surgical approaches. **A,** (.__.) Midline abdominal. **B,** (xxx) Pfannenstiel low transverse. **C,** (ooo) Transverse flank. **D,** (---) Left paramedian with cranial flank extension.

lows the intestines to fall anteriorly and decreases the amount of retraction needed to perform a retroperitoneal approach. The thoracolumbar spine should be approached from the left if possible, as the inferior vena cava is protected by the aorta throughout most of the procedure. Surgical misadventures involving the aorta are easier to repair than those involving the inferior vena cava. Should an incidental venotomy occur, this should be repaired with 4-0 Prolene with a taper needle. A simple running stitch is adequate.

The majority of adult patients with scoliosis will undergo an anterior release of multiple thoracic and lumbar vertebrae, if the curves are rigid and correction is desirable. The best approach to obtain maximal visualization of these vertebrae is a transpleural retroperitoneal approach. The patient should be placed in a supine position, with a soft roll under the right hip and shoulder. The pleura is usually entered through the rib two levels cranial to the uppermost vertebra to be operated on.

Instrumentation

There are several anterior instrumentation devices available, but the three most frequently used at Johns Hopkins Hospital are the Zielke, Yuan I plate, and Kostuik-Harrington systems. Surgeons who are comfortable with inserting these devices know that they will be prepared to handle any situation that may require anterior instrumentation. Selby documents a higher rate of arthrodesis when internal fixation is used on the spine.[45] In addition, most surgeons believe that patients can be mobilized earlier, which results in improved respiratory status, prompt recovery, and accelerated rehabilitation. Unfortu-

nately, inserting the devices requires increased operative time, and accompanying this is increased blood loss and incidence of infection. Operative risks now include increased chances of neurologic damage and instrumentation failure. A careful assessment of the patient's degree of osteoporosis should be included in the preoperative evaluation because the instrumentation construct is only as strong as the bone into which it was inserted. Severe osteoporosis may dictate the use of methylmethacrylate to augment the screw fixation in the vertebral body. Insertion techniques for the anterior instrumentation devices listed above will be described in the following paragraphs. Initially, it is helpful to use the instrumentation on a spine model prior to inserting the device in a patient.

Zielke Instrumentation The literature supports the use of this system with thoracolumbar and lumbar curves that do not require fusion at the lumbosacral joint. The adult patients with scoliosis should be mobile on bending films and the lumbar lordosis should be preserved.[23,29,41] In the adult, the entire curve should be spanned, but in an adolescent fewer levels may require instrumentation. The insertion technique is discussed below in a stepwise manner.

1. The levels to be fused should be exposed using the technique previously described.

2. The intervertebral disc and vertebral end plates are removed back to the posterior longitudinal ligament using a scalpel, rongeur, and various sizes of chisels.

3. An adequate exposure is required so that vertebral screws can be inserted toward the junction of the opposite pedicle and vertebral body.

4. If the entire disc is removed, a depth gauge can be inserted to determine the exact diagonal width of the vertebral body. Two millimeters should be added to this measurement because most patients with this diagnosis have spondylitic lipping near the end-plate region of the vertebrae.

5. One staple is placed into the end vertebrae furthest from the apex. The initial hole is made with a staple starting tool. Special efforts should be made not to insert the staple tine into the disc space.

6. The appropriate-length screw is inserted through a beveled washer (concave up) into the vertebral body. Side-opening screws are preferred over top-opening screws.

7. A 3.2-mm diameter threaded rod is inserted into the closed Zielke screws and laid into the open-head Zielke screws. Nuts are positioned on the rod to lie on the compression side of the screw head (opposite from curve apex) and on both sides of the end vertebral screw head.

8. The screws of the screw head should always be inserted from the convex side of the scoliosis as the eventual compression/derotation placed on the vertebra will reduce the scoliosis as well as improve the rate of arthrodesis. Screws placed too anteriorly result in increasing the kyphotic deformity when compression is applied.

9. An outrigger device is then attached to the ends of the rod to improve lumbar lordosis or decrease thoracolumbar kyphosis.

10. Autogenous morsalized cortical cancellous bone (rib) or iliac crest is placed between the vertebrae prior to tightening the instrumentation into the final position.

11. A compressor is placed between the two head screws, and when the desired correction is obtained, the nuts on the compression side are tightened. This process is carried sequentially and symmetrically from the apex outward.

12. If the bone is osteoporotic, it may be necessary to place methylmethacrylate into the vertebrae prior to inserting the screws. Using low-viscosity or cooled methylmethacrylate will delay cement hardening and improve placement accuracy.

The Zielke instrumentation can be used from T9 to L5. Minimal scoliotic correction will be obtained with use above this level because the disc spaces are narrower. Thoracic curves do not require external support, but thoracolumbar and lumbar curves will benefit from a total-contact molded orthosis. Several authors have reported curve corrections between 60% and 70%, and fortunately the loss of correction over 1 year is less than 5%.[28,30,41] Rotational deformity improves a minimum of one grade using

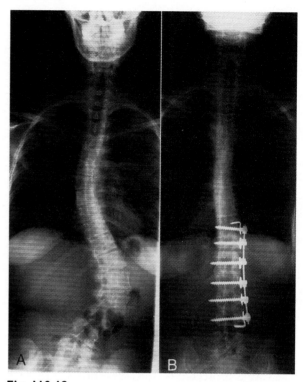

Fig. 110-12

Zielke instrumentation. *(From Kostuik JP: The Adult Spine, Principles and Practice, vol 2, New York, 1991, Raven Press.)*

the Nash-Moe method of classification.[38] Figure 110-12 shows the device inserted in a 75-degree left thoracolumbar curve.

Kostuik-Harrington Device This system represents a modification of the Harrington device used posteriorly on the spine for over 35 years. The system can be used for distraction, compression, or stabilization. It is primarily used in the treatment of thoracolumbar kyphotic and lumbar (flat-back) deformities.[27] Prior to the enlargement of the screw diameters, breakage occurred in 12.5% of the screws. However, no neurovascular injuries or pseudarthrosis were reported.

Problems Specific to Adult Scoliosis

Adult patients with scoliosis often present with rigid scoliotic curves, severe imbalance, osteopenia, degenerative spinal stenosis, chronic pain and iatrogenic lumbar kyphosis (flat-back deformity). The majority of rigid deformities are still seen with idiopathic scoliosis, as most congenital curves with significant imbalance are treated at a younger age. Occasionally, the rigidity in the curve is secondary to a prior surgical fusion. Treatment of these patients must include osteotomy through a surgical or congenital fusion.

In the past, surgery was performed posteriorly with three to four osteotomies, rib releases on the concavity, and rib resections on the convex side. Following posterior and occasionally anterior releases, the patient was placed in a halo-pelvic or halo-femoral traction while in a circoelectric bed at 30 degrees dependency or a halo wheelchair device. The second stage of the operation involved performing a posterior fusion and instrumentation approximately 2 weeks later. Fortunately, the segmental spinal instrumentation devices (Cotrel-Dubousset instrumentation, Isola, etc.) allow for immediate correction and stabilization. Therefore, immobilization and traction devices and delayed surgical procedures are not required. Obviously, it is more difficult to correct congenital versus idiopathic scoliosis.

Paralytic Curves

The patient with paralytic scoliosis often presents in a wheelchair with significant deformity and back pain secondary to pelvic obliquity, thoracolumbar kyphosis, or lumbar hyperlordosis. It is common knowledge that a collapsing scoliosis may lead to respiratory dysfunction. Equally important, but not as life threatening is the patient's loss of socialization, which accompanies severe flexion deformities. Patients with severe paralytic scoliosis demonstrate difficulties with personal hygiene, which tends to stress interpersonal relationships. Pulmonary function is improved by lifting the diaphragm into a position where it can function more effectively. Some authors feel that you can estimate how effective this operation would be by placing the patient in a halo-dependent traction and performing respiratory function tests. Patients who represent significant operative risks should be considered for a custom seating device.

We have recommended that circumferential fusion procedures be performed to eliminate the need for prolonged immobilization. The patient is fitted with a high plastic (back) corset (front) brace with crossed padded shoulder straps and encouraged to transfer to a chair or wheelchair as soon as possible.

Scoliosis in the Aged

Elderly patients will often present with rigid curves, spinal stenosis, and osteopenic bone. It is tempting to perform posterior fusion/instrumentation procedures alone and not attempt to reduce the curve.

However, we have found that these patients can be treated in a manner somewhat similar to a young patient with surgical or congenitally fused scoliotic curves. This is due to the more recent use of Cotrel-Dubousset or Zielke instrumentation in contrast to the Harrington instrumentation device. Individuals in whom a preservation of lumbar lordosis is demonstrated can be treated by an anterior Zielke fusion and instrumentation. Depending on the degree of osteopenia, methylmethacrylate can be used to enhance screw fixation.

The major indication for surgery in this age group is still pain. It is not unusual for patients to demonstrate clinical evidence of nerve-root impingement, which if present must be explored thoroughly during the posterior procedure. Unfortunately, more than 50% of patients will exhibit some degree of chronic pain postoperatively, but the radiculopathy is usually relieved if the root is decompressed. Our experience has demonstrated that the greatest curve correction can be obtained with either the Zielke or the Cotrel-Dubousset system. Potential complications associated with this type of surgery are varied. They include adult respiratory distress syndrome, pleural effusions, coagulopathy, infection, partial or complete paralysis, instrumentation dislodgement or failure, pseudearthrosis, and iatrogenic hypolordosis. Infection rates will increase with prolonged operative time, excess room traffic, breaks in sterile technique, no preoperative antibiotics, and inadequate hemostasis. Infection rates greater than 2% to 3% should be analyzed closely.

Adult patients with scoliosis who have had previous fusions will often have increased degenerative changes at the level adjacent to the fusion. Prior studies have shown that the risks of this occurring is proportional to the number of lumbar segments fused. Failed nonoperative treatment usually results in surgical extension of the fusion. Spinal stenosis can accompany this degenerative process and must be considered prior to formulating a surgical plan. Preoperative radiographic studies (CT myelogram and MRI) will, in addition to a thorough history and physical examination, demonstrate these stenoses. The operative approach varies according to the planned procedure. If an arthrodesis to the sacrum is not required, either a posterior or anterior fusion extension will suffice. However, if the extension includes a lumbosacral arthrodesis a circumferential fusion is required. We prefer an anterior fusion and instrumentation as well as posterior fusion and instrumentation using bone-screw fixation. At present we are placing interbody autografts anteriorly between L5 and S1 and then placing two AO 6.5-

mm cancellous screws from the anterosuperior aspect of the L5 vertebra to the anterior surface of the S1 vertebrae. These screws should pass through the body of the S1 vertebrae. The Cotrel-Dubousset method is used for the posterior instrumentation, as this allows for derotation of the vertebra and possible accentuation of the lumbar lordotic curve.

Iatrogenic Flat-Back Deformities

Harrington instrumentation has proven to be unsatisfactory when performing a lumbosacral fusion because it produces lumbar hypolordosis, as a result of distraction, in a high percentage of patients. The decreased lumbar lordosis is tolerated by the young adult but results in low-back fatigue and chronic pain with increasing age. Severe flattening of the lumbar spine flexes the trunk forward. In an effort to stand upright the patient compensates by flexing his/her hips and knees. Remaining in this position for an extended period results in a flexion contracture at the joints. Flat-back syndrome can occur when distraction instrumentation arises from either the L5 or S1 vertebrae, and a thoracolumbar junction kyphosis of 15 degrees or greater is present (especially if associated with hypokyphosis of the thoracic spine). A considerable amount of emphasis is placed on pseudarthrosis as a cause of chronic low-back pain. However, patients will continue to experience pain if the hypolordotic curve is not corrected at the same time as the pseudarthrosis is fused. We prefer a concurrent two-stage anterior and posterior fusion with instrumentation.

Restoration of the lumbar lordosis with fused iatrogenic (flat-back) syndrome may require wedge osteotomies in the fusion mass in addition to the anterior and posterior instrumentation.

Mobile thoracolumbar scoliotic curves are treated with Zielke instrumentation and anterior interbody fusions followed by Cotrel-Dubousset posterior fusion and instrumentation. This staged treatment allows for correction of the scoliosis as well as improvement in the lumbar lordosis. Rigid thoracolumbar scoliosis curves are usually treated by multiple-level anterior discectomies and interbody bone chip fusions followed by Cotrel-Dubousset instrumentation. If the curve extends down to the sacrum, we use Yuan I-beam plates between L4 and L5 and two 6.5-mm cancellous screws between L5 and S1 (Fig. 110-13). Wedge-shaped tricortical grafts are placed between the lower lumbar vertebrae prior to placement of the instrumentation. The pseudarthrosis rate appears to be significantly decreased when these two-staged procedures are performed.

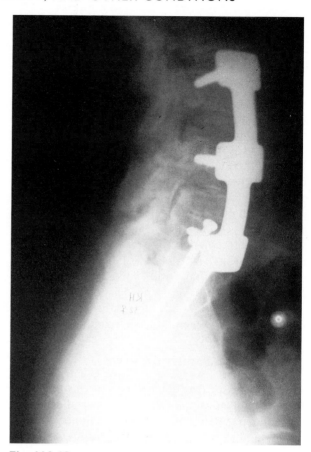

Fig. 110-13

Example of anterior discectomy at L3-L4, L4-L5, and L5-S1, followed by instrumentation. Posterior fusion and instrumentation followed anterior procedure.

It is important to identify the nerve roots at the level of the osteotomy. Imbalance in the anterior-posterior plane may require a quadrilateral wedge osteotomy both anteriorly and posteriorly. The technique is similar to a Smith-Peterson procedure for ankylosing spondylitis. Concurrently, the opening-wedge osteotomy is done through the intervertebral disc at the same level as a closing-wedge osteotomy through the posterior bone elements or fusion. If there has been a previous anterior fusion this must be osteotomized. A tricortical graft is inserted in the anterior osteotomy while the posterior osteotomy side is allowed to collapse. AO contoured plates can be placed posteriorly to reduce rotation, while Kostuik-Harrington instrumentation can be placed anteriorly to open up the osteotomy maximally. A minimum of two screws should be placed above and below the posterior osteotomy site. Common complications of this procedure include neurologic injury, nonunion, failure of pain relief, and recurrence of deformity.

Degenerative Adult Scoliosis

Patients with de novo degenerative adult scoliosis (or collapsing scoliosis) are usually in their late 50s, have osteoporosis, have decompression fractures, and have scoliosis ranging between 7 and 50 degrees. Back pain was usually the presenting symptom of most adults diagnosed with new-onset scoliosis. Osteomalacia was implicated as a causative factor in one study, but these scoliotic curves were usually mild and demonstrated no rotation. In a 1982 study on scoliosis in the elderly, it was concluded that there was little correlation between osteoporosis, degeneration, and curve progression.[42] Epstein et al.,[12] Benner and Ehni,[3] and Grubb et al.[14] concluded that scoliosis can arise de novo, can have a degenerative course, and can result in severe back pain. Grubb et al. attempted to differentiate the adults with preexisting scoliosis from those with new curves and found that the mean age of the degenerative group was 60 and the female:male ratio was 1:1.[14] Patients with idiopathic scoliosis average 42 years old and are primarily female. Interestingly, both groups had low-back pain with radiation into the buttock region, but the degenerative group demonstrated clinical symptoms of spinal stenosis in 90% of the cases. In particular, pain was exacerbated by hyperextension. In contrast to the usual spinal stenosis patient, pain was not decreased by sitting but rather by supporting their weight with their arms.

In Grubb et al.'s study, radiography demonstrated idiopathic curves from 34 to 78 degrees and degenerative curves from 15 to 53 degrees. Interestingly, the average 9-degree deformity per vertebral segment was the same. This is explained by the degenerative scoliosis usually spanning over fewer vertebral levels. Lateral translation was much more common in the degenerative scoliosis group. The adult-onset degenerative scoliosis group rarely demonstrated increased pain on provocative discogram studies despite radiographic documentation of profoundly degenerated discs, whereas pain by discography was common in the idiopathic adult-onset scoliosis group.

Conservative treatment for patients with degenerative adult scoliosis include nonsteroidal antiinflammatory medications and low-back and abdominal strengthening exercises. Low-impact aerobic exercises and range-of-motion flexibility exercises have become popular. Exercises promoting hyperextension are discouraged for patients showing clinical signs of spinal stenosis.

Braces are prescribed for temporary relief from back pain. Many studies have shown that, other than limited range of motion, they do not support the spine. Female patients who are premenopausal should be encouraged to exercise a minimum of 20 minutes four times a week. Postmenopausal women should be placed on hormonal replacement and daily calcium supplements if their spine appears radiographically osteoporotic.

The primary reason for surgical treatment of adult degenerative scoliosis continues to be pain. Pain secondary to radiculopathy and spinal stenosis is treated with decompression procedures followed by fusion. Fusions are not always required if one nerve root is being compressed and the facet joint can be maintained. A degenerative disc that appears collapsed on lateral roentgenography usually represents a segment with minimal motion and does not necessarily signify instability or the need for automatic fusion. In fact it is the wide disc with surrounding vertebral degenerative changes, near the suspected radiculopathy, that may require a fusion.

Overview

Adult scoliosis is often due to degeneration, osteoporosis, and osteomalacia and often follows multilevel posterior spinal decompression procedures. These patients present with rigid curves, spinal stenosis, and osteopenic bone. The major indication for surgery is pain, especially when the pain has plateaued at a level unacceptable to the patient, represents more than an annoyance, and significantly alters the quality of life. Potential complications of surgery include respiratory distress syndrome, pleural effusions, coagulopathy, infection, partial or complete paralysis, pseudoarthrosis, and iatrogenic hypolordosis.

Degenerative scoliosis (collapsing scoliosis) is one of the most common causes of adult scoliosis. Patients are in their late 50s, have osteoporosis, have compression fractures, have scoliosis ranging between 7 and 50 degrees, and report low-back pain. Spinal stenosis symptoms and increased pain with hyperextension are usually noted. Surgical treatment focuses on a posterior spinal decompression followed by a fusion. The fusion should include vertebrae that demonstrate rotatory subluxation, displacement with wedging, and severe degenerative arthritis and all levels that are pain generators. Hemisacralization and an oblique L5 vertebra indicate the need to include an L5-S1 fusion. A fusion/instrumentation procedure is not always required if one or two roots are responsible for the pain and can be decompressed without creating instability.

Spinal instrumentation procedures have resulted in accelerated degenerative changes at the level adjacent to the fusion. These regions must be evaluated closely on patients who present with pain but have already undergone fusion with instrumentation procedures. Extension of fusion/instrumentation operations has become one of the most common reasons for reoperation in centers that specialize in spinal reconstruction surgery. Fortunately, the use of contoured instrumentation with multiple fixation has resulted in a significant decrease in flat-back syndrome. Lumbosacral fusion is very difficult to attain. Increased success has been found with circumferential fusion and sacral instrumentation using four ala screws. The learning curve for spinal reconstruction surgery is steep but with specialized training, experience, and multidisciplinary support the rewards are significant.

References

1. Allen BL Jr, Ferguson RL: The Galveston technique for L-rod instrumentation of the scoliotic spine, *Spine* 7:276, 1982.
2. Balderston RA, Winter RB, Moe JH, et al.: Fusion to the sacrum for nonparalytic scoliosis in the adult, *Spine* 11:824, 1986.
3. Benner B, Ehni G: Degenerative lumbar scoliosis, *Spine* 4:548, 1979.
4. Bradford DS: Adult scoliosis: current concepts of treatment, *Clin Orthop* 229:70, 1988.
5. Brodsky AE, Binder WF: Lumbar Discography: its value in diagnosis and treatment of lumbar disc lesions, *Spine* 4:110, 1979.
6. Byrd JA III, Scoles PV, Winter RB, et al.: Adult idiopathic scoliosis treated by anterior and posterior spinal fusion, *J Bone Joint Surg* 69A:843, 1987.
7. Coe JD, Becker PS, McAfee PC, Gurr KR: Neuropathy with spinal instrumentation, *J Orthop Res* 7:359, 1989.
8. Cotrel Y: *Instrumentation for surgery of the spine*, 1986, Freud Publishing House, Ltd.
9. Cotrel Y, Dubousset J, Guillaumat M: New universal instrumentation in spinal surgery, *Clin Orthop* 227:10, 1988.
10. Denis F: Cotrel-Dubousset instrumentation in the treatment of idiopathic scoliosis, *Orthop Clin North Am* 19:291, 1988.
11. Dwyer AF: Experience of anterior correction of scoliosis, *Clin Orthop* 93:191, 1973.
12. Epstein JA, Epstein BS, Jones MD: Symptomatic lumbar scoliosis with degenerative changes in the elderly, *Spine* 4:542, 1979.
13. Goldner JL, Urbaniak Jr, McCollum DE: Anterior disc excision and interbody spinal fusion for chronic low back pain, *Orthop Clin North Am* 2:543, 1971.
14. Grubb SA, Lipscomb HJ, Coonrad RW: Degenerative adult onset scoliosis, *Spine* 13:241, 1988.
15. Haher JE, Devlin V, Freeman B, Rondon B: Long term effects of sublaminar wires on the neural canal, *Orthop Trans* 11:106, 1987.
16. Hall JE: Dwyer instrumentation in anterior fusion of the spine, *J Bone Joint Surg* 63A:1188, 1981.
17. Harrington PR, Dickson JH: An eleven-year clinical investigation of Harrington instrumentation: a preliminary report on 578 cases, *Clin Orthop* 93:113, 1973.
18. Herndon WA, Sullivan JA, Yneve DA, et al.: Segmental spinal instrumentation with sublaminar wires, *J Bone Joint Surg* 69:851, 1987.
19. Herring JA, Wenger DR: Segmental spinal instrumentation: a preliminary report of 40 consecutive cases, *Spine* 7:285, 1982.
20. Hoover NW: Indications for fusion at the time of removal of intervertebral disc, *J Bone Joint Surg* 50:189, 1968.
21. Jackson RP, Simmons EH, Stripinis D: Incidence and severity of back pain in adult idiopathic scoliosis, *Spine* 8:749, 1983.
22. Johnson JR, Holt RT: Combined use of anterior and posterior surgery for adult scoliosis, *Orthop Clin North Am* 19:361, 1988.
23. Johnston CE II, Happel LT Jr, Norris R, et al.: Delayed paraplegia complicating sublaminar segmental spinal instrumentation, *J Bone Joint Surg* 68:556, 1986.
24. Kaneda K, Fujiya N, Satoa S: Results with Zielke instrumentation for idiopathic thoracolumbar and lumbar scoliosis, *Clin Orthop* 205:195, 1986.
25. Kostuik JP: *Adult scoliosis*. Frymoyer JW, editor: *The adult spine, principles and practice*, New York, 1991, Raven Press, Ltd.
26. Kostuik JP: Decision making in adult scoliosis, *Spine* 4:521, 1979.
27. Kostuik JP, Bentivoglio J: The incidence of low back pain in adult scoliosis, *Spine* 6:268, 1981.
28. Kostuik JP, Carl A, Ferron S: Anterior Zielke instrumentation for spinal deformity in adults, *J Bone Joint Surg* 71:898, 1989.
29. Kostuik JP, Hall BB: Spinal fusions to the sacrum in adults with scoliosis, *Spine* 8:489, 1983.
30. Kostuik JP, Maurais GR, Richardson WJ: Primary fusion to the sacrum using Luque instrumentation for adult scoliotic patients, *Orthop Trans* 13:30, 1989.
31. Kostuik JP, Worden HR, Salo P: Long term functional outcome following surgery for adult scoliosis, presented at the American Orthopedic Association meeting, Boston, 1990.
32. Louis DK, Ponsetti IV: Long term follow-up of patients with idiopathic scoliosis not treated surgically, *J Bone Joint Surg* 51:425, 1969.
33. Luque ER: Segmental spinal instrumentation for correction of scoliosis, *Clin Orthop* 163:192, 1982.
34. Luque ER: The anatomic basis and development of segmental spinal instrumentation, *Spine* 7:256, 1982.
35. Moe JH, Purcell GA, Bradford DS: Zielke instrumentation (VDS) for the correction of spinal curvature: analysis of results in 66 patients, *Clin Orthop* 180:133, 1983.
36. Nachemson A: A longterm follow-up study of nontreated scoliosis, *J Bone Joint Surg* 50A:203, 1969.
37. Nachemson A: Adult scoliosis and back pain, *Spine* 4:513, 1979.
38. Nash CL Jr, Moe JH: A study of vertebral rotation, *J Bone Joint Surg* 51A:223, 1969.
39. Nilsonne U, Lunderen KD: Longterm prognosis in idiopathic scoliosis, *Acta Orthop Scand* 39:455, 1968.

40. O'Brien JP: The role of fusion for chronic low back pain, *Orthop Clin North Am* 14:639, 1983.

41. Ogiela DM, Chan DPK: Ventral derotation spondylodesis: a review of 22 cases, *Spine* 11:18, 1986.

42. Robin GC, Span Y, Steinberg R, et al.: Scoliosis in the elderly: a follow-up study, *Spine* 7:355, 1982.

43. Saands AR Jr, Eisberg HB: The incidence of scoliosis in the state of Delaware, *J Bone Joint Surg* 37A:1243, 1955.

44. Simmons EH, Segil CM: An evaluation of discography in the localization of symptomatic levels in discogenic disease of the spine, *Clin Orthop* 108:57, 1975.

45. Selby DK: Internal fixation with Knodt rods, *Clin Orthop* 203:179, 1986.

46. Thompson GH, Wilber RG, Shaffer JW, et al.: Segmental spinal instrumentation in idiopathic scoliosis: a preliminary report, *Spine* 10:623, 1985.

47. Weinstein SL, Ponsetti IV: Curve progression in idiopathic scoliosis, *J Bone Joint Surg* 65A:447, 1983.

48. Winter RB: Combined Dwyer and Harrington instrumentation and fusion in the treatment of selected patients with painful adult idiopathic scoliosis, *Spine* 3:135, 1988.

49. Zielke K, Stunkat R, Beaujean F: Venture Derotations-Spondylodese, *Arch Orthop Unfauchir* 85:257, 1976.

Chapter III

Clinical Cervical Deformity and Postlaminectomy Kyphosis

Edward D. Simmons

Peter N. Capicotto

Classification

Evaluation

Imaging

Postlaminectomy Kyphosis

    incidence
    pathogenesis
    management: prevention of deformity
    management: established deformity
    postoperative management

Degenerative Cervical Kyphosis with Myeloradiculopathy

    surgical treatment
    alternative surgical procedures

Kyphosis Secondary to Tumor

Neuromyopathic Flexion Deformity

Surgical Techniques

    keystone anterior fusion
    Dewar posterior cervical fusion

Torticollis

    techniques of C1-C2 fusion
    alternative procedures

Deformities of the cervical spine, including post-laminectomy kyphosis, present some of the most challenging and difficult problems spine surgeons may confront. This chapter will deal mainly with adult deformities, excluding spondyloarthropathies. It will also cover surgical intervention for torticollis.

Classification

A classification scheme exists that is similar to that used for the thoracic and lumbar spine (see box below).

Classification for Cervical Deformity

- Congenital
  Klippel-Feil
- Inflammatory
  Septic
  Rheumatoid
  Seronegative spondyloarthropathies
- Posttraumatic/traumatic
- Tumor—primary, metastatic
- Iatrogenic/postlaminectomy kyphosis
- Neuromyopathic flexion deformity

Evaluation

In assessing cervical deformities one must know the patient's entire medical history, including a detailed account of neurologic disorders, tumors, previous surgery, radiation, or trauma to the cervical spine. Systemic arthropathies also need to be identified and evaluated.

The rapidity with which the deformity developed should be known. Was it over a short period of time, as may occur with fractures in ankylosing spondylitis, or has it been gradual, occurring over years, as in simple spondylosis or myopathic deformities?

Is the deformity associated with pain? The quality and location may help in determining the etiology. Is there associated pain or neurologic signs in the upper or lower extremities suggesting a myeloradiculopathy? This will determine the sequence and type of operative procedure required.

Finally, the impact of the deformity on the patient's daily function must be known. For example, the inability to masticate or episodic choking are frequent problems in those with chin-on-chest deformity. Severe anxiety due to restricted field of vision and inability to ambulate safely may warrant operative correction.

The physical should include a detailed neurologic examination and assessment of degree of the deformity by the chin-brow to vertical angle as described by Simmons (Fig. 111-1). Also the amount of passive and active correction that exists must be evaluated.

Imaging

Imaging should include a standard cervical spine series with supervised flexion-extension views if there are neurologic abnormalities. Particular attention must be paid to the C1-C2 complex and the cervicothoracic junction. Tomography is useful in these regions.

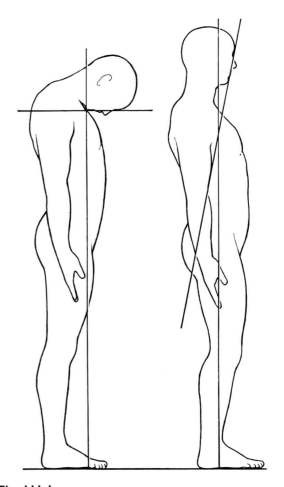

Fig. 111-1

Measurement of the chin-brow to vertical angle. With the neck in its neutral or fixed position and with knees and hips extended, the angle between vertical and a line tangent to the chin and brow is measured. *(Redrawn from Simmons EH, Bradley D: Neuromyopathic flexion deformities of the cervical spine, Spine 13:756, 1988.)*

CT scanning should be used when assessing osseous destruction and postmyelographically in cases in which neurologic deficits exist.

MRI is used to identify extradural or intradural processes and is helpful in assessing regional spread of soft-tissue masses.

Postlaminectomy Kyphosis

Since the advent of laminectomy for spinal tumors by MacEwen,[51] there has always been a concern over the potential for instability of the laminectomized spine. Following laminectomy of the cervical spine, the most common deformity that occurs is kyphosis. It may be a sharp angular type or a gentle curve. Often with unilateral facetectomies there may be associated scoliosis. Lonstein found that approximately two thirds of patients with kyphotic deformities also had an element of scoliosis postlaminectomy.[47] In 1974 Sim et al. described a swan-neck deformity following extensive laminectomy.[63] This was characterized by progressive subluxation and kyphosis accompanied by a compensatory lordosis cephalad to the laminectomy site. They noted that the most severe angular deformities occurred at the cervicothoracic junction, while bilateral laminectomies of the fourth to the sixth cervical vertebrae led to moderate deformities.

Incidence

The incidence of postlaminectomy deformity has always been a point of controversy. Reports vary from 30% to 80%.[47] Since the writings of Haft et al.[40] and Bette and Engelhardt,[13] it has been known that postlaminectomy deformities are much more common in the child and adolescent.[75] Rogers[62] and Jenkins[44] noted that instability was rare in adults. In a literature review of four series Lonstein noted an incidence of 49% in 251 children undergoing multilevel laminectomy for a variety of reasons.[47] Bell et al. noted a 38% incidence of kyphosis and a 15% incidence of hyperlordosis or swan neck in 132 children after cervical laminectomy.[10] Aronson et al. found a 95% incidence of instability when laminectomy was combined with suboccipital decompression for Arnold-Chiari malformations.[5] Interestingly however, isolated suboccipital decompressions have not led to deformity.

Yasouka et al., reporting on 58 patients who underwent multilevel laminectomy for conditions that in themselves would not produce deformity, found a 46% incidence in those aged less than 15 years and a 6% incidence in those 15 to 24 years old.[81] How-

ever, kyphosis developed in all patients after cervical laminectomy. This review is important because many of the previous reports dealt with patients whose underlying diagnoses were mixed, including conditions that by themselves potentiated or caused deformity.

The true incidence of postlaminectomy deformity in adults is even less clear. Laminectomy remains one of the most common approaches for myeloradiculopathy over multiple segments. Fortunately, the presence of spondylosis is thought to add some stability. Despite this, the presence of preoperative instability or kyphosis is potentiated postoperatively and can lead to a severe progressive deformity.

Thus, the incidence of postlaminectomy kyphosis is thought to depend on: (1) age, (2) underlying diagnosis—that is tumors or intrinsic cord abnormalities that produce instability or deformity themselves, (3) preoperative curvature of the cervical spine or existing instability, and (4) degree of posterior resection—cervical laminectomy with preservation of facets is well tolerated in adults and less so in children, in whom more dynamic factors are acting upon growing structures. Jenkins,[44] Albouker et al.,[3] and others[30,75] have not encountered postoperative deformity in adult patients undergoing cervical laminectomy and limited foraminotomy. Epstein[28,29] recommended that not more than one fourth to one third of the facets be excised. Biomechanical experiments have shown that bilateral facetectomy of greater than 50% significantly decreases the resistance to flexion-axial loading and rotation.[22,60,85] Besides the width of the decompression, the length may also become a risk factor. Yasouka,[81] Fraser,[35] and Mikawa[52] and their colleagues found no correlation between the number of laminae removed and postoperative instability. However, numbers were small in their series. Katsumi et al.,[45] in analyzing cervical instability resulting from laminectomy for spinal cord tumor, found a C2 laminectomy to be a definite risk factor even in adults. Nolan and Sherk have found that the head and neck extensors (semispinalis, cervicis, and capitis) insert into the arch of the axis.[55] Thus, they advocate preserving the arch of C2 to maintain the dynamic head and neck extensors. It has been shown clinically that extensor myopathies or neuropathies can lead to deformities even in the intact spine.[68] Thus, theoretically, disruption of the extensors and their insertions surgically could potentiate an instability pattern.

Pathogenesis

Pal and Sherk demonstrated that in axial loading 64% of the load is transmitted distally through the intact lateral masses; the remainder of the load is borne through the anterior column.[56] Despite its lordotic posturing, however, gravity normally exerts a flexion moment on the cervical spine. This flexion moment is greatest at the cervico-thoracic junction. Under normal conditions the posterior osseous and ligamentous complex resist these flexion and compression forces. Disruption of these structures leads to loss of the counteractive force. This unstable situation eventually may ultimately lead to deformity. Gentle kyphotic deformities may result with isolated laminectomy and its intended disruption of the posterior elements.

In children deformities are potentiated by the vertebral wedging that occurs as a result of excess anterior compression and eventual growth plate arrest. In a similar manner, radiation for spinal tumors leads to anterior growth arrest and exacerbation of kyphotic deformities.

Another mechanical factor that has been cited by Fielding and Hawkins for the increased incidence of deformity in children has been the more horizontally oriented facets compared to adults.[32] These resist translational motions poorly and with violation of the facet capsule a sharp angular kyphosis occurs. If unilateral laminectomy or facetectomy is performed a kyphoscoliosis may result.

Management: Prevention of Deformity

Following multiple level cervical laminectomy, we agree with Yasouka et al. that those under 25 years of age should be evaluated for a minimum of 6 years postoperatively on an annual basis at least.[80] Even in adults, especially those with bilateral facetectomy, multilevel laminectomy inclusive of C2 or other risk factors, it would be wise to have annual follow-up for several years. Halo bracing may be effective in childhood and adolescence, but plays little role in preventing deformity in the adult. Once deformity is present in the adult or child, bracing should be replaced by fusion.

Treatment is thus directed at prevention of deformity or progression once identified. Prophylactic stabilization may be performed at the time of decompression. Lonstein and Yasouka recommended delaying prophylactic fusion until 1 week postoperatively.[47,80,81] They thought this prevented hematoma formation and cord compression, especially if durotomy had been performed. A variety of posterior stabilization techniques have been described. Callahan et al. recommended facet wiring and onlay iliac or rib grafts in adults, especially those with preexisting deformities or evidence of instability (Fig. 111-

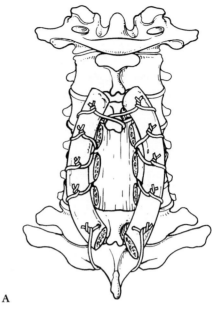

A

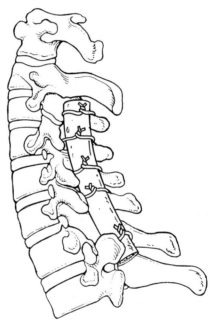

B

Fig. 111-2

Facet fusions postlaminectomy with rib or iliac graft wired into place. Following periosteal exposure and currettement of facet joints, 24-gauge wire is passed through the inferior facet and either rib or iliac strut graft is wired into the lordotic contour. The fusion should extend into at least one intact level. **A,** posterior view. **B,** lateral view demonstrating lordotic curve. *(Redrawn from Callahan RA, Johnson RM, Morgolis, RN, et al.: Cervical facet fusion for control of instability following laminectomy, J Bone Joint Surg 69A:991, 1977.)*

2).[18] This technique may be modified using Luque segmental fixation (Fig. 111-3). The fusion should include one level below and extend to the exposed facet joint above the laminectomy. The indications

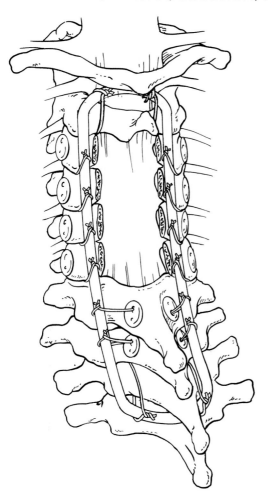

Fig. 111-3

Stabilization postlaminectomy using segmental facet and spinous process wires with contoured Luque rectangle. This technique is useful in cases where correction of deformity occurs and in those requiring long fusions, especially in patients in whom autografts may be mechanically deficient.

for fusion in children are not well defined. A treating physician must weigh the patient's life expectancy and risk factors for progression prior to embarking on an additional stabilization procedure.

Anterior fusion may be used in cases with nearly deficient facets or it may be used to supplement posterior fusion. One must realize that anterior grafts alone may be unstable and fail to provide immediate stability.

Management: Established Deformity

Once deformity is present it is progressive, and prompt surgical intervention needs to be considered. Lonstein and Cho have demonstrated the failure of bracing in preventing deformity even in the pediatric population.[49]

Treatment should begin with gentle halo traction. During this period close observation must be rendered, particularly in those with preoperative neurologic deficits. Often patients have had preoperative radiation and intramedullary or intradural procedures that may lead to a compromised spinal cord reserve capacity. Traction must be discontinued if a neurologic deficit develops or progresses.

The preferred surgical approach is anterior, particularly in severe fixed deformities. It not only allows decompression and osteotomy of the rigid fused kyphotic spine, but places the graft under compression favoring osseous union. In addition it has been pointed out by Lonstein[48] that posterior procedures may technically be difficult. This is because of scarring with increased risk of incidental durotomy and the small area available for instrumentation and grafting.

A variety of techniques exist for anterior fusion. They include the Smith-Robinson,[71] Bailey-Badgley,[8] Cloward,[19] and Simmons keystone[67] techniques and Whitecloud's fibular strut.[77] The preferred technique utilizes a corticocancellous strut following corpectomies. Multiple interbody fusions have proven to be unstable in similar conditions with associated significant nonunion rates.[9,72] In situations such as short sharp angular kyphosis requiring corpectomies and possible osteotomies of less than three bodies, our preferred technique is an autogenous keystone type graft because of its inherent stability and high union rate (Fig. 111-4). With involvement of three or more vertebral bodies Whitecloud and LaRocca[77] have demonstrated success in using fibular autograft in a dovetail type of construct for cervical myelopathy (Fig. 111-5). They thought the graft provided structural support while incorporating fairly rapidly with a 100% union rate. Zdeblick and Bohlman demonstrated the success of a similar technique whereby the fibular ends are rounded and seated entirely within troughs made in the vertebral bodies (Fig. 111-6).[83] The difficulty with fibular grafts is at the cervicothoracic junction, where most deformities take place. Here the thoracic spine turns posteriorly, making an interference fit with a straight fibular graft difficult. A keystone type of graft at this position using allograft iliac crest bone from the iliac wing will allow contouring of the graft, enabling it to match the reversal of kyphosis at the cervicothoracic junction. Besides the ability to select a properly shaped graft, other advantages include the avoidance of graft-site pain, hematoma, cluneal or lateral femoral cutaneous nerve damage, and infections. One has to factor in the delayed incorporation rate and the possibility of disease transmission when using allografts. Wittenberg et al.

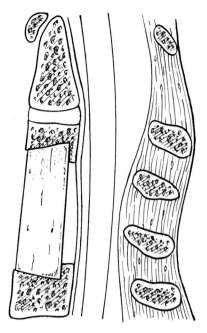

Fig. 111-4

Keystone iliac or fibular strut. Release of traction locks the graft in place. It is important to leave a lip of posterior cortex intact to prevent posterior extrusion.

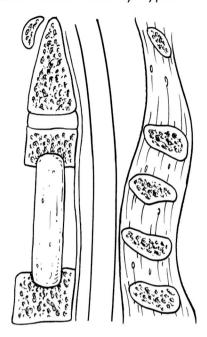

Fig. 111-6

Bohlman's technique of countersinking graft. The wide portion of the graft is placed posteriorly. *(Redrawn from Zdeblich T, Bohlman H: Cervical kyphosis and myelopathy, J Bone Joint Surg 71A:170, 1989.)*

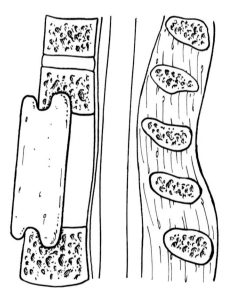

Fig. 111-5

Whitecloud technique. Dovetailing of fibular graft minimizes chance of extrusion while providing stability following multilevel corpectomy. *(Redrawn from Wood EG III, Hanley EN: Types of anterior cervical grafts, Ortho Clin North Am 23:475, 1992.)*

have demonstrated the biomechanical superiority of fibular autografts and allografts to those of anterior and posterior iliac crests.[79] However, they also thought that all three graft types may still provide sufficient strength in vivo. Several studies have

demonstrated no adverse effect of the preservation process on mechanical properties.[70,79] Clinically, many surgeons have reported favorable results with allografts in anterior cervical surgery.[16,42,84] In patients who require long struts we recommend additional posterior stabilization with autogenous grafting.

Circumferential fusion provides additional stability, thus preventing recurrence of deformity. Nakata et al. reported higher fusion rates with circumferential fusion.[54] They found a 90% union rate compared to 75% and 50% for anterior or posterior procedures alone, respectively.

With the introduction of anterior cervical spine plating systems, immediate postoperative stability may be realized. Plates may obviate the need for additional posterior stabilization and the need for halo immobilization postoperatively. Biomechanical data indicate that plating definitely adds stability, yet it is thought to be inferior to an additional posterior stabilization.[2,20,53,73,76] Evidence has suggested clinically that, even with traumatic posterior disruption, certain anterior plating devices provide adequate stability obviating the need for halos, despite biomechanical evidence to the contrary.[36] Their role in postlaminectomy kyphosis remains to be defined.

Postoperative Management

One must consider the age, location and degree of deformity, patient's compliance, and construct stability prior to recommending the length of bed rest and immobilization. At present, we would recommend a halo cast or vest for at least 4 months in an ambulatory setting.

Degenerative Cervical Kyphosis with Myeloradiculopathy

Infrequently, cervical spondylosis will present with gross kyphotic deformity. Physical examination will usually reveal loss of rotation, flexion, and extension with associated crepitation. Pain and tenderness are seldom major symptoms. Although the true incidence of associated myeloradiculopathy is not known, it does occur and would be the major indication for surgical intervention in degenerative disease with kyphosis.

As explained by Batzdorf,[6] spondylosis consists of annular protrusion secondary to degenerative changes of the intervertebral discs. Loss of water content, decreased disc height, and anterior wedging may set the stage for progressive collapse and kyphosis. With repetitive micro or macro trauma the posterior elements become incompetent, allowing for further wedging of both disc and osteopenic bone. The effect of vascular disturbances at both the cord and the vertebral body level in this cascade is not well understood and actually may play a significant role. This is in contrast to Hadley, who thought in the absence of macro trauma that the cervical spine maintains its normal lordotic posturing despite advanced spondylosis.[39]

The development of myeloradiculopathy is dependent on both mechanical and vascular factors extrinsic to the cord.[1,57] Congenital cervical stenosis with a canal size of less then 13 mm is a major predisposing factor.[4,25] This, coupled with chondroosseous spurs and abnormal motion, as pointed out by Robinson, is the basic etiology of myelopathy.[61]

Although the canal is narrowed in extension, with flexion (despite a slight increase in canal diameter) the cord itself becomes stretched and flattened over the anterior osteophytes. This leads to both mechanical compression as well as the vascular insufficiency culminating in a myeloradiculopathy.

Once myelopathy occurs, complete remission never occurs. The course can be variable, and despite numerous studies, precise prognostication of those who will or will not have progression is difficult.[11] Thus, treatment must be based on degree of neurologic impairment, documented progression, specific disability, age, and general medical condition of the patient.

Surgical Treatment

The specific approach to surgical treatment of multilevel myelopathy has been a source of considerable controversy. Laminectomy with or without posterior fusion, laminoplasty, vertebrectomy, or multilevel discectomy and interbody fusions all have clinical, biologic, and mechanical data to support their use. However, in cases with associated kyphosis the pendulum swings strongly in favor of anterior vertebrectomy and strut grafting. Epstein, a proponent of laminectomy, does not advise posterior decompression alone in kyphotic deformities.[28] Elegant work by Batzdorf and Batzdorf demonstrated the inadequacy of posterior decompression to allow clearance of anterior osteophytes in the kyphotic spine.[7] Tencer et al. demonstrated the lack of posterior dural deflection with anterior impingement in the kyphotic thoracic spine.[74] This was thought to demonstrate the lack of true decompressive effect by laminectomy.

Thus, the recommended approach would be anterior decompression with keystone iliac or fibular strut grafting. Preoperative traction may be effective, since this is usually a fairly stiff curve and in some cases a compression arthrodesis has developed. Intraoperatively, halo traction of approximately 5 kg would be sufficient. Spinal cord monitoring is routinely used. We prefer a right-sided approach, and if decompressing over three levels, a longitudinal incision along the anterior border of the sternocleidomastoid would be used in lieu of a transverse incision. We have preferred the right-sided approach for a right-handed surgeon because this avoids the thoracic duct if decompression is carried out at the cervicothoracic junction. However, one has to be concerned with the recurrent laryngeal nerve and its aberrancies prior to embarking on the right-sided approach.

Decompression should be back to but not through the posterior longitudinal ligament. For decompressing the posterior vertebral cortex a diamond burr or curettes may be used. After release and decompression, the neck is gently extended along with increasing weight of traction. Postoperatively a four poster brace is used for any patient who has had a two-level corporectomy or less. A halo is recommended for all others for at least 12 weeks.

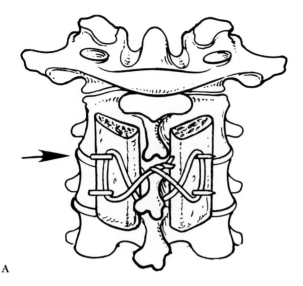

A

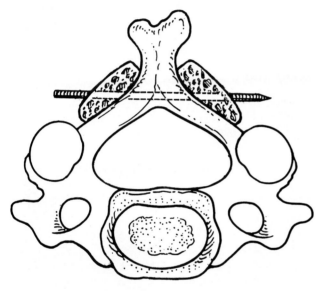

B

Fig. 111-7

Dewar Fusion. **A,** The combination of figure eight tension band wiring and bone plates provides immediate stability. **B,** Compere pin should be placed as low as possible in the spinous process.

Alternative Surgical Procedures

The indications for anterior cervical instrumentation remain to be elucidated in this disease. We have used it in patients with poor interference fit in whom dislodgment of the graft is of particular concern and fusions extend three or more levels.

The Dewar posterior cervical fusion is our preferred technique when contemplating a circumferential fusion in those who have had a previous anterior procedure.[12,23] This technique offers a superior rigidity and a high rate of fusion (Fig. 111-7).[64]

If posterior elements are nonexistent, facet fusion with Luque segmental wiring or lateral mass plating may be required. (Figs. 111-8 and 111-9).

Kyphosis Secondary to Tumor

Tumors of the cervical spine are rare. Deformities can range from torticollis, as seen in osteoid osteoma, to kyphosis or kyphoscoliosis, or even spondyloptosis and fixed atlantooccipital subluxation.[32,59] Tumors of the cervical spine in children are likely to be benign, whereas those in adults are more likely to be metastatic.

Metastatic lesions usually cause symptoms prior to gross destruction and rarely present with deformity. Similar to the thoracic and lumbar spine the vertebral body is commonly the initial site of spread. Radiographically, the initial finding is that of pedicle destruction.

Less common but of similar importance are primary tumors. These include the benign tumors, osteoid osteoma, aneurysmal bone cyst, and giant-cell tumors as well as malignant tumors, of which multiple myeloma is the most common.

Perhaps the most common tumor discussed in regard to deformity is neurofibromatosis. It is estimated that 30% of patients who have von Recklinghausen disease with spinal involvement will have abnormalities of the cervical spine.[82] Craig and Govender reported on eight patients in whom cervical kyphosis of up to 90 degrees was the dominant feature.[21] The vast majority had complete destruction or deficiencies of the vertebral bodies. They had best results with anterior strut grafting. This was done with and without a posterior procedure. Winter et al. recommended anterior and posterior fusions in those with dystrophic kyphoscoliosis and neurofibromatosis of the thoracic spine.[78]

Fielding et al. reported on 20 patients in whom corpectomy was used to treat a cervical tumor.[34] Thirteen had additional posterior stabilization, seven of which were done prior to the anterior procedure.

Bohlman et al., in their review of primary neoplasms of the cervical spine, recommended anterior and posterior resection if two-column instability existed.[14] They also recognized that total excision is not feasible but intralesional excision should be used to decompress neural and vascular structures.

In any type of pathologic fracture with kyphosis, two-column instability may exist. The recommended treatment would be determined by the degree of deformity and the neurologic status. For patients with mild to moderate kyphotic deformities without

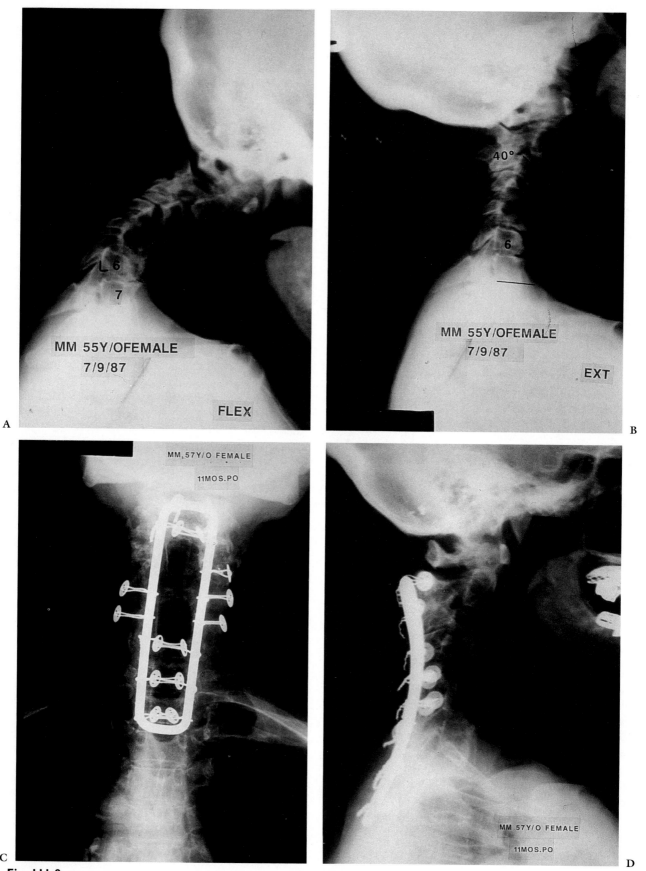

Fig. 111-8

56-Year-old female post C3-C7 laminectomy and subsequent C4-C5 discectomy and fusion without relief of myelopathy. She had developed a progressive cervical kyphosis. **A** and **B,** demonstrate the flexibility of this deformity by flexion extension views. **C** and **D,** demonstrate postoperative radiographs following staged anterior decompression of C3-C4, C5-C6, C6-C7 with secondary posterior Luque segmental instrumentation and fusion.

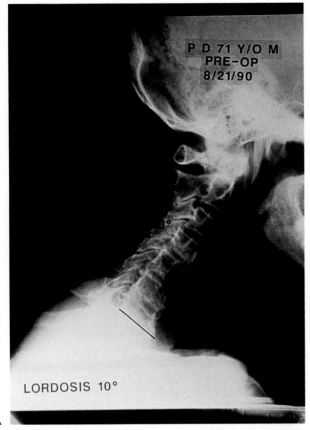

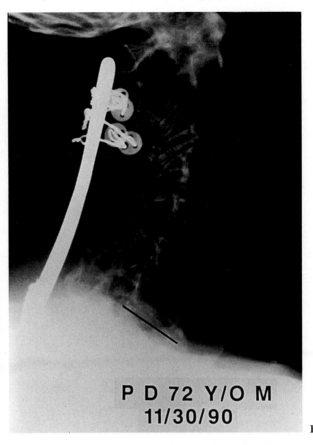

Fig. 111-9

A, 71-Year-old male with myelopathy and flexion deformity. **B,** After laminectomies and foraminotomies C4, C5, C6, and C7 normal lordosis was reestablished using Luque segmental instrumentation and autogenous iliac crest graft. This allows cord to float posteriorly.

myelopathy, a 5- to 7-day period of halo traction with gradual reduction would be attempted. Following acceptable reduction, a posterior arthrodesis would be performed extending at least one level above and one level below the planned anterior arthrodesis (Fig. 111-10). For those situations, a Luque rectangle with facet wiring, spinous process wiring, or even sublaminar wires have worked well. If lateral masses are intact, lateral mass plates may be also used. In younger patients with good quality iliac crest a Dewar type fusion works well providing the posterior elements are not involved with tumor themselves. Following the posterior procedure an anterior procedure would be performed. It is elected to perform the posterior procedure first in order to secure stability prior to embarking on the anterior procedure. Patients with severe deformity and myelopathy may tolerate traction poorly. In such cases it may be beneficial to decompress and strut graft anteriorly, obtaining gentle correction and then a fusing posteriorly according to the same guidelines.

Allograft iliac or fibular strut can be used also in those with a limited lifespan, but we recommend autogenous bone grafting posteriorly. This may be supplemented with morselized allogeneic bone graft. Hanley and Enneking have shown that allograft struts will incorporate over a long period.[27,42]

Methylmethacrylate has been used to obtain immediate stability in tumor surgery. We would recommend that cement be used only in those with a limited lifespan and that it be used anteriorly under compression. Numerous reports have been written on the hazards and the biologic ill effects that methylmethacrylate can have when used, especially under tension.[24,50]

The circumferential procedure may be staged or performed at one setting. Postoperatively if fixation is rigid a four-poster or Somi-type brace may be used. No hesitation should exist to use halos if stability is still questionable.

Again, the effectiveness of anterior plating is not widely known and may prove to obviate the need for a posterior procedure.

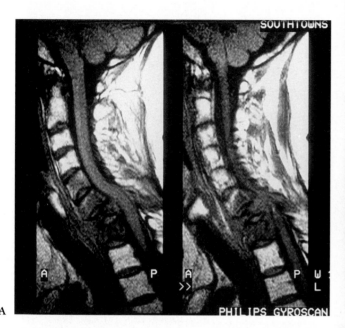

A

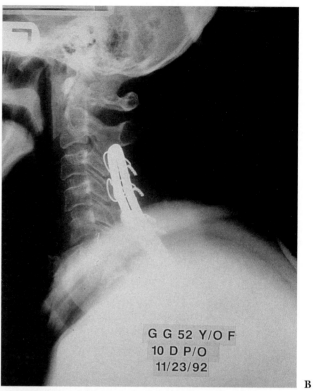

B

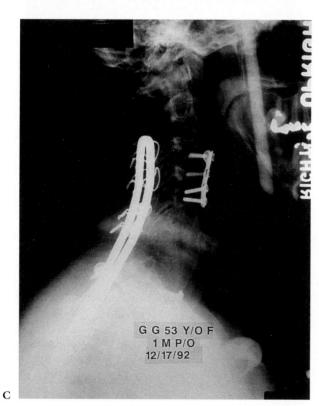

C

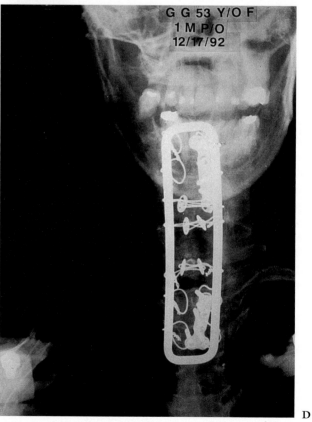

D

Fig. 111-10

Metastatic breast cancer with pathologic fracture and local kyphosis causing myeloradiculopathy. **A,** MRI demonstrates cord deformation. **B,** Following preoperative reduction with halo-traction, posterior instrumentation and fusion from C3-T3 was performed. **C** and **D,** Following the posterior procedure a mutlilevel vertebrectomy and fusion C5-T1 using allograft iliac crest contoured to the lordotic segment was performed. Plates were used to achieve additional stability.

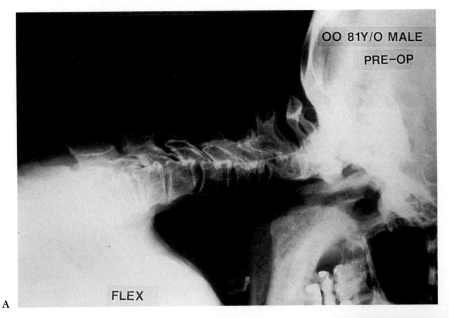

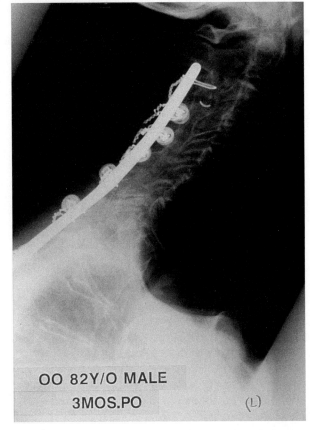

Fig. 111-11
Neuromyopathic flexion deformity chin-brow vertical angle measured 60° clinically. **A,** Lateral C-spine x-ray demonstrated deformity located mainly in lower cervical and cervical-thoracic junction. **B,** Postoperative lateral radiograph following C3 to T3 posterolateral fusion and Luque instrumentation. Patient went on to solid fusion.

Neuromyopathic Flexion Deformity

A small subset of patients will have a chin-on-chest deformity on the basis of a neuropathic or myopathic condition. Simmons and Bradley reported first on six patients with severe flexion deformities without a history of ankylosing spondylitis, trauma, or laminectomy.[68] Degenerative changes were variable, as was the rapidity with which deformity developed. The recommendation was that if cases are suspected, blood studies, electromyograms, and muscle biopsies should be performed. In conditions such as myasthenia gravis, treatment of the underlying disorder may be enough if the deformity is not fixed. In spasm-producing disorders such as Parkinson disease, anterior muscle release and halo support may be enough.

In myopathies of long duration with fixed deformity and/or inactive extensor muscles, a short duration of halo traction with or without anterior release, followed by posteroinferior facet resection and fusion with Luque rectangle and Drummond buttons is the preferred technique (Fig. 111-11). The fusion should be of sufficient length to prevent deformity above. Postoperatively patients are protected in a halo for 3 months followed by bracing for an additional 1 to 3 months in a four-poster or Philadelphia collar–type brace.

Surgical Techniques

Keystone Anterior Fusion

After a standard anterior approach has been made and the correct levels identified a number 15 blade is used to enter the disc spaces involved. Once the disc spaces are emptied, a special set of shoulder chisels are used to create a keystone configuration. Alternatively, an oscillating saw or burr can be used to fashion the keystone bed, particularly in myelopathic patients with congenital stenosis. If no decompression is required the posterior cortex of all the vertebrae involved are left intact. At this point with a rigid kyphotic deformity they may require resection back to the posterior longitudinal ligament in order to obtain some correction. Care must be taken to place the osteotomy site in the central position and that the side walls are cut in the true anterior and posterior planes in order to avoid damage to neural or vascular structures.

The dimensions of the keystone osteotomy are recorded and a rectangular-shaped graft is taken from the iliac crest. After measuring to fit into the distracted space of the osteotomy site, the superior and inferior ends of this tricortical graft are then beveled approximately 14 to 18 degrees. Repeat anterior and posterior measurements are made to ensure that no canal encroachment has occurred and that the graft is driven into place with the neck in distraction. This can be accomplished by halter traction or by the caspar cervical retractor. Cancellous bone is packed around the edges. X-ray studies may be performed at this point. The wound is then closed over a Penrose drain.

The advantages of the keystone technique for this type of procedure is that it provides a large surface area to encourage fusion. Simmons and Bhalla showed that it has approximately 30% more surface area than a Cloward technique type of fusion.[67] The keystone configuration in addition is inherently more stable in resisting extrusion with hyperextension and has demonstrated a much greater stability to lateral bending than a Cloward-type fusion. Light and Simmons,[46] using the keystone technique reported a 100% fusion rate in one-level discectomy and fusions. They also reported an 86% fusion rate for two-level keystone fusions and an 80% fusion rate for three-level keystone fusions.

Complications

Complications are those of anterior cervical surgery and include neurologic injury at both cord and root level, vertebral artery injury if decompression is carried out too widely, and respiratory obstruction post-extubation in those who are myelopathic.[26] Delayed union or nonunion of the graft, graft extrusion, or collapse can also occur. There are inherent risks to the approach alone. On the right side a recurrent laryngeal nerve may be damaged, leading to hoarseness. This has been reported to occur in 10% to 11% of cases, most of them being transient.[43] If you are working at the cervicothoracic junction, a pneumothorax must be carefully avoided, and if one does occur a chest tube should be placed. When approaching from the left side, to avoid the recurrent laryngeal nerve, one must be aware that the thoracic duct empties into the trunk of the subclavian artery, which may be injured when working low in this area. If this does occur, ligation of the thoracic duct should be undertaken. Finally, cervical spinal fluid leaks especially when decompressing for myelopathy is a definite concern. If this occurs, initial steps should be taken for a fascial or muscle patch with abundant gelfoam and a lumbar subarachnoid drain placed to shunt cervical spinal fluid.

"Dewar" Posterior Cervical Fusion

The Dewar technique has proven useful in conditions such as posttraumatic instability or kyphosis. Other indications for its use include (1) instability associated with tumors provided that the posterior elements are intact, (2) nonunions, and (3) circumferential fusions following anterior strut grafting.

The posterior neck is prepared and draped widely to allow percutaneous pin passage well lateral to the incision. A standard posterior approach is used. After meticulous stripping of the spine, the posterior wing of the iliac crest is split to form double corticocancellous grafts. The cancellous surfaces are carefully shaped to conform to the posterior arches and spinous processes in firm apposition.

Threaded Compere pins, varying from 3/32 in. to 7/64 in. in size, are passed percutaneously through the graft on one side, then through the spinous process and the graft on the opposite side, extending a distance adequate to allow for wire fixation around the end of the pin. The pin is then cut to appropriate size leaving enough length protruding from each side to allow for wire fixation. A 20- or 22-gauge wire is placed around the ends of the threaded pins in a figure-eight fashion, enhancing fixation of the grafts to the spine. Additional cancellous bone graft is then placed over the spine on each side of the main strut grafts.

The technique is relatively simple and produces an effective biologic autograft form of internal fixation. The same procedure can be extended for multilevel fusion. One clinical and biomechanical study showed increased stiffness versus the Rogers wiring technique.[64]

Complications

Complications can include loss of reduction secondary to loss of fixation, although this is rare. One must be certain to tighten wires securely, to use wire of sufficient strength, and to avoid kinking or nicking wire. Last but not least, care must be used in placing the Compere pins, avoiding intracanal placement.

Torticollis

The most important aspect of managing torticollis is understanding the differential diagnosis (see box). Congenital conditions associated with torticollis include Klippel-Feil syndrome, congenital wryneck or muscular torticollis, occipitocervical dysplasias, and pterygium coli. The acquired conditions include central nervous system or posterior fossa tumors, ocular dysfunction (abducens nerve palsy), trauma, and inflammatory conditions (i.e., adenitis, osteomyelitis, or juvenile rheumatoid arthritis). Torticollis has also been seen secondary to rheumatoid arthritis and ankylosing spondylitis. Rotational deformity or torticollis is a condition seen mainly in childhood.[58] However, isolated cases in adults have been reported.[31] There have been a few case reports on torticollis secondary to retropharyngeal abscess or Grisel syndrome.[17,37]

In cases with atlantoaxial subluxation or dislocation, the patient will present with a painful torticollis. Unlike the congenital muscular torticollis type, the patient with atlantoaxial subluxation will display a spasm of the sternocleidomastoid on the side contralateral to the rotational deformity.

If the subluxation is severe or chronic, attempts at reduction have a poor prognosis. If the C1-C2 subluxation cannot be reduced, fusion is recommended. Surprisingly, despite fusing in situ the cosmetic deformity may spontaneously correct itself to a moderate degree.

There have been reports on lateral mass collapse in rheumatoid arthritis and ankylosing spondylitis as well as juvenile rheumatoid arthritis leading to torticollis.[41,66] Usually the main symptom is pain, with deformity and dysfunction secondarily. In patients with lateral mass collapse all have been predomi-

Differential Diagnosis for Torticollis

- Congenital
  Congenital muscular torticollis
  Congenital cervical scoliosis
  Occipitocervical anomalies
  Pterygium coli
  Klippel-Feil syndrome

- Acquired
  Traumatic
    Subluxation
    Dislocation
    Fractures
  Neoplastic
    Cerebellar tumors
    Cord tumors
    Vertebral tumors
  Inflammatory
    Intervertebral discitis
    Cervical lymphadenitis
    Ankylosing spondylitis
    Juvenile rheumatoid arthritis
    Rheumatoid arthritis
  Others
    Syringomyelia
    Atlantoaxial rotary displacement

nantly unilateral at either the C1 or C2 level. The head is tilted to the side of the collapse and rotated away. The indication for surgery here is intractable pain. Despite conservative therapy and following fusion in situ the deformity may again correct to a moderate degree.

Techniques of C1-C2 Fusion

A posterior C1-C2 fusion seems to be the safest and most reliable procedure. The posterior methods include (1) Gallie technique with a modified H graft, (2) Brooks technique with a dural bone block graft and dural sublaminar wires, (3) transarticular fixation with screws, and (4) Halifax clamp-type device. Our preferred fusion is with a Gallie technique with a modified H graft (Fig. 111-12).[65] The posterior midline approach is used, which will minimize bleeding. The C2 spinous process is identified by finger palpation. The soft tissues are cleared subperiosteally over C1 and C2. The C2-C3 interspinous ligament must not be damaged during the dissection. Careful stripping of C1 with a Cobb or pusher should not proceed further than 1.5 to 2.0 cm lateral to the midline. This will avoid damaging the vertebral

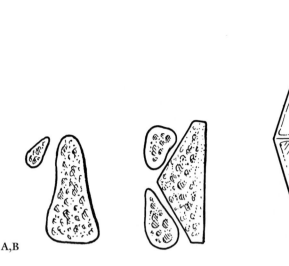

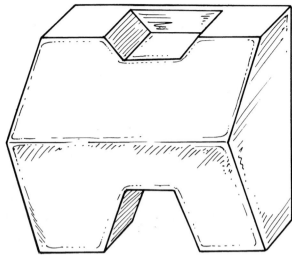

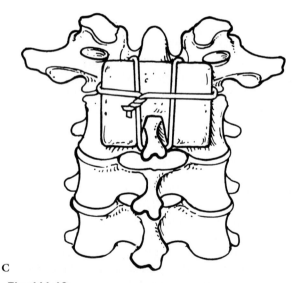

C

Fig. 111-12

Gallie fusion. **A,** The modified graft harvest from the posterior iliac crest. The graft is fashioned to allow maximum bony contact. **B,** A lateral view demonstrates the wedge shape nature of the graft. **C,** Posterior view demonstrating the graft in position. Wire is looped through the C2-C3 interspinous ligament which must be preserved. The wire passes over the C1 lamina then turns inferiorly and is tied over the graft. *(Redrawn from Simmons EH: Ankylosing spondylitis and rheumatoid arthritis. In Lauren CA, et al., editors: An atlas of orthopaedic surgery, Chicago, 1989, Year Book Medical Publishers.)*

artery and vein as it swings over the top of C1. Care is taken then in stripping the ligamentum flavum from the anterior surface of C1 and in passing the wires around the arch of C1.

Gallie uses a modified **H** graft harvested from the posterior iliac crest. A single 22-gauge wire is passed below the C2 spinous process through the C2-C3 interspinous ligament. The two ends are carried upward posterior to the graft and around the notch in its superior portion then under the arch of C1 on each side of the graft. The two ends of wire are tied over the posterior aspect of the graft, locking them into position and pulling back the arch of C1. Passing the wires through the C2-C3 ligament is an important step to prevent dislodgment of the wire.

The grafts should be taken just anterior to the posterosuperior iliac spine, where the crest has a normal external convex cortical surface. This allows enough cancellous bone so contouring the graft can take place to fit well apposed to the posterior arches of C1 and C2. An inverted **V** is cut into the inferior margin of the graft allowing it to sit astride the C2 spinous process. Cancellous chips are placed in the lateral gutters. When passing the wires the ends should be bent back on themselves to avoid dural penetration and a gentle curve should be bent into the end, allowing it to hug the anterior cortex of C1 as it passes around the lamina.

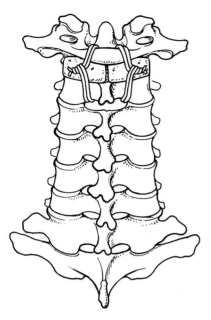

Fig. 111-13

Brooks wedge compression technique. The technique requires passage of double wires. The added stability may obviate the need for halo-immobilization. *(Redrawn from Grub D, et al.: Biomechanical evaluation of four different posterior atlantoaxial fixation techniques, Spine 17:480, 1992.)*

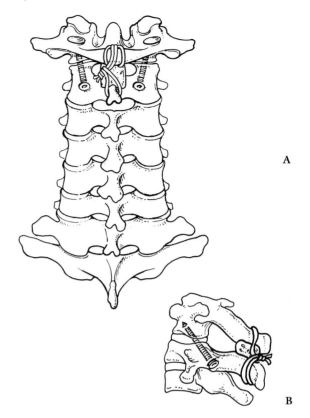

Fig. 111-14

C1-C2 transarticular fixation and posterior interspinous bone block graft and wiring. **A,** Following reduction, transarticular C1-C2 screws are placed and joints packed with cancellous bone. Fixation and grafting may be enhanced by an intraspinous graft as demonstrated here or by a Brook's or Gallie technique. **B,** Lateral view of the transarticular technique. *(Redrawn from Aebi M: Surgical treatment of cervical spine fractures by AO spine technique. In Bridwell K, Dewald RL, editors: The textbook of spinal surgery, New York, 1991, J.B. Lippincott.)*

The patient should then be treated with a halo for approximately 10 to 12 weeks until the graft consolidates.

Complications

Complications have been reported. Nonunions are rare. Simmons and Fielding reported that 1 of 51 patients had a nonunion associated with a lack of halo immobilization postoperatively.[69] Simmons and Fielding also reported on 2 of 30 patients in whom the fusion extended up to the occiput. The potential risk for neurologic injury exists, but seldom has been reported.

Alternative Procedures

Other variations of the posterior C1-C2 fusion include the Brooks wedge compression fusion (Fig. 111-13).[15] This technique was thought to enhance stability and the subsequent fusion rate. It requires passage of sublaminar wires below both C1 and C2 off the midline. With the passage of two wires around both laminae the potential for neurologic injury increases. The advantages that have been cited are its higher fusion rate as reported by some and

the fact that it may obviate the need for postoperative halo immobilization.

A biomechanical study by Grob et al. demonstrated the superiority of the transarticular screw fixation with posterior wiring and grafting (Fig. 111-14) for C1-C2 instability.[38] All four types of constructs, which included the Halifax clamp system (Fig. 111-15), the Gallie fusion, the Brooks fusion, and the transarticular screw with posterior wiring significantly decreased motion in extension, flexion, rotation, and lateral bending compared to the injured and intact spine. However, we still continue to recommend a Gallie fusion because of its simplicity and its excellent success. Other methods may be considered if the patient is felt possibly to be noncompliant with halo use or unable to use halo postoperatively.

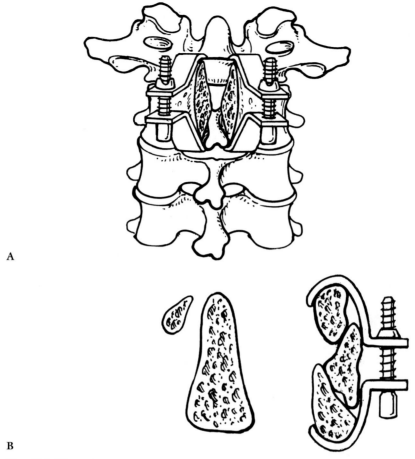

A

B

Fig. 111-15

Halifax clamp C1-C2 arthrodesis. **A,** Posterior view of C1-C2 fusion with Halifax clamp. The technique avoids penetration of the spinal canal. **B,** The wedge graft adds stability reducing the chance of rotational displacement of the clamp. *(Redrawn from Moskovich R, Crockard HA: Atlantoaxial arthrodesis using interlaminar clamps: an improved technique. Spine 17:261, 1992.)*

References

1. Adams CBT, Logue V: Studies in cervical spondylotic myelopathy II, *Brain* 94:569, 1971.
2. Aebi M, Zuber K, Manchesi D: Anterior plating for cervical injuries, *Spine* 16:538, 1991.
3. Albouker J, et al.: Les myelopathies cervicales d'origine rachidienne, *Neurochirurgie* 11:88, 1965.
4. Arnold JG Jr: The clinical manifestations of spondylochondrosis (spondylosis) of the cervical spine, *Ann Surg* 141:872, 1955.
5. Aronson DD, Kahn RJ, Canady A: *Cervical spine instability following suboccipital decompression and cervical laminectomy for Arnold-Chiari syndrome,* Presented at the 56th meeting of the American Academy of Orthopaedic Surgeons, Las Vegas, NV, 1989.
6. Batzdorf U: *Complex cervical myelopathies.* Frymore JW, editor: *The adult spine: principles and practice,* New York, 1991, Raven Press Ltd., p 1207.
7. Batzdorf U, Batzdorf A: Analysis of cervical spine curvature in patients with cervical spondylosis, *Neurosurgery* 22:827, 1988.
8. Bailey RW, Badgley CE: Anterior fusion of the cervical spine, *J Bone Joint Surg* 42A:565, 1960.
9. Bell DG, Bailey SI: Anterior cervical fusions for trauma, *Clin Orthop Relat Res* 128:155, 1977.
10. Bell DF, Walker JL, O'Connor G: *Spinal deformity following multiple level cervical laminectomy in children,* Presented at the 56th annual meeting of the American Academy of Orthopaedic Surgeons, Las Vegas, NV, 1989.
11. Bernhardt M, et al.: Cervical spondylotic myelopathy, *J Bone Joint Surg* 75A:119, 1993.
12. Bernstein AJ, et al.: *The "Dewar" posterior cervical fusion: description and comparative results,* Presented at the 54th annual meeting of the American Academy of Orthopaedic Surgeons, San Francisco, CA, 1993.
13. Bette H, Engelhardt H: Folgezustande von Laminektomien an der harswierbelsaule, *Z Orthop* 85:564, 1955.
14. Bohlman HH, et al.: Primary neoplasms of the cervical spine: diagnosis and treatment of twenty-three patients, *J Bone Joint Surg,* 68A:483, 1986.

15. Brooks AL, Jenkins ED: Atlantoaxial arthrodesis by the wedge compression method, *J Bone Joint Surg* 60A:279, 1978.

16. Brown MD, Malinin TI, Davis PB: A roentgenographic evaluation of frozen allografts versus autografts in anterior cervical spine fusions, *Clin Orthop Relat Res* 119:231, 1976.

17. Buchwald CHR, Nissen F, Thomsen J.: View from within: radiology in focus, parapharyngeal abscess and torticollis, *J Laryngol Otol* 104:829, 1990.

18. Callahan RA, Johnson RM, Margolis RN, et al.: Cervical facet fusion for control of instability following laminectomy, *J Bone Joint Surg* 59A:991, 1977.

19. Cloward RB: The anterior approach for removal of ruptured cervical disks, *J Neurosurg* 15:602, 1958.

20. Coe JD, et al.: Biomechanical evaluation of cervical spine stabilization methods in a human cadaveric model, *Spine* 14:1122, 1989.

21. Craig JB, Govender S: Neurofibromatosis of the cervical spine: a report of eight cases, *J Bone Joint Surg* 74B:575, 1974.

22. Cusier JF, et al.: Biomechanics of cervical spine facetectomy and fixation techniques, *Spine* 13:808, 1988.

23. Davey JR, et al.: A technique of posterior cervical fusion for instability of the cervical spine, *Spine* 10:722, 1985.

24. Dunn EJ: The role of methylmethacrylate in the stabilization and replacement of tumors of the cervical spine: a project of the Cervical Spine Research Society, *Spine* 2:15, 1977.

25. Edwards WC, LaRocca H: The development segmented sagittal diameter of the cervical spinal cord in patients with cervical spondylosis, *Spine* 8:20, 1983.

26. Emery SE, Smith MD, Bohlman HH: Upper airway obstruction after multilevel cervical corpectomy for myelopathy, *J Bone Joint Surg* 73A:544, 1991.

27. Enneking WF, Mindell ER: Observations on massive retrieved human allografts, *J Bone Joint Surg* 73A:1123, 1991.

28. Epstein JA: The surgical management of cervical spinal stenosis, spondylosis and myeloradiculopathy by means of the posterior approach, *Spine* 13:864, 1988.

29. Epstein JA, et al.: A comparative study of the treatment of cervical spondylotic myeloradiculopathy: experience with 50 cases treated by means of extensive laminectomy, foraminotomy and excision of osteophytes during past 10 years, *Acta Neurochir* (Wien) 61:89, 1982.

30. Fager CA: Results of adequate posterior decompression in the relief of spondylotic cervical myelopathy, *J Neurosurg* 38:684, 1973.

31. Fielding JW, Hawkins RJ: Atlanto-axial rotatory fixation (fixed rotatory subluxation of the atlanto-axial joint), *J Bone Joint Surg* 59A:37, 1977.

32. Fielding JW, Hawkins RJ: *Roentgenographic diagnosis of the injured neck*, AAOS Instruct Course Lect 25:149, 1976.

33. Fielding JW, Hensinger RN, Hawkins RJ: The cervical spine. In Lovell WW, Winter RB, editors: *Pediatric orthopaedics*, ed 3, Philadelphia, 1990, JB Lippincott.

34. Fielding JW, Pyle RN, Fietti VG: Anterior cervical vertebral body resection and bone-grafting for benign and malignant tumors: a survey under the auspices of the Cervical Spine Research Society, *J Bone Joint Surg* 61A:251, 1979.

35. Fraser RD, Shikuta J, Nakamura T: Analysis of cervical instability resulting from laminectomy for removal of spinal cord tumor, *Spine* 14:1172, 1989.

36. Garvey T, Eismont F, Roberti L: Anterior decompression, structural bone grafting, caspar plate stabilization for unstable cervical spine fractures and/or dislocations, *Spine* 17:S431, 1992.

37. Grisel P: Enucleation de l'atlas et torticollis nasopharyngean, *Presse Med* 38:50, 1930.

38. Grob D, et al.: Biomechanical evaluation of four different posterior atlantoaxial fixation techniques, *Spine* 17:480, 1992.

39. Hadley LA: Roentgenographic studies of the cervical spine, *Am J Roetngenol* 52:173, 1944.

40. Haft H, Ransohoff J, Carter S: Spinal cord tumors in children, *Pediatrics* 23:1152, 1959.

41. Halla JT, Sohrab F, Hardin J: Nonreducible rotational head tilt and atlantoaxial lateral mass collapse: clinical and roentgenographic features in patients with juvenile rheumatoid arthritis and ankylosing spondylitis, *Arch Intern Med* 143:471, 1983.

42. Hanley EN, et al.: Use of allograft bone in cervical spine surgery, *Semin Spine Surg* 1:262, 1989.

43. Heeneman H: Vocal cord paralysis following approaches to the anterior cervical spine, *Laryngoscope* 83:17, 1973.

44. Jenkins DHR: Extensive cervical laminectomy—long term results, *Br J Surg* 60:852, 1973.

45. Katsumi Y, Honmu T, Nakamura T: Analysis of cervical instability resulting from laminectomies for removal of spinal cord tumor, *Spine* 14:1172, 1989.

46. Light K, Simmons EH: Simmons keystone anterior cervical discectomy and fusion, *Surg Rounds Orthop*, October:13, 1989.

47. Lonstein JE: *Post laminectomy kyphosis.* In Chou SN, Selsekey EL, editors: *Spinal deformities and neurological dysfunction*, New York, 1978, Raven Press.

48. Lonstein JE: Spinal stability after tumor resection by laminectomy, *Spine State Art Rev* 2:383, 1988.

49. Lonstein JE, Cho JL: Treatment of post-laminectomy spine deformity, *Orthop Trans* 10:32, 1986.

50. McAffee PC: Failure of stabilization of the spine with methylmethacrylate: a retrospective analysis of twenty-four cases, *J Bone Joint Surg* 68A:1145, 1986.

51. MacEwen W: The surgery of the brain and spinal cord, *BMJ* 2:302, 1888.

52. Mikawa Y, Shikata J, Tamamurot: Spinal deformity and instability after multilevel cervical laminectomy, *Spine* 12:6, 1987.

53. Montesano PX, et al.: Biomechanics of cervical spine internal fixation, *Spine* 16:S10, 1991.

54. Nakata Y, et al.: *Post-laminectomy spine deformity*, Presented at the 27th annual meeting of the Scoliosis Research Society, Kansas City, MO, September 1992.

55. Nolan JP Jr, Sherk HH: Biomechanical evaluation of the extensor musculature of the cervical spine, *Spine* 13:9, 1988.

56. Pal GP, Sherk HH: The vertical stability of the cervical spine, *Spine* 13:447, 1988.

57. Parke WW: Correlative anatomy of cervical spondylotic myelopathy, *Spine* 13:831, 1988.

58. Phillips WA, Hensinger RN: The management of rotatory atlanto-axial subluxation in children, *J Bone Joint Surg* 71A:664, 1989.

59. Raskas DS, et al.: Osteoid osteoma and osteoblastoma of the spine, *J Spinal Disord* 5:204, 1992.

60. Raynor RD, Pugh J, Shapiro I: Cervical facetectomy and its effect on spine strength, *J Neurosurg* 63:278, 1985.

61. Robinson RA, et al.: Cervical spondylotic myelopathy: etiology and treatment concepts, *Spine* 2:89, 1977.

62. Rogers L: The surgical treatment of cervical spondylolytic myelopathy—mobilization of the complete cervical cord into an enlarged canal, *J Bone Joint Surg* 43B:3, 1961.

63. Sim FH, et al.: Swan-neck deformity following extensive cervical laminectomy: a review of twenty-one cases, *J Bone Joint Surg* 56A:504, 1974.

64. Simmons ED, et al.: *Biomechanical comparison of the Dewar and Rogers cervical spine techniques*, Presented at the European Spinal Deformities Society meeting, Lyon, France, June 1992.

65. Simmons EH: *Alternatives in surgical stabilization of the upper cervical spine in early management of acute spinal cord injury*, New York, 1982, Raven Press.

66. Simmons EH: *Surgery of the spine in rheumatoid arthritis and ankylosing spondylitis.* In Evarts CM, Editor: *Surgery of the musculoskeletal system*, vol 2, New York, 1983, Churchill Livingstone.

67. Simmons EH, Bhalla SK: Anterior cervical discectomy and fusion: a clinical and biomechanical study with eight year follow-up, *J Bone Joint Surg* 51B:225, 1959.

68. Simmons EH, Bradley DD: Neuro-myopathic flexion deformities of the cervical spine, *Spine* 13:756, 1988.

69. Simmons EH, Fielding JW: Atlanto-axial arthrodesis, *J Bone Joint Surg* 49:1022, 1967.

70. Smeather JE, Joanes DN: Dynamic compressive properties of human lumbar intervertebral joints: a comparison between fresh and thawed specimens, *J Biomech* 21:425, 1988.

71. Smith GW, Robinson RA: The treatment of certain cervical-spine disorders by anterior removal of the intervertebral disc and interbody fusion, *J Bone Joint Surg* 40A:607, 1958.

72. Stauffer ES, Kelly EG: Fracture-dislocations of the cervical spine. Instability and recurrent deformity following treatment by anterior interbody fusion, *J Bone Joint Surg* 59A:45, 1977.

73. Sutterlin CE III, et al.: A biomechanical evaluation of cervical spine stabilization methods in a bovine model: static and cyclical loading, *Spine* 13:795, 1988.

74. Tencer AF, Allen BF, Ferguson RL: A biomechanical study of thoracolumbar spinal fractures with bone in the canal: Part I, The effect of laminectomy, *Spine* 10:580, 1986.

75. Teng P: Spondylosis with compression of spinal cord and nerve roots, *J Bone Joint Surg* 42A:392, 1960.

76. Ulrich C, et al.: Biomechanics of fixation systems to the cervical spine, *Spine* 16:54, 1991.

77. Whitecloud TS, LaRocca H: Fibular strut graft in reconstructive surgery of the cervical spine, *Spine* 1:33, 1976.

78. Winter RB, et al.: Spine deformity in neurofibromatosis: a review of one hundred and two patients, *J Bone Joint Surg* 61A:677, 1979.

79. Wittenburg RH, et al.: Compressive strength of autologous and allogenous bone grafts for thoracolumbar and cervical spine fusion, *Spine* 15:1073, 1990.

80. Yasouka S, et al.: Pathogenesis and prophylaxis of post-laminectomy deformity of the spine after multiple level laminectomy: difference between children and adults, *Neurosurgery* 9:145, 1975.

81. Yasouka S, Peterson HA, MacCarty CS: Incidence of spinal column deformity after multilevel laminectomy in children and adults, *J Neurosurg* 57:441, 1982.

82. Yong-Hing K, Kalamchi A, MacEwan D: Cervical spine abnormalities in neurofibromatosis, *J Bone Joint Surg* 61A:695, 1979.

83. Zdeblick TA, Bohlman HH: Cervical kyphosis and myelopathy, *J Bone Joint Surg* 71A:170, 1989.

84. Zdeblick TA, Ducker T: The use of freeze dried allograft bone for anterior cervical fusions, *Spine* 16:726, 1991.

85. Zdeblick TA, et al.: Cervical stability after foraminotomy, *J Bone Joint Surg* 74A:22, 1992.

Section 5
Other Conditions

112 Arthritic Spinal Deformity—
 Ankylosing Spondylitis

Edward H. Simmons

113 Paget's Disease

Alexander G. Hadjipavlou
Philip H. Lander

Chapter 112
Arthritic Spinal Deformity— Ankylosing Spondylitis
Edward H. Simmons

Atlantoaxial Instability

    surgical stabilization

Atlantooccipital Disability Spondylodiscitis

    case reports

Flexion (Kyphotic) Deformities of the Spine

    indications for surgical correction
    assessment of the deformity

Kyphotic Deformity of the Lumbar Spine

    technique of lumbar osteotomy
    evolution of the author's technique for lumbar resection-extension osteotomy in ankylosing spondylitis

Kyphotic Deformity of the Thoracic Spine

Kyphotic Deformity of the Cervical Spine

    selection of patients for cervical osteotomy
    occult fractures as a cause of kyphotic deformity
    technique of cervical osteotomy

Muscle Disease as a Cause of Kyphotic Deformity in Ankylosing Spondylitis

A major cause of severe spinal disability associated with seronegative spondylitic arthropathy is related to ankylosing spondylitis. Ankylosing spondylitis as a seronegative arthritis is a disease of unknown etiology, although an immune response in patients with a genetic predisposition is postulated.[4,9]

As a systemic disease, ankylosing spondylitis may have extraarticular manifestations, including iridocyclitis,[8] aortitis,[7,8,66] cardiac conduction abnormality,[8,66] arachnoiditis,[22,65] and cauda equina syndrome.[6,44] It has a recognized association with ulcerative colitis,[32] regional enteritis,[32] psoriasis,[32] multiple sclerosis,[17] Reiter's disease,[32] and Behçet's disease.[32]

Clinicians assessing patients presenting with back pain should be well aware that ankylosing spondylitis affects the spine. It results in ossification of the annulus fibrosis and adjacent vertebral ligaments—evident in its later stages.[8] The disease causes a loss of the normal anterior vertebral body concavity producing "squaring" of vertebrae, and formation of bridging syndesmophytes.[8] Loss of the normal cervical and lumbar lordosis may occur in increasing thoracic kyphosis, resulting in severe flexion deformity of the spine.[49]

Ankylosing spondylitis has often been described as "rheumatoid spondylitis." However, it should be recognized that it is a different disease with different serology. Ankylosing spondylitis is more common in males, with a predilection to affect the spine and major joints, whereas rheumatoid arthritis is more common in females, with a predilection to affect the joints of the appendicular skeleton.

In its early stages ankylosing spondylitis is a disease of the young male. It presents with insidious onset of low-back pain that is worse in the morning and better with activity. It is not uncommon for the low-back symptoms to be interpreted as "disc disease" and in some instances, inappropriate surgery may be carried out for "low-back pain" mistakenly thought to be discogenic.

The incidence of patients with clinical manifestation of ankylosing spondylitis is two to three per thousand, representing a significant patient population in a country the size of the United States.

A detailed review of the histories of North American patients referred to the author for correction of deformity, shows that the average time from onset of symptoms to diagnosis is 5.5 years.

The clinician should be alert to the presentation of low-back pain of insidious onset in a young male that is worse in the morning and better as the day progresses, and should not relegate the patient to a routine diagnosis of "low-back pain." Decreased lengthening of the spine on forward bending as indicated by tape measure, decreased lateral bending of the spine, decreased chest expansion, and sacroiliac or costochondral tenderness should be looked for as part of the examination. Early radiographic changes in the sacroiliac joints, squaring of lumbar vertebrae, positive bone scan related to the sacroiliac joints and a positive HLA-B27 antigen test complete the diagnosis. However, the most important diagnostic tool is an intelligent, thinking clinical observer.

In ankylosing spondylitis the main presenting clinical problems are gross, fixed deformities. In rheumatoid arthritis the main problems are local destruction and instability. However, atlantoaxial subluxation and dislocation may occur in both diseases.

Atlantoaxial Instability

The recognition of atlantoaxial instability in patients with rheumatoid arthritis and ankylosing spondylitis requires a constant awareness and careful monitoring by the clinician in treating patients with these diseases.

In ankylosing spondylitis, a solid column of bone below may place increased stress at the craniocervical junction. With the additional attritional effects of inflammation of the transverse ligament and associated hyperemia of its bony attachments, atlantoaxial subluxation and dislocation may occur. In certain patients the joint may subluxate and then subsequently stabilize in the subluxed position without significant symptoms. However, the possibility of significant instability at C1-C2 should be recognized in planning surgery under general anesthesia on any patient with ankylosing spondylitis in whom manipulation of the neck might be required during intubation or positioning. Routine flexion and extension lateral radiography should be performed before any procedures are performed.

The incidence would appear greater in rheumatoid arthritis, being reported in 25% to 90% of patients depending on diagnostic criteria.* In rheumatoid arthritis, the types of involvement that occur in decreasing frequency are (1) atlantoaxial subluxation, (2) atlantoaxial subluxation combined with subaxial subluxation, (3) subaxial subluxation, and (4) superior migration of the odontoid process combined with any of the first three abnormalities.

In ankylosing spondylitis the most frequent problems are (1) atlantoaxial subluxation, (2) subaxial fracture deformity, and (3) occipital-atlantal destruction and deformity.

*References 5, 10, 31, 38, 41, and 42.

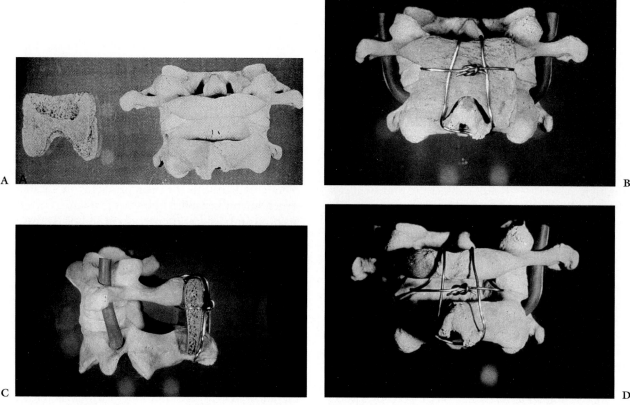

Fig. 112-1

A, Gallie modified H graft shown in skeletal model. Deep cancellous surface of graft is contoured from posterior iliac crest to fit over posterior arches of C1 and C2. It sits astride spinous process of C2. **B,** Posterior view of C1-C2 showing graft in position with cortical surface posteriorly. Gallie wire passes under spinous process of C2, through interspinous ligament of C2-C3 and upward over graft on each side, coming out below arch of C1 laterally. It is tied firmly posteriorly. **C,** Lateral view of model showing position of H graft and Gallie wire pulling back C1 into normal relationship with C2. Importance of preserving the C2-C3 interspinous ligament, which will help to stabilize wire below spinous process of C2, will be appreciated. **D,** Posterior view without graft to show configuration of wire.

Surgical Stabilization

Where there is gross symptomatic atlantoaxial instability, particularly when associated with long-tract signs in a patient with ankylosing spondylitis, surgical stabilization is very definitely required. Although different techniques have been described to achieve this, in my experience it is most effectively and safely achieved by a Gallie-type posterior atlantoaxial arthrodesis.* W.E. Gallie used a modified H graft shaped from the posterior iliac crest and contoured it to fit over the posterior aspect of the arches of C1 and C2, sitting astride the spinous process of C2. A single wire of 22-gauge stainless steel is passed inferior to the spinous process of C2 through the interspinous ligament between C2 and C3. The two

*References 33, 47, 51, 52, 61, and 63.

ends of the wire are carried upward posterior to the graft around a notch cut in its upper border, and under the arch of C1 on each side of the graft. The ends of the wire are tied over the posterior aspect of the graft, locking it into position and reducing the arch of C1 into normal relationship with the arch of C2 (Fig. 112-1). A useful and somewhat essential instrument is a wire-tightening apparatus such as that developed by the late R.I. Harris.[18] The wire tightener grasps the wire and allows forceful tension on it while tying the knot quite firmly in the narrowing confines of the wound by gentle hand pressure (Fig. 112-2).

The cancellous surface of the graft is contoured to fit over the curved posterior surfaces of the arches of C1 and C2, so that the graft will be in intimate contact with the vertebrae (Fig. 112-3). It should be emphasized that in addition to the main graft, a

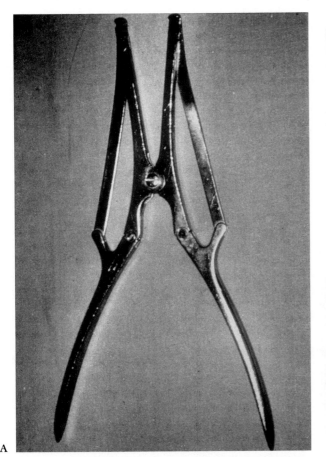

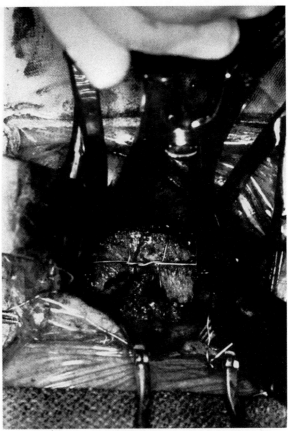

Fig. 112-2

A, Harris wire tier allows wire to be grasped and tightened firmly in depths of wound. **B,** Operative view showing use of wire tier to fix graft into position. First knot is tightened approximating graft against two vertebra. First knot is fixed with needle driver and second loop of square knot added, knot being firmly tightened by tier.

very important part of the grafting technique is to place cancellous bone chips over the laminae on both sides lateral to the main graft and under its edges as far laterally as possible. The procedure immobilizes the involved segment. It avoids the necessity of an occipital-cervical fusion for lesions at the atlantoaxial junction, preserving the very important function of the atlantooccipital joints, which in a patient with ankylosing spondylitis may be the only remaining mobile joint in the cervical spine. The technique does require external immobilization to be certain of success. In my experience this has not presented a problem in patients with ankylosing spondylitis, and this technique is preferred over other forms of internal fixation that are not necessarily secure in osteopenic bone. A halo cast or a well-fitting halo vest is most effective for this. If this is done, success is almost certain.[14,47,51,60] The anatomy of the area should be understood. The relationship of the ver-

tebral arteries and neural elements must be recognized. Care is taken in dissecting the ligamentum flavum from the anterior surface of the posterior arch of C1. A curved guide may be inserted around the arch of C1, or the end of the wire may be bent backward on itself, preparing a blunt end that may be directed around the arch by a needle driver.

Atlantooccipital Disability

In some patients with ankylosing spondylitis major disability may arise from destructive changes at the atlantooccipital joints. In many patients this is the last joint in the spine to be involved. Destructive changes may occur with severe pain associated with minimal persisting motion. When the symptoms do not respond to medical therapy and bracing, stabilization by occipital-cervical fusion may be required.

In some patients, destructive changes at the at-

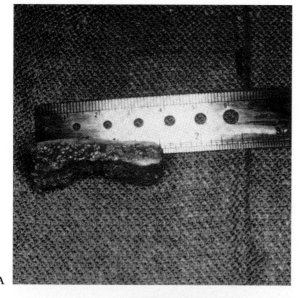

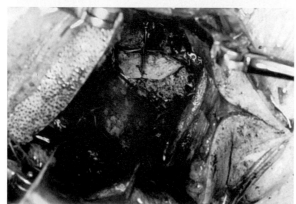

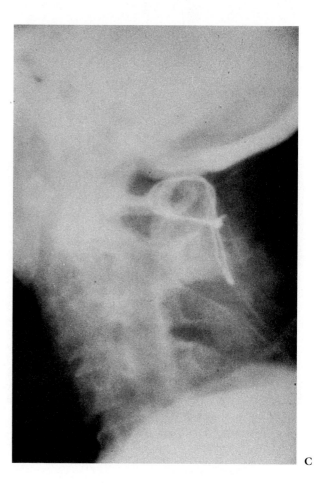

Fig. 112-3

A, Axial view of modified H graft showing contour of deep cancellous surface, shaped to fit over underlying vertebrae. **B,** Operative view with main graft supplemented by adequate cancellous bone placed laterally over laminae on both sides. **C,** Postoperative lateral radiogram showing relationship of graft with restoration of normal relationship of C1 to C2.

lantooccipital joints may give rise to deformity as well as pain. The deformity is most commonly anterior subluxation, but rotatory or lateral angulatory deformity may occur as well. If the deformity is major and the pain not responsive to conservative management, gradual reduction of the deformity can be achieved by halo-dependent traction along the line of the neck and then stabilization with occipital-cervical fusion with the head and neck in normal alignment (Fig. 112-4). The use of internal fixation with occipital-cervical plates for occipital-cervical fusion has its proponents. However, my preference for patients with ankylosing spondylitis is a modified Dewar technique,[12,13,53] fixing double onlay cortical and cancellous iliac grafts to the base of the skull and the upper cervical spine, reinforced by multiple cancellous grafts (Fig. 112-5). After the base of the skull is stripped, a wire is passed through holes in the skull to be used to fix the grafts against the skull. Double iliac cortical and cancellous onlay grafts are contoured to fit over the posterior arches of the upper cervical vertebrae (usually down to C4), the cancellous surfaces of the graft being contoured to fit over the posterior arches.

The grafts are shaped to fit accurately against the skull and are held firmly in this position. They are fixed to the posterior arches of the cervical vertebrae by passing threaded Compere wires percutaneously from one side of the neck penetrating the graft on one side of the spine through the base of the spinous process and then through the graft on the opposite side. The Compere wire is cut free on the side of its

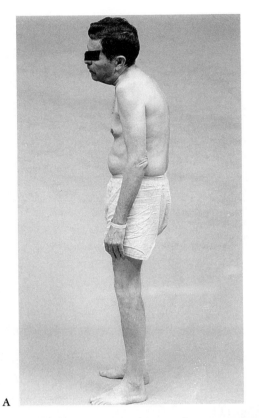

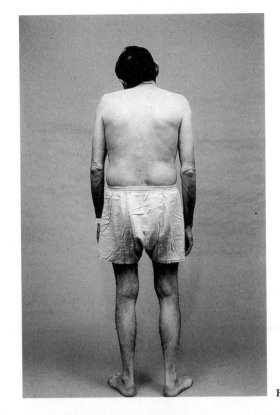

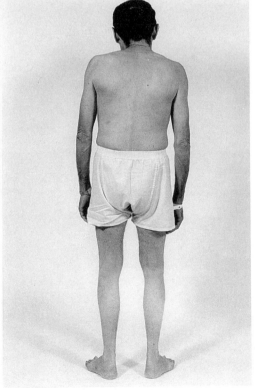

Fig. 112-4

A and B, Lateral and posterior views of patient with severe painful torticollis associated with destruction of the atlantooccipital joints. Patient had undergone three operations for "low-back pain" during earlier stages of disease represented by scars in lumbar area. C, Following halo-dependent traction and reduction of deformity in situ, occipital cervical fusion was carried out with halo-vest immobilization. Postoperative lateral radiogram shows successful fusion. D, Posterior postoperative view of patient who is completely relieved of pain with correction of deformity.

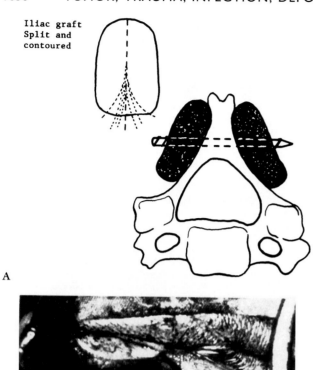

Iliac graft
Split and
contoured

A

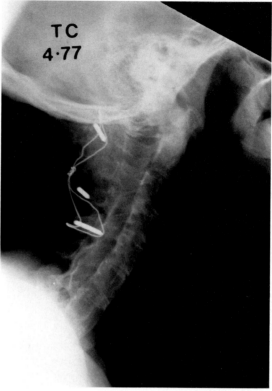

TC
4·77

D

Fig. 112-5

A, Axial diagram showing technique of insertion of threaded pins through Dewar onlay graft on one side, through base of spinous process, and graft on the opposite side. Contouring of cancellous surface of grafts allows them to be applied closely to posterior arches of the spine. Figure-eight encircling wire adds to fixation. Further cancellous and cortical onlay grafts are placed laterally on both sides. **B,** Operative view with Dewar onlay cortical and cancellous grafts in position. Grafts are fixed to upper cervical spine posterior arches with transfixing threaded Compere pins. Over-tying loop of stainless steel wire that has been passed through skull keeps grafts in firm contact with skull and compresses them against posterior aspect of spine. **C,** Operative with showing additional cancellous and cortical onlay bone grafting reinforcing main grafts, extending from skull to cervical spine. **D,** Postoperative lateral radiogram showing technique of fixation with wire passing through outer table of skull and threaded Compere pins in position. There is solid fusion from occiput to cervical spine.

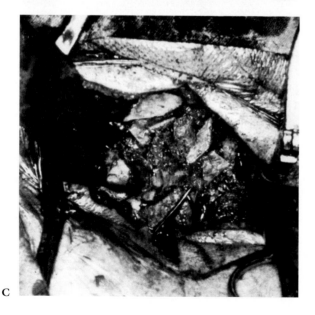

B

C

entrance lateral to the graft. The wire that has been passed through the skull is used to fix the grafts against the skull as well as to tie the grafts over the posterior arches by passing the wire around the ends of the threaded Compere wires. Further multiple cancellous grafts are used to reinforce the main grafts, being placed between the skull and the cervical spine about the main grafts (see Fig. 112-5, *B, C, D,* and *E*).

Postoperative immobilization by a well-fitted halo cast or a well-fitted halo vest for a period of 3 months is necessary to protect the area of fusion from abnormal stress, because the rest of the spine is entirely rigid.

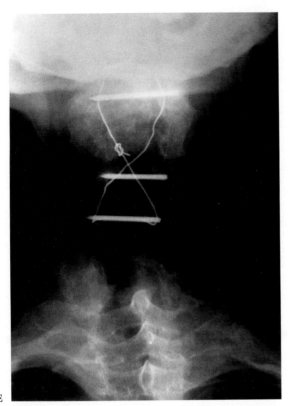

Fig. 112-5, cont'd

E, Postoperative anterior posterior radiogram showing configuration of wire loop, threaded pins, and graft. Neck must be prepared and draped well laterally to allow threaded pins to be inserted percutaneously from lateral aspect of neck through graft on that side, spinous process, and graft on opposite side. Pins are divided lateral to graft on side of their insertion and excess portion removed.

Spondylodiscitis

The early erosive sclerotic changes of bone adjacent to the sacroiliac joints in ankylosing spondylitis are well recognized. Less well recognized is the fact that similar erosive sclerotic changes may on occasion involve the intervertebral disc and adjacent bone producing a lesion termed "spondylodiscitis." These erosive lesions of the disc space and adjacent bone were first reported by Andersson in 1937.[3] In 1960 Wholey et al. reported on biopsy of the lesions showing chronic inflammatory change without evidence of infection. They reported that spontaneous healing could occur without specific treatment. They considered that the lesion was just another manifestation of ankylosing spondylitis.[69] In 1963 Coste et al. further reported on the lesion being an inflammatory process as a manifestation of the disease.[11] In 1969 Kanefield et al. on the basis of three patients studied suggested that the lesion could represent delayed union or nonunion of fractures occurring in ankylosing spondylitis.[25] However, this suggestion is not supported by the evidence available. Little and others have shown that it most frequently presents as an asymptomatic abnormality on routine radiographic examination.[31,43]

The ossified spine in ankylosing spondylitis is susceptible to fracture, and the findings are usually fairly typical and distinct from those noted in spondylodiscitis. It is consistently noted at surgery on an ossified spine in ankylosing spondylitis that the ossified interspinous ligaments, ligamentum flavum, and disc are much harder and stronger in caliber than the bone itself. It should be recognized that fractures are more prone to occur through the vertebral body rather than the disc space. They are usually associated with a significant traumatic incident with acute onset of pain.

Spondylodiscitis as a manifestation of the inflammatory disease arises as a destructive lesion of the disc space and is frequently asymptomatic, being noted on routine radiographic studies. However, it may become symptomatic with minor injury or stress. Significant destruction anteriorly with loss of bony substance makes the posterior elements more vulnerable to injury and even to stress fracture if they were previously ossified. These facts should be considered when deciding whether the true nature of the lesion is a fracture, pseudarthrosis, or spondylodiscitis with or without superimposed injury, in a particular patient.

The radiographic appearance of spondylodiscitis is fairly typical (Fig. 112-6). Erosion of the subchondral bony plates widens the disc space. The surrounding bone becomes sclerotic and radiodense. Either erosion or sclerosis may be more prominent. The reported incidence of spondylodiscitis is 5% to 6%.[31,43,46] It occurs most frequently in the lower thoracic spine. Approximately half the lesions present with back pain, and a little over half are discovered on routine radiologic examination; these lesions are asymptomatic.[31] Generally, the lesions follow a benign course and usually respond to conservative management.

Case Reports

Figure 112-7 illustrates the typical findings of a fracture pseudarthrosis. The patient was a 56-year-old barber with longstanding ankylosing spondylitis, but without major complaint until about 2.5 years earlier. At that time he suffered a major injury when the jack of his car slipped while he was changing a tire and the car fell on him. He had severe pain with increasing painful deformity aggravated by any mo-

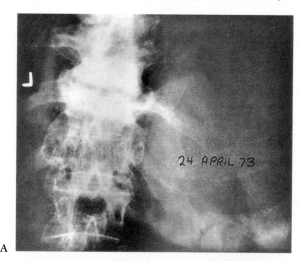

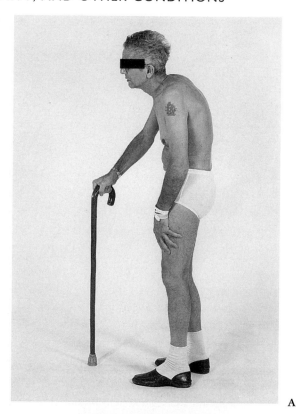

A

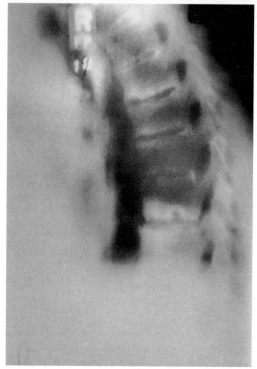

B

Fig. 112-6

A and **B** Anteroposterior and lateral radiograms of patient with ankylosing spondylitis showing typical areas of spondylodiscitis. Significant lesion is seen in lower thoracic spine—most frequent location. Typical erosive sclerotic changes involve vertebral end plates and adjacent disc space.

tion. Radiograms show a typical area of pseudarthrosis through the upper vertebral body of L1 with no involvement of the disc space (Figs. 112-7, *B, C,* and *D*). Because of his deformity the lesion was under shear stress with the weight of his upper body anterior to the lesion. He was treated with extension osteotomy of the midlumbar spine under local anesthesia, correcting the trunk deformity, shifting the weight of his upper trunk posterior to the lesion, and transferring shear stress at the fracture site to

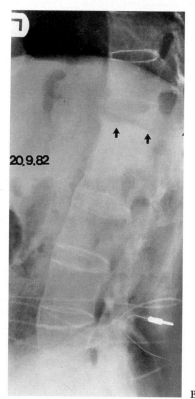

B

Fig. 112-7

A, Fifty-six-year-old male with painful thoracolumbar kyphotic deformity following significant spinal injury. He had pain in keeping with fracture pseudarthrosis. **B,** Lateral radiogram showing transverse sheer fracture through upper body of L1 through posterior elements. The $2\frac{1}{2}$ year duration of the lesion is in keeping with pseudarthrosis.

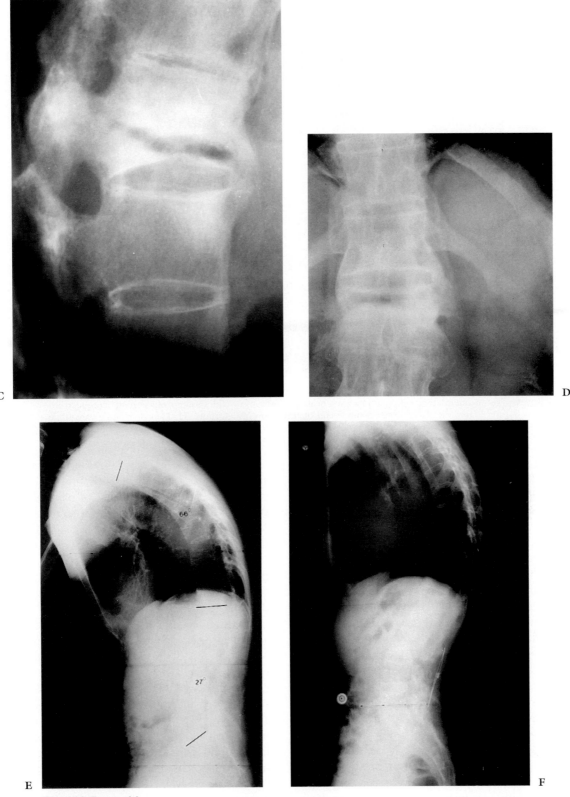

Fig. 112-7, cont'd

C, Close-up view indicating involvement of vertebral body and not disc space. **D,** Anteroposterior view showing typical fracture pseudarthrosis without significant bone destruction. **E,** Three-foot lateral standing radiogram showing weight-bearing line of body anterior to fracture site producing shear stress. **F,** Lateral 3-ft postoperative standing radiogram demonstrating correction of spinal deformity by lumbar extension osteotomy with weight-bearing line posteriorly with area of pseudarthrosis under compression allowing spontaneous healing.

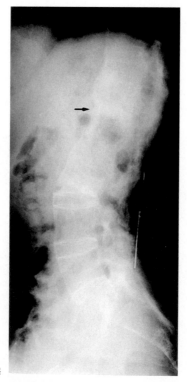 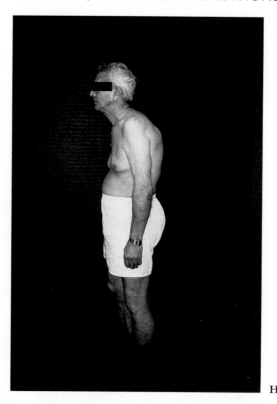

G   H

Fig. 112-7, cont'd

G, Postoperative lateral radiogram showing healing of osteotomy with spontaneous healing of pseudarthrosis after lesion was placed under compression of correction of deformity. **H,** Lateral standing view of patient with normal spinal alignment. Patient had complete relief of preoperative painful symptoms.

horizontal compression force, which allowed spontaneously healing of the nonunion (Figs. 112-7, *E, F, G,* and *H).*

In contrast Fig. 112-8 shows a 58-year-old physician with a 22-year history of ankylosing spondylitis. For 3 to 4 years he had noted increasing kyphotic deformity of his thoracolumbar spine but was able to function adequately. Nine months earlier he had minimal stress on stepping down some steps forcefully, suffering pain the lower thoracic spine. This was mild at first but increased progressively with increasing flexion deformity. Radiography demonstrated a typical area of spondylodiscitis at the T12-L1 level. The destructive lesion involved the disc space, in keeping with preexisting spondylodiscitis. His chief symptom was increasing pain interfering with his practice and activities of daily living. The lesion was under flexion-shear strain due to his kyphotic deformity with the weight-bearing line of his upper trunk anterior to the lesion producing angulatory stress. His deformity was corrected by resection-extension osteotomy of the midlumbar spine under local anesthesia shifting the weight-bearing line posterior to the osteotomy site. This transferred the shear forces acting on the area of spondylodisci-

tis to compression forces, and following this the lesion went on to spontaneous healing. The deformity was fully corrected with relief of pain, allowing return to normal work activities with a normal posture (Figs. 112-8, *E, F,* and *G).* An assessment of the radiographic appearances of these two examples illustrates their differences. The fracture has involved the bone; the spondylodiscitis has involved the disc space with a greater degree of erosive change and less tendency to repair.

The incidence of spondylodiscitis in patients with advanced disease may be greater than the literature would suggest. Its recognition requires an awareness of its presence. One group of 124 patients who had radiograms available of the entire spine that were suitable for study were reviewed. The patients had all been referred for evaluation and surgical correction of spinal deformity. Of these patients, 28 (23%) had radiologic evidence of spondylodiscitis.[61] This higher incidence may be attributable to the severity of the cases analyzed. Progressive kyphotic deformity was the chief symptom in 23 of the 28 cases. Nine of the patients described a traumatic episode that produced increasing pain and deformity in the area of spondylodiscitis. The lesions were found from T7

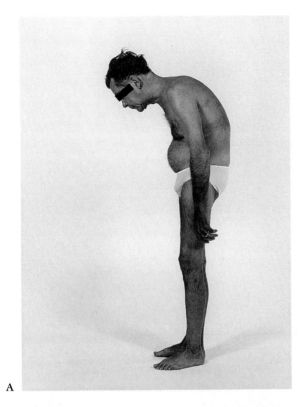

A

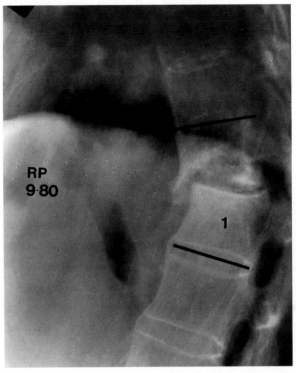

B

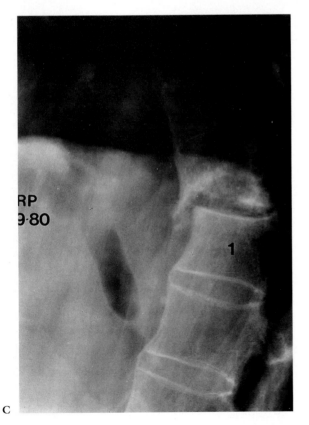

C

Fig. 112-8

A, Fifty-eight-year-old physician with increasing painful kyphotic deformity with apex at thoracolumbar junction. **B,** Lateral radiogram demonstrating destructive spondylodiscitis at T12-L1. Note end-plate destruction and bone absorption. **C,** Anteroposterior radiogram showing involvement of disc space.

Continues.

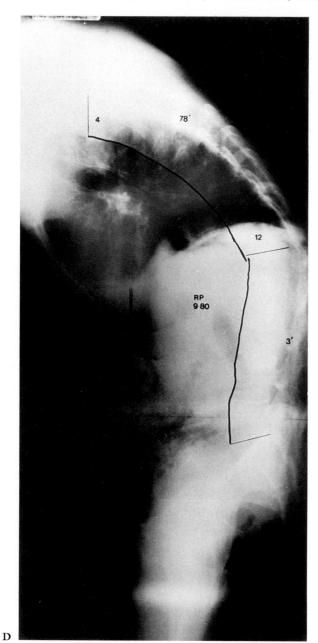

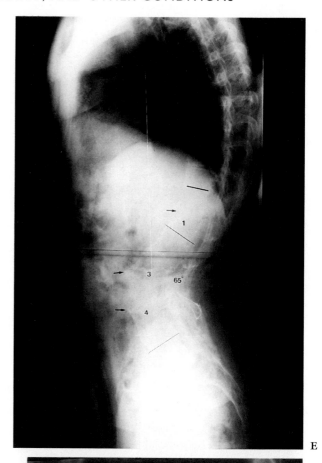

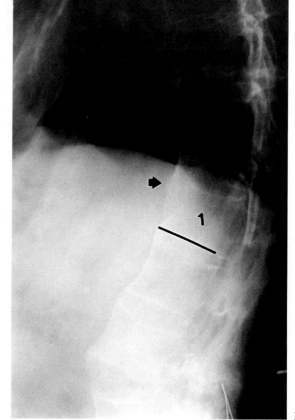

Fig. 112-8, cont'd

D, Three-foot standing lateral radiogram showing weight-bearing line well anterior to level of destructive spondylodiscitis. **E,** Standing lateral postoperative radiogram following resection-extension osteotomy of midlumbar spine. Note that weight-bearing line has been shifted posteriorly, converting sheer force to compression force at site of spondylodiscitis. **F,** Close-up lateral radiogram of T12-L1 4 months postoperatively, showing healing of spondylodiscitis by change of force from shear to compression.

to L5, most commonly at T11-L1. Twenty-four of the 28 patients had surgical correction of the main deformity. When the spondylodiscitis was in the area of the deformity, correction of the deformity resulted in fusion at the site of the spondylodiscitis. As the weight-bearing line of the upper body was shifted posteriorly, the shear forces acting on the area of spondylodiscitis were transferred to compression, resulting in healing of the lesion. Occasionally, surgical stabilization may be required for intractable pain in patients without deformity. When this occurs, there is usually an associated fracture or disruption of the posterior fused spine at the same level. The risks of an anterior approach in a patient with spondylodiscitis should be known. These patients breathe only with their diaphragm. Resection and stabilization may be done in lesions above the diaphragm, but it should not be disturbed if it is at all possible. Figure 112-9 shows the radiograms of a patient with longstanding ankylosing spondylitis who presented with severe pain from an unrecognized area of spondylodiscitis occurring postoperatively following hip replacement arthroplasty. Extensive destructive spondylodiscitis is evident at T9-T10, with breakdown of the posterior fusion. The symp-

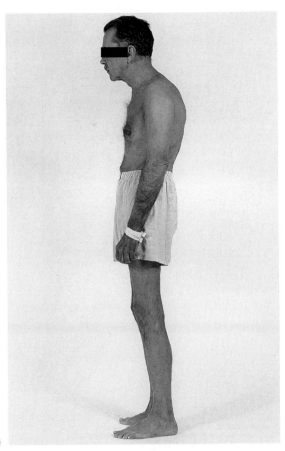

Fig. 112-8, cont'd

G, Postoperative lateral view of patient relieved of pain with correction of deformity.

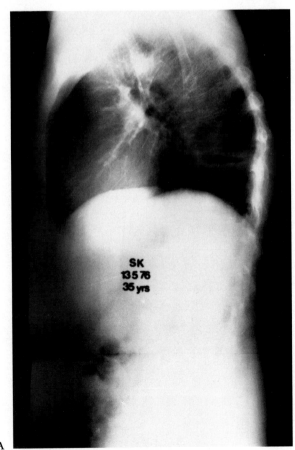

Fig. 112-9

A, Thoracic spine lateral radiogram showing extensive destructive change of spondylodiscitis at T9-T10. Patient had been asymptomatic, but suffered immediate severe pain following total hip arthroplasty likely due to breakdown of posterior fusion by movements of patient during surgery.

Continues.   **A**

Fig. 112-9, cont'd

B, Extent of end-plate destruction and bone absorption is evident in close-up lateral view. Radioluscent line is noted in posterior fusion mass. **C,** Operative view showing excision of area of spondylodiscitis with fibular strut grafts in position. **D,** Operative view showing completion of anterior grafting with additional onlay cancellous and cortical bone graft. **E,** Twenty-one-month postoperative lateral radiogram following successful fusion and normal spinal alignment. Patient was relieved of pain and back working on assembly-line with motor car company. **F,** Anteroposterior postoperative radiogram 21 months postoperatively.

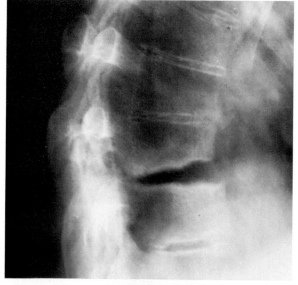

B

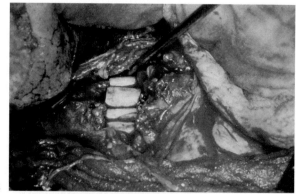

C

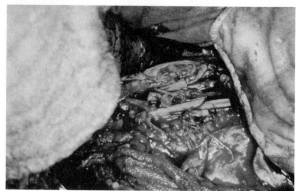

D

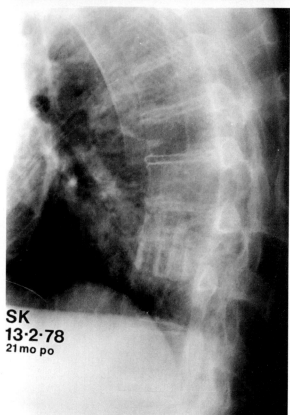

E

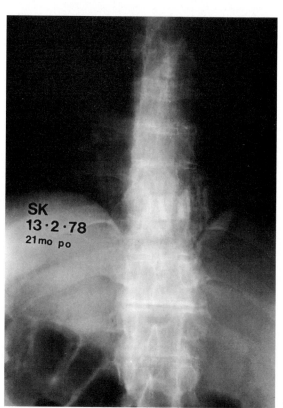

F

toms were undoubtedly provoked by movement of the patient's trunk during and after surgery. Anterior transthoracic resection of the area of spondylodiscitis was required with fibular strut grafting. This gave relief of pain with the patient going on to a solid fusion, returning to full-time work on an assembly line. If anterior resection is required, all the inflammatory tissue should be resected back to healthy bone with the anterior grafts placed in bone, free of the destructive change of spondylodiscitis (Fig. 112-10).

Flexion (Kyphotic) Deformities of the Spine

It is well recognized that severe flexion deformities of the spine may occur in patients with ankylosing spondylitis. Despite emphasis on earlier recognition and current advances in medical treatment, patients

are seen with advanced kyphotic deformities of the trunk who are very severely disabled and who present a major challenge for definitive surgical correction of their deformity.

Indications for Surgical Correction

The indications for surgical correction of kyphotic deformity are variable and depend on the extent of the deformity, the degree of functional embarrassment, the age and general condition of the patient, the feasibility of correction, and above all else, the earnest desire of the patient to accept the risks and rehabilitative measures required for correction.

Assessment of the Deformity

In assessing patients for possible surgical correction, it is essential to recognize the primary site of the deformity, for if any major correction is to be carried out, the correction must be done in the area of the

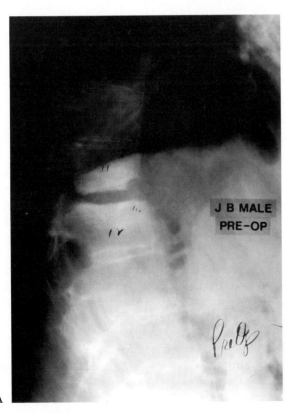
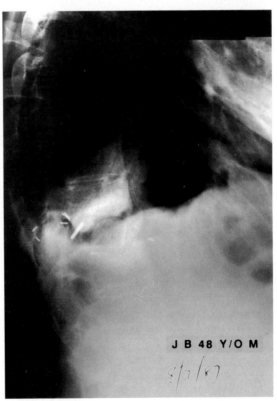

A

B

Fig. 112-10

A, Lateral radiogram of 51-year-old male with a 29-year history of ankylosing spondylitis. For 1 year he had severe increasing pain at thoracolumbar junction. Destructive changes of ankylosing spondylitis are noted with widening of disc space, sclerosis of opposing vertebral surfaces, and absorption of bone anteriorly. Patient had no gross kyphotic deformity, and lesion was above diaphragm. **B,** Lateral postoperative radiogram showing anterior grafting but with still areas of involved disc space and bone remaining.
Continues.

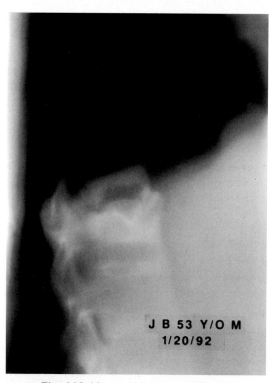

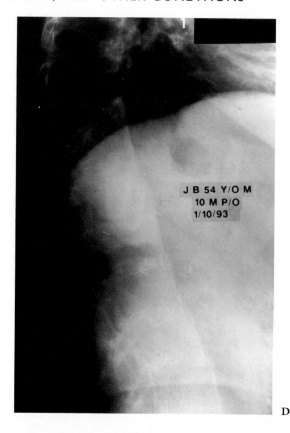

Fig. 112-10, cont'd

C, Lateral tomogram 4.5 years postoperatively showing absorption of graft and lack of stability anteriorly. D, Lateral radiogram of thoracic spine 10 months postoperatively following further complete excision of disease tissue back to healthy bone with fibular strut grafting supplemented by rib grafts. Patient has gone on to further evidence of solid union with complete relief of preoperative pain. This emphasizes importance of completely excising granulomatous destructive tissue associated with spondylodiscitis if anterior grafting is required.

main deformity. Patients who present because of apparent spinal deformity may have their main deformity in the hip joints, the lumbar spine, the thoracic spine, or it may be primarily cervical in situation (Fig. 112-11). Accurate assessment and measurement of trunk kyphotic deformity is required when planning treatment and to assess its results. The most reliable measure of trunk deformity is the chin-brow to vertical angle. This is a measure of the angle formed by a line from the brow to the chin through the vertical, when the patient stands with the hips and knees extended, and the neck in its neutral or fixed position (Fig. 112-12 on p. 1672).

Kyphotic Deformity of the Lumbar Spine

This was the first type of kyphotic deformity corrected surgically in ankylosing spondylitis, reported by Smith-Petersen et al. in 1945.[64] The initial procedure as reported by Smith-Petersen et al. was done under general anesthesia with the patient lying prone. This was further reported by LaChappelle,[26] Herbert,[19,20] Nunziata,[40] Wilson and Turkell,[71] Law[27-29] and others.* To avoid difficulties with the use of the prone position for a patient with kyphotic deformity, Adams recommended that surgery be done with patients on their sides, and he used a three-point rack to manipulate the spine for correction.[2]

Some have recommended a two-stage or double-exposure procedure with division of the longitudinal ligament anteriorly. In my experience this is not required, and correction can be consistently done from the posterior approach alone. It should be appreciated that a major and consistent complication of lumbar osteotomy is gastric dilatation and abdominal ileus. When the spine is extended with the

*References 2, 15, 16, 24, 35 to 37, 45, 48, 53, and 70.

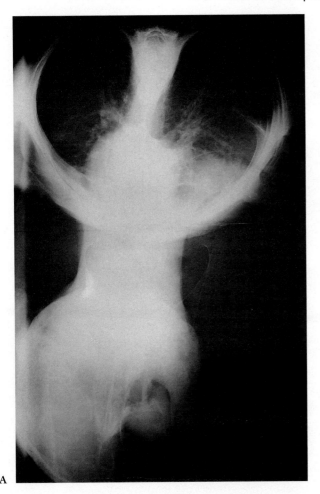

A

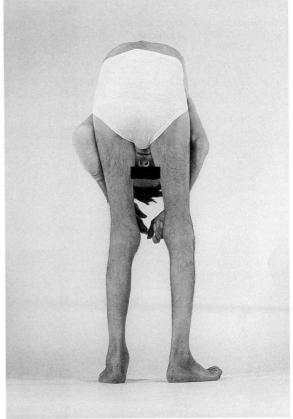

B

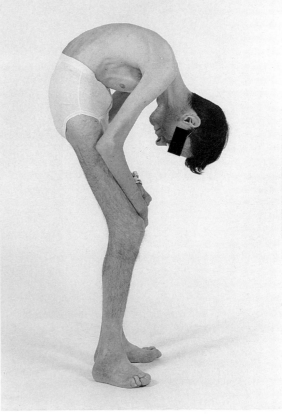

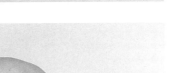

C

Fig. 112-11

Thirty-six-year old male with 18-year history of ankylosing spondylitis demonstrating complexity of spinal deformity and its assessment. **A,** Anteroposterior standing radiogram of patient's spine. Thorax resembles CT axial view. **B** and **C,** Posterior and lateral standing views of patient. He could see only backward, and to move about, he had to walk backward. Lateral view shows chin-brow to vertical angle of 134 degrees. He has combined deformities of thoracic kyphosis, lumbar kyphosis, some cervical kyphosis, and hip-flexion deformities.

Continues.

Fig. 112-11, cont'd

D, Lateral standing radiogram showing neck flexion deformity, thoracic kyphosis of 68 degrees, complete loss of lumbar lordosis with superimposed 47 degrees of lumbar kyphosis and finally hip-flexion deformities. **E,** Anteroposterior radiogram of pelvis showing fused hip joints. Patient was treated with bilateral total hip replacement arthroplasties at one sitting, under regional anaesthesia. **F,** Anteroposterior view of hip joints followed total replacement arthroplasties. **G,** Lateral standing view of patient following bilateral hip arthroplasties. His deformity was improved, but he could now see neither backward nor forward for walking. **H,** Postoperative standing lateral radiogram of spine following resection-extension osteotomy of 104 degrees at L3-L4 done under local anesthesia. Weight-bearing line is shifted well posterior to osteotomy site. **I,** Close-up lateral radiogram of lumbar spine showing extent of lumbar osteotomy. Patient had associated spondylodiscitis above area of osteotomy, which went on to heal spontaneously. **J,** Standing lateral postoperative view of patient showing correction of major deformities. He still has some flexion of knees and neck and is able to stand and look ahead. He walks in a normal fashion and is able to enjoy normal daily activities with his family.

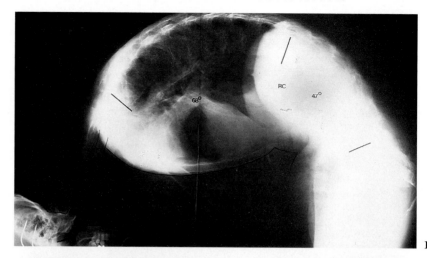

D

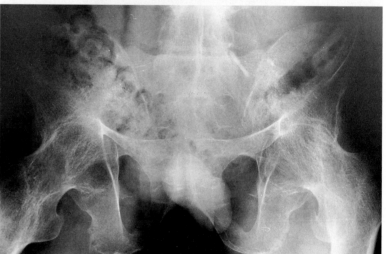

E

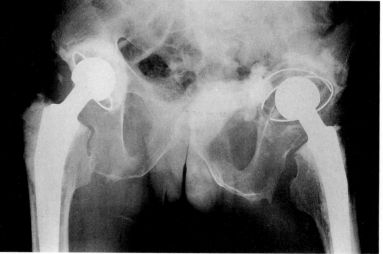

F

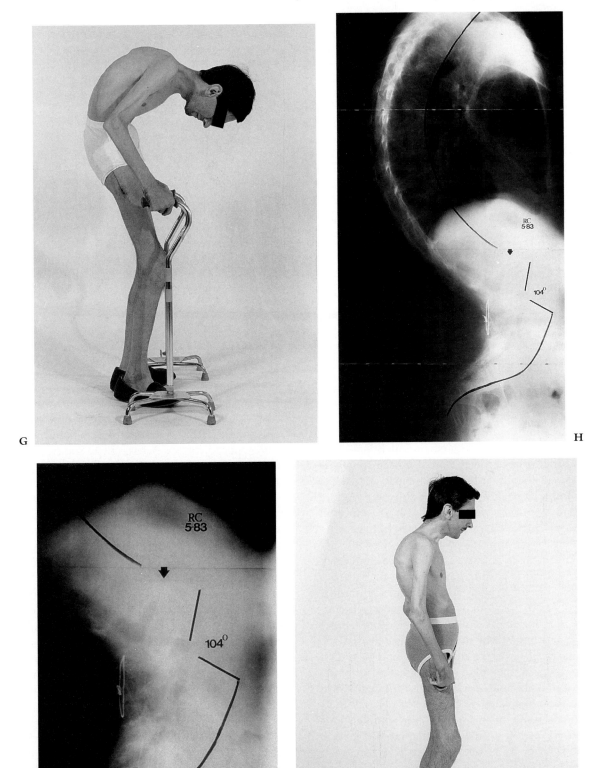

Figure 112-11

For legend see opposite page.

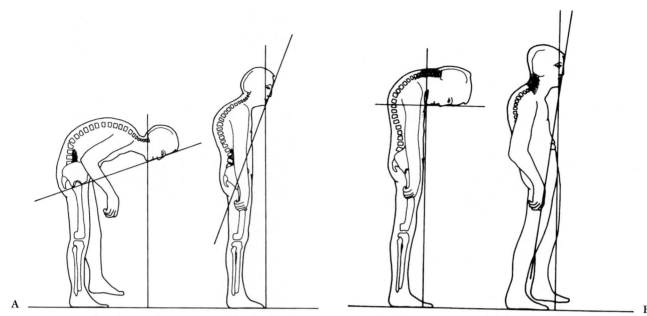

Fig. 112-12

A and B, Measurement of degree of kyphotic deformity of spine in ankylosing spondylitis using the chin-brow to vertical angle. This angle is formed by a line from brow to chin to vertical, measured with patient standing with hips and knees extended and neck in its fixed or neutral position (see p. 1668).

costal margin moving away from the pelvis, the superior mesenteric artery is stretched over the third part of the duodenum, producing a functional block to the outlet of the stomach predisposing to gastric dilatation. If this hazard is not anticipated, patients may vomit a large amount. With a stiff rigid neck in the supine position, there is major risk of aspiration, which could prove fatal. It is necessary to have a nasogastric tube in position postoperatively with suction drainage until intestinal motility is established and the patient is passing gas. Early workers recognized the risk of general anesthesia in the performance of lumbar osteotomy.[15,24] A review of the results of all reported cases of lumbar osteotomy under general anesthesia prior to 1969 indicated that the mortality was 8% to 10% and that neurologic deficit of some degree, including paraplegia, had an incidence of 30%. In analyzing the causes of death, two thirds appeared related to the use of general anesthesia. As a result of this, the author routinely carried out correction on the lumbar spine under local anesthesia from 1969 on. This was found to be a safe, reliable, and practical procedure.[49-51,53,70]

With improvement in anesthesia, particularly the ability to carry out fiberoptic intubation with the patient awake and the development of spinal cord monitoring, the risks of surgery under general anesthesia have markedly decreased. The author's current technique is for the patient to be intubated while awake. With the endotracheal tube in position the patient is able to stand and place himself/herself on an adjusted Tower table with the hips and knees flexed and supports adjusted for the pelvis, chest, and head. These are adjusted until the patient is comfortable, avoiding any strain on the neck or elsewhere. When comfortable, the patient gives an OK signal with the hand, and general anesthesia is commenced. Spinal cord monitoring is done throughout the procedure. It is important to have valid preoperative tracings for comparison with the findings during surgery. The use of general anesthesia makes the resection easier to perform and allows easier undercutting of the pedicles above and below, with a more thorough decompression of the L3 nerve roots. When the hips are extended to produce anterior osteoclasis and extension of the lumbar spine, the knees should be kept flexed to avoid any sciatic nerve tension that would alter the evoked spinal responses if posterior tibial nerve stimulation is used at the ankles (Fig. 112-13).

The initial recommendation of Smith-Peterson et al.[64] was to carry out a posterior wedge resection of the midlumbar spine in a V fashion, with fracturing of the anterior longitudinal ligament. A midline resection was carried upward and outward through the superior facet of the vertebrae above and the inferior facet of the vertebrae below in an oblique fashion. The obliquity of the osteotomy was to allow locking of the vertebrae following correction in an effort to prevent displacement. This technique is the basis for the author's current procedure.

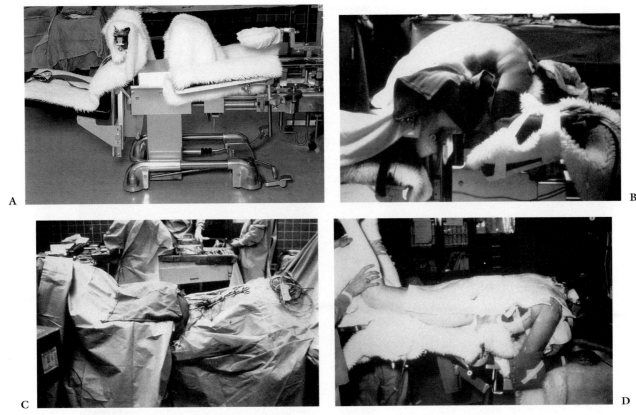

Fig. 112-13

A, Tower table prepared for lumbar osteotomy under general anesthesia, viewed from side. Supports for knees, hips, pelvis, and head may be adjusted for deformity. Patient is intubated while awake, allowing patient to position himself/herself on table while awake. **B,** Side view, showing patient on table. With patient awake, adjustments are made so that head is supported in comfortable position, with eyeballs free of pressure. Chest and pelvic supports are adjusted until comfortable, with abdomen free. Part of patient's weight is borne by knees, with knees and hips flexed. When patient gives an OK sign with fingers, general anesthesia is commenced. **C,** Operative view, with correction of the kyphotic deformity after resection-extension osteotomy of lumbar spine. Hips are extended, spine fracturing anteriorly with resected defect closing posteriorly. Knees are kept flexed to avoid stretching sciatic nerves with possible interference with spinal cord monitoring. Spinal cord monitoring is done throughout procedure, with stimulation of the posterior tibial nerves at ankle. Following closure of defect, instrumentation and grafting is completed. **D,** Postoperative view of patient following application of posterior plaster shell to support patient evenly when turned supine. Note complete correction of deformity with knees flexed.

Technique of Lumbar Osteotomy

Patients are selected who have primarily a lumbar kyphotic deformity with loss of lumbar lordosis. This is determined by clinical and radiologic assessment. The angle of correction that will be required is indicated by measurement of the chin-brow to vertical angle. This angle is transposed to a lateral radiograph of the lumbar spine with the apex of the angle at the posterior longitudinal ligament of the L3-L4 disc space (Fig. 112-14).

The L3-L4 level is one usually selected (on rare occasions, L4-L5) by the author. It represents the apex of the normal lumbar lordosis. It is below the termination of the spinal cord. It is at or below the bifurcation of the aorta.

One of the concerns that has been raised about extension osteotomy of the lumbar spine is the possibility of injury to the major vessels, particularly the abdominal aorta.[2,30,68] All the reported cases of major vascular injury associated with resection-extension osteotomy of the lumbar spine for ankylosing spondylitis have been reviewed, and the level at which the osteotomy was performed in each case was documented by the author. It is noted that in all cases with injury to the abdominal aorta the osteotomy was done at T12-L1, L1-L2, or L2-L3. There is no reported case of aortic injury with osteotomy performed at L3-L4 or L4-L5. One hundred sixteen consecutive lumbar osteotomies performed by the author were also reviewed. Of these, 113 were done at L3-L4, 2 at L4-L5, and only 1 at

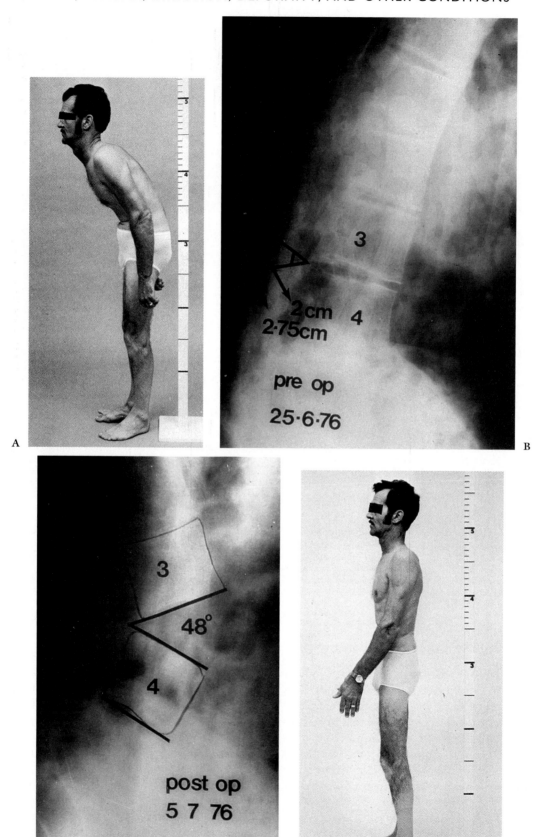

Fig. 112-14

For legend see opposite page.

Fig. 112-14

A, Lateral view of patient standing with hips and knees extended, showing preoperative flexion deformity of lumbar spine with patient's eyes closed and neck in neutral position—chin-brow to vertical angle measured 42 degrees. **B,** Preoperative lateral radiogram demonstrating planned angle of resection at L3-L4 with amount of bone removal indicated. **C,** Lateral postoperative radiogram showing extension correction of 48 degrees demonstrating anterior osteoclasis and closure of posterior resection defects. **D,** Lateral postoperative view of patient showing incomplete correction of preoperative deformity *(From Simmons EH: Kyphotic deformity of the spine in ankylosing spondylitis,* Clin Orthop 128:65, 1977.)

L2-L3. There was no incidence of major arterial injury. The presence of previous radiation or atheromatous change did not result in major vessel injury. The extent of correction was also not a factor. Correction ranged from 40° to 140°, with an overall average of 58° (see Fig. 112-11). The reasons for greater vascular safety of osteotomies done at L3-L4 or L4-L5 are the increased mobility of the aortic bifurcation and iliac arteries related to lower limb motion, the segmental vessels of L5 arise from the internal iliac arteries, and the segmental vessels of L5 and L4 are smaller vessels than higher segmental arteries. The reasons for greater vascular risk of osteotomies at higher levels are that the aorta becomes less mobile proximally; the renal arteries arise at L2-L3, adding to fixation of the aorta; and the segmental vessels increase in size proximally.

The only vascular injury encountered by the author was an inferior vena caval thrombosis extending above the renal veins. This occurred in a markedly obese male who had undergone previous extension osteotomy at L2-L3 but still had major deformity. The thrombosis was likely related to the weight of his corpulent abdomen resting on his stretched vena cava after extension correction. The patient did well in the early postoperative interval, but 4 to 5 days postoperatively gradually increasing edema developed, which became massive and extended up to the midchest, with his scrotum "the size of a football." There was no change in arterial pulses or evidence of arterial insufficiency. Routine Doppler studies of his lower extremities did not reveal the diagnosis initially, it being established by nuclear venography. With the increased intraspinal venous pressure neurologic deficit developed on the basis of venous stasis of the conus, as described by Aboulker et al.[1] The neurologic deficit was maximal when the edema was greatest. Most of the patients with this disease are relatively thin, which is likely the reason that this has not been encountered in other cases. There was no change in arterial pulses or evidence of arterial insufficiency.

Evolution of the Author's Technique for Lumbar Resection-Extension Osteotomy in Ankylosing Spondylitis

Earlier Technique

Initially the operation was done under local anesthesia. This avoided pulmonary complications and mortality related to pulmonary complications. It provided the best of intraoperative monitoring of neurologic, vascular, and other vital functions.[48,49,52,53] The results of the first 64 cases done under local anesthesia were reported by D.J. Wills in 1985.[70] Stabilization of the osteotomy when performed under local anesthesia was initially based on a **V**-shaped locking osteotomy with plaster shells and a turning frame for 6 to 8 weeks. Later, wire-loop fixation of the osteotomy site was added to increase comfort (Fig. 112-15). A Luque rectangle was then used with Drummond buttons and wires and Colrel-Dobousset instrumentation was also used, this all being possible with the procedure done under local anesthesia. Regardless of whether or not internal fixation is used and regardless of what type of fixation is used, the most important factor in the successful maintenance of correction is to correct the deformity completely, shifting the weight-bearing line posterior to the osteotomy site so that gravity will maintain and tend to increase correction with stimulation of bone formation through the weight-bearing lines of the fusion masses posterolaterally. Postoperative management used well-molded posterior and anterior plaster body shells extending from head to knee in which the patient could be firmly strapped for turning with the use of a circoelectric bed, later a Stryker turning frame, and finally a Roto-rest bed.[34,36,39]

Current Technique

The author's current technique of fiberoptic intubation with the patient awake was described above.

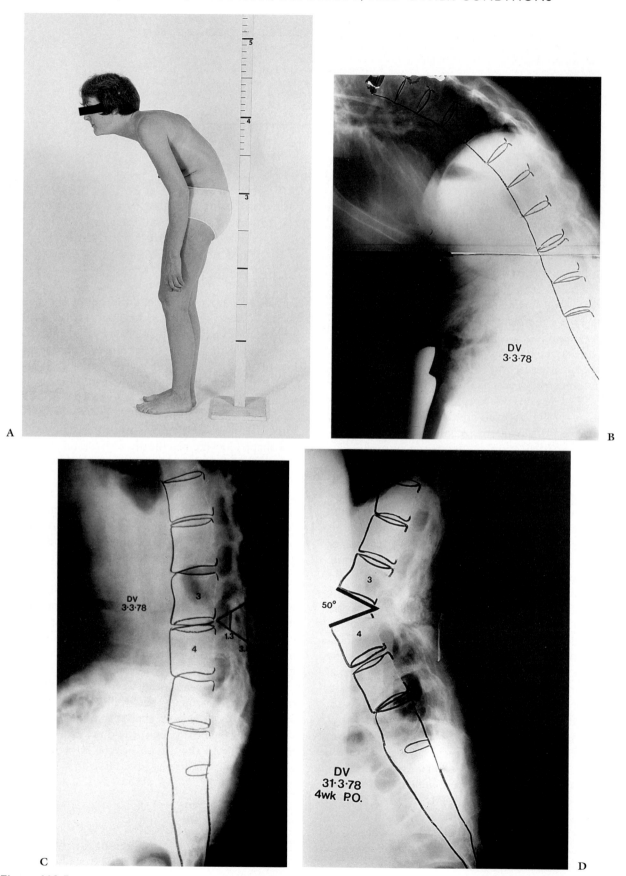

Figure 112-5

For legend see opposite page.

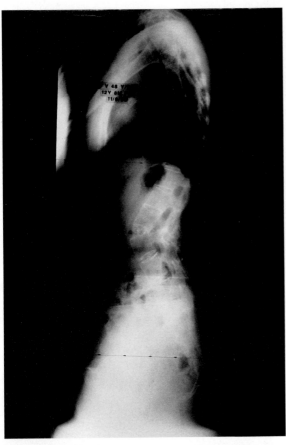

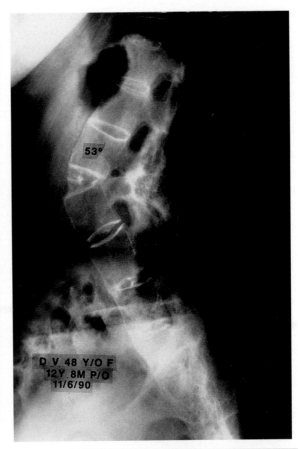

E

F

Fig. 112-15

A, Lateral standing view of female patient with primarily lumbar kyphotic deformity. Patient tends to flex knees and hyperextend neck to compensate for deformity. Weight-bearing line is well anterior to midlumbar spine. **B,** Preoperative standing lateral radiogram showing complete loss of lumbar lordosis. **C,** Lateral radiogram of lumbar spine showing loss of lumbar lordosis with sacrum in vertical position. Planned resection osteotomy at L3-L4 is indicated. **D,** Lateral postoperative radiogram of lumbar spine showing extension correction of 50 degrees. Weight-bearing line is posterior to osteotomy site. **F,** Lateral standing 3-ft radiogram of the spine 12 years postoperatively showing maintenance of correction with weight-bearing line posterior to osteotomy site reducing bone formation posteriorly. **F,** Lateral standing postoperative radiogram of lumbar spine showing solid union with bone hypertrophy posteriorly. Effect of gravity has maintained correction and if anything added to it. Extension angle now measures 53 degrees. **G,** Postoperative lateral view of patient showing complete correction of deformity. Only internal fixation used was wire loop at ossified interspinous ligaments above and below. Patient being treated with plaster molds in recumbent position on circoelectric bed for 6 weeks followed by immobilization in plaster body cast.

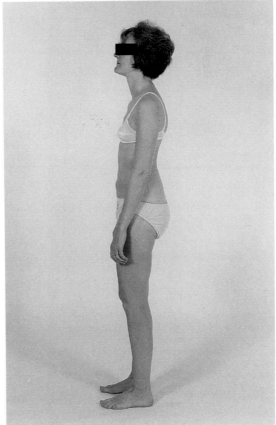

G

The patient is placed on an adjusted Tower table while awake. Anesthesia is commenced when the patient is comfortable. Spinal cord monitoring is carried out throughout the procedure. Bone screws are inserted into the pedicles at the appropriate levels above and below the planned osteotomy site. The posterior resection is done with the laminae and pedicles undercut to avoid nerve-root and dural sac impingement. The hips are extended with anterior osteoclasis and closure of the posterior osteotomy. The screw-rod (TSRH) instrumentation is completed. Posterolateral and posterior bone grafting is done using the removed morselized bone, which is usually quite generous. A well-molded posterior plaster shell is applied extending from head to knee. The patient is strapped into the shell and transferred in the shell to a Roto-rest bed. It is important to recognize that this is an essential part of the procedure. Following extension osteotomy the rigid thoracic kyphosis will be more prominent than the pelvis, and if the patient is lying on a flat surface, gravity will tend to push the thorax forward and allow the pelvis and lower lumber spine to come posteriorly. If the trap door of the bed is removed for a bowel movement, the spine would be unsupported. A well-contoured rigid posterior plaster shell provides a contoured well-fitted surface on which the rigid trunk can lie protecting the osteotomy site (Fig. 112-16). A nasogastric suction tube is placed before the patient leaves the operating room. It is maintained until the patient is passing gas, with normal gastric function.

The advantages of the current technique are that it allows easier and more liberal decompression. It provides more rigid internal fixation with less risk of displacement, easier and more rapid mobilization, and probably greater comfort for the patient. Its disadvantages are increased operative time, the altered anatomy for screw insertion into the pedicles and the potential risks of bone screws. At this time it would appear that the advantages outweigh the disadvantages, and to date it has provided excellent results (Figs. 112-17 and 112-18).

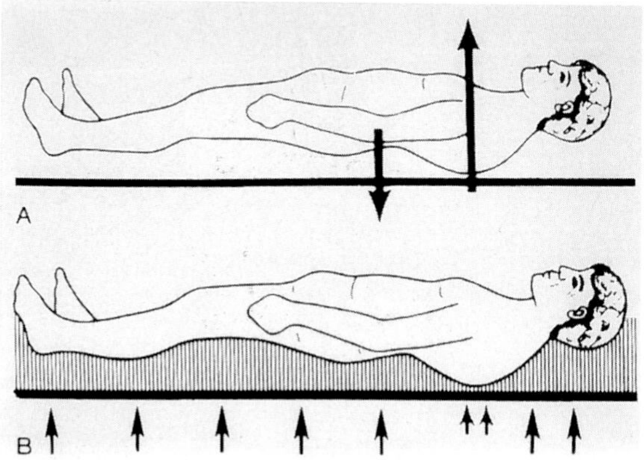

Fig. 112-16

A, Diagrammatic outline of patient's contour following extension correction of lumbar spine. It is important to appreciate that patient's spine is rigid. Illustration shows the areas of relative pressure contact when the corrected spine is placed in supine position. Pressure against thoracic hump tends to push it forward with lumbar spine tending to translate posteriorly. **B,** Diagram showing effect of a well-molded rigid plaster shell providing equal support throughout spine, avoiding any uneven contact pressure forces, which would favor displacement.

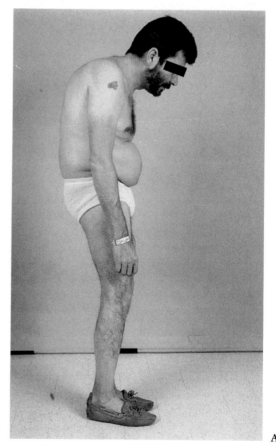

A

Fig. 112-17

A, Lateral view of 41-year-old male with 21-year history of ankylosing spondylitis. He had suffered major kyphotic deformity for 10 years, which prevented him from working for 5 to 6 years. Chin-brow to vertical angle measured 55 degrees.

Continues.

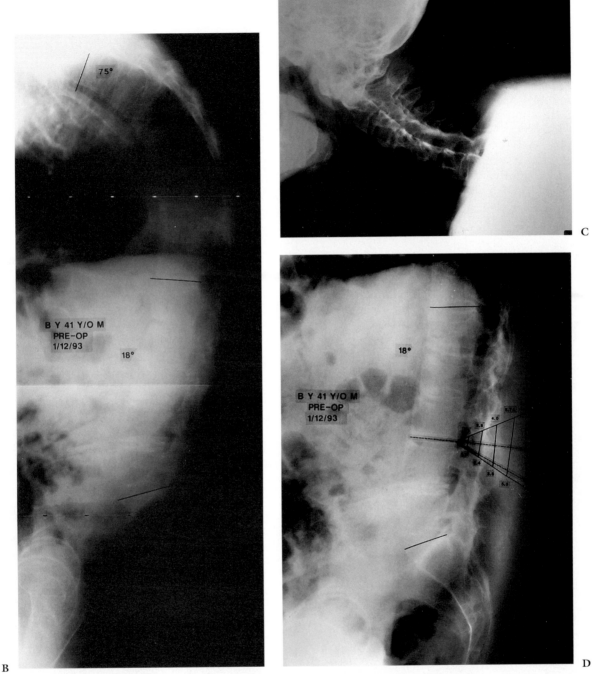

Fig. 112-17, cont'd

B, Lateral standing 3-ft film of spine showing increased thoracic kyphosis measuring 75 degrees but decreased lumbar lordosis measuring 18 degrees. Weight-bearing line is well anterior to the midlumbar spine. **C,** Lateral standing radiogram of cervical spine showing compensatory increase in cervical lordosis with ossification from C2 distally. **D,** Preoperative lateral radiogram of lumbar spine showing planned resection-osteotomy at L3-L4 of 50 degrees to 55 degrees.

Continues.

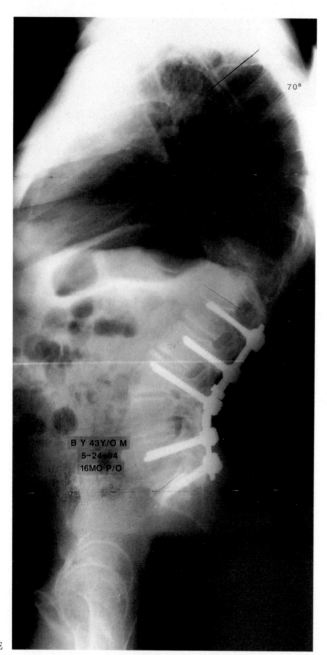

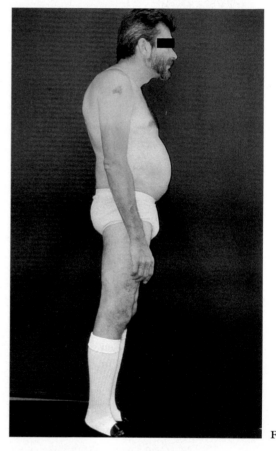

Fig. 112-17, cont'd

E, Lateral standing 3-ft radiogram 16 months postoperatively showing healed osteotomy with lumbar lordosis measuring 74 degrees. Thoracic kyphosis is corrected slightly to 70 degrees. Spine is in balance. Main weight-bearing line is posterior to osteotomy site. **F,** Standing lateral view of patient 16 months postoperatively. Patient has returned to normal lifestyle. His correction prompted uninformed observer to state that his wife was living with "a different man."

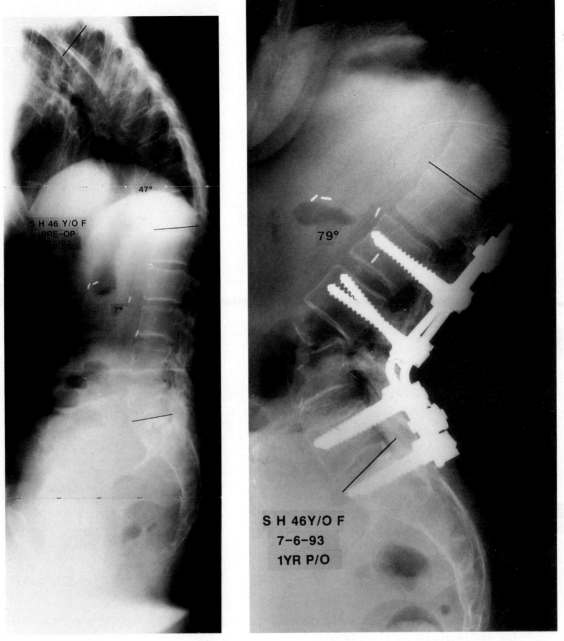

Fig. 112-18

A, Standing lateral 3-ft radiogram of 45-year-old female with 20-year history of Crohn's disease and 16-year history of ankylosing spondylitis. She had combined kyphotic deformity of her spine with a chin-brow to vertical angle of 65 degrees. This amount of correction was planned. **B,** Lateral radiogram of lumbar spine 1 year postoperatively showing extension correction allowed with stable fixation using transpedicular screw fixation. Lumbar lordosis of 79 degrees has been created.

Continues.

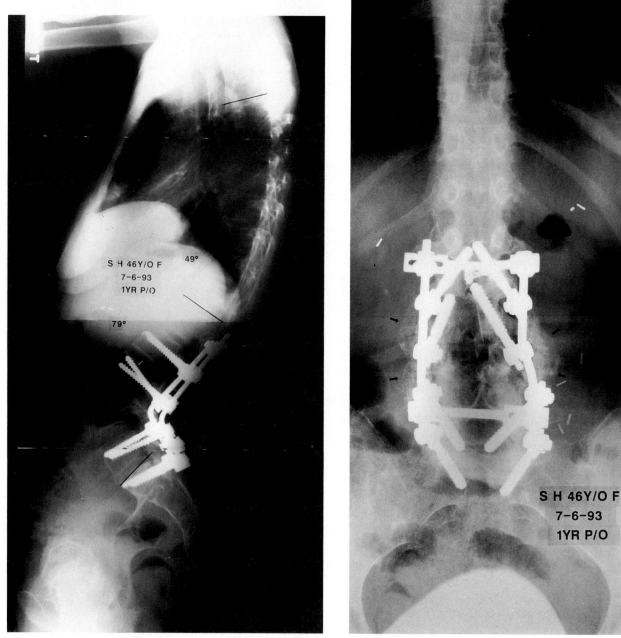

Fig. 112-18, cont'd

C, Standing lateral 3-ft radiogram of spine 1 year postoperatively showing weight-bearing line well posterior to osteotomy site with patient's chin-brow to vertical angle being restored to normal range. **D,** Anteroposterior radiogram 1 year postoperatively showing hypertrophy of fusion masses along lines of stress posterolaterally. Anterior defect is slow to fill in due to lack of stress.

Kyphotic Deformity of the Thoracic Spine

Some increase in thoracic kyphosis is fairly common in patients with spinal deformity associated with ankylosing spondylitis. However, it is unusual for the thoracic kyphosis to be an isolated deformity requiring correction that is confined to that area.

Patients with thoracic kyphosis can be classified into two groups. In the first group there is major increase in thoracic kyphosis, but in addition there is an associated loss of lumbar lordosis with a rigid spine. If the thoracic kyphosis is mild or moderate and the lumbar spine flattened and rigid, restoration of spinal balance and overall correction of spinal deformity may be accomplished in this group by a compensating extension osteotomy of the lumbar spine. With sufficient extension of the lumbar spine, compensation can be achieved for the thoracic kyphosis allowing a horizontal gaze and erect posture (see (Fig. 112-17). Patients in the second group have thoracic kyphotic deformity but maintain a normal or even increased (compensatory) cervical and lumbar lordosis. This necessitates surgery directed primarily to the thoracic kyphosis. This presents significant problems. A single major angular correction of the thoracic spine could cause significant spinal cord or even vascular injury.[2,30,68]

The spinal canal is relatively small in the thoracic region. The spinal cord and nerve roots have little mobility, and the blood supply to the thoracic spinal cord is the most precarious. The same principles that have been adapted to rigid kyphotic deformity in Scheuermann's disease or congenital thoracic kyphosis have to be followed. This employs combinations of preoperative traction and staged anterior and posterior osteotomies with intervertebral traction and posterior instrumentation. When employing these surgical principles it is feasible to obtain satisfactory correction of primary kyphotic deformity of the thoracic spine secondary to ankylosing spondylitis.

Patients with primarily thoracic kyphosis who have maintained a normal or increased lumbar and cervical lordosis can be further separated into two subgroups, according to the rigidity of the thoracic spine. The first subgroup is distinguished by having incomplete ossification of the thoracic spine or extensive areas of destructive spondylodiscitis resulting in areas of relative mobility. The second subgroup has a rigid thoracic kyphosis with essentially complete ossification.

In the first subgroup with incomplete ossification of the thoracic spine or areas of destructive spondy-lodiscitis, preliminary correction may be obtained by halo-dependent traction, followed by multiple posterior resection osteotomies and compression instrumentation. The halo-dependent traction is continued, followed by a second-stage anterior resection of the areas of spondylodiscitis and the disc spaces with anterior strut grafting (Fig. 112-19).

The more common second subgroup involves patients with rigid thoracic kyphosis and relatively complete ossification. A first-stage anterior transthoracic procedure is required. A right-sided thoracotomy approach is used, with removal of the rib at the level of the apex of the deformity in the midaxillary line. The pleura is incised lateral to the spine and reflected medially. The ossified disc spaces are resected completely from the right to the left side of the spine back to the posterior annulus and longitudinal ligament. The resected disc spaces are packed with morselized portions of the removed bone, complemented by iliac crest bone graft where necessary. The disc spaces are resected in the area of main deformity. The diaphragm is not disturbed, recognizing that these patients depend almost entirely on diaphragmatic breathing for respiration. Halo-dependent traction is carried out postoperatively.

A second stage posterior procedure is than required 7 to 10 days later. Multiple V-shaped resection osteotomies are carried out at each level involved in the thoracic kyphosis, resecting the ossified ligamentum flavum and adjacent portions of the laminae upward and outward through the fused facets and foramina, removing enough bone to allow adequate correction following closure. Bilateral compression instrumentation is applied, gradually closing the osteotomy sites and correcting the deformity (Fig. 112-20). Despite the feasibility and the satisfactory results that have been obtained with the combined procedure, it should be recognized that combined anterior and posterior procedures under general anesthesia in patients with this disease are more hazardous than a single-stage extension correction of the lumbar spine that is done under general or local anesthesia, and particularly the latter. Tracheostomy has been required in almost a third of these patients, with its attendant problems. However, if the primary deformity is thoracic with a normal lordosis above and below, the risks have to be accepted if the deformity is to be corrected. The safety of the correction is enhanced by the fact that multiple osteotomies are performed in the thoracic region so that correction at any one level is minimal, yet the accumulative effect allows significant correc-

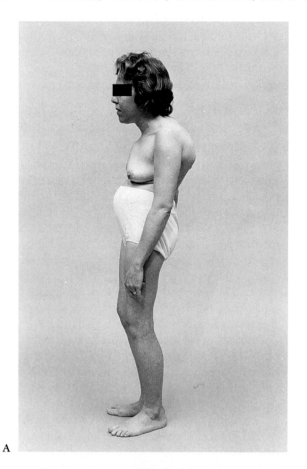

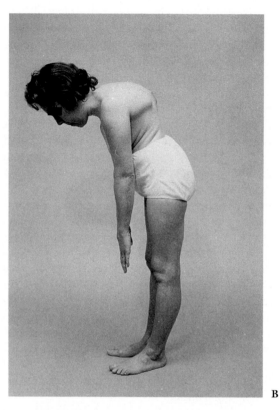

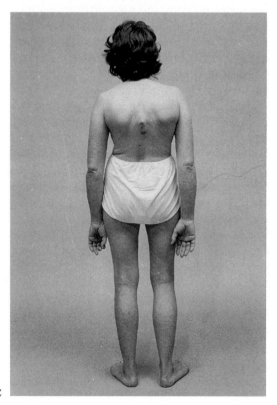

Fig. 112-19

A, B, and **C,** Standing lateral, lateral flexion, and posterior views of 32-year-old female with severe thoracic kyphosis associated with ankylosing spondylitis and steroid therapy. She had suffered a decrease in height of 6 in. with rib impingement against pelvis. She had skin pressure changes over the apex of her thoracic gibbus.

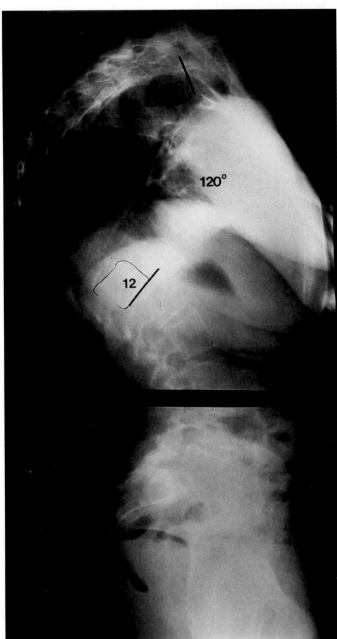

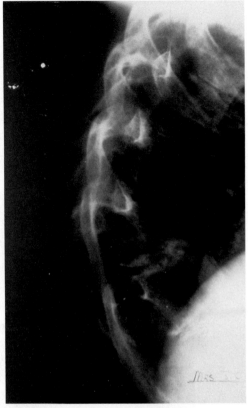

Fig. 112-19, cont'd

D, Standing lateral radiogram demonstrating thoracic kyphosis of 120 degrees with exaggerated lumbar lordosis. **E,** Lateral radiogram of apex of thoracic deformity showing destructive spondylodiscitis. **F,** Operative view of resection of areas of spondylodiscitis with prepared trough from T6 to T11 for strut graft placement.

Continues.

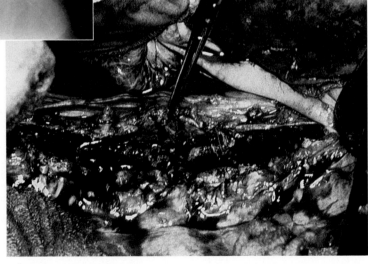

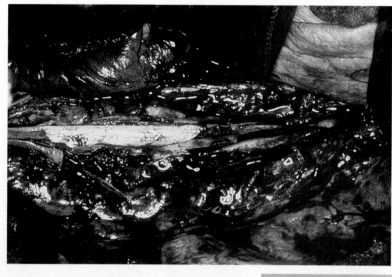

G

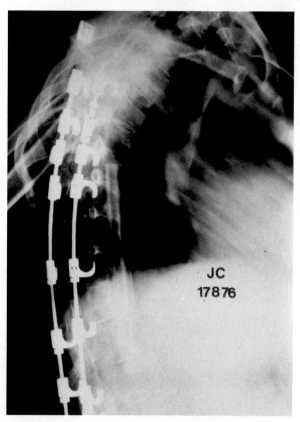

H

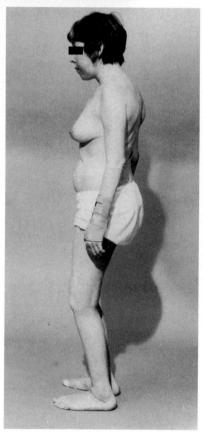

I

Fig. 112-19, cont'd
G, Operative view showing fibular strut graft from T6 to T11 with onlay rib grafts. **H,** Lateral postoperative radiogram showing strut graft and posterior compression instrumentation. Areas of spondylodiscitis are healed. **I,** Lateral standing postoperative view of patient showing correction of deformity. Patient had increase in height of 5 in.

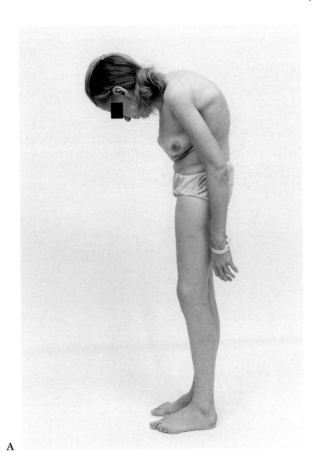

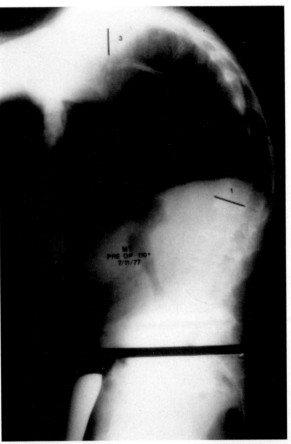

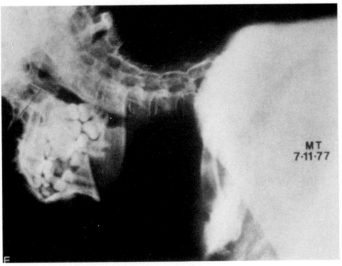

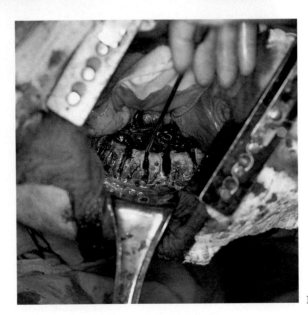

Fig. 112-20

A, Lateral view of 34-year-old female presenting with rigid thoracic kyphosis with normal cervical and lumbar lordosis. She had lost 5 in. in height. **B,** Standing lateral 3-ft preoperative radiogram demonstrating thoracic kyphosis of 110 degrees with normal lumbar lordosis. **C,** Preoperative lateral radiogram of cervical spine showing normal or increased cervical lordosis. **D,** Operative view of complete anterior transthoracic resection of disc spaces from one side to other.

Continues.

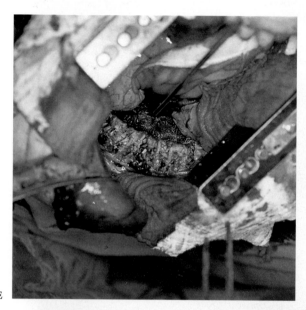

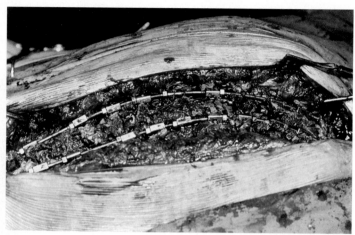

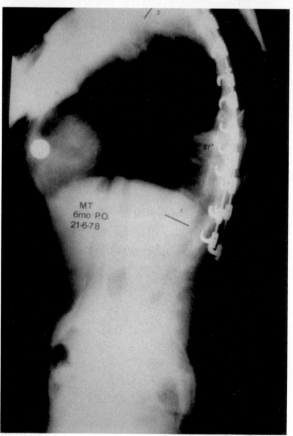

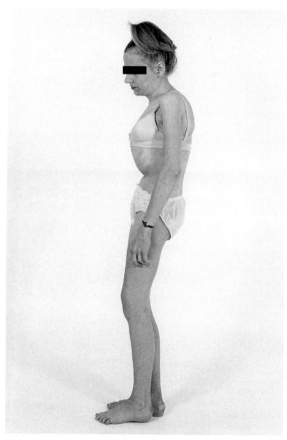

Fig. 112-20, cont'd

E, Operative view of autogenous rib grafting of resected disc spaces. F, Operative view of multiple posterior osteotomies with bilateral compression instrumentation and fusion. Resections of ossified ligamentum flavum was carried out at each level passing upward and laterally through fused posterior joint.
G, Lateral postoperative standing 3-ft radiogram showing restoration of normal spinal alignment following
correction of thoracic kyphotic deformity. H, Lateral postoperative view of patient showing correction of
major deformity. Ribs are lifted out of pelvis.

tion. Anterior and posterior osteotomies with interval traction allow correction while the patient is awake, reducing neurologic risk. The use of spinal cord monitoring, particularly for the posterior instrumentation, allows greater safety in carrying out reasonable correction in a critical area (Fig. 112-21).

Kyphotic Deformity of the Cervical Spine

A few patients with ankylosing spondylitis present with kyphotic deformity primarily in the cervical spine. This deformity may be severely disabling, with marked restriction of the field of vision and interference with skin care and shaving under the chin, progressing to marked interference with opening of the mouth, with acute angulation of the neck and chin-on-chest deformity. There may be major difficulty in swallowing, with episodes of choking, which in some patients is the chief symptom for which they request correction of the deformity. Because of its relative infrequency, orthopedic surgeons are less familiar with the techniques required for correction and the potentially greater hazards. There is no major review available of all attempts to carry out osteotomy of the cervical spine under general anesthesia. In my experience, verbal communication related to isolated attempts made at various centers has indicated a high rate of disastrous complications, including death. For the few severely afflicted patients with this particular deformity, the principles related to its possible correction proven on the basis of experience and the indications for it should be clearly understood.

Selection of Patients for Cervical Osteotomy

In assessing patients for correction of cervical kyphotic deformity, a very important differentiation

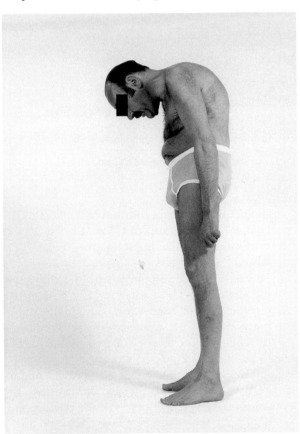

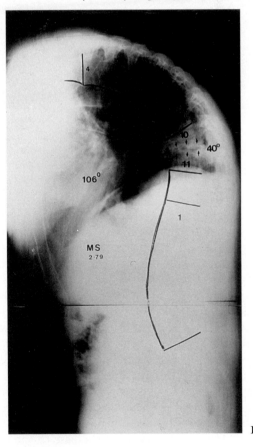

Fig. 112-21

A, Preoperative lateral view showing primarily thoracic deformity in 48-year-old surgeon. Cervical and lumbar lordosis is normal. **B,** Preoperative standing lateral 3-ft radiogram showing fixed kyphosis of 106 degrees with normal lumbar lordosis. Spine was rigid, without any correction obtained with halo-dependent traction despite localized area of spondylodiscitis. Anterior osteotomies and grafting followed by halo-dependent traction and then posterior osteotomies with posterior compression instrumentation were carried out.

Continues.

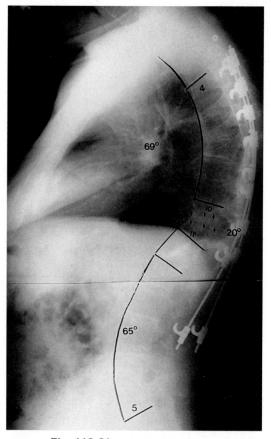

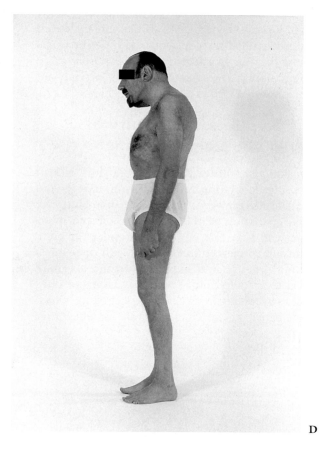

C   D

Fig. 112-21

C, Standing lateral postoperative 3-ft radiogram showing correction of thoracic kyphosis from 106 degrees to 69 degrees balanced by lordosis of 65 degrees. Area of spondylodiscitis has healed. **D,** Lateral postoperative view of patient showing correction of major kyphotic deformity. Patient was able to return to practice of surgery and normal lifestyle.

should be made between patients with longstanding fixed and relatively painless deformity from those who present with recent painful progressive deformity. Patients with longstanding ankylosing spondylitis who go on to sudden painful increasing kyphotic deformity of the neck, even after minimal or what is thought to be insignificant trauma, should be considered as having a fracture of the cervical spine until proven otherwise. The areas of injury to be suspected are at the base of the neck at the cervical-thoracic junction, or less commonly at the craniocervical junction. Fractures of the spine in ankylosing spondylitis resemble fractures of an osteoporotic tubular long bone with a transverse shear pattern. They tend to occur at the base of the neck due to the leverage effect of the weight of the head and a fused cervical spine.[56] The fractures are very commonly missed due to the fact that they can be produced by minor injury and the difficulty in demonstrating them on routine radiographic examination. The fractures are usually obscured by the

shoulders, varying in location from C6 to T2, most commonly in the area of C7 to T1. Their outline is even more indistinct in osteoporotic bone.[56] The obscured fracture undergoes gradual erosion and compression collapse anteriorly, with the chin approaching the chest. The patient usually notices that the position of the head varies during the day, being more elevated on awakening in the morning, with the chin approaching the chest as the day progresses (Fig. 112-22).

On occasion the patient may present holding the head with the hands to ease the distress. There is usually localized tenderness at the fracture site. It is important to recognize the presence of fracture at the cervical-thoracic junction by the use of lateral tomography and not to disregard the patient's reported symptoms. When the fracture is still in its painful mobile state, patients do not require cervical osteotomy. A cranial halo should be applied with traction initially applied along the line of the neck slowly restoring the alignment of the neck to its nor-

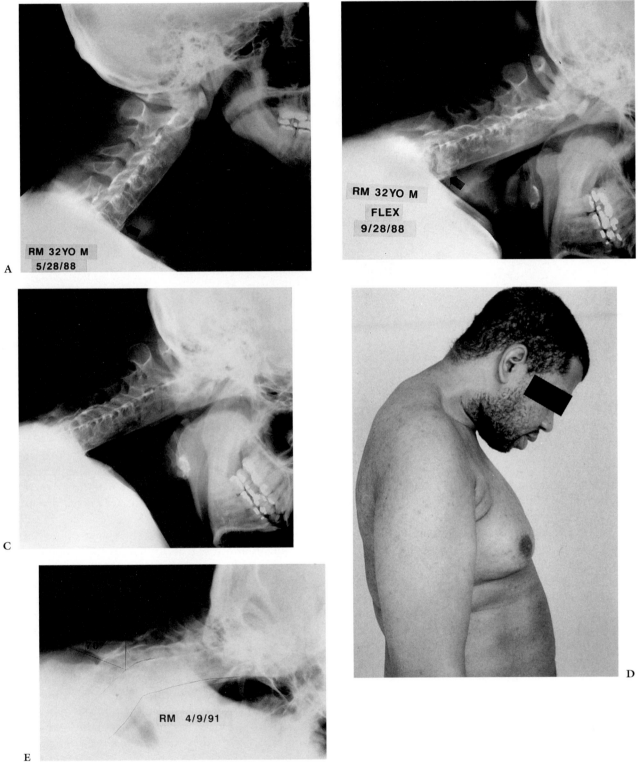

Fig. 112-22

A, Lateral x-ray film done in emergency department of cervical spine of 32-year-old male with a known history of ankylosing spondylitis who presented with pain in neck after minor injury. Radiogram was thought to be "normal," and patient was advised that he had no major bony injury but a "sprain." Undetected area of fracture is indicated by *arrow.* **B,** Lateral radiogram of same patient 4 months later, showing development of kyhotic deformity of cervical spine. Area of fracture erosion is indicated by *arrow.* Patient was treated with collar support. **C,** Lateral radiogram of cervical spine 1 year after injury. By this time patient had gone on to relief of pain with fixed painless kyphotic deformity following healing of fracture with chin-on-chest deformity. **D,** Lateral view of patient presenting with painless fixed kyphotic deformity of cervical spine following missed fracture at base of neck and healing with chin approaching chest. **E,** Preoperative lateral tomogram outlining 70 degrees wedge resection, which was required for extension osteotomy.

continues.

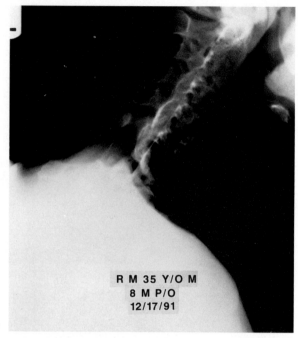

R M 35 Y/O M
8 M P/O
12/17/91

F

Fig. 112-22, cont'd

F, Lateral radiogram of cervical spine showing healed osteotomy 8 months postoperatively. G, Postoperative lateral standing view of patient showing correction of deformity with normal chin-brow to vertical angle. Early recognition of fracture would have prevented progression of deformity and need for osteotomy correction.

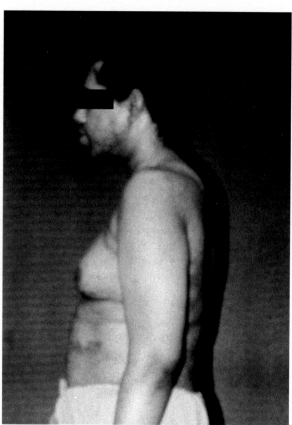

G

mal position. This is most easily and efficiently accomplished with the use of a circoelectric bed. The line of pull is easily adjusted and changed on the bed, and the patient can be tilted toward the vertical, maintaining the traction. A normal chin-brow to vertical angle can usually be restored, or at least the alignment can be returned to the preinjury state.

Following the restoration of satisfactory alignment, the patient should be immobilized in a well-molded halo cast for 4 months. The rigid immobilization of a very well-molded halo cast is recommended, rather than a less substantial halo vest. A routine halo vest usually does not supply adequate immobilization for these patients with a solid column of bone above and below the fracture site. The cast should be very well applied, being molded over the iliac crests and under the costal cage, so that it does not move independently of the patient's movements. In my experience, if rigid immobilization is provided in this union consistently occurs during the period of immobilization, which is usually followed by a shorter interval of bracing (Fig. 112-23).

If in a rare instance spontaneous healing did not occur, then posterior fusion fixation or even anterior fusion with a Keystone graft[57] would have to be con-

sidered. Although they occur most commonly at the base of the neck, shear fractures may occur at any level. With significant initial displacement, patients may present with evidence of spinal cord injury, and this may occur rapidly during the course of the early treatment, as a result of displacement.

It should be recognized that patients with ankylosing spondylitis suffering fracture dislocations of the cervical spine are prone to disastrous results if conventional methods of treatment are used for fracture dislocations without ankylosing spondylitis. The spine above and below the fracture site in these patients is rigid. Any movement of the trunk translates motion to the fracture site. A common comment of relatives of patients when they first see them in the emergency department often immobilized on a fracture board, is that "the neck is straight," whereas before the injury the patient had a well-recognized kyphotic deformity. It should be recognized that the patient has an extension displacement at the fracture site if lying flat. The patient or the relative should be questioned concerning the preinjury alignment of the neck and attempts made to simulate this position with support and the early application of a halo with gentle traction along what was believed to be

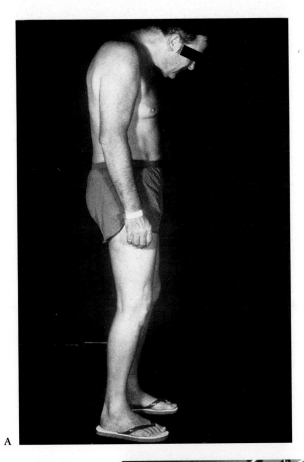

A

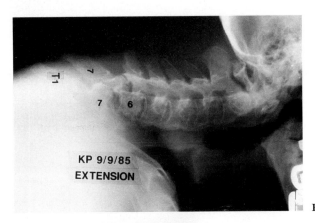

B

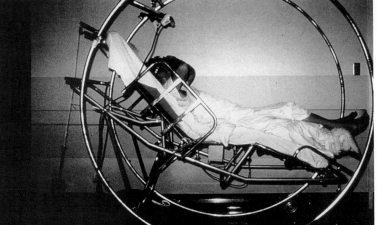

C

Fig. 112-23

A, Standing lateral view of 55-year-old executive referred for cervical osteotomy. Patient had sustained minor injury to neck 9 months previously and had gone on to painful cervical kyphotic deformity. **B,** Lateral radiogram of patient showing cervical kyphotic deformity, emphasizing difficulty of visualization of fracture at the C7-T1 level. Patient had pain on attempted motion of neck. **C,** Technique of halo-dependent traction, which is used to reduce fracture deformity gradually. Traction is applied along line of neck in both sagittal and coronal planes, restoring alignment to preinjury position. Some improvement in preinjury chin-brow to vertical angle may be obtained if indicated.

Continues.

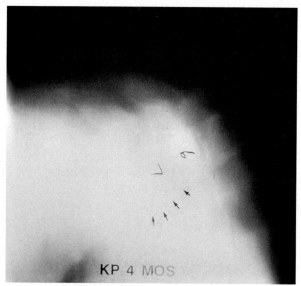

D

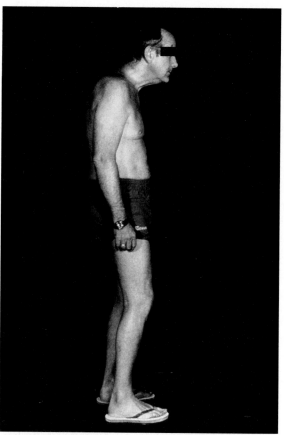

E

Fig. 112-23, cont'd

D, Lateral radiogram of cervical spine showing healing of missed fracture with new bone formation anteriorly following reduction with halo-dependent traction and immobilization in halo cast for 4 months. **E,** Postreduction and fracture unilateral view of patient showing correction of deformity and normal chin-brow to vertical angle. Osteotomy was not required despite duration of fracture deformity.

the normal alignment, with the patient then being protected with a halo vest. Ideally, this should be done before any radiographic studies are carried out to avoid displacement while the studies are being done. Lateral tomography is the most valuable and essential radiographic assessment on initial presentation, concerning the recognition and alignment of the fracture, along with other routine radiographic studies.[56]

When incomplete spinal cord injury has occurred and is associated with incomplete reduction, open reduction and internal fixation is indicated to protect the cord from further injury caused by motion at the fracture site magnified by the solid segments above and below. Accurate reduction of spinal canal alignment, in itself, allows decompression of the spinal cord. The dangers of attempted operative reduction under general anesthesia should be recognized.

Movement of the neck required for intubation with a rigid upper cervical spine can cause further spinal cord injury. Transferring patients in the operating room and positioning them also present some risk under general anesthesia. In my experience, these patients are most safely operated on while awake and in the sitting position. After stabilization of the neck in a halo jacket, surgery is performed in the sitting position. Traction is applied along the line of the neck, adding to the support of the patient and the immobilization provided by the halo vest. The posterior cervical spine is exposed under local anesthesia, with the fracture accurately reduced and fixed internally. In my experience this is most quickly and efficiently accomplished by passing threaded Compere wires percutaneously through the bases of the spinous processes above and below with an encircling stainless steel wire. It is thought that this is an appropriate indication of the use of methylmethacrylate, which is used to fix the spine, with methylmethacrylate bridges on each side incorporating the threaded pins (Fig. 112-24).

This technique provides instant fixation relieving pain at the fracture site and it maintains accurate alignment of the spinal canal until healing occurs anteriorly. If further decompression is thought to be indicated, this can be done in the midline with the methylmethacrylate bridges placed on each side of the decompression. However, the restoration of accurate alignment is undoubtedly the main factor in the decompression. It has been my practice that following the surgery, the halo vest is changed to a well-molded halo cast to supply more rigid immobilization. Again, the cast should be molded over the iliac crests and below the costal cage to prevent upward and downward excursion. This is used for 4 months.

The craniocervical junction is the other area where lesions may occur, causing patients to present with painful neck flexion deformity. C1-C2 subluxation may present with painful neck kyphotic deformity with or without neurologic symptoms. This can be treated with halo-traction reduction and posterior atlantoaxial arthrodesis as already described. Erosive fractures through the posterior arch of C1 may be associated with C1-C2 subluxation, and de-

structive arthritis at the atlantooccipital joints may result in a painful kyphotic deformity. A lateral radiogram of the cervical spine will show a relatively normal lordosis with flexion at the craniocervical junction, with the mandible approaching the cervical spine. These lesions should be recognized as the cause of the kyphotic deformity, with the deformity corrected by halo traction initially along the line of the neck, restoring normal alignment, followed by posterior stabilization. For destructive change at the occipital-atlantal joints and erosive fractures through the arch of C1, occipital-cervical fusion is required with excision of the posterior fragmented arch of C1 (see Figs. 112-4 and 112-25).

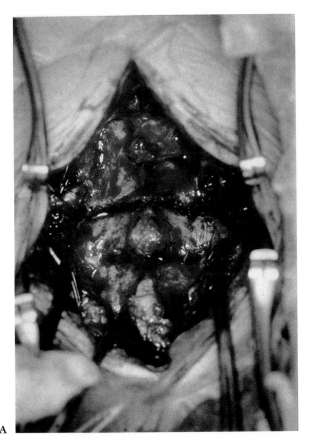 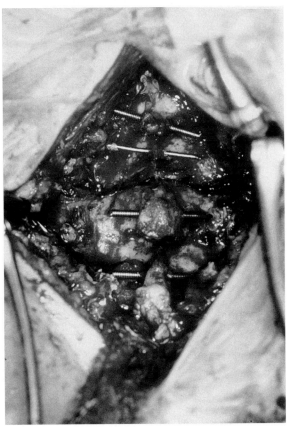

A   B

Fig. 112-24

A, Operative view of posterior aspect of cervical spine of 32-year-old male suffering ankylosing spondylitis with displaced fracture dislocation of C6-C7 with partial quadriplegia following automobile accident. Position of fracture was improved by placing patient in halo vest simulating his preoperative alignment. Some displacement persisted. Patient was operated on in sitting position under local anesthesia. Halo vest supported his head, with head being suspended along line of neck for cervical traction adding to immobilization. Under local anesthesia fracture has been reduced with C5 and C6 spinous processes exposed above and spinous processes of C7 and T1 below with their associated laminae. **B,** Posterior operative view showing reduction of fracture dislocation with threaded Compere pins in position through posterior arches of C5, C6, C7, and T1. Threaded pins were inserted percutaneously from left side of the neck, traversing bases of spinous processes, wires then being cut lateral to spine.

Continues.

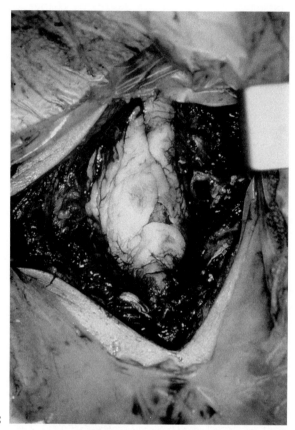

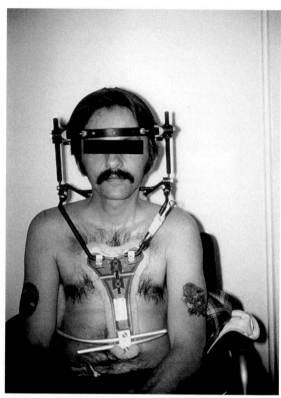

C

D

Fig. 112-24, cont'd

C, Posterior view of spine following methylmethacrylate fixation incorporating Compere pins and spinous processes. This maintained reduction with instant fixation of unstable shear fracture dislocation. Immobilization provides protection to injured spinal cord, thus facilitating recovery. It prevents damaging effects of any further motion at fracture site until bony healing occurs. If midline decompression is required, bridges of methylmethacrylate may be placed laterally on each side, leaving midline free. Use of local anesthesia allows best of spinal cord monitoring and avoids any possible injury due to manipulation of neck in course of endotracheal intubation and use of general anesthesia. **D,** Early postoperative view of patient. Accurate reduction, internal fixation, and adequate external immobilization allow early active rehabilitation. Patient went on to full recovery in lower limbs, with residual central cord involvement of upper extremities.

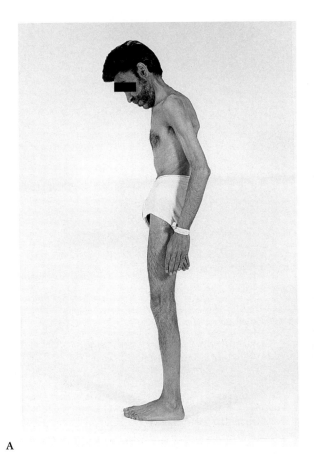

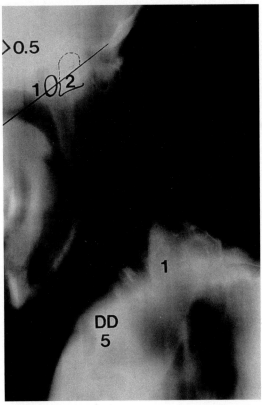

A

B

Fig. 112-25

A, Lateral presenting view of male referred for cervical osteotomy. He had a painful chin-on-chest deformity. Patient used hands to hold head when sitting to control pain. **B,** Lateral tomogram showing approximation of chin to cervical spine but also demonstrating normal cervical lordosis with normal alignment at cervical thoracic junction. Neck is flexed at occipital-atlantal joints; C1-C2 relationships are normal. There was destructive change at occipital-atlantal joints. At surgery, posterior arch of C1 was eroded and loose, likely causing dural irritation with any attempt at extension.

Continues.

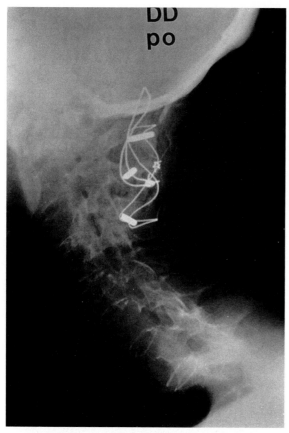

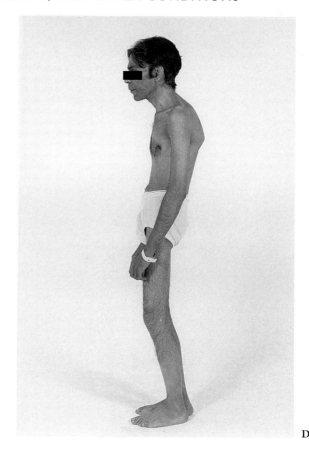

C

D

Fig. 112-25, cont'd

C, Lateral radiogram of cervical spine following surgical treatment. This consisted of graduated reduction of deformity with halo traction, operative excision of loose posterior arch fragment of C1 and posterior occipital-cervical fusion. This was done using double onlay cortical and cancellous iliac grafts fixed to skull and upper cervical spine using Dewar technique, augmented with cancellous grafts. **D,** Lateral view of patient postoperatively, showing restoration of normal chin-brow to vertical angle. Patient's pain was relieved by solid arthrodesis.

Occult Fractures as a Cause of Kyphotic Deformity

Occult or unrecognized fractures at the cervical-thoracic junction go on to gradual erosion and collapse anteriorly until the chin reaches the chest. They ultimately heal in this position with disappearance of pain, leaving the patient with a fixed painless flexion deformity. Patients with this deformity require osteotomy for correction. In a previous review of 39 patients referred for cervical osteotomy, it was found that 36% showed evidence of previous fracture. A fracture contributed significantly to the final kyphotic deformity in 31%. Unfortunately, it had been diagnosed previously in only 14% of those who presented with a fracture.[56,59] In a more recent review of a group of 38 patients, it was found that 18 (47%) had evidence of a previous fracture, and in only 1 had the fracture been recognized prior to pre-sentation for osteotomy.[21] These observations emphasize the fact that early recognition of the fracture and adequate immobilization are essential if the risk of increased late fixed deformity is to be avoided.

Technique of Cervical Osteotomy

The surgical correction of major fixed kyphotic deformity of the cervical spine in ankylosing spondylitis by resection-extension osteotomy involves an anatomic area of major potential risk in patients with major systemic disease and associated medical risks. In considering osteotomy correction of deformity, it is prudent to understand these risks fully and to follow basic established principles to allow major correction of deformity with least risk to the patient.

Since 1966 the author has followed a consistent and reliable technique that has allowed a very gratifying correction of deformity with risks entirely in keeping with major surgery on patients with this disease, related to other areas of their skeleton. Following the recommendation of Urist,[67] surgery is performed under local anesthesia with the patient in the sitting position. This avoids most anesthetic hazards. It provides the most accurate of all forms of spinal cord monitoring and assessment of vital functions with the patient awake. It avoids any major neurologic complication during surgery. The patient is able to assist with anatomic localization during the decompression, which is of real value to the surgeon. The patient is able to recognize when there is irritation to the C8 nerve root and communicate distribution of the pain to the surgeon. The level between the C7 and T1 vertebrae is selected for correction (Fig. 112-26). As Mason et al.[39] and Urist[67] pointed out, this level is more adaptable to surgical correction than any other level in the cervical region. The spinal canal is relatively wide at this level, and the cervical spinal cord and eighth cervical nerve roots have reasonable flexibility. Any deficit caused by injury to the eighth cervical nerve root will cause less disability than other roots.

Anatomic Considerations

Anatomically, it is fortunate that the vertebral artery and veins usually pass in front of the transverse process of the seventh vertebrae and enter the cervical spine through the transverse foramen at the sixth cervical vertebra. The relationship of these vessels above the level of the first thoracic vertebra protects them from likelihood of injury during osteotomy at the C7-T1 level (Fig. 112-27). Adequate decompression must be carried out posteriorly with subsequent fracturing of the ossified anterior longitudinal ligament and disc space anteriorly, with extension of the spine at the cervical-thoracic junction (Fig. 112-28). Attention to detail preoperatively, operatively, and postoperatively is essential for safety and success.

Preoperative Preparation

An important and essential preoperative measure is the application of a well-molded plaster body jacket incorporating the supports for the halo unit, applied 1 to 2 days preoperatively. The cast must be well molded below the costal margins and over the iliac crests so that it will not move upward and downward to any significant degree. It should be trimmed so that the patient is comfortable sitting and using the upper extremities. A halo is fitted to the skull, with the patient allowed to be up and about with the halo and cast in place, adjusting to both. The halo is used partly to control the position of the head during the procedure and to serve as a basis for immediate stabilization of the spine after extension correction. A dental-type chair is used for the procedure. This allows the patient to sit comfortably, with the height of the chair easily adjusted for the surgeon's conven-

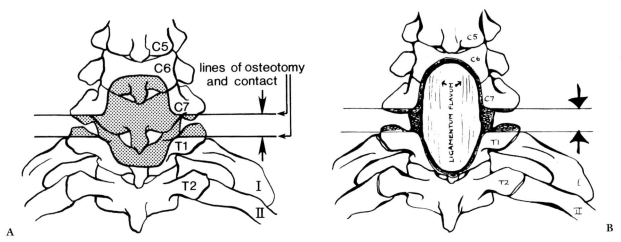

Fig. 112-26

A, Outline of area of posterior resection of the cervical-thoracic spine. This involves entire posterior arch of C7, inferior arch of C6 and superior arch of T1; amount varies with degree of correction required. Fused posterior joints of C7-T1 are resected completely through laterally. Lines of resection are beveled away from each other in keeping with angle of correction required so that following correction surfaces will be parallel and in contact. **B,** Diagrammatic view showing extent of midline and lateral resections. Inferior pedicles of C7 and superior pedicles of T1 should be undercut to avoid impingement of C8 nerve roots following extension. Laminar surfaces are undercut above and below to avoid impingement against dura following extension. *(From Simmons EH: Kyphotic deformity of the spine in Ankylosing Spondylitis, Clin Orthop 128:65, 1977.)*

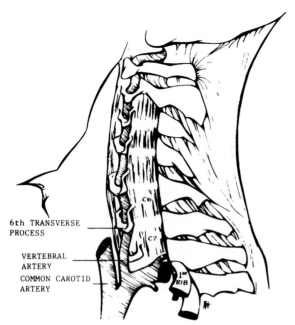

Fig. 112-27

Anatomic diagram demonstrating position of vertebral artery and veins in front of the transverse process of seventh vertebra and their entry into spine via transverse foramen of sixth vertebra. (*From Simmons EH: Kyphotic deformity of the spine in Ankylosing Spondylitis, Clin Orthop 128:65, 1977.*)

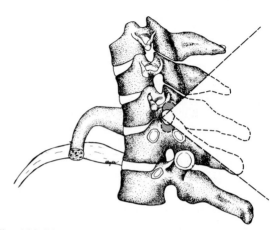

Fig. 112-28

Lateral diagrammatic view of area of posterior resection at C7-T1 level. Shaded areas indicate where pedicles should be undercut to avoid eighth-nerve-root impingement following extension correction.

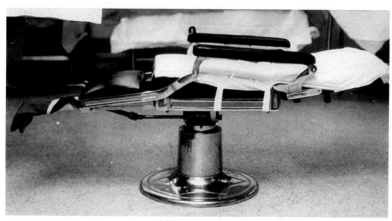

Fig. 112-29

Type of dental chair used for cervical osteotomy. Chair can be elevated to height comfortable for surgeon. It can be extended to horizontal position as demonstrated if this should be required.

ience. It will also allow the patient to be placed in a recumbent position, if this should be required during the procedure (Fig. 112-29). The patient should have had an opportunity to discuss the procedure in detail with the surgeon preoperatively.

Involvement and Organization of the Anesthesia Team

The patient should have an opportunity to meet the operating room staff and in particular the anesthe-sia staff prior to the surgery. An important part of anesthetic management is a knowledgeable, experienced staff who can converse with the patient freely during the procedure, providing understanding and reassurance. Exposure is carried out posteriorly with local anesthetic infiltration (1% lidocaine and epinephrine 1:200,000). The soft tissues should be dissected from the spine carefully, so as not to disturb the spinous process bony anatomy.

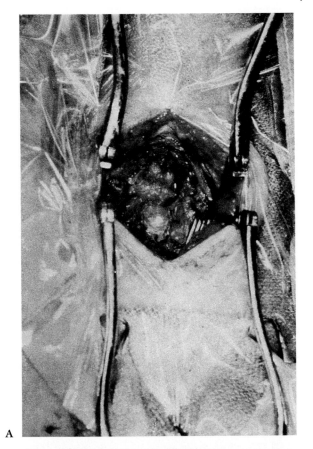

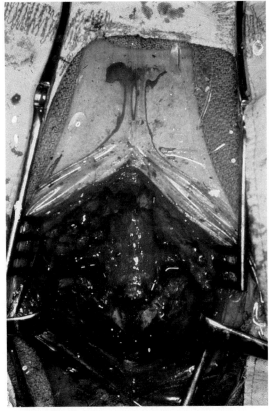

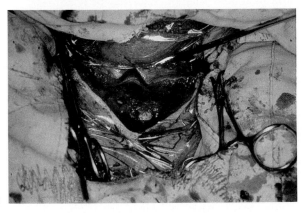

Fig. 112-30

A, Posterior exposure of spine demonstrating last bifid spinous process of C6 seen in upper end of wound. **B,** Posterior view of midline decompression and decompression of C8 nerve roots. **C,** Operative view of wound following extension correction with anterior osteoclasis. Vertical wound has become transverse. Lateral masses are together on each side.

and the upper portion of the spinous process and laminae of T1. The spine is stripped well, before resection and the bone is preserved for grafting.

Identification of Level

If careful dissection is carried out, the last bifid spinous process of C6 is usually easily identified (Fig. 112-30, *A*). This is a fairly consistent anatomic landmark unless there has been previous fracture. If any difficulty is encountered or doubt entertained, radiographic confirmation of the level should be obtained. This may require identification of a level higher up in order to produce a recognizable image on a lateral radiogram. The spinous process and laminae of C7 are entirely removed, along with the inferior portion of the spine and lower laminae of C6

Extent of Posterior Decompression

The entire posterior arch of C7 and at least the inferior half arch of C6 and the superior half arch of the T1 are removed depending on the amount of extension correction required. The remaining arches of C6 and T1 should be undercut to avoid impingement following extension. This opens the spinal canal widely; the dura and spinal cord are protected with cotton pads. The areas of the pedicles of C7 and T1 are noted, and the eighth-nerve-root canals are identified. The patient is frequently able to assist in confirming the localization by indicating any paresthesias along the distribution of the eighth nerve root as the nerve root is retracted or displaced. Bone is removed symmetrically over the C8 nerve-root canals on both sides, resecting the fused area of the posterior joints and decompressing the eighth nerve roots thoroughly.

Planning the Degree of Operative Correction

The amount of bone to be resected is planned preoperatively and is indicated by the angle of correction desired. This is assessed by the preoperative chin-brow to vertical angle. When the patient stands with the hips and knees extended, the angle formed by a line from the brow to the chin to the vertical is measured with the patient's neck in either its fixed or neutral position. An angle of this amount is transposed to a lateral radiogram or tomogram of the cervical spine with the apex at the posterior longitudinal ligament at the C7-T1 level. The posterior part of the angle is centered over the posterior arch of C7. This gives an indication of the amount of bone to be resected in the area of the fused posterior joints, at the base of the pedicles in the spinal canal, at the level of the laminae, and at the level of the spinous processes. The resection lines are beveled upward from below and downward from above so that following correction the two surfaces will be parallel and in apposition (Fig. 112-30, B). The inferior margins of the bases of the pedicles of C7 and the superior margins of the bases of the pedicles of T1 are removed sufficiently and undercut to avoid impingement or a pincher effect on the eighth cervical nerve roots following extension correction of the cervical spine. Less discomfort to the patient will occur if removal of the pedicles is commenced away from the nerve root and working toward it and then at the last removing the thin remaining portion of bone adjacent to the root. If possible, a recess should be cut into the bases of the pedicles of C7 and T1 to accommodate the C8 nerve roots and avoid pressure on them when the neck is extended. The amount of bone to be resected should be carefully assessed preoperatively as noted on the lateral radiogram or tomogram. The lateral masses should be resected symmetrically on both sides and completely through to their lateral margin to allow easy extension and good bony contact following correction.

Supplemental oxygen is frequently administered by the anesthetist during the procedure either by face mask or nasal catheter. The patient is encouraged to enjoy music of his/her choice provided by a radio or tape player. This and a continuous cheerful conversation between the anesthetist and the nurse-anesthetist are very important parts of anesthetic management. When done well, the amount of discomfort or concern expressed by the patient is minimal. Fentanyl and midazolam (Versed) are used by the anesthetist to supplement local anesthesia as indicated. Pulse oximetry, CO_2 analyzer, and systemic blood gas levels are used to monitor the patient. A Doppler apparatus is routinely fixed to the patient's chest to detect any possibility of air embolism. A basin of saline-soaked sponges is kept available by the scrub nurse to be placed into the wound if there is any suspicion of air embolism; this is very rarely needed. When the planned decompression has been completed in a symmetrical fashion, the deep muscular sutures are placed in the wound and left untied. A drain is inserted. The patient is given a small dose of short-acting barbiturate, either Brevital sodium (methohexital sodium) or, more currently, propofol (Diprivan). This is administered slowly by the anesthetist while conversing with the patient. When the anesthetist indicates that it has had its effect, the neck is extended by the surgeon. This is done by grasping the halo through the drapes, tilting the head backward while endeavoring to keep the head and upper cervical spine in their normal relationship so that the stress occurs at the base of the neck and not in the upper cervical spine. A physical sense of fracture will be appreciated by the surgeon and an audible snap or crack may be heard. The neck is extended carefully until a sense of resistance occurs. Palpation will indicate that the lateral masses have come together posteriorly on each side (see Fig. 112-30, C). Supplemental 100% oxygen is given until the patient is fully awake, and this should occur readily. The patient is then able to confirm normal neurologic function of the extremities with the ability to move the upper and lower extremities, including hands and feet, without sensory complaint. The head is held firmly in the corrected position by the surgeon, while unscrubbed assistants stabilize the head by connecting the anterior supports for the halo to the cast. Portions of bone that have been removed during the decompression are placed posterolaterally on both sides over the approximated lateral masses. The midline defect is left free. The deep closing sutures are then tied with the suction drain in position. The importance of placing the sutures before the extension correction will then be appreciated, as the vertical wound has been changed to a transverse one, making the insertion of the sutures into the deep muscles more difficult. The skin is usually closed with interrupted silk sutures. The surgeon can then assess the degree of correction and make any adjustments or alterations in the position of the head by adjusting the anterior supports. After the dressings have been applied, the posterior supports for the halo are applied, rigidly immobilizing the osteotomy site. In my experience, when this is completed the patients have been consistently able to stand and walk to their circoelectric bed, which is turned to the vertical to allow them to back into it easily. The bed is then tilted to the horizontal with the patient supine. It is usually partly flexed, depending on the patient's choice for comfort. The surgeon should avoid overcorrection of the deformity, particularly in patients with a rigid cervical spine and no significant motion at the occipital-cervical junction. Patients must have a compromise between being able to look straight ahead when standing and walking and still being able to work at a desk. If they have some persisting motion in the upper cervical spine, this will usually allow full correction with restoration of the chin-brow to vertical angle to 0 degrees; the remaining motion allows them to flex slightly when at a desk (Figs. 112-31 and 112-32).

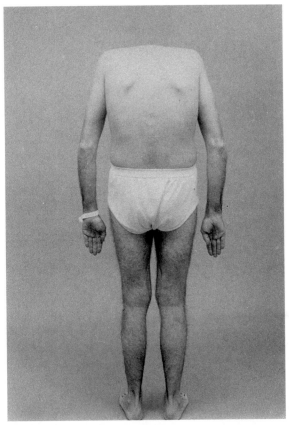

Fig. 112-31

A, B, and C, Posterior, lateral, and anterior views of male presenting with severe kyphotic deformity confined to cervical spine. Note that head is not visible from posterior aspect. Chin is rigidly fixed against chest, restricting field of vision and ability to open mouth.

continues.

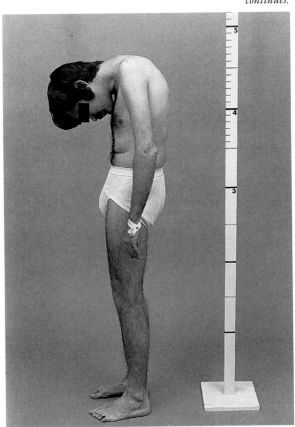

B

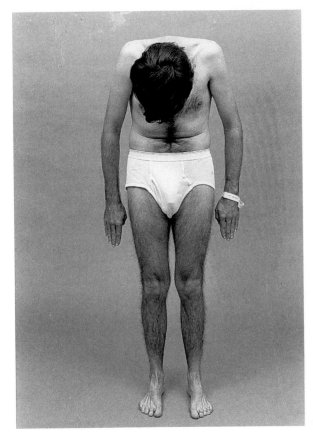

C

A

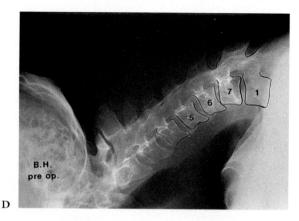

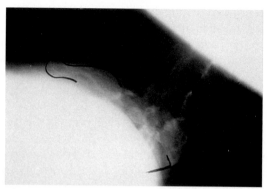

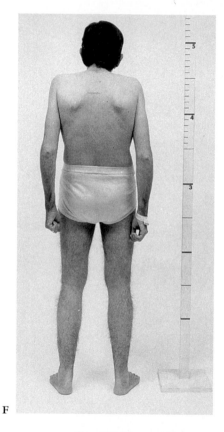

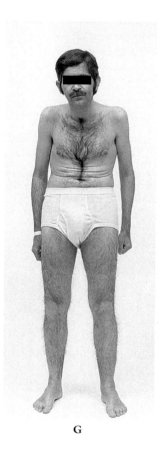

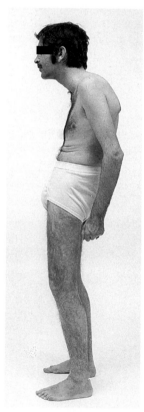

Fig. 112-31, cont'd

D, Preoperative lateral radiogram of cervical spine showing fusion of posterior joints with fixed previous subluxation of C6-C7. **E,** Lateral postoperative radiogram following extension correction. **F, G,** and **H,** Posterior, lateral, and anterior views of patient showing restoration of head to normal functional alignment with normal chin-brow to vertical angle. Patient had restoration of ability to see ahead, open mouth for normal dental hygiene, swallow, and shave.

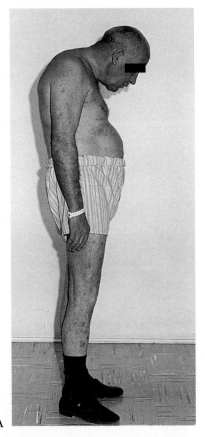
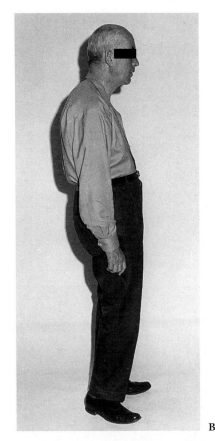

Fig. 112-32

A, Preoperative lateral view of male presenting with kyphotic deformity of cervical spine resulting from ankylosing spondylitis associated with psoriasis. **B,** Postoperative lateral view of patient demonstrating restoration of normal chin-brow to vertical angle.

It should be noted that excessive force is not required to straighten the neck, provided there has been an adequate and complete decompression posteriorly. When the spine does not fracture fairly easily, the surgeon should be certain that there is not a bridge of bone left laterally and that the operative level is at C7-T1 and not below in the upper thoracic area. Ordinarily, an attempt is made to obtain full or nearly full correction at the time of the procedure. However, on occasion this may be limited by tightness of the musculature anteriorly or by apprehension on the part of the patient, or even the surgeon, that overcorrection may be occurring. Stabilization can be carried out in what is felt to be a reasonable position, and the degree of correction then assessed postoperatively. If any further correction is desired, this can be achieved about 7 days postoperatively, when the soft tissues have had an opportunity to stretch. At that time the patient may be placed supine and with midazolam and fentanyl sedation; the supports for the halo may be detached with the head supported by the surgeon, allowing further gradual ex-

tension until the desired position is reached. The head is then stabilized in the new position.

Postoperative Management

Patients are nursed in the immediate postoperative interval on a circoelectric bed. This is ideal, as it allows the patient to be brought up to the vertical position easily, so that they can stand and walk about and return to the recumbent position without difficulty. When sufficiently comfortable and mobile so that they are able to get in and out of a regular bed, patients are transferred to a hospital bed, usually with a trapeze attachment. When initially applying the halo cast, it is helpful to have shoulder straps, or these may be applied postoperatively. If a patient loses weight, the straps tend to prevent the cast from moving distally, avoiding the weight being transferred to the osteotomy site. Also, a type of halo unit should be used that will allow some graduated careful lengthening of the distance between the halo and the cast, if symptoms due to the weight of the cast

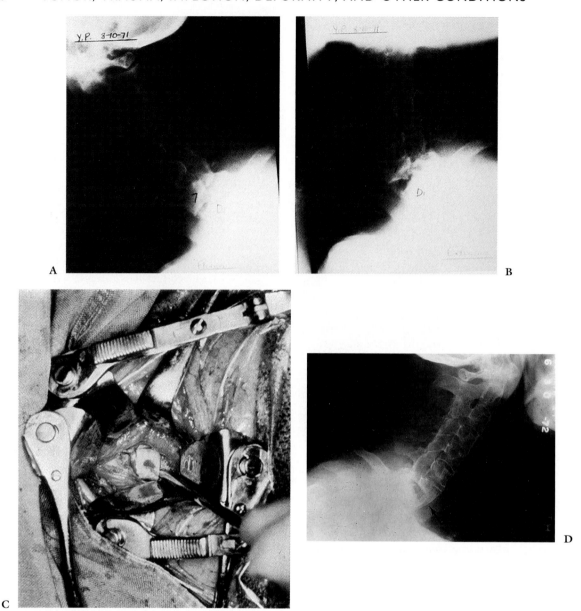

Fig. 112-33

A, and B, Flexion and extension lateral views of 50-year-old physician indicating nonunion following cervical osteotomy. C, Operative view of anterior keystone fusion at C7-T1 level performed under local anesthesia. D, Lateral postoperative radiogram de-monstrating solid bony union with incorporation of keystone graft.

occur. This can frequently relieve any late C8 nerve-root discomfort or paresthesias. The patients are immobilized in a halo cast for 4 months, at which time it is removed and radiographic studies are done, including lateral tomography centered at C7-T1. Evidence of clinical union is assessed with lack of pain on attempted motion. Further splinting using a Somi brace is carried out for an additional 2 months or until there is certain evidence of solid bony union on the basis of clinical and radiographic assessment.

Results and Complications

As a result of the success achieved and relative freedom of major complications, the same technique has been followed in a consistent fashion without any major deviation since 1966, in a total of 130 patients.[21,48-51,53-55,61] The results have been exceedingly gratifying, with a relatively small amount of complications considering the nature of the deformity and associated disease process. General systemic complications have been less than is reported for major replacement arthroplasty in patients with the same disease process. There has been no major spinal cord injury. Union appears to occur readily in most patients. However, in four patients nonunion occurred, an incidence of 3%. Three nonunions were successfully treated with an anterior cervical fusion at the C7-T1 level using a keystone iliac strut graft,[57] one of these being done under local anesthesia (Fig. 112-33). One patient required both anterior and posterior fusion to obtain solid union. It would appear that patients on steroids or high doses of nonsteroidal antiinflammatory drugs have more risk, and this should be corrected if possible. The most common postoperative neurologic complaint is some degree of transient C8 paresthesia or even signs, occurring in 10%. This can usually be eased by gentle distraction between the halo and the cast. They gradually resolve, even when there is some transient weakness, as stabilization of the osteotomy occurs. Only one patient has required further decompression of the eighth nerve root with improvement; the patient now plays golf without difficulty. Although there has been no major permanent injury to the spinal cord, one dramatic intraoperative experience occurred, demonstrating the need for surgery to be performed under local anesthesia. A 70-year-old man presented with a chin-on-chest deformity associated with a previously unrecognized fracture that had healed with his chin on the chest. His chief complaint was a fear of choking, having had several episodes of difficulty with swallowing. At the time of surgery under local anesthesia, dense scarring about the dura related to his previous trauma was noted. As decompression was completed in the midline the patient suffered increasing weakness of his lower extremities, his left upper extremity, and finally, difficulty with speech. The dura was exceedingly tense, with dense scarring about it. It was split longitudinally down to the arachnoid. When this was done, there was an immediate return of neurologic function in the lower extremities and return of normal speech. The procedure was continued, and as decompression was completed on the left he again began to experience weakness of his right lower limb. The dura was split further distally, again with immediate recovery of neurologic function. Following this the operation was completed without difficulty and the patient went on to a satisfactory result without neurologic deficit (Fig. 112-34).[23] This experience is in keeping with the report of McKenzie and Dewar[34] describing the results of laminectomy for cord compression associated with kyphoscoliosis. In their review of the literature and their own cases, they reported that the only patients who did not be-

come worse after laminectomy or who had any benefit, were those who had an extensive splitting of the dura. The authors related neurologic deficit to the compression affect of the dura in kyphosis after the posterior laminae were removed. They recommended splitting of the dura both longitudinally and transversely. Surgeons embarking on this type of surgery should be familiar with this recommendation. If the problem occurs, adequate splitting of the dura should be carried out not only longitudinally, but probably transversely as well.

During the operative procedure in one patient a sudden cardiac arrest occurred. The chair was flattened and the patient responded quite well to resuscitation, with no permanent deficits. The possibility of air embolism was considered; however, there was no gross venous bleeding and aspiration of the heart revealed no air. The cause of the cardiac arrest is unknown. To detect any possibility of air embolism, routine monitoring is done with a Doppler apparatus fixed to the patient's chest. One 79-year-old female patient died 21 days postoperatively from pulmonary embolism. One patient suffered a fatal pulmonary embolism while in the hospital, prior to surgical correction. It should be recognized that pulmonary embolism can occur in these patients as in other types of surgery, justifying appropriate preoperative assessment and prophylaxis. One patient suffered a perforated peptic ulcer just before his planned discharge from hospital. As a result of this, he suffered a respiratory arrest and finally fatality related to surgical treatment of his perforation. It should be recognized that these patients have frequently been on nonsteroidal antiinflammatory medication and even steroids. They have an increased tendency toward peptic ulceration, which can have very serious consequences in these patients. They breathe only with their diaphragm, and any intraabdominal catastrophe is more likely to be lethal. In recognition of this, patients are now routinely placed on ranitidine (Zantac) preoperatively and postoperatively.

The average desired angle of correction has been 60 degrees. The average measured amount of local anesthetic used has been 54 ml of 1% lidocaine with 1:200,000 epinephrine.

In 21 patients cervical osteotomy was combined with lumbar osteotomy for major deformity in both areas.[55] In a third of these patients, the procedures were done on separate admissions because of subsequent development of deformity in the other area. In two thirds, the procedures were performed during the same admission, with the patients initially presenting with severe combined deformity in both areas. In these patients the cervical osteotomy is

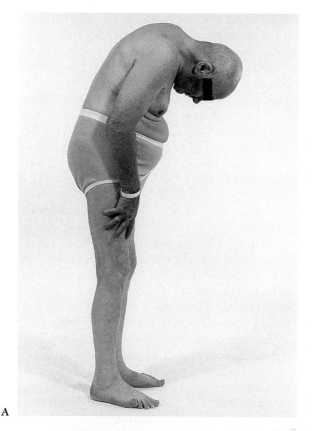

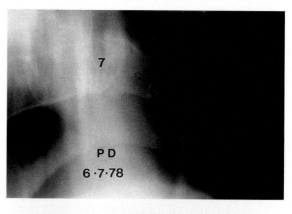

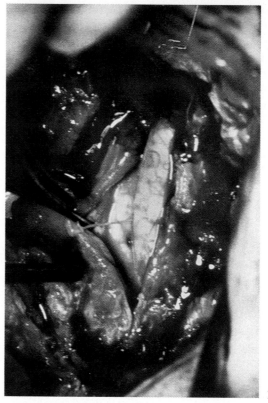

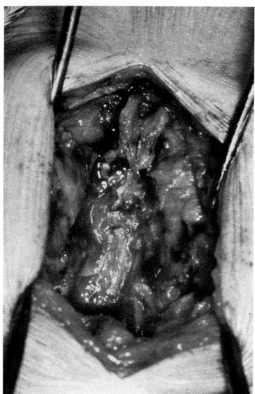

Fig. 112-34

A, Lateral view of 70-year-old male presenting with severe neck kyphotic deformity accentuated by unrecognized fracture 3 years previously. Patient's chief symptom was difficulty swallowing causing fear of choking. **B,** Lateral tomogram showing previous compression at C7-T1. **C,** Operative view following bony decompression showing extensive scarring of dura. **D,** Operative view demonstrating excision of scar and dura down to arachnoid. It was later necessary to split dura further at lower end of operative site as result of recurrent neurologic symptoms. Symptoms and signs were relieved.

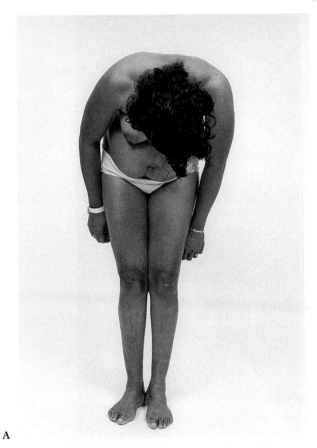

A

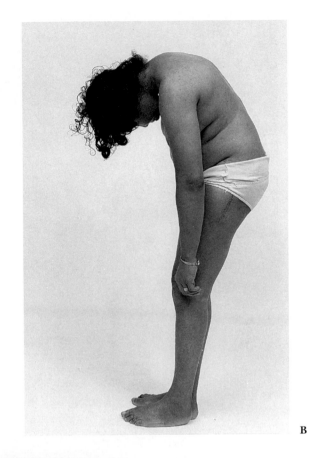

B

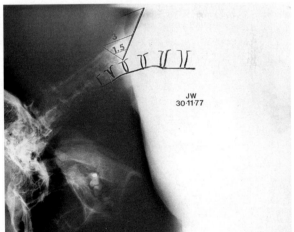

C

D

Fig. 112-35

Post reduction lateral view of patient following, union showing correction of deformity and normal chin-brow to vertical angle. **A,** and **B,** Anterior and lateral views of 33-year-old woman with severe arthritic disease since her teens. She had undergone hip arthroplasty, and her neck deformity was complicated by unrecognized fracture of cervical spine, which added to her deformity. Her field of vision was markedly restricted. **C,** Lateral standing radiogram showing combined kyphotic deformities of cervical and lumbar spine. **D,** Preoperative lateral radiogram of cervical spine indicating planned extension-resection.

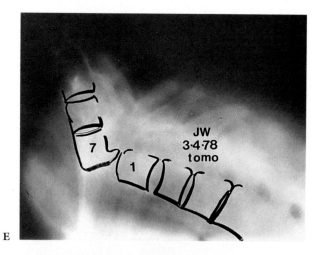

E

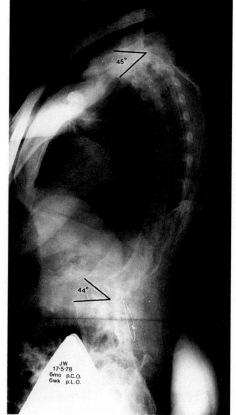

F

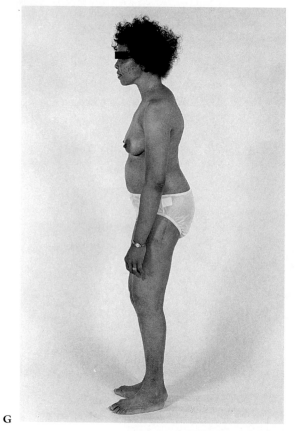

G

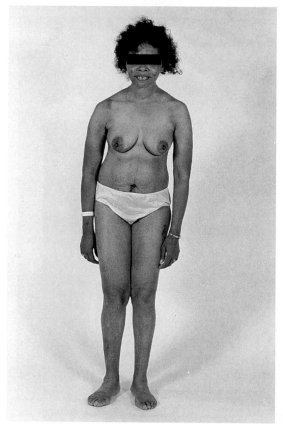

H

Fig. 112-35, cont'd

E, Postoperative lateral tomogram showing cervical extension osteotomy correction. **F,** Standing 3-ft postoperative radiogram showing combination of extension osteotomies of cervical and lumbar spine. Weight-bearing line of trunk is posterior to lumbar resection site. **G** and **H,** Postoperative lateral and anterior views demonstrating correction of combined deformities. Patient had normal field of vision and resumed social work activities. She has normal chin-brow to vertical angle.

done first, followed by lumbar osteotomy 10 days later. In 17 of the patients, both procedures were done under local anesthesia. When this was done, the patient was placed on the side with the posterior portion of the plaster being removed in the lumbar area to allow lumbar osteotomy to be performed. The remaining plaster immobilized the cervical spine. After the lumbar osteotomy was performed, the lower portion of the cast was completed in the new position (Fig. 112-35, and see Fig. 112-38). More recently, the cervical osteotomy has been done first under local anesthesia, followed by lumbar extension osteotomy done under general anesthesia with fiberoptic intubation done while the patient is awake, as described earlier (Fig. 112-36).

Resection-extension osteotomy of the cervical spine for severe fixed kyphotic deformity when carried out with the technique described and when care-

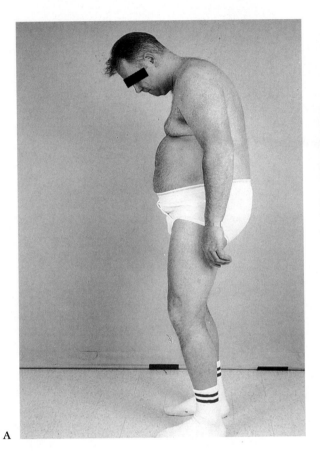

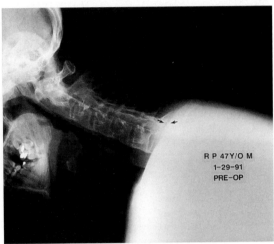

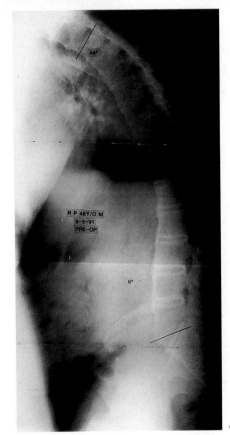

Fig. 112-36

A, Lateral standing view of 47-year-old male with 22-year history of ankylosing spondylitis. He had suffered injury to neck 10 years previously with unrecognized fracture. When he stood with his knees extended his chin-brow to vertical angle measured 75 degrees. **B,** Preoperative standing lateral radiogram of cervical spine showing previous healed fracture of C7. **C,** Lateral standing 3-ft preoperative radiogram showing lumbar lordosis reduced to 6 degrees with thoracic kyphosis of 48 degrees.

Continues.

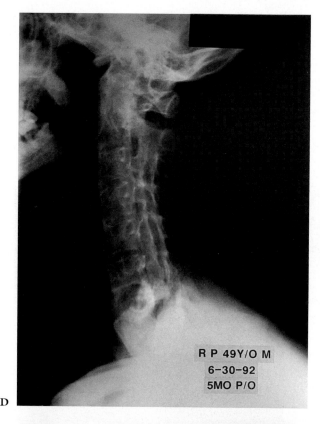

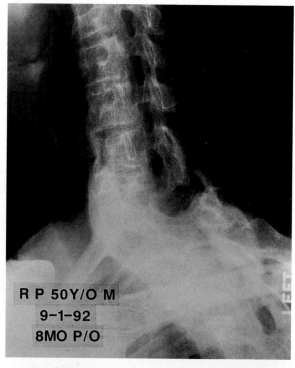

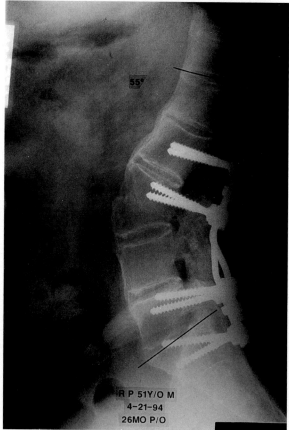

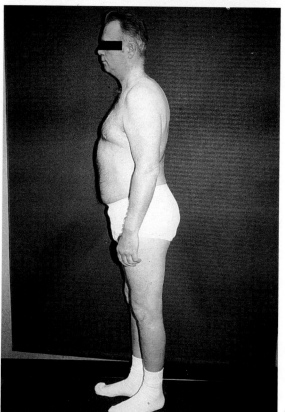

Fig. 112-36, cont'd

D, Postoperative lateral radiogram of cervical spine showing healed extension osteotomy at C7-T1 5 months postoperatively. **E,** Oblique view of cervical-thoracic junction showing extent of bony union 8 months postoperatively. **F,** Postoperative lateral view of lumbar spine showing extent of osteotomy correction and solid bony union 26 months postoperatively. **G,** Postoperative lateral standing view of patient showing complete correction of deformities with normal chin-brow to vertical angle.

fully planned and executed, is a valid technique, with acceptable risks and providing major benefits to patients. It should be emphasized that the essential factor in the technique is the performance of surgery under local anesthesia with the patient awake. This provides the surgeon with the most accurate continual monitoring of the patient's neurologic and vital functions, allowing instant responsive action if any dysfunction should occur.

The author has been consulted concerning various instances in which disastrous complications occurred with attempts at cervical osteotomy using other techniques, which warrant the following observations and recommendations. When a major complication has occurred under general anesthesia it has unfortunately not been recognized until sometime following the procedure, when the patient was awake and quadriparesis was noted. Recovery following this has often been minimal, indicating the need for the very accurate monitoring allowed by local anesthesia. Attempts at posterior instrumentation to stabilize the osteotomy have been attempted. Posterior instrumentation is useful for deformities that are not rigid, allowing diffuse correction to be carried out similar to scoliosis. However, for a solid spine with a one-level extension osteotomy of major magnitude, it would be very difficult to insert instrumentation due to the configuration of the wound, with the osteotomy in its depth and the approximation of the skull to the upper thoracic spine. When the use of instrumentation has been associated with major spinal cord dysfunction postoperatively, the instrumentation has been blamed for the deficit, which may or may not be the cause. In some instances the operative procedure has been reported to have gone well until an attempt was made to apply a halo cast postoperatively, at which time displacement occurred with spinal cord compression. It would seem essential that a well-molded cast be applied preoperatively, with the halo in position, so that the osteotomy can be instantly stabilized following extension correction. Attempts to carry out extension osteotomy in the midcervical region, in the area of the vertebral arteries, have resulted in major difficulties associated with vertebral artery insufficiency with patients failing to regain consciousness. From an anatomic standpoint, and considering the fused nature of the spine, it would seem evident that the osteotomy should be done below the area of entry of the vertebral arteries into the cervical spine. Finally, it would seem evident that resection-extension osteotomy of the cervical spine in ankylosing spondylitis is not an operation to be done by a committee. It should be done by a knowledgeable, experienced surgeon who is aware of the risks, has taken appropriate steps to avoid them, and will accept full responsibility for the entire surgical treatment.

Muscle Disease as a Cause of Kyphotic Deformity in Ankylosing Spondylitis

As stated previously, ankylosing spondylitis has well-defined extraarticular manifestations, including neurologic abnormalities of cardiac conduction defects, arachnoiditis, cauda equina syndrome, and an association with multiple sclerosis.

In the author's early experience with the orthopedic management of these patients, the main concern was the treatment of patients with gross fixed deformity. It was accepted that the deformity was a manifestation of inflammatory disease of the spine, accompanied by osteopenia, painful kyphotic deformity, and later ossification. Little thought was given to other possible mechanisms for the deformity, such as involvement of the extensor muscles of the spine.

Patients were referred to the author for correction of kyphotic deformities of the neck, which on assessment were proven not to be due to ankylosing spondylitis, but to myopathic flexion deformities of the cervical spine. These patients exhibited electrodiagnostic abnormality of the extensor muscles in keeping with myopathy, muscle biopsy changes, and laboratory findings of extensor muscle disease. The results of this study were reported in 1988.[58]

It had been a consistent finding at operation on patients with spinal deformity associated with ankylosing spondylitis that the extensor muscles were usually pale and somewhat atrophied compared to the extensor muscles of a normal patient. The recognition of myopathic kyphotic deformities of the neck in patients without ankylosing spondylitis suggested the possibility of similar pathogenesis for the deformity in those with the disease.

Patients with ankylosing spondylitis were seen with major kyphotic deformity of the cervical spine that was not fixed and responded to halo-dependent traction. Electromyographic studies, creatine kinase studies, and isometric muscle biopsies illustrated severe extensor muscle disease with atrophy of Type I and Type II muscle fibers (Fig. 112-37). A prospective study was then carried out on all patients presenting for correction of kyphotic deformity in ankylosing spondylitis. Consistent abnormality of the extensor muscles of the spine was noted. The findings were in keeping with a denervating process of the paraspinal extensor muscles typical of neuro-

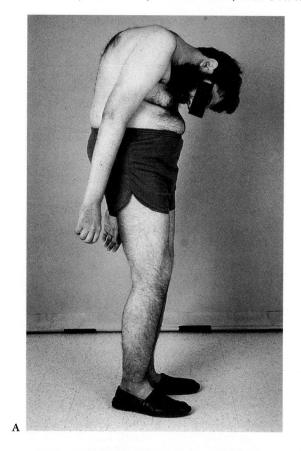

A

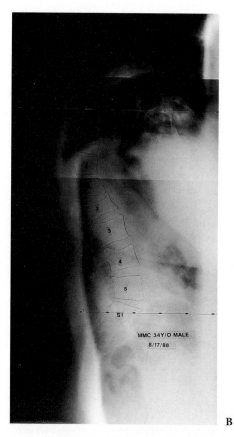

B

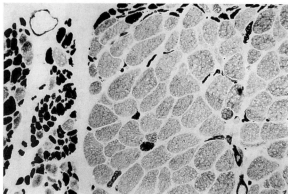

C

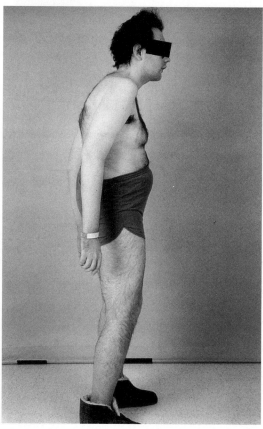

D

Fig. 112-37

A, Lateral view of 34-year-old male referred for surgical correction for cervical kyphotic deformity. He had 4-year history of ankylosing spondylitis followed by rapid progression of kyphotic deformity. His chin-brow to vertical angle was 97 degrees. **B,** Standing lateral radiogram of patient demonstrating severe osteopenia, multiple compression fractures, his chin on chest, and thoracic kyphosis of 100 degrees. Lack of fusion suggested possibility of correction with traction treatment and raised questions about pathogenesis of the deformity. **C,** Isometric muscle biopsy from paracervical extensor muscles showing abnormality of small scattered angular fibers, majority of which reacted as Type II fibers in ATPase stain. Findings were in keeping with neuropathic atrophy. Biopsy of gluteal musculature revealed similar findings. Electromyographic studies were interpreted as being consistent with nonspecific neuropathic abnormality. **D,** Lateral view of patient 5 months after correction with halo-dependent traction, including 4 months in a halo cast. Patient was treated concurrently with calcium, vitamin D and calcitonin.

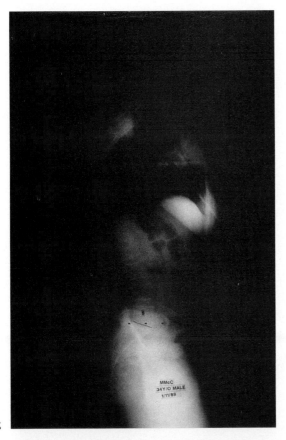

E

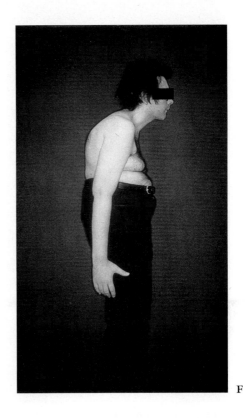

F

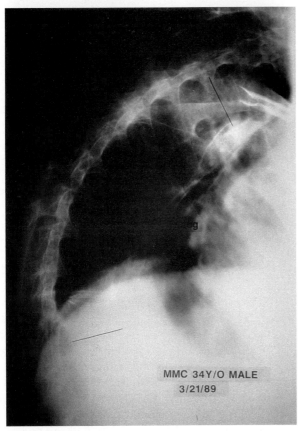

G

Fig. 112-37, cont'd

E, Lateral 3-ft radiogram 5 months following initiation of treatment showing correction of deformity and increase in bone density. **F,** Lateral view of patient 1 year after initiation of treatment. Recurrence of deformity is noted in thoracic spine associated with weakness of extensor musculature. Fortunately, correction is maintained in cervical spine, which showed progressing ossification. **G,** Lateral radiogram of thoracic spine showing increased kyphotic deformity.

Continues.

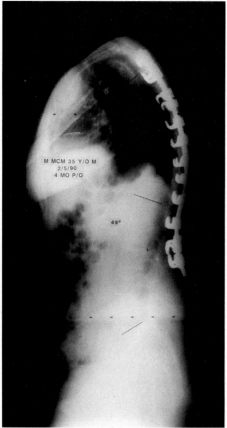

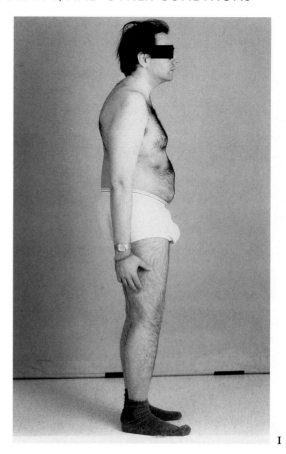

H   I

Fig. 112-37, cont'd

H, Postoperative lateral radiogram following Cotrel-Dubousset instrumentation with correction of thoracic kyphosis. **I,** Final lateral postoperative view of patient showing correction of thoracic kyphotic deformity and maintenance of correction of severe cervical kyphosis.

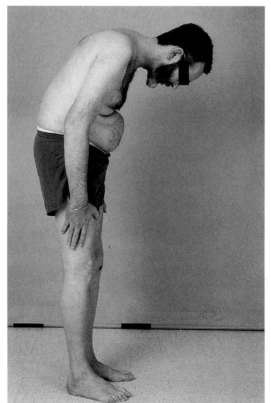

Fig. 112-38

A, Lateral view of 47-year-old male with severe spinal kyphosis restricting field of vision and difficulty swallowing. His chin-brow to vertical angle was 82 degrees. He had obvious combined kyphotic deformity of cervical spine and lumbar spine.

continues.

pathic atrophy. The results of the initial study were reported in 1991.[62]

These findings have been consistent in an ongoing study of all patients since that time (Fig. 112-38). It would appear that chronic denervation of the spinal extensor musculature is related to the pathogenesis of kyphotic deformity in ankylosing spondylitis. Extensor muscle involvement may have prognostic significance in patients with ankylosing spondylitis. It is possible that patients at risk for spinal deformity could be identified at an earlier stage of their disease. Conceivably more aggressive medical management could be indicated to slow the progression of the disease and decrease the likelihood of deformity. Strengthening exercises of the extensor musculature and bracing would be more indicated in patients who had early detection of extensor muscle involvement. Further prospective studies of patients with and without deformity will be re-

A

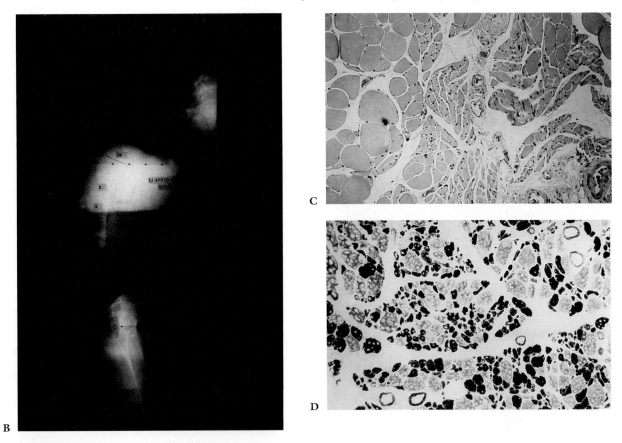

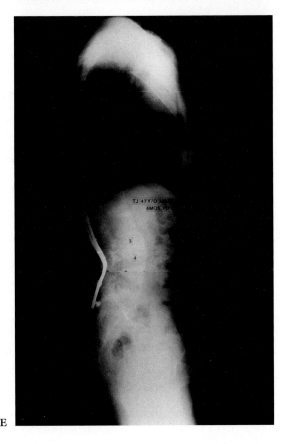

Fig. 112-38, cont'd

B, Lateral standing 3-ft radiogram showing lumbar lordosis reduced to 3 degrees with thoracic kyphosis of 57 degrees. Cervical extension-resection osteotomy was performed, followed by lumbar extension osteotomy. **C,** Biopsy of cervical extensor musculature. Muscle was pale and atrophic in appearance. It was poorly contractile to tactile stimulation. Musculature shows grouped atrophy of small angular fibers indicating chronic denervation. **D,** Histologic studies showing target fibers with central pale area surrounded with rim of increased enzyme activity. Numerous target fibers were visualized. Changes are in keeping with severe atrophic process suggestive of chronic denervation. EMG studies were consistent with neuropathic change. **E,** Lateral standing 3-foot radiogram of spine 4 months postoperatively showing extension osteotomy correction of lumbar spine. Note weight-bearing line shifted posterior to osteotomy site. Cervical osteotomy was done under local anesthesia with patient in sitting position. This was followed by extension osteotomy of lumbar spine also under local anesthesia with use of Luque segmental instrumentation and Drummond buttons for fixation.

Continues.

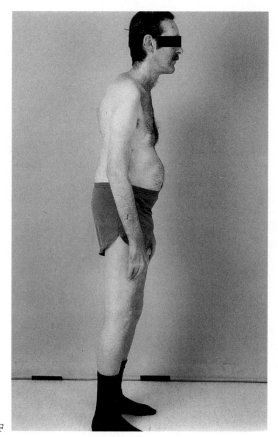

F

Fig. 112-38, cont'd

F, Postoperative lateral standing view of patient indicating normal chin-brow to vertical angle. Patient has been able to return to normal lifestyle.

quired to establish this. Physicians should be aware of paraspinal muscle involvement as part of the systemic disease process in ankylosing spondylitis.

The author would like to acknowledge the very significant contribution of, and express his gratitude to, Mary E. Smith in her assistance in preparation of the manuscript.

References

1. Aboulker J, Aubin ML, Leriche H, et al.: L'hypertension veineuse intra-rachidienne par anomalies multiples du systeme cave, *Acta Radiol Suppl* 347:395, 1975.
2. Adams JC: Technique, dangers, and safeguards in osteotomy of the spine, *J Bone Joint Surg* 34B:226, 1952.
3. Andersson O: Rontgenbilden vid spondylarthrosis ankylopoetica, *Nord Med* 14:2000, 1937.
4. Attern J, Hockberg M: Epidemiology and genetics of ankylosing spondylitis, *J Rheumatol* (Suppl 16):22, 1988.
5. Bland JH: Rheumatoid arthritis of the cervical spine, *J Rheumatol* 3:319, 1974.
6. Bove EA, Glasgow GL: Cauda equina lesions associated with ankylosing spondylitis: report of 3 cases, *BMJ* 2:24, 1961.
7. Buckley BH, Robert WC: Ankylosing spondylitis and aortic regurgitation: description of the characteristic cardio-vascular lesion from study of 8 necropsy patients, *Circulation* 18:1014, 1978.
8. Calin A: *Ankylosing spondylitis.* In Kelly WN, Harris ED, Ruddy S, Sledge CB, editors: *Textbook of rheumatology.* Philadelphia, 1981, W.B. Saunders, p 1017.
9. Calin A, Elwood J, Rigg S, et al.: Ankylosing spondylitis: an analytic review of 1500 patients: the changing pattern of disease, *J Rheumatol* 15:1234, 1988.
10. Conlon PW, Isdale IC, Rose BS: Rheumatoid arthritis in the cervical spine: an analysis of 333 cases, Ann *Rheumatol Dis* 25:120, 1966.
11. Coste F, Delbarre F, Cayla J, et al.: Spondylites destructives dans la spondylarthrite ankylosante, *Press Med* 71:1013, 1963.
12. Davey JR, Rorabeck CH, Bailey SI, et al.: A technique of posterior cervical fusion for instability of the cervical spine, *Spine* 10:722, 1985.
13. Dewar FP: Personal communication, 1955.
14. Donovan MM: *Efficacy of rigid fixation of fractures of the odontoid process—historical review of treatment and retrospective analysis of 54 cases,* doctoral thesis, Houston, 1977, University of Texas.
15. Emneus H: Wedge osteotomy of spine in ankylosing spondylitis, *Acta Orthop Scand* 39:321, 1968.
16. Goel MK: Vertebral osteotomy for correction of fixed flexion deformity of the spine, *J Bone Joint Surg* 50A:287, 1968.
17. Hanrachan P, Russell A, McLean P: Ankylosing spondylitis and multiple sclerosis: an apparent association, *J Rheumatol* 15:1512, 1988.
18. Harris RI: New investigations: instrument for tightening knots in steel wire, *Lancet* 1:504, 1944.
19. Herbert JJ: Vertebral osteotomy for kyphosis, especially in Marie-Strumpell arthritis: a report on 50 cases, *J Bone Joint Surg* 41A:291, 1959.
20. Herbert JJ: Vertebral osteotomy, technique, indications and results, *J Bone Joint Surg* 30A:680, 1948.
21. Hruska JS, Simmons EH: *Review of cervical extension osteotomy in ankylosing spondylitis,* Orthopaedic Residents Annual Graduation Presentation, State University of New York at Buffalo, May 27, 1994.
22. Isenbery DA, Smith ML: Muscle disease in systemic lupus erythematosus: a study of its nature, frequency, and cause, *J Rheumatol* 18:917, 1981.
23. Jackson RP, Simmons EH: Dural compression as a cause of paraplegia during operative correction of cervical kyphosis in ankylosing spondylitis, *Spine* 16:846, 1991.
24. Kallio KE: Osteotomy of the spine in ankylosing spondylitis, *Ann Chir Gynaecol* 52:615, 1963.
25. Kanefield DG, Mullins BP, Freehafer AA, et al.: Destructive lesions of the spine in rheumatoid ankylosing spondylitis, *J Bone Joint Surg* 51A:1369, 1969.
26. LaChapelle EH: Osteotomy of the lumbar spine for correction of kyphosis in a case of ankylosing spondylarthritis, *J Bone Joint Surg* 28A:270, 1959.
27. Law WA: Lumbar spinal osteotomy, *J Bone Joint Surg* 41B:270, 1959.
28. Law WA: Osteotomy of the spine, *J Bone Joint Surg* 44A:1199, 1962.
29. Law WA: Osteotomy of the spine, *Clin Orthop* 66:70, 1969.

30. Lichtblau PO, Wilson PD: Possible mechanism of aortic rupture in orthopaedic correction of rheumatoid spondylitis, *J Bone Joint Surg* 38A:123, 1956.

31. Little H, Urowitz MB, Smythe HA, et al.: Asymptomatic spondylodiscitis: an unusual feature of ankylosing spondylitis, *Arthritis Rheum* 17:487, 1974.

32. McEwen CD, Tata D, Ling C, et al.: Ankylosing spondylitis and spondylitis accompanying ulcerative colitis, regional enteritis, psoriasis, and Reiter's disease, *Arthritis Rheum* 14:291, 1971.

33. McGraw RW, Rusch RM: Atlanto-axial arthrodesis. *J Bone Joint Surg* 55B:482, 1973.

34. McKenzie KG, Dewar FP: Scoliosis with paraplegia, *J Bone Joint Surg* 31B:162, 1949.

35. McMaster PE: Osteotomy of the spine for fixed flexion deformity, *J Bone Joint Surg* 44A:1207, 1962.

36. McMaster PE: Osteotomy of the spine for fixed flexion deformity, *Pacific Med Surg* 73:314, 1965.

37. McMaster MJ, Coventry MB: Spinal osteotomy in ankylosing spondylitis, *Mayo Clin Proc* 48:476, 1973.

38. Martel W, Duff IF, Preston RE, et al.: The cervical spine and rheumatoid arthritis: correlation of radiographic clinical manifestations, *Arthritis Rheum* 7:326, 1964 (abstract).

39. Mason C, Cozen L, Adelstein L: Surgical correction of flexion deformity of the cervical spine, *Calif Med* 79:244, 1953.

40. Nunziata A: Osteotomia de la columna: operacio de Smith-Petersen, *Prensa Med Argent* 35:1536, 1948.

41. Pellicci PM, Ranawat CS, Tsarairis P, et al.: Progression of rheumatoid arthritis of the cervical spine, *J Bone Joint Surg* 63A:342, 1981.

42. Ranawat CS, O'Leary P, Pellicci PM, et al.: Cervical spine fusion in rheumatoid arthritis, *J Bone Joint Surg* 61A:1003, 1979.

43. Rosen PS, Graham DC: Ankylosing spondylitis (a clinical review of 128 cases), *Arch Intern Am Rheumatol* 5:158, 1962.

44. Russell ML, Gorder DA, Orgryzlo MA, et al.: The cauda equina syndrome of ankylosing spondylitis, *Ann Intern Med* 78:551, 1973.

45. Scudese VA, Calabro JJ: Vertebral wedge osteotomy, *JAMA* 186:104, 1963.

46. Schultz KP: Destruktive Veranderungen an Wirbelkorpern bei der Spondyliarthritis Ankylopoetica, *Arch Orthop Unfall Chir* 64:116, 1968.

47. Simmons EH: *Alternatives in the surgical stabilization of the upper cervical spine.* In Tator CH, editor: *Early management of acute spinal cord injury,* New York, 1982, Raven Press, p 393.

48. Simmons EH: *Ankylosing spondylitis: surgical considerations,* In Rothman-Simeone editor: *The Spine,* ed 3, Philadelphia, 1992, Saunders, p 1447.

49. Simmons EH: Kyphotic deformity of the spine in ankylosing spondylitis, *Clin Orthop* 128:65, 1977.

50. Simmons EH: *Surgery of rheumatoid arthritis,* Philadelphia, 1971, J.B. Lippincott Co., p 100.

51. Simmons EH: *Surgery of rheumatoid arthritis.* In Cruess RL and Mitchell Evarts NS, editor *Surgery of the spine in rheumatoid arthritis and ankylosing spondylitis,* Philadelphia, 1971, J.B. Lippincott, p 93.

52. Simmons EH: *Surgery of the spine in rheumatoid arthritis and ankylosing spondylitis.* In Evarts CM,

editor: *Surgery of the musculoskeletal system,* vol 2, New York, 1983, Churchill Livingstone, p 85.

53. Simmons EH: Surgery of the spine in ankylosing spondylitis and rheumatoid arthritis. In Chapman M, editor: *Operative orthopaedics,* vol 3, Philadelphia, 1988, J.B. Lippincott Co., p 2077.

54. Simmons EH: The surgical correction of flexion deformity of the cervical spine in ankylosing spondylitis, *Clin Orthop* 86:132, 1972.

55. Simmons EH: *The surgical correction of flexion deformity of the cervical spine.* In Cervical Spine Research Society, editors: *Ankylosing spondylitis in the cervical spine,* ed 2, Philadelphia, 1989, J.B. Lippincott Co., p 573.

56. Simmons EH, Bernstein AJ: *Fractures of the spine in ankylosing spondylitis,* In Floman Y, Farcy J-P, Argenson C, editors: *Throacolumbar spine fractures,* New York, 1993, Raven Press, Ltd.

57. Simmons EH, Bhalla SK: Anterior cervical discectomy and fusion (keystone technique), *J Bone Joint Surg* 51B:225, 1969.

58. Simmons EH, Bradley DD: Neuro-myopathic flexion deformity of the cervical spine, *Spine* 13:756, 1988.

59. Simmons EH, Duncan CP: Fracture of the cervical spine in ankylosing spondylitis: an analysis of its influence on severe deformity presenting for spinal osteotomy, *Orthop Trans* 3:126, 1979.

60. Simmons EH, Fielding JW: Atlanto-axial arthrodesis, *J Bone Joint Surg* 49A:1022, 1967.

61. Simmons EH, Goodwin CB: Spondylodiscitis: a manifestation of ankylosing spondylitis, *Orthop Trans* 8:165, 1984.

62. Simmons EH, Graziano GP, Heffner R Jr: Muscle disease as a cause of kyphotic deformity in ankylosing spondylitis, *Spine* 16, pp 5351-5360, 1991.

63. Simmons EH, Mouradian WH: Unusual malunion of the odontoid process, *J Bone Joint Surg* 59A:552, 1977.

64. Smith-Petersen MN, Larson CB, Aufranc OE: Osteotomy of the spine for correction of flexion deformity in rheumatoid arthritis, *J Bone Joint Surg* 27:1, 1945.

65. Thomas DJ, Kendall MJ, Witfield ABW: Nervous system involvement in ankylosing spondylitis, *J Neurol Neurosurg Psychiatry* 41:559, 1978.

66. Tucker CR, Fowles RE, Calin A, et al.: Aortitis in ankylosing spondylitis: early detection of aortic root abnormalities with 2-dimensional echocardiography, *Am J Cardiol* 9:680, 1982.

67. Urist MR: Osteotomy of the cervical spine: report of a case of ankylosing rheumatoid spondylitis, *J Bone Joint Surg* 41A:833, 1958.

68. Weatherley C, Jaffray D, Terry A: Vascular complications associated with osteotomy in ankylosing spondylitis: a report of two cases, *Spine* 13:43, 1988.

69. Wholey MH, Pugh DG, Bickel WH: Localized destructive lesions in rheumatoid spondylitis, *Radiology* 74:54, 1960.

70. Wills DG: Anesthetic management of posterior lumbar osteotomy, *Can Anesth Soc J* 83:248, 1985.

71. Wilson MJ, Turkell JH: Multiple spinal wedge osteotomy: its use in the case of Marie-Strumpell spondylitis, *Am J Surg* 77:777, 1949.

Chapter 113

Paget's Disease

Alexander G. Hadjipavlou
Philip H. Lander

Etiology

Histopathology

Prevalence and Distribution

Prevalence of Low-Back Pain and
Spinal Stenosis

Pathomechanics of Back Pain and
Spinal Stenosis

    spinal pain (back and neck pain)
    spinal stenosis

Other Associated Conditions

    malignant transformation
    rheumatic and arthritic conditions
      in Paget's disease

Treatment

    bisphosphonates
    calcitonin
    gallium nitrate
    mithramycin (plicamycin)
    ipriflavone

Treatment of Back Pain

Treatment of Spinal Stenosis

Methods for Monitoring Antipagetic
Drug Treatment

Summary

Etiology

Paget's disease of bone is a monoostotic or polyostotic nonhormonal osteometabolic disorder. Over a century after the original disease was described by Paget in 1877 and despite recent intensive studies and widespread interest, the etiology still remains obscure.

The proclivity to sarcomatous transformation, the variability of osteoblasts (size, shape, and staining), the peculiarity of osteoclasts (size and number of nuclei up to 100, seen also in giant-cell tumors), and control of the disease by antimitotic agents such as plicamycin (also known as mithramycin) suggest that the disease may be a benign neoplasm of the mesenchymal osteoprogenitor cells, as was postulated by Rasmussen and Bordier in 1973.[83]

More recent reports claim that the disease may be caused by a viral infection[10,98]; however, these claims are only circumstantial evidence of electron microscopic, immunologic, and epidemiologic studies. Electron microscopy of osteoclasts reveals viral intranuclear inclusion structures resembling those of an RNA-type virus related to measles or subacute sclerosing panencephalitis. We have observed similar virus-like structures in our cases[45] (Fig. 113-1). Immunologic studies show the presence of specific viral antigens in osteoclasts and cells grown from Paget's bone.[71]

Some reports have indicated that Paget's disease of the bone is a zoonosis because it is associated with ownership of either dogs or cats. These epidemiologic studies have suggested that canine distemper, a paramyxovirus closely related to measles, can contaminate human osteoclast cells, contributing to the development of Paget's disease.[54,75] However, Siris et al.[100] found no risk factors for development of Paget's disease that relate to prior dog or cat ownership, thus exonerating these pets.

Histopathology

Histopathologically, Paget's disease of bone is characterized by two pathologic entities: an osseous lesion and a bone marrow fibrosis. The former is characterized by the so-called mosaic appearance (Fig. 113-2), the hallmark of pagetic cellularity is the variable size of osteoblasts and large osteoclasts (Fig. 113-3) with multiple nuclei (up to 100).[83] Bone marrow fibrosis is not associated with anemia because bone marrow hemopoietic activity can expand to the appendicular skeleton,[21] thus compensating for the extensive bone marrow fibrosis.

Prevalence and Distribution

Paget's disease is found more commonly in populations of Anglo-Saxon origin. It is rare to find Paget's disease in China, Japan, Iran, India, Scandinavia, Africa, or the Middle East[8]; however, Singer[97] mentioned that 10% of his patients in the Los Angeles area are of African decent. A survey of Paget's disease of bone in Johannesburg, South Africa, revealed an unexpected prevalence of 1.3% among the black and 2.4% among the white population.[42] These findings suggest that Paget's disease of bone may not be

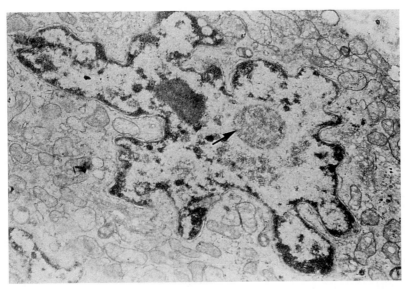

Fig. 113-1

Electron microscopic examination of portion of osteoclastic cell showing a nucleus. Arrow points to osteoclastic inclusions not bound to membrane arranged in paracrystalline array 15 nm in diameter.

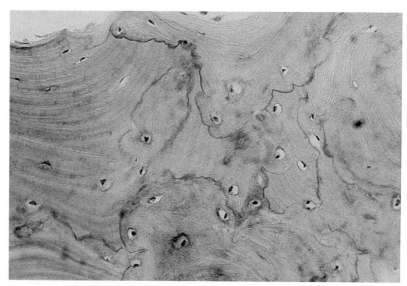

Fig. 113-2

Mosaic appearance of bone in Paget's disease formed by cement lines of sequential reformation of new bone without formation of typical haversian systems.

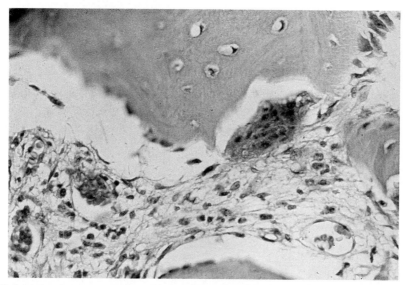

Fig. 113-3

Dense fibrous tissue with large osteoclast containing numerous nuclei eroding bone spicule. Osteoblasts are aligned to adjacent new bone matrix.

uncommon in some Africans. Autopsy reports indicate that the overall prevalence of Paget's disease is 3% to 3.7%,[19,94] with a tendency to increase with age. At the age of 90, the expected prevalence is about 10%.[94] Radiographic studies revealed a prevalence of 3.5%.[80] According to Siris et al.,[101] Paget's disease often occurs in more than one member of a family. A positive family history in parents or siblings was reported in 12.3% of cases and 2.1% of controls. The prevalence of Paget' disease was approximately seven times as high in relatives of cases as in relatives of controls.

Prevalence of Low-Back Pain and Spinal Stenosis

The spine is the second most commonly affected site in Paget's disease[5,21,69] and predisposes these patients to low-back pain and spinal stenosis.[4,48,52,109]

Hartman and Dohn[52] have shown that 15.2% of patients with Paget's disease had involvement of the vertebrae, and 26% of these patients had symptoms of spinal stenosis. Franck et al.[32] reported the incidence of back pain in Paget's disease as 11%, Altman et al.[5] reported 34%, and Rosenkrantz et al.[89] reported 43%. The causal relationship between vertebral Paget's disease and back pain has even been disputed by Altman et al.[5], who attributed the low-back pain in Paget's disease to coexisting osteoarthritis of the spine in 22 of 25 patients (88%) and to Paget's disease alone in 3 patients (12%). Guyer and Shepherd[43] think that Paget's disease rarely causes back pain; however, in our population[48] 33% of the patients with Paget's disease demonstrated pagetic involvement of their spine; 54% of these patients suffered back pain and 30% had clinical symptoms of spinal stenosis.

Pathomechanics of Back Pain and Spinal Stenosis

Paget's disease of bone can be defined as an abnormal disturbance of bone remodeling,* which in turn leads to abnormal modeling.† This disturbance of bone remodeling changes the bone texture and gives rise to the four phases of the disease as seen radiologically; that is, the osteolytic, mixed (Fig. 113-4), osteoblastic (Fig. 113-5), and the inactive osteosclerotic phase with normal or decreased bone scan activity.[60]

Spinal Pain (Back and Neck Pain)

Facet arthropathy can be produced by abnormal pagetic remodeling and modeling changes, causing the joint to become hypertrophic and incongruous with destruction of articular cartilage, as may occur in other pagetic joints.[47,67] Pagetic facet arthropathy is a major contributing factor to both back pain and spinal stenosis. The more severe the facet arthropathy, the greater the likelihood the patient will suffer clinical spinal stenosis and/or back pain. However, this does not necessarily preclude the presence of severe facet arthropathy remaining asymptomatic.[48] Back pain in Paget's disease may also be attributed to hypervascularity (engorgement) of the vertebral body caused by the abnormal and rapid

*Frost[34] has defined remodeling as a constant bone renewal or turnover without changes in the size and shape of bone.
†Bone modeling is a process that determines the shape and geometry of the bone[33] and, in Paget's disease, leads to bone expansion and deformities.[60]

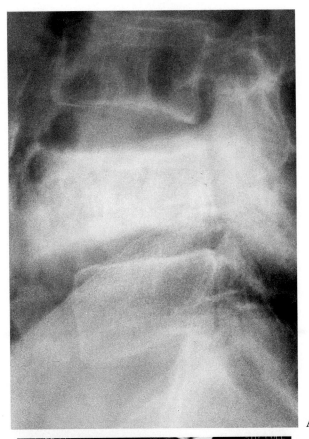

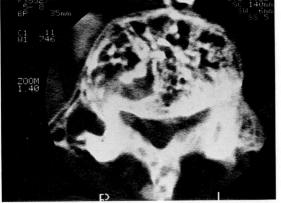

Fig. 113-4
A, Lateral radiograph. Mixed-phase Paget's disease of L4 vertebra. **B,** CT scan. Mixed-phase Paget's disease of L4 vertebra with thickened cortex and trabeculae. Wide marrow space of fat density. Note expansion of body and neural arch.

pagetic remodeling process,[12,51] invasion of the vertebral disc space by the pagetic process,[59] or spinal stenosis.[109] We may hypothesize that microfractures of the pagetic vertebral bodies, especially in the osteolytic or mixed phase, can also lead to back pain. In our series, the most common type of spinal pain was mechanical or arthritic and was found in 27% of

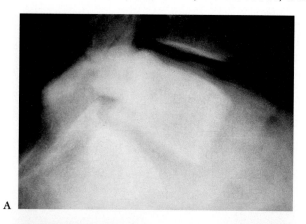

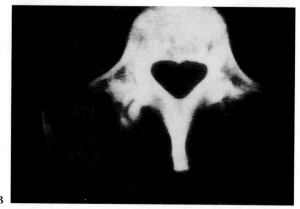

Fig. 113-5

A, Lateral radiograph. Osteoblastic phase Paget's disease of L5. **B,** CT scan. There is a dense trabecular pattern with a wide cortex.

the patients. Constant spinal pain attributed to Paget's disease alone was present in 13%, a combination of mechanical or arthritic back pain in association with pagetic pain was present in 14%, and the remaining 46% reported no spinal pain. Pagetic back pain is characterized by a deep, dull, rather constant ache or pain unrelated to activity and not relieved by rest or nonsteroidal antiinflammatory medications. This is in contrast to so-called mechanical back pain, which improves with rest and worsens with activity or any sustained position. Arthritic pain is manifested by variable aching and stiffness during inactivity and improves with walking.[48]

Spinal Stenosis

Pagetic spinal stenosis can be caused either by posterior expansion of the vertebra body alone (Fig. 113-6) (least common), by expansion of the neural arch and the facet joints, or a combination of these.[48,109] One third of the patients with spinal involvement in our series had evidence of clinical spinal stenosis symptoms.[48] Clinical spinal stenosis can be characterized as central or lateral stenosis. Lateral spinal stenosis is manifested by a constant or intermittent leg pain of variable intensity with a specific radicular distribution associated with paresthesia. This pain is made worse by walking, improves with rest, and may be associated with motor weakness, reflex changes, and sensory changes according to the nerve root involved. Clinical central stenosis is characterized by weakness in the legs, cramps, and changeable amounts of pain provoked by walking variable distances. Objective clinical signs usually are absent. A combination of central and lateral stenosis may also be present. Central stenosis with myelopathy is associated with upper-motor-neuron manifestations.

Several authors have mentioned that neural involvement is more commonly associated with Paget's disease of the thoracic spine[52,58,95] or the cervical spine[66] than the lumbar spine. This was attributed to the large size of the spinal cord relative to the capacity of the vertebral canal; therefore, the same proliferation of bone in all vertebrae would result in compression of the cervical and thoracic thecal sacs sooner than it would in the lumbar spine.[95] In our series, involvement of the cervical spine tended to predispose to clinical spinal stenosis (Fig. 113-7) with myelopathy.[48] Ten distinct mechanisms have been implicated as producing neural element dysfunction in the spines of patients affected by Paget's disease of bone: (1) compression of the neural element by the pagetic bone overgrowth[24,48,58]; (2) compression of the neural elements by pagetic intraspinal soft tissue[48,50]; (3) ossification of the epidural fat similar to ankylosing spondylitis[18]; (4) neural ischemia produced by blood diversion, causing the so-called "arterial steal phenomenon"[17,52,53,79]; (5) interference with blood supply to the cord by compression of the nutrient artery by the expanding pagetic bone,[95] or other factors not well defined[65]; (6) vertebral fracture or atlantoaxial subluxation[95,107]; (7) platybasia may result in impingement on the medulla[20]; (8) spinal cord compression can also be caused by epidural hematoma from spontaneous bleeding[61,87]; (9) formation of syringomyelia was also reported as a complication of Paget's disease of the spine, especially after cranial settling caused by basilar invagination[29,39]; and (10) rarely, neurocompression can be caused by pagetic sarcomatous degeneration.[55] Bone compression by the expanding pagetic vertebrae is by far the most common cause of neural dysfunction[48] and was first reported by Wyllie in 1923.[108] However, severe CT scan stenosis may remain without evidence of clinical spinal stenosis. This suggests an adaptability of the thecal sac and its neural elements

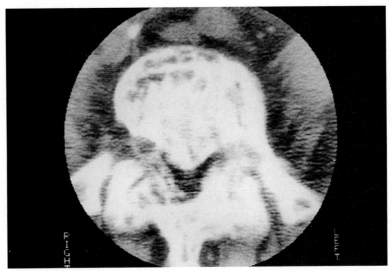

Fig. 113-6
Axial CT scan showing posterior expansion of vertebral body compromising spinal canal.

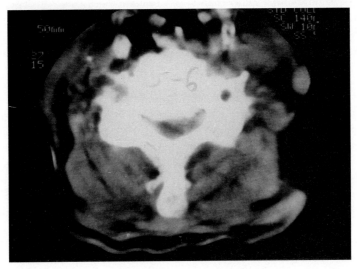

Fig. 113-7
CT scan cervical spin (C5). Pagetic expansion of body has caused spinal canal stenosis with compression of spinal cord.

to severe spinal stenosis without significant loss of function, as pointed out by Schwarz and Reback in 1939.[95]

The mechanism of neural ischemia is, however, still theoretical and supported only by circumstantial evidence, namely, that patients with spinal cord symptomatology respond to calcitonin treatment better than patients with spinal nerve root lesions[20]; that some patients have a progressive deterioration of neural function without evidence of myelographic block not easily explained by mechanical effect alone[92]; that neurologic signs do not always correlate with the site of skeletal involvement; and that rapid clinical improvement occurs in some patients with medical treatment alone. These observations suggest that neural dysfunction in Paget's disease may also result from mechanisms other than mere bone encroachment on the neural element,* such as deprivation of blood supply from the neural elements by the rapidly remodeling hypervascular pagetic bone—"steal phenomenon."

In conclusion, the altered remodeling unit in Paget's disease of bone results in abnormal bone

*References 26, 51, 53, 56, 79, 104, and 108.

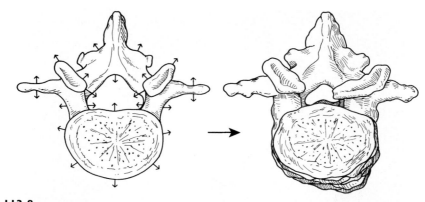

Fig. 113-8

Bone modeling of vertebra can be depicted diagrammatically to demonstrate tendency of bone expansion toward all directions, leading to hypertrophic facet osteoarthropathy and spinal stenosis.

modeling, producing structural changes precipitating or leading to facet osteoarthropathy and spinal stenosis (Fig. 113-8). In the majority of cases, therefore, the clinical picture of pagetic spinal stenosis and facet osteoarthropathy is not expected to differ from that of degenerative spondylosis of the spine (see Fig. 113-8). A minority of patients, however, exhibit constant spinal pain attributed to the pagetic pathologic remodeling process. Because the natural history of Paget's disease affecting the spine is progressive with bone proliferation, vertebral expansion, and structural changes (see Fig. 113-8), preventive therapy is obviously recommended.

Other Associated Conditions

Malignant Transformation

Malignant transformation is the most dreaded complication of Paget's disease of bone. Fortunately, this complication is relatively rare, occurring in about 0.7% of patients in our series of patients with Paget's disease.[49] We have not seen any patient with sarcomatous degeneration in the spine in our series. In Schajowicz et al.'s series,[93] in 62 patients with sarcomatous transformation, five occurred in the spine. These observations suggest that the incidence of malignant transformation in the spine is even more rare and represents about 7% of all sarcomatous degeneration in Paget's disease.[93] Huang et al.[55] described the clinical presentation of Paget's sarcomatous transformation in the spine as dismal, with pain being the cardinal feature. The course is a rapid downhill deterioration with eventual neurocompression. Surgical decompression offers little, if any, true relief of pain. The longest survival was just over 5 months.[55]

Rheumatic and Arthritic Conditions in Paget's Disease

Forestier's disease, or disseminated idiopathic skeletal hyperostosis (DISH) can frequently affect the population of patients with Paget's disease of bone. However, care should be taken not to confuse DISH with Paget's extraosseous bone formation.[14] The incidence of DISH in Paget's disease of bone was reported to range between 14%[48] and 30%.[4] Pagetic tissue may invade the hyperostotic lesions produced by DISH and transform them into pagetic exostosis (Figs. 113-9 and 113-10). Other rheumatic and arthritic conditions such as psoriatic or ankylosing spondylitis may coexist and may be responsible for the clinical presentation.[5,32] Paget's disease has also been noted to be associated with an increased incidence of gout[32] and pseudogout.[81] These conditions, however, are not clearly implicated in the production of back pain.[48] One has to keep in mind that treatment with sodium etidronate may be responsible for accumulation of pyrophosphate crystals in the synovial joint, producing pseudogout.[37]

Treatment

Paget's disease can be reasonably managed with a common sense approach based on an understanding of the principles of the disease behavior (see Fig. 113-8). Abnormal bone remodeling leads to structural changes (abnormal modeling) with bone expansion, spinal stenosis, and facet arthropathy. Prevention of these abnormalities should be the goal of treatment. Five classes of drugs are available for medical treatment of Paget's disease—bisphosphonates, calcitonin, mithramycin (plicamycin), gallium nitrate, and ipriflavone. Only sodium etidronate of the

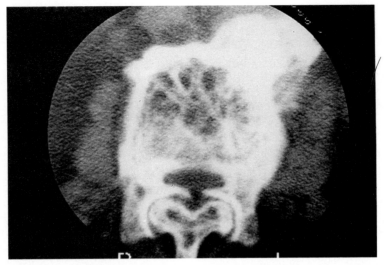

Fig. 113-9

Axial CT scan of thoracic vertebra showing spinal stenosis caused by expansion of lamina, facets, and pedicles. There is also large hyperostosis on left side of vertebra arising from anterolateral vertebral body.

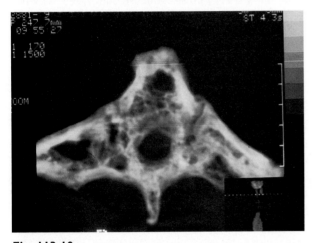

Fig. 113-10

Axial CT of thoracic vertebra showing multidirectional expansion of Paget's disease with transformation of flowing hyperostosis of Forestier (DISH) and contiguous with pagetic vertebral body. Note wide marrow spaces and thick cortices.

bisphosphates and injectable calcitonin are available for clinical use in the United States. The rest of these medications are obtainable only for experimental protocols. Patients who are asymptomatic with inactive biochemical and imaging parameters do not require treatment. However, patients who are asymptomatic with activity as shown by biochemical markers and positive bone bloodflow and scan should be treated until there is normalization of these indices.

Bisphosphonates

Bisphosphonates are compounds characterized by two carbon-phosphorus (P-C-P) bonds that were previously erroneously called "diphosphonates."[31] Several bisphosphonates have been investigated, but for the clinical setting, the following forms of bisphosphonates are available: 1,hydroxyethylene-1,1-bisphosphoric acid, or EHDP, or HEBP etidronate; dichloromethylidene bisphosphonic acid, or Cl_2MBP, or clodronate; 3-amino-1-hydroxypropylidene-1,1-bisphosphonic acid, or aminopropylidine AHPrBP, or APD, or pamidronate; aminohexane disphosphonate, or AHDP; chloro-4-phenylthiomethylene bisphosphonate; aminohydroxybutylidene bisphosphonate, or 4-amino-1-hydroxybutylidene-1,1disphosphonate, or ABDP.

According to Fleisch,[31] the mechanism of action of bisphosphonates on bone consist of inhibition of normal calcification by interfering with calcium phosphate crystal growth. In vitro, they bind strongly to hydroxyapatite crystals and inhibit both their formation and dissolution. Etidronate in sufficient dose inhibits bone mineralization and may result in osteomalacia. Cl_2MBP displays relatively little inhibiting activity on bone mineralization. The bisphosphonates also inhibit bone resorption at a cellular level and after a certain time, bone formation decreases as well, probably because of the well-known coupling between bone formation and resorption. CL_2MBP and HEBP inhibit prostaglandin synthesis in bone cells; prostaglandins are powerful bone resorbers. Numerous other cellular effects of bisphosphonates have been described, such as an increase in the production of alkaline phosphatase; an increase or decrease in the synthesis of proteoglycans; inhibition of multiplication of bone macrophages that are osteoclast precursors; and decrease in lactic acid production, which plays an important role in crystal dissolution. Intravenous administration of 4-amino-1-hydroxybuthilidene-1,1bisphosphonate (AHButBP), or 3-amino-1-hydroxypropylidene-1,1-bisphosphonate (AHPrBP), or 6-amino-1-hydroxyhexylidene-1,1-bisphosphonate (AHHexBP) induces an acute-phase response (APR) irrespective of the underlying disease, manifested by a fall in the number of circulating lymphocytes and serum zinc concentration and in a rise in C-reactive protein (CRP); a febrile reaction occurs in 30% of patients. This APR occurs within 28 to 30 hours of intravenous administration of bisphosphonates and disappears 2 to 3 days later, despite continuous treatment. It seems that these phenomena occur because bisphosphonates interact with macrophage-like cells resident in the skeleton and stimulate interleukin-1 release, which is responsible for the appearance of APR. At the same time, these cells are rendered insensitive to further stimulation for several months.[1]

Disodium Etidronate or EHDP

The usual dose of disodium etidronate, or EHDP, is 5 mg/kg per day for 6 months or 10 mg/kg per day for 3 months, or 20 mg/kg per day for 1 month. Etidronate is effective in most patients. It is important that the drug be taken on an empty stomach, at least 2 hours before eating, and to avoid dairy products for 5 to 6 hours for better absorption. Higher-dose or more prolonged therapy may result in osteomalacia and pathologic fractures.[40,44,99] Combination treatment of 1α-hydroxyvitamin D$_3$ with disodium etidronate in order to prevent the mineralization defect caused by the bisphosphonate was not successful in the treatment of Paget's disease.[82] Treatment with disodium etidronate should aim at reducing the serum levels of alkaline phosphatase by 40% to 50% at 3 months with subsequent adjustment of dosage upward or downward according to the response[30]; and it should be repeated cyclically every 6 months until normalization of bone remodeling markers. If EHDP is ineffective after 6 months of treatment, or if it becomes resistant after a few treatments, then we recommend other agents such as Cl$_2$MBP, APD, or calcitonin. A study comparing oral clodronate (Cl$_2$MBP) 600 mg daily and etidronate 5 to 10 mg/kg per day for 6 months

shows that the proportion of patients responding to etidronate was less, and clodronate had a more sustained response.[41]

Clodronate or Dichloromethylene Disphosphonate

Clodronate, or dichloromethylene disphosphonate, is a very potent bisphosphonate and its action on the skeleton consists of inhibition of bone resorption without mineralization defect.[26,86] The inhibitory effect on bone resorption is mediated mainly through cytotoxic effect on osteoclasts.[86] The clinical response seems to be better than that achieved with EHDP or calcitonin.[26] The recommended dose is 800 to 1600 mg per day orally for 6 months,[16,23,26,41] with a prolonged remission expected to last about 1 to 2 years after withdrawal of the drug.[11,16,23] Bickerstaff et al.[11] have shown that clodronate can also reverse progression of pagetic deformities. Unfortunately, there has been an association of leukemia in three patients treated with clodronate, and this observation has halted the release of the drug for clinical practice except for clinical investigation.[41]

Pamidronate 3-Amino-1Hydroxypropylidene-1,Bisphosphonate or APD (AHPrBP)

Pamidronate, or 3-amino-1-hydroxypropylidene-1,1 bisphosphonate, or APD, is a very effective drug in the treatment of Paget's disease and can even be used when salmon calcitonin, or sodium etidronate, or plicamycin becomes ineffective. This drug has a prolonged biochemical response and can reverse the alkaline phosphatase activity to normal or nearly normal values in severely symptomatic patients or patients with polyostotic Paget's disease. Except for transient hypocalcemia, no other recognizable side effect has been reported.[13,28,64] APD is administered in an intravenous and an oral form. Because of the profound effects on mineral and bone metabolism, close monitoring is required during intravenous treatment with ADP.[28] The intravenous administration is given at a dose ranging from 15 to 25 mg for 5 to 7 consecutive days or a single dose of 60 mg in 0.9% saline infusion over 2 hours.[13,102,105] The suppression period of bone turnover after intravenous administration of this biphosphonate has not been established with certainty. Vega et al.[105] reported a relapse greater than 30% and a short suppression period averaging 2 to 3 months, whereas Dodd et al.[25] and Thiebaud et al.[102, 103] reported a long sustained remission up to 12 months. The oral form given at a high dose of 1200 mg per day over

5 consecutive days induces a rapid decline of biochemical indices. APD is effective in healing lytic lesions[25,63] as opposed to EHDP-treated patients who demonstrated significant deterioration in bone texture in 50% of the lytic lesions.[25] Although APD is a useful means to suppress the bone turnover rapidly, it merits further studies to determine the optimal dose, the length of treatment, and the need to combine the oral with intravenous therapy for prolonged remission.[105]

Chloro-4-Phenylthiomethylene Bisphosphonate

Chlorothiomethylene bisphosphonate has a relatively rapid action, with marked clinical improvement observed from the first month of treatment. No resistance to medication or mineralization defect were recorded. The drug can be taken orally at a dose of 200 to 400 mg daily for 6 months. The average drop in alkaline phosphatase levels actively at 6 months after the onset of treatment was $42 \pm 4\%$ ($p < 0.01$) for the 200 mg and $48 \pm 9\%$ ($p < 0.01$) for the 400 mg dose.[85]

Aminohexane Disphosphonate (AHDP)

Aminohexane disphosphonate (AHDP) is another bisphosphonate that was tried successfully in Paget's disease, with neither adverse effects on mineralization nor significant side effects. The oral dose is 400 mg daily for 1 to 3 months and the intravenous dose is 25 to 50 mg daily for 5 days. This drug provides a long suppression of biochemical indices (up to 18 months). AHDP was also used successfully in patients in whom resistance to treatment developed after sodium etidronate treatment.[6,22]

Aminohydroxybutylidene Bisphosphonate (ABDP)

Aminohydroxybutylidene bisphosphonate, or 4-amino-1-hydroxybutylidene-1,1-disphosphonate, or ABDP, is one of the latest bisphosphonates.[78] This drug is administered intravenously at a dose of 5 mg per day for 4 to 5 days and has a profound inhibition of bone resorption. At 12 days, marked significant decrease of bone biochemical markers was observed.[73]

Calcitonin

Three forms of calcitonin are available—porcine, salmon, and human synthetic for intramuscular or subcutaneous administration. Salmon calcitonin is also available in suppositories and intranasal spray. The potency of salmon and porcine calcitonin is expressed in MRC (Medical Research Council) units. The dose for porcine calcitonin is 1 to 22 MRC units per kg of body weight, whereas that of salmon calcitonin is 50 to 160 MRC units,[7] given either daily or three times a week in a single or divided dose for a prolonged period—6 to 12 months. The dose of human synthetic calcitonin is 0.25 to 0.5 mg per day by subcutaneous injections.[99] Human calcitonin can be used when salmon calcitonin becomes ineffective because of antibody formation against calcitonin.

Salmon calcitonin has been introduced as a nasal spray or suppository at a dose of 200 to 400 units for the nasal spray and 300 units for suppositories. The noninjectable form is still used experimentally in the United States. It seems that injection of salmon (100 IU) calcitonin is more effective than nasal spray (200 IU). Nasal spray of calcitonin was ineffective in three patients with severe Paget's disease as compared to the injectable form.[38] The fall in serum alkaline phosphatase after a 3-month period of nasal calcitonin is expected to average 33% of pretreatment values.[35] The ease of administration and the patient acceptance makes this form of drug a reasonable alternative for geriatric patients.[35] The exposure to intranasal synthetic salmon calcitonin of patients who previously had been treated with parenteral calcitonin may cause secondary antibody response and clinical resistance.[62]

Calcitonin acts directly on the osteoclasts with immediate inhibition of osteoclastic activity and marked reduction in the number of osteoclasts.[15] Calcitonin enhances the production of 1,25-dihydroxyvitamin D_3.[36] Calcitonin also promotes the renal excretion of phosphate, calcium, sodium, and water.[46] O'Donoghue and Hoskins[74] in 1987 reported that the response to salmon calcitonin (100 MRC units thrice weekly) and disodium etidronate (EHDP 400 mg daily) given for 6 months was almost similar. The reduction in alkaline phosphatase was 53% and 56%, respectively. Combination therapy produced a 71% reduction in alkaline phosphatase, which is significantly greater than in the noncombined treatment. More sustained control of the disease activity was achieved with EHDP given either alone or in combination, with the combination retaining the advantage obtained during treatment. However, Rico et al.[88] cautioned against the combination treatment of calcitonin and bisphosphonates (EHDP) because they think that EHDP may diminish the calcitonin effect, which is more active than EHDP.

Gallium Nitrate

Gallium nitrate is a new drug in the treatment of Paget's disease. The response duration is variable, lasting from 6 to 42 weeks. The drug is administered either intravenously at a dose of 2.5 mg/kg body weight per day in 5% glucose for 7 consecutive days or by subcutaneous injections at a dose of 0.25 to 0.5 mg/kg body weight per day for 14 days. The effectiveness of treatment is proportioned to the dose of the drug administered. Response to intravenous treatment was more marked than to subcutaneous injection.[106] Treatment with gallium nitrate significantly reduces serum levels of alkaline phosphatase and urinary excretion of hydroxyproline. Hydroxyproline fall precedes the alkaline phosphatase suppression, suggesting that suppression of osteoclastic bone resorption (reduced hydroxyproline) precedes that of bone reformation by osteoblasts (alkaline phosphate). Transient hyperparathyroidism has also been recorded secondary to the drop in the serum calcium levels during treatment. The effects of gallium seem to be long-lasting.[68] The treatment is still experimental, and larger trials are required to evaluate the safety and effectiveness of this drug. Gallium uptake is dependent on cellular function. The exact mechanism is unknown but may be related to a similar inhibitory effect of calcitonin on osteoclasts.[70]

Mithramycin (Plicamycin)

Mithramycin action on bone resorption is through osteoclastic toxicity. This inhibits the DNA directed RNA synthesis of osteoclasts.[90] Mithramycin has a quick response on bone remodeling and dramatic normalization of bone scan activity.[51,90] Mithramycin (plicamycin) is indicated for severe cord compression, especially when the disease is in the osteolytic phase.[44,51] The recommended dose is 15 μg/kg per day, administered in an intravenous glucose injection over 6 to 8 hours, for 5 days. The same regimen should be repeated after a 7-day interval. Mithramycin is toxic to the liver, kidneys, and platelets. Monitoring of the patient receiving plicamycin should include a platelet count, hematocrit, measurement of blood urea nitrogen, and liver-function tests every second day. We did not encounter permanent kidney, liver, or bone marrow complications in the regimen described. Mithramycin may predispose to hypokalemia that may result in death, especially in patients with predisposing cardiac disease receiving diuretics.[9] Patients may die of bleeding diathesis with larger doses (37.5 to 50 μg/kg) given for cancer therapy.[57]

Ipriflavone

Ipriflavone (7-isoproxy-3-phenyl-4h-1-bonzopyran-4-one) is an isoflavone that has been found to have a beneficial effect on Paget's disease of bone.[2] At a dose of 600 mg daily for 30 days, there was a significant alleviation of pagetic bone pain and improvement of biochemical bone markers. The drug was well tolerated, and only some mild gastrointestinal intolerance was reported.[77] The drug apparently acts indirectly on bone, inhibiting bone resorption by stimulating the release of calcitonin.[72] This drug is still experimental and is available only in Europe.

Treatment of Back Pain

For patients with low-back pain and Paget's disease, suppressive therapy with EHDP (disodium etidronate) was beneficial in 36% of patients in one report.[4] This suggests that unless a well-defined lesion is related to the low-back pain, antipagetic therapy is not expected to be beneficial. As our statistics have shown, only 12% of patients demonstrated pain clearly due to Paget's disease. The rest have either mechanical or arthritic back pain, or a combination of these with pagetic pain. If antipagetic medical therapy is ineffective within 3 months, a concomitant nonsteroidal antiinflammatory drug and other treatment methods for back pain should be prescribed, especially when the presenting back pain is mechanical or arthritic in nature. The asymptomatic patient with active Paget's disease as shown by biochemical indices and scintigraphic imaging may progress to a symptomatic stage. In these patients, treatment with cyclic administration of disodium etidronate may prevent the complications of pagetic pain and spinal stenosis.

Treatment of Spinal Stenosis

Treatment of pagetic spinal stenosis symptoms should start with medical antipagetic therapy. Calcitonin, mithramycin, and sodium etidronate have been reported either to improve or to reverse completely the clinical symptoms of spinal stenosis[3,17,84]; however, relapse of spinal stenosis symptomatology after medical antipagetic treatment is not uncommon[27]; therefore, patients should be closely monitored and cyclical therapy should be continued if necessary. If the symptoms persist in spite of normalization of bone markers (alkaline phosphates, hydroxyproline, osteocalcin, and bone scan), surgery may be an alternative treatment.

Table 113-1 summarizes our experience with surgical treatment for Paget's spinal stenosis in our patients. The results of surgery have shown variable improvement in 85%,[92] with frequent relapses or failures that may improve with subsequent medical antipagetic therapy.[3,17,84] As shown in the table, three of our patients who showed either partial or temporary improvement after laminectomy were treated with further antipagetic medical treatment (one patient was treated with calcitonin, one with a combi-

Table 113-1

Outcome of surgically treated patients

Patient Number	Treatment	Outcome	Pathology	Complications	Additional Antipagetic Treatments	Comments
LUMBAR SPINE						
1	Failed antipagetic treatment before surgery Laminectomy	Successful	Epidural pagetic soft tissue	None	Not necessary	Sustained
2	No previous treatment Laminectomy	Partial improvement	Stenosis caused by laminar and facet expansion	Profuse bleeding	Salmon calcitonin	Marked improvement sustained
3	No previous treatment Laminectomy	Marginal improvement	Stenosis caused by laminar and facet expansion	Profuse bleeding	Mithramycin followed by salmon calcitonin	Marked improvement sustained
4	No previous treatment Laminectomy	Failed	Stenosis caused by laminar and facet expansion	Torrential bleeding	Mithramycin followed by cyclical salmon calcitonin	Marginal improvement sustained with continued antipagetic treatment
CERVICAL SPINE						
5	Failed antipagetic treatment before surgery Vertebrectomy, fusion, and instrumentation	Successful	Stenosis caused by posterior vertebral expansion	None	Cyclical etidronate	Sustained
6	Failed antipagetic treatment before surgery Laminectomy	Failed Remained paraparetic	Stenosis caused by posterior vertebral expansion	Further worsening, almost paraplegic	Mithramycin followed by calcitonin	Minimal improvement
7	Laminectomy of first cervical vertebra	Marginal improvement	Compression of spinal cord by pagetic soft tissue of 1st cervical vertebra	None	Cyclical etidronate	Marked improvement sustained

(con't)

Table 113-1, cont'd

Outcome of surgically treated patients

Patient Number	Treatment	Outcome	Pathology	Complications	Additional Antipagetic Treatments	Comments
THORACIC SPINE						
8	Treatment with massive steroid administration which fails Vertebrectomy, fusion, and instrumentation	Failed	Cord compression and paraplegia by pathological fracture of seventh thoracic vertebra	Died. Cardiorespiratory failure, profuse bleeding	Post-operative salmon calcitonin	Paraplegic for 2 weeks before surgery

nation of calcitonin and mithramycin, and one with cyclic etidronate). They had a marked improvement of their symptomatology with sustained relief. In patient 7 the spinal stenosis was caused by pagetic soft tissue compressing the medulla at the C1 level. He underwent laminectomy and widening of the foramen magnum with marginal improvement and was placed on cyclical treatment with etidronate with subsequent marked and sustained improvement. Relapse of spinal stenosis symptomatology after medical treatment is not uncommon.[27] This type of patient should be closely monitored and continued on cyclical therapy until normalization of biochemical bone indices. From our experience and other reports, spinal surgery for pagetic spinal stenosis may fail to reverse the neurologic deficit completely[14] and may be associated with serious complications such as a mortality rate of 11%[92] and dangerous profuse, if not massive bleeding.[91] As can be seen in Table 113-1, three of our patients suffered profuse bleeding. Therefore, we advise a preoperative radionuclide bone blood flow of the affected spinal region to assess the vascularity of bone. We have found this test reliable and reproducible.[12] If there is an increased vascularity, we strongly recommend a course of medical antipagetic treatment until normalization of the bone blood flow. In our experience, this may take 2 to 3 months with calcitonin therapy or 2 to 3 weeks with mithramycin treatment. The most recent intravenous drugs such as gallium nitrate or the new generation of bisphosphonates can also be used. In emergency situations, embolization of the region may be indicated. Because of the expected torrential bleeding during laminectomy, the use of cell saver is strongly recommended.[91] In one of our patients, no. 4, decompression of the lumbar spine was per-

formed for spinal stenosis symptomatology (Fig. 113-11). The patient bled profusely during surgery, as was mentioned previously, and subsequently a huge hematoma developed that was organized in a thick scar tissue. If this patient had been treated with antipagetic therapy before surgery, the surgical decompression would have been less traumatic and more effective.

Surgery for spinal stenosis, when indicated, should be tailored to the pathology responsible for neural compression. If the compression is caused by posterior expansion of vertebral bodies, an anterior approach with corpectomy and fusion would be indicated. If neural compression is caused by the posterior vertebral elements, then posterior decompression would be the approach of choice. In one of our patients (no. 6) a delayed laminectomy was performed for a rapidly progressive cervical myelopathy caused by cervical C5-C6 vertebral expansion posteriorly into the cervical spinal canal compressing the spinal cord. This type of surgery failed to decompress the cord, and the patient's condition deteriorated. Anterior decompression would have been more appropriate in this situation. Another patient (no. 5) with a similar situation whose cord was compromised because of posterior vertebral expansion underwent an anterior approach with corpectomy with marked improvement of his myelopathy (Fig. 113-12). A patient with osteopenic Paget's disease of the thoracic spine (no. 8) sustained a spontaneous wedge fracture of T4 with increased kyphosis and posterior expansion of the vertebral body compressing the cord and producing paraparesis (Fig. 113-13). This patient was admitted as an emergency to the hospital. Unfortunately, he was treated with large doses of cortisone and a wait-and-see policy was

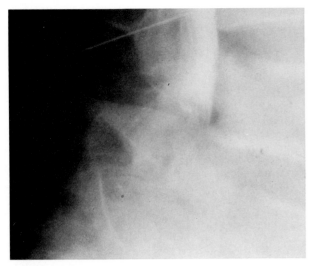

Fig. 113-11
Lateral myelogram of lumbar spine with complete obstruction of thecal sac at L3.

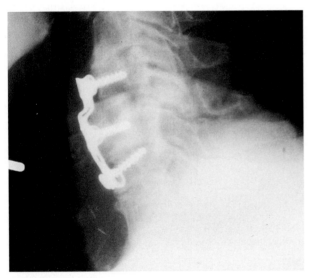

Fig. 113-12
Postoperative corpectomy of C6 with bone graft stabilized by anterior plate.

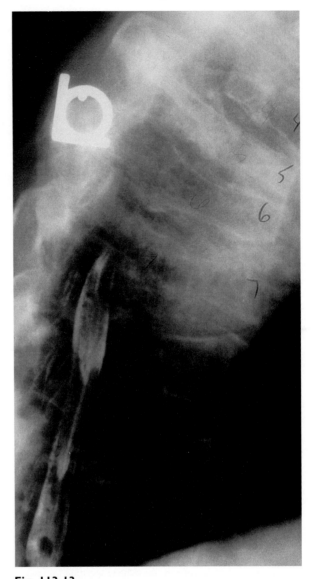

Fig. 113-13
Lateral radiograph of dorsal spine showing kyphosis and partial compression of body of T7 affected with Paget's disease with complete myelographic block at T4.

adopted. This type of bone compression by bone impingement and kyphosis does not respond solely to cortisone therapy. Complete paraplegia developed and the patient was referred to us 2 weeks later. A thoracotomy and anterior decompression with bone graft and stabilization with Kostuik-Harrington instrumentation was performed. During surgery, the patient had profuse bleeding, but decompression was successful; however, the patient died 2 weeks later from cardiorespiratory arrest. An acute onset of spinal cord compression seems to bear a graver prognosis than the more gradual development of symp-

toms, which tend to respond better to surgical decompression.[96]

We think that surgery is indicated if well-applied medical antipagetic treatment fails to improve the symptomatology of spinal stenosis, if during conservative therapy there is a deterioration of the neurologic deficit, and when neural compression is secondary to fractures, dislocations, epidural hematoma, syringomyelia, platybasia, or sarcomatous transformation.

Antipagetic medical therapy is rewarding in treating pagetic back pain and spinal stenosis syndrome. Decompression for spinal stenosis should be insti-

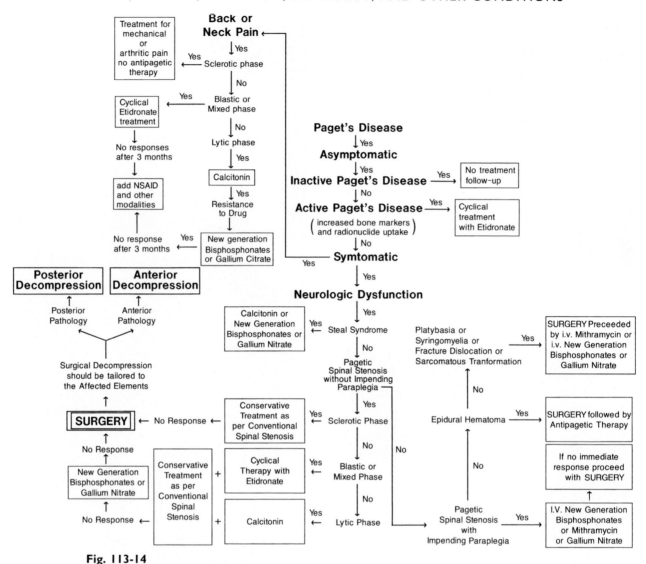

Fig. 113-14

Self-explanatory algorithmic approach for management of spinal manifestations of Paget's disease of bone.

tuted promptly after failure of antipagetic medical therapy. In these circumstances, procrastination may lead to irreversible myelopathy or radiculopathy.

Methods for Monitoring Antipagetic Drug Treatment

The effect of treatment is best monitored by the patient's clinical response and scintigraphic images, including radionuclide bone blood flow before and 3 months after treatment (Radionuclide bone blood flow can be used to monitor the vascularity and therefore the potential bleeding of the region before proceeding with surgery especially in an emergency situation before and after completion of intravenous antipagetic therapy); conventional bone scan 6 months after treatment and 12 months thereafter depending on the behavior of the pagetic lesion; and the 24-hour retention scan, which is a more quantitative radionuclide assessment and can be used as an adjunct to the bone scan.[12] Radiographic images should be obtained before and every 1 to 2 years thereafter to monitor the modeling (bone expansion) and remodeling changes (phase of the disease activity). A hematologic profile, serum eletrolytes, and kidney and liver function tests are helpful to assess the overall medical condition of the patient with Paget's disease of the spine who are within the geriatric age group,[48] and especially when administering antipagetic drugs such as mithramycin or the new-generation bisphosphonates. Bone remodeling biochemical markers are useful to monitor the effect of treatment on the bone remodeling process. These should be assessed before treatment and every 3 to 6 months thereafter, depending on the activity of the pagetic lesion and the drug used.

Summary

In summary, Paget's disease of the spine is characterized by numerous variables encompassing the different stages of bone remodeling and modeling activities, the diversity of clinical manifestations of spinal pain and the neurologic dysfunction of several etiologic factors. From the therapeutic perspective, the different surgical interventions and several antipagetic drugs currently available are not specifically tailored to a particular disease process. These variables prompted us to design a detailed algorithmic approach with a comprehensive toxonomy based on pathomorphology and clinical manifestations of this osteometabolic disorder (Fig. 113-14). The algorithmic approach is consistent with conventional wisdom and permits definition, simple decision, and a piecemeal solution for problems in a predetermined path. If the results of the tests are not suggestive of any specific diagnosis, or the treatment fails, then it takes the user to a preordained path that is signposted, and a new decision is analyzed stepwise until a final specific outcome is reached.

References

1. Adami S, Bhalla AK, Dorizzi R, et al.: The acute-phase response after bisphosphonate administration, *Calcif Tissue Int* 41:326, 1987.
2. Agnusdei D, Cemporeale A, Gonnelli S, et al.: Short-term treatment of Paget's disease of bone with ipriflavone, *Bone Miner* 19(Suppl):35, 1992.
3. Alexandre C, Trillet M, Meunier P, et al.: Traitement des paraplégics pagétiques par les disphosphonates, *Rev Neurol* (Paris) 135:625, 1979.
4. Altman RD, Brown M, Gargano F: Low back pain in Paget's disease of bone, *Clin Orthop* 217:152, 1987.
5. Altman RD, Collins B: Musculoskeletal manifestation of Paget's disease of bone, *Arthritis Rheum* 23:1121, 1980.
6. Atkins RM, Yates AJ, Gray RE, et al.: Aminohexane disphosphonate in the treatment of Paget's disease of bone, *J Bone Miner Res* 2:273, 1987.
7. Avramides A: Salmon and porcine calcitonin treatment of Paget's disease of bone, *Clin Orthop Relat Res* 127:78, 1977.
8. Barry HC: *Paget's disease of bone,* Edinburgh, 1969, Churchill Livingstone.
9. Bashiz Y, Tomson LR: Cardiac arrest associated with hypocalcemia in a patient receiving mithromycin, *Postgrad Med J* 64:289, 1988.
10. Baslé MF, Rebel A, Fournier JG, et al.: On the trail of paramyxoviruses in Paget's disease of bone, *Clin Orthop* 217:9, 1987.
11. Bickerstaff DR, Douglas DL, Burke PH, et al.: Improvement in the deformity of the face in Paget's disease treated with diphosphonates, *J Bone Joint Surg* 72B:132, 1990.
12. Boudreau RJ, Lisbona R, Hadjipavlou A: Observations on serial radionuclide blood flow studies in Paget's disease, *J Nucl Med* 24:880, 1983.
13. Cantrill JA, Buckler HM, Anderson DC: Low dose intravenous 3-amino-1-hydroxy-prohylidene-1, 1-bisphosphonate (APD) for the treatment of Paget's disease of bone, *Ann Rheum Dis* 45:1012, 1986.
14. Cartlidge N, McCollum JPK, Ayyar RDA: Spinal cord compression in Paget's disease, *J Neurol Neurosurg Psychiatry* 35:825, 1970.
15. Chambers TJ, McSheehy PMJ, Thomson BM, et al.: The effect of calcium regulation hormones and prostaglandins on bone resorption by osteoclasts disaggregated from neonatal rabbit bones, *Endocrinology* 60:234, 1985.
16. Chapuy MC, Charhon SA, Meunier PJ: Sustained biochemical effects of short treatment of Paget's disease of bone with dichloromethylene disphosphonate, *Metab Bone Dis Relat Res* 4:325, 1983.
17. Chen JR, Richard SCR, Wallach S, Avramides A, et al.: Neurologic disturbances in Paget's disease of bone: response to calcitonin, *Neurology* 29:448, 1979.
18. Clarke PR, Williams HI: Ossification in extradural fat in Paget's disease of the spine, *Br J Surg* 62:571, 1975.
19. Collins DH: Paget's disease of bone: incidence and subclinical forms, *Lancet* 2:51, 1956.
20. Curran JE: Neurological sequelae of Paget's disease of the vertebral column and skull bone, *Austral Radiol* 19:15, 1975.
21. Danais S, Hadjipavlou A: Etude scintighaphique comparative des lésions osseuses et de la moelle osseuse dans la maladie de Paget, *Union Med Can* 106:1100, 1977.
22. Delmas PD, Chapuy MC, Edouard C, et al.: Beneficial effects of aminohexane disphosphonate in patients with Paget's disease of bone resistant to sodium etidronate, *Am J Med* 83:276, 1987.
23. Delmas DP, Chapuy MC, Iignon E, et al.: Long term effects of dicholoromethylene disphosphonate in Paget's disease of bone, *J Clin Endocrinol Metab* 54:837, 1982.
24. Direkze M, Milnes JN: Spinal cord compression in Paget's disease, *Br J Surg* 57:239, 1970.
25. Dodd GW, Ibbertson HK, Fraser TR, et al.: Radiological assessment of Paget's disease of bone after treatment with bisphosphonate EHDP and APD, *Br J Radiol* 60:849, 1987.
26. Douglas DL, Duckworth T, Kanis JA, et al.: Biochemical and clinical responses to dichloromethylene disphosphonate (Cl$_2$MDP) in Paget's disease of bone, *Arthritis Rheum* 23:1185, 1980.
27. Douglas DL, Duckworth T, Kanis JA, et al.: Spinal cord dysfunction in Paget's disease of bone: has medical treatment a vascular basis? *J Bone Joint Surg* 63B:495, 1981.

28. Drake S, Massie JD, Postelwaite AE, et al.: Pomidronate sodium and calcitonin-resistant Paget's disease: Immediate response in a patient, *Arch Intern Med* 149:401, 1989.

29. Elisevich K, Fontaine S, Bertrand C: Syringomyelia as a complication of Paget's disease, *J Neurosurg* 67:611, 1987.

30. Evans RA: Paget's disease of bone: comments by eight specialists, Princeton, NJ, 1988, *Excerpta Medica*.

31. Fleisch H: Experimental basis for the use of bisphosphonates in Paget's disease of bone, *Clin Orthop* 217:72, 1987.

32. Franck WA, Bress NM, Singer FR, et al.: Rheumatic manifestations of Paget's disease of bone, *Am J Med* 56:592, 1974.

33. Frost H: *Bone modeling and skeletal modeling errors*. In *Orthopedic lectures*, vol 4, Springfield, IL, 1973[b], Charles C Thomas.

34. Frost HM: *Bone remodeling and its relationship to metabolic bone diseases*. In *Orthopedic lectures*, vol 3, Springfield, IL, 1973[a], Charles C Thomas.

35. Gagel RF, Logan C, Melette LE: Treatment of Paget's disease of bone with salmon calcitonin nasal spray, *J Am Geriatr Soc* 30:1010, 1988.

36. Galante L, Colston KW, MacAuley SJ, et al.: Effect of calcitonin on vitamin D metabolism, *Nature* 238:271, 1972.

37. Gallagher SJ, Boyle IT, Capell HA: Pseudogout associated with the use of cyclical etidronate therapy, *Scott Med J* 36:49, 1991.

38. Gonzales D, Vega E, Ghiringhelli G, et al.: Comparison of the acute effect of the intranasal and intramuscular administration of salmon calcitonin in Paget's disease, *Calcif Tissue Int* 41:313, 1987.

39. Goodman SJ: Syringomyelia in Paget's disease, *J Neurosurg* 67:790, 1987.

40. Gray RE: Paget's disease of bone: comments by eight specialists, Princeton, NJ, 1988, *Excerpt Medica*.

41. Gray RE, Yates JP, Preston CJ, et al.: Duration of effect of oral disphosphonate therapy in Paget's disease of bone, *Q J Med* 64:755, 1987.

42. Guyer PB, Chamberlain AT: Paget's disease of bone in South Africa, *Clin Radiol* 39:51, 1988.

43. Guyer PB, Shepherd DFC: Paget's disease of lumbar spine, *Br J Radiol* 53:286, 1980.

44. Hadjipavlou A: Paget's disease of bone: comments by eight specialists, Princeton, NJ, 1988, *Excerpta Medica*.

45. Hadjipavlou A, Begin LR, Abitbol JJ: Observations morphologiques, histochimique et ultrastructurales de culture cellulaires in vitro d'os pagetique et normal, *Union Med Can* 115:746, 1986.

46. Hadjipavlou A, Brooks EE: Etude de l'action de la calcitonin sur le rein, *Union Med Can* 105:915, 1976.

47. Hadjipavlou A, Lander P, Srolovitz H: Pagetic arthritis: pathophysiology and management, *Clin Orthop* 208:15, 1986.

48. Hadjipavlou A, Lander P: Paget's disease of the spine, *J Bone Joint Surg* 73A:1376, 1991.

49. Hadjipavlou A, Lander P, Srulovitz H, Enker P: Malignant transformation in Paget's disease of bone, *Cancer* 70:2802, 1992.

50. Hadjipavlou A, Shaffer N, Lander P, Srolovitz H: Pagetic spinal stenosis with extradural pagetoid ossification: a case report, *Spine* 13:128, 1988.

51. Hadjipavlou A, Tsoukas G, Siller T, et al.: Combination drug therapy in treatment of Paget's disease of bone: clinical and metabolic response, *J Bone Joint Surg* 59A:1045, 1977.

52. Hartman JT, Dohn DF: Paget's disease of the spine with cord or nerve root compression, *J Bone Joint Surg* 48A:1079, 1966.

53. Herzberg L, Bayliss E: Spinal cord syndrome due to compressive Paget's disease of bone: a spinal artery steal phenomenon reversible with calcitonin, *Lancet* 2:13, 1980.

54. Holdaway IM, Ibberston HK, Wattie D, et al.: Previous pet ownership and Paget's disease, *Bone Miner* 8:53, 1990.

55. Huang TL, Cohen NJ, Sahgal SA, et al.: Osteosarcoma complicating Paget's disease of the spine with neurologic complication, *Clin Orthop* 14:260, 1979.

56. Kay HD, Levy-Simpson S, Riddoch G, et al.: Osteitis deformans with roentgenologic section, *Arch Intern Med* 53:208, 1934.

57. Kennedy BJ: Metabolic and toxic effects of mithromycin during tumor therapy, *Am J Med* 48:494, 1970.

58. Klenerman L: Cauda equina and spinal cord compression in Paget's disease, *J Bone Joint Surg* 48B:365, 1966.

59. Lander P, Hadjipavlou A: Intradiscal invasion of Paget's disease of the spine, *Spine* 16:46, 1991.

60. Lander P, Hadjipavlou A: A dynamic classification of Paget's disease, *J Bone Joint Surg* 68B:431, 1986.

61. Lee KS, McWhorter JM, Angelo JN: Spinal epidural hematoma associated with Paget's disease, *Surg Neurol* 30:131, 1988.

62. Levy F, Muff R, Dotti-Sigrist S, et al.: Formation of neutralizing antibodies during intranasal synthetic salmon calcitonin treatment of Paget's disease, *J Clin Endocrinol Metab* 7:541, 1988.

63. Maldaque B, Malghem J: Dynamic radiologic patterns of Paget's disease of bone, *Clin Orthop* 217:125, 1987.

64. Mallette LE: Successful treatment of resistant Paget's disease of bone with pamidronate, *Arch Intern Med* 149:2765, 1989.

65. Mathé JF, Delobel R, Resche F, et al.: Syndromes medullaire au cours de la maladie de Paget: Role du facteur vasculaire, *Nouv Presse Med* 5:2619, 1976.

66. Mawhinney R, Jones R, Worthington BJ: Spinal cord compression secondary to Paget's disease of the axis, *Br J Radiol* 58:1203, 1985.

67. Merkow RL, Lane JM: Paget's disease of bone, *Orthop Clin North Am* 21:171, 1990.

68. Matkovic V, Apseloff G, Shepard DR, et al.: Use of gallium nitrate on bone: a pilot study, *Lancet* 335:72, 1990.

69. Meunier PJ, Salson C, Mathieu L, et al.: Skeletal distribution and biochemical parameters of Paget's disease, *Clin Orthop* 217:37, 1987.

70. Mills BG, Masuoka LS, Graham CC Jr, et al.: Gallium-67 citrate localization in osteoclast nuclei of Paget's disease of bone, *J Nucl Med* 29:1083, 1988.

71. Mills BG, Singer FR: Critical evaluation of viral antigen data in Paget's disease of bone, *Clin Orthop* 217:16, 1987.

72. Nakamura S, Mozimoto S, Takamoto S, et al.: Effect of ipriflavone on bone mineral density and calcium related factors in elderly females, *Calcif Tissue Int Suppl* 1:30, 1992.

73. O'Doherty DP, Bickerstaff DR, McCloskey EV, et al.: Treatment of Paget's disease of bone with aminohydroxybutylidene bisphosphonate, *J Bone Miner Res* 5:483, 1990.

74. O'Donoghue DJ, Hoskins DJ: Biochemical response to combination of disodium etidronate with calcitonin in Paget's disease, *Bone* 8:219, 1987.

75. O'Driscoll JB, Buckler HM, Jeacurk J, et al.: Dogs, distemper, and osteitis deformans: a further epidemiological study, *Bone Miner* 11:204, 1990.

76. Paget J: On a form of chronic inflammation of bone (osteitis deformans), *Trans R Med Chir Soc Lond* 60:36, 1877.

77. Passeri M, Bioudi M, Costi D, et al.: Effect of ipriflavone on bone mass in elderly osteoporotic women, *Bone Miner Suppl* 19:57, 1992.

78. Pedrazzoni M, Pelumuezi E, Ciotti G, et al.: Short-term effects on bone and mineral metabolism of 4-amino-1-hydroxybutylidene-1,1-disphosphonate (ABDP) in Paget's disease of bone, *Bone Miner* 7:301, 1989.

79. Porrini AA, Maldonado-Cocco JA, Morteo GO: Spinal artery steal syndrome in Paget's disease of bone, *Clin Exp Rheumatol* 5:377, 1987.

80. Pygott F: Paget's disease of bone: the radiological incidence, *Lancet* 1:1170, 1957.

81. Radi I, Epiney J, Reiner M: Chondrocalcinose et maladie osseuse de Paget, *Rev Rheum* 37:385, 1970.

82. Ralston SH, Boyce BF, Cowan RA, et al.: The effect of 1-alpha-hydroxyvitamin D_3 on the mineralization defect in disodium etidronate treated Paget's disease: a double-blind randomized clinical study, *J Bone Miner Res* 2:5, 1987.

83. Rasmussen H, Bordier P: The physiological cellular basis of metabolic bone disease, *N Engl J Med* 284:25, 1973.

84. Ravichandran G: Neurologic recovery of paraplegia following use of salmon calcitonin in a patient with Paget's disease of spine, *Spine* 4:37, 1979.

85. Reginster JY, Dezoisy R, Lecart MP, et al.: (Chloro-4 phenyl)thiomethyne bisphosphonate in Paget's bone disease, *Acta Belg Med Phys* 12:47, 1989.

86. Reitsma PH, Teitelbaum SL, Bijvoet OLM, et al.: Differential action of bisphosphonates (3-amino-1-hydroxypropylidene)-1,1-bisphosphonate (ADP) and disodium dichloromethylidene bisphosphonate (Cl$_2$MDP) on rat macrophage-mediated bone resorption *in vitro*, *J Clin Invest* 70:927, 1982.

87. Richter RL, Semble EL, Turner RA, et al.: An unusual manifestation of Paget's disease of bone: spinal epidural hematoma presenting as acute cauda equina syndrome, *J Rheumatol* 17:975, 1990.

88. Rico H, Hernandez ER, Younes M, et al.: Biochemical assessment of acute and chronic treatment of Paget's bone disease with calcitonin and calcium with or without bisphosphonate, *Bone* 9(1):63, 1988.

89. Rosenkrantz JA, Wolf J, Kaicher JJ: Paget's disease (osteitis deformans), *Arch Intern Med* 90:610, 1952.

90. Ryan WG: Treatment of Paget's disease of bone with mithramycin, *Clin Orthop* 127:106, 1977.

91. Ryan MD, Taylor TKF: Spinal manifestations of Paget's disease, *Aust N Z J Surg* 62:33, 1992.

92. Sadar SE, Walton RJ, Grossman HH: Neurological dysfunction in Paget's disease of the vertebral column, *J Neurosurg* 37:661, 1972.

93. Schajowicz F, Araujo SE, Berestein M: Sarcoma complicating Paget's disease of bone: a clinicopathological study of 62 cases, *J Bone Joint Surg* 65B:299, 1983.

94. Schmorl G: Über osteitis deformans Paget, *Virchows Arch Anat Physiol* 283:694, 1932.

95. Schwarz GA, Reback S: Compression of the spinal cord in osteitis deformans (Paget's disease of the vertebrae), *Am Roentgenol Radi Ther* 42:345, 1939.

96. Siegelman SS, Levine SA, Walpin L: Paget's disease with spinal cord compression, *Clin Radiol* 19:421, 1968.

97. Singer RF: *Paget's disease of bone*, New York, 1977, Plenum Medical Book Co.

98. Singer FR, Mills BG: The etiology of Paget's disease of bone, *Clin Orthop* 127:37, 1977.

99. Siris ES: Paget's disease of bone: comments by eight specialists, Princeton, NJ, 1988, *Excerpta Medica*.

100. Siris ES, Kelsey JL, Flaster E, et al.: Paget's disease of bone and previous pet ownership in the United States: dogs exonerated, *Int J Epidemiol* 19:455, 1990.

101. Siris ES, Ottman R, Flasher E, et al.: Familial aggregation of Paget's disease of bone, *J Bone Miner Res* 6:495, 1991.

102. Thiébaud D, Jaeger P, Gobelet C, et al.: A single infusion of the bisphosphonate AHPrBP (APD) as treatment of Paget's disease of bone, *Am J Med* 85:207, 1988.

103. Thiébaud D, Jaeger P, Burchardt P: Paget's disease of bone treated in five days with AHPrBP (APD) per OS, *J Bone Miner Res* 2:45, 1987.

104. Turner JWA: Spinal complications of Paget's disease (osteitis deformans), *Brain* 63:321, 1940.

105. Vega E, Gonzales D, Ghiringhelli G, et al.: Intravenous aminopropylidene bisphosphonate (APD) in the treatment of Paget's bone disease, *J Bone Miner Res* Aug 2:267, 1987.

106. Warrell RP Jr, Bosco B, Weinerman S, et al.: Gallium nitrate for advanced Paget's disease of bone, effectiveness and dose: response analysis, *Ann Intern Med* 113:847, 1990.

107. Whalley N: Paget's disease of the atlas and axis, *J Neurol Neurosurg Psychiatry* 9:84, 1946.

108. Wyllie WG: The occurrence in osteitis deformans of lesions of the central nervous system with a report of four cases, *Brain* 46:336, 1923.

109. Zlatkin MB, Lander PH, Hadjipavlou A, Levine JS: Paget's disease of the spine: CT with clinical correlation, *Radiology* 160:155, 1986.

Appendix A

Dynamic Lumbar Stabilization Exercises*

Arthur H. White

---

*Taken from San Francisco Spine Institute: Dynamic lumbar stabilization video program.

The Neutral Position

Each individual should establish their own "neutral position." Neutral spine does not necessarily mean zero degrees of lordosis but rather the most comfortable position for the individual.

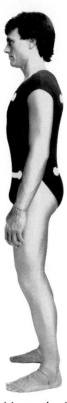

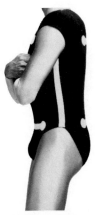

The abdominal muscles should be contracted to "corset" and maintain this position. Sometimes it is helpful for the patient to feel the abdominal musculature with his or her fingers to make sure the muscles are tight.

The patient should stand with knees slightly bent, and weight distributed evenly. Using the abdominal muscles to tilt the pelvis, the lumbar spine should be flexed and extended until the balanced position of optimal function and stability is attained.

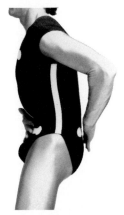

The hips play an important role in maintaining the neutral spine position. Rotate the pelvis forward and backward until a balanced, pain-free, midrange position is attained. The hips should rotate as if there were a round hinge inserted directly into the hip socket. This imaginary hinge can be dialed forward or backward to bend the body or reposition the spine.

Make sure the hips and shoulders are square. The patient should imagine the spine, hips, and shoulders as a single unit. This stabilized unit should be maintained even though the rest of the body may move in a variety of postures and activities.

Abdominal Bracing

Purpose: To gain awareness of the contraction of the abdominal muscles while holding a neutral spine posture.

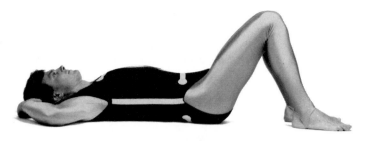

A, Find the neutral position. Tighten the abdominal muscles, paying particular attention to the lower abdomen. Contract the abdominal muscles to keep the spine in the neutral position.

B, Feel the corseting effect of the abdominal muscles.

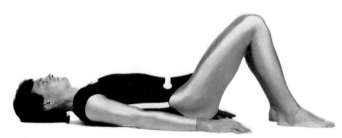

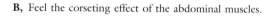

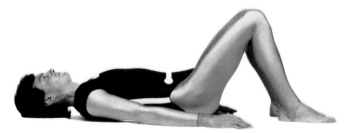

Abdominal bracing with arms and unsupported legs. Purpose: To strengthen the abdominal muscles. This is the more advanced exercise of this type.

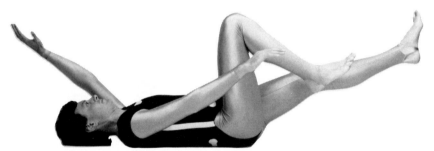

A, Find the neutral position and brace the abdominal muscles.

B, Relax the neck and shoulders as the arms and legs are lifted off the floor. Gradually straighten the leg while raising the arm on the same side.

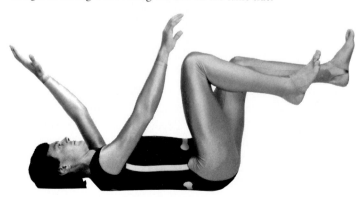

C, There should be no tightness in the lower back while performing this exercise. The only tightness should be in the abdominal muscles.

Fig. A-4

Supine leg thrusts. Purpose: To strengthen the lower abdominal muscles.

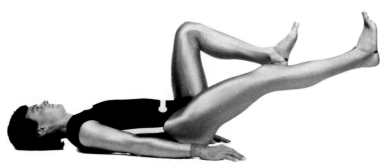

A, Hold the neutral position. Lift both legs off the floor and gently thrust them forward one at a time. Contract the abdominal muscles with each leg thrust. Do not thrust the pelvis forward as this will bend the spine or lift it off the floor.

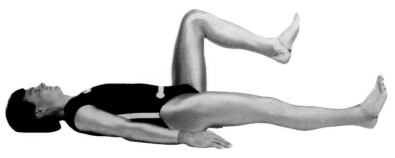

B, Continue to breathe throughout the exercise, relaxing the upper body while moving the legs smoothly in a continuous motion.

Fig. A-5

Partial sit-ups. Purpose: To strengthen the abdominal muscles.

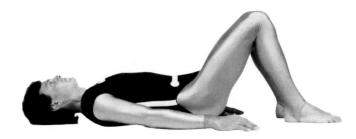

A, Start from the neutral position.

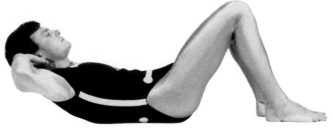

B, Use the abdominal muscles to raise the upper back off the floor. Rise only enough to clear the shoulder blades. Hold the lift at the top of the movement for a count of three. Do not thrust the body off the floor or lift the head with the arms. Keep the feet flat on the floor. Feel the contractions only in the abdominal muscles. Let the motions be smooth and relaxed.

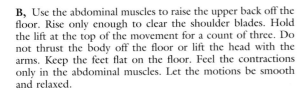

Fig. A-6

Bridging. Purpose: To strengthen the abdominal, buttocks, and lower back muscles while challenging the ability to hold neutral spine position.

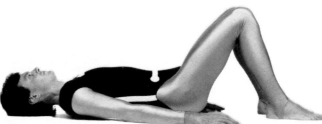

A, Tighten the abdominal muscles to hold the lower spine in a stable position.

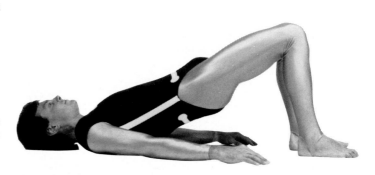

B, Using the buttocks muscles, slowly rise off the surface without bending the lower back. Use the abdominal and buttocks muscles to keep the pelvis elevated. Relax the shoulders and neck while holding the position being sure to breathe evenly.

Fig. A-7

Bridging with leg extension. Purpose: To strengthen the abdominal, buttocks, and lower back muscles. This is a more advanced level of this exercise.

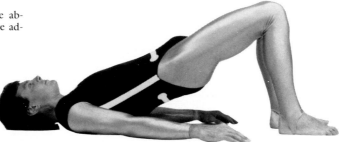

A, Stabilize the lower spine. Using the buttocks muscles, slowly raise the trunk off the floor. Make sure the lower abdominal muscles are holding the lower trunk while lifting the legs one at a time.

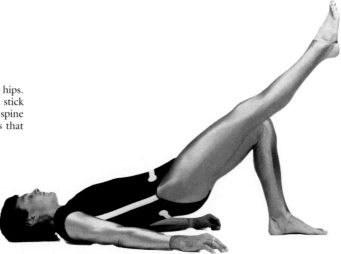

B, Extend the leg from the knee hinge without moving the hips. The arms, neck, and shoulders should be relaxed. Placing a stick across the hips will help maintain the stabilization of the spine and lower trunk. If the stick dips or rolls off, this indicates that the pelvis is not stabilized.

Fig. A-8

Prone arm and leg lifts. Purpose: To strengthen the arm, shoulder, and leg muscles.

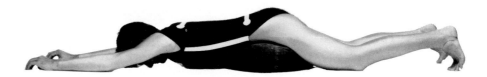

A, Use the abdominal muscles to stabilize the position. It is sometimes necessary to place a bolster under the pelvis for comfort.

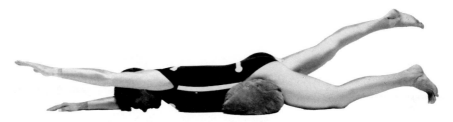

B, Lift one arm and the opposite leg. The trunk should not move. Keep the motion controlled and smooth.

Fig. A-9

Quadruped arm raises. Purpose: To strengthen the lower back and arm muscles while increasing awareness of the neutral spine.

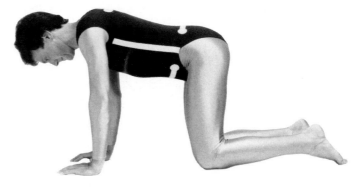

A, Tighten the abdominal muscles to stabilize the lower spine.

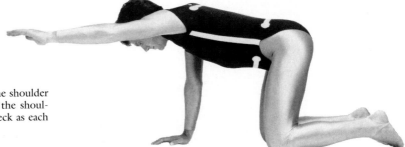

B, Raise one arm, then the other. Move only from the shoulder while keeping the back and hips steady. Do not let the shoulders rise up or twist. Keep breathing and relax the neck as each arm is raised and lowered.

Fig. A-10

Quadruped arm and leg raises. Purpose: To practice stabilization and strengthen the arm and leg muscles.

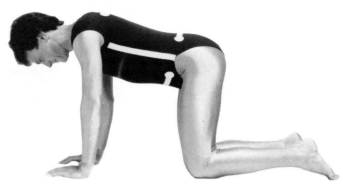

A, Relax the neck and tighten the abdominal muscles to stabilize the spine in the neutral position.

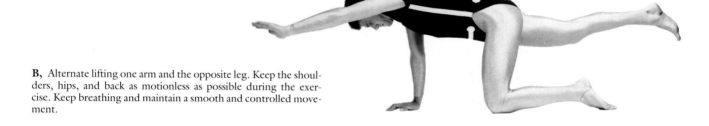

B, Alternate lifting one arm and the opposite leg. Keep the shoulders, hips, and back as motionless as possible during the exercise. Keep breathing and maintain a smooth and controlled movement.

Fig. A-11

Forward lunges. Purpose: To strengthen the abdominal, leg, and buttocks muscles and practice balance and stabilization.

B, Keep the back straight while moving smoothly down and up. Use the abdominal muscles to keep the spine in a neutral position during the entire move. Relax the neck and shoulders and keep breathing evenly while alternating legs.

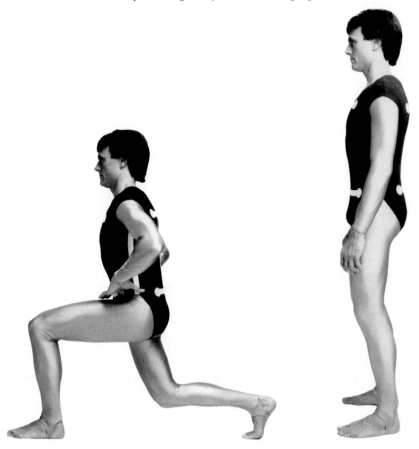

A, Stabilize the lower spine with the abdominal muscles; step toward and bend the knee to lower the trunk.

Fig. A-12

Backward lunges. Purpose: To strengthen the abdominal, leg, and buttocks muscles and practice balance and stabilization.

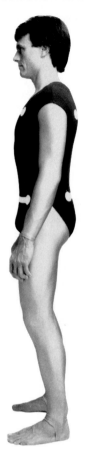

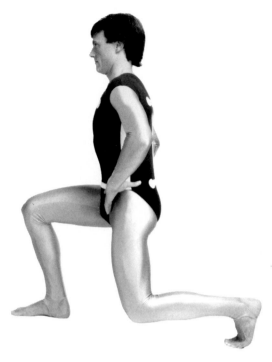

B, Step backward and lower the trunk. Stabilize the upright position with the abdominal muscles. Keep the motion smooth and controlled. The trunk should remain square and straight during the entire move.

A, Find the neutral postion.

Fig. A-13

Straight back bends. Purpose: To strengthen the lower back and abdominal muscles and practice correct bending.

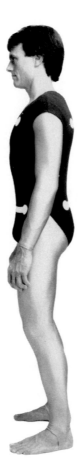

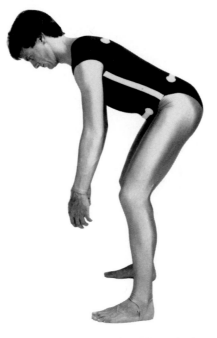

B, Keep the back straight and use the buttocks muscles while bending forward. All the motion should take place from the hip. Use the abdominal muscles to hold the spine while moving smoothly forward.

A, Tighten the abdominal muscles to stabilize the position.

Appendix B
Practical Guide to Billing
Bobbi Buell

Introduction

At this moment, getting paid for your services is the hardest part of being in health care. And yet, it is the most important factor in the economic survival of your practice. Even if major health-care reform is enacted in the very near future, reimbursement will remain the key practice management issue of the decade. How your practice deals with reimbursement will be instrumental to being viable as a single entity or as an acquisition candidate for a larger group practice or health maintenance organization (HMO). Thus, in this appendix, we offer some tips to remain or become profitable and to expedite collection of all revenues to which you are entitled. Before we start, there are three major caveats to being realistic about reimbursement for your services.

First of all, the days of charge-based reimbursement are almost over. What you charge has less, little, or nothing to do with what you will collect these days. It used to be that Medicare, Workers' Compensation, commercial, and other payers based payment on charges. Although some insurance companies base payment on charges, fees must be usual, reasonable, and customary (URC). This means that your charges must be within one standard deviation of those of your local peers. On the other hand, Medicare, Workers' Compensation, preferred provider organizations (PPOs), and some of the managed-care companies operate on fee schedules. This means that you will be paid based on coding. Three types of codes are used—ICD-9-CM coding for the patient diagnosis; CPT (Current Procedural Terminology) for the service delivered; and HCPCS (HCFA Common Procedural Coding System) for supplies and medicines used. The latter is used mostly by Medicare. Therefore, it doesn't matter what you charge, you'll get paid via a fee for a certain CPT or HCPCS code, if your diagnosis code is appropriate for the procedure performed. More about this later.

What all of this "alphabet soup" means is that someone in your practice should be coding accurately. This is what will pay off now, and in a post–health-care reform world for spine practices.

Second, the days of leaving everything to the practice manager or to your clerical staff are now behind you. In surgical specialties, a physician in the practice must get involved with coding and other aspects of reimbursement. In our experience, the bigger practice management disasters occur because physicians have delegated coding, denial response, and receivables managment without proper oversight. Although we know that there is an "opportunity cost" (i.e., not being in the operating room) to physicians who manage practice operations, there is a bigger cost to your practice if cash flow or revenue optimization veer out of control. Thus, a clinician must be involved with reimbursement management. Hopefully, the following sections will explain further why this is true.

Finally, it is important to take a holistic approach to reimbursement management. In too many practices, we perceive that practitioners are seeking a "magic bullet" that will banish all of their reimbursement woes. Unfortunately, the process is very laborious. Many different steps must occur before a service is paid correctly. Each one of these steps in a practice that performs complex and sometimes controversial services—like psychiatric services for spinal ailments or surgeries that require co-surgeons—must be executed perfectly. If they are not, there will be a definitive financial impact. The steps to creating better reimbursement in your practice are

- Pay attention to the information gathered at registration in your practice.
- Make sure that eligibility for benefits and authorization is obtained before performing any procedure.
- Document the services performed clearly and concisely.
- Code each case correctly and aggressively.
- Make sure your charges are optimal for your payer mix.
- Bill each claim efficiently and correctly.
- Pursue denials with determination.
- Stay up-to-date on all changes.

More detail about these important steps is outlined in the following sections.

Pay Attention to Information Gathered at Registration

Registration (sometimes called "Reception") is one of the most important areas in your practice. This is true for both marketing and reimbursement reasons. As consultants, we often notice that this area is neglected because the most inexperienced personnel are placed here. This is a major mistake for the following reasons.

- *Demographic data is vital to billing the patient.* Receptionists and other office workers have been told that it is important to be polite and to minimize waiting time in the reception area. In most cases, the receptionist concentrates on insurance information. However, patient demographics are often either erroneous or incomplete. This is a big problem because patient portions (copayments) are now and will be a good portion of the reimbursement amount. Thus, if you cannot find or contact the patient, you are going to see high dollar amounts in your receivables.

- *Registration time is collection time.* We encourage practices to collect as much money at the time of service as possible. Copayments should be collected from patients when the amount can be calculated correctly. Self-pay patients (those who do not have coverage) can pre-pay for surgical or nerve-block services. Patients may be also pay for services for which they have no coverage. For full-service spine practices, this might include psychiatric, chiropractic, and pain-management services. The receptionist is the primary screener for collection at the time of service. If this role is not fulfilled correctly, your receivables and bad debt percentage will be higher than desirable.

- *Reception screens insurance for practice participation.* One of the most problematic areas we see in practices is that Reception thinks that, if a patient is insured, the practice will take assignment of benefits. Thus, the patient starts treatment with a basic misconception. If your practice does not take assignment for Medicare or other insurance companies, the patient needs to know from the outset what the payment arrangements will be. Even more important, patients insured under managed-care programs need to be told if, for some reason, the practice does not contract with their program. Then, the patient will need to get a referral from the primary-care physician, or they may have to be treated by a participating physician, or will have to pay cash. This is a key step to better payment and to better patient relations.

- *Finally, Reception sets up your basic payment understanding with the patient.* If your Reception area misleads a patient as to what his or her obligation will be with the practice, this will be difficult, and sometimes costly, to repair. Also, conditions of payment and forms are signed in this area. If patients or your business office is misinformed here, it will impact reimbursement over the course of the patient's treatment and, possibly, for some period thereafter.

We recommend that you place persons in Reception who already have billing experience. Less-experienced employees should be made billing clerks under direct supervision of a more experienced biller. Further, we believe anyone in Reception should get feedback regarding billing problems generated by them.

Verify Benefits/Eligibility and Get Services Authorized Before Treatment

If your practice does not verify that coverage exists and is authorized for treatment rendered, then there is no reason to expect that payment will be forthcoming. Not obtaining verification of eligibility or authorization for treatment is one of the biggest mistakes a practice can make. This is due to the fact that insurance companies can subsequently deny an entire course of treatment without benefit of appeal. So, here are some tips to ensure your practice does not fall into a very expensive trap.

- *First find out how long the patient has had back problems.* Many spine surgeons are tertiary-case specialists, meaning that the patient has seen one or more specialists in the past. All insurance companies have policies regarding "preexisting" conditions. Where we have seen major losses is when the back problem predates the patient's policy. Be sure to verify that the patient's coverage predates the back problem.

- *Ascertain what the ceiling is on patients' coverage for a single problem.* Back problems often last for a number of years. This often entails multiple surgeries; multiple treatment modalities; and big dollar figures for the insurance company. Sometimes, policies have an annual or lifetime payment "cap" in them. Your practice needs to know the amount and current status of the cap.

- *Obtain authorization for every form of service your practice delivers.* Unauthorized surgery is almost always not paid. Every practice has some level of compliance in this area. However, we believe that every service you deliver (other than examinations in the office or consultations for new patients) should be preauthorized by the insurance company. This includes a long course of medical back treatment, physiatry, chiropractic, and pain management (nerve blocks, etc.). When your practice obtains authorization, the following items should be obtained with the authorization: the authorization number; the name of the person giving authorization; the telephone number of that person; the date and time of the authorization; and the authorizing entity, if different from the insurance company. We would also like to mention that authorization does not mean that you will automatically get paid. If the patient is not eligible for services rendered or the case is later considered not medically necessary, there may be no payment. The persons authorizing services and the insurance company are often two different entities.

We recommend that verification of eligibility, determination of benefits, and authorization be documented somewhere, either in your computer system or in the patient chart, for quick retrievability.

Document Services Delivered Carefully and Concisely

When we consult to hospital medical records departments, we are acutely aware that physicians hate charting in medical records. Until about 1989, we definitively agreed with physicians that, in terms of their practices, charting was an exercise in bureaucracy. However, because much reimbursement now hinges on coding, your documentation should be regarded with the same care as the procedures you perform. Here are some hints as to how you can get the greatest benefits from good documentation.

- *Make sure to dictate every relevant detail of the procedure in Operative Reports.* We also recommend that you name every procedure in the report heading. This way, whoever codes and/or reads the report will be able to code accurately what was done. Physicians should familiarize themselves with the CPT codes for laminectomies, arthrodesis, grafts, and hardware placement so that your reports give important clues as to the codes that should be used. Even if you code your own records, insurance companies often request them prior to paying the bill. And remember that the persons reading these reports for payments are not often clinically educated.
- *When procedures that have no listed CPT code or something unusual happens during the surgery, be sure to be even clearer with documentation.* In each of these cases, we believe that practices will get paid more if it is clearly stated how this procedure differs from the listed or normal procedures. Also, if cases take an inordinately long time in the operating room, total operating time should be listed in the operative report.
- *If examinations and/or consults are dictated, try to dictate them in CPT Evaluation and Management format.* The most important factors in CPT payment are level of history, physical, and medical decision making. Thus, if notes are dictated in this manner, the level of coding can be easily determined by your staff or an outside auditor. There is, however, some confusion as to the documentation requirements for medical decision making. Medical decision making is the number

of diagnoses involved in the care; the risk to the patient; and the amount of medical data that must be assimilated before treatment can take place. This should be dictated into your examination or consultation notes.

- *Be sure to state clearly the reason for which the patient is being seen and/or treated every time the patient encounters the practice.* We have found that diagnosis coding is very important to obtaining payment for spinal surgeries. If, for example, an anterior and posterior procedure is performed, instability should be coded. Also, if a patient develops a urinary-tract infection postoperatively and the surgeon works it up and/or treats it, it should be stated. If the case is coded this way, there will be additional revenues for the practice. Higher-level visits and consults can be billed if the patient has multiple problems. However, these problems must be clearly documented and coding using ICD-9-CM.
- *Finally, documentation is the best and only defense in a Medicare audit.* Medicare audits work on a sampling basis. If the auditor finds that notes are not in the chart for services performed and/or for all facets of a spinal procedure, the auditor will make an assumption as to how many times this occurred over the audit period, and this will be the amount owed to the Medicare Carrier. Thus, all services rendered should not only be documented by the physician, but filed logically in charts for quick reference.

The objective of this section has been to increase understanding that medical records should be handled with care in the practice and that every note and report must convey services rendered in detail.

IV. Code Each Record Correctly and Optimally

In spine practices, we found that it is very effective for a surgeon to get directly involved with the CPT and ICD-9-CM coding. However, this is a good idea only if the involved clinician is properly trained by professional coders and has the tools at his or her disposal to do an adequate job of coding. Do not make the assumption that coding logically reflects clinical practice. This is definitely not always the case.

CPT Coding

CPT coding is the basis of payment for most payers, except Medicaid and/or Workers' Compensation in certain areas. Thus, it is mandatory that someone in the practice is knowledgeable about all coding systems. The following sections outline how an experienced coder can enhance practice revenues.

- *For major procedures, never code without an operative report.* This rule should never be violated for spine surgeries that involve multiple codes. Examples include multilevel laminectomies, anterior and posterior repairs, re-do's, corpectomies, and arthrodesis. Coders should be taught to read through the entire report before assigning codes. This is true even if the operating surgeon codes the case. Busy surgeons may not remember all billable procedures done. This practice will pay off, even if very few cases are corrected in a calendar year.

- *Be aggressive in coding.* We certainly do not support fradulent coding or flagrant abuse of published carrier guidelines. We do, however, strongly recommend that every service that can possibly be paid is coded. If there is a doubt, code the service. Let the carrier decide to deny the service. For example, the surgeon has a re-do on a spinal patient. There may be a question as to whether to code the re-exploration of fusion when there is no definitive documentation. We suggest coding this because it can be assumed that the fusion was explored or else a reparative procedure would not have been performed.

- *Understand CPT modifiers as they apply to surgery.* One of the big problems that we see in spine practices is the lack of modifiers placed on surgeries. Also, we see poor utilization of modifiers. Here are some helpful hints about some modifiers:

- *Modifier -51 (Multiple Procedures)* should be used wisely. This is the modifier for multiple procedures. We used to tell practices that take insurance assignment not to use this modifier and let the carrier reduce the service. However, in the past year or so, we have seen claims rejected for lack of this modifier. Remember that this modifier is *not* necessary or preferable (except for Workers' Compensation in some areas) for procedures that are reduced by definition. Examples of this include laminectomies/fusions at additional levels, graft harvesting, and each level of a discogram.

- *Modifier -22 (Unusual Services)* can be used in cases in which something unusual happens. This normally pays about 20% more than the allowable. However, because of the payment factor, this modifier has been overutilized and some insurance companies (like Medicare) rarely pay on it. The way to get paid on this modifier is to document carefully what unusual event took place during the procedure; how long it took to perform services related to the unusual event; and how much postoperative care was involved with the unusual event, if any. Do not use this modifier if no code exists.

- *Modifier -24, -25, and -57 (Global Em Modifiers)* are used to bill services additional to the global surgery charge. Modifier -24 is used if an additional service takes place in the postoperative period. If an entirely nonrelated service is rendered during the recovery period, use this modifier and ICD-9-CM code to get paid for an additional evaluative service. Modifier -25 is used when a separately identifiable EM service is rendered during the preoperative period *or* on the day of service for a minor procedure. For example, a patient comes to your office for an evaluation of back pain. In the course of the visit, you find that the patient also has bursitis of the shoulder, and you give the patient a shot of cortisone in the shoulder. Modifier -25 would be used on the office visit or consult. Otherwise, this service may be denied. The -57 modifier is used if your initial surgical evaluation of the patient is done within 24 hours of surgery. So, if a patient traumatically fractures the spine and is brought in through the Emergency Department, and they are evaluated by you pre-operatively, use -57 for the preoperative consult or visit.

- *Modifiers -78, -79, -58 (Global Surgery Modifiers)* are used for surgeries performed in the global surgery period. These are attached to surgical codes. Modifier -78 is used for reparative procedures in the global period. This modifier is *only* used if the re-do is performed by the operating surgeon. Modifier -79 is used if another, nonrelated procedure is performed by the operating surgeon. Modifier -58 is used if a staged procedure or an extension of the first procedure is done in the global period. For example, a patient has a surgery for scoliosis. In the global period, Harrington rods are placed. The second procedure will include Modifier -58

- *Modifiers -76 and -77 (Repeat Procedures)* are used when the same procedure is performed. This is more likely to happen in spine surgeries than in most other types of procedures. Modifier -76 is used for the same procedure by the same physician. Modifier -77 is used for the same procedure done by a different physician. These modifiers should be used in conjunction with good ICD-9-CM coding for rejection prevention and for optimal payment outside the global period.

- *Modifiers -62 (Co-surgeon)* is used when two surgeons perform the same case. This modifier pays more frequently when two surgeons are of differing specialties. When two spinal surgeons are co-surgeons, particularly if they are in the same practice, it may be wise to bill one as an assistant and one as the primary rather than as co-surgeons. The reason for this is that, with co-surgery, two surgeons generally split 125% of the global fee. With an assistant plus primary, the practice receives 116-120%. However, the risk of denial is not as great. The practice should evaluate these options based on its payer mix and rejection rate.

These are just the most prevalent problems in coding modifiers for spine surgery. We strongly suggest that all practices read Appendix A in *CPT* to gain a full understanding of the applications of all modifiers.

- *Understand what is included in every CPT code. Insurance companies are increasingly reducing fees for "unbundling" of codes.* The best defense against "unbundling" is to understand what "(separate procedure)" means and what is included in the CPT code descriptions. (Separate procedure) in CPT notation means that the designated procedure can only be coded this way if it is not performed in conjunction with other procedures. To code this separately constitutes "unbundling" and this will not be paid by most insurance companies. This edit can be appealed if (separate procedure) are performed via a separate incision. You must enclose a report to explain this to the carrier. "Unbundling" can also occur when descriptions of CPT codes are not read thoughtfully as they are coded. For example, corpectomies always include the discectomies on the levels above and below the operative site. To bill these discectomies separately would be unbundling. Finally, Medicare has their own edits as to what procedures can be billed together. These are called "rebundling edits" and they are published by Medicare carriers once every year or so. For a copy of these, contact your carrier.

- *Understand completely the descriptions of Evaluation and Management services.* Since 1992, the description for visits and consults ("EM services") have changed drastically. Many offices for whom we consult have not yet updated their charge tickets and/or not modified their behavior to fulfill the criteria of the revised EM descriptors. For new patients of initial services, there are three major factors that contribute to higher level visits. These are the level of documentation of the history, physical, and medical decision making. For established patients, only two aspects of these criteria are necessary. Where most spine practices undercode is in the level of medical decision making involved in their patient care. Medical decision making is predicated on the number of diagnoses or options available to the patient; the amount of data the treating physician has to assimilate prior to treating the patient; and the risk of morbidity or mortality involved in the decision. For most spine patients, the complexity of decision making is rather high because of the number of treatment modalities available in spine care and because of the risk of significant morbidity. When making a choice of EM codes, be sure that the complexity of decision making is realistically documented and coded.

- *Remember that EM services can be "upcoded" for counseling patients and their families.* If more than 50% of an EM service is spent in counseling the patient and/or the family, the service can be coded solely according to time criteria. The only caveat is that the time spent on counseling, the reason for it, and the outcome must be documented in the medical record. Spine care practices often counsel patients on the impact of disability upon their lives; handling pain; and about various options available to them. However, in our consultations, we rarely see this incorporated into coding.

- *Do not code the same level of service for most or all office visits.* Medicare profiles physicians on their levels of EM service. If 99213 or 99214 are the only office visits billed, you will be audited. Apply criteria to each case's documented service and this problem can be avoided. If this seems overly time-consuming, bear in mind that, in our experience, Medicare audit has never cost a surgical practice less than $10,000.

There are many other "pearls of wisdom" we could have imparted to spine-care practices regarding CPT coding. However, we believe that the above problems are the most frequently encountered data quality and/or reimbursement issues. If there is a problem that we have not covered herein, please contact Documedics at (800)-795-CODE.

ICD-9-CM Coding

ICD-9-CM coding became a factor in physician payment in 1989. However, physician practices still believe that it is not worth the time and effort to become familiar with diagnosis coding. As reimbursement experts, we strongly disagree with this logic. ICD-9-CM coding can make a material difference in reimbursement from all insurance companies, with the possible exception of some Workers' Compensation carriers. Here are some ways in which ICD-9-CM coding can be utilized to increase payment.

- *Use the appropriate code for every encounter with your practice.* For example, if a patient comes in for "back pain," do not code degenerative disc disease unless this diagnosis is confirmed. On the other hand, when billing for complex surgeries, use the specific code for which the patient had surgery. Vague codes such as lumbar strain can cause rejections for surgeries.

- *Code to the highest level of known specificity—to the fourth or fifth digit if possible.* This conveys the most complete reason that the service delivered was medically necessary. Specificity of ICD-9-CM coding can prevent rejections and appeals and can support the claim without attachment of an operative report to every surgery claim. Poor ICD-9-CM coding will definitely elicit medical necessity denials and costly appeals.

- *Code only comorbid diagnoses that are applicable to the current treatment plan.* We believe that the inclusion of comorbids can increase the level of EM coding. However, use of unrelated diagnoses, like V10.0—history of cancer—may have the oppposite effect and can cause coverage problems. Try to be honest and ask if the diagnosis used impacts the treatment plan.

- *When billing higher-level EM services, always use more than one diagnosis code, if possible.* This is a shorthand way of telling the insurance company that complex decision making was used to treat a patient.

- *When using CPT modifiers, make sure that the ICD-9-CM diagnosis justifies the use of the modifier.* For example, let's say a patient developed hypotension during spine surgery. Thus, a modifier -22 was used to describe that the procedure took 2 hours longer owing to the measures performed to stablize the patient. In addition to the modifier -22, the ICD-9-CM for intraoperative hypotension should be used.

- *Do not use your fee ticket (superbill) for ICD-9-CM coding.* Having ICD-9-CM codes on the superbill tempts office staff to use only codes that appear there rather than correct codes. In spine practices, there are too many ways to lose money through ICD-9-CM coding for coding to be performed in this manner. Use an ICD-9-CM coding book or ICD-9-CM software for coding.

- *Be aware that ICD-9-CM coding will have more of an impact on your practice in a managed-care environment.* The way we currently interpret health-care reform bills indicates that ICD-9-CM coding will be the basis by which health alliances or other purchasers of your services will evaluate the quality and/or utilization in the practice. For example, if the code for lumbar spondylisthesis is given, the services associated with that diagnosis will be assessed against treatment protocols to ensure that quality and cost are within parameters established by the contracting entity. This is why it is smart to use ICD-9-CM wisely now.

These are but a few of the myriad of possible uses of ICD-9-CM coding in spine practices. To become more familiar with the ICD-9-CM coding, have a member of your staff contact the medical record director of your nearest hospital or clinic. They probably know where classes are being offered at the lowest cost.

Make Sure Your Charges Are Optimal for All Payors

We recently interviewed one of the major insurance companies. They will pay up to 90% of Usual, Reasonable, and Customary (UCR) charges. However, owing to the fee schedules of practices, they usually pay about 56% of UCR charges, on average. This means that 34% of charges are "left on the table" by practices that do not set their fees in a rational way. Here are some directions on how to do this.

- *Use a rational tool to set your fees.* Do not set fees based on rumors or actual fees from another practice. Use a rational fee schedule to set fees. In 1994, we recommend that you use the Resource Relative Value Scale (RBRVS). The reason that we recommend this is twofold. First, it is cheap. It is available through the Federal Government at about $5.00 per copy. Just ask for the *Federal Register* with the physician fee schedule. It is usually released in late November. The second reason is that we believe that RBRVS may be the standard for many managed-care payers in the future. The major warning for practices using RBRVS is to not price below Medicare or below community standards. Ascertain the Medicare conversion factor (1994 conversion factor is about $35.00 for surgical services and $33.25 for EM) from the *Federal Register* and set fees 40% to 60% above the fee schedule, depending on what the market will bear.

- *Monitor EOMBs to see what is being paid by insurance companies.* We constantly see practices getting paid at 100% of charges and not raising their fees. On the other hand, we also see practices having a collection rate of less than 40% on charges. This is usually due to either (1) too many claims rejections; or (2) charges that are set too high. The only way you can determine which is the problem is to monitor your EOMBs carefully. We strongly recommend that a physician examine at least a sample every month to be in touch with the payment patterns in the practice.
- *Do not discuss fees with other spine care practices in your area.* This is dangerous because the Federal Trade Commission considers collusion between providers to be price-fixing. Also, we strongly recommend not taking the advice of hardware or pharmaceutical vendors as to how fees should be set for certain procedures. It is in their best interest to maintain high charges for services involving their products. It is not necessarily in your best interest.

Bill Effectively and Correctly

It is wise to remember that, in the days before Medicare Physician Payment Reform, it was not necessary to pay attention to cash flow. This meant that bills could remain unpaid indefinitely. However, with more fee schedule–based payment and contracted rates, cash flow is increasingly important. Although our consulting practice is not focused on billing, we would like to share a few facts that we have assimilated in spine practices.

- *Pay attention to your days in receiveables.* If more than 10% to 20% of receiveables are over 90 days outstanding on average, there is a problem with billing and collections. Although we can not guess what the problem might be, it may be well to first examine how patient portions are collected and how aggressively they are pursued. Collections are important to the practice and, if these are not pursued or written off in a timely fashion, this will increase days in receiveables.
- *Bill electronically, if possible.* Because so many spine claims cannot be billed electronically owing to the necessity of report submission, it is mandatory that every possible claim be submitted electronically. Electronic submission can reduce receiveables by 10 to 14 days, depending on the insurance company. It is vital because of the complexity of spinal surgeries that every

claim that can be submitted electronically is submitted via modem or computer program.
- *Do not bill separate services on the same claim.* To avoid rejections and appeals, we recommend that separate services be billed on separate claims. For example, if an anterior and a posterior procedure are done the same day, but with different surgical teams and/or in different operating room scenarios, these procedures should be billed on different claims. The same holds true if two surgeons in the same practice perform cosurgery. And, if there is reason to believe that EM services might be rejected if billed in conjunction with a surgery, bill them separately.
- *Claims should be "clean" when billed.* By clean claims, we mean that the demographics, coding, and physician information is correct. The best way to submit clean claims a majority of the time is to (1) code records correctly, and (2) purchase computer software that edits claims for missing or illogical demographic data. If claims are not "clean" upon submission, it takes an additional 60 days, on average, to collect cash. This makes the computer software affordable, if costs and benefits are assessed correctly.
- *Do not trust billing services with your cash flow.* Unfortunately, we have seen billing services take advantage of their clients' lack of business acumen. Practices using billing services should demand reports outlining days in receiveables, collection rates on fees charged, and denial/rejection rates on claims processed. In addition, based on negative experience, we strongly recommend that coding should not be left in the hands of a billing service unless they can prove that their personnel are qualified to perform this task.

Pursue Denials with Determination

Insurance companies make money if a claim is rejected and the billing practice does not respond. We have walked into far too many practices where denials are left in a desk drawer with no response. An important fact to remember is that insurance companies may reject claims for totally unsubstantiated reasons. This is particularly true of Medicare carriers. To avoid losing unnecessary dollars, we suggest following these steps.

- *Determine the reason for denial.* We have seen denials in which the practice has responded to the medical necessity of the surgery when the actual problem was the lack of coverage for the patient. In this case, the patient is liable and the insurance company should not be involved. Read the EOMB carefully and determine whether any clues are available. If not, contact the insurance company and see if further information can be obtained. Sometimes, a claim can simply be rebilled without pursuing the arduous appeal process.

- *Do the appropriate research before responding to the denial.* If your practice is performing unusual or "state of the art" procedures, make sure that you submit the latest research from objective sources (medical journals, compendia, etc.) to substantiate your treatment. If claims are denied owing to carrier policy, call the insurance company to obtain written proof of the policy and, if necessary, dispute it, if patient care is involved.

- *Do not vent frustrations in the denial response letter.* Today, virtually everyone is frustrated with the health-care system, with the Congress, with RBRVS, and with the confusion in medical billing. However, when trying to recover denied payment, we suggest that these opinions should not be shared with the insurance company.

- *All denial letters should be signed by a physician in the practice.* The reason is that this can and usually does not put the claim into physician review. If the treatment rendered was truly reasonable and necessary, a physician is more likely to understand this than a clerk or a utilization review person. Also, we recommend that, for public-pay patients (Medicare and Medicaid), letters for second-level appeals involving payment issues be copied to your congressman and/or to your district office of the Healthcare Financing Administration (HCFA). We have found that, when the claim should be paid, these copies bring action.

- *If the claim is worth a high dollar amount, pursue denials until told not to do so.* For Medicare claims, if the claim is rejected at the second level of appeal or by a peer-review organization (PRO), it can go to an administrative law judge for a final opinion. For other insurance companies, appeals can be pursued through the clerk and, then, the medical director level. If this does not produce results, go to the patient or patient's employer and state that the insurance company did not pay a medically necessary claim. A persuasive employer argument for spine practices is that the patient's disability would have been extended without whatever service was rendered

Often, the employer will then pressure the insurance company into paying the claim. If all else fails, bringing an attorney into the process can help. However, we suggest a cost/benefit analysis before using attorneys.

Finally, we recommend keeping a file as to what strategies worked in terms of retrieving lost monies in the practice. This way, there is no need to "reinvent the wheel" the next time a claim is rejected.

Stay Up to Date

Reimbursement policies are changing almost daily. Coding changes annually. Billing procedures are slated to be revolutionized over the next 5 years. In our view, payment can easily be lost if services are billed using outdated forms, codes, or procedures. To keep current, here are some things that should be adopted by all spine-care practices.

- *Update your code books annually.* This means both ICD-9-CM and *CPT.* in addition to buying the updates, a physician should read the updates to *CPT* that are pertinent to your practice. This will ensure that documentation continues to support coding conventions. Make sure all physicians are equally updated in coding changes annually.

- *Read the Medicare Bulletin whenever it is released.* Someone in the practice should be assigned the task of reading this information and disseminating it to the rest of the practice as necessary. Yes, we know that they are boring. Read them before bedtime.

- *Send personnel to coding and reimbursement seminars.* If the practice is large enough, consultants will educate the practice on-site. If not, many organizations sponsor these seminars. It is important that someone in the practice obtains this information and distributes it to the appropriate parties.

- *Subscribe to publications that provide maximum information about coding and/or payment.* As consultants, we read 8 to 10 publications per month. There are many publications that arrive in your mail daily. Some recommendations include:

St. Anthony's *Coding for Physician Reimbursement,* published by St. Anthony Publishing, Inc., (800)-632-0123.

Part B News, published by United Communications, Inc., (301)-816-8950.

Documedics' *DataExpress,* published by Documedics, (800)-795-2633, (this is not an unbiased opinion).

Summary

We believe that, in light of the existing regulatory environment, payment will not improve over the next several years. Thus, we strongly recommend that, if there is reason to believe that reimbursement controls are not intact in your practice, a manager or consultant be hired to ensure that revenues are flowing smoothly. This will be an expenditure that will pay for itself over and over again in the years to come.

Index

Index

A

AANS (American Association of Neurological Surgeons), 993
AAOS; *see* American Academy of Orthopaedic Surgeons
Aarskog syndrome, 1565
AATB (American Association of Tissue Banks), 892, 893
Abacus Concepts, 130
Abbott, Jim, 504
Abdominal bracing, illustrated, 1740
ABDP (aminohydroxybutylidene bisphosphonate), 1727, 1729
ABG (autologous bone graft), 883
Ablative procedures
  cancer pain treatment with, 589
  defined, 585
  FBSS treatment with, 585, 587–588
  summarized, 585
Accessory process, 814
ACDF (anterior cervical discectomy with fusion), 1372–1373, 1390
Acetaminophen (APAP)
  adult scoliosis treated with, 1616
  as peripherally acting analgesic, 512
  use of for acute pain, 511
ACL (anterior cruciate ligament), 1293
Acquired immune deficiency syndrome; *see* AIDS
Active range of motion (AROM), 532
Activities of daily living (ADLs), 531, 532, 533
  rehabilitation from spinal-cord injury and, 1537–1538
Acupuncture, 565
Acute anulus tear, low-back pain and, 42–43
Acute conservative care, 370–373
  guidelines for, 369–370
Acute pain, 114
  chronic versus, 510–511
ADA; *see* Americans with Disabilities Act
Adamkawitz, artery of, 1468
Adenosine triphosphate (ATP), 380–381
Adhesions, postoperative, graft materials to prevent, 899–907
ADLs; *see* Activities of daily living
Administrative component of multidisciplinary team, 266
Adolescent idiopathic scoliosis, 1578
Adult scoliosis, 1612–1631
  in the aged, 1627–1628
  degenerative, 1629
    illustrated, 1618
  history of, 1613–1614
  illustrated, 1618, 1619, 1620
  nonoperative care and, 1616
  patient evaluation and selection and, 1614–1616
  problems specific to, 1626–1629
  surgical treatment of
    complications of, 1624
    indications for, 1592, 1616–1617
    planning for, 1617–1618

Adult scoliosis,—cont'd
  surgical treatment of,—cont'd
    risks of, 1617
    techniques in, 1618–1626
Adult structure, development of, 793
Adverse neural tissue tension (ANTT), 458–460, 466, 468
Aerobic capacity testing, 490
Aerobic conditioning, work hardening in, 490–491
Aerobic exercise, 405
  prevention of bone loss with, 856
Agency for Health Policy Reform, guidelines for acute conservative
    care developed by, 369–370
Aging
  chemonucleolysis and, 996
  congenital kyphosis and, 1573
  "degenerative spiral" and, 89
    illustrated, 90
  disc degeneration and, 87, 89, 90, 143–144
  osteoporosis and, 848
  scoliosis and, 1627–1628
  spinal coordination and, illustrated, 128, 130
  spinal-cord injuries and, 1530, 1540
AHDP (aminohexane disphosphonate)
  treatment of Paget's disease with, 1727, 1729
AHPrBP (pamidronate 3-amino-1 hydroxypropylidene-1, 1 bisphos-
    phonate)(APD), treatment of Paget's disease with, 1727,
    1728–1729
AIDS
  blood loss during spine surgery and, 951
  transmission of during bone transplants, 1102
  see also HIV infection
Ainsworth, Mary, 559
Alar ligament, 821, 1319, 1320
  illustrated, 1319
Albee, Fred, 779, 781, 1056, 1101, 1158, 1234
Albright, Tenley, 650
Alcohol overuse
  low-back pain and, 58
  osteoporosis and, 856
  spinal surgery and, 924, 974–975
  tissue donation excluded by, 893
ALIF; *see* Anterior lumbar interbody fusion
Alkaline phosphatase, 286–287
Allen-Ferguson classification of cervical spine injuries, 1487–1489,
    1498
Allodynia, 23
Allograft(s), 881–884
  antigen-extracted (AAA), 883–884
  bone banking and; *see* Bone banking
  defined, 881
  femoral cortical-cancellous composite, 1130–1133
    illustrated, 1132

Allograft(s),—cont'd
    freeze drying in, 882, 895
    freezing in, 882, 895–896
    treatment of with radiation, heat, or chemicals, 882–883,
        894–895
    see also Bone graft(s)
ALM (anterior laparoscopic microdiscectomy), "report card" on,
    1081
ALPS (anterior locking plate system), 1236, 1239–1240
Alternative care sub-specialties, 369
AMA; see American Medical Association
American Academy of Orthopaedic Surgeons (AAOS), 993
    instability defined by, 1513
    intraoperative fluoroscopy recommended by, 1189
American Academy of Pediatrics, 1446
American Association of Neurological Surgeons (AANS), 993
American Association of Tissue Banks (AATB), 892, 893
American College of Sports Medicine, 395
American Heart Association guidelines for Cardiopulmonary Resusci-
    tation (CPR), 1439
American Hockey Association, 684
American Journal of Public Health, The on undertreatment of pain,
    497
American Medical Association (AMA)
    Guidelines of, to the Evaluation of Permanent Impairment, 241,
        532
    normal ranges of motion of spine identified by, 257
American Medical Electronics, Inc., 1297, 1300, 1301
American Neurologic Association, 783
American Occupational Therapy Association (AOTA), 490
American Orthopedic Association, 779
American Psychiatric Association, use of DSM-III-R advocated by to
    express diagnoses, 542
American Spinal Injury Association (ASIA) Motor Index Score, 1512,
    1531
Americans with Disabilities Act (ADA), 257
    case study regarding, 479–484
    ergonomic intervention and, 473
    impact of on society, 492
    job analysis and, 474
Aminohexane disphosphonate (AHDP), treatment of Paget's disease
    with, 1727, 1729
Aminohydroxybutylidene bisphosphonate (ABDP), treatment of
    Paget's disease with, 1727, 1729
AMS plate, 862
Anabolic steroids
    osteoporosis management and, 860
    see also Steroid(s)
Analgesia
    patient-controlled; see Patient-controlled analgesia
    "selective spinal," 600
    stimulation-produced (SPA), 574
    see also Analgesics
Analgesic discography, 220
Analgesics, 512–523
    antidepressants as, 521–523
    antihistamines as, 523
    caffeine added to, 523
    centrally acting, 516–518
    dosing intervals and, 511
    muscle relaxants as, 519–520
    peripherally acting, 512–516, 1616
    sedative-hypnotics as, 518–519
    treatment of sprains with, 1442
Anatomic procedures
    cancer pain treatment with, 588
    defined, 585
    FBSS treatment with, 585, 586
    summarized, 585

Andrews frame, 960–962, 1032, 1036
    illustrated, 960, 961, 962, 1033
Anesthesia
    airway management and, 942–944
    autonomic dysreflexia and, 946–947
    in cervical spine surgery, 939–949
    discography plus, 97
    in endoscopic thoracic spine surgery, 1012–1013
    epidural, headaches and, 335
    hypothermia and, 946
    induction of, 944–945
    intraoperative management and, 942–948, 972–973
    local, microsurgery and, 1040
    maintenance of, 944–945
    monitoring and, 947–948
    positioning of patient and, 947, 952
    postoperative considerations and, 948
    preoperative evaluation of patient and, 940–942
    spinal shock and, 945–946
    temperature maintenance and, 946
    use of succinycholine and, 945
Anesthesiologist(s)
    multidisciplinary program and, 266, 267
    preoperative evaluation of patient by, 940–942
    see also Anesthesia
Aneurysmal bone cysts, 1459
Anger, chronic low-back pain and, 544
Angle of minimum kyphosis, 532
Ankylosing spondylitis
    atlantoaxial disability and, 1655–1659
    atlantoaxial instability and, 1653–1655
    kyphotic deformities in, 1667–1718
        muscle disease as cause of, 1713–1718
        see also Kyphotic deformity(ies)
    Smith-Peterson procedure for, 1628
    spondylodiscitis and, 1659–1667, 1667
    torticollis and, 1645
Anulus fibrosus, 143, 799, 800–801, 839–840, 1324
    illustrated, 1324–1325
Anspach Company, 1037
Anspach drill, 1037
Anterior arch, 814
Anterior atlantooccipital membrane, 821
Anterior cervical discectomy with fusion (ACDF), 1372–1373, 1390
Anterior cervical fusion, 1402–1403, 1414–1418
    anterior plate fixation technique in, 1418
    Bailey-Badgley, illustrated, 1417
    Cloward, illustrated, 1417
    Robinson technique in; see Robinson fusion technique
    Smith-Robinson, illustrated, 1417, 1423
    vertebral body reconstruction technique in, 1416, 1418
        illustrated, 1419–1422
Anterior cervical plate fixation, 1429–1433
    complications of, 1432–1433
    indications for, 1429
    surgical approach to, 1430–1432
Anterior cruciate ligament (ACL), 1293
Anterior discectomy, 1234
    illustrated, 1423
Anterior horn cell, illustrated, 243
Anterior interbody fusion
    choice of exposure for, 1113–1114
    contraindications for, 1114
    with fibular graft for high-grade spondylolisthesis, 1292–1293
    history of, 780–781, 1127
    indications for, 1113, 1129, 1137–1139, 1234, 1291–1292,
        1573
    lumbar; see Anterior lumbar interbody fusion
    morbidity criteria for, 1140–1144

Anterior interbody fusion,—cont'd
    potential complications of, 1122–1125, 1127–1128
    results of, 1135–1156
        illustrated, 1146–1156
    surgical technique in, 1114–1121, 1129–1133, 1292–1293
    team approach to, 1114
Anterior laparoscopic microdiscectomy (ALM), "report card" on, 1081
Anterior locking plate system (ALPS), 1236, 1239–1240
Anterior lumbar interbody fusion (ALIF)
    advantages of, 1128
    biomechanics of, 1127
    combined anterior and posterior fusion versus, 1128–1129
    contraindications for, 1114
    disc excision in, 1118–1119
        illustrated, 1118, 1119
    exposure for
        anterior abdominal wall, 1114–1115
            illustrated, 1114–1115
        choice of, 1113
        retroperitoneal, 1115–1116
            illustrated, 1116, 1117
        vertebral disc, 1116, 1118
            illustrated, 1117, 1118
    history of, 1127
    indications for, 1113, 1291–1292
    instrumentation used with, 1233–1249
    morbidity criteria for, 1140–1144
    potential complications of, 1122–1125, 1127–1128, 1248
    results of, 1135–1156
        illustrated, 1146–1156
    risks specific to, 1122–1125, 1127–1128
    role of, 1128
    surgical technique in, 1114–1121, 1292–1293
    team approach to, 1114
    see also Anterior interbody fusion
Anterior plate fixation technique, 1418
Anterior reduction of bilateral jumped facets, 1502
Anterior scalene muscle, 1331
Anterior screw fixation, 1433–1435
Anterior vertebrectomy and fusion, 1373–1374
Anterior wedge compression fractures, 1498
Anterior-posterior stenosis, 1085
Anterolisthesis, 1267–1268
    illustrated, 1268, 1270
Anteroposterior fusion; see Simultaneous combined anterior and posterior fusion
Anteroposterior standing and stretch, illustrated, 1580
Antibiotics
    treatment of spinal infection with, 1550
    use of during discography, 234
Anticonvulsants for pain of spinal origin, 524
Antidepressants, 521–523
    commonly used
        biochemical activity of, 521
        relative side effects of, 522
    use of, 522
Antigen-extracted allogeneic bone, 896–897
Antigen-extracted allograft, 883–884
Antigenicity, use of chymopapain and, 995
Antihistamines, 523
Antiinflammatory medication; see Nonsteroidal antiinflammatory drugs (NSAIDs)
ANTT; see Adverse neural tissue tension
Anxiety
    clinical symptoms of, 924
    defined, 922
    DSM-III-R criterion for, 924
    patient with chronic spine pain and, 260–261, 544

Anxiety,—cont'd
    psychologic cascade and, 37
AO cervical plates, 1479
AO contoured plates, 1628
AO Fixateur Interne, 1518, 1521
AO Orozco plate, 1429, 1431–1432
    illustrated, 1431
AO screws, 1201, 1429
    illustrated, 1624
AOTA (American Occupational Therapy Association), 490
APAP; see Acetaminophen
APD (pamidronate 3-amino-1 hydroxypropylidene-1, 1 bisphosphonate)(AHPrBP), treatment of Paget's disease with, 1727, 1728–1729
APF; see Simultaneous combined anterior and posterior fusion
APLD; see Automated percutaneous lumbar discectomy
Aquatic stabilization exercises, 734–742
Arachnoiditis
    imaging of, 164, 167
    as risk of posterior spine surgery, 1108
Arch
    anterior, 814
    posterior, 814
    vertebral; see Vertebral arch
Archimedes, 731
Arm and leg lifts
    prone, illustrated, 1743
    quadruped, illustrated, 1744
Arm raises, quadruped, illustrated, 1743
Armstrong plate, 862, 1236
Arnold-Chiari deformity, 1570
AROM (active range of motion), 532
Arterial supply to vertebrae, 11
Artery(ies)
    of Adamkawitz, 1468
    intersegmental, 796
    vertebral supply from, 11
Arthritis
    of the hips or knees, lumbar DDD pain and, 57
    as indication for cervical spine fusion, 1396
    Paget's disease and, 1726
    rheumatoid; see Rheumatoid arthritis
    spinal deformity and, 1652–1719
Arthritis Self-Management Program, 353
Arthrodesis
    illustrated, 1642, 1648
    indications for, 1396, 1641
    posterior, Gallie-type, 1654
    without instrumentation, results of, 1425
    see also Cervical fusion
Arthrogram
    sacroiliac, 301
    zygapophyseal, 303, 311
Arthroscopic discectomy, 1263–1264
    biportal, 1007–1009
    history of, 776–777
Arthroscopic foraminal decompression, 1011–1012
Arthroscopic interbody fusion of lumbar spine; see Arthroscopic lumbar interbody fusion
Arthroscopic lumbar interbody fusion, 1055–1066
    indications for use of, 1056–1057
    instruments used in, 1058–1059
    limitations of, 1057
    operative technique in, 1059–1064
    potential use of bone substitutes and bone morphogenetic protein for, 1064–1065
    potential use of titanium cage in, 1065
Arthroscopic microdiscectomy, 776–777, 1002–1016
    advantages of, 1003–1004

Arthroscopic microdisectomy,—cont'd
   biportal, 1007–1009
   instrumentation for, illustrated, 1005
   in lumbar spine, 1003–1010
   operative technique in, 1004–1009
   outcome analysis and, 1010
   postoperative management and, 1010
   preoperative planning for, 1004
   in thoracic spine, 1010–1012
Arthroscopic microsurgical discectomy
   biportal, 1081
   uniportal, 1080
Articular facet, 811
Articular pillar, 813
Articular processes, 811
   illustrated, 9
Articulating clamp, 1201, 1205, 1208–1209, 1214
   illustrated, 1202
ASA; see Aspirin
Asahi Kohgaku Company, 1070
ASIA (American Spinal Injury Association) Motor Index Score,
      1512, 1531
Aspirin (ASA)
   absorption of enhanced by caffeine, 523
   as peripherally acting analgesic, 512
   preoperative use of, 1253
Asthma
   risk of infection increased with, 968
   spinal surgery in patients with, 973
Atlantal ligament, 1318, 1320
Atlantoaxial disability, 1655–1659
Atlantoaxial instability, 1653–1655
Atlantoaxial joints, 1312, 1318–1320
Atlantoaxial ligament, 1318
Atlantoaxial membrane, 1318
Atlantooccipital disability, 1655–1659
Atlantooccipital joints, 813, 1312, 1316–1318
Atlantooccipital membrane, 821, 1318
   illustrated, 1319
Atlas, 813–814, 1312–1315
   illustrated, 813–814, 1312–1313, 1314
   prenatal development of, 1310–1311
      illustrated, 1310
"Atlas-dens interval," 1320
ATP (adenosine triphosphate), 380–381
Attachment
   clinical implications of, 561–562
   defined, 559
   neuropsychology of, 561
   research in, 560–561
   security of, 560, 561
   theory of, 558–563
Attorney, workers' compensation injuries and, 30–31
Augmentative procedures
   cancer pain treatment with, 588–589
   defined, 585
   FBSS treatment with, 585, 586–587
   summarized, 585
Autograft(s), 871–881
   advantages of, 871
   in arthroscopic spine fusion, 1064–1065
   complications of, 875–880
   defined, 871
   iliac crest
      anterior, 872–873
      posterior, 873–875
   sites for, 880–881
   see also Bone graft(s)
Autologous bone graft (ABG), 883

Automated percutaneous lumbar discectomy (APLD),
      1017–1027
   chemonucleolysis versus, 1021
   complications of, 1023
   contraindications to, 1019
   future predictions regarding, 1024–1025
   history of, 1018
   indications for use of, 1018–1019
   laminotomy versus, 1022
   manual percutaneous discectomy versus, 1021–1022
   open discectomy versus, 1022
   patient selection for, 1019–1021
   percutaneous laser discectomy versus, 1022
   "report card" on, 1080
   results of, 1023–1024
   technique of, 1022–1023
Autonomic dysreflexia, 946–947
   as complication of spinal-cord injury, 1534
Avitene, 906
Axial subluxation, 940–941
Axis, 813–814, 1315–1316
   illustrated, 813–814, 1314, 1315–1316
   pars interarticularis of, 1315–1316
   prenatal development of, 1310–1311
      illustrated, 1310

B
Back bends, illustrated, 1745
Back school, 352, 370, 395, 417
Backward lunges, illustrated, 1745
Bagby basket, 1225
Bailey-Badgley fusion, 784, 1636
   illustrated, 1417
BAK titanium cage, 1065
Ball bridging, illustrated, 405
Ballet; see Dance
Baltimore Therapeutic Equipment, Inc., 488, 490
Barr, Joseph, 775, 783, 785
Basbaum, Allan I., 502
Baseball, 608–626
   biomechanics of, 609
   hitters in
      clinical correlation of hitting and, 612–624
      electromyographic analysis of, 609–612
      with lumbar spine injuries, treatment of, 624
      pitchers in, electromyographic analysis of torque transfer in, 614
Basic elements of performance (BEPs), 530, 532, 533
Basic multicellular unit (BMU), 282, 284, 285, 286
   illustrated, 282
   osteoporosis and, 848
Basildon (Gardner) frame, 955
Basini, Ron, 234
Basketball, 627–634
   spine injuries in, 628–630
      criteria for return to play after, 633
      mechanisms of, 628
   spine stabilization in, 630–632
      exercise programs for, 632–633
Batson system, 1544
Baxter Laboratories, 993
Baxter V. Mueller, 1034
Beaver blade, 1037, 1039
Beaver Company, 1037
Beecher, Henry K., 501
Behavioral medicine, multidisciplinary, models for, 931, 937
Behcet's syndrome or disease, 1653
   low-back pain and, 49

Bend (bending)
  lateral, spinal coordination and, 128–129
  left versus right, spinal coordination and, 129
    illustrated, 130
"Bend test," 1579, 1582
  illustrated, 1579, 1583, 1584, 1605, 1606, 1607
Bent knee pull
  conduct of during physical examination, 77
Bentham, Jeremy, 497
BEP (basic elements of performance), 530, 532, 533
Bicycling, 635–640
  anatomy and pathophysiology of, 637–638
  back pain and, 636
  bicycle design and, 636–637
  conditioning and training in, 639–640
  proper fit of bike to rider and, 638–639
Bilateral decompression for spinal stenosis, 1040–1041
Billing
  authorization of services and, 1748–1749
  coding and, 1747, 1749–1752, 1754
  denials of payment and, 1753–1754
  documentation of services and, 1749
  guide to, 1746–1755
  information at registration and, 1747–1748
  keeping current and, 1754
  Medicaid and, 1749
  Medicare and, 1747, 1749, 1751, 1752, 1753
  usual, reasonable, and customary charges (URC) and, 1747,
    1752
  verification of benefits and, 1748–1749
  workers' compensation and, 240, 1747, 1749, 1752
Biochemical assessment, 290–291
Biochemical markers for bone metabolism, 286
Biodex, 489
Biofeedback, 262–263, 565, 566
Biopsy
  bone, 291–294
  see also Spinal tumor(s), biopsy of
Bio-Vascular, Inc., 906
Biportal arthroscopic microdiscectomy, 1007–1009
Biportal arthroscopic microsurgical discectomy, 1081
Bisphosphonates
  osteoporosis management and, 859
  treatment of Paget's disease with, 859, 1726, 1727–1729
Blade(s)
  Beaver, 1037, 1039
  Taylor, 1036
    illustrated, 1034
Blastemal vertebral column, 796
Blocked vertebra, illustrated, 1558
Blocks
  diagnostic; see Diagnostic blocks
  tricortical iliac, 1129–1130
Blood
  conservation techniques and, 970–972
  loss of during surgery, 951–952, 970–972, 1108, 1122
Blood count(s), 276–277
  white, 276
Blood vessels, use of chymopapain and, 994
BMD; see Bone mineral density
BMP; see Bone morphogenetic protein
BMU; see Basic multicellular unit
Body mechanics, proper, illustrated, 401
Boeing study, 240
Bohlman's technique of countersinking graft, 1636
  illustrated, 1637
Bohlman's triple-wire fixation, 1500
  illustrated, 1501
Bonding osteogenesis, 885

Bone(s)
  antigen-extracted allogeneic, 896–897
  biopsy of, 291–294
  cutting of, 1257–1258
  demineralized, 896–897
  grafting of; see Bone graft(s)
  heterologous, 884
  impaction of, 1092–1093, 1258–1260
    illustrated, 1092, 1093, 1259, 1260
    instruments for, illustrated, 1258
  implanting of; see Bone implant(s)
  Kiel, 884
  long, fracture of, as complication of spinal-cord injury,
    1536–1537
  metabolism of, bone markers for, 286–289
  microsurgical removal of, 1037
  processing of, for bone grafts, 882–883, 894–895
  tumors of; see Spinal tumor(s)
Bone banking, 891–898
  tissue recovery and, 893–894
Bone cyst, aneurysmal, 1459
Bone graft(s), 870–885
  allograft; see Allograft(s)
  in arthroscopic spine fusion, 1064–1065
  autograft; see Autograft(s)
  autologous (ABG), 883
  biomechanical properties of, 882
  bone banking and; see Bone banking
  "clothespin," 1158
  complications of, 875–880, 1376
  corticocancellous, illustrated, 1398, 1416
  Dewar onlay, illustrated, 1658
  donor selection and screening for, 893
  dowel; see Dowel graft(s)
  fat; see Fat graft(s)
  femoral ring, 1122
  fibular; see Fibular bone graft
  free-fat; see Free-fat graft(s)
  free-vascularized, 881
  H, modified, 1654
  heterograft, 884
  heterologous bones and, 884
  horseshoe-shaped, 1415
  iliac crest
    anterior, 872–873, 1479
    posterior, 873–875
  incidence of, 892
  in lumbar fusion, 1121–1122, 1130–1133, 1236
  pelvic instability and, 879–880
  placement of, 1120–1121
  processing of bone for, 882–883, 894–895
  Robinson-type, 1372
  sites for, 880–881
    preparation of, 1119–1120
  in treatment of degenerative spondylolisthesis,
    1276–1277
  tricortical, 1415
  without additional instrumentation, 1244
  xenograft; see Xenograft(s)
Bone implant(s), 884–886
  in arthroscopic spine fusion, 1064–1065
  methylmethacrylate cement and, 886–887
  nonmetallic, 885–886
  synthetic, 884–886
  titanium mesh, 884–885
Bone marker(s)
  of bone formation, 286–288
  for bone metabolism, 286–289
  of bone resorption, 288–289

Bone mass reduction, 849–850
  prevention of, 856–862
  spine fractures and, 855
Bone mineral density (BMD)
  fluoride therapy and, 861
  menopause and, 849, 855
  spine fracture and, 855
Bone modeling, 284–285
  defined, 284
  Paget's disease and, illustrated, 1726
  pathophysiology of, 285–286
Bone morphogenetic protein (BMP), 883–884
  rapid bone formation and, 896
  use of in arthroscopic spine fusion, 1064–1065
Bone remodeling
  Paget's disease and; see Paget's disease
  pathophysiology of, 285–286
Bone resorption, bone markers for, 288–289
Bone scan(s), 277–279, 289–290
  illustrated, 277, 278
  spinal infection and, 1546
  see also Radiography
Bone screw fixation systems; see Screw system(s)
Bone screws; see Screw(s)
Bone tumors; see Spinal tumor(s)
Bonica, John J., 500
Boots Pharmaceuticals, 993
Boston brace, 1285, 1287
Bowel dysfunction, as complication of spinal-cord injury,
  1533–1534
Boyd, Janet, 505–506
BPTT (brachial plexus tension test), 459
Brace(s)
  Boston, 1285, 1287
  Hudson, 1120
  Milwaukee; see Milwaukee brace
  Minerva, 1388
"Brachial plexopathy," 1449
Brachial plexus neuropraxia, 1449–1450
Brachial plexus tension test (BPTT), 459
Branched primary afferent, 91–92
Breast cancer
  metastatic lesions of, 278
  osteoporosis and, 858
Bridging, 1742
  ball, illustrated, 405
  with leg extension, illustrated, 404, 1742
Brooks fusion technique, 1399, 1645
  illustrated, 1400, 1401, 1647
  modified, 1399–1401
Brown fat, 901
Browne-Sequard syndrome, 1531
Browning, Kurt, 650
Brown-Sequard syndrome, 863
Brucella aspergillus, 1549
11-BS (11-Point Box Scale), 365
BTE
  function of, 488, 490
  illustrated, 479
Buckling, 439–440
  illustrated, 440
Buoyancy, swimming and, 731–733
Burman, Michael, 1068
Burners, 1446, 1449–1450
"Burning hands syndrome," 1447
Burst fracture(s), 1498
  C1, 1493
  illustrated, 1412, 1521–1522, 1524–1525
  treatment of, 1247–1248, 1521–1525

Burton, C. V., 1231
Butterfly hemivertebra, illustrated, 1558

C
C1 burst fractures, 1493
Cable systems
  Dwyer; see Dwyer cable system
  kyphosis and, 1234
Caffeine, enhancement of analgesics with, 523
CAGE questionnaire, 58
  preoperative substance abuse screening with, 975
Calcification, rate of, 293
  illustrated, 292
Calcitonin
  deficiency in, osteoporosis and, 850
  hormonal and biochemical assessment and, 290–291
  osteoporosis management and, 859
  treatment of Paget's disease with, 1726, 1727, 1729
  treatment of spinal stenosis with, 1730
Calcitonin gene-related peptide (CGRP), 221
Calcium
  deficiency in
    bone formation and, 294
    osteoporosis and, 848, 849, 856
  osteoporosis management and, 860
Calisthenics, 701
Callahan fusion technique, 1408–1409
  illustrated, 1410–1411
Camerius, Joachim, 747
cAMP (cyclic adenosine monophosphate), 291
Camper's fascia, 904
Canal compromise, fractures of vertebral body and, 1498–1499
Canal stenosis, 158, 1447–1449
  assessment of, illustrated, 1448
  illustrated, 155
Cancer
  breast; see Breast cancer
  as cause of primary low-back pain, 49, 57–58
  lymphoma, illustrated, 1461, 1463
  pain from, neurosurgical treatment for, 586, 588–589
  see also Metastatic disease
Cardiac abnormalities, congenital scoliosis and, 1564–1565
Cardiac complications, spinal-cord injury and, 1534
Cardiac disease, spinal surgery in patients with, 973
Cardiopulmonary Resuscitation (CPR), 1439
Cardiovascular system
  exercise and, 382–383, 386
  idiopathic scoliosis and, 1583
Carl Zeiss, Inc., 1032
C-arm fluoroscopy
  discography and, 226, 231
  during surgery, 952, 1063
    positioning of patient and, 1004–1005
Cartilage, "fetal," 799–800
Cartilage plates, 799, 800
Cascade
  debilitation; see Deconditioning cascade
  deconditioning; see Deconditioning cascade
  defined, 3
  "motion," 729, 730
  psychologic; see Psychologic cascade
  socioeconomic; see Socioeconomic cascade
  structural degenerative; see Structural degenerative cascade
Caspar distractor(s), 1416
  screw-post, 1373
Caspar retractor, 1416
Caspar trapezoidal plate system, 1429, 1431–1432

Catheter(s)
  Fogarty, 878
  Foley, 969, 1512
Cauda equina,1031, 93, 778, 830
  mechanical compression of, 98–99
Caudal epidural steroids, 323
  preparations for injections of, 324
  techniques for use of, 328–330
Caudal regression, 1565
C1-C2 dislocation, 1493
C2-C3 intraarticular blocks, 307
C1-C2 posterior cervical fusion, 1399–1402
  Brooks technique in, 1399, 1645
    illustrated, 1400, 1401, 1647
C1-C2 posterior cervical fusion—cont'd
    modified, 1399–1401
  Gallie technique in, 1399, 1401–1402, 1502, 1645–1647
    illustrated, 1402, 1646
  with Halifax clamp-type device, 1645, 1647
    illustrated, 1648
  with transarticular fixation, 1645
    illustrated, 1647
C1-C3 posterior cervical fusion, 1402
  illustrated, 1403
CCN, solution to socioeconomic cascade and, 31
CD instrumentation system, 862, 1164, 1236, 1244, 1520, 1593
CeDaR Surgical, Inc., 956
CeDaR Surgical Platform, 956–960
Cell(s)
  horn, illustrated, 243
  osteoblastic, 284
  Schwann, 94
Centers for Disease Control and Prevention (CDC) guidelines
    monitoring and preventing wound infections, 967, 968
Central canal stenosis, 158
  illustrated, 155
Central cord lesion, 1531–1532
Central stenosis, 1085
  decompressions for, 1088–1090
Centrally acting analgesics, 516–518
Cephalocaudal stenosis, 1085
Cerebral palsy, paralytic scoliosis associated with, illustrated, 1596, 1597
Cerebrospinal fluid (CSF) leaks, 336, 1041–1042, 1375
Cervical anomalies, illustrated, 1561
Cervical cord, 142
  neuropraxia of, with transient quadriplegia, 1446–1449
Cervical deformity(ies), 1632–1650
  classification of, 1633
  evaluation of, 1633
  imaging of, 1632–1634
  kyphotic, 1689–1713
  neuromyopathic flexion, 1643
Cervical degenerative joint disease (DJD) in dancers, 647
Cervical disc disease
  anatomy of, 1352
  cervical spondylitic myelopathy as; see Cervical spondylitic myelopathy
  cervical spondylitic radiculopathy as; see Cervical spondylitic radiculopathy
  diagnosis of, 1352–1354
  as indication for cervical spine fusion, 1396
  nonoperative treatment of, 1354
  nonradicular nonmyelopathic neck pain as, 1354
  operative treatment of; see Cervical disc surgery; Cervical spondylotic surgery
  see also Cervical spondylosis
Cervical disc injury(ies), 1442–1446
  biomechanics and kinematics of, 1442–1445

Cervical disc injury(ies),—cont'd
  epidemiology of, 1442–1443
Cervical disc puncture, 231
  illustrated, 232
Cervical disc surgery, 1354–1357
  anterior approaches to, 1356–1357, 1372–1377
  complications associated with, 1362
  laminotomy/discectomy as; see Laminotomy/discectomy
  posterior approaches to, 1358–1367
  for spondylosis; see Cervical spondylotic surgery
Cervical discectomy
  anterior, fusion with (ACDF), 1372–1373, 1390
  complications of, 1374–1376
  literature review regarding, 1376–1377
Cervical discography, 225–226, 231
  classification system of, illustrated, 1355
  diagnosing neck pain with, 1354
  illustrated, 232
  pain response in, 231, 233
Cervical epidural steroids, 324, 326
  techniques for use of, 331
Cervical facet injection, illustrated, 1353
Cervical fusion
  anterior; see Anterior cervical fusion
  complications of, 1418, 1424
  history of, 1395
  indications for, 1395–1396
  occipitoatlantal, 1397–1399
    illustrated, 1397, 1398, 1399
  posterior
    C1-C3, 1402
      illustrated, 1403
    C1-C2; see C1-C2 posterior cervical fusion
    Dewar, 1502
    interspinous; see Posterior cervical interspinous fusion
  techniques in
    in lower cervical spine, 1403–1404, 1406–1418
    in upper cervical spine, 1396–1403
Cervical kyphosis
  degenerative, 1638–1639
  illustrated, 1382
  postlaminectomy; see Postlaminectomy kyphosis
  secondary to tumor, 1639, 1641–1642
Cervical kyphotic deformity(ies), 1382, 1689–1713
Cervical laminaplasty, 1363–1365, 1385, 1387–1388
  complications in, 1365
  illustrated, 1365, 1388
  technique in, 1363–1365, 1387–1388
Cervical laminectomy, 1362–1363, 1385
  complications in, 1363
  illustrated, 1363, 1386
  sectioning of dentate ligaments following, illustrated, 1364
Cervical medial branch blocks, 307–309
  illustrated, 308, 309
Cervical osteotomy
  postoperative management and, 1705–1706
  results and complications of, 1706–1713
  selection of patients for, 1689–1698
  technique of, 1698–1705
Cervical pain, 16–17
Cervical spinal stenosis, 1446–1449
Cervical spine
  anatomy of, 142–143, 1381–1382
    clinical, 1306–1334
    developmental, 1307–1312
      congenital abnormalities and, 1311–1312
      early, 1307–1309
        illustrated, 1307–1309
      postnatal, 1311

Cervical spine,—cont'd
  anatomy of, 142–143, 1381–1382,—cont'd
    prenatal, 1309–1311
      illustrated, 1309, 1310
  anomalies in, illustrated, 1561
  anterior instrumentation of, 1428–1436
  anterior relationships of, 1333–1334
    illustrated, 1334
  case study of, 135
  coupled motion in, 133–135
    definitions used in study of, 135
  deformity of; see Cervical deformity(ies)
  development of, 793
  epidemiology and, 17–18
  fracture of; see Cervical spine fracture(s)
  function of, 810
  imaging of, 142–143, 146–147, 158–159
  injuries to; see Cervical spine injuries
  kyphotic deformities of, 1382, 1689–1713
  lower, 1320–1327
    illustrated, 1321
    injuries to, 1498
    intervertebral joints of, 1323–1327
  motion of, 18–19
  musculature of, 826–827, 1330–1333
    anterior, 1331–1332
      illustrated, 1331
    posterior, 1332–1333
      illustrated, 1333
  natural history and, 17
  neural relationships with, 1327–1330
  posterior exposure of, illustrated, 1338
  sagittal sections through, illustrated, 1329
  spinal manipulative therapy (SMT) and, 446
  sports injuries of, 1437–1454
  structural degenerative cascade and, 16–23
    discogenic phase of, 19–20
    stabilization phase of, 20–22
    summarized, 22
  surgical treatment of; see Cervical spine surgery
  upper
    injuries to, 1490–1498
    posterior exposure of, illustrated, 1339
    relationship of, illustrated, 1339
  vertebrae of; see Cervical vertebra(ae)
Cervical spine fracture(s), 1442–1446, 1486–1509
  Allen-Ferguson classification of, 1487–1489, 1498
  epidemiology of, 1442–1443
  kinematics of, 1443–1445
  mechanics of, 1443–1445, 1487–1490
  stabilization techniques for, outline of, 1503–1504
  treatment for
    outline of options in, 1490, 1491–1492
    selected cases of, 1505–1507
    surgical, 1500–1502
  types of, 1491–1492
Cervical spine injuries
  lower, 1498
  upper, 1490–1498
  see also Cervical spine fracture(s)
Cervical spine surgery
  anesthesia in, 939–949
  anterior instrumentation of, 1428–1436
  approach(es) to, 1335–1350
    anterior, 1339–1349
      anteromedial (Smith-Peterson), 1339–1340
        illustrated, 1340
      to C1-C3, 1341
      to cervicothoracic junction, 1347–1349
        illustrated, 1349

Cervical spine surgery,—cont'd
  approach(es) to, 1335–1350,—cont'd
    retropharyngeal, 1344–1345
      illustrated, 1344, 1345, 1346
    anterolateral retropharyngeal (Whitesides-Henry), 1345–1347
      hockey-stick-shaped incision for, illustrated, 1347
      illustrated, 1347
      to os odontoideum, illustrated, 1348
    posterior, 1336–1339
      anatomy for, illustrated, 1337
      to C3-C7, 1336–1338
        illustrated, 1336
      exposure of, illustrated, 1338
      to occiput and C1-C2, 1338–1339
        illustrated, 1338, 1339
    transoral, 1341–1344
      anatomic relationships of, illustrated, 1341
      case report of, 1342–1344
      for resection of odontoid, illustrated, 1342–1343
      to upper cervical spine, illustrated, 1341
  of cervical disc; see Cervical disc surgery; Cervical spondylotic surgery
  fusion as; see Cervical fusion
  history of, 782–785
  for kyphotic deformities of the cervical spine, 1689–1713
  laminaplasty as; see Cervical laminaplasty
  laminectomy as; see Cervical laminectomy
  open, 1305–1454
  osteotomy as; see Cervical osteotomy
  Smith-Robinson approach to, 1372
  treatment of cervical deformity and, 1644–1645
  treatment of spinal tumors and, 1479–1481
  see also Spine surgery
Cervical spondylosis, 20, 1352, 1359
  diagnostic evaluation of, 1369–1370
  history of, 1380
  illustrated, 1371, 1381
  pathology of, 1369
  preoperative planning and, 1370–1372
  surgical treatment of; see Cervical spondylotic surgery
  see also Cervical spondylotic myelopathy; Cervical spondylotic radiculopathy
Cervical spondylotic myelopathy (CSM), 1354
  natural history of, 1380–1381
  surgical treatment for
    indications for, 1383
    results of, 1390–1392
    techniques in, 1383–1388
    see also Cervical spondylotic surgery
Cervical spondylotic radiculopathy (CSR), 1354
  natural history of, 1380
  surgical treatment for
    indications for, 1383
    results of, 1389–1390
    techniques in, 1384–1388
    see also Cervical spondylotic surgery
Cervical spondylotic surgery, 1372–1377
  complications of, 1374–1376
  literature review regarding, 1376–1377
  posterior approach to, 1379–1393
  results of, 1389–1392
  see also Cervical spondylotic myelopathy
Cervical sprains, 1442
Cervical vertebra(ae), 812–814, 1320–1323
  anterior approach to, illustrated, 1415
  degenerated, 1330
    illustrated, 1330
  fifth, illustrated, 1321
  illustrated, 812
  lower five, illustrated, 1321

Cervical zygapophyseal joint block(s), 300
Cervicothoracic junction, surgical approach to, 1347–1349
Cervicothoracic stabilization training (CTST), 414, 416–420
   exercise program of, 420–435
C-*fos* protooncogene, 98–99
CGRP (calcitonin gene-related peptide), 221
Chance fracture, 1518
   illustrated, 1519–1520
Chatteck Corporation, 489
Chemical(s)
   involved in pain transduction, 24–25
      summarized, 25
   treatment of allografts and xenografts with, 883
   see also Drugs; Medication
Chemonucleolysis, 991–1001, 1076–1077
   automated percutaneous lumbar discectomy versus, 1021
   complications of, 997
   contraindications to, 995, 996
   future predictions regarding, 1000
   history of, 992
   operative technique in, 997–1000
   patient selection for, 995–996
   "report card" on, 1080
   see also Chymopapain
Chest stretch, illustrated, 399
Chest x-ray
   preoperative, 965
   see also Radiography
Chest-wall deformities, congenital scoliosis and, 1565, 1570
Childhood, psychological risk factors of, 59
Chiropractor(s)
   appropriate practice parameters and, 438
   as part of multidisciplinary program, 268
Chisel, Cloward, 1276
Chloro-4-phenylthiomethylene bisphosphonate, treatment of Paget's
      disease with, 1727, 1729
Chondrosarcomas, 1459–1460
CHOP frame, 958, 959
Chopin block, 1167
   illustrated, 1168
Chopin plate, 1168
Chordoma, 1459
Chronic obstructive pulmonary disease (COPD)
   risk of infection increased with, 968
   spinal surgery in patients with, 973
Chronic pain
   acute versus, 510–511
   attachment theory and, 558–563
   cognitive-behavioral treatment for; *see* Cognitive-behavioral treatment
   diathesis-stress model of, 540
   gate control model of, 549
   neurosurgical approaches to, 584–590
   of nonmalignant origin (CNMP), 516
   operant behavioral model of, 548–549
   programs for treatment of, 936–937
   psychogenic model of, 547–552
   psychological conceptualizations of, 547
Chymodiactin; *see* Chymopapain
ChymoFAST test, 1000
Chymopapain
   biochemistry and toxicology of, 993–995
   clinical trials of, 995, 1076–1077
   complications in use of, 997
   contraindications to, 996
   FDA approval and, 992–993, 997, 1076, 1077
   history of clinical use of, 992
   indications for use of, 995–996
   pharmaceutical and regulatory history of, 992–993
   "report card" on, 1080
   treatment of intervertebral discs with; *see* Chemonucleolysis

Ciccone, Donald S., 504
Cigarette smoking; *see* Smoking
Circumferential lumbar fusion; *see* Simultaneous combined anterior
      and posterior fusion
Clamp(s)
   articulating, 1201, 1205, 1208–1209, 1214
      illustrated, 1202
   Halifax, 1645, 1647
      illustrated, 1648
   Kocher, 874, 1118
   saddle, in Wiltse system, 1184–1185
      illustrated, 1186
Clay-shoveler's fractures, 1445, 1451
Cline, Henry, 774, 785
Clodronate (dichloromethylene disphosphonate), treatment of Paget's
      disease with, 1727, 1728
Clostridium difficile, 974
"Clothespin" graft, 1158
Cloward, Ralph, 225, 780, 781, 784, 895, 1056, 1101, 1102, 1165
Cloward chisel, 1276, 1288
Cloward frame, 955
Cloward fusion, 1376, 1636, 1644
   illustrated, 1417
Cloward laminar spreader, 1227, 1372
   illustrated, 1228
Cloward retractor, 1034, 1037, 1228
   illustrated, 1034
CMAP (compound muscle action potential), 193
CNMP (chronic pain of nonmalignant origin), 516
Cobb angle, 1580, 1587, 1594
   technique of measurement of, illustrated, 1580
Cobb dissector, 1253
Cobb elevator, 1013, 1235, 1253, 1275
Cobb measurement, 1565, 1573, 1574, 1590
Coccyx, 810, 815
   illustrated, 815
Codman & Shurtleff, 1034
Cognitive-behavioral treatment, 546–557
   education and, 553
   essential components of, 553
   evaluation and, 552–553
   future directions of, 555
   model of, 549–550
   research support for, 550–552
"Cold" lesions, 277
Collagen, 886
Collapsing scoliosis; *see* Adult scoliosis, degenerative
Combined stenosis, 1085
Compensatory curve(s), 1580–1581
   illustrated, 1597
Compere pins, 1644, 1645
   illustrated, 1680, 1696
Compere wires, 1656, 1658, 1694
Complete neurologic injury, 1513
Compound muscle action potential (CMAP), 193
Compression fracture(s), 1514, 1515, 1518
   anterior wedge, 1498
Compression injury, 122
   illustrated, 122
Compressive extension injury, 1487
   illustrated, 1489
Compressive flexion injury, 1487
   illustrated, 1488
Computed tomography (CT), 141
   of anterior interbody fusion
      illustrated, 161
   of arachnoiditis, 164, 167
      illustrated, 167, 168
   arthroscopic microdiscectomy preoperative planning
      and, 1004

Computed tomography (CT),—cont'd
of central canal stenosis, 158
illustrated, 155
of cervical spine, 146–147
deformities of assessed with, 1632–1650, 1633–1634
congenital scoliosis evaluated with, 1565
degenerative spondylolisthesis and spinal stenosis evaluated with, 1279
illustrated, 1280
of developmental lumbar stenosis, 153, 155
illustrated, 154
of disc degeneration, 144–147
of disc extrusion, illustrated, 146
of disc herniation, 145, 147, 164
of disc protrusion, 145
illustrated, 144
of disc sequestration, 145–146
illustrated, 145
of discitis, 168–169
discography versus, 221, 234
of dural tear, 171
of epidural abscess, 178
of epidural fibrosis, 161–162, 164
illustrated, 162
foraminal stenosis best demonstrated with, 1271
idiopathic scoliosis evaluated with, 1583, 1585
leg pain evaluated with, 273
of lumbar spine, 144–146
lumbar stenosis evaluated with, 152–153
with multiplaner reformations (CT/MPR), 141
of neural foraminal stenosis, illustrated, 157, 159
osteomyelitis diagnosed with, 1546–1547
of posterior element fracture, illustrated, 181
of postoperative spine, 160–162, 164, 167–169, 171
of postoperative stenosis, 164
preoperative evaluation with, 1032, 1139
preoperative preparation and, 1032
of pseudomeningocele, 171
pyogenic infection detected with, 176
quantitative (QCT); see Quantitative computed tomography
radiologists and, 268
of solid posterolateral fusion mass, 160–161
illustrated, 160
of spinal fusion, 167–168
illustrated, 169
of spinal infection, 175–179
spinal stenosis diagnosed with, 1085
spinal tumor surgery and, 1458
spinal-cord injuries determined with, 1532
of spine tumors, 171–172, 175
spondylolysis detected with, 159–160
of thoracic spine, 146–147
through TFC, illustrated, 1230
titanium versus stainless steel and, 1226
of vertebral body fracture, illustrated, 180
of zygapophyseal joint, 313
see also Radiography
Concentric muscle contraction, 378
Congenital curves, illustrated, 1559
Congenital deformity(ies), 1554–1576
classification of, 1555–1560, 1571–1575
evaluation of patient with, 1563–1564, 1571
natural history of, 1560, 1562–1563
radiographic evaluation of, 1565–1566
resulting from failure of formation, 1556–1557, 1571–1574
illustrated, 1556, 1557, 1558
resulting from failure of segmentation, 1557, 1559–1560, 1574–1575
illustrated, 1558, 1559, 1560–1561

Congenital deformity(ies),—cont'd
treatment of
orthotic, 1566
surgical, 1566–1571, 1572–1575
Congenital kyphoscoliosis, 1575
Congenital kyphosis
classification of, 1571–1575
evaluation of patient with, 1571
illustrated, 1556, 1559, 1568–1569, 1572, 1574
in older patients, 1573
treatment of, 1572–1575
see also Congenital deformity(ies)
Congenital lordosis, 1575
illustrated, 1559
Congenital scoliosis, 1311, 1555–1571, 1613
embryology specific to, 1555
etiology of, 1555
evaluation of patient with, 1563–1564
illustrated, 1556, 1557, 1558, 1561, 1562
natural history of, 1560, 1562–1563
radiographic evaluation of, 1565–1566
treatment of
orthotic, 1566
surgical, 1566–1571
see also Congenital deformity(ies)
Congenital spondylolisthesis, 1293
defined, 1281
illustrated, 1281
Conservative care; see Conservative treatment
Conservative treatment, 347–770
aggressive, 395
cookbook for, 370
nonoperative, 368, 369–370
aggressive, 395
phases of, 370
psychosocial, chronic pain and, 373
surgical decision-making and, 909
time frames for, 368–369
Contact osteogenesis, 885
Contraves electromagnetic stand, 1033
illustrated, 1030
Controlled falling, 617
Convergence-projection theory, 92
illustrated, 91
COPD; see Chronic obstructive pulmonary disease
Cornua of the sacral, 815
Coronal plane, 1579
Corpectomy, 1429, 1430
Cortical "trap door" in bone grafting, 873
Corticocancellous bone graft, illustrated, 1398, 1416
Corticosteroids
cysts treated with, 1268
epidural; see Epidural corticosteroids
oral; see Oral corticosteroids
use of, 510
Cortisol, 291
normal values of, 292
Costovertebral joint(s), 823–824
illustrated, 823
Cotrel-Dubousset bone screw system, 1482
Cotrel-Dubousset system, 782, 1181
adult scoliosis treatment with, 1613, 1617, 1618, 1620–1623, 1624, 1627, 1628
use of in surgery to treat kyphotic deformity, 1675
illustrated, 1715, 1716
Cotrel-Dubousset transpedicular screws, 863
Coumadin, 1535
Cousins, Michael, 600

Cousins, Norman, 500
CPR (Cardiopulmonary Resuscitation), 1439
Craig Bone Biopsy Set, 1014
Craig needle, 777, 1468
Craniocervical joint(s), 820–821
   illustrated, 820
Craniovertebral ligaments, illustrated, 1317, 1319
Crawford needle, 330
C-reactive protein (CRP), 275–276
Crock, Harry, 222, 1034, 1040–1041, 1101, 1102, 1292
Crock chisels, 1292
Crock curette, 1119
   illustrated, 1119
Crock dowels, 1292
Crock instrumentation, 780, 781
Crohn's disease, 1681
Cross links in internal fixation systems, 1183–1184
   illustrated, 1179, 1180
CRP (C-reactive protein), 275–276
Cruciate ligament, 821
Cruciform ligament, 1319
   illustrated, 1319
Cryptococcus neoformans, 1549
CSM; see Cervical spondylotic myelopathy
CSR; see Cervical spondylotic radiculopathy
CT; see Computed tomography
CT discography, 220, 221–222, 224–225
CT/MPR (computed tomography with multiplaner reformations),
   141
CTST; see Cervicothoracic stabilization training
Culture of Pain, The, 500
Curette(s)
   Crock, 1119
   Epstein, 1039
   Oswestry, 1119
   Scoville, 1105
Curve(s)
   compensatory, 1580–1581
      illustrated, 1597
   congenital, illustrated, 1559
   lumbosacral, illustrated, 1561
   paralytic, 1627
   primary, 1580–1581
      double, illustrated, 1584
Curve patterns, 1581
Cybex 6000 dynamometer, illustrated, 534
Cybex EDI-320, illustrated, 533
Cybex Liftask, 489, 534
Cyclic adenosine monophosphate (cAMP), 291
Cyst, bone, 1459

D

Dallas discogram scale, 222, 224
   illustrated, 222
Dallas Pain Drawing, 918, 922
   illustrated, 929, 932, 935
Dallas Pain Questionnaire (DPQ), 918, 926
   illustrated, 919–923, 928, 930, 931, 933, 934, 936
   laser discectomy patients and, 1050–1051
Dance, 641–648
   back injury in
      diagnosis and treatment of, 645–647
      risk factors for, 642–645
   dance medicine and, 647–648
   neck strain and, 647
   therapeutic exercises for, 645–646
Dandy, Walter, 775
Danek system, 1181

DBM; see Demineralized bone matrix
DCP plates, 1236, 1237
DCS (dorsal column stimulation), 574
DDAVP (Demopressin), 970, 971
DDD; see Degenerative disk disease
DDT (Dispositif de Traction Transversale) device, 1623
Debilitation, workers' compensation injury and, 29
Debilitation cascade; see Deconditioning cascade
Decompensation
   saggital plane, illustrated, 1596
   spinal; see Spinal decompensation
Decompression(s)
   anterior
      lumbar, 1235–1236
      of spinal cord, 1573
   for central stenosis, 1088–1090
   direct, via posterolateral technique, 1523
   dissection and, 1253–1257
   fusion after, 1275
   indications for, 1087–1088
   intracapsular lateral, "report card" on, 1081–1082
   lateral, intracapsular, "report card" on, 1081–1082
   for lateral and far-out stenosis, 1091–1098
   lumbar, 1235–1236, 1251–1260
   microsurgical discectomy and, 1028–1045
   midline posterior, 1272–1273
      illustrated, 1273
      stability and, 1287
   paralateral
      "report card" on, 1082
      for subarticular stenosis, 1097–1098
   paraspinal, "report card" on, 1082
   patient selection for, 1087–1088
   posterior, 843, 1272
   soft-tissue; see Soft-tissue decompression(s)
   for subarticular stenosis, 1090
      paralateral approach for, 1097–1098
      transverse approach for, 1093–1097
   without bony resection, 1574
Deconditioning
   consequences of, 390
   mental, 538–539
   workers' compensation injury and, 29
Deconditioning cascade
   physical correlates of, 528–536
   see also Deconditioning syndrome
Deconditioning syndrome, 48–49
   defined, 531
   physical correlates of, 528–536
   psychosocial correlates of, 537–545
Deep tendon reflexes, testing of, 76
Deep venous thrombosis (DVT), spinal-cord injury and, 1535–1536
"Defense scoliosis," 73
Deformity; see Spinal deformity(ies)
Degenerative cervical kyphosis with myeloradiculopathy, 1638–1639
Degenerative disc disease (DDD)
   anterior discectomy and, 1234
   arthritis of the hips or knees and, 57
   of cervical spine; see Cervical disc disease
   as indication for cervical spine fusion, 1396
   low-back pain and, 43, 57
   surgical decision-making for, 908–914
   see also Cervical disc disease
Degenerative joint disease (DJD), 647
Degenerative scoliosis
   degenerative spondylolisthesis and, 1277–1278
      illustrated, 1277
"Degenerative (aging) spiral," 89
   illustrated, 90

Degenerative spondylolisthesis, 779, 1266–1279
  conservative care for, 1268
  defined, 1267, 1281–1282
  degenerative scoliosis and, 1277–1278
    illustrated, 1277
  fusion selection for, 1274–1275
  indications for surgical treatment of, 1271–1272
  isthmic spondylolisthesis versus, 1267
  operative treatment of, 1272–1277
    midline approach to, 1272–1273
  pathologic process of, 1267–1268
  prevalence and etiology of, 1267
  radiologic assessment of, 1268, 1270–1271
    illustrated, 1270, 1271
  signs and symptoms of, 1267
DeJeune, Joseph Jules, 774, 777–778
della Francesca, Piero, pain depicted by, 498–499, 506
Demineralized bone, 896–897
Demineralized bone matrix (DBM), 883
  collagen and, 886
Demopressin (DDAVP), 970, 971
Denis, Frances, 1514, 1520
Dens
  defined, 1316
  illustrated, 1319
  osteosynthesis of, 1402–1403
Densitometry, assessment of osteoporosis with, 854–855
Dentate ligaments, 1364
Depression
  defined, 922
  patient with chronic spine pain and, 260–261, 544
  psychologic cascade and, 38
  symptoms of, 925
Dermatomal pain, 273
Dermatomes, 833–835
  defined, 834
  illustrated, 834
Descartes, René, model of pain depicted by, 497–498, 499, 506
Descending modulation, 23
Designs-for-Vision, 1029
Detraining; see Deconditioning
Dewar onlay graft, illustrated, 1658
Dewar posterior cervical fusion, 1413, 1502, 1639, 1641,
    1644–1645
  illustrated, 1639
  technique in, modified, 1656
DEXA (dual energy x-ray absorptiometry), 855
  illustrated, 854
Diabetes, spinal surgery in patients with, 974
Diagnosis(es)
  decision making and, 41–51
  of low-back pain, differential, 42
Diagnostic block(s)
  of cervical medial branch, 307–308
    illustrated, 308, 309
  controversies surrounding, 314–316
  of lateral atlantoaxial joint, 300–301, 310
    illustrated, 310
  of lumbar medial branch, 304–305
    illustrated, 304, 305
  of sacroiliac joint, 301, 311
  specificity of, 314
  of spinal synovial joints; see Spinal synovial joint blocks
  of third occipital nerve, 309
  validity of, 314
  workers' compensation injury testing and, 242
  of zygapophyseal joint; see Zygapophyseal joint block(s)
Diagonal curls, illustrated, 398

Diaphragm, 827
Diathesis-stress model of chronic pain, 540
Dichloromethylene disphosphonate (clodronate), treatment of Paget's
    disease with, 1727, 1728
Didronel, 1537
Dilke study regarding epidural steroid injections, 337–338
Direct current stimulation in spinal fusion, 1297–1300
  clinical efficacy of, 1298–1299
  cost of and procedural codes for, 1300
  indications for use of, 1299
  surgical procedures for implantation in, 1299–1300
Disabled individual, reasonable accommodation for, 478, 479
Disc(s)
  anatomy of, 85–87
  biochemistry of, 87
  cervical
    injury to; see Cervical disc injury(ies)
    normal, illustrated, 17, 1352
    puncture of; see Cervical disc puncture
  clinical biomechanics of, 839–841
  defined, 839
  degeneration of; see Disc degeneration
  degradation of; see Disc degeneration
  development and growth of, 793–795
  excision of, 1037, 1039–1040, 1118–1119
  fragments of, posterior, evacuation of, 107
  herniation of; see Disc herniation
  injuries to, 757
  internal disruption of; see Internal disc disruption
  intervertebral; see Intervertebral disc
  lumbar
    development of, 795
    illustrated, 18
    puncture of; see Lumbar disc puncture
    see also Lumbar discography
  nutrition of, illustrated, 12
  puncture of, 226–229
  surgical treatment of; see Disc surgery
  thoracic, herniated, 1015
  venous drainage of, 11–12
Disc degeneration, 151
  aging and, 87, 89, 90, 143–144
  discogram of, 223
    illustrated, 224
  illustrated, 151
  imaging of, 143–151, 223
    illustrated, 224
  smoking and, 352
  see also Cervical disc disease; Degenerative disc disease
Disc herniation
  defined, 841
  imaging of, 145, 147, 149–150, 164, 166
  intervertebral, soft, 1326
  at level of spondylolisthesis, 1287
  recurrent
    illustrated, 166
    scar versus, 162, 164
  surgical procedures for, 841, 1015, 1041, 1287; see also Discec-
    tomy
  see also Disc degeneration
"Disc pain," 85
Disc surgery
  limited removal of disc in, curettage of disc space versus, 1041
  retained disc fragments in, 1041
  selection of, 1042
    by analysis of pain generators, 984–989
  see also Discectomy
Disease; see Chymopapain

Discectomy
    anterior, 1234
        illustrated, 1423
    arthroscopic; *see* Arthroscopic discectomy
    cervical; *see* Cervical discectomy
    history of, 776–777, 1003
    laser; *see* Laser discectomy
    microlumbar, 1029
    microsurgical; *see* Microdiscectomy; Microsurgical discectomy
    minimally invasive, 990–1073
        evolution of, 1047–1048
    open, automated percutaneous lumbar discectomy versus, 1022
    percutaneous; *see* Percutaneous discectomy
Discharge planning, 978
Discitis
    as complication of discography, 234
    imaging of, 168–171
    postoperative, 168–169, 171
Discography, 219–238
    analgesic, 220
    antibiotic injection during, 234
    cervical; *see* Cervical discography
    complications of, 233–234
    computed tomography (CT) versus, 234
    contraindications to, 233
    CT, 220, 221–222, 224–225
    defined, 220
    historical background of, 220–226
    indications to, 233
    lumbar; *see* Lumbar discography
    magnetic resonance imaging (MRI) versus, 234–235
    plus anesthesia, 97
    preoperative evaluation with, 1139–1140
    provocation, 220, 235
    techniques of, 226–233, 1139–1140
    utility of, 235
    validity of, 234
DISH; *see* Disseminated idiopathic skeletal hyperostosis
Dislocation(s)
    C1-C2, 1493
    facet, 1499
        bilateral, anterior reduction of, 1502
    fracture, 1514, 1518–1520
    hyperextension fracture and, 1500
    occipitoatlantal, 1490
    of vertebral body, 1499
Disodium etidronate (EHDP)(HEBP etidronate)
    treatment of back pain with, 1730
    treatment of Paget's disease with, 1727, 1728
    treatment of spinal stenosis with, 1730
Disorder(s)
    lumbar spine; *see* Lumbar spine, disorders of
    paralytic, classification of, 1593
Dispositif de Traction Transversale (DDT) device, 1623
Dissection
    decompression and, 1253–1257
    electrosurgical, 1253, 1256–1257
    subperiosteal, 1253, 1337–1338
        illustrated, 1338
Dissector(s)
    Cobb, 1253
    Penfield, 1037, 1399, 1407
Disseminated idiopathic skeletal hyperostosis (DISH), Paget's disease and, 1726
    illustrated, 1727
Dissociative movement therapy (DMT), 658
    illustrated, 660
Distance osteogenesis, 885

Distractive extension injury, 1487
    illustrated, 1489
Distractive flexion injury, 1487
    illustrated, 1488
Disturbed mineralization, 294
Diuretics, thiazide, osteoporosis management with, 861
Diving, cervical spine injuries in, 1446
DJD (degenerative joint disease), 647
DMT; *see* Dissociative movement therapy
Dohring, S., 1069
Doppler apparatus, 1702, 1707
Dorsal column stimulation (DCS), 574
Dorsal horn, 25
Dorsal rami of spinal nerves, 831–832
Dorsal rhizotomy, 587
Dorsal root ganglion (DRG)
    chemicals involved in pain transduction and, 25
    as modulator of low-back pain, 94–99
    neuropeptides in, 96
Dorsal-root ganglionectomy, 587–588, 596
Double primary curve, illustrated, 1584
Double primary curve patterns, 1581
Double thoracic major curve patterns, 1581
Dowel graft(s)
    femoral, 1122
    illustrated, 1121
    patellar, 1122
Down syndrome, 942
Doxinate, 1534
DPA (dual-photon absorptiometry), assessment of osteoporosis with, 854–855
DPQ; *see* Dallas Pain Questionnaire
DRG; *see* Dorsal root ganglion
Drugs
    abuse of
        low-back pain and, 47–48
        spinal surgery and, 924, 974–975
        tissue donation excluded by, 893
    health education and, 355
    neuroleptic, for pain of spinal origin, 524
    nonsteroidal antiinflammatory; *see* Nonsteroidal antiinflammatory drugs
    spinally-administered; *see* Spinally administered narcotic (SAN) infusion therapy
    treatment of Paget's disease with, 859, 1726–1730, 1734–1735
    see also Chemical(s); Corticosteroids; Medication; Steroid(s)
Drummond buttons, 863, 1643, 1675
Drummond wire, 863
DSM-III-R
    American Psychiatric Association advocates use of, 542
    psychological factors affecting physical condition under, 48
    somatoform pain disorder described by, 47
Dual energy x-ray absorptiometry (DEXA), 855
    illustrated, 854
Dual-photon absorptiometry (DPA), assessment of osteoporosis with, 854–855
Dumbbell tumors, 1609
Dunn device, 1236
    vascular injuries with, 1248
Duodenal ulcer, development of low-back pain and, 58
Dural tear
    imaging of, 171
    as risk of posterior spine surgery, 1108
DVT (deep venous thrombosis), spinal-cord injury and, 1535–1536
Dwyer, Allen, 1162, 1297, 1298

Dwyer cable system, 782, 1162, 1200
  urologic complications and, 1248
  use of for anterior spinal instrumentation, 1234, 1241
Dwyer instrumentation, 782, 1613
Dynamic muscle contraction, isotonic contraction versus, 378
Dynamometer, 125
Dyspepsia
  development of low-back pain and, 58
  NSAID use and, 514
Dysplastic spondylolisthesis; see Congenital spondylolisthesis

E
Eagleston, Richard, 735
EBI Medical Systems, Inc., 1297, 1299
Eccentric muscle contraction, 378
ECG (electrocardiography), preoperative, 965–966
Echo time (TE), 141–142
Education
  barriers to, 354–355
  of patient; see Patient education
  pre- and postsurgical, 925–926
  as primary treatment of low-back pain, 347–358
  of public, 271, 1080
Educational therapy, 350–354
Edward rod sleeves, 1521
EEOC; see Equal Employment Opportunity Commission
Effective intersegmental mobility (EISM)
  effects of age on spinal coordination and, 130
  effects of gender on spinal coordination and, 129
  in recovery from flexion, 126–128
    illustrated, 127, 133
EHDP (disodium etidronate)(HEDP etidronate)
  treatment of back pain with, 1730
  treatment of Paget's disease with, 1727, 1728
  treatment of spinal stenosis with, 1730
EISM; see Effective intersegmental mobility
Ejaculation, retrograde, as complication of lumbar fusion,
    1123–1124, 1127
Electrical stimulation for spinal fusion
  direct current stimulation in; see Direct current stimulation in
    spinal fusion
  history of, 1297
  mechanism of action of, 1297
  see also Pulsed electromagnetic field (PEMF) in spinal fusion
Electrocardiography (ECG), preoperative, 965–966
Electrodes, 206
  placement of, in SCS, 578–580, 591–592
Electrodiagnostic studies, 191–203
  accuracy of, 199
  establishing or confirming clinical diagnosis with, 200
  indications for, 199–200
  limitations of, 200–201
  medical-legal documentation with, 200
  of nerve injuries, 200
  report of, 201
Electroencephalogram (EEG)
  10–20 system of, illustrated, 207
  discogram versus, 206
  electrodes used in, 206
Electroknife hot loop, 1252, 1256–1257
  illustrated, 1252
Electromagnetic spectrum, illustrated, 1302
Electromyography (EMG), 192
  analysis of baseball hitters with, 609–612
  analysis of torque transfer in baseball pitchers with, 614
  examination in radiculopathy with, 193–194, 196, 198,
    200–201, 209–211

Electromyography (EMG),—cont'd
  golf injury diagnosed by, 676
  H reflex versus, 194
  motor potential (MEP) studies versus, 205
  muscular endurance measured by, 534–535
  needle; see Needle EMG
  single-fiber (SFEMG), 198–199
  somatosensory evoked potential (SEP) studies versus, 205
Electrophysiologic testing; see Electrodiagnostic studies
Electrosurgical dissection, 1256–1257
  illustrated, 1253
Elekta Instruments, 1035
Elevator
  Cobb, 1013, 1235, 1253, 1275
  Penfield, 1384
Ellis, William, 668
Elongated spondylolisthesis; see Isthmic spondylolisthesis
Elsberg, Charles, 775
Elyot, Sir Thomas, 747
EMG; see Electromyography
Employer, workers' compensation injuries and, 30
Employment and Rehabilitation Institute of California (ERIC), Work
    Tolerance and Screening Battery of, 488
Endocrine problems, spinal surgery in patients with, 974
Endoscopic nucleotomy, 1072–1073
Endoscopic thoracic spine surgery, 1012–1015
  anesthesia in, 1012–1013
  complications of, 1014–1015
  technique in, 1013–1014
End-plate fracture, 223
Endurance, measurement of, 534–535
Energy metabolism, 380–382
Engel, George L., 503, 559
Enterobacteriaceae, 176
Entitlement, chronic low-back pain and, 544
EPIC Progressive Lifting Capacity (PLC) test, illustrated,
    247
Epidural abscess
  as complication of discography, 234
  imaging of, 178–179
Epidural anesthesia, headaches and, 335
Epidural corticosteroids
  treatment for herniated nucleus pulposus with, 44
  treatment of acute anulus tear with, 42
  see also Epidural steroids; Steroid(s)
Epidural cortisone injections (ESI), 757
Epidural fibrosis, 161–162
  illustrated, 162
Epidural scar, as complication specific to posterior lumbar interbody
    fusion, 1108
Epidural steroids, 322–343
  caudal; see Caudal epidural steroids
  cervical; see Cervical epidural steroids
  complications in use of, 335–336
  contraindications for use of, 328
  controversies surrounding, 339–340
  defined, 323
  efficacy of, 336–339
  historical background of, 323–326
  indications for use of, 327–328
  lumbar; see Lumbar epidural steroids
  rationale for use of, 326–327
  risks in use of, 335–336
  sacral; see Sacral epidural steroids
  side effects of, 335
  techniques for use of, 328–335
Epstein, J. A., 1069–1070
Epstein curettes, 10399

EPT; *see* Estrogen replacement therapy
Equal Employment Opportunity Commission (EEOC)
  claims related to back disabilities and, 474
  job analysis and, 475
Erector spinae, 828–829
Ergonomic intervention, 472–485
  job analysis in, 474–476
ERIC (Employment and Rehabilitation Institute of California), Work
    Tolerance and Screening Battery of, 488
Erickson, Milton, 567
Erythrocyte sedimentation rate (ESR), 275–276, 1545, 1549, 1550
Escherichia coli, 234, 1544
ESI (epidural cortisone injections), 757
ESR (erythrocyte sedimentation rate), 275–276, 1545, 1549, 1550
Essential function analysis, 475
Estrogen replacement therapy (EPT)
  bone loss prevention and, 856
  incidence of fractures and, 858
  osteoporosis and, 848, 850, 856, 858
Eugonomics, 1082
Ewing's sarcoma, 278, 1459
Excessive pain behavior, 261
Exercise(s)
  aerobic; *see* Aerobic exercise
  in cervicothoracic stabilization training (CTST), 420–435
    illustrated, 425–433
  interscapular muscle strengthening, 435
  osteoporosis and, 856
  position of, 422
  progression of, 422, 423–424
  regional, 422
  resistance; *see* Resistance exercise
  shoulder girdle muscle strengthening, 434
  stabilization; *see* Stabilization exercises
  therapeutic; *see* Therapeutic exercise(s)
  trunk, 402
  upper-extremity muscle strengthening, 435
  see also Weight training
Exercise response, 382–386
Exhaustion, psychologic cascade and, 38
Extraforaminal stenosis, 1085

F
F wave, 195
FABER (flexion, abduction, and external rotation) testing, 79, 1615
Facet dislocation, 1499
Facet fusion
  illustrated, 1410, 1640, 1641
  posterolateral; *see* Posterolateral facet fusion
Facet joint(s), 9, 15–16
  anatomy of, 87–89
  biochemistry of, 89
  in cervical versus lumbar spine, 793–795
  development of, 793–795, 803–804
    illustrated, 802, 803
  injury to, 756–757, 1499
  pain in, 90
Facet syndrome, 46, 90
Facet-joint fixation, 1160
Failed back surgery syndrome (FBSS), 160
  ablative procedures and, 587–588
  anatomic procedures and, 586
  augmentative procedures and, 586–587
  spinal cord stimulation (SCS) and, 574, 575, 591
  spinal stenosis as cause of, 164
Falling, in martial arts, 696–697, 703
  illustrated, 697, 707

Farfan, Harry, 614
"Far-out" stenosis, 1085
  methods of decompression for, 1091–1098
  spondylolisthesis and, 1287
Fast-twitch ("Type II" or "white") muscle fibers, 379–380
Fat graft(s)
  illustrated, 902, 903, 904
  nature of, 900–901
  obtaining, 903–905
  see also Free-fat graft(s)
Fatigue resistance, measurement of, 534–535
FBSS; *see* Failed back surgery syndrome
FCE; *see* Functional capacity evaluation
FDA; *see* Food and Drug Administration
Fear
  chronic low-back pain and, 544
  psychologic cascade and, 37
Federal Trade Commission, fees and, 1753
Fees; *see* Billing, 1746–1755
Femoral cortical-cancellous composite allograft, 1130–1133
  illustrated, 1132
Femoral dowel grafts, 1122
Femoral ring grafts, 1122
Femoral stretch test, conduct of during physical examination, 77
Ferguson view, 1229
"Fetal cartilage," 799
Fever, associated with low-back pain, 57
FFA (free fatty acids), 382
Fibrosis
  barriers to, 900
    synthetics as, 906
  preservation of ligamentum flavum and, 1040
  retroperitoneal, as complication of fixation device use, 1248
  sources of, 900
Fibular bone graft, 881, 1130, 1292–1293
  illustrated, 1292
  see also Whitecloud fibular strut technique
Figure skating, 649–666
  epidemiology and, 650–651
  functional restoration program for, 655–662
  injury prevention in, 664–665
  jump in, biomechanics of, 653–655
  lift in, biomechanics of, 651–652
  return-to-play issues in, 662, 664
  stabilization exercises in, 658–662
    illustrated, 659, 660–662, 663–664
  weight training in, 662
Film, plain, radiographic analysis and, 1546
Fine, Perry, 112, 113, 114
Fixation; *see* Internal fixation
Flat-back deformity; *see* Iatrogenic flat-back deformity
Flexibility, assessment of, 1583
Flexion
  flexion, abduction, and external rotation (FABER) testing and,
    79, 1615
  normal/recovery from, spinal coordination and, 126–128, 133
Flexion deformities; *see* Kyphotic deformity(ies)
Flexion-distraction injuries, 1514, 1518
Flexion-distraction technique, illustrated, 442
Fluoride, osteoporosis management and, 860–861
Fluoroscopy
  C-arm; *see* C-arm fluoroscopy
  intraoperative, 1189–1190
Fogarty catheter, 878
Foley catheter, 969, 1512
Food and Drug Administration (FDA)
  chymopapain use and, 992–993, 997, 1076, 1077
  classification of transcranial stimulation (TCS) as experimental by, 205

Food and Drug Administration (FDA),—cont'd
  Drug Bulletin of, 993
  implantable direct current bone growth stimulator approved by,
    1299
  intrathecal narcotics for nonmalignant pain approved by, 600
  Investigational Device Exemption (IDE) USA study of Ray TFC
    by, 1230–1231
  spinal instrumentation use and, 1082
  Wiltse system and, 1187
Football, 667–674
  brachial plexus neuropraxia in, 1449–1450
  burners in, 1449–1450
  "burning hands syndrome" and, 1447
  history of, 668
  injuries in, 668
    cervical spine, 1445, 1446, 1505–1506
    immobilization of patient and, 1438, 1440
      illustrated, 1441
    literature related to, 669–670
    mechanism of, 668–669
    on-field examination and, 1438–1440
    prevention of, 670–671
    radiographic evaluation and, 1440
    transport of patient and, 1438, 1440
      illustrated, 1441
  rehabilitation and stabilization training in, 671–672
Foramen(ina)
  intervertebral, 811–812
  neural, 143
  transverse, 142, 813
  vertebral, 811
Foramen transversarium, 813
Foraminal decompression
  arthroscopic, 1011–1012
  treatment of high-grade spondylolisthesis and, 1288
Foraminal stenosis, 1085
  computed tomography as best demonstration of, 1271
  degeneration of intervertebral disc and, 1267–1268
  distribution of pain and, 1287
  evaluation of, isthmic spondylolisthesis and, 1286
Foraminotomy(ies)
  laminotomy and, 1384
  multiple, illustrated, 1387
Fordyce, W. E., 917
Forestier's disease; *see* Disseminated idiopathic skeletal
    hyperostosis
Forward lunges, illustrated, 1744
Foundation for Informed Decision Making
  educational materials developed by, 351
  patient education candidate guidelines of, 351
Fracture(s)
  burst; *see* Burst fractures
  cervical spine; *see* Cervical spine fracture(s)
  chance, 1518
    illustrated, 1519–1520
  clay-shoveler's, 1445, 1451
  compression; *see* Compression fracture(s)
  diagnosis of, 180, 181
  end-plate, 223
  estrogen and, 858
  hangman's; *see* Hangman's fracture(s)
  Jefferson, 1314, 1395, 1451, 1493
  lateral mass, 1499
    illustrated, 1500
  of long bones, as complication of spinal-cord injury, 1536–1537
  occipital condyle, 1493
    illustrated, 1494
  occult, as cause of kyphotic deformity, 1698

Fracture(s),—cont'd
  odontoid, 1495
    illustrated, 1496
  osteoporosis and, 848
  pedicle, of C2; *see* Hangman's fracture(s)
  of posterior elements, 1499
  spine, bone mineral density (BMD) and, 855
  spinous process, 757
  teardrop, 1444–1445, 1498
  thoracolumbar spine; *see* Thoracolumbar spine fracture(s)
  three-part two-plane fracture, 1444–1445
    illustrated, 1444
  unrecognized, as cause of kyphotic deformity, 1698
  of vertebral body, 1498–1500
    with canal compromise, 1498–1499
Fracture dislocations, 1514, 1518–1520
Frame(s), 955, 956–962
  Andrews; *see* Andrews frame
  for arthroscopic microdiscectomy, 1004
    illustrated, 1005
  Basildon (Gardner), 955
  CeDaR, 956–960
    illustrated, 957
  CHOP, 958
  Cloward, 955, 958
  Hall, 955
  Hall-Recton, 1620
  Hastings, 956
  Hicks, 956
  Kambin, 955, 958
  Norfolk, 955
  Pronease, 958
  Relton, 955
  Stryker, 947, 1396, 1675
  Tarlov, 956, 958
Frankel classification system, 1512–1513, 1521, 1525,
    1531
Free fatty acids (FFA), 382
Free fragment, 145–146, 149, 1037
Free-fat graft(s), 900–903
  fate of, 901–903
  nature of, 900–901
  see also Fat graft(s)
Free-vascularized bone grafts, 881
Freeze drying, bone storage and, 882
Freezing, bone storage and, 882
Freud, Sigmund, 567
"Front-back" stenosis, 1085
FRS (Functional Rating Scale), 363
Functional activities assessment, 407
  illustrated, 409
Functional capacity
  assessment of, 414–416
  defined, 488
  job analysis and, 478
  physical capacity versus, 533
  workplace demands versus, 492
  see also Functional capacity evaluation
Functional capacity evaluation (FCE), 125, 254–255
  illustrated, 256
  normative data on, 257
  surgical decision-making and, 910–911
Functional gym stabilization evaluation, 407–410
  illustrated, 408
Functional Measurement Laboratory, 488, 490
Functional Rating Scale (FRS), 363
Functional restoration, 491–492
  figure skating and, 655–662

Functional-economic rating scale, 1043
Fusion
    after decompression, 1275
    anterior
        interbody; *see* Anterior interbody fusion
        plate fixation technique in, 1418, 1624–1626
    arthroscopic; *see* Arthroscopic lumbar interbody fusion
    Bailey-Badgley, illustrated, 1417
    biomechanics of, 843–844
    Bohlman technique in, 1409
    Brooks technique in; *see* Brooks fusion technique
    Callahan technique in; *see* Callahan fusion technique
    cervical; *see* Cervical fusion
    circumferential lumbar; *see* Circumferential lumbar fusion
    Cloward, illustrated, 1417
    congenital scoliosis treated with, 1567–1570
    Cotrel-Dubousset approach to, 1620–1623
    Dewar technique in; *see* Dewar posterior cervical fusion
    electrical stimulation used for; *see* Electrical stimulation for spinal
        fusion
    facet; *see* Facet fusion
    Gallie technique in; *see* Gallie fusion technique
    Garber-Meyer technique in, 1409
    of hemivertebrae, 1569–1570
    history of, 779–781
    imaging of, 167–168, 169
    interbody
        anterior; *see* Anterior interbody fusion
        arthroscopic; *see* Arthroscopic lumbar interbody fusion
        indications for, 1113
        posterior; *see* Posterior interbody fusion
    Keystone technique, 1636, 1644
    length of, congenital deformity and, 1567, 1573
    long-segment, illustrated, 1601
    lumbar; *see* Lumbar fusion
    neurocentral, 804
    oblique wiring technique in; *see* Oblique wiring fusion technique
    occipitoatlantal, 1397–1399
        illustrated, 1397, 1398, 1399
    occipitocervical, illustrated, 1397, 1398
    posterior
        interbody; *see* Posterior interbody fusion
        with internal fixation, 1567, 1620–1623
        plate fixation technique in, 1413
        plating technique in, 1413–1414
        in situ, 1567
    reexploration of, 1570
    "report card" on, 1082
    Robinson technique in; *see* Robinson fusion technique
    Rogers technique in; *see* Rogers fusion technique
    simultaneous combined anterior and posterior; *see* Simultaneous
        combined anterior and posterior fusion
    single-stage instrumentation and, 1587–1588
    Smith-Robinson, illustrated, 1417, 1423
    for spondylolisthesis
        degenerative, 1274–1275
        isthmic, 1286–1287, 1291–1293
    staged reconstruction and, 1590, 1592
    triple-wire technique in; *see* Triple-wire fusion technique
    vertebral body reconstruction technique in, 1416, 1418
        illustrated, 1419–1422

G
Galen, 348, 747, 774
Gallie fusion technique, 1399, 1401–1402, 1502, 1645–1647
    illustrated, 1402, 1646
Gallie wire, 1654

Gallie-type posterior atlantoaxial arthrodesis, 1654
Gallium nitrate, treatment of Paget's disease with, 1726, 1730
Galveston technique, 1168, 1620
Ganglion, dorsal root; *see* Dorsal root ganglion
Garber-Meyer fusion technique, 1409
Gardner three-pin head holder, 1396
Gardner-Wells apparatus, 1360
Gardner-Wells tongs, 1373, 1396, 1414
Garner, Matt, 1230
Gastrocnemius stretch, 400
Gastroenterologic disorders, spinal surgery in patients with, 974
Gastrointestinal abnormalities, congenital scoliosis and, 1565
Gate control, 500, 574
    defined, 23
Gate control model of pain, 549, 917
Gelfoam, 874, 906, 951, 971, 1032, 1034, 1037, 1042, 1122,
        1164, 1277, 1361, 1482
Gelpi retractor, 1291
    illustrated, 1095, 1291
Gender, effects of, on spinal coordination, illustrated, 129
General Electric CT scanner, 1230
Genitourinary abnormalities, congenital scoliosis and, 1564
German Athletic Association, 747
Giant-cell tumors, 1459
Gill procedure, 1287, 1291
Glucocorticosteroids, for pain of spinal origin, 523–524
Glycosylated hydroxylysine, 288
Goldenhar syndrome, 1565
Golf, 675–682
    "back savers" in, 680–681
    injuries in, 676
        incidence and etiology of, 676
        prevention of, 676–681
    swing in, 678–680
    warmup in, 676–678
Golf Digest, 680
Gonadal hormones, normal values of, 291
Government, health education and, 355
Graft, bone; *see* Bone graft(s)
Graft resorption, as complication specific to posterior lumbar inter-
        body fusion, 1108
Graft retropulsion, as complication specific to posterior lumbar inter-
        body fusion, 1108
Grafton, 1014
Gram-negative infections, 1544
Granulomatous disease of the spine, 1549–1550
Graphics tablet, illustrated, 596
Gray's Anatomy, 117
Greenwald, Howard P., 503
Grisel syndrome, 1645
Gross motion analysis systems, 125
Growth hormone, 291
    normal values of, 292
    osteoporosis management and, 861–862
"Guillotine mechanism," 1443
Gunshot wounds, 1490
Gymnastics, cervical spine injuries in, 1446

H
H graft, modified, illustrated, 1654, 1656
H reflex, 194–195
Hadler, Nortin M., 504
Halifax clamp, 1414, 1504, 1645, 1647
    illustrated, 1648
Hall frame, 955
Hall-Recton frame, 1620
Halo immobilization, 783, 1376

Halo traction, 947
Hamstring stretch, illustrated, 399, 678
Hand-held bender, illustrated, 1191
Hangman's fracture(s), 1316, 1402, 1496–1498
    illustrated, 1497–1498
Harrington, Paul, 782, 1159, 1161
Harrington compression system, 1518
Harrington distractor, 1502
Harrington hooks, 782, 1197, 1198
Harrington instrumentation, 782, 912, 1242, 1245, 1300, 1520,
        1521, 1523
    adult scoliosis treated with, 782, 1613, 1618–1619, 1627, 1628
    osteoporosis treatment with, 862
Harrington rods, 781, 782, 844–845, 948, 1159, 1409, 1479, 1520,
        1523, 1594, 1613
    illustrated, 1175
    Kostuik-Harrington device and, 782, 1242
    Vermont Spinal Fixator and, 1197, 1198, 1200
    Wiltse system versus, 1187
Harris, R. I., 1654
Harris wire tightener, 1654
    illustrated, 1655
Harvard Program in Medical Anthropology, 502
Harvey Cushing Society, 784, 1101
Hastings frame, 956
Haverfield-Scoville retractor, 1034, 1036
HCFA Common Procedural Coding System (HCFA), 1747
HCPCS (HCFA Common Procedural Coding System), 1747
Head, sports injuries of, 1437–1454
Headache
    cerebrospinal fluid (CSF) leakage and, 336
    as side effect of steroid use, 335, 336
    spinal manipulative therapy (SMT) and, 447
Health
    defined, 350
    education in; see Education
Healthy People 2000, 353
Heart rate (HR), response of to incremental work, 382
    illustrated, 383
Heat, treatment of allografts and xenografts with, 883
HEBP etidronate (disodium etidronate)(EHDP)
    treatment of back pain with, 1730
    treatment of Paget's disease with, 1727, 1728
    treatment of spinal stenosis with, 1730
Heisman, John W., 668
Heithoff, Kenneth, 1230, 1231
Helms, Clyde, 1231
Hemangioma, 1459
    illustrated, 1461
Hemivertebra(ae)
    butterfly, illustrated, 1558
    excision and fusion of, 1569–1570
    fully segmented, incarcerated, illustrated, 1558
    illustrated, 1556, 1563
    multiple, illustrated, 1557
    unsegmented, illustrated, 1557
Hensen node, 796
Hepatitis
    immunization for, 969
    issue donation excluded by, 893
    postoperative complications and, 969
    screening for, 1615
    testing superficial pain sensation and, 78
Herbert screws, 1347
Hernia
    bone grafts and, 879
    as risk specific to anterior lumbar interbody fusion, 1128
Herniated nucleus pulposus (HNP)
    dancers and, 642, 646

Herniated nucleus pulposus (HNP),—cont'd
    low-back pain and, 43–45
    manual therapy and, 466
    straight leg raise in diagnosis of, 76
Herniated thoracic discs, endoscopic spine surgery and, 1015
Heterografts, 884
Heterologous bones, 884
Heterotopic ossification, as complication of spinal-cord injury, 1537
Hibbs, Russel A., 779, 781, 1101, 1234
Hibbs retractors, 959, 1116, 1263
    illustrated, 958, 1117
Hicks frame, 956
"High jumper's neck," 1446
High-grade spondylolisthesis, 1287–1293
    surgical techniques in treatment of, 1288–1293
Hines, Ben, 612
Hippocrates, 348, 438, 774, 782
Histomorphometric assessment, normal values of, 293
Histomorphometry, bone biopsy for, 291–294
Hitters
    electromyographic analysis of, 609–612
    with lumbar spine injuries, treatment of, 624, 626
Hitting, in baseball, biomechanics of, 609
HIV infection
    blood loss during spine surgery and, 970
    postoperative complications and, 969
    rise of tuberculosis within inner cities and, 1550
    risk of in dance community, 647
    screening for, 942, 1615
    testing superficial pain sensation and, 78
    tissue donor selection and, 893
    transmission of during bone transplants, 892, 1102, 1109
HLA-B27 antigen test, 1653
HNP; see Herniated nucleus pulposus
Hockey; see Ice hockey
Holdsworth, Sir Frank, 1514
Holt-Oram syndrome, 1565
Homework for patients, 554
Hooks
    Harrington, 782, 1197, 1198
    Weiss, 1198
Hope, psychologic cascade and, 39
Hormonal assessment, 290–291
Hormone(s)
    gonadal, 291
    growth, 291, 292
        osteoporosis management and, 861–862
    parathyroid (PTH), 284, 285, 290
        osteoporosis management and, 861
    thyroid, 291, 292
Horn, Thomas J., 124
Horner's syndrome, 1333, 1425
Horseshoe headrest, 1384
Horseshoe-shaped bone graft, 1415
Hot wire RF cutting loop, 1252, 1256–1257
    illustrated, 1252
HR; see Heart rate
Hudson brace, 1120
Human locomotion
    importance of lordosis in, 121
    role of spine in, 119–121
Human performance
    measurement of, 531–532
    quantification of, 532–535
Hydrostatic pressure, swimming and, 733
Hydroxyproline, 288
Hyperalgesia, defined, 23–24
Hyperextension fracture/dislocation, 1500
Hyperextension injuries, 1499–1500

Hyperplasia, 388
Hypnosis, 262–263
  defined, 566
  see also Hypnotherapy
Hypnotherapy, 565, 566–572
  defined, 566
  evaluations for, 569
  selection of patients for, 568–569
  specific treatment approaches in, 569–571
  treatment outcome and, 571–572

I

I plate device, 1236
  biomechanics of, 1244
  Syracuse; see Syracuse I plate
IASP; see International Association for the Study of Pain
Iatrogenic flat-back deformity, 1626, 1628
  management of, 1245
Iatrogenic lumbar kyphosis; see Iatrogenic flat-back deformity
Ice hockey, 683–686
  cervical spine injuries in, 1446
  drills in, 685–686
  skating in, biomechanics of, 684
  stabilization training in, 685
IDD; see Internal disc disruption
IDE (Investigational Device Exemption); see Food and Drug Administration
Idiopathic scoliosis, 1578–1593, 1613
  adolescent, 1578
  etiology and natural history of, 1578
  illustrated, 1586–1587, 1589–1590, 1591
  infantile, 1578
  juvenile, 1578
  lumbar, illustrated, 1583
  neurologic examination and, 1583
  pathogenesis of, 1578–1579
  physical examination of patient with, 1581–1585
    illustrated, 1581
  quantitation of structural changes and, 1583, 1585
  terminology of, 1579–1585
  thoracic, illustrated, 1582
  thoracolumbar, illustrated, 1582
  three sisters with, illustrated, 1579
  treatment of, 1583–1593
Iliocostalis muscle, 829, 1332
Imaging
  determination of spinal-cord injuries with, 1532–1533
  of leg pain, 273
  magnetic resonance; see Magnetic resonance imaging
  radionuclide, of bone, 289–290
  of spinal tumors, 1458
  of spine, 140–190
  workers' compensation injury testing and, 241–242
  see also Computed tomography; Discography
Imhoptep, 774
Immobilization
  halo, 783, 1376
  in sports injuries, 1438, 1440
    illustrated, 1441
  see also Traction
Impaction; see Bone(s), impaction of
Impotence, as complication of lumbar fusion, 1123, 1127
Inaccessible zone, 1251–1252
  illustrated, 1252
  working inside, 1260–1261
Incomplete neurologic injury, 1513
Inconsolability, 261
Infantile idiopathic scoliosis, 1578

Infection(s)
  as cause of primary low-back pain, 57
  as complication of internal fixation, 1181, 1248
  as complication of SAN, 605
  gram-negative, 1544
  hepatitis; see Hepatitis
  HIV; see HIV infection
  as indication for cervical spine fusion, 1396
  postoperative, 1042, 1248
  spinal; see Spinal infection(s)
  surgical wound
    factors affecting, 967
    prevention of, 967, 968
  urinary tract, as complication of spinal-cord injury, 1533
Infectious myelitis, imaging of, 179
Infectious spondylitis, imaging of, 175–178
Inferior laminectomy, illustrated, 1261
Inflammatory agents, pain production and, 988
Information overload, as barrier to health education, 354
Infrahyoid (strap) muscles, 1332
Infrared lasers, 1047
Inglehart, Tammi, 658
Inguinal pain, as complication of lumbar fusion, 1124
Injury(ies)
  compressive extension, 1487, 1489
  compressive flexion, 1487, 1488
  distractive extension, 1487, 1489
  distractive flexion, 1487, 1488
  facet joint, 756–757, 1499
  flexion/distraction, 1514, 1518
  hyperextension, 1499–1500
  lateral flexion, 1487, 1489
  nerve; see Nerve injury(ies)
  neurologic, 1513
  prevention of, 477
    in figure skating, 664–665
    in football, 670–671
    in golf, 676–681
    in running, 713–714
    in wrestling, 769–770
  simple unicolumn, 1514, 1515
  to spinal cord; see Spinal-cord injury(ies)
  sport-specific; see Sports injury(ies)
  thoracolumbar; see Thoracolumbar spine fracture(s)
  "three-column," 1498
  vascular; see Vascular injury(ies)
  vertical compression, 1487, 1488
  work-related; see Workers' compensation injury
  see also Fracture(s); Spine injury(ies)
Inner-city drug users, infection and, 1544
Innervation
  of intervertebral disc and peridiscal ligaments, 85–87
  of lumbar spine, illustrated, 85
  of motion segment, 11
    illustrated, 11
Instability, 47
  defined, 1251, 1513
  as risk of posterior spine surgery, 1108
Institute of Medicine, 350
Instrument(s)
  for bone impaction, illustrated, 1258
  for for microsurgical spinal surgery, 1005, 1034–1035, 1036–1037, 1039, 1058–1059
  see also Instrumentation; specific instruments
Instrumentation
  for arthroscopic microdiscectomy, illustrated, 1005
  cable system; see Cable systems
  in cervical spine surgery, 1428–1436
  complications with, 1179–1180, 1248, 1275

Instrumentation,—cont'd
  failure of, 1179–1180, 1248
  in lumbar spine surgery
    anterior, 1233–1249
    posterior, 1173–1195
  of pelvis, 1592
  plate system; *see* Plate systems
  rod system; *see* Rod systems
  screw system; *see* Screw system(s)
  single-stage, fusion and, 1587–1588
  see also specific devices
Insurance company(ies)
  health education and, 355
  workers' compensation injuries and, 30, 348
Interbody graft displacement, as complication of lumbar fusion,
    1124–1125
Interference screws, 1122
Internal disc disruption (IDD), 16, 45, 223
  as cause of low-back pain, 222
  illustrated, 223, 224
Internal fixation, 1174–1175
  anatomic strategies of, 1157–1172
  anterior cervical plate; *see* Anterior cervical plate fixation
  anterior fusion and
    indications for, 1234
    technique in, 1236–1237
  anterior screw; *see* Anterior screw fixation
  complications of, 1176–1181, 1248
  of disc space, 1164–1166
  facet-joint, 1160
  future trends in, 1168–1170
  history of, 781–782, 1234
  instrumentation in; *see* Instrumentation
  lamina and, 1159–1160
  lateral mass plate, 1500
    illustrated, 1501
  of lumbosacral spine, 844–845
  lumbrosacral-junction, 1166–1168
  odontoid screw, 1433
  pedicle, 1160–1162, 1163
  prevention of cervical deformity and, 1635–1636
  spinous process and, 1158
  treatment of idiopathic scoliosis and, 1588–1590
    illustrated, 1589–1590
  Vermont Spinal Fixator (VSF) and; *see* Vermont Spinal Fixator
  vertebral body and, 1162–1164
  Wiltse system of; *see* Wiltse spinal internal fixation system
International Association for the Study of Pain (IASP)
  pain defined by, 501
  painful sensations defined by, 78
International Skating Union, 650
International Society for the Study of Lumbar Spine, 1070
Interscapular muscle strengthening exercises, 435
Intersegmental arteries, 796
Interspinal muscles, 1332
Interspinous ligament, 819
Intervertebral disc(s) (IVD), 10–11, 811, 817–818
  aging of, illustrated, 1325
  degeneration of, 147, 149, 1326
    degenerative spondylolisthesis and, 1267
    effect of on selection of disc surgery, 988
  development and growth of, 793–795, 799–801
    changes in disc nutrition and, 801–803
    illustrated, 800, 801
  function of, 817
  hydrostatic pressure of, effect of on selection of disc surgery, 987
  illustrated, 10, 817, 985, 1324–1325
  injuries to, 630
  postoperative reduction of height of, effect of on selection of disc
    surgery, 987–988

Intervertebral foramen(ina), 811–812
  illustrated, 812
Intervertebral joints, 1323–1327
Intraarticular cervical zygapophyseal joint blocks, 305–307
Intraarticular lumbar zygapophyseal joint blocks, 302–304
Intraarticular steroids, zygapophyseal joint pain and, 316
Intracapsular lateral decompression, "report card" on, 1081–1082
Intracorp, solution to socioeconomic cascade and, 31
Intraoperative fluoroscopy, 1189–1190
Intraspinal meningoceles, 1609
Intraspinal opioids, 518
  postoperative pain management and, 976
Intraspinal synovial cyst
  illustrated, 1269
  as source of stenosis, 1268
Invasive procedures for pain of spinal origin, 586
Investigational Device Exemption (IDE); *see* Food and Drug Admin-
    istration
Ipriflavone
  osteoporosis management and, 862
  treatment of Paget's disease with, 1726, 1730
Ischemic peripheral vascular disease, SCS treatment for pain from,
    576
Isernhagen, Susan, 234
Isokinetic muscle contraction, 378
Isokinetic tests, 534
Isola instrumentation system, 862, 863, 1181, 1520, 1593, 1613,
    1627
  illustrated, 1591
Isola plate, 1167
Isola spinal implants, 1587
Isolation
  psychiatric consultation and, 261
  psychologic cascade and, 38
Isometric cervical strength measurements, 533
Isometric lateral flexion, illustrated, 425
Isometric muscle contraction, 378
Isometric test, 534
Isotechnologies B-200, 489
Isotonic muscle contraction, dynamic contraction versus, 378
Isthmic spondylolisthesis
  defined, 1281
  degenerative spondylolisthesis versus, 1267
  high-grade; *see* High-grade spondylolisthesis
  illustrated, 1281, 1283, 1284, 1289
  incidence and pathogenesis of, 1282
  natural history of, 1282
  nonoperative treatment of, 1285–1286
  physical findings of, 1283
  radiographic analysis and measurement of, 1283–1285, 1289
  surgical treatment of, 1286–1287
    paraspinal approach to, 1290–1291
Ito, Midori, 653
Itrel II, illustrated, 581
IV drug abuse, infection and, 1549
IVD; *see* Intervertebral disc(s)
"Izzo strap," 682
  illustrated, 681

J
Jahn, Friedrich Ludwig, 747
JAMAR isometric grip strength tool, 241, 246
Japanese Orthopaedic Association scoring system, 1048, 1377
Jarcho-Levin syndrome, 1559, 1565
Jefferson fractures, 1314, 1395, 1451, 1493
Jehovah's Witnesses, 971
Jensen, Mark P., 504
Job analysis
  application of, 476–479

Job analysis,—cont'd
  defined, 474
  tools and equipment used in, 475–476
Johnson, Ben, 658
Joint(s)
  atlantoaxial, 1312, 1318–1320
  atlantooccipital, 813, 1312, 1316–1318
  contracture of, as complication of spinal-cord injury, 1535
  costovertebral, 823–824
  craniocervical; see Craniocervical joint(s)
  dysfunction of; see Joint dysfunction
  examination of, 79
  facet; see Facet joint(s)
  intervertebral, 1323–1327
  lateral atlantoaxial, 813
    diagnostic block of, 300–301
  of Luschka, 17, 19, 142, 1322, 1324, 1326, 1330, 1352
    illustrated, 1325
  median atlantoaxial, 814
  neurocentral, 1352
  sacrococcygeal, 821–822
  spinal, 816–826
    synovial, diagnostic block of, 298–321
  uncovertebral; see Uncovertebral joint(s)
  zygapophyseal; see Zygapophyseal joint(s)
Joint dysfunction, local findings associated with, 440
Jones, Arthur, 245
Journal of the American Medical Association, 763, 1076, 1077
Jump, in figure skating, biomechanics of, 653
Juvenile idiopathic scoliosis, 1578
Juvenile kyphosis (Scheuermann's disease), 73, 730, 766, 806, 807,
    1602–1605, 1683
  examination and, 1602–1603
  family history of, spondylolysis and, 61
  illustrated, 1603–1605
  treatment of, 1603–1605

K
Kambin, Parviz, 1070
Kambin frame, 955
Kaneda instrumentation system, 782, 1163, 1236, 1242–1244
  adult scoliosis treated with, 1620
  biomechanics of, 1244
  illustrated, 1164, 1243
  kyphosis treated with, 1245
  lumbar scoliosis treated with, 1245
  osteoporosis treatment and, 862, 863
Kerrison punch, 1090, 1091, 1097, 1364, 1387, 1430
  illustrated, 1095
Kerrison rongeur, 878, 1015, 1035, 1037, 1235, 1236, 1276, 1360,
    1362, 1384, 1385, 1523
Keystone anterior fusion, 784, 1636, 1644
Kicking
  in martial arts, 702
    illustrated, 703, 706, 707
  in soccer, 722–723
Kiel bone, 884
Kim, Y-S, 1230
Kin-Com, 489
Kirkaldy-Willis degenerative process, 12, 16, 19, 395, 438
  illustrated, 16
Kirschner wire, 1061
Kittner ("peanut gauze"), 1340, 1356
Kittner sponge, 1013
Klenerman study regarding epidural steroid injections, 338, 339
Klippel-Feil syndrome, 1311, 1370, 1451, 1452, 1560, 1565, 1645
Knodt hooks, 1198
Knodt instrumentation system, 912
Knodt rods, 781, 844–845, 1159, 1186

Knoringer screws, 1403
  illustrated, 1404
Kocher clamp, 874, 1118
Kostuik-Harrington device, 782, 1242
  adult scoliosis treated with, 1620, 1625, 1626, 1628
  biomechanics of, 1244
  illustrated, 1242
  kyphosis treated with, 1245
  lumbar scoliosis treated with, 1245
  osteoporosis treatment and, 862, 863
  Paget's disease treated with, 1733
  in spinal tumor surgery, 1481
Krebs cycle, 381
Kugelberg-Welander disease, illustrated, 1598
"K-W" degenerative process; see Kirkaldy-Willis degenerative process
Kyphoscoliosis
  congenital, 1575
  illustrated, 1607
Kyphosis
  angle of minimum, 532
  cervical; see Cervical kyphosis
  congenital; see Congenital kyphosis
  iatrogenic lumbar; see Iatrogenic flat-back deformities
  juvenile; see Juvenile kyphosis
  postlaminectomy; see Postlaminectomy kyphosis
  posttraumatic; see Posttraumatic kyphosis
  use of cable systems and, 1234
  Zielke device and, 1242
Kyphotic deformity(ies)
  in ankylosing spondylitis, 1667–1718
  of cervical spine, 1382, 1689–1713
  of lumbar spine, 1668–1682
  measurement of, illustrated, 1672
  of thoracic spine, 1683–1689

L
"Lactate threshold," 385
Lactic acid metabolism
  exercise and, 385–386, 387
Laminae, 811
Laminaplasty, cervical; see Cervical laminaplasty
Laminectomy
  cervical; see Cervical laminectomy
  history of, 775–776, 785
  inferior, illustrated, 1261
  lateral, 1091–1093
    illustrated, 1260, 1261
  limited exposure, illustrated, 1254–1256
  "report card" on, 1081
  superior, illustrated, 1261
Laminotomy
  automated percutaneous lumbar discectomy versus, 1022
  decompression of degenerative spondylolisthesis with, 1272
  foraminotomy and, 1384
Laminotomy/discectomy, 1359–1362
  complications of, 1361
  illustrated, 1360
  results of, 1361
  technique in, 1360–1361
Lane, William A., 777
Lanke, Fritz, 779, 781
Laparoscopic techniques, 1263–1264
Laryngoscope, 783
Laser(s)
  infrared, 1047
  "poor man's," 1256–1257
  surgical, 1047; see also Laser discectomy
  ultraviolet, 1047
  visible-light, 1047

Laser discectomy, 1046–1054
  clinical application of, 1050–1051
  experimental basis for, 1048–1050
  primary, "report card" on, 1050–1051
  technique of, 1051–1053
Laser particle surgical face mask, 1257
Laser surgery; see Laser discectomy
Lateral atlantoaxial joint, 813
Lateral atlantoaxial joint blocks, 300–301, 310
  illustrated, 310
Lateral bend, spinal coordination and, 128–129
Lateral cervical muscles, 826–827
Lateral flexion injury, 1487
  illustrated, 1489
Lateral intraarticular blocks, 306–307
Lateral laminectomy, 1091–1093
  illustrated, 1260, 1261
Lateral mass, 813
Lateral mass fracture, 1499
  illustrated, 1500
Lateral mass plate fixation, 1500
  illustrated, 1501
Lateral recess stenosis, 1085
  evaluation of, isthmic spondylolisthesis and, 1286
Lateral stenosis, 1085
  methods of decompression for, 1091–1098
Latissimus pull exercise, illustrated, 406
Lavin, Marilyn Aronberg, 498
Lee, Casey, 1132
Leg pain, 372–373
  back pain and, 53–55
  imaging of, 273
  spinal nerve root compression and and, 93
Leg thrusts, 1741
Leksell rongeur, 1418
Lesion(s)
  central cord, 1531–1532
  "cold," 277
  manipulable, 438–440
  metastatic, imaging of, 175, 278
  spinal cord; see Spinal-cord lesion(s)
Lewis, Carl, 658
Lhermitte's sign, 1369
Lido Back System, 489
Lido Lift, 489
Lift testing, 489, 534
Lifting
  in dance, 644
  in figure skating
    biomechanics of, 651–652
  power; see Weight lifting
  role of muscles in, 118
  weight; see Weight lifting
  in wrestling, 765
Ligament(s)
  alar, 821, 1319, 1320
  atlantal, 1318, 1320
  atlantoaxial, 1318
  craniovertebral, illustrated, 1317, 1319
  cruciate, 821, 1293
  cruciform, 1319
    illustrated, 1319
  dentate, 1364
  interspinous, 819
  longitudinal; see Longitudinal ligament(s)
  peridiscal, innervation of, 85–87
  posterior, 819–820
  transverse, 821, 1318, 1320
    illustrated, 1319

Ligamentous strain, 628–629
Ligamentum flavum, 330, 819, 839, 841, 1318
  as barrier material, 905
  preservation of, 1040
Ligamentum nuchae, 819, 1320
Link America, 1035
Link-Beatty rongeur, 1035, 1037
  illustrated, 1034
Locomotion, human; see Human locomotion
Loeser, John D., 502, 539–540
Long term opioid (LTO), 516–518
Longissimus muscle, 829, 1332
Longitudinal ligament(s)
  anterior, 142, 143, 818, 1318, 1323
  posterior, 142, 143, 818, 841, 1320, 1323
    ossification of (OPLL); see Ossification of posterior longitudinal
      ligament
Lordosis, 121
  congenital; see Congenital lordosis
Loredan, 489
Loss, terror of, psychologic cascade and, 37
Loupes, 1029, 1257, 1372
Low-back neurons, illustrated, 112
Low-back pain (LBP)
  acute anulus tear and, 42–43
  alcohol overuse and, 58
  anatomy, biochemistry, and physiology of, 84–103
  avoidance of, 487
  back sprain and, 47
  back strain and, 47
  cancer as cause of, 49, 57–58
  childhood psychological risk factors and, 59
  chronic
    idiopathic, 104–115
    see also Deconditioning syndrome
  cigarette smoking and, 58
  cost of, 348, 368
  defined, 529
  degenerative disc disease and, 43, 57
  diffuseness of, 106–109
  disability from; see Low-back pain disability
  duodenal ulcer and, 58
  dyspepsia and, 58
  etiology of, 273
  fever associated with, 57
  herniated nucleus pulposus, 43–45
  idiopathic
    causes of, 838
    chronic, 104–115
  infection as cause of, 57
  leg pain and, 53–55
  management of, osteoporosis and, 863–864
  mechanical, 841–843
  mechanical etiology of, 121–123, 273, 838–839
  medical causes of, 42, 49, 273, 274–275, 838
  medication used for; see Medication(s)
  motor vehicle accidents and, 60
  nonspecific, 47–50, 370–372
  Paget's disease and, 1722–1724
  psychogenic origin of, 113–114
  radiculopathy and, 45
  severely disabling, 47
  sexual history and, 58
  single-fiber electromyography (SFEMG) and, 199
  skin markers and, 129–131
  specific, 372–373
  spinal manipulative therapy (SMT) for, 445–446
  substance-abuse disorder and, 47–48, 58
  sympathetic mechanisms and, 111–113

Low-back pain (LBP),—cont'd
  systemic medical illness as cause of, 273
  treatment for, illustrated, 32, 33
  workers' compensation patients and, 28–33
  see also Pain
Low-back pain disability
  chronic
    assessment and treatment implications of, 542–544
    psychiatric illness and, 542
    psychosocial concomitants of, 542
  physical and mental deconditioning model of, 540–541
Low-back strain, 645–646
LTO (long term opioid), 516–518
Lumbago, 91
Lumbar curve patterns, 1581
Lumbar disc puncture, 226–229
  illustrated, 227, 228, 229
Lumbar discography, 220–225
  grading system for, illustrated, 230
  illustrated, 230
Lumbar epidural steroids, 323–324
  preparations for injections of, 325
  techniques for use of, 330–331
Lumbar fusion
  arthroscopic; see Arthroscopic lumbar interbody fusion
  bilateral lateral, implantation of stimulation device in,
      1299–1300
  interbody
    anterior; see Anterior lumbar interbody fusion
    posterior; see Posterior lumbar interbody fusion
Lumbar humps, 1579, 1581
Lumbar medial branch blocks, 304–305
  illustrated, 304, 305
Lumbar osteotomy, 1673–1675
Lumbar pathoanatomy, approaches to, 1250–1265
Lumbar resection-extension osteotomy, 1675–1682
Lumbar scoliosis
  illustrated, 1583
  management of, 1245
Lumbar spinal stenoses, 1084–1099
Lumbar spine
  anatomy of, 143
  case studies on, 131–133
  clinical biomechanics of, 837–846
  development of, 793
  discography and, 220–222
  disorders of
    ergonomic intervention and, 472–485
    mechanical etiology of, 121–123
    taking and interpreting history of, 52–70
      family history and, 61
      motor vehicle accidents and, 60
      past medical history and, 61–67
      review of symptoms (ROS) in, 57–58
      vocational history and, 59–60, 67–69
  function of, 810
  imaging of, 143, 144–146, 153–157
  inaccessible zone in; see Inaccessible zone
  injuries to; see Spine injury(ies); Thoracolumbar spine
      fracture(s)
  innervation of, illustrated, 85
  internal fixation of; see Internal fixation
  kyphotic deformities of; see Lumbar kyphosis
  motion of, database for, 126–129
  pain analysis and, 124
  spinal manipulative therapy (SMT) and, 445–446
  stabilization exercises for, 1738–1745
  structural degenerative cascade and, 9–16
  surgical treatment of; see Lumbar spine surgery

Lumbar spine surgery
  anterior
    history of, 1234
    indications for, 1234–1235
    instrumentation in, 1233–1249
    technique in, 1235–1237
    see also Anterior lumbar interbody fusion
  arthroscopic microdisectomy as; see Arthroscopic microdisectomy
  automated percutaneous discectomy as; see Automated percuta-
      neous lumbar discectomy
  chemonucleolysis as; see Chemonucleolysis
  clinical biomechanics of, 837–846
  decompression of soft tissue in, 1251–1260
  extension versus flexion of during, 953
  fusion as; see Lumbar fusion
  historical review of, 838
  inaccessible zone in; see Inaccessible zone
  internal fixation in; see Internal fixation
  for kyphotic deformities of the lumbar spine, 1668–1682
  laparoscopic techniques in, 1263–1264
  minimally invasive, 990–1073
  open, 1074–1304
  paralateral approach to, 1261–1263
    illustrated, 1262
    prone-sitting frame for, illustrated, 1263
  positioning patient for; see Operative position
  posterior
    instrumented, 1173–1195
    see also Posterior lumbar interbody fusion
  procedures in, 841–845, 1299–1300
  stereotactical techniques in, 1264
  treatment of spinal tumors and, 1481–1482
  see also Fusion; Spine surgery
Lumbar transforaminal steroids, 331–333
Lumbar vertebra(ae), 814
  illustrated, 814
Lumbar zygapophyseal joint block(s), 299
Lumbosacral curve, illustrated, 1561
Lumbosacral spine, internal fixation of, 844–845
Lumbosacral-junction fixation, 1166–1168
Lunges
  backward, illustrated, 1745
  forward, illustrated, 1744
Luque rectangle, 844, 1399, 1481, 1643, 1675
  illustrated, 1636
Luque rods, 782, 844, 1481
  with Galveston technique, 1168, 1620
    illustrated, 1169
  Wiltse system versus, 1187
Luque segmental fixation, 1635–1636, 1639
  illustrated, 1636, 1640, 1641
Luque system, 1593, 1613
Luque wires, 782, 1197, 1198
Luschka
  joints of; see Joint(s) of Luschka
  nerve of; see Sinovertebral nerve
Lymphoma, malignant, illustrated, 1461, 1463
Lytic spondylolisthesis; see Isthmic spondylolisthesis

M
Macelroy retractor, 960
Machida Medical Instrument Company, 1070
MacNab, Ian, 1069
Magerl's posterior screw fixation, 782, 1345, 1503
Magnetic resonance imaging (MRI), 141–142
  of anterior interbody fusion, illustrated, 161
  of arachnoiditis, 164, 167
    illustrated, 167, 168

Magnetic resonance imaging (MRI),—cont'd
  arthroscopic microdiscectomy preoperative planning and, 1004
  assessing cervical deformities with Cervical deformity(ies), 1634
  of central canal stenosis, 158
    illustrated, 156, 158
  of cervical cord astrocytoma, 172
  of cervical spine, 142–143
  of compression fracture, illustrated, 181
  congenital scoliosis evaluated with, 1565–1566
  of developmental lumbar stenosis, 153, 155
    illustrated, 154
  of disc degeneration, 144, 147–151
    illustrated, 147
  of disc extrusion, 149, 151, 153
    illustrated, 148
  of disc herniation, 149–150, 164
    illustrated, 147, 166
  of disc protrusion, 149, 164
    illustrated, 147, 152
  of disc sequestration, 149, 151
    illustrated, 150
  of discitis, 169, 171
    illustrated, 170, 176–177
  discography versus, 221, 234–235
  of dural tear, 171
  early detection of vertebral osteomyelitis with, 1547
  of epidural abscess, 178–179
    illustrated, 178
  of epidural hematoma, 184
    illustrated, 183
  of hemorrhagic metastatic lung carcinoma, 174
  infectious myelitis found with, 179
  leg pain evaluated with, 273
  of lumbar spine, 143
  lumbar stenosis evaluated with, 152–153
  of metastatic lesions, 175, 273
  of neural foraminal stenosis, illustrated, 157, 159
  osteomyelitis detected with, 176–178
    vertebral, illustrated, 1547–1548
  of posterior element fracture, 181
  of postoperative fibrosis with seroma, 165
  of postoperative granulation tissue, illustrated, 163
  of postoperative spine, 160–161, 167, 169, 171
    illustrated, 163, 165–167, 168, 170
  of postoperative stenosis, 164
  posttraumatic myelomalacia evaluated with, illustrated, 183
  preoperative evaluation with, 1032, 1139
  preoperative preparation and, 1032
  of pseudomeningocele, 171
  pyogenic infection detected with, 176
  radiologists and, 268
  spinal cord evaluated with, illustrated, 182
  spinal fusion and, 168
  of spinal infection, 175–179
  spinal stenosis diagnosed with, 1085
  spinal-cord injuries determined with, 1532–1533
  spine trauma diagnosis with, 180–182, 180–184, 184
  of spine tumors, 171–175
    illustrated, 172, 173–174
    surgery on, 1458
  spondylolisthesis detected with, 160
  spondylolysis detected with, 159–160
  of thoracic neurofibroma, 173
  of thoracic spine, 143
  titanium versus stainless steel and, 1226
  tuberculous spondylitis detected with, 178
  of vertebral body fracture, illustrated, 180
  workers' compensation injury testing and, 241–242
  see also Radiography

Malignancy; see Cancer
Malingering, 543
Mallampati classification, 941
Mamillary process, 814
Manipulable lesion(s), 438–440
  theoretical pathomechanics of, 439
Manipulation; see Spinal manipulative therapy
Mann-Whitney U test, 1447
Manual therapy (MT)
  assessment in, 464–467
    case study to illustrate, 464–466
  clinical trial related to, 452–453
  examination process in, 453–464
  in spinal rehabilitation, 451–470
  treatment with, 467–468
  see also Spinal manipulative therapy
Manuel de Orthopedie Vertebrale, 783
Marcaine, 1040
Marcus Aurelius, 774
Martial arts, 687–710
  aspects of that are healthful to spine, 693–697
  calisthenics in, 701
  defined, 688
  practices in, that may be hazardous to spine, 697–708
  spine principles relevant to, 688–692
MAST questionnaire, 975
Maximal voluntary contraction (MVC), 387
Maximum manual muscle test (MMT), 609
Maximum medical improvement (MMI), 492
Mayfield headrest, 1360, 1396
  "horseshoe," 1620
  pinholder, 1384
MBF; see Muscle blood flow
McCoy Incomplete Sentences, 918, 922
McCulloch, John, 1000
McCulloch retractor system, 1034
McGill Pain Questionnaire (MPQ), 55–56, 363–364
  SCS and, 575, 592, 595
    illustrated, 595
MDMP (Multimodal Disability Management Program), 544–545
Mechanical low-back pain, 841–843
Mechanical pain, medical spinal pain versus, 273
Median atlantoaxial joint, 814
Medical evaluation, 272–280
  review of systems in, 273–274
  specialized testing in, 275–277
Medical management
  arthritis and, 353
  of failed spine surgery, 1245, 1247
  of iatrogenic flat-back deformity, 1245
  of lumbar scoliosis, 1245
  of osteoporosis; see Osteoporosis, management of
  of pain; see Pain management
  of postoperative pain, 978
  posttraumatic kyphosis and, 1244–1245
  of spinal cord-injured patients, 1529–1541
  of spine pathology, 348–350
Medical Record, 1068
Medical specialist, workers' compensation injuries and, 29–30
Medical spinal pain, mechanical pain versus, 273
Medical-legal situations, electrophysiologic testing and, 200
Medicare
  audits by, 1749, 1751
  fee schedules of; see Billing
Medication(s)
  antiinflammatory; see Nonsteroidal antiinflammatory drugs (NSAIDs)
  excessive reliance on, 261
  intraoperative, 1032

Medication(s),—cont'd
  management of osteoporosis with, 856, 858–862
  for pain of spinal origin, 509–527
    categories of, 510
    dosing intervals in use of, 511
    selection of, 511
  see also Chemical(s); Drugs; Steroid(s)
Meditation, 262–263
Medtronic Pices Quad leads, illustrated, 578
Medtronic Pices Quad Plus leads, illustrated, 578, 579
Medtronic Resume electrode, 577
Medtronic Resume lead, 579
  illustrated, 580
Medtronic Synchromed infusion pump, illustrated, 600, 601
Med-X, 489
Melzac, Ronald, 500, 506, 574, 917
Membrane
  atlantooccipital, 821
  tectorial, 818
Mendelson, George, 504
Meningomyelocele, paralytic scoliosis associated with, illustrated, 1600–1601
Menopause
  bone mineral density (BMD) and, 849, 855
  osteoporosis and, 848, 849
Mental deconditioning, 538–539
  model of, 540–541
    illustrated, 541
Mersilene tapes, 1601
Mesmer, Franz, 566–567
Metabolism
  of bones, bone markers for, 286–289
  use of chymopapain and, 994
Metastatic bone tumors, 1458, 1460
Metastatic disease
  imaging of, 172, 174, 175, 273
  low-back pain and, 49
  PMMA as preferred supplement to fixation in, 1480–1481
  spinal tumors and, 1458, 1460, 1463, 1465
  see also Cancer
Methylmethacrylate cement, 886–887, 1641; see alsp Polymethyl-methacrylate
Meyerding retractor, 1275
Microdiscectomy
  anterior laparoscopic, "report card" on, 1081
  arthroscopic; see Arthroscopic microdisectomy
  defined, 1081
  illustrated, 1254–1256
  "report card" on, 1081
  see also Microsurgical discectomy; Microsurgery
Microlumbar discectomy, 1029
Microscope, operating; see Operating microscope
Microsurgery
  future predictions regarding, 1044
  local anesthesia and, 1040
  outpatient, 1040
  postoperative management in, 1040
  potential complications of, 1041–1042
  principles of, 1031
  results of, 1042–1044
  technique of, 1032–1041
    operative, 1036–1040
    "standard" techniques versus, 1029–1031
Microsurgical discectomy
  arthroscopic; see Arthroscopic microsurgical discectomy
  defined, 1081
  future predictions regarding, 1044
  history of, 775–776, 1029
  indications for, 1029

Microsurgical discectomy,—cont'd
  local anesthesia and, 1040
  outpatient, 1040
  postoperative management in, 1040
  potential complications of, 1041–1042
  "report card" on, 1081
  results of, 1042–1044
  and spinal decompression, 1028–1045
  technique of, 1032–1041
    operative, 1036–1040
    "standard" techniques versus, 1029–1031
  see also Microdiscectomy; Microsurgery
Midas Rex Company, The, 1037
Midas Rex drill, 1037
Middleton, George, 774, 785, 1047
Midline posterior decompression, 1272–1273
  illustrated, 1273
  stability and, 1287
MIL (Million Questionnaire), 363
Million Questionnaire (MIL), 363
Milwaukee brace, 1566, 1610
  illustrated, 1585
Minerva brace, 1388
Minimally invasive spine care, 1077–1082
  criteria to compare procedures in, 1078, 1079
  report card rating system of, 1078–1080
  spectrum of, summarized, 1078
Minimally invasive surgery of the spine, 990–1084
Minnesota Department of Labor and Industry, 240
Minnesota Multiphasic Personality Inventory (MMPI), 54, 80, 262, 538–539
  description of, 926–927
  preoperative patient assessment with, 965
  profile of, illustrated, 539, 928, 931
  SCS treatment and, 575
  surgical candidate evaluation with, 918, 921, 926, 1615
Mitchell, S. Weir, 506–507
Mithramycin
  treatment of Paget's disease with, 1726, 1730
  treatment of spinal stenosis with, 1730
Mixter, Jason, 775, 783, 785
MMI (maximum medical improvement), 492
MMPI; see Minnesota Multiphasic Personality Inventory
MMT (maximum manual muscle test), 609
Modulock system, 1244, 1520
Moire photography, 1583
Mood disorders, DSM-III-R classifications of, 924
Morbidity, patients proposed for anterior lumbar fusion and, 1140–1144
Morphine pump
  illustrated, 600, 601
  pain control with, 599–606
  problems with, 605
  see also Spinally administered narcotic (SAN) infusion therapy
Morquio's syndrome, 942
Morscher screws, 1418
"Motion cascade," 729
  illustrated, 730
Motion segment(s)
  anatomy of, 9–10
    illustrated, 9, 10
  arterial supply of, illustrated, 11
  buckling responses of, 439
  cervical, lumbar motion segments versus, 793–795
  degeneration of, illustrated, 21
  development and growth of, 793–795
  innervation of, 11
    illustrated, 11
  lumbar, cervical motion segments versus, 793–795

Motion segment(s),—cont'd
  neuroanatomic definition of, illustrated, 88
  progressive degeneration of, 14–15
  spinal, defined, 839
  venous drainage of, illustrated, 12
Motor evoked potential (MEP), 205, 212–214
  anatomic and physiologic basis of, 213
  indications to, 214
  stimulation techniques in, 213
Motor examination, conduct of during physical examination, 74–76
Motor Index Score, 1512
Motor unit action potential (MUAP)
  changes in parameters of, 193
  in nerve-conduction studies, 194
Motor vehicle accidents (MVA), spine injury in, 57, 60
Movement science skills, 251
Movement testing, 457–458
MPQ; see McGill Pain Questionnaire
MRI; see Magnetic resonance imaging
MUAP; see Motor unit action potential
Muller, Fredrick, 747
Multidisciplinary behavioral medicine models, 931, 936
Multidisciplinary evaluation, 265–271
  defined, 265
  team for, 265–269
Multidisciplinary program
  composition of, 266–269
  defined, 266
  education and, 270–271
  establishment of, 269–270
  for treatment of chronic pain, 936–937
Multifidus muscle, 827–828, 1332
Multimodal Disability Management Program (MDMP), 544–545
Multiple hemivertebra, illustrated, 1557
Multiple myeloma, 1459
Multiple pterygium syndrome, 1565
Multiple Tasks Obstacle Course, 488, 490
Multiple thoracic anomalies, illustrated, 1564
Muscle(s)
  anterior scalene, 1331
  blood flow in; see Muscle blood flow
  of cervical spine; see Cervical spine, musculature of
  clinical testing of, 75
  contraction of, 378–379
  contracture of, as complication of spinal-cord injury, 1535
  contusion of, 628–629
  disease of, as cause of kyphotic deformity in ankylosing spondylitis, 1713–1718
  endurance of, measurement of, 534–535
  energy metabolism and, 380–382
  fibers of, 379–380
  iliocostalis, 829, 1332
  infrahyoid (strap), 1332
  interscapular, exercises for strengthening of, 435
  interspinal, 1332
  length of, evaluation of, 463–464
  longissimus, 829, 1332
  multifidus, 827–828, 1332
  overwork of, 389
  postvertebral, 827–830
  potential force generation by, illustrated, 377
  prevertebral, 827
  rectus capitis
    anterior, 1331
    posterior, 1332
  role of, in lifting, 118
  semispinalis, 828
  semispinalis cervicis, 1332
  shoulder girdle, exercises for strengthening of, 434

Muscle(s),—cont'd
  skeletal, 376–380
  splenius, 829–830, 1332
  sternocleidomastoid, 1331
  strain of, 628–629, 1442
  strap (infrahyoid), 1332
  strength of; see Muscle strength
  suboccipital, 1332
  unisegmental, 826
  upper trapezius, 1332
  upper-extremity, 435
  used in baseball hitting, 609–614
  used in baseball pitching, 614–620
  of vertebral column, 826–830
Muscle balance in figure skating, 655, 656–658
Muscle blood flow (MBF), 383
  exercise and, 383, 386–387
Muscle flexibility in figure skating, 655–658
Muscle relaxants, 519–520
  commonly used, 519
Muscle strength
  evaluation of, 463–464
  grading of, 74
  increasing, 406, 435
MVA (motor vehicle accidents), spine injury in, 57, 60
MVC (maximal voluntary contraction), 387
Mycobacterium tuberculosis, 1549
Myeloradiculopathy with degenerative cervical kyphosis, 1638–1639
Myeloscopy
  degenerative spondylolisthesis and spinal stenosis evaluated with, 1279
    illustrated, 1280
  equipment used in, 1070–1072
  evaluation of congenital scoliosis with, 1565–1566
  historical aspects of, 1068–1070
  preoperative evaluation with, 1139
  technique used in, 1070–1072
Myofacial strain, 756
Myopathic scoliosis, 1613
Myotomes, 833–835
  defined, 833–834
  illustrated, 835

N
NASS; see North American Spine Society
National Back Injury Network, 252
  guidelines for acute conservative care developed by, 369–370
  solution to socioeconomic cascade and, 31
National Collegiate Athletic Association (NCAA), 668, 669, 1447
National Council Against Health Fraud (NCAHF), 565
National Federation of State High Schools (NFSHSA), 669
National Football Head and Neck Injury Register, 669, 1442, 1443, 1444, 1445
National Football League (NFL)
  injuries in, 670
  Management Council of, 671
National Health and Medical Research Council of Australia, report on epidural steroids commissioned by, 340
National Institute of Occupational Safety and Health (NIOSH)
  ergonomic intervention and, 473
  lifting test guidelines of, 534
National Institutes of Health (NIH), 848
National Operating Committee on Standards for Athletic Equipment (NOCSAE), 668, 670, 1438, 1442
National Osteoporosis Foundation, 848
Nautilus, 245
NCAA (National Collegiate Athletic Association), 668, 669, 1447
NCV; see Nerve condition velocity

Neck
    "high jumper's," 1446
    injuries of, in wrestling, 765–767
    pain in; see Neck pain
    triangles of, illustrated, 1340
Neck pain (NP)
    defined, 529
    diagnosis of, 1352–1354
    generators of, 1353
    nonradicular nonmyelopathic, 1354
    Paget's disease and, 1723–1724
    see also Cervical disc disease
Neck strain in dancers, 647
Needle(s)
    Crawford, 330
    Tuohy, 330
Needle EMG, 195–198
    findings of for specific radiculopathies, 197
Neoplastic conditions, treatment of, 1247–1248
Nerve(s)
    afferent, primary, 24
    injuries to; see Nerve injuries
    of Luschka; see Sinovertebral nerve
    peripheral; see Peripheral nerve(s)
    "pinched," 1449
    sinovertebral (SVN); see Sinovertebral nerve
    spinal; see Spinal nerves
    third occipital, diagnostic block of, 309
    tissue of, use of chymopapain and, 994
    "vertebral," 833
    of vertebral column, 830–835
Nerve condition velocity (NCV)
    motor evoked potential (MEP) studies versus, 205
    somatosensory evoked potential (SEP) studies versus, 205
Nerve injuries
    bone grafts and, 876–877
    as complication fixation device use, 1248
    electrophysiologic testing and, 200
Nerve lesions, electrophysiologic testing and, 200
Nerve root(s), 92–94
    anatomy of, 192–193
        illustrated, 192
    compression of, 92–94, 193
        neurophysiologic changes after, 92
    injection of, illustrated, 1354
    injury to, 1108
        as complication specific to posterior lumbar interbody fusion,
            1106
    mechanical pressure on, effect of on selection of disc surgery,
        985–986
    spinal cord and, 830
    tension signs and, 76–77
Nerve-conduction studies, 194
Nerve-conduction velocity (NCV), examination in radiculopathy with,
    209, 210
Nerve-tension sensitivity in martial arts, 704–705
Neural foramina, 143
Neural injury, as complication of fixation device use, 1177, 1248
Neural processes, 796
Neural tube, 796
Neurobiologic Mechanisms in Manipulative Therapy, 453
Neurocentral fusion, 804
Neurocentral joints, 1352
Neurofibramatosis, scoliosis in, 1606–1610
    classification of, 1606, 1608
    etiology and natural history of, 1606
    illustrated, 1606, 1607, 1608, 1609, 1610
    radiographic evaluation of, 1609–1610
    treatment of, 1610

Neurofibroma, imaging of, 172, 173
Neuroleptic drugs, for pain of spinal origin, 524
Neurologic deficit
    postoperative, 1041
    surgical timing and, 911
Neurologic injury, 1513
Neurologic status, Frankel classification of, 1512–1513, 1521, 1525
Neuromuscular scoliosis; see Paralytic scoliosis
Neuromyopathic flexion deformity, 1643
Neuron(s)
    low-back, illustrated, 112
    spinal; see Spinal neuron(s)
Neuronal plasticity, 109–111
Neuropathic pain, defined, 24
Neuropeptides, in dorsal root ganglion, 96
Neuropraxia
    brachial plexus, 1449–1450
    of cervical cord with transient quadriplegia, 1446–1449
Neurosurgical procedures
    ablative; see Ablative procedures
    anatomic; see Anatomic procedures
    augmentative; see Augmentative procedures
    to relieve chronic pain, 584–590
Neutral spine
    in dance, 645
    defined, 396
    illustrated, 397, 1739
    stabilization training and, 396–398, 1739
New England Journal of Medicine, 775, 1513
    NASCIS II study in, 1487
New England Surgical Society, 775
New Zealand Report, objective assessment of chiropractic by, 438
Newton's law(s)
    first, human locomotion and, 120
    third, Jefferson fractures and, 1314
NFL; see National Football League
NFSHSA (National Federation of State High Schools), 669
NIH (National Institutes of Health), 848
NIOSH; see National Institute of Occupational Safety and Health
Nociceptive-specific (NS) spinal neurons, 109
Nociceptor(s)
    defined, 24, 539–540
    reflex activation of, 92
NOCSAE (National Operating Committee on Standards for Athletic
            Equipment), 668, 670, 1438, 1442
Node(s)
    Hensen, 796
    Schmorl; see Schmorl nodes
Nonradicular nonmyelopathic neck pain, 1354
Nonspecific low-back pain, 47–50, 370–372
Nonsteroidal antiinflammatory drugs (NSAIDs)
    bicycling and, 639
    dosing suggestions for, 513
    dyspepsia occurrence with use of, 514
    as first choice of medication, 511
    history of ulcers and, 58
    inflammation reduced by, 510
    isthmic spondylolisthesis and, 1283
    as peripherally acting analgesic, 512–516
    postoperative pain management and, 978
    preoperative use of, 966, 967, 1253
    side effects of, 514–516
    spinal manipulative therapy (SMT) and, 444
    treatment for acute anulus tear with, 42
    treatment for adult scoliosis with, 1616
    treatment for herniated nucleus pulposus with, 44
    treatment for low-back pain with, 348, 355
    treatment of sprains with, 1442
    use of, summarized, 516

Nontranspedicular screw fixation systems, 1175–1176
Norfolk frame, 955
Normal flexion/recovery from flexion, spinal coordination and, 126–128, 130
Normal lateral bend, spinal coordination and, 128–129
North American Journal of Medicine and Surgery, 774
North American Spine Society (NASS)
    Back Pain Questionnaire of
        on Baseline Medical Employment History, and Work Status, 67–69
        on Baseline Medical History, Expectations and Outcomes, 61–67, 360, 364
    continuing education and format for presentation of research findings provided by, 271
    Executive Committee of, position statement of, on discography, 221
    national low-back educational program recommended by, 353
    Outcome Committee of, Oswestry Low Back Pain Questionnaire (OSW) revised by, 362
    quantification of pain and, 56
Notochord, 796
NP; *see* Neck pain
NRS (Numerical Rating Scale) 11 or 101, 55, 364
NS (nociceptive-specific) spinal neurons, 109
NSAIDs; *see* Nonsteroidal antiinflammatory drugs
Nuclear medicine imaging of the spine; *see* Bone scan(s)
Nucleus pulposus, 143, 799, 800, 839, 840–841, 1324
    herniated; *see* Herniated nucleus pulposus
    illustrated, 13, 1324, 1325
Numerical Rating Scale (NRS) 11 or 101, 55, 364
Nuprin Pain Report, 503
Nurse practitioner, as part of multidisciplinary program, 268

O

Objective functional testing, 246–248
OBLA (onset of blood lactate), 385
Oblique wiring fusion technique, 1407–1408
    illustrated, 1409
Occipital condyle fracture, 1493
    illustrated, 1494
Occipitoatlantal dislocations, 1490
Occipitoatlantal fusion, 1397–1399
    illustrated, 1397, 1398, 1399
Occipitocervical fusion, illustrated, 1397, 1398
Occiput
    atlas, axis and, 1312–1320
    prenatal development of, 1310
Occult fractures, as cause of kyphotic deformity, 1698
Occupational Safety and Health Administration (OSHA), 473
Occupational therapy, work hardening in, 490
Odontoid, resection of, 1342–1344
Odontoid fractures, 1495
    illustrated, 1496
Odontoid hypoplasia, 940
Odontoid process, 813
    congenital abnormalities and, 1311
Odontoid screw fixation, 1433
Olympus Camera Company, 1070
OMPT; *see* Orthopedic manual physical therapist
Onik, Gary, 1023, 1048, 1053, 1070
Onset of blood lactate (OBLA), 385
Open discectomy, automated percutaneous lumbar discectomy versus, 1022
Operant behavioral model of pain, 548–549, 917
Operating microscope(s)
    advantages of, 1029–1031, 1257–1258

Operating microscope(s),—cont'd
    disadvantages of, 1031
    first use of, 775
    illustrated, 1030, 1031
    inexperience using, 1041
    Zeiss; *see* Zeiss operating microscope
Operative position, 947, 950–963, 1032
    access to operative field and, 951
    anesthesia access and, 947, 952
    blood loss and, 951–952
    extension versus flexion of lumbar spine and, 953
    positioning techniques for, 953–962, 1620, 1621, 1624–1625
    protection of peripheral nerves and, 952
    protection of pressure points and, 952–953
    radiograph access and, 952
Opioids
    as centrally acting analgesics, 516–518
    intraspinal, 518
    long term (LTO), 516–518
        chronic pain of nonmalignant origin and, 517–518
        use of, 519
OPLL; *see* Ossification of the posterior longitudinal ligament
Opportunity, psychologic cascade and, 39
Optifuse; *see* Ray Threaded Fusion Cage
Oral corticosteroids
    treatment for herniated nucleus pulposus with, 44
    treatment of acute anulus tear with, 42
    see also Steroid(s)
Orozco H plate design, 1429
Orthopedic manual physical therapist (OMPT)
    palpation of spine by, 460–463
    role of, 452
    see also Manual therapy
Orthopedic Systems, Inc., 960, 962, 1032
Orthotics
    as adjunct to independent living, 1538
    treatment of congenital deformity with, 1566
Os odontoideum, surgical approach to, illustrated, 1348
OSHA (Occupational Safety and Health Administration), 473
Osseous homeostasis, 282–285
Ossification
    heterotopic, as complication of spinal-cord injury, 1537
    of the posterior longitudinal ligament (OPLL), 158, 784, 1363, 1369
        illustrated, 1375
        laminaplasty for, 1383
Osteoblastic cells, 284
Osteoblastoma, 1458–1459
Osteocalcin, 287–288
Osteochondromas, 1458
Osteoclasts, 284–285
Osteogenesis, 885
Osteoid osteoma, 1458–1459
Osteomalacia, 285
Osteometabolic bone disease
    assessment of, 281–296
    laboratory investigation of, 286–294
Osteomyelitis, vertebral; *see* Pyogenic vertebral osteomyelitis
Osteopaths, as part of multidisciplinary program, 268
Osteopenia, 285–286
Osteoporosis, 847–869
    biomechanics of, 850–851
    bone mass reduction in, 849–850
    classification and etiology of, 848–849
    clinical presentation of, 851
    decay of skeleton in, 849
    defined, 285, 848
    high turnover, 286
    laboratory assessment of, 851–855

Osteoporosis,—cont'd
    magnitude of the problem of, 848
    management of, 855–864
        algorithm for, 857
        prevention of bone loss and, 856–862
    management of back pain and, 863–864
    model of pain in, illustrated, 851
    origin and severity of, algorithm to determine, 852
    pathology of, 850
    risk factors for, 849
    surgical treatment for, 862–863
Osteosarcoma, 1459
Osteosynthesis of the dens, 1402–1403
Osteotomy
    cervical; see Cervical osteotomy
    lumbar, 1673–1675
    lumbar resection-extension, 1675–1682
OSW (Oswestry Low Back Pain Questionnaire), 247, 362
Oswestry curette, 1119
    illustrated, 1119
Oswestry Low Back Pain Questionnaire (OSW), 247, 362
Ottolenghi, Carlos, 1072
Outcome
    assessment of
        instruments for, 361–363
        problems with, 360–361
    monitoring of, 444
    studies of, evaluation of, 359–366
Overtraining, 389–390
Oxygen consumption, exercise and, 384–385
    illustrated, 383, 384

P

PACT (performance assessment and capacity test), 247
PAD (purified protein derivative), 647
Paget's disease, 276, 278, 285, 286, 287–288, 289, 290, 1720–1737
    defined, 1723
    etiology of, 1721
    histopathology of, 1721
    illustrated, 1722, 1723, 1724, 1725, 1727, 1733
    malignant transformation and, 1726
    osteosarcoma and, 1459
    prevalence and distribution of, 1721–1722
    rheumatic and arthritic conditions in, 1726
    spinal stenosis and, 1722–1723, 1724–1726, 1730–1734
    treatment of
        algorithmic approach to, 1734
        with drugs, 859, 1726–1730, 1734–1735
        with surgery, 1731–1734
Pain
    acupuncture and, 565
    acute, 114
        chronic versus, 510–511
    analysis of, 124
    applied neurophysiology of, 23–26
    avoidance of, 487
    back
        bicycling and, 636
        management of, osteoporosis and, 863–864
        Paget's disease and, 1722–1724
        steroid use and, 327–328
        see also Low-back pain
    biocultural model of, 496–508
    biofeedback and, 565, 566
    biomechanics of, 56–57
    biophysical conceptualizations of, 539–540
        illustrated, 540
    at bone graft donor-site, 877–878

Pain,—cont'd
    cancer; see Cancer
    Cartesian principles and, 498, 499
    cervical, 16–17
    change in, evaluation of, 363–365
    chronic; see Chronic pain
    culture and, 505–507
    defined, 78, 501, 540
    definitions and explanations of essential terms regarding, 23–24
    dermatomal, 273
    "disc," 85
    exacerbation of, as side effect of steroid use, 336
    excessive pain behavior and, 261
    in facet joints, 90
    gate control theory of, 500, 549, 574
    indications for electrophysiologic testing and, 199–200
    inflammatory agents and, 988
    inguinal, 1124
    leg; see Leg pain
    location of, 53–55
    low-back; see Low-back pain
    management of; see Pain management
    meaning of, 496–508
    medical spinal, mechanical versus, 273
    medication used for; see Medication(s)
    models of, 917
    modulation of, 92–99
    multiple voices of, 504–505
    neck; see Neck pain
    neuropathic, 24
    onset of, 57
    osteoporosis and, 851
    pathways of, 92–99
    pattern of, 273
    persistent, 114
    postoperative, 975–978
    psychologic aspects of, 58–59
    psychologic conceptualizations of, 547
    psychologic factors and, 47–48
    quality of, 56
    quantification of, 55–56, 363–365
    radicular, 273
        steroid use and, 327
    referred; see Referred pain
    reproduction of, illustrated, 441
    role of c-fos protooncogene and, 98–99
    sclerotomal, 273
    sensitization and; see Sensitization
    sympathetically maintained, 575
    theories of, 917
    transcutaneous electrical nerve stimulation and, 565
    transduction of, chemicals involved in, 24–25
        summarized, 25
    undertreatment of, 497
    vocational history and, 59–60
    ways of understanding, 498
    "working through," 543
Pain and Impairment Relationship Scale (PAIRS), 504
Pain as Human Experience: An Anthropological Perspective, 502
Pain avoidance, 487
Pain behavior(s), 548
    defined, 540
Pain Beliefs Questionnaire, 504
Pain control
    morphine pump used for, 599–606
    see also Pain management
Pain drawing, 364
    Dallas; see Dallas Pain Drawing
    illustrated, 596, 929, 932, 935

Pain management
    back pain and, 863–864
    by electrical implant, 573–583, 591–598
    postoperative, 975–978
    spinal cord-injured patient and, 1536
    see also Pain control
Pain Rating Index (PRI), 55, 363
"Pain-prone personalities," 6
PAIRS (Pain and Impairment Relationship Scale), 504
PAIVM; see Passive accessory intervertebral movement
Palpation of the spine, 78–79, 460–463
Pamidronate 3-amino-1 hydroxypropylidene-1, 1 bisphosphonate
        (APD)(AHPrBP), treatment of Paget's disease with, 1727,
        1728–1729
Paralateral decompression, "report card" on, 1082
Paralytic curves, 1627
Paralytic disorders, classification of, 1593
Paralytic scoliosis, 1593–1602, 1613
    comprehensive care and, 1598
    illustrated, 1594, 1595, 1596–1598, 1599, 1600–1601
    natural history of, 1593–1598
    physical examination of patient with, 1598
        illustrated, 1599
    treatment of, 1600–1602
Paraplegia
    paralytic scoliosis due to, illustrated, 1594
    see also Spinal-cord injury(ies)
Paraspinal decompression, "report card" on, 1082
Paratenon, as barrier material, 905
Parathyroid hormone (PTH), 284, 285, 290
    osteoporosis management and, 861
Paraxial mesoderm, 796
Parkinson's disease, 1643
Pars interarticularis
    of the axis, 1315–1316
    defects involving; see Spondylolysis
    repair of, 1288–1289
Partial sit-up (PSU), 407–410
    illustrated, 1741
Pascal's law, 1324
Passive accessory intervertebral movement (PAIVM), 462
    illustrated, 462, 463
Passive physiologic intervertebral movements (PPIVMs), 462–463
    illustrated, 463
Passive range of motion (PROM), 532
Past medical history, lumbar spine disorders and, 61–67
Pasteur, Louis, 1544
Patellar dowel grafts, 1122
Pathologic (Type V) spondylolisthesis, 1282
Patient(s)
    with chronic pain; see Chronic pain
    cooperation of, 937
    education of; see Patient education
    expectations of
        as barrier to health education, 354
        surgical decision-making and, 912
    fees to; see Billing
    homework for, 554
    with injury to spinal cord; see Spinal cord-injured patient(s)
    multiple-trauma, spinal fractures in, 1525–1526
    with pain; see Pain
    with "pain-prone personalities," 6
    perioperative care of; see Perioperative care
    physical examination of; see Physical examination
    positioning of for spine surgery; see Operative position
    preoperative; see Preoperative patient(s)
    psychologic cascade and, 36–39, 495–606
    satisfaction of, evaluation of, 365
    smoking by; see Smoking

Patient(s),—cont'd
    socioeconomic cascade and, 27–34, 471–494
    with spine pain
        medical evaluation of, 272–280
        multidisciplinary evaluation of, 265–271
        psychiatric evaluation of, 259–264
        see also Pain
    with structural degenerative disease, 346–470
    as surgical candidates, assessment of, 918–936
    surgical decision-making and, 912
    with work-related injury; see Workers' compensation injury
Patient education, 270–271
    candidates for, 351
    cervicothoracic stabilization training and, 417
    in cognitive-behavioral concepts, 553
    goals for, 352
    physician guidelines for, 352
    as primary treatment of low-back pain, 347–358
Patient-controlled analgesia (PCA), 517
    order sheet for, illustrated, 977
    postoperative pain management and, 976–977
Paul of Agena, 774, 783
PCA; see Patient-controlled analgesia
"Peanut gauze" (Kittner), 1340, 1356
Pedicle(s), 811
    cervical, 142
    thoracic, 143
Pedicle awl, illustrated, 1191
Pedicle feeler, illustrated, 1191
Pedicle fixation, 1160–1162, 1163
Pedicle fractures of C2; see Hangman's fracture(s)
Pedicle tap, illustrated, 1191
Pelvis
    instability of, bone grafts and, 879–880
    instrumentation of, 1592
    motion of for range of loads, illustrated, 129
    strapping of in strength testing, 125
PEMF; see Pulsed electromagnetic field
Penfield dissector, 1037, 1399, 1407
Penfield elevator, 1384
Penrose drain, 1373, 1644
People in Pain, 502–503
People With Pain Speak Out, 505–506
PEP (Preoperative Evaluation Program), 933–936
Percutaneous discectomy
    automated; see Automated percutaneous lumbar discectomy
    history of, 776–777, 1018
    laser, 1022
    manual, automated percutaneous discectomy versus, 1021–1022
Perdriolle method, 1580, 1583
Performance assessment and capacity test (PACT), 247
Perfusion test, 290
Periannular structures, anatomic status of, effect of on selection of
        disc surgery, 986–987
Peridiscal ligaments, innervation of, 85–87
Perioperative care, 964–983
Peripheral circulation, exercise and, 383
Peripheral deafferentation conditions, SCS treatment for, 576
Peripheral nerve(s)
    injury to, SCS treatment for, 575
    protection of, positioning of patient during surgery and, 952
Peripheral-joint dysfunction, 729
Peripherally acting analgesics, 512–516
Persistent pain, 114
Persistent sensitization, 113
Pfannenstiel incision, 1624
    illustrated, 1625
Phenothiazines, for pain of spinal origin, 524
Philadelphia collar, 1344, 1409, 1430, 1493, 1495, 1643

Phychiatrist, as part of multidisciplinary program, 267
Physical capacity
    assessment of, 414–416
    defined, 488
    functional capacity versus, 533
    quantification of, 489
Physical examination, 71–81, 274–275, 455–460
    aims and goals of, 456
    analysis of subjective data/plan of, 456
    assessment after, 466–467
    detailed spinal motion and, 124
    inspection of patient during, 73–74
    movement testing in, 457–458
    neurologic examination and, 1512–1513
    observation of patient during, 72–73, 456–457
    on-field, in sports, 1438–1440
    possible sequence for, 72
    preoperative, by anesthesiologist, 941
    sensory examination during; see Sensory examination
    of spinal cord-injured patient, 1530–1532
    systemic examination during, 79
Physical therapist(s)
    orthopedic manual; see Orthopedic manual physical therapist
    as part of multidisciplinary program, 268
    role of in spinal function evaluation, 251
    teamwork between physician and, 251, 257
Physical therapy (PT)
    algorithmic methods of, 252–253
    diagnosis with, functional evaluations in, 253–257
    structural evaluation components and, 251, 252
    treatment with
        for acute anulus tear, 42–43
        in dance, 645–646
        for work-related injuries, 251, 252
    in work hardening, 490
Physician(s)
    expectations of, as barrier to health education, 354–355
    primary care, as part of multidisciplinary team, 266–267
    referring, education of, 270
    teamwork between physical therapist and, 251, 257
Physician assistant, as part of multidisciplinary program, 268
Physician extender, as part of multidisciplinary program, 268
PILE; see Progressive Isoinertial Lifting Evaluation
"Pinched nerve," 1449
"Pin-hole" stenosis, 1085
Pitchers, electromyographic analysis of torque transfer in, 614
Pituitary rongeur, 1418
Plain film, radiographic analysis and, 1546
Plate system(s), 1166–1168, 1236, 1237, 1239–1241, 1429–1433
    cervical spine fractures and, 1503, 1504
    illustrated, 1237, 1238, 1239, 1240, 1241, 1429, 1431, 1432
    see also specific devices
Plato, 506
PLD (primary laser discectomy), "report card" on, 1050–1051
Plicamycin; see Mithramycin
PLIF; see Posterior lumbar interbody fusion
PLT (progressive lifting capacity) test, 247
Plyometric muscle contraction, 378–379
PMMA; see Polymethylmethacrylate
PNF; see Proprioceptive neuromuscular facilitation
POF; see Position of optimal function
11-Point Box Scale (11-BS), 365
Poliomyelitis
    first attempts at spine surgery for, 779
    paralytic scoliosis due to, illustrated, 1594
POLT; see Position of optimal load tolerance
Polymethylmethacrylate (PMMA)
    reconstruction of spine with, 1461–1465, 1479–1483
        illustrated, 1466–1467, 1468, 1480

Polymethylmethacrylate (PMMA),—cont'd
    treatment of osteoporosis and, 862
    treatment of surgical complications with, 1624
    see also Methylmethacrylate cement; Spinal tumor surgery, techniques in
POOF; see Position of optimal function
Pool, J. Lawrence, 1068
"Poor man's" laser, 1256–1257
Poor posture, 414
    illustrated, 415, 416
Position of optimal function, 414, 655, 656, 658, 659, 660, 662
    cervicothoracic stabilization training and, 417, 422, 426
    illustrated, 415
Position of optimal load tolerance (POLT), 688, 697, 701, 707,
        708
    illustrated, 691, 701, 702, 703, 707
Posterior arch, 814
Posterior atlantoaxial screw fixation, 1403
    illustrated, 1405–1406
Posterior atlantooccipital membrane, 821
Posterior cervical interspinous fusion, 1396–1404, 1406–1414
    oblique wiring technique in; see Oblique wiring fusion technique
    Rogers technique in; see Rogers fusion technique
Posterior fusion with internal fixation, 1567, 1620–1623
Posterior in situ fusion, 1567
Posterior indirect reduction, 1521–1523
Posterior interbody fusion
    history of, 780
    lumbar; see Posterior lumbar interbody fusion
    morbidity criteria for, 1140
Posterior intraarticular blocks, 305–306
Posterior ligaments, 819–820
Posterior lumbar interbody fusion (PLIF), 1100–1111
    advantages of, 1103, 1224
    comparative options to, 1104
    complications of, 1108, 1176–1181
    disadvantages of, 1224–1225
    history of, 1101–1102
    indications for, 1102–1103
    instrumentation used with, 1173–1195
    morbidity criteria for, 1140–1141
    predictions regarding, 1108–1109
    results with, literary review of, 1108, 1109
    technique of, 1104–1106
        illustrated, 1105, 1106, 1107, 1108, 1109
Posterior plate fixation fusion technique, 1413
Posterior plating fusion technique, 1413–1414
Posterior spinal decompression, 843
Posterior-anterior (P-A) pressures, 462
    illustrated, 462
Posterolateral facet fusion
    Bohlman technique in, 1409
    Callahan technique in; see Callahan fusion technique
    Dewar technique in, 1413
    Garber-Meyer technique in, 1409
    posterior plate fixation technique in, 1413
    posterior plating technique in, 1413–1414
    triple-wire technique in; see Triple-wire fusion technique
Posterolateral fusion, morbidity criteria for, 1140
Postlaminectomy kyphosis, 1634–1638
    established deformity and, 1636–1637
    incidence of, 1634
    pathogenesis of, 1634–1635
    postoperative management and, 1638
    prevention of deformity and, 1635–1636
    surgical intervention and, 1636–1637
Postoperative complications, prevention of, 967–970
Postoperative fibrosis; see Fibrosis
Postoperative instability, as indication for cervical spine fusion, 1396

Postoperative neurologic deficit, 1041
Postoperative spine, imaging of, 160–171
Postoperative (Type VI) spondylolisthesis, 1282, 1293–1294
Postsympathectomy syndrome, as complication of lumbar fusion, 1124
Posttraumatic kyphosis
    management of, 1244–1245
    treatment of, 1514
        illustrated, 1246, 1516
Posttraumatic progressive myelopathy (PTPM), 182
Posture
    inspection of during physical examination, 73–74
    poor; see Poor posture
    reeducation regarding, 417–418
        illustrated, 418
Postvertebral muscles, 827–830
    illustrated, 827, 828, 829
Pott's disease, 779, 780, 1056, 1549
    anterior surgery and, 1234
    first attempts at surgery and, 779
Power lifting; see Weight lifting
PPIVMs; see Passive physiologic intervertebral movements
PPO (preferred provider organizations); see Billing
Preferred provider organizations (PPO); see Billing
Pregnancy
    as contraindication to treatment with chemonucleolysis, 996
    preoperative testing for, 966
Preoperative Evaluation Program (PEP), 933, 936
Preoperative patient(s)
    anesthesiologist's evaluation of, 940–942
    psychologic assessment of, 261, 918–936, 965
    testing of, 965–967, 1139–1140
Press-ups, performance of during physical examination, 80
Pressure points, protection of, positioning of patient during surgery and, 952–953
Prevertebral muscles, 827
Prevertebral space, 142–143
PRI (pain Rating Index), 55, 363
PRIDE (Productive Rehabilitation Institute of Dallas for Ergonomics), 395, 534, 539
Primary afferent nerves, 24
Primary care, defined, 487
Primary care physician, as part of multidisciplinary team, 266–267
Primary curves, 1580–1581
Primary laser discectomy (PLD), "report card" on, 1050–1051
Primtec Company, 1070
Principles of Morals and Legislation, 497
Process
    accessory, 814
    articular, 811
    mamillary, 814
    neural, 796
    odontoid, 813
    spinous, 811, 1316, 1322–1323
    transverse, 811
    uncinate, 812
Procollagen Type I, 288
Productive Rehabilitation Institute of Dallas for Ergonomics (PRIDE), 395, 534, 539
Progressive Isoinertial Lifting Evaluation (PILE), 246–247, 489, 534
    use of, illustrated, 535
Progressive lifting capacity (PLC) test, 247
Prolo functional-economic rating scale, 1043
PROM (passive range of motion), 532
Prone arm and leg lifts, illustrated, 1743
Prone knee bend, conduct of during physical examination, 77

Pronease frame, 958
Proprioceptive neuromuscular facilitation (PNF), 395
    techniques of, illustrated, 403
Prostrate specific antigen (PSA), 276–277
Provocation discography, 220, 235
PSA (prostrate specific antigen), 276–277
Pseudarthrosis
    anterior lumbar interbody fusion and, 1128, 1129
    as complication of internal fixation, 1180–1181, 1248
    as complication specific to posterior lumbar interbody fusion, 1108
    graft-related complications and, 1376
    smoking as cause of, 1301
Pseudoarthrosis; see Pseudarthrosis
Pseudomeningocele, imaging of, 171
Pseudomonas aeruginosa, 1544
Psoas abscess, as complication of lumbar fusion, 1125
Psoas major, 827
PSU; see Partial sit-up
Psychiatric evaluation
    case example of, 263
    follow-up of, 263
    of patient with chronic spine pain, 259–264
    selection of consultant for, 261–262
    structure of, 262
Psychiatrist, multidisciplinary program and, 266, 267–268
Psychologic cascade, 6, 35–40, 495–606
    background of, 36
    illustrated, 4, 37
    sources of, 36
Psychologic difficulties, history of, 261
Psychologic evaluation, 262
    of surgical candidates
        assessment guidelines for, 918–936
        purpose of, 916
        reasons for referral for, 917–918
Psychologic preparation for surgery, 915–938
Psychologic scoliosis, 799
Psychology of Pain, The, 503
PT; see Physical therapy
PTH (parathyroid hormone), 284, 285, 290
PTPM (posttraumatic progressive myelopathy), 182
Public, education of, 271
Puka chisels, 1105
Pulmonary complications, as complication of spinal-cord injury, 1534–1535
Pulmonary disease; see Chronic obstructive pulmonary disease
Pulmonary function, idiopathic scoliosis and, 1583
Pulmonary malformations, congenital scoliosis and, 1565
Pulsed electromagnetic field (PEMF) in spinal fusion
    advantages and disadvantages of, 1301–1302
    clinical efficacy of, 1300–1301
    cost of and procedural codes for, 1302
    electromagnetic spectrum and, illustrated, 1302
    indications for use of, 1301
    patients who smoke and, 1129, 1301
    safety of, 1302
Purified protein derivative (PAD), 647
Pyogenic spondylitis, imaging of, 175–176
Pyogenic vertebral osteomyelitis, 1547, 1549
    illustrated, 1545
    laboratory analysis and, 1544–1545
    microbiology and, 1544
    pathophysiology of, 1544
    radiographic analysis of, 1546–1547
Pyridinium cross-links (pyridinoline), 289
Pyridinoline (pyridinium cross-links), 289

Q

QCT; *see* Quantitative computed tomography

Quadratus lumborum, 827

Quadriplegia
    paralytic scoliosis due to, illustrated, 1599
    transient, 1446–1449
    see also Spinal-cord injury(ies)

Quadriplegic hand, surgical reconstruction of, 1539

Quadruped alternate leg lift, 403

Quadruped arm and leg raises, illustrated, 1744

Quadruped arm raises, illustrated, 1743

Quadruped single arm lift, 400

Quantitative computed tomography (QCT), assessment of osteoporosis with, 854

Quantitative radionuclide scanning, 290

Quebec Task Force on Spinal Disorders
    diagnostic testing for work-related injuries and, 242
    on effectiveness of back school, 352
    guidelines for acute conservative care developed by, 369–370
    multidisciplinary evaluation recommendations of, 271
    solution to socioeconomic cascade and, 31–32

Quigley, Matthew, 1020

R

Radial tear, 144

Radiation, treatment of allografts and xenografts with, 882–883

Radicular pain, 273
    steroid use and, 327

Radiculopathy(ies)
    clinical and electrophysiologic presentations of, 197, 199
    electrodiagnostic studies and, 193–194, 196, 198, 200–201, 209–211
    low-back pain and, 45
    somatosensory evoked potential (SEP) evaluation of, 209–211

Radiofrequency (RF), 141

Radiofrequency facet denervation, 588

Radiofrequency percutaneous rhizotomy, 864

Radiofrequency system, 1521

Radiogallium scanning, 290

Radiography
    analysis and measurement of isthmic spondylolisthesis with, 1283–1285
    assessment of degenerative spondylolisthesis with, 1268, 1270–1271
    assessment of osteoporosis with, 852–854
    evaluation of athlete with neck injury with, 1440
    evaluation of congenital deformities with, 1565–1566
    evaluation of congenital scoliosis with, 1565–1566
    intraoperative, 1035–1036
    positioning of patient during surgery and, 952
    preoperative, 965
    in spinal assessment, 124
    see also Chest x-ray, 965

Radiologist, spinal, as part of multidisciplinary program, 268

Radiology; *see* Radiography

Radionuclide bone imaging, 289–290

Ramus meningeus nervorum spinalium; *see* Sinovertebral nerve

Randomized, controlled trials (RCT), 360

Randomized, double-sided, controlled, and prospective (RDCP) studies, 1076

Range of motion (ROM)
    inspection of during physical examination, 74
    measurement of, 489
    spinal coordination versus, 119
    use of in spinal assessment, 119, 124–125

Rating of perceived exertion (RPE) scale, 388

Ray, Charles D., 905

Ray Threaded Fusion Cage (TFC), 1225–1231
    advantages of, 1225–1231
    follow-up after implantation of, 1229–1230
    illustrated, 1225, 1229
    implantation technique with, 1227–1229
    instrumentation used during implantation of, illustrated, 1226, 1228
    outcome with, 1230–1231
    patient selection for, 1227

Raylor retractor, 959
    illustrated, 958, 1253

"Razorback," 1581

RBRVS (Resource Relative Value Scale), 1752, 1754

RCT (randomized, controlled trials), 360

RDCP (randomized, double-sided, controlled, and prospective studies), 1076

Reasonable accommodation
    for disabled individual, 478
    job modification for, 479

Reconditioning, work hardening in, 490

Recording
    electrodes used in, 206
    in somatosensory evoked potential (SEP), 205–206

Rectus capitis muscle
    anterior, 1331
    posterior, 1332

"Red" (slow-twitch or "Type I") muscle fibers, 379–380

Reduction
    of high-grade spondylolisthesis, 1288
    posterior indirect, 1521–1523

Referred pain, 90–92, 273
    convergence-projection theory and, 91, 92
    defined, 24
    diffuseness of low-back pain and, 106–109
    somatic, steroid use and, 327
    theories of, 91–92
        illustrated, 91

Referring physician, education of, 270

Reflex sympathetic dystrophy (RSD)
    low-back pain and, 111–114
    SCS treatment for, 575

Reflex sympathetic syndrome, as complication of lumbar fusion, 1124, 1128

Reflex testing, 76, 194–195

Refraction of light in water, swimming and, 734

Regional exercises, 422

Rehabilitation
    activities of daily living (ADLs) and, 1537–1538
    in dance, 645–646
    in football, 671–672
    job analysis as basis for, 478
    of patients with spinal-cord injuries, 1537–1538
    postoperative, 978
    pre- and postsurgical, 925–926
    in running, 714–715
    in snow skiing, 718–719
    in soccer, 725
    spinal; *see* Spinal rehabilitation
    in swimming, 735–742
        contraindications for, 741
    vocational, 490

Reiter's syndrome (disease), 1653
    low-back pain and, 49

Relaxation, 141
    techniques in, 262–263
        postoperative pain management and, 976

Relton frame, 955

Remodeling unit, illustrated, 282, 283

Repetition time, 141–142
Replam hydroxyapatite-porites (RHAP), 885
Research
  in attachment theory, 560–561
  spinal, 271
  support of, for cognitive-behavioral perspective of chronic pain, 550–552
Resection(s)
  bony, 1574
  tissue, guiding principles in, 1251
Resistance exercise, 422, 426
  response to, 387–388
Resource Relative Value Scale (RBRVS), 1752, 1754
Respiratory system, exercise and, 383–384, 386
Retractor(s)
  Cloward; see Cloward retractor
  Gelpi, 1291
    illustrated, 1095, 1291
  Haverfield-Scoville, 1034, 1036
  Hibbs, 958, 1116, 1117, 1263
  Macelroy, 960
  McCulloch, 1034
  Meyerding, 1275
  Raylor, illustrated, 958, 1253
  Sawbill, 959
    illustrated, 958
  Taylor, 874, 1034, 1276
    illustrated, 1253, 1254–1256
Retrograde ejaculation, as complication of lumbar fusion, 781, 1123–1124, 1127
Retroperitoneal fibrosis, as complication of fixation device use, 1248
RF (radiofrequency), 141
RF system, 1521
RHAP (replam hydroxyapatite-porites), 885
Rheumatoid arthritis
  atlantoaxial instability and, 1653–1655
  as indication for cervical spine fusion, 1396
  Paget's disease and, 1726
  tissue donation excluded by, 893
  torticollis and, 1645
Rheumatoid spondylitis; see Ankylosing spondylitis
Rheumatologist, as part of multidisciplinary program, 268
Rhizotomy
  dorsal, 587
  radiofrequency percutaneous, 864
Rhythmic stabilization, illustrated, 403
Rib humps, 1579, 1581
  illustrated, 1579
Ride Across America, 639
Ring apophysis, 811
Risser sign, 804
Robinson fusion technique, 1370, 1376, 1414–1416, 1424
  illustrated, 1417
Robinson-Smith approach, 783–784, 1372, 1376, 1391
Robinson-type grafts, 1372, 1376
Rod(s)
  Harrington; see Harrington rods
  Knodt, 741, 844–845, 1159, 1186
  Luque; see Luque rods
  in Wiltse system, 1184
    illustrated, 1185, 1186
Rod systems, 1236, 1241–1244
  management of specific conditions with, 1245, 1247–1248
  see also specific devices
Roentgenography; see Radiography
Rogers, William, 785, 1403
Rogers fusion technique, 1395, 1403–1404, 1406, 1409, 1507, 1645

Rogers fusion technique,—cont'd
  modified, 1406–1407, 1408
    illustrated, 1406–1408
Rogozinski instrumentation system, 1613
Roland Adaptation of Sickness Impact Profile (ROL-SIP), 362–363
ROL-SIP (Roland Adaptation of Sickness Impact Profile), 362–363
ROM; see Range of motion
Roman chair extensions, illustrated, 404
Rongeur(s)
  Kerrison, 878, 1015, 1034, 1037, 1235, 1236, 1276, 1360, 1362, 1384, 1385, 1523
  Leksell, 1418
  Link-Beatty; see Link-Beatty rongeur
  pituitary, 1418
Roosevelt, Theodore, 668
Rotational prominence, 1579
Rotatory atlantoaxial subluxation, 1495–1496
Rothman, Richard H., 905, 960
Roto-rest bed, 1675, 1678
Roy, Rajan, 501
RPE (rating of perceived exertion scale), 388
RSD; see Reflex sympathetic dystrophy
Rugby, cervical spine injuries in, 1445–1446
Running, 711–715
  injuries in
    biomechanics of, 712–713
    prevention of, 713–714
  rehabilitation in, 714–715
Rusk, H. A., 1068

S
S1 transforaminal steroids, 334–335
Sacral epidural steroids, 323
Sacral hiatus, 815
"Sacral sparing," 1531–1532
Sacral vertebra(ae), 810, 814–815
  illustrated, 815
Sacrococcygeal joints, 821–822
Sacroiliac joint(s), 824–826
  diagnostic block of, 301, 311
    illustrated, 312
  illustrated, 824, 825
Sacroiliac stability, 880
Sacrum, malignant lymphoma of, illustrated, 1461, 1463
Saddle clamp in Wiltse system, 1184–1185
  illustrated, 1186
"Safe triangle" for steroid injection, 331
"Safe zone of Steele," 1327
Safety hazard evaluations, 476–477
Safeway, Inc., solution to socioeconomic cascade and, 31
Saggital plane, 1579
  alignment of, illustrated, 1579
Saggital plane decompensation, illustrated, 1596
Saggital plane imbalance, illustrated, 1598
Sagittal rotation (slip angle), 1284–1285
  illustrated, 1285
SAID (specific adaptation to imposed demand), 388
Salmonella, 176
Salvail, Eve, 505
SAN; see Spinally administered narcotic (SAN) infusion therapy
San Francisco Spine Institute, 988
  guidelines for acute conservative care developed by, 369–370
Sarcomere, 376, 377, 378
  schematic representation of, illustrated, 376
Sawbill retractor, 959
  illustrated, 958
SCAPF; see Simultaneous combined anterior and posterior fusion

Scar, epidural, as complication specific to posterior lumbar
    interbody fusion, 1108
Scarpa's layer, 904
Schanz pins, 1198
Schedule for Rating Permanent Disabilities, 241
Scheuermann's disease or kyphosis; *see* Juvenile kyphosis
Schmorl nodes
    development of, influences on, 805–806, 1602
        illustrated, 806
    multiple
        juvenile kyphosis and, 806, 807
Schwann cells, 94
"Sciatic scoliosis," 73
Sclerotomal pain, 273
Sclerotomes, 1307–1308
    illustrated, 1308
Scoliosis
    adult; *see* Adult scoliosis
    in ballet dancers, 647
    collapsing; *see* Adult scoliosis, degenerative
    congenital; *see* Congenital scoliosis
    "defense," 73
    degenerative; *see* Degenerative scoliosis
    first attempts at surgery and, 779
    idiopathic; *see* Idiopathic scoliosis
    lumbar; *see* Lumbar scoliosis
    myopathic, 1613
    in neurofibromatosis; *see* Neurofibramatosis, scoliosis in
    neuromuscular; *see* Paralytic scoliosis
    paralytic; *see* Paralytic scoliosis
    psychologic, 799
    "sciatic," 73
    symptomatic spondylolisthesis and, 1283
    Zielke device and, 1241–1242
Scoliosis Research Society, classification of paralytic disorders by,
    1593
Scoville curettes, 1105
Screener, 578
    illustrated, 580
Screw(s)
    AO, 1201, 1429
        illustrated, 1624
    Cotrel-Dubousset, 863
    design of, 1201, 1204, 1207–1208, 1212–1214
    failure rate of, 1179
    Herbert, 1347
    insertion of, 1189–1191
    interference, 1122
    in internal fixation systems, 1181–1184, 1201–1202, 1205,
        1207–1208, 1209, 1212–1214
    Knoringer, 1403
        illustrated, 1404
    Morscher, 1418
    Sherman, 1201
    Steffee, 863
    strengths of, 1208, 1209
    stresses on, 1183
    in transpedicular screw systems, 1181–1184
    in Vermont Spinal Fixator, 1201–1202, 1205, 1207–1208, 1209
    in Wiltse system, 1184
        illustrated, 1185
    Zielke, 1626
    see also Screw system(s)
Screw bolting, 1182–1183
Screw plate, 1181, 1182
Screw system(s), 1482
    cervical spine fractures and, 1503, 1504
    complications in, 1176–1181, 1434–1435

Screw system(s),—cont'd
    history of, 785
    nontranspedicular, 1175–1176
    transpedicular; *see* Transpedicular screw fixation system(s)
SCS; *see* Spinal cord stimulation
Secondary care
    clinical dilemmas in delivery of, 492–493
    defined, 487
    measures of work and physical capacities and, 488
    quantification in, 492
Secondary gains, 6, 48
Secure Base, A, 560
Sedative-hypnotics, 518–519
    use of, 519
Segmental sensory stimulation, 206
Selby, David, 1251
Selby I system, 1185–1186
    illustrated, 1187
Selby II system, 1186
    illustrated, 1188
"Selective spinal analgesia," 600
Semispinalis muscle, 828, 1332
Sensitization
    defined, 24
    persistent, 113
    recruitment of nociceptive afferents and, 111
    of spinal neurons, 109–111
Sensory examination, 77–79
    definitions of terms regarding, 78
    dermatomal sensory distribution and, 78
SEP; *see* Somatosensory evoked potential
Seronegative spondyloarthropathies, 49–50
Serum sickness syndrome, as complication of lumbar fusion, 1124
Sexual dysfunction, as complication of spinal-cord injury, 1536
Sexual history, low-back pain and, 58
SFEMG (single-fiber electromyography), 198–199
SGPs (stress-generated potentials), 1297
Shaffer, Ben, 609
Shakespeare, William, 774
Sharpey fibers, 800
Sherman screws, 1201
Shinko Medical Instrument Company, 1070
Shoulder girdle muscle strengthening exercises, 434
Shumway, David "Cactus," 656, 658
SI joints, examination of, 79
SIADH (syndrome of inappropriate antidiuretic hormone),
    1570–1571
Sickness Impact Profile (SIP), 362
    Roland Adaptation of (ROL-SIP), 362–363
Simeone, Frederick A., 960
Simmons, Edward, 785
Simmons keystone technique, 1636, 1644
Simple unicolumn injuries, 1514, 1515
Simultaneous combined anterior and posterior fusion (SCAPF), 1104
    anterior fusion alone versus, 1128–1129
    history of, 781
    as treatment for congenital scoliosis, 1567–1568
    as treatment for isthmic spondylolisthesis, 1291–1293
Single-fiber electromyography (SFEMG), 198–199
Single-photon absorptiometry, assessment of osteoporosis with, 854
Sinovertebral nerve (SVN), 85–86
    illustrated, 85
SIP; *see* Sickness Impact Profile
Sitting pressure sores, as complication of spinal-cord injury, 1536
Sit-ups; *see* Partial sit-up
Skating
    figure; *see* Figure skating
    in hockey; *see* Ice hockey

Skeletal muscle, 376–380
Skeleton, decay of in osteoporosis, 849
Skiing; see Snow skiing
Skin, inspection of during physical examination, 73
Skin markers, low-back pain and, 129–131
Skin ulcers, as complication of spinal-cord injury, 1535
Slip angle (sagittal rotation), 1284–1285
    illustrated, 1285
Slow-twitch ("Type I" or "red") muscle fibers, 379–380
SLR; see Straight leg raise (SLR)
Smith, Alban Gilpin, 774
Smith, Edwin, 774, 782
Smith, G. Richard, 503
Smith, George, 335
Smith, Lyman, 992
Smith Laboratories, 993, 1076–1077
Smith-Peterson procedure, 1628
Smith-Robinson fusion technique, 1356, 1372, 1376, 1391, 1636
    illustrated, 1417, 1423
Smoking
    as cause of pseudarthrosis, 1301
    disc degeneration and, 352
    estrogen replacement therapy and, 858
    low-back pain and, 58
    postoperative complications and, 968
    risk of osteoporosis and, 849, 856
    success of spine surgery and, 924, 973, 1082, 1128, 1129, 1133,
        1301
SMT; see Spinal manipulative therapy
Snow skiing, 716–720
    biomechanics of, 717
    injury in
        back, evaluation of, 718
        mechanism of, 717
    rehabilitation in, 718–719
Soccer, 721–726
    activities in, 722–725
    injuries in, 722
    rehabilitation techniques in, 725
Social Context of the Chronic Sufferer, The, 501
Social Security Disability system, 240, 543
    low-back pain disability claims and, 349
Socioeconomic cascade, 27–34
    defined, 28
    illustrated, 4, 6–7, 27–34, 28, 32
    patient within, 471–494
    players in, 29–31
    result of, 31
    solution to, 31–33
    workers' compensation patients and, 28–33
Soft tissue
    flexibility training and, 418, 419–420
    imaging of, 161–162
    injury to
        tests for, 240
        treatment for, 243–245
    see also Soft-tissue decompression(s)
Soft-tissue decompression(s)
    concepts in, 1251–1260
    dissection and, 1253–1257
    making the incision in, 1252–1253
    planning the approach in, 1252–1253
Solidity, 900
Somatization, malingering versus, 543
Somatization Disorder in the Medical Setting, 503
Somatoform pain disorder, 47
Somatosensory evoked potential (SEP), 205–212
    anatomic and physiologic basis of, 207–208

Somatosensory evoked potential (SEP),—cont'd
    clinical interpretation of, 208–209
    evaluation of radiculopathies with, 209–211
    functional versus organic complaints and, 211
    history of, 205
    illustrated, 205, 208, 209
    indications to, 209–211, 1609
    intraoperative monitoring and, 211–212
    stimulation and recording techniques of, 205–207
Somi collar, 1409, 1418, 1641
Somites, 796
    illustrated, 796, 1307
Southern Pacific Railway Company
    costs of workers' compensation injuries controlled by, 30
    solution to socioeconomic cascade and, 31
Southwick-Robinson approach, 1502
Specific adaptation to imposed demand (SAID), 388
Specific gravity of water, swimming and, 733
Spence's rule, 1493
    illustrated, 1495
SpF Spinal Fusion Stimulator, 1297
SpF 2T device, 1299–1300
Spina bifida, 799, 1312
Spinal abnormalities, congenital scoliosis and, 1564
Spinal balance, 1579
Spinal canal
    abnormalities in, congenital scoliosis and, 1570
    contents of, illustrated, 1328
Spinal coordination, 118–119
    defined, 118
    effects of age on, illustrated, 128
    effects of loading on, 126–129
    range of motion (ROM) versus, 119
Spinal cord
    afferent divergence and convergence within, 106–109
    anterior decompression of, 1573
    chemicals involved in pain transduction and, 25
    injury to; see Spinal-cord injury(ies)
    nerve roots and, 830
    patient with injury to; see Spinal cord-injured patient(s)
Spinal cord stimulation (SCS)
    clinical assessment of, 592, 594
    clinical literature on, summarized, 593–594
    complications of, 576–577
    defined, 574
    efficacy of, 576
    experimental assessment of, 594–595
    future applications of, 580, 582
    indications to, 575–576, 591
    lead and generator placement in, 578–580, 591–592
    outcome measurement of, illustrated, 595
    pain management by, 573–583, 591–598
    patient evaluation and, 577
    stimulator adjustment in, 595–596
    trial testing and, 577
Spinal cord-injured patient(s)
    activities of daily living (ADLs) of, 1537–1538
    adjunct to independent living of, 1538–1539
    ambulation by, 1537–1538
    community reentry of, 1539–1540
    life expectancy of, 1540
    management of, 1529–1541
    nutritional support for, 1536
    pain management and, 1536
    physical examination of, 1530–1532
    preventing medical complications in, 1533–1537
    rehabilitation of, 1537–1538
    standing and, 1537

Spinal cord-injured patient(s),—cont'd
  wheelchair use by, 1537
  see also Spinal-cord injury(ies)
Spinal curvature flexibility, 1580
Spinal decompensation, 1579
  illustrated, 1595, 1596, 1597
Spinal deformity(ies), 1553–1719
  arthritic, 1652–1719
  of cervical spine; *see* Cervical deformity(ies)
  congenital; *see* Congenital deformity(ies)
  flat-back; *see* Iatrogenic flat-back deformity
  flexion; *see* Kyphotic deformity(ies)
  kyphotic; *see* Kyphotic deformity(ies)
  neuromyopathic flexion, 1643
Spinal disorders
  ergonomic intervention and, 472–485
  see also Cervical spine; Lumbar spine; Thoracic spine
Spinal epidural abscess, 1549
Spinal fusion; *see* Fusion
Spinal infection(s), 1543–1552
  imaging of, 175–179
  laboratory analysis of, 1544–1545
  microbiology and, 1544
  pathophysiology of, 1544
  radiographic analysis of, 1546–1547
  as risk of posterior spine surgery, 1108
  treatment of, 1550
Spinal instability
  defined, 841
  mechanical low-back pain and, 841–843
  posterior spinal decompression and, 843
Spinal joints, 816–826
  synovial, diagnostic block of; *see* Spinal synovial joint blocks
Spinal manipulative therapy (SMT)
  case management with, 440
  clinical relevance of, 445–447
  contraindications to, 442
  effectiveness of, 445
  historical review of, 438
  outcome monitoring in, 444
  patient selection for, 440–442
  procedure-patient matching in, 442, 444
  profile of optimum case for response to, 446
  relationship of, to other subspecialties, 444–445
  techniques of, illustrated, 442, 443
  validity and basis of, 437–450
  see also Manual therapy
Spinal motion, 532–533
Spinal nerves, 830–831
  dorsal rami of, 831–832
    illustrated, 831
  "pinched," 1449
  ventral rami of, 832
Spinal neuron(s)
  nociception-induced sensitization of, 109–111
    illustrated, 110
  nociceptive-specific (NS), 109
  recordings from, illustrated, 107, 108
  wide-dynamic-range (WDR), 108, 109–111
Spinal radiologist, as part of multidisciplinary program, 268
Spinal rehabilitation
  activities of daily living (ADLs) and, 1536–1538
  role of manual therapy in, 451–470
Spinal research, 271
Spinal shock, 1531
  anesthesia and, 945–946
Spinal stenosis(es), 46
  anatomy and variations of, 1085–1087

Spinal stenosis(es),—cont'd
  anterior-posterior, 1085
  bilateral decompression for, 1040–1041
  canal; *see* Canal stenosis
  central; *see* Central stenosis
  cephalocaudal, 1085
  cervical, 1446–1449
  combined, 1085
  degenerative spondylolisthesis and, 1268, 1270–1271
  extraforaminal, 1085
  "far-out"; *see* "Far-out" stenosis
  foraminal; *see* Foraminal stenosis
  "front-back," 1085
  imaging of, 151–157, 158–159, 164, 1085
  lateral; *see* Lateral stenosis
  lateral recess; *see* Lateral recess stenosis
  lumbar, 1084–1099
  Paget's disease and, 1722–1723, 1724–1726, 1730–1734
  "pin-hole," 1085
  postoperative, 164
  SEP findings in, illustrated, 213
  subarticular; *see* Subarticular stenosis
  surgical treatment of, 777–778, 1040–1041, 1731–1734
  transient quadriplegia and, 1446–1449
  "up-down," 1085
Spinal stereotaxia, 1264
Spinal strength tests, 533–534
Spinal synovial joint blocks, 298–321
  arthrologic approach to, 300
  controversies surrounding, 314–316
  historical background of, 299–301
  indications to, 311–312
  interpretation of, 313–314
  neurosurgical approach to, 299–300
  prevalence of, 316
  selection of procedure for, 312–313
  specificity of, 314
  techniques of, 301–311
  treatment and, 316–317
  validity of, 314
Spinal tumor(s)
  anterior, illustrated, 1464
  biopsy of, 1465, 1468
    illustrated, 1469–1470
  decompression of, 1015
  diagnostic decision making and, 1463–1465
  dumbbell, 1609
  endoscopic spine surgery and, 1015
  imaging of, 171–175
  as indication for cervical spine fusion, 1395
  kyphosis secondary to, 1639, 1641–1642
  metastatic, 1458, 1460
  presentation of, 1460–1463
  primary
    benign, 1458–1459
    malignant, 1458, 1459–1460
  surgical treatment of; *see* Spinal tumor surgery
  "winking owl" sign and, 1460
    illustrated, 1462
Spinal tumor surgery, 1457–1484
  in cervical spine, 1479–1481
  complications in, 1482–1483
  diagnostic decision making and, 1463–1465
  future considerations in, 1483
  history of, 1458–1460
  in lumbar spine, 1481–1482
  surgical approaches to, illustrated, 1470–1478

Spinal tumor surgery,—cont'd
  techniques in, 1465–1482
  in thoracic spine, 1481
Spinal-cord injury(ies)
  determination of by imaging techniques, 1532–1533
  Frankel classification of, 1531, 1533
  pain management and, 1536
  prevention of medical complications and, 1533–1537
  recovery of complete lesions from, 1532
  see also Spinal cord-injured patient(s)
Spinal-cord lesions
  completeness of, velocity of injury and, 1530
  SCS treatment for, 576
Spinalis, 828
Spinally administered narcotic (SAN) infusion therapy,
      599–606
  case studies regarding, 603–604
  complications of, 604–605
  history of, 600
  implantation of
      prerequisites for, 601–602
      procedure for, 602–603
        illustrated, 602–603
  patient selection for, 600–601
  rationale for, 600
Spinal-Stim PEMF Spinal Fusion System Model 8500, 1297,
      1300, 1301
  illustrated, 1302
Spine, 784
Spine
  anatomy of, 809–836
  assessment of, 123–126
  biomechanics of, 116–138
  cervical; see Cervical spine
  coordination of; see Spinal coordination
  curvature of, 121; see also Curve(s)
  decompression of, 843; see also Decompression(s)
  defined, 810
  deformities in; see Spinal deformity(ies)
  electrodiagnostic evaluation of, 191–203
  evolution of, 117
  imaging of, 140–190
      nuclear medicine; see Bone scan(s)
      see also Imaging
  infection in; see Spinal infection(s)
  injuries to; see Spine injury(ies)
  knowledge of, development of, 117–118
  lumbar; see Lumbar spine
  lumbosacral, internal fixation of, 844–845
  manipulation of; see Spinal manipulative therapy
  martial arts practices hazardous to, 697–708
  neutral; see Neutral spine
  osteoporosis of; see Osteoporosis
  pain in; see Pain
  palpation of, 78–79, 460–463
  postoperative; see Postoperative spine
  role of, in human locomotion, 119–121
  "short-segment" defects in, 1197
  stability of, classification of spinal injuries and, 1513–1525
  thoracic; see Thoracic spine
  total, stabilization of, 416
  transmitting forces through, 695–696
  tuberculosis of; see Pott's disease, 1549
  tumors of; see Spinal tumor(s)
Spine care
  comprehensive field of, 1082
  information regarding, 1076, 1077
  minimally invasive; see Minimally invasive spine care
  "report card" rating of, 1078–1082

Spine injury(ies)
  in ballet, 642–645
  baseball hitters with, 624, 626
  in basketball, 628–630
  classification of, spinal stability and, 1513–1525
  in dance, 642–647
  in diving, 1446
  in figure skating, 654–655
  flexion/distraction, 1514, 1518
  in football; see Football
  in gymnastics, 1446
  in rugby, 1445–1446
  running and, 712
  simple unicolumn, 1514, 1515
  in snow skiing, 717, 718
  in soccer, 722
  to spinal-cord; see Spinal-cord injury(ies)
  in swimming, 728–731
  during weight lifting, 755–758, 1446
  in wrestling, 765–767, 768–769, 1446
  see also Injury(ies); Sports injury(s)
Spine pain; see Pain
Spine pathology, medical and surgical management of,
      348–350
Spine surgery
  anesthesia in, 939–949, 972–973
  arthroscopic microdisectomy as; see Arthroscopic
      microdisectomy
  for atlantoaxial disability, 1655–1659
  for atlantoaxial instability, 1654–1655
  blood loss during, 951–952
  of cervical spine; see Cervical spine surgery
  complications following, prevention of, 967–970
  congenital deformities treated with, 1566–1571,
      1572–1575
  degenerative disease (DDD) and, 908–914
  discectomy as; see Discectomy
  endoscopic, 1012–1015
  failed, management of, 1245, 1247
  fusion as; see Fusion
  history of, 773–791
  idiopathic scoliosis treated with, 1585–1593
  internal fixation as; see Internal fixation
  for kyphotic deformities of the spine, 1667, 1668–1682
  laminectomy as; see Laminectomy
  laminotomy as; see Laminotomy
  laparoscopic techniques in, 1263–1264
  laser; see Laser discectomy
  of lumbar spine; see Lumbar spine surgery
  microsurgical techniques in, 1032–1041
      "standard" techniques versus, 1029–1031
  minimally invasive, 990–1084
  osteoporosis and, 862–863
  osteotomy as; see Osteotomy
  positioning patient for; see Operative position
  principles of, 1031
  psychologic preparation for, 915–938
  selection of, by analysis of pain generators, 984–989
  spinal stenosis treated with; see Spinal stenosis
  spondylodiscitis and, 1659–1667, 1668
  spondylolisthesis treated with; see Spondylolisthesis
  stereotactical techniques in, 1264
  of thoracic spine; see Thoracic spine surgery
  treatment of spinal disease with, 1550
  tumors and; see Spinal tumor surgery
  wound infection factors and, 967
  see also Minimally invasive spine care; Spinal tumor surgery;
      Surgery; Surgical decision-making
Spine trauma, imaging in, 180–184

Spine tumors; *see* Spinal tumors
SpineCare model
   of aggressive nonoperative care, 395
   of stabilization training, 396
Spinoscope, 125, 126, 129
Spinous process, 811, 1316, 1322–1323
Spinous process fractures, 757
Splenius cervicis muscle, 1332
Splenius muscle, 829–830
Spondylitis
   ankylosing; *see* Ankylosing spondylitis
   pyogenic, imaging of, 175–176
Spondylodiscitis, 1659–1667, 1667
Spondylolisthesis
   classification of, 1281–1282
   degenerative; *see* Degenerative spondylolisthesis
   detection of, 160
   dysplastic; *see* Congenital spondylolisthesis
   elongated; *see* Isthmic spondylolisthesis
   high-grade; *see* High-grade spondylolisthesis
   history of, 1281
   isthmic; *see* Isthmic spondylolisthesis
   lytic; *see* Isthmic spondylolisthesis
   pathologic (Type V), 1282
   postoperative (Type VI), 1282, 1293–1294
   surgical treatment of, 47, 160
      basketball and, 629–630
      dance and, 642, 646–647
      history of, 778–779
      wrestling and, 766
   traumatic; *see* Traumatic spondylolisthesis
   Type I; *see* Congenital spondylolisthesis
   Type II; *see* Isthmic spondylolisthesis
   Type III; *see* Degenerative spondylolisthesis
   Type IV; *see* Traumatic spondylolisthesis
   Type VI (postoperative), 1282, 1293–1294
Spondylolysis
   basketball and, 629–630
   dance and, 642, 646–647
   defined, 159
   detection of, 159–160
   wrestling and, 766
Spondylosis, cervical; *see* Cervical spondylosis
Spondylothoracic dysplasia, illustrated, 1560–1561
Sports injury(ies), 607–770
   in baseball, 608–626
   in basketball, 627–634
   in bicycling, 635–640
   of cervical spine, 1437–1454
   in dance, 641–648
   in diving, 1446
   in figure skating, 649–666
   in football, 667–674, 1437–1454, 1505–1506
   in golf, 675–682
   in gymnastics, 1446
   of head and cervical spine, 1437–1454
   in ice hockey, 683–686
   immobilization of patient in, 1438, 1440
      illustrated, 1441
   in the martial arts, 687–710
   on-field examination and, 1438–1440
      protocol for, illustrated, 1439
   radiographic evaluation and, 1440
   return to play after, 1451–1452
   in rugby, 1445–1446
   in running, 711–715
   in snow skiing, 716–720
   in soccer, 721–726
   in swimming, 727–745

Sports injury(ies),—cont'd
   transport of patient and, 1438, 1440
      illustrated, 1441
   in weight lifting, 746–761, 1446
   in wrestling, 762–770, 1446
   see also specific sport
Sprains, cervical, 1442
Sprengel deformity, 1563, 1565
SSI system, 1593
Stabilization
   exercise programs for; *see* Stabilization exercises
   postlaminectomy, illustrated, 1636
   in power lifting, 758–759
   rhythmic, illustrated, 403
   techniques of, for cervical spine fractures, 1503–1504
   of total spine, 416
Stabilization continuum, 399–400
Stabilization exercises, 397–403, 420–435
   in basketball, 632–633
   dynamic lumbar, 1738–1745
   for figure skaters, 658–662, 660–662
      illustrated, 659, 660–662, 663–664
   specific, 403–406
   in swimming, 734–742
      illustrated, 735, 737–740
   see also Stabilization training; Therapeutic exercises; Weight training
Stabilization training
   cervicothoracic (CTST), 414, 416–420
      exercise program of, 420–435
   defined, 395
   diagnosis and, 396
   evaluation and, 396, 407–410
   flexibility and, 398–399
   in football, 671–672
   in ice hockey, 685
   neutral spine concepts and, 396–398
   phases of progression in, 400–403
   specific exercises in, 403–406
   SpineCare model of, 395
Stable zone, 1580
Staged reconstruction and fusion, 1590, 1592
Staphylococcus aureus, 176, 234, 967, 1544, 1549
Staphylococcus epidermitis, 234
Statsview, 130
Steffee, Arthur, 782
Steffee instrumentation system, 845, 862
Steffee transpedicular screws, 863
Steinman pin, 1293, 1468, 1481, 1622
Stenosis; *see* Spinal stenosis
Stereotaxia, spinal, 1264
Stern, Elias, 1068
Sternbach, Richard A., 503
Sternocleidomastoid muscle, 1331
Steroid(s)
   anabolic, osteoporosis management and, 860
   controversies surrounding, 339–340
   efficacy of, 336–339
   epidural; *see* Epidural steroids
   intraarticular; *see* Intraarticular steroids
   risks in use of, 335–336
   side effects of, 335
   "steroid response" and, 339
   transforaminal; *see* Transforaminal steroids
   see also Corticosteroids
"Steroid response," 339
Stimulation-produced analgesia, 574
"Stinger," 1449
Stookey, Brian, 783
Straight back bends, illustrated, 1745

Straight leg raise (SLR)
    performance of during physical examination, 76–77, 80
    use of in human performance quantification, 532
Strains, muscle, 628–629, 1442
Strap (infrahyoid) muscles, 1332
Strength testing in functional capacity evaluation, 125
Stress, psychiatric consultation and, 261
Stress-chronic pain cycle, illustrated, 538
Stress-generated potentials (SGPs), 1297
Stretching
    illustrated, 419, 420, 421, 700
    in martial arts, 700
    in weight lifting, illustrated, 753, 754
Structural degenerative cascade, 5–6, 8–26
    in cervical spine, 16–23
    defined, 5
    degenerative process in
        beginnings of, 12–14
        discogenic phase of, 19–20
        instability phase of, 14
        stabilization phase of, 20–22
    illustrated, 4
    Kirkaldy-Willis process in; see Kirkaldy-Willis degenerative
        process
    in lumbar spine, 9–16
    progressive degeneration of motion segment in, 14–15
Structural degenerative disease, 346–470
Stryker frame, 947, 1396
Stryker turning frame, 1675
Subarticular stenosis, 1085
    decompressions for, 1090
Sublaminar wires, 1159–1160
Suboccipital muscles, 1332
Subperiosteal dissection, 1253, 1337–1338
    illustrated, 1338
Substance-abuse disorder
    low-back pain and, 47–48, 58
    tissue donation excluded by, 893
    see also Drugs, abuse of
Succinycholine, contraindications to use of, 945
Sudeck atrophy, 286
Suffering, defined, 540
Sullivan, Cindy, 657
Summers, Jay D., 503–504
Sumo shoulder flies, illustrated, 407
Sunnybrook Cord Injury Scale, 1512
Superior laminectomy, illustrated, 1261
Supine leg thrusts, 1741
Surgeons, multidisciplinary program and, 266, 267
Surgery
    basic surgical concepts and, 909–910
    choice of, 912–914
    goals of, 910
    herniated nucleus pulposus and, 44–45
    necessity of, 910
    nonsurgical decisions and, 909
    psychologic preparation for, 261, 915–938, 965
    spine; see Spine surgery
    timing of, 911–912
    tumors and; see Spinal tumor surgery
    see also Surgical decision-making
Surgical decision-making, 908–914
    accurate diagnosis and, 909
    basic surgical concepts and, 909–910
    choice of surgery and, 912–914
    in degenerative spondylolisthesis, 1271–1272
    outcome predictors and, 930
    political and social issues regarding, 909

Surgical decision-making,—cont'd
    psychologic assessment of surgical candidates and,
        918–936
    spinal tumors and, 1463–1465
    surgical timing and
        neurologic deficit and, 911
        socioeconomic factors and, 912
Surgical decompression; see Decompression
Surgical Dynamics, Inc., 956, 1231, 1254
Surgical lasers, 1047
Surgical management of spine pathology, 348–350
Surgical microscope; see Operating microscope(s)
Surgical telescopes, 1029n
Surgicel, 874, 1013, 1121
    use of, illustrated, 1121
SVN; see Sinovertebral nerve
Swimming, 727–745
    peripheral-joint mechanics and general spinal abnormalities in,
        729–731
    prone, 741
    spinal injury in
        biomechanics of, 728–729
        diagnosis and treatment of, 731
    stabilization exercises in, 734–742
        illustrated, 735, 737–740
    stroke technique in, 742
    supine, 742
    water and, 731–734
Swing
    in baseball, 611, 613–614
    in golf, 678–681
Swiss gym ball, 426
    illustrated, 426, 433
Sympathetic causalgia, as complication of lumbar fusion,
    1124
Sympathetic trunks, 832–833
Symptom magnification, malingering versus, 543
Synchromed infusion pump, illustrated, 600, 601
Syndrome of inappropriate antidiuretic hormone (SIADH),
    1570–1571
Synovial cyst, intraspinal; see Intraspinal synovial cyst
Synovial joints, diagnostic block of; see Spinal synovial
    joint blocks
Synthetic bone implants, 884–886
    nonmetallic, 885–886
Syracuse I plate, 782, 1237
    illustrated, 1237, 1238, 1239
Systemic examination, 79

T
Tacoma Monorail System, illustrated, 1169, 1170
Tacoma plates, 1167, 1168
    illustrated, 1168
Tallis, Ray, 500
Tarlov seat, 956, 958
Tartrate-resistant acid phosphatase, 288
Task performance testing, 490
Taylor, Vern, 653
Taylor blade, 1036
    illustrated, 1034
Taylor retractor, 874, 1034, 1276
    illustrated, 1253, 1254–1256
TCS; see Transcranial stimulation
TE (echo time), 141–142
Teacher, John, 774, 785, 1047
Teardrop fracture, 1444–1445, 1498

Tectorial membrane, 818, 1320
    illustrated, 1319
TEF (trunk extension-flexion unit), 489
Temperature of water, swimming and, 734
TENS; *see* Transcutaneous electrical nerve stimulation
Terror of loss, psychologic cascade and, 37
Tertiary care
    clinical dilemmas in delivery of, 492–493
    defined, 487
    measures of work and physical capacities and, 488
    quantification in, 492
Texas Scottish Rite system, 1181
TFC; *see* Ray Threaded Fusion Cage
Thecal sac, illustrated, 9
Therapeutic exercise(s)
    in dance, 645–646
    duration of, 388–389
    frequency of, 389
    intensity of, 388
    measuring response to, 245–246
    mode of, 389
    muscular overwork and, 389
    overtraining and, 389–390
    physiologic basis of, 375–393
    prescription of, 388–389
    resistance, response to, 387–388
    stabilization, specific, 403–406
    as treatment for soft-tissue work-related injuries, 243–245
    upper-body versus lower-body, 386–387
    see also Stabilization exercises
Therapy
    educational, 350–354
    estrogen replacement; *see* Estrogen replacement therapy
    manual; *see* Manual therapy
    narcotic infusion; *see* Spinally administered narcotic (SAN) infusion therapy
    occupational, 490
    physical; *see* Physical therapy
    spinal manipulative; *see* Spinal manipulative therapy
Thiazide diuretics, osteoporosis management with, 861
Third occipital nerve blocks, 309
Thomas, Lewis B., 992
Thomas Test, 80
Thoracic anomalies, illustrated, 1561, 1564
Thoracic cord, 143
Thoracic curve patterns, 1581
Thoracic hemivertebrae, illustrated, 1563
Thoracic kyphosis, 1683–1689
Thoracic scoliosis, illustrated, 1582
Thoracic spine
    anatomy of, 143
    anomalies in, illustrated, 1561, 1564
    function of, 810
    imaging of, 143, 146–147
    injuries to; *see* Thoracolumbar spine fracture(s)
    kyphotic deformities of; *see* Thoracic kyphosis
    spinal manipulative therapy (SMT) and, 447
    surgical treatment of; *see* Thoracic spine surgery
Thoracic spine surgery
    arthroscopic foraminal decompression as, 1011–1012
    arthroscopic microdisectomy as; *see* Arthroscopic microdisectomy
    endoscopic; *see* Endoscopic thoracic spine surgery
    history of, 785–786
    for kyphotic deformities of the thoracic spine, 1683–1689
    treatment of spinal tumors and, 1481
    see also Spine surgery
Thoracic vertebra(ae), 811–812
    illustrated, 811, 812

Thoracic zygapophyseal joint block(s), 301, 310–311
Thoracolumbar curve patterns, 1581
Thoracolumbar scoliosis, illustrated, 1582, 1589–1590, 1618
Thoracolumbar spine fracture(s), 1510–1528
    classification of, spinal stability and, 1513–1525
    history of, 1511
    initial patient management and, 1511–1512
    in multiple traumatized patients, 1525–1526
    neurologic status and, 1512–1513
Thoracolumbarsacral orthosis (TLSO)
    injuries to thoracic spine and, 1513, 1518, 1521
    treatment of scoliosis and, 1590, 1592, 1610
Threaded Fusion Cage (TFC); *see* Ray Threaded Fusion Cage
Threat, feeling of by patient, 37–38
"Three-column" injury, 1498
Three-part two-plane fracture, 1444–1445
    illustrated, 1444
Thromboembolic disease, postoperative, 969–970
Thyroid hormone, 291
    normal values of, 292
Tibia, as site for bone graft, 880
Tilt angle, 1580
Tissue banking, 892
Tissue healing, 487
Tissue resections, guiding principles in, 1251
Titanium cage(s)
    posterior lumbar interbody fusions by, 1223–1332
    use of in minimally invasive arthroscopic lumbar fusion, 1065
    see also Ray Threaded Fusion Cage
Titanium locking screw plate system (TLSP), 1429, 1430–1431
Titanium mesh implants, 884–885
TLSO; *see* Thoracolumbarsacral orthosis
TLSP (titanium locking screw plate system), 1429, 1430–1431
Tool design, 477–478
Torsion injury, 122–123
Torso rotation unit, 489
Torticollis, 1645–1648
    differential diagnosis for, 1645
Total peripheral resistance (TPR), 386
Tower table, 1672, 1678
    illustrated, 1673
TPR (total peripheral resistance), 386
Traction
    halo, 947
    during intubation, 943
    treatment of adult scoliosis with, 1616
    treatment of congenital scoliosis with, 1570
    see also Immobilization
Transcranial stimulation (TCS), 205
    motor evoked potential (MEP) and, 212–214
Transcutaneous electrical nerve stimulation (TENS), 565
    adult scoliosis and, 1616
    history of, 574
    postoperative use of, 974, 978
Transforaminal steroids, 326
    efficacy of, 339
    lumbar, 331–333
    S1, 334–335
    techniques for use of, 331–335
Transient quadriplegia, 1446–1449
Transpedicular screw fixation, 1176
Transpedicular screw fixation system(s), 1176
    issues related to, 1183–1184
    screw bolting design of, 1181, 1182–1183
        illustrated, 1182, 1183

Transpedicular screw fixation system(s),—cont'd
    screw plate design of, 1181–1182
        illustrated, 1182
Transverse ligament, 821, 1318, 1320
    illustrated, 1319
Transverse process, 811
"Trap door" in bone grafting, 873
Trauma, 1485–1542
    gunshot wounds and, 1490
    as indication for cervical spine fusion, 1395
    see also Fracture(s)
Traumatic spondylolisthesis, 1282, 1293
    C2; see Hangman's fracture(s)
    defined, 1293
Travaux de Neurologie Chirurgicale, 783
Treatise of Man, 497
Treatment
    cognitive-behavioral; see Cognitive-behavioral treatment
    conservative; see Conservative treatment
    education as, 347–358; See also Education; Patient
        education
    financial disincentives to, 543
    with manual therapy (MT), 467–468
    by multidisciplinary team, 268–269
    randomized, controlled trials (RCT) and, 360
    selection of, 368
    surgical; see Surgery
Tricortical bone graft, 1415
Tricortical iliac block, 1129–1130
Triple-wire fusion technique, 1408, 1409, 1423, 1500
    illustrated, 1411–1413, 1501
Trunk bracing mechanism in martial arts, illustrated,
    691
Trunk exercises, 402
Trunk extension-flexion unit (TEF), 489
Trunk stability and movement, in martial arts, 695
Trunk strength measures, 489
Trunks, sympathetic, 832–833
TSRH system, 1164, 1236, 1244, 1520, 1593
    kyphosis treated with, 1245, 1678
        illustrated, 1246
Tuberculosis
    HIV-postitive patients and, 1550
    inner-city drug users (IVDA) and, 1544
    of the spine; see Pott's disease
    tissue donation excluded by, 893
Tuberculous spondylitis, 178
Tumor; see Spinal tumor(s)
Tumor nodules, imaging of, 172
Tuohy needle, 330
Turbulence in water, swimming and, 734
Type I end plate changes, 149–150
"Type I" (slow-twitch or "red") muscle fibers, 379–380
Type I spondylolisthesis; see Congenital spondylolisthesis
Type II end plate changes, 149–150
    illustrated, 151
"Type II" (fast-twitch or "white") muscle fibers, 379–380
Type II spondylolisthesis; see Isthmic spondylolisthesis
Type IV spondylolisthesis; see Traumatic spondylolisthesis
Type V (pathologic) spondylolisthesis, 1282
Type VI (postoperative) spondylolisthesis, 1282, 1293–
    1294

U

Ultrasonography, assessment of osteoporosis with, 855
Ultraviolet lasers, 1047
ULTT; see Upper limb tension test

Uncinate processes, 812
Uncovertebral joint(s), 818, 822, 1352, 1353
    development of, 794
Uniportal arthroscopic microsurgical discectomy, 1080
Unisegmental muscles, 826
United States Department of Health and Human Services, practice
    guidelines on acute pain management published by,
    975–976
United States Figure Skating Association, 650
United States Food and Drug Administration; see Food and Drug
    Administration
United States Masters Swimming, 728
United States Preventive Services Task Force, 858
United States Public Health Service, 353
Unrecognized fractures, as cause of kyphotic deformity, 1698
"Up-down" stenosis, 1085
Upjohn, 971
Upper limb tension test (ULTT), 459–460
    illustrated, 459, 460, 461
Upper trapezius muscle, 1332
Upper-extremity muscle strengthening exercises, 435
Urinalysis, 276
Urologic dysfunction
    as complication of fixation device use, 1248
    as complication of spinal-cord injury, 1533–1534

V

Valsalva maneuver, 1424
Variable load tolerance range (VLTR), 688, 701
    illustrated, 691
VAS (visual analog scale), 55, 364
Vascular injury(ies)
    bone grafts and, 878–879
    as complication of fixation device use, 1177–1178, 1248
    Dunn device and, 1248
    during lumbar fusion, 1108, 1122–1123, 1128
    during microsurgery, 1042
Venous drainage
    of disc, 11–12
    of motion segment, 12
Ventral rami of spinal nerves, 832
Verbal Rating Scale (VRS), 364–365
Vermont Spinal Fixator (VSF), 1181, 1196–1222
    characteristics of, 1197
    clinical experience with, 1215
    complications with use of, 1180
    components of, illustrated, 1199
    design of, 1197–1202
    history of, 1197
    methods of use of, 1203–1205
    results with, 1205–1210
    screw failure rate with, 1179
Vertebra(ae)
    arterial supply to, 11
    blocked, illustrated, 1558
    bone modeling of, Paget's disease and, illustrated, 1726
    cervical; see Cervical vertebra(ae)
    homologies of, 815–816
    lumbar; see Lumbar vertebra(ae)
    sacral, 810
    thoracic; see Thoracic vertebra(ae)
    see also Hemivertebra
Vertebra prominens, 1322
Vertebral arch, growth of, neural influences on, 799
Vertebral body, 811
    cervical, 142
    dislocation of, posterior element fracture and, 1499

Vertebral body,—cont'd
  fractures of, 1498–1500
  injuries to, 757–758, 1498–1500
  thoracic, 143
Vertebral body reconstruction fusion technique, 1416, 1418
  illustrated, 1419–1422
Vertebral canal, 811
  illustrated, 812
Vertebral column
  development and growth of, 793, 796–799
    asymmetric, vascular influences and, 798–799
    blastemal stage of, 796
    cartilaginous stage of, 796–797
    in length, 804–806
    maturation of, regional differences in, 804
    mechanical and postural influences on, 805
    osseous stage of, 797
    sexual diphorphism in, 805
  function of, 810
  muscles of, 826–830
  nerves of, 830–835
  regions of, 810–811
Vertebral foramen(ina), 811
"Vertebral nerve," 833
Vertebral osteomyelitis; see Pyogenic vertebral osteomyelitis
Vertebrectomy
  in anterior cervical spine, 1373–1374
  in anterior lumbar spine, 1235
Vertical compression injury, 1487
  illustrated, 1488
Viscosity of water, swimming and, 734
Visible-light lasers, 1047
Visual Analog Scale (VAS), 55, 364
Visual Numerical Scale (VNS), 55, 364
Visualization techniques, 262–263
Vitamin D, 291
  bone modeling and, 284
  deficiency in, 276, 294
    osteoporosis and, 848, 850, 856, 860, 861
VNS (visual numerical scale), 55, 364
Vocation evaluation centers, 478
Vocational history, lumbar spine disorders and, 59–60, 67–69
Vocational rehabilitation, work hardening in, 490
von Recklinghausen disease, 1606, 1639
VRS (Verbal Rating Scale), 364–365
VSF; see Vermont Spinal Fixator

W
Wackenheim's line, 1490
  illustrated, 1493
WADDELL (Waddell Disability Index), 363
Waddell Disability Index (WADDELL), 363
Waddell signs, 80–81
Wall, Patrick D., 500, 501, 503, 574, 917
Warren, John Collins, 506
Water, properties, 731–734
WCA (Work Capacity Assessment), 407
WDR (wide-dynamic-range spinal neurons), 108, 109–111
Weber study, 44, 352
  illustrated, 45
Weight lifting, 746–761
  biomechanics of, 750–752
  defined, 747
  different styles of, 748–750
  history, 747–748
  spine injuries in, 755–758, 1446

Weight lifting,—cont'd
  training methods of, 752–755
  see also Weight training
Weight training, 405–406
  defined, 747
  for figure skaters, 662
Weiss hooks, 1198
West 2, 489
Westergren technique, 275
Wheelchair, as adjunct to independent living, 1538
White, Arthur H., 252, 843, 905, 1273
White blood cell count, 276
White fat, 901
"White" (fast-twitch or "Type II") muscle fibers, 379–380
Whitecloud fibular strut technique, 784, 1636
  illustrated, 1637
Wide-dynamic-range (WDR) spinal neurons, 108, 109–111
Williams, David A., 504
Williams, Robert, 775–776, 1029, 1048, 1053
Wills, D. J., 1675
Wilson frame, 955
Wiltse, Leon, 778, 779, 843, 1000, 1069, 1080, 1261, 1273, 1281, 1285, 1287, 1288, 1290, 1291
Wiltse spinal internal fixation system, 845, 1181
  advantages of, 1185
  clinical results of, 1192–1193
  components of, 1184–1185
    illustrated, 1185, 1186
  illustrated, 1184, 1187, 1188, 1189
  indications for, 1188–1189
  mechanical testing of, 1187
  modifications of, 1185–1186
  surgical technique in use of, 1189–1192
"Winking owl" sign, 1460
  illustrated, 1462
Wire(s)
  Compere, 1656, 1658, 1694
  Drummond, 863
  Gallie, 1654
  hot; see Hot wire RF cutting loop
  Kirschner, 1061
  Luque, 782, 1197, 1198
  sublaminar, 1159–1160
  triple; see Triple-wire fusion technique
Wisconsin Cancer Pain Initiative, 505
Wolff's law, 14, 16, 1297
Work capacity
  assessment of, 407
  evaluation of, 255, 257
  measurement of, 488
  quantification of, 489–490
Work Capacity Assessment (WCA), 407
Work conditioning, 937
Work Evaluation Systems Technology, 489
Work hardening, 478, 490–491, 937
  defined, 490
Work simulation, defined, 491
Workers' compensation injury
  barriers to returning to work following, 240
  diagnosing patient with
    diagnostic tests for, 239–249
    physical therapy approach to, 250–258
  electrophysiologic testing and, 200
  evaluation of disability from, 241
  fees charged for treatment of; see Billing
  imaging and, 241–242
  insurance company and, 240
  objective functional testing and, 246–249

Workers' compensation injury,—cont'd
  patients with, unsubsidized injured workers versus,
    492–493
  physical therapy and, 250–258
  socioeconomic cascade and, 28–33
  surgical decision-making and, 910–911
  treatment for, 243–245
    measuring response to, 245–246
    response to, as diagnostic test, 242–243
Work-related injury; *see* Workers' compensation injury
Workstation design, 477
Work-task evaluation, 253–254
Wrestling, 762–770
  "burners" in, 1446
  neck and back injuries in, 765–767, 768–769, 1446
    evaluation of, 767
    treatment of, 769

X

Xenograft(s)
  defined, 884
  treatment of with radiation, heat, or chemicals,
    882–883
  see also Bone graft(s)
X-ray; *see* Chest x-ray
X-TREL system, illustrated, 582

Y

Yaksh, Tony, 501
YMCA study, 397
Yuan I plate instrumentation, 782, 1625
  illustrated, 1624
Yuan I-beam plates, 1628

Z

Z plate, 1237, 1239
  illustrated, 1239, 1240, 1241
Zander, Gustaf, 244–245
  equipment designed by, illustrated, 245, 246
Zborowski, Mark, 502–503
Zeiss operating microscope, 1032–1033
  illustrated, 1030
Ziegfeld, Florence, 747
Zielke instrumentation system, 845, 1162–1163, 1181, 1236,
    1241–1242, 1613, 1619–1620
  adult scoliosis treated with, 782, 1625–1626, 1627, 1628
    illustrated, 1626
  illustrated, 1241
  kyphosis treated with, 1245
  lumbar scoliosis treated with, 1245
Zielke screws, 1626
Zimmer anterior fixation device, 1525
"Zinger," 1449
Zollinger-Ellison syndrome, 290
Zung Anxiety Scale, 55
Zygapophyseal joint(s), 15–16, 811
  in cervical spine versus in lumbar spine, 793–795
  development of, 793–795, 803–804
    illustrated, 802, 803
  diagnostic block of; *see* Zygapophyseal joint block(s)
  illustrated, 313, 812
  regional differences in, 818–819
    illustrated, 819
Zygapophyseal joint block(s), 299–300, 301–304, 305–317
  cervical, 300
    intraarticular, 305–307
  illustrated, 302, 303, 306, 307, 308
  lumbar, 299
    intraarticular, 302–304
  thoracic, 301, 310–311